INDEX-HANDBOOK OF OTOTOXIC AGENTS, 1966–1971

INDEX-HANDBOOK OF OTOTOXIC AGENTS
1966–1971

E. Louisa Worthington, Lois F. Lunin, Miriam Heath, Francis I. Catlin
*of the Information Center for Hearing, Speech, and Disorders of Human
Communication, The Johns Hopkins Medical Institutions, Baltimore, Maryland*

THE JOHNS HOPKINS UNIVERSITY PRESS
Baltimore and London

The Information Center for Hearing, Speech, and Disorders of Human Communication,
a part of the Neurological Information Network of the National Institute of
Neurological Diseases and Stroke, is supported by contract number NIH 71-2281.

The Johns Hopkins University Press, Baltimore, Maryland 21218
The Johns Hopkins University Press Ltd., London

Library of Congress Catalog Card Number 72-12349
ISBN 0-8018-1438-3

29979

TABLE OF CONTENTS

FOREWORD

Ototoxicity has a long, if unfortunate, history. As early as 1822, the Duke of Wellington, then 53, was treated by a "quack specialist" who tried to cure him of deafness by syringing the affected ear with a strong solution of caustic. Shortly thereafter the Duke noticed extraordinary sensitivity of hearing: "...The noise of a carriage passing along the street was like loudest thunder, and anyone that spoke to me seemed to be shrieking at me at the very top of his voice." When he was seen the next day by Dr. Hume, a medical "veteran" of Waterloo, this physician noted "...and when he got up he staggered like a drunken man". Similarly, the potential dangers of other ototoxic agents such as quinine, arsenic, alcohol, aniline, and oil of chenopodium have long been recognized.

Interest in ototoxic agents revived during the antibiotic period. The successful use of penicillin prompted an intensive search for other antimicrobials. Streptomycin was first publicly announced by Schatz, Waksman and Bugie in 1944, and subsequently the family of streptomyces antibiotics produced about ten, most of them aminoglycosides, known or thought to be toxic to the inner ear. In 1946, it is noteworthy that the Committee on Therapeutics and Other Agents of the National Research Council reported in the Journal of the American Medical Association their findings on 1,000 cases treated with streptomycin. Included in their report were 33 instances of vertigo and 6 of deafness, yet for the next decade these neurologic disturbances continued to be reported in the scientific literature.

Other antibiotics have caused damage to the cochlea and vestibular apparatus. One of these, capreomycin, was introduced for tuberculosis therapy in 1961. Chloramphenicol in high doses can produce sensorineural hearing loss, and a rare case of hearing loss and vertigo due to ampicillin has been reported. A new antibiotic, tobramycin, has produced ototoxic effects in animals, and there is now speculation about the potential danger of spectinomycin, an antibiotic chemically related to streptomycin.

Moreover, other groups of agents may also cause ototoxicity. Recently, both transient and permanent ototoxic effects due to two diuretics, ethacrynic acid and furosemide, have been reported. Transient effects have also been noted after high doses of salicylates, including aspirin.

Voltaire described a physician as "one who pours drugs of which he knows little into a body of which he knows less". Certainly the physician of today knows much about both the body and the drugs. But even today damage to the ear is caused unwittingly due to either the unawareness of the physician to the dangers of new drugs, or to a failure to recognize that many drugs can be toxic under certain conditions, such as the presence of renal dysfunction, or with rapid absorption of the drug, or with advanced age.

One of the purposes of this Index-Handbook, with its analysis of the current literature on ototoxic agents, is to alert the physician to the potential dangers of new drugs as well as the hazards of known drugs under conditions which enhance the risk of ototoxicity. Another is to provide an overview of the current research on ototoxicity for the research scientist. It is hoped that this compilation will be of value to all who work with ototoxic agents, to whom this volume is dedicated.

PREFACE

The growth of scientific research since World War II with the resulting "information explosion" has necessitated the investigation and development of modern methods of handling published materials. This has generated a new emphasis on the analysis and synthesis of information with its subsequent availability and dissemination.

An important development in information methods has been the establishment of the Neurological Information Network by the National Institute of Neurological Diseases and Stroke. This Network consists of a group of interrelated information centers that help interested investigators, clinicians, administrators, and educators keep up-to-date with developments in neurological and sensory research.

The Information Center for Hearing, Speech, and Disorders of Human Communication, a member of the national Neurological Information Network, is located at The Johns Hopkins Medical Institutions. Its mission is to identify, locate, analyze, store, retrieve, repackage, synthesize, and disseminate information and to develop new methods for information transfer in hearing, language, speech, and communication disorders. The Information Center is staffed by scientists of the faculty of The Johns Hopkins University School of Medicine and by information specialists. The Center maintains close cooperation with the Medical Division of the University's Computing Center, the National Library of Medicine, and other information centers in the Neurological Information Network.

This INDEX-HANDBOOK OF OTOTOXIC AGENTS stems from the charge to the Information Center to develop new methods of information transfer and was initiated for the purpose of collecting, analyzing, and repackaging detailed information, experimental and clinical, concerning the effects of ototoxic agents on the auditory and vestibular systems. It is based on the assumption that existing indexing methods often do not meet the needs of scientists and clinicians for detailed, informative data. The intent here is to provide detailed data and present it in a uniform way so that the user can obtain the information he needs immediately and can easily compare the results of one study with another. In addition, if the user does wish to consult the original papers, his search is minimized since the information presented in the Index-Handbook pinpoints with precision the pertinent papers. Moreover, if the user wishes to study variables other than those used as subject headings in the Index-Handbook, he can request such a search directly from the Information Center.

The development of the project and the sources used in its preparation appear as Appendix III.

Because this INDEX-HANDBOOK OF OTOTOXIC AGENTS is a new project, the Center is particularly eager to receive comments from users regarding the organization, format, and content of entries. We would also like to hear about the uses to which this Index-Handbook has been put.

A list of other Information Center products and services can be obtained by writing to: Information Center for Hearing, Speech, and Disorders of Human Communication, 310 Harriet Lane Home, The Johns Hopkins Medical Institutions, Baltimore, Md., 21205.

PROJECT PARTICIPANTS

This book was designed and compiled by the following members of the Information Center staff:

        Mrs. Lunin, Program Director
        Dr. Catlin, Scientific Director
        Mrs. Heath, Head, Analysis and Processing Unit
        Miss Worthington, Information Specialist, Literature Search Unit

ACKNOWLEDGEMENTS

We are most grateful for the expert help of Beth Damon Coonan, who keypunched
the material for the Index-Handbook, and Marion McMillan, who assisted in
searching the literature for papers on ototoxic agents.

The papers analyzed in the Index-Handbook were located in the following
facilities:

        Information Center for Hearing, Speech, and Disorders of Human
            Communication, Baltimore, Maryland
        Welch Medical Library, The Johns Hopkins Medical Institutions,
            Baltimore, Maryland
        Francis A. Countway Library of Medicine, Boston, Massachusetts
        Lucien Howe Library, Massachusetts Eye and Ear Infirmary,
            Boston, Massachusetts
        National Library of Medicine, Bethesda, Maryland

The cover illustration for the Index-Handbook was prepared by the Department
of Art as Applied to Medicine of The Johns Hopkins University School of
Medicine, from an original drawing by Max Broedel.

The computer processing was done in the Computing Center of The Johns Hopkins
University School of Medicine.

HOW TO USE THE INDEX-HANDBOOK

The INDEX-HANDBOOK OF OTOTOXIC AGENTS is arranged in two sections: 1) Mini-Abstract Section and 2) Citation Section. In addition, there are two indexes: 1) Index to Mini-Abstracts by Page Number and 2) Author to Document Number Index. Additional information may be found in the three appendices.

RAPID SEARCH GUIDE

To search for a SUBJECT

1. Begin with the Table of Contents to find the page number of the subject heading.

2. Go to the Mini-Abstract Section and scan the mini-abstracts under the subject heading.

3. If desired, go to the Citation Section to locate the citations for the papers on the subject.

To search for an AUTHOR

1. Begin with the Author to Document Number Index to find the document numbers of papers by the author.

2. Go to the Citation Section to find the subject of the papers in the titles of the references.

   Note:
   If the subject of the papers is indicated in the titles, see 3A.
   If the subject of the papers is not indicated in the titles, see 3B.

3A. Go to the Table of Contents to find the page number of the subject heading and then
    Go to the Mini-Abstract Section and scan the mini-abstracts under the subject heading.

3B. Go to the Index to Mini-Abstracts by Page Number to find the pages on which the data may be found in the Mini-Abstract Section.

MINI-ABSTRACT SECTION

The mini-abstracts contain the analyzed data for 732 papers on ototoxic agents arranged under subject headings listed in the Table of Contents. In Part I, the mini-abstracts are in numerical order. In Parts II and III, the mini-abstracts are arranged according to the ototoxic agents. Mini-abstracts with no ototoxic agent entry are listed first, followed by single-agent entries in alphabetic order according to the ototoxic agent. Mini-abstracts with multiple-agent entries follow in numerical order. A mini-abstract will appear in each appropriate subject section.

The following is a diagram of a mini-abstract. The numbers 1 to 10 refer to the explanation that follows the diagram.

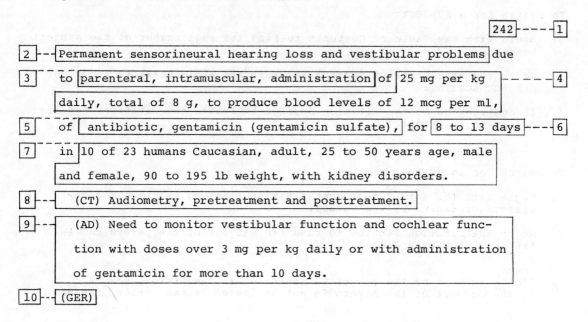

1   Document number
     The number assigned to each paper at the time it was analyzed. Each mini-abstract and citation bear the same document number.

2   Type of effect of ototoxic agents
     Physiological and/or structural effects; cochlear and/or vestibular location are indexed. Negative ototoxic effects are indicated when pertinent.

3   Route of administration
     The three primary administrative routes (oral, parenteral, and topical) are further subdivided into specified methods, sites, or vehicles.

4   Dosage
     Daily and total dosages, as well as the levels of ototoxic agents in the blood and inner ear, are indexed as reported by the authors. Abbreviations for weights and measures may be found at the beginning of the Mini-Abstract Section.

5   Ototoxic agents
     Specific ototoxic agents are indexed as reported in the papers. Different forms of an agent are indicated in parentheses following the generic terms. The class category, e.g., antibiotics, is used when the specific agent is not reported.

6   Duration of administration
     The period of administration or of exposure is indexed as reported.

7   Species affected by ototoxic agents
     Specific aspects of the species, human or animal, affected by ototoxic
     agents are indexed in the following order: race/species, age, sex,
     weight and condition.

     The following age categories were established for humans:

                         Fetus   2 months to term
                         Newborn infant   Birth to 4 weeks
                         Infant   5 weeks to 2 years
                         Child   3 to 12 years
                         Adolescent   13 to 18 years
                         Adult   19 to 64 years
                         Aged   65 years and older

     Age categories for animals were established as: fetus, newborn infant,
     young, adult.

8   Controls
     Controls for experimental and clinical studies are shown by the code
     (CT) and are indented.

9   Additional information
     Additional data, such as significance of findings, conclusions, secon-
     dary effects of ototoxic agents, and other data thought pertinent, are
     shown by the code (AD) and are indented.

10   Language
     The language of the paper is shown at the end of each mini-abstracts.
     The abbreviations for languages may be found at the beginning of the
     Mini-Abstract Section.

11   Codes used in the mini-abstracts
     The following codes have been devised to indicate relationships among
     the data indexed in the mini-abstracts:

         (CT) - Controls, as described in (8)
         (AD) - Additional information, as described in (9)
         (SQ) - Sequential   )   relationships among routes of adminis-
                  or   )   tration, dosage, ototoxic agents and/or
         (SM) - Simultaneous)   duration of administration
         (CB) - Indicates that two or more ototoxic agents have been
                administered in combination in one vehicle.
         (IB) - Indicates that an inhibitor has been administered with
                the ototoxic agent in order to decrease or prevent oto-
                toxic effects.

                            CITATION SECTION

The Citation Section contains the bibliographic data for the 732 papers
indexed in the Mini-Abstract Section.

The following is a diagram of a citation in the Index-Handbook format. The
numbers 1 to 9 refer to the explanation that follows the diagram.

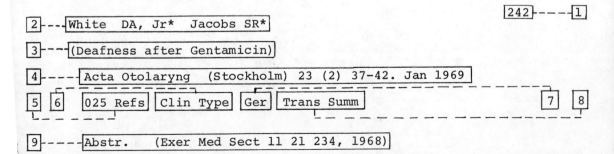

1 Document number

2 Author(s)

3 Title
Translated titles are in parentheses.

4 Publication data
A list of journal abbreviations may be found in Appendix I.

5 Number of references
The number 000 indicates an absence of references or lack of information about the number of references.

6 Type of paper

Art - article	Monogr - monograph
Rev - review	Exp - experimental
Clin - clinical	Histol - histological

7 Language

Bul - Bulgarian	Jap - Japanese
Cz - Czech	Nor - Norwegian
Dan - Danish	Pol - Polish
Dut - Dutch	Rum - Rumanian
Eng - English	Rus - Russian
Fin - Finnish	Ser - Serbo-Croatian
Fr - French	Sl - Slovene
Ger - German	Sp - Spanish
Hun - Hungarian	Sw - Swedish
It - Italian	

8 Translation of summary
The notation Trans Summ indicates that a translation of the summary was used as the basis for analysis of the paper.

9 Abstract
An abstract in a secondary source was used as the basis for the analysis when it was not possible to use either the original language text or a translation of the summary of the paper.

INDEX TO MINI-ABSTRACTS BY PAGE NUMBER

The Index to Mini-Abstracts by Page Number provides a reference from the document number of each paper to a page on which the mini-abstract for the paper may be found.

AUTHOR TO DOCUMENT NUMBER INDEX

The Author to Document Number Index provides a reference from the authors to the document numbers in the Citation Section. All of the authors for each paper are listed.

MINI-ABSTRACT SECTION

ABBREVIATIONS USED IN MINI-ABSTRACT SECTION

Weights and Measures

cc - cubic centimeter(s)
cm - centimeter(s)
ED - effective dose(s)
g - gram(s)
kg - kilogram(s)
l - liter(s)
lb - pound(s)
m - meter(s)

M - molar
mc - millicurie(s)
mcg - microgram(s)
mg - milligram(s)
ml - milliliter(s)
mM - millimole(s)
ppm - parts per million

Languages

Bul - Bulgarian
Cz - Czech
Dan - Danish
Dut - Dutch
Eng - English
Fin - Finnish
Fr - French
Ger - German
Hun - Hungarian
It - Italian

Jap - Japanese
Nor - Norwegian
Pol - Polish
Rum - Rumanian
Rus - Russian
Ser - Serbo-Croatian
Sl - Slovene
Sp - Spanish
Sw - Swedish

Abbreviated Index Terms

ATP - adenosine triphosphate
comp w - compared with
decr - decrease, reduction
EEG - electroencephalography,
        electroencephalogram

ENG - electronystagmography,
        electronystagmogram
incr - increase
PTS - permanent threshold shift
TTS - temporary threshold shift

Part I OTOTOXIC AGENTS

235
Effect on hair cells of vestibular apparatus and organ of Corti due to ototoxic drugs in humans and animals.
   (AD) Suggested role of hair cells of vestibular apparatus and organ of Corti as sensory meters with relative resistance to drugs.
   (AD) Literature review of effects of drugs on sensory endings. (ENG)

281
Vestibular neuritis due to ototoxic agents in humans. (SER)

352
Severe hearing loss due to ototoxic drugs in humans, newborn infant.
   (AD) Comment on previous report on ototoxicity in premature infants.
   (AD) Discussion of decr in congenital hearing loss and prelingual hearing loss due to ototoxic drugs and other etiologic factors. (ENG)

386
Possible damage to inner ear due to topical administration in ear drops of ototoxic drugs for long period in humans.
   (AD) Discussion of clinical use and possible toxic effects of ear drops.
   (GER)

398
Effect on auditory threshold due to parenteral, subcutaneous, administration of ototoxic drugs in 4 animals, dogs, 1 to 2 years age, 7 to 10 kg weight, conditioned.
   (CT) Determined standard deviation of auditory threshold in dogs by measurement of changes without administration of drugs.
   (CT) Measurement of auditory threshold before and after administration of drugs. (ENG)

407
Hearing loss due to ototoxic drugs in humans.
   (AD) Discussion of cochleotoxic effects of ototoxic drugs. (FR)

419
Hearing loss and vestibular problems due to antibiotic, streptomycin, in humans with various disorders.
Hearing loss and vestibular problems due to other ototoxic drugs in humans with various disorders.
   (AD) Discussion of cochleo-vestibulotoxic effects of ototoxic drugs used in therapy for various disorders. (GER)

442
Degeneration of inner ear due to ototoxic drugs in humans.
   (AD) Changes in inner ear due to virus infections comp w changes due to ototoxic drugs or circulation problems. (ENG)

479
Auditory system problems due to ototoxic drugs in humans.
   (AD) Discussion of drugs with possible toxic effects on ear. (FR)

499
Sensorineural hearing loss due to ototoxic drugs in humans.
   (AD) Management of hearing loss includes prevention of ototoxicity due to drugs. (ENG)

505
Congenital hearing loss due to ototoxic drugs in humans, newborn infant.

(AD) Discussion of etiology of congenital hearing loss.   (ENG)

717

Hearing loss in fetus due to ototoxic drugs in humans treated during pregnancy.
   (AD) Discussion of etiology of hearing loss in risk children.   (GER)

ANALEPTICS
Amphetamine

413

Decr in threshold of detection of acoustic stimuli of shorter duration than
16 msec due to 0.4 g of analeptic, caffeine, in humans, adult, and animals.
Decr in threshold of detection of acoustic stimuli of longer duration than 16
msec due to 0.015 to 0.02 g of analeptic, amphetamine, in humans, adult, and
animals. (RUS)

417

No significant effects on threshold at any frequency due to 5 mg of analep-
tic, amphetamine (dextro-amphetamine sulfate), in humans, adult, range of 22
to 38 years age, male and female, with no history of auditory system problem.
   (CT) Audiometry before and 65 minutes after administration of drug.
   (CT) Same method using placebo in 12 subjects, control group.
   (CT) Same method using no drug in 12 subjects, control group.
   (AD) Study to determine effects, toxic or therapeutic, of amphetamine on
   auditory threshold of humans.   (ENG)

444

Changes in cochlear function and vestibular function due to analeptic, caf-
feine, in animals and humans.
Changes in cochlear function and vestibular function due to analeptic, amphe-
tamine, in animals and humans.
Changes in cochlear function and vestibular function due to sedatives and
tranquilizers in animals and humans.
   (AD) Suggested mechanism of action of drugs.
   (AD) Literature review of ototoxic effects of drugs.   (IT)

Caffeine

413

Decr in threshold of detection of acoustic stimuli of shorter duration than
16 msec due to 0.4 g of analeptic, caffeine, in humans, adult, and animals.
Decr in threshold of detection of acoustic stimuli of longer duration than 16
msec due to 0.015 to 0.02 g of analeptic, amphetamine, in humans, adult, and
animals. (RUS)

444

Changes in cochlear function and vestibular function due to analeptic, caf-
feine, in animals and humans.
Changes in cochlear function and vestibular function due to analeptic, amphe-
tamine, in animals and humans.
Changes in cochlear function and vestibular function due to sedatives and
tranquilizers in animals and humans.
   (AD) Suggested mechanism of action of drugs.
   (AD) Literature review of ototoxic effects of drugs.   (IT)

Dimorpholamine

276

Decr in vestibular responses due to parenteral, intramuscular, administration
of 250 mg per kg of antibiotic, streptomycin (streptomycin sulfate), in 10 or
25 injections in 13 animals, guinea pigs, 250 to 300 g weight.
Decr in vestibular responses for several hours due to parenteral, intraperitoneal, administration of 1.5, 3.0, or 4.5 mg of analeptic, dimorpholamine,
in 17 animals, guinea pigs, 250 to 300 g weight. (GER)

ANALGESICS

SALICYLATES

115

Permanent cochleo-vestibulotoxic effects due to antibiotics, aminoglycoside, in humans.
Transient cochlear impairment due to salicylates in humans.
Ototoxic effects due to antimalarial, quinine, in humans.
Ototoxic effects due to chemical agent, nicotine, in humans.
   (AD) Report on ototoxic effects of various drugs.
   (AD) Need for audiometry and vestibular function tests with clinical use
   of ototoxic drugs.   (FR)

249

Cochleo-vestibulotoxic effects due to antibiotics, aminoglycoside, in humans.
Cochlear impairment due to antimalarial, quinine, in humans.
Transient cochlear impairment and vestibular problems due to salicylates in humans.
   (AD) Occurrence of ototoxic effects with different dosages due to indivi-
   dual responses to drugs.
   (AD) Need for observation and tests with clinical use of ototoxic drugs.
   (FR)

384

Usually transient hearing loss and no structural damage to organ of Corti, stria vascularis, and spiral ganglion due to oral or topical administration of salicylates in humans.
Hearing loss due to antimalarial, quinine, in humans.
Usually permanent hearing loss due to antimalarial, chloroquine, in humans.
Transient and permanent hearing loss and possible damage to hair cells of organ of Corti due to diuretic, ethacrynic acid, in humans.
Sensorineural hearing loss due to cardiovascular agent, hexadimethrine bromide, in humans with kidney disorder.
Sensorineural hearing loss and damage to organ of Corti due to topical ad-ministration of antineoplastic, nitrogen mustard, in humans.
Sensorineural hearing loss due to high doses of antibiotic, chloramphenicol, in humans.
Primary vestibular problems due to antibiotic, streptomycin, in humans.
Hearing loss due to high doses usually of antibiotic, streptomycin, in hu-mans.
   (AD) Early detection of hearing loss by audiometry prevents permanent
   damage.
High frequency hearing loss and severe damage to outer hair cells and slight damage to inner hair cells of organ of Corti due to antibiotic, kanamycin, in humans.
Sensorineural hearing loss due to parenteral, oral, and topical administra-tion of antibiotic, neomycin, in humans with or without kidney disorders.
Degeneration of hair cells of organ of Corti and of nerve process due to antibiotics, aminoglycoside, in animals.
   (AD) Literature review of physiological and structural cochleo-vestibulo-
   toxic effects of ototoxic drugs.
   (AD) Discussion of suggested mechanism of ototoxicity and routes of drugs
   to inner ear.
Bilateral sensorineural hearing loss due to oral administration of antibio-tic, neomycin, in 4 of 8 humans with liver disease.
Bilateral sensorineural hearing loss due to oral administration of range of doses of antibiotic, neomycin (SM), in 2 of 5 humans with liver disease.
Bilateral sensorineural hearing loss due to diuretics (SM), in 2 of 5 humans with liver disease.
Transient progression of previous hearing loss due to parenteral, intra-venous, administration of diuretic, ethacrynic acid (SM), in 1 injection in 1 of 5 humans with liver disease.
   (CT) Normal cochlear function in 6 humans, control group, with liver
   disease and not treated with neomycin or diuretics.
   (CT) Normal cochlear function in 13 humans, control group, with liver
   disease and treated with diuretics but not with neomycin.

(AD) Hearing loss confirmed by audiometry.
(AD) Reported that hearing loss due to neomycin or diuretics in humans
with liver disease not related to dosage.
(AD) Clinical study of effects of treatment with neomycin and diuretics in
humans with liver disease.
Bilateral sensorineural hearing loss and vertigo due to antibiotic, ampicil-
lin, in 1 human, adolescent, 17 years age, female, with tonsillitis.
(AD) Cited case report.
Severe sensorineural hearing loss and vertigo due to topical administration
in ear drops of antibiotic, framycetin, in 1 human, adult, 42 years age,
male, with previous slight high frequency hearing loss.
(AD) Cited case report.
Atrophy of hair cells of organ of Corti and hearing loss due to antibiotic,
dihydrostreptomycin, in humans with tuberculous meningitis.
(AD) Cited study.
Loss of inner hair cells and damage to outer hair cells due to 18 g of anti-
biotic, neomycin, for 18 days in 1 human.
(AD) Cited case report. (ENG)

401

Possible TTS(auditory) of 24 hours duration due to high doses of salicylates
in humans.
Obstruction of capillaries of spiral vessels of basilar membrane due to high
doses of salicylates in humans.
(AD) Same obstruction of capillaries due to sound stimulation.
(AD) TTS(auditory) possibly due to obstruction of capillaries by salicy-
lates or sound.
Susceptibility to PTS(auditory) due to salicylates in humans exposed to
noise.
(AD) Conclusions based on animal experimentation. (ENG)

438

Suppression of microphonic potentials of saccule due to topical, intraluminal, administration of antibiotic, streptomycin, in animals, goldfish.
Suppression of microphonic potentials of saccule due to topical, intraluminal, administration of antibiotic, kanamycin, in animals, goldfish.
Suppression of microphonic potentials of saccule due to topical, intraluminal
or extraluminal, administration of 0.5 mg of chemical agent, cyanide, in
animals, goldfish.
Suppression of microphonic potentials of saccule due to topical, intraluminal
or extraluminal, administration of 0.1 mg of antimalarial, quinine, in animals, goldfish.
Suppression of microphonic potentials of saccule due to topical, intraluminal
or extraluminal, administration of 2 mg of anesthetic, procaine, in animals,
goldfish.
No effect on microphonic potentials of saccule due to topical administration
of salicylates in animals, goldfish. (ENG)

448

Significant decr in ATP levels of Reissner's membrane but no change in P-
creatine due to parenteral, intraperitoneal, administration of high doses,
400 mg per kg, of salicylate in animals, guinea pigs, young, about 200 g
weight.
Incr in ATP of cochlear nerve and incr in P-creatine of stria vascularis due
to parenteral, intraperitoneal, administration of high doses, 400 mg per kg,
of salicylate in animals, guinea pigs, young, 200 g weight.
(CT) Same method using 0.9 percent saline in 3 guinea pigs, control group.
(AD) Suggested that ototoxicity of salicylate possibly due to impairment
of energy metabolism of Reissner's membrane. (ENG)

596

Tinnitus due to high doses of salicylates in humans.
(AD) Tinnitus early symptom of salicylate intoxication in some cases.
(AD) Discussion of etiology, symptoms, diagnosis and evaluation, treat-
ment, and prevention of salicylate intoxication. (ENG)

597

Hearing loss due to salicylates in humans.

Hearing loss due to antimalarial, quinine, in humans.
Hearing loss due to antibiotic, streptomycin, in humans.
Tinnitus due to chemical agent, camphor, in humans.
Tinnitus due to chemical agent, tobacco, in humans.
Tinnitus due to cardiovascular agent, quinidine, in humans.
Tinnitus due to chemical agent, ergot, in humans.
Tinnitus due to chemical agent, alcohol, methyl, in humans.
   (AD) Discussion of toxic effects of drugs. (ENG)

627

Sensorineural hearing loss and vestibular problems due to parenteral, oral,
and topical administration of antibiotics in humans with and without kidney
disorder.
Degeneration of cochlea due to parenteral, intratympanic, administration of
antibiotic, neomycin, in animals, guinea pigs.
Transient sensorineural hearing loss due to high doses of salicylates in
humans.
Sensorineural hearing loss due to antimalarial, quinine, in humans.
Sensorineural hearing loss due to chemical agent, tobacco, in humans.
Sensorineural hearing loss due to sedative, alcohol, in humans.
   (AD) Discussion of ototoxicity of various drugs as 1 etiology of sen-
   sorineural hearing loss in adults. (ENG)

686

Decr in ATP and p-creatine of organ of Corti, spiral ganglion, cochlear
nerve, stria vascularis, and Reissner's membrane only after 3 days of exposure due to range of doses of salicylate in animals, guinea pigs.
   (AD) Results of study suggest that ototoxicity of salicylates not due to
   impairment of energy metabolism of cochlea. (ENG)

706

Ototoxic effects due to chemical agents and heavy metals in humans.
   (AD) Literature review of ototoxic effects of nicotine, carbon monoxide,
   carbon tetrachloride, mercury, arsenic, and lead.
Cochleo-vestibulotoxic effects, functional and structural, due to antibiotics
in humans.
   (AD) Literature review of ototoxicity of streptomycin, dihydrostreptomy-
   cin, neomycin, kanamycin, gentamicin, capreomycin, rifampicin, viomycin,
   isoniazid, aminosidine, and framycetin.
Hearing loss due to salicylates in humans.
Hearing loss due to antimalarial, quinine, in humans.
Hearing loss due to diuretic, ethacrynic acid, in humans.
   (AD) Literature review of effects of various ototoxic agents. (IT)

Acetylsalicylic acid, Aspirin

007

Permanent unilateral sensorineural hearing loss and transient vertigo and
tinnitus due to oral administration of range of 0.6 to 0.9 g of salicylate,
aspirin, for every 2 hours for 3 days in 1 human, adult, 19 years age, female, with pain after tooth extraction.
   (AD) Literature review showed 2 other case reports of hearing loss due to
   aspirin. (ENG)

021

Transient bilateral sensorineural hearing loss due to unspecified method of
administration of as much as 5.2 g daily of salicylate, acetylsalicylic acid,
for unspecified period in 1 human, aged, 76 years age, female, with rheumatoid arthritis.
   (AD) Improvement in hearing after cessation of treatment with acetylsalicylic acid.
   (AD) Suggested that damage to stria vascularis due to presbycusis and not
   due to acetylsalicylic acid. (ENG)

105

Transient bilateral incr in pure tone threshold but without tone decay and
without difference limen and decr in duration of nystagmus and in slow phase
velocity of nystagmus due to oral administration of incr doses to about 6 to

8 g per day, until subjective hearing loss observed, of salicylate, aspirin
(CB), in 12 humans, adult and aged, range of 23 to 68 years age, with rheuma-
toid arthritis.
Combined administration of magnesium aluminum hydroxide (CB) in 12 humans,
adult and aged, range of 23 to 68 years age, with rheumatoid arthritis.
   (CT) Withdrawal of salicylates before treatment for standardization of
   salicylate level.
   (CT) Audiometry and vestibular function tests before, during, and after
   treatment with salicylate.
   (AD) Serum salicylate level determined when subjective hearing loss reported.
Transient sensorineural hearing loss but no damage to hair cells of organ of
Corti or to membranous labyrinth due to oral administration of high doses, as
high as 7 to 10 g per day, of salicylates for long period in 1 human, Caucasian, adult, 62 years age, female, with previous progressive hearing loss.
Transient sensorineural hearing loss but no damage to organ of Corti, spiral
ganglion, or membranous labyrinth due to oral administration of high doses,
as high as 5 g per day, of salicylate, aspirin, for 15 years in 1 human,
adult, 61 years age, female, with rheumatoid arthritis.   (ENG)

113

Transient sensorineural hearing loss but no vestibular problems due to 0.5 to
1.0 g 4 times daily of solution of salicylate, acetylsalicylic acid, in 8 (16
percent) of 50 humans after tonsillectomy.
   (AD) Audiology and vestibular function tests to determine ototoxic effects.   (DAN)

128

Transient tinnitus due to oral administration of 2 tablets every 4 hours or
more frequently, to produce serum salicylate level of 92 mg per 100 ml, of
salicylate, aspirin, for about 6 days in 1 human, Caucasian, adolescent, 14
years age, female, self treatment for upper respiratory system infection.
Tinnitus and dizziness due to oral administration of about 5 bottles of 100
tablets each, to produce serum salicylate levels of 72 mg per 100 ml after 3
to 4 hours, 59 mg per 100 ml after 6 to 7 hours, 150 mg per 100 ml after 14
to 15 hours, of salicylate, aspirin, in 1 dose in 1 human, Caucasian, adult,
19 years age, female, suicide.
Loss of equilibrium due to oral administration of 62.5 mg per teaspoon of
colic medicine of salicylate in 1 human, Caucasian, infant, 3 months age,
male, with colic.
   (AD) Low serum salicylate level in infant.
   (AD) Discussion of 3 case reports of salicylate ototoxicity.   (ENG)

143

Transient unsteady gait and dizziness due to oral administration of high
doses, 12 to 30 tablets per day, of salicylate, aspirin, in 1 human, adult,
44 years age, male, self treatment for pain after accident.
   (AD) EEG abnormal for 5 weeks.   (ENG)

186

Diplacusis due to antibiotics, aminoglycoside, in humans.
Diplacusis due to antimalarial, quinine, in humans.
Diplacusis due to salicylate, aspirin, in humans.
Diplacusis due to chemical agent, carbon monoxide, in humans.
   (AD) Report on etiology of diplacusis with comment on ototoxic drugs.
   (ENG)

188

Possible hearing loss due to antibiotics in humans, child, treated when
newborn infant.
   (AD) Reported that 23 percent of 46 children with idiopathic hearing loss
   treated with antibiotics in neonatal period.
   (CT) Reported that 2 percent of 54 children with normal hearing treated
   with antibiotics in neonatal period.
Possible hearing loss in fetus due to salicylate, aspirin, in humans, female,
during pregnancy.
   (AD) Ingestion of salicylate, aspirin, during pregnancy by mothers of 2
   percent of total of 118 children with hearing loss.

(CT) Ingestion of salicylate, aspirin, during pregnancy by mothers of 0 of 54 children with normal hearing.
(AD) Study of etiology of hearing loss in children.   (ENG)

219

Cochleo-vestibulotoxic effects due to antibiotics in humans.
Transient and permanent sensorineural hearing loss due to diuretic, etha- crynic acid, in humans.
Transient sensorineural hearing loss, tinnitus, and vertigo due to salicy- late, aspirin, in humans.
Transient and permanent sensorineural hearing loss and dizziness due to antimalarial, quinine, in humans.
Sensorineural hearing loss due to antimalarial, chloroquine, in humans.
Sensorineural hearing loss, tinnitus, and vertigo due to chemical agents in humans.
   (AD) Literature review of ototoxic drugs with clinical and histopathologi- cal correlations.
   (AD) Comment on ototoxicity of some chemical agents.
   (AD) Review of theories of mechanism of action of ototoxic drugs.   (ENG)

305

Dizziness, vertigo, tinnitus, and hearing loss due to oral administration of 50, 100, 150, and then 200 mg, incr daily doses each week, of anti-inflamma- tory agent, indomethacin, for 4 weeks in 7 of 24 humans, adult and aged, range of 23 to 69 years age, male and female, with rheumatoid arthritis.
Dizziness, vertigo, tinnitus, and hearing loss due to oral administration of 1.6, 3.2, 4.8, and then 6.4 g, incr daily doses each week, of salicylate, acetylsalicylic acid, for 4 weeks in 18 of 24 humans, adult and aged, range of 23 to 69 years age, male and female, with rheumatoid arthritis.
   (AD) Comparative study of effectiveness of indomethacin and acetylsalicy- lic acid in treatment of rheumatoid arthritis.   (ENG)

315

Dysacusis due to oral administration of 9 tablets for 4 days, 6 tablets for 7 days, and 3 tablets for 2 days, each tablet containing 500 mg of salicylate, aspirin (aspirin aluminum), for total of 13 days in 1 of 19 humans, adult, 21 years age, female, with rheumatoid arthritis.
Tinnitus and dysacusis due to oral administration of 6 tablets for 3 days, 12 tablets for 2 days, 8 tablets for 2 days, and 9 tablets for 15 days, each tablet containing 500 mg of salicylate, aspirin (aspirin aluminum), for total of 22 days in 1 human, adult, 37 years age, female, with rheumatoid arthri- tis.
   (AD) Loss of appetite also due to administration of aspirin (aspirin aluminum) for 22 days.   (ENG)

333

Vestibular problems due to antibiotic, streptomycin, in humans.
Severe cochlear impairment due to antibiotic, dihydrostreptomycin, in humans.
Loss of hair cells in organ of Corti and hearing loss due to antibiotics, aminoglycoside, in humans.
Hearing loss in fetus due to antimalarial, quinine, in humans, female, treated during pregnancy.
Transient hearing loss due to high doses of salicylate, aspirin, for long period in humans.
   (AD) Discussion of possible cochleo-vestibulotoxic effects of ototoxic drugs.
   (AD) Ototoxic effects related to concurrent disorders, dosage, duration of treatment, and age of individuals.   (ENG)

345

Transient hearing loss and vestibular problem due to salicylate, aspirin, in humans.
Decr in cochlear microphonic and action potential and decr in malic dehydro- genase in endolymph and perilymph due to salicylate, aspirin, in humans.
   (AD) Suggested that cochleo-vestibulotoxic effects of salicylates due to electrophysiological and biochemical changes and not structural changes.
Primary distribution in stria vascularis and spiral ligament due to salicy- late, aspirin, in humans.

(AD) Possible but not definite location of toxic activity of aspirin.
High concentration in inner ear after 5 to 7 hours due to parenteral, intraperitoneal, administration of salicylate, sodium salicylate, in animals,
cats.
(AD) Report on clinical use and ototoxic effects of aspirin.   (ENG)

355
Tinnitus and hearing loss due to previous oral administration of (SQ) 4.5 g
daily of salicylate, (SQ) aspirin, in 4 of 6 humans with rheumatoid arthritis.
Tinnitus and hearing loss due to oral administration of (SQ) 3.6 g daily of
salicylate, (SQ) aspirin, for short period, 2 weeks, in 1 of 6 humans with
rheumatoid arthritis.
No ototoxic effects due to oral administration of 0.3, 0.6, and 0.9 g daily
of anti-inflammatory agent, (SQ) ibuprofen, for short period, 2 weeks, in 6
humans with rheumatoid arthritis.
No ototoxic effects due to range of 200 to 1200 mg daily, average of 600 mg
daily, of anti-inflammatory agent, ibuprofen, for long period, 3 months to
over 12 months, in 27 humans, adult, 60.6 years average age, male and female,
with rheumatoid arthritis.
(AD) Comparative study of effectiveness of aspirin and ibuprofen in treatment of rheumatoid arthritis.   (ENG)

359
Hearing loss due to oral administration of 400, 600, or 800 mg of anti-inflammatory agent, ibuprofen, for 2 weeks in 2 of 30 humans, adult and aged, 30
to 79 years age, female and male, with rheumatoid arthritis.
Unspecified ototoxic effects due to oral administration of 2.4, 3.6, or 4.8 g
daily of salicylate, aspirin, for 2 weeks in 18 of 30 humans, adult and aged,
30 to 79 years age, female and male, with rheumatoid arthritis.
(AD) Comparative study of ibuprofen, aspirin, and placebo in treatment of
rheumatoid arthritis.   (ENG)

361
Transient dizziness and tinnitus due to oral administration of 750 mg daily
of anti-inflammatory agent, ibuprofen, for 5 days in 1 of 9 humans, adult and
aged, 37 to 67 years age, male and female, with rheumatoid arthritis.
(AD) Ibuprofen therapy discontinued after 5 days.
Hearing loss and tinnitus due to oral administration of 5 g daily of salicylate, aspirin, for 1 week in 3 of 9 humans, adult and aged, 37 to 67 years
age, male and female, with rheumatoid arthritis.
(AD) Comparative study of ibuprofen, aspirin, and prednisolone in treatment of rheumatoid arthritis.   (ENG)

373
Possible progressive sensorineural hearing loss due to antibiotics, aminogly-
coside, in humans.
Possible transient hearing loss due to high doses of salicylate, aspirin, in
humans.
Possible transient hearing loss due to high doses of antimalarial, quinine,
in humans.
Possible hearing loss due to diuretic, ethacrynic acid, in humans.
Bilateral sudden deafness due to antibiotic, kanamycin, in 4 humans, adult,
34 years average age, male and female.
(AD) Hearing loss due to ototoxic drugs usually progressive.
(AD) Sudden deafness due to ototoxic drugs possible in some cases, as in
humans with kidney disorder.
(AD) Literature review on etiology of sudden deafness.   (ENG)

411
Total bilateral hearing loss and within 48 hours, unilateral hearing loss,
due to oral ingestion of 46 tablets of salicylate, aspirin, in 1 dose in 1
human, in suicide attempt.
Vestibular problems due to oral ingestion of 46 tablets of salicylate, aspirin, in 1 dose in 1 human, in suicide attempt.
(AD) Case report of cochleo-vestibulotoxic effects of high dose of aspirin
in suicide attempt.   (FR)

423

More severe and more rapid progression of presbycusis due to antimalarial,
quinine, in humans, adult and aged.
More severe and more rapid progression of presbycusis due to antibiotics,
aminoglycoside, in humans, adult and aged.
More severe and more rapid progression of presbycusis due to salicylate,
aspirin, in humans, adult and aged.
More severe and more rapid progression of presbycusis due to chemical agent,
carbon monoxide, in humans, adult and aged.
   (AD) Discussion of factors resulting in more severe and more rapid progression of presbycusis.   (FR)

562

Decr in microphonic potential of saccule due to topical, intraluminal, administration of antibiotic, streptomycin, in animals, goldfish.
Decr in microphonic potential of saccule due to topical, intraluminal, administration of antibiotic, kanamycin, in animals, goldfish.
Permanent decr in microphonic potential of saccule due to topical, intraluminal or extraluminal, administration of 0.5 mg per ml of chemical agent,
cyanide, in animals, goldfish.
Permanent decr in microphonic potential of saccule due to topical, intraluminal or extraluminal, administration of 0.1 mg per ml of antimalarial,
quinine, in animals, goldfish.
No effect on microphonic potential of saccule due to salicylate, aspirin, in
animals, goldfish.
Some decr in microphonic potential of saccule due to 2 mg per ml of anesthetic, procaine, in animals, goldfish.
   (AD) Study of effects of various agents on microphonic potential of saccule of goldfish.   (JAP)

566

Gradual decr in cochlear microphonics and decr in endocochlear potentials,
but not significant, due to salicylate, acetylsalicylic acid, in animals,
guinea pigs, 250 to 400 g weight.
Severe decr in cochlear potentials due to 2.0 mM of chemical agent, cyanide
(potassium cyanide), in animals, guinea pigs, 250 to 400 g weight.
   (AD) Study of effects of various agents on cochlear potentials.   (ENG)

621

Primarily vestibular problems due to antibiotic, streptomycin, in humans.
Primarily hearing loss but also vestibular problems due to antibiotic, dihy-
drostreptomycin, in humans.
Primarily hearing loss but also vestibular problems due to antibiotic, kana-
mycin, in humans.
Primarily hearing loss but also vestibular problems due to antibiotic, neomy-
cin, in humans.
Primarily hearing loss but also vestibular problems due to antibiotic, genta-
micin, in humans.
Vertigo and ataxia due to antituberculous agent, isoniazid, in humans.
Hearing loss due to salicylate, aspirin, in humans.
Hearing loss and vertigo due to antimalarial, quinine, in humans.
Nystagmus due to barbiturates in humans.
Vestibular problems due to analgesic, morphine, in humans.
Nystagmus due to sedative, alcohol, in humans.
Nystagmus and hearing loss due to chemical agent, carbon monoxide, in humans.
Ototoxic effects due to antineoplastic, nitrogen mustard, in humans.
Ototoxic effects due to chemical agent, aniline, in humans.
Ototoxic effects due to chemical agent, tobacco, in humans.
Nystagmus due to chemical agent, nicotine, in humans.
Vestibular problems due to anticonvulsants in humans.
Vestibular problems due to anesthetics in humans.
Vestibular problems due to diuretics in humans.
   (AD) Inclusion of comprehensive list of ototoxic agents.   (SP)

649

Transient tinnitus, hearing loss, or dizziness due to oral administration in
tablets of 1.4 g, in 4 tablets, in 3 initial doses at 7 hour intervals and
then daily, to produce high serum levels of 20.5 to 28.0 mg per 100 ml, of

salicylate, aspirin, for 2 to 3 weeks in 9 of 20 humans, adolescent, adult,
and aged, 15 to 70 years age, female and male, with bone and joint disorders.
   (AD) Report on use of new sustained release aspirin in treatment of bone
   and joint disorders.   (ENG)

694

Vertigo and tinnitus due to oral administration in 3 tablets of 750 mg daily
of anti-inflammatory agent, (SQ) monophenylbutazone, for 5 days in 1 of 10
humans, male, with rheumatoid arthritis.
Previous oral administration in 3 tablets of 840 mg daily of salicylate, (SQ)
acetylsalicylic acid, for 2 weeks in 1 of 10 humans, male, with rheumatoid
arthritis.   (ENG)

Salicylic acid

168

Appearance of salicylate in blood vessels of stria vascularis and spiral
ligament after 15 minutes due to parenteral, intravenous and intraperitoneal,
administration of 6.6 to 49.5 mc per kg, tritium-labelled solution, of salicylate, salicylic acid, in 5 animals, guinea pigs, albino, adult, 300 to 320
g weight.
Concentration of salicylate in stria vascularis and spiral ligament and
diffusion into organ of Corti and Rosenthal's canal after 1 hour due to
parenteral, intravenous and intraperitoneal, administration of 6.6 to 49.5 mc
per kg, tritium-labelled solution, of salicylate, salicylic acid, in 5 animals, guinea pigs, albino, adult, 300 to 320 g weight.
Small amount of salicylate after 6 hours and no salicylate after 13 hours in
cochlea due to parenteral, intravenous and intraperitoneal, administration of
6.6 to 49.5 mc per kg, tritium-labelled solution, of salicylate, salicylic
acid, in 5 animals, guinea pigs, albino, adult, 300 to 320 g weight.
   (AD) Autoradiographical study to determine mechanism of salicylate ototoxicity by localization of tritiated salicylate in cochlea of guinea pigs.
   (AD) Salicylate levels in cochlea due to vascular route and diffusion into
   cochlear duct and not due to accumulation in specific areas.   (ENG)

312

Transient bilateral sensorineural hearing loss of 60 and 50 decibels due to
topical, direct site, administration of ointment with 5 percent of salicylate, salicylic acid, for 3 times daily in 2 humans, female, with psoriasis.
(ENG)

Sodium salicylate

082

Transient threshold shift due to parenteral, intraperitoneal, administration
of 300 mg per kg (equivalent to 65 aspirin tablets for 70 kg man),in saline
solution, of salicylate, sodium salicylate, in 1 injection in animals, guinea
pigs.
   (CT) Electrophysiological measurement of hearing sensitivity before and
   after salicylate injection.
Transient threshold shift due to parenteral, intraperitoneal, administration
of 100 to 250 mg per kg of salicylate, sodium salicylate, in animals, guinea
pigs, conditioned.   (ENG)

166

Decr in succinic dehydrogenase concentration, in particular in stria vascularis and outer hair cells of organ of Corti, and decr in esterases and
sulfhydryl compounds due to parenteral, subcutaneous, administration of 100
mg per kg daily, in 2 ml distilled water, of salicylate, sodium salicylate,
for 28 days in animals, guinea pigs.
   (CT) Study of guinea pigs, control group, not treated with sodium salicylate.
   (AD) Report on relationship between changes in metabolism in inner ear due
   to sodium salicylate and auditory system problems.   (GER)

189

Threshold shift due to parenteral, intraperitoneal, administration of 300 mg
per kg of salicylate, sodium salicylate, in 1 dose in 4 animals, cats.

Small threshold shift of about 3 decibels due to parenteral, intraperitoneal, administration of 125 mg per kg daily of salicylate, sodium salicylate, for total of 28 injections in 4 animals, cats.
Threshold shift due to parenteral, intraperitoneal, administration of (SQ) 300 mg per kg of salicylate, sodium salicylate, in (SQ) 1 dose in 6 animals, guinea pigs.
Small threshold shift of about 4 decibels due to parenteral, intraperitoneal, administration of (SQ) 150,225, or 300 mg per kg daily of salicylate, sodium salicylate, for (SQ) total of 10 injections in 6 animals, guinea pigs.   (ENG)

205

Changes in biochemical composition of endolymph and perilymph due to parenteral, intraperitoneal, administration of 350 mg per kg of salicylate, sodium salicylate, in 1 injection in 6 animals, cats.
   (CT) Same method using 10 ml saline solution in 3 cats, control group.
Decr in cochlear microphonic and neural potential due to parenteral, intraperitoneal, administration of 350 mg per kg of salicylate, sodium salicylate, in 1 injection in 7 animals, cats.
   (CT) Baseline cochlear microphonic and neural potential obtained.
   (AD) Suggested that hearing loss in salicylate intoxication due to biochemical changes in cochlea.   (ENG)

284

Hearing loss due to antibiotics, aminoglycoside, in humans.
Hearing loss due to salicylate, sodium salicylate, in humans.
Hearing loss due to antimalarial, quinine, in humans.
   (AD) Discussion of clinical use and cochleotoxic effects of ototoxic drugs in humans.   (FR)

345

Transient hearing loss and vestibular problem due to salicylate, aspirin, in humans.
Decr in cochlear microphonic and action potential and decr in malic dehydrogenase in endolymph and perilymph due to salicylate, aspirin, in humans.
   (AD) Suggested that cochleo-vestibulotoxic effects of salicylates due to electrophysiological and biochemical changes and not structural changes.
Primary distribution in stria vascularis and spiral ligament due to salicylate, aspirin, in humans.
   (AD) Possible but not definite location of toxic activity of aspirin.
High concentration in inner ear after 5 to 7 hours due to parenteral, intraperitoneal, administration of salicylate, sodium salicylate, in animals, cats.
   (AD) Report on clinical use and ototoxic effects of aspirin.   (ENG)

OTHER ANALGESICS

Clonixin

353

Dizziness due to oral administration of 600 mg of analgesic, clonixin, in 1 dose in 2 of 24 humans, adult and aged, 21 to 68 years age, male and female, 126 to 210 lb weight, treated after surgery.
Hearing loss due to parenteral, intramuscular, administration of 6 mg of analgesic, morphine (morphine sulfate), in 1 dose in 1 of 24 humans, adult and aged, 21 to 68 years age, male and female, 126 to 210 lb weight, treated after surgery.
   (AD) Comparative study of effectiveness of oral clonixin and parenteral morphine in treatment after surgery.   (ENG)

Fentanyl

265

Hearing loss due to analgesic, fentanyl (SM), in humans, treated before ultrasound therapy for Meniere's disease.
Hearing loss due to tranquilizer, droperidol (SM), in humans, treated before ultrasound therapy for Meniere's disease.
   (AD) More severe hearing loss with simultaneous use of droperidol and fentanyl than with use of local anesthetic only.   (ENG)

310

Transient decr in vestibular function due to parenteral, intravenous, administration of 2 ml of tranquilizer, droperidol (CB), for 2 minutes in 18 of 21
humans, adolescent and adult, female and male.
Transient decr in vestibular function due to parenteral, intravenous, administration of 2 ml of analgesic, fentanyl (CB) (fentanyl citrate), for 2
minutes in 18 of 21 humans, adolescent and adult, female and male.
   (CT) Caloric tests, pretreatment and posttreatment.   (DAN)

703

No nystagmus due to parenteral, intramuscular, administration of 0.150 mg of
analgesic, fentanyl, in 5 animals, rabbits, 2.5 to 3 kg weight.
Positional nystagmus within 15 to 30 minutes due to parenteral administration
of 4 ml per kg of 96 percent solution of sedative, alcohol, in 8 animals,
rabbits, 2.5 to 3 kg weight.
Positional nystagmus within 15 to 30 minutes due to parenteral administration
of 4 ml per kg of 96 percent solution of sedative, (SQ) alcohol, in 11 animals, rabbits, 2.5 to 3 kg weight.
Partial or total suppression of positional nystagmus due to parenteral,
intramuscular, administration of 0.150 mg of analgesic, (SQ) fentanyl, in 6
of 11 animals, rabbits, 2.5 to 3 kg weight.
Decr in positional nystagmus due to parenteral, intramuscular, administration
of 0.08 to 0.10 mg of analgesic, (SQ) fentanyl, in 5 of 11 animals, rabbits,
2.5 to 3 kg weight.   (IT)

Morphine

353

Dizziness due to oral administration of 600 mg of analgesic, clonixin, in 1
dose in 2 of 24 humans, adult and aged, 21 to 68 years age, male and female,
126 to 210 lb weight, treated after surgery.
Hearing loss due to parenteral, intramuscular, administration of 6 mg of
analgesic, morphine (morphine sulfate), in 1 dose in 1 of 24 humans, adult
and aged, 21 to 68 years age, male and female, 126 to 210 lb weight, treated
after surgery.
   (AD) Comparative study of effectiveness of oral clonixin and parenteral
   morphine in treatment after surgery.   (ENG)

621

Primarily vestibular problems due to antibiotic, streptomycin, in humans.
Primarily hearing loss but also vestibular problems due to antibiotic, dihy-
drostreptomycin, in humans.
Primarily hearing loss but also vestibular problems due to antibiotic, kana-
mycin, in humans.
Primarily hearing loss but also vestibular problems due to antibiotic, neomy-
cin, in humans.
Primarily hearing loss but also vestibular problems due to antibiotic, genta-
micin, in humans.
Vertigo and ataxia due to antituberculous agent, isoniazid, in humans.
Hearing loss due to salicylate, aspirin, in humans.
Hearing loss and vertigo due to antimalarial, quinine, in humans.
Nystagmus due to barbiturates in humans.
Vestibular problems due to analgesic, morphine, in humans.
Nystagmus due to sedative, alcohol, in humans.
Nystagmus and hearing loss due to chemical agent, carbon monoxide, in humans.
Ototoxic effects due to antineoplastic, nitrogen mustard, in humans.
Ototoxic effects due to chemical agent, aniline, in humans.
Ototoxic effects due to chemical agent, tobacco, in humans.
Nystagmus due to chemical agent, nicotine, in humans.
Vestibular problems due to anticonvulsants in humans.
Vestibular problems due to anesthetics in humans.
Vestibular problems due to diuretics in humans.
   (AD) Inclusion of comprehensive list of ototoxic agents.   (SP)

ANESTHETICS

550

Decr in cochlear potentials due to parenteral, intraperitoneal, administra-

tion of 15 mg per kg of anesthetics (CB) in 2 groups of 15 animals, guinea
pigs, pigmented and albino, 300 g weight.
Decr in cochlear potentials due to parenteral, intraperitoneal, administration of 15 mg per kg of sedative, barbiturate (CB) in 2 groups of 15 animals,
guinea pigs, pigmented and albino, 300 g weight.   (IT)

621

Primarily vestibular problems due to antibiotic, streptomycin, in humans.
Primarily hearing loss but also vestibular problems due to antibiotic, dihy-
drostreptomycin, in humans.
Primarily hearing loss but also vestibular problems due to antibiotic, kana-
mycin, in humans.
Primarily hearing loss but also vestibular problems due to antibiotic, neomy-
cin, in humans.
Primarily hearing loss but also vestibular problems due to antibiotic, genta-
micin, in humans.
Vertigo and ataxia due to antituberculous agent, isoniazid, in humans.
Hearing loss due to salicylate, aspirin, in humans.
Hearing loss and vertigo due to antimalarial, quinine, in humans.
Nystagmus due to barbiturates in humans.
Vestibular problems due to analgesic, morphine, in humans.
Nystagmus due to sedative, alcohol, in humans.
Nystagmus and hearing loss due to chemical agent, carbon monoxide, in humans.
Ototoxic effects due to antineoplastic, nitrogen mustard, in humans.
Ototoxic effects due to chemical agent, aniline, in humans.
Ototoxic effects due to chemical agent, tobacco, in humans.
Nystagmus due to chemical agent, nicotine, in humans.
Vestibular problems due to anticonvulsants in humans.
Vestibular problems due to anesthetics in humans.
Vestibular problems due to diuretics in humans.
    (AD) Inclusion of comprehensive list of ototoxic agents.   (SP)

Cocaine

613

Significant decr in cochlear microphonic due to topical administration to
round window of 10 percent concentration of anesthetic, cocaine, in 15
minutes in animals, guinea pigs, 400 to 600 g weight.
Less, but permanent, decr in cochlear microphonic due to topical administration to round window of 2 percent concentration of anesthetic, tetracaine, in
15 minutes in animals, guinea pigs, 400 to 600 g weight.
    (AD) Need for careful consideration in use of topical anesthetic within
    middle ear.
    (AD) Suggested that cocaine not be used within middle ear.   (GER)

Garrot

190

Sudden deafness and tinnitus due to topical administration of anesthetic,
garrot, in 1 human, adult, 36 years age, female, with previous hearing loss.
    (AD) Need for careful consideration in use of topical garrot in humans
    with history of auditory system problems or vestibular problems.   (FR)

Lidocaine

152

Transient moderate dizziness due to parenteral, intravenous, administration
of 1.0 mg per kg of 1 percent concentration of anesthetic, lidocaine, for 30
seconds in 23 humans.
Transient severe dizziness and tinnitus due to parenteral, intravenous,
administration of 1.5 mg per kg of 1 percent concentration of anesthetic,
lidocaine, for 30 seconds in 6 humans.
    (CT) Same study without lidocaine injection in 9 humans, control group.
    (AD) Auditory system problems due to lidocaine reported in previous stu-
    dies.   (ENG)

443

Decr in summating potential and threshold shift due to topical administration

to round window of 2 percent solution of anesthetic, tetracaine, in animals, guinea pigs.
Decr in summating potential and threshold shift due to topical administration to round window of 4 percent solution of anesthetic, lidocaine, in animals, guinea pigs.
   (AD) More changes in summating potential and threshold due to tetracaine than to lidocaine.
   (AD) Partial recovery of summating potential after 60 minutes in guinea pigs treated with lidocaine.   (GER)

                                                                                    553
Tinnitus and distortion of sound due to parenteral, rapid intravenous, administration to arm of 2.5 mg per kg of 0.5 percent concentration of anesthetic, lidocaine, in 1 injection, with release of tourniquet 5 minutes after injection, in 9 of 10 humans, unpaid subjects.   (ENG)

                                                                                    646
Possible vertigo and tinnitus due to parenteral, intravenous, administration of 2 percent solution of anesthetic, lidocaine, in humans with heart disorder.   (ENG)

                                    Procaine

                                                                                    418
Hearing loss within 2 to 3 minutes after injection and tinnitus due to parenteral, intravenous, administration of anesthetic, procaine (procaine hydrochloride), in 30 humans with normal hearing and treated for disorders.
   (AD) Study of effect on hearing loss and tinnitus of manual compression of neurovascular bundle.
   (AD) No effect on tinnitus or hearing loss of manual compression of neurovascular bundle before and during injection of procaine.
   (AD) Disappearance of tinnitus due to unilateral manual compression of neurovascular bundle after injection of procaine in 23 subjects.
   (AD) Suppression of tinnitus only during manual compression of neurovascular bundle in other subjects.
   (AD) Less effect on hearing loss of manual compression of neurovascular bundle after injection of procaine.   (FR)

                                                                                    438
Suppression of microphonic potentials of saccule due to topical, intraluminal, administration of antibiotic, streptomycin, in animals, goldfish.
Suppression of microphonic potentials of saccule due to topical, intraluminal, administration of antibiotic, kanamycin, in animals, goldfish.
Suppression of microphonic potentials of saccule due to topical, intraluminal or extraluminal, administration of 0.5 mg of chemical agent, cyanide, in animals, goldfish.
Suppression of microphonic potentials of saccule due to topical, intraluminal or extraluminal, administration of 0.1 mg of antimalarial, quinine, in animals, goldfish.
Suppression of microphonic potentials of saccule due to topical, intraluminal or extraluminal, administration of 2 mg of anesthetic, procaine, in animals, goldfish.
No effect on microphonic potentials of saccule due to topical administration of salicylates in animals, goldfish.   (ENG)

                                                                                    562
Decr in microphonic potential of saccule due to topical, intraluminal, administration of antibiotic, streptomycin, in animals, goldfish.
Decr in microphonic potential of saccule due to topical, intraluminal, administration of antibiotic, kanamycin, in animals, goldfish.
Permanent decr in microphonic potential of saccule due to topical, intraluminal or extraluminal, administration of 0.5 mg per ml of chemical agent, cyanide, in animals, goldfish.
Permanent decr in microphonic potential of saccule due to topical, intraluminal or extraluminal, administration of 0.1 mg per ml of antimalarial, quinine, in animals, goldfish.
No effect on microphonic potential of saccule due to salicylate, aspirin, in animals, goldfish.

Some decr in microphonic potential of saccule due to 2 mg per ml of anesthetic, procaine, in animals, goldfish.
   (AD) Study of effects of various agents on microphonic potential of saccule of goldfish.   (JAP)

Tetracaine

266
Effect on enzymes of cochlea and vestibular apparatus due to topical adminis-
tration to bulla of 0.2 ml of 2 percent solution of anesthetic, tetracaine
(tetracaine hydrochloride), in animals, guinea pigs.
   (CT) Study of guinea pigs, control group, not treated with tetracaine.
   (GER)

351
No observed ototoxic effects due to topical administration of 1 drop of
chemical agent, dimethyl sulfoxide (CB), in humans as anesthetic for myringotomy.
No observed ototoxic effects due to topical administration of 1 drop of
anesthetic, tetracaine (CB) (tetracaine hydrochloride), in humans as anesthetic for myringotomy.   (ENG)

389
Damage to epithelial cells of round window due to 1 percent solution of
anesthetic, tetracaine, in animals, guinea pigs, 250 to 500 g weight.   (GER)

443
Decr in summating potential and threshold shift due to topical administration
to round window of 2 percent solution of anesthetic, tetracaine, in animals,
guinea pigs.
Decr in summating potential and threshold shift due to topical administration
to round window of 4 percent solution of anesthetic, lidocaine, in animals,
guinea pigs.
   (AD) More changes in summating potential and threshold due to tetracaine
   than to lidocaine.
   (AD) Partial recovery of summating potential after 60 minutes in guinea
   pigs treated with lidocaine.   (GER)

613
Significant decr in cochlear microphonic due to topical administration to
round window of 10 percent concentration of anesthetic, cocaine, in 15
minutes in animals, guinea pigs, 400 to 600 g weight.
Less, but permanent, decr in cochlear microphonic due to topical administration to round window of 2 percent concentration of anesthetic, tetracaine, in
15 minutes in animals, guinea pigs, 400 to 600 g weight.
   (AD) Need for careful consideration in use of topical anesthetic within
   middle ear.
   (AD) Suggested that cocaine not be used within middle ear.   (GER)

ANTIBIOTICS

032
Progressive permanent sensorineural hearing loss due to topical administration of unspecified doses of antibiotics for long period in 1 human, child, 6
years age, female, with severe burns on 80 percent of body.   (ENG)

039
Damage to endorgan of cochlea and vestibular apparatus due to parenteral or
oral administration of high doses of antibiotics for long periods in humans.
No reported ototoxic effects due to topical administration of unspecified
doses of antibiotics for unspecified period in humans.   (ENG)

065
Prevention of destruction of organ of Corti due to low doses of antibiotics
(IB) in animals, guinea pigs, with administration of vitamin B and amino
acids.
   (AD) Need for histological studies to determine method for prevention of
   ototoxicity.   (FR)

066

Hearing loss due to various methods of administration of antibiotics in
humans with acute otitis media.   (RUS)

083

Cochleo-vestibulotoxic effects due to parenteral, oral, and topical administration of antibiotics in humans, with normal kidney function and with kidney
disorder.
      (AD) Literature review of ototoxic effects of antibiotics.
      (AD) Recommended dosage and duration of dosage of antibiotics discussed.
      (ENG)

087

High frequency hearing loss and tinnitus due to antibiotics in humans, parti-
cularly infant and aged, and humans with kidney disorder.
Degeneration in hair cells of organ of Corti due to antibiotics in humans.
Vertigo and unsteady gait due to antibiotic, streptomycin, in humans.
Bilateral damage to vestibular apparatus due to antibiotic, streptomycin, in
humans.
      (AD) Literature review of physiological and structural cochleo-vestibulo-
      toxic effects of antibiotics.
      (AD) Degree of damage determined by dosage and duration of dosage of
      antibiotics.   (ENG)

099

Hearing loss due to antibiotics in humans, adult and child, male and female,
with kidney disorder.   (HUN)

109

Damage to hair cells in organ of Corti due to topical administration of 300
mg per kg of antibiotic, kanamycin, in 14 injections in animals, guinea pigs.
Severe degeneration of hair cells of organ of Corti and membranous labyrinth
due to topical administration to middle ear of low doses of antibiotics in
animals, guinea pigs.
      (AD) Report on studies of several years on cochleo-vestibulotoxic effects
      due to antibiotics.   (ENG)

115

Permanent cochleo-vestibulotoxic effects due to antibiotics, aminoglycoside,
in humans.
Transient cochlear impairment due to salicylates in humans.
Ototoxic effects due to antimalarial, quinine, in humans.
Ototoxic effects due to chemical agent, nicotine, in humans.
      (AD) Report on ototoxic effects of various drugs.
      (AD) Need for audiometry and vestibular function tests with clinical use
      of ototoxic drugs.   (FR)

118

Nystagmus and unsteady gait due to unspecified doses of antibiotics (SM) in 1
human, adult, 47 years age, male, with epilepsy.
Simultaneous administration of anticonvulsant, primidone (SM), in 1 human,
adult, 47 years age, male, with epilepsy.
Simultaneous administration of antihistamine, dimenhydrinate (SM), in 1
human, adult, 47 years age, male, with epilepsy.   (ENG)

123

Sensorineural hearing loss and vestibular problems due to range of doses of
antibiotics in humans.
      (AD) Report on cochleo-vestibulotoxic effects of antibiotics used clini-
      cally.   (ENG)

127

Ototoxic effects due to antibiotics in humans with kidney tuberculosis.
      (AD) Literature review of ototoxic effects of streptomycin, viomycin,
      kanamycin, and capreomycin.   (GER)

132

Sensorineural hearing loss due to antibiotics in humans.

(AD) Study of iatrogenic hearing loss.   (GER)

135

Vertigo and sensorineural hearing loss due to antibiotics, aminoglycoside, in humans.
 (AD) Possible permanent damage due to low doses of streptomycin, dihydros-treptomycin, or kanamycin.
 (AD) Report on etiology of vertigo.   (ENG)

149

Damage to organ of Corti due to antibiotics in humans.
 (AD) Discussion of ototoxicity in humans based on animal experimentation.
 (FR)

154

Ototoxic effects due to antibiotics in humans with tuberculosis.
 (AD) Literature review of some new antituberculous agents of 1968.   (GER)

182

Sensorineural hearing loss, from frequency at 8000 cps to speech range, due to antibiotics in humans.
 (AD) Specific audiometric configuration for hearing loss due to antibio-tics.
 (AD) Use of level of 15 db at 8000 cps for detection of hearing loss due to antibiotics.   (ENG)

186

Diplacusis due to antibiotics, aminoglycoside, in humans.
Diplacusis due to antimalarial, quinine, in humans.
Diplacusis due to salicylate, aspirin, in humans.
Diplacusis due to chemical agent, carbon monoxide, in humans.
 (AD) Report on etiology of diplacusis with comment on ototoxic drugs.
 (ENG)

188

Possible hearing loss due to antibiotics in humans, child, treated when newborn infant.
 (AD) Reported that 23 percent of 46 children with idiopathic hearing loss treated with antibiotics in neonatal period.
 (CT) Reported that 2 percent of 54 children with normal hearing treated with antibiotics in neonatal period.
Possible hearing loss in fetus due to salicylate, aspirin, in humans, female, during pregnancy.
 (AD) Ingestion of salicylate, aspirin, during pregnancy by mothers of 2 percent of total of 118 children with hearing loss.
 (CT) Ingestion of salicylate, aspirin, during pregnancy by mothers of 0 of 54 children with normal hearing.
 (AD) Study of etiology of hearing loss in children.   (ENG)

193

Sensorineural hearing loss and structural damage to cochlea due to low doses of antibiotics in humans.
 (AD) Report on clinical and pathological effects possible with use of antibiotics.
 (AD) Toxic levels in blood possible due to low doses in therapy.
 (AD) Need for audiometry, vestibular function tests, and determination of blood levels of antibiotics during treatment.   (SER)

201

Vertigo and sensorineural hearing loss due to antibiotics, aminoglycoside, in humans.
 (AD) Report on risks in clinical use of different antibiotics.
 (AD) Need for audiometry and vestibular function tests in antibiotic therapy over long period.
 (AD) Cochleo-vestibulotoxic effects due to daily and total dosage of antibiotics.   (FR)

202

Risk of cochleo-vestibulotoxic effects due to antibiotics, aminoglycoside, in
humans, child, treated for tuberculosis and in particular with kidney disor-
ders.
   (AD) Good prognosis for vestibular problems in children.
   (AD) Need for early detection of hearing loss in children.
   (AD) Comment on maximum doses of antibiotics. (FR)

210

Risk of cochleo-vestibulotoxic effects due to oral or parenteral administration of antibiotics, aminoglycoside, in humans with normal kidney function
and with kidney disorder.
Risk of cochleo-vestibulotoxic effects due to topical administration of low
doses of antibiotics, aminoglycoside, in humans.
   (AD) Literature review of auditory system problems due to aminoglycoside
   antibiotics.
   (AD) Need to determine dosage of antibiotics on basis of body weight,
   kidney function, and age.
   (AD) Need for audiometry, vestibular function tests, determination of
   blood levels, and tests of kidney function during treatment with antibiotics. (SW)

219

Cochleo-vestibulotoxic effects due to antibiotics in humans.
Transient and permanent sensorineural hearing loss due to diuretic, etha-
crynic acid, in humans.
Transient sensorineural hearing loss, tinnitus, and vertigo due to salicy-
late, aspirin, in humans.
Transient and permanent sensorineural hearing loss and dizziness due to
antimalarial, quinine, in humans.
Sensorineural hearing loss due to antimalarial, chloroquine, in humans.
Sensorineural hearing loss, tinnitus, and vertigo due to chemical agents in
humans.
   (AD) Literature review of ototoxic drugs with clinical and histopathologi-
   cal correlations.
   (AD) Comment on ototoxicity of some chemical agents.
   (AD) Review of theories of mechanism of action of ototoxic drugs. (ENG)

221

Cochleo-vestibulotoxic effects due to antibiotics, aminoglycoside, in humans
with tuberculosis of genitourinary system.
   (AD) Need for multiple antibiotic therapy in tuberculosis but risk of
   ototoxic effects. (IT)

222

Cochleo-vestibulotoxic effects due to antibiotics in humans treated for
tuberculosis.
   (AD) Report on ototoxic effects of antibiotics used in tuberculosis chemotherapy and control of ototoxic effects. (GER)

240

Ototoxic effects due to topical administration to inner ear of antibiotics,
aminoglycoside, in 200 animals, guinea pigs, 250 g weight, with positive
Preyer reflex.
   (CT) Study of guinea pigs, control group.
   (AD) Comparative study of ototoxicity of aminoglycoside antibiotics.
   (GER)

244

Hearing loss and damage to organ of Corti due to antibiotics, aminoglycoside,
in humans.
   (AD) Literature review of ototoxic effects of different aminoglycoside
   antibiotics. (GER)

249

Cochleo-vestibulotoxic effects due to antibiotics, aminoglycoside, in humans.
Cochlear impairment due to antimalarial, quinine, in humans.
Transient cochlear impairment and vestibular problems due to salicylates in
humans.

(AD) Occurrence of ototoxic effects with different dosages due to indivi-
dual responses to drugs.
(AD) Need for observation and tests with clinical use of ototoxic drugs.
(FR)

260

High antibiotic levels in perilymph due to topical administration to inner
ear of antibiotics in animals, guinea pigs.
(AD) Antibiotic levels in perilymph due to topical administration comp w
levels due to intramuscular administration.
(AD) Neomycin levels due to topical route higher than levels due to intramuscular route.   (GER)

264

Cochleo-vestibulotoxic effects due to antibiotics in humans.
(AD) Comment on complications due to antibiotics after head and neck
surgery.   (ENG)

272

Hearing loss and damage to organ of Corti due to antibiotics in humans.
(AD) Literature review of ototoxic effects of antibiotics used in therapy.
(FIN)

279

Transient inhibition of endorgan of ampulla of semicircular canal due to
range of doses of antibiotics, aminoglycoside, in animals, frogs.
(CT) Study of frogs, control group.
(AD) In vitro study of effect of antibiotics on function of ampullar
endorgan of semicircular canal of frog.   (IT)

284

Hearing loss due to antibiotics, aminoglycoside, in humans.
Hearing loss due to salicylate, sodium salicylate, in humans.
Hearing loss due to antimalarial, quinine, in humans.
(AD) Discussion of clinical use and cochleotoxic effects of ototoxic drugs
in humans.   (FR)

294

Hearing loss and vestibular problems due to antibiotics in humans, adult,
male and female, with chronic kidney disorder.   (RUS)

357

Hearing loss due to antibiotics in 60(5.4 percent) of 1100 humans treated for
different disorders.   (RUS)

410

Damage to organ of Corti of fetus due to antibiotics in humans, female,
during pregnancy.
(AD) Discussion of etiology of damage to organ of Corti in fetus.   (FR)

422

Hearing loss due to antibiotics in humans, female, treated during pregnancy
or for disorders of genitourinary system.   (RUS)

423

More severe and more rapid progression of presbycusis due to antimalarial,
quinine, in humans, adult and aged.
More severe and more rapid progression of presbycusis due to antibiotics,
aminoglycoside, in humans, adult and aged.
More severe and more rapid progression of presbycusis due to salicylate,
aspirin, in humans, adult and aged.
More severe and more rapid progression of presbycusis due to chemical agent,
carbon monoxide, in humans, adult and aged.
(AD) Discussion of factors resulting in more severe and more rapid progression of presbycusis.   (FR)

441

Ototoxic effects due to antibiotics in humans.

(AD) Monogr on production of antibiotics, mechanism of action, clinical
use, toxicity, and other aspects.   (RUS)

458

Damage to cochlear function and vestibular function and structural damage to
cochlea and vestibular apparatus due to antibiotics in animals, guinea pigs.
   (AD) Use of Preyer reflex, vestibular function tests, and measurement of
   cochlear microphonics to determine ototoxic effects of antibiotics on
   function of inner ear.
   (AD) Histological study to determine structural damage to inner ear.
   (ENG)

462

Damage to hair cells of organ of Corti, stria vascularis, nerve process,
spiral ganglion, limbus, and cochlear wall due to antibiotics in animals,
guinea pigs.
   (AD) Ototoxic effects result of retention of antibiotics in inner ear
   longer than in blood due to slower elimination.
   (AD) More active cells of cochlea more sensitive to ototoxic antibiotics.
   (AD) Neomycin most ototoxic, followed by kanamycin, viomycin, streptomycin, and capreomycin.
   (AD) Study of effect of inhibitors, nialamide, pantothenic acid, methylated compounds, and vitamin B on ototoxicity of antibiotics.
   (AD) Electrophysiological and histological study of cochleo-vestibulotoxic
   effects of antibiotics in guinea pig.   (ENG)

506

Damage to hair cells of vestibular apparatus and cochlea due to antibiotics
in humans and animals.
   (AD) Discussion of relationship between elimination of drugs and damage to
   ear.
   (AD) Need for careful consideration in use of aminoglycoside antibiotics.
   (ENG)

521

Hearing loss due to antibiotics in humans, child, with infections.
   (AD) Analysis of ototoxic effects due to antibiotics.   (RUS)

523

Cochleo-vestibulotoxic effects due to topical, parenteral, or oral administration of antibiotics, aminoglycoside, in humans.   (NOR)

545

Ototoxic effects due to antibiotics in humans with disorders.
   (AD) Literature review of clinical use and toxic effects of antibiotics.
   (IT)

549

Cochleo-vestibulotoxic effects due to antibiotics in humans with disorders.
(RUS)

592

Ototoxic effects due to antibiotics in humans.
   (AD) Discussion of effects of some drugs used in otolaryngology.   (CZ)

608

Possible hearing loss due to antibiotics in humans with disorders.
   (AD) Evaluation of degree of hearing loss due to antibiotics possible with
   pretreatment and posttreatment audiometry.   (HUN)

609

Possible ototoxic effects due to antibiotics in humans with genitourinary
system infections.
   (AD) Literature review of antibiotic therapy of genitourinary system
   infections.   (GER)

627

Sensorineural hearing loss and vestibular problems due to parenteral, oral,

and topical administration of antibiotics in humans with and without kidney
disorder.
Degeneration of cochlea due to parenteral, intratympanic, administration of
antibiotic, neomycin, in animals, guinea pigs.
Transient sensorineural hearing loss due to high doses of salicylates in
humans.
Sensorineural hearing loss due to antimalarial, quinine, in humans.
Sensorineural hearing loss due to chemical agent, tobacco, in humans.
Sensorineural hearing loss due to sedative, alcohol, in humans.
   (AD) Discussion of ototoxicity of various drugs as 1 etiology of sen-
   sorineural hearing loss in adults. (ENG)

                                                                    630
Ototoxic effects due to antibiotics in humans treated for infection. (ENG)

                                                                    638
Hearing loss due to antibiotics in humans with disorders. (RUS)

                                                                    640
Ototoxic effects due to antibiotics in humans with tuberculosis.
   (AD) Literature review of chemotherapy of tuberculosis with comment on
   toxic effects of drugs. (GER)

                                                                    689
Hearing loss due to antibiotics in humans with tuberculosis. (POL)

                                                                    704
Functional damage to cochlea evident before changes in structure due to
antibiotics in animals.
   (AD) Need for correlation of various methods, morphological, electrophy-
   siological, and biochemical, in study of function of inner ear.
   (AD) Literature review of various methods of study of auditory system.
   (ENG)

                                                                    706
Ototoxic effects due to chemical agents and heavy metals in humans.
   (AD) Literature review of ototoxic effects of nicotine, carbon monoxide,
   carbon tetrachloride, mercury, arsenic, and lead.
Cochleo-vestibulotoxic effects, functional and structural, due to antibiotics
in humans.
   (AD) Literature review of ototoxicity of streptomycin, dihydrostreptomy-
   cin, neomycin, kanamycin, gentamicin, capreomycin, rifampicin, viomycin,
   isoniazid, aminosidine, and framycetin.
Hearing loss due to salicylates in humans.
Hearing loss due to antimalarial, quinine, in humans.
Hearing loss due to diuretic, ethacrynic acid, in humans.
   (AD) Literature review of effects of various ototoxic agents. (IT)

                                                                    712
Ototoxic effects due to antibiotics in humans in surgery. (HUN)

                                                                    713
Inhibition of oxygen consumption of cochlea due to antibiotics in animals,
guinea pigs.
   (AD) In vitro study using microrespirometer of effect of antibiotics on
   oxygen consumption in guinea pig cochlea. (JAP)

                              Actinomycin

                                                                    457
Tinnitus and progressive sensorineural hearing loss due to parenteral, intramuscular, administration of antibiotic, (SQ) streptomycin, for 10 days in 1
human, adult, 38 years age, female, with infections and later development of
kidney disorder.
Tinnitus and progressive sensorineural hearing loss due to 13.2 g of antibiotic, (SQ) kanamycin, for 11 days in 1 human, adult, 38 years age, female,
with infections and kidney disorder.
Hearing loss due to antimalarial, (SQ) quinine, in 1 human, adult, 20 years

age, male, with various infections and later development of kidney disorder.
Hearing loss due to 400 mg 2 times daily, total dose of 6.5 g, of antibiotic,
(SQ) kanamycin (SM), for 8 days in 1 human, adult, 20 years age, male, with
various infections and later development of kidney disorder.
Hearing loss due to 150 mg 2 times daily, total dose of 2400 mg, of antibiotic, (SQ) colistin (SM), for 8 days in 1 human, adult, 20 years age, male,
with various infections and later development of kidney disorder.
Tinnitus, total bilateral hearing loss, and vestibular problems due to parenteral, intramuscular, administration of 4.0 g daily, total of 21 g, of antibiotic, (SQ) kanamycin (SM), for 5 days in 1 human, adult, 20 years age,
male, with infections and kidney disorder.
Tinnitus, total bilateral hearing loss, and vestibular problems due to 0.6 g
daily, total dose of 1.3 g, of antibiotic, (SQ) colistin (SM), for 2 days in
1 human, adult, 20 years age, male, with infections and kidney disorder.
Tinnitus, total bilateral hearing loss, and vestibular problems due to 2 g
and then 8 g per 24 hours in divided doses, total dose of 26.5 g, of antibiotic, (SQ) chloramphenicol, for 9 days in 1 human, adult, 20 years age, male,
with infections and kidney disorder.
Bilateral hearing loss due to 1 g daily of antibiotic, actinomycin (SM), for
5 days in 1 human, adult, 62 years age, male, with infections and kidney
disorder.
Bilateral hearing loss due to unknown dose of antibiotic, kanamycin (SM), for
5 days in 1 human, adult, 62 years age, male, with infections and kidney
disorder.
Bilateral hearing loss and vestibular problems due to parenteral administration of high doses of antibiotic, (SQ) neomycin, for total of 21 days in 1
human, adult, 25 years age, male, with infection from wound.
Previous administration of unspecified doses of antibiotic, (SQ) streptomycin, in 1 human, adult, 25 years age, male, with infection from wound.
Later administration of antibiotic, (SQ) chloramphenicol, in 1 human, adult,
25 years age, male, with infection from wound.
Tinnitus and rapidly progressive bilateral hearing loss due to parenteral,
intramuscular, administration of 0.5 g every 12 hours of antibiotic, (SQ)
streptomycin, for 5 days in 1 human, adult, 21 years age, male, with infection from wound.
Tinnitus and rapidly progressive bilateral hearing loss due to parenteral,
intramuscular, administration of 200 mg daily, total of 6.8 g, of antibiotic,
(SQ) colistin (SM), in 1 human, adult, 21 years age, male, with infection
from wound.
Tinnitus and rapidly progressive bilateral hearing loss due to parenteral
administration of unspecified doses of antibiotic, (SQ) neomycin (SM), for
about 35 days in 1 human, adult, 21 years age, male, with infection from
wound.
Tinnitus and progressive bilateral hearing loss due to parenteral administration of 2 l per 24 hours of 1 percent solution of antibiotic, (SQ) neomycin,
for 10 days in 1 human, adult, 26 years age, male, with infection from wound.
   (AD) Hearing loss confirmed by audiometry.
Previous administration of 500 mg four times a day of antibiotic, (SQ) ampicillin, in 1 human, adult, 26 years age, male, with infection from wound.
Bilateral sudden deafness due to administration in dialysis fluid of less
than 150 mg of antibiotic, neomycin (SM), in 1 human, adult, 44 years age,
female, with kidney disorder.
Bilateral sudden deafness due to 50 mg of diuretic, ethacrynic acid (SM), in
1 human, adult, 44 years age, female, with kidney disorder.
   (AD) Hearing loss confirmed by audiology.
Tinnitus and progressive bilateral hearing loss beginning after 8 days of
treatment due to parenteral administration of 1 l every 4 hours for 3 days
and then every 8 hours for 10 days of 1 percent solution of antibiotic,
neomycin, in 1 human, adult, 20 years age, male, with infection from wound.
   (AD) Hearing loss confirmed by audiology.
Tinnitus and bilateral sensorineural hearing loss due to parenteral, intramuscular, administration of 1 g and then 0.5 g every 12 hours of antibiotic,
streptomycin (SM), for 15 days in 1 human, adult, 23 years age, male, with
infection from wound.
Tinnitus and bilateral sensorineural hearing loss due to topical administration by irrigation of 1 percent solution every 12 hours of antibiotic, neomycin (SM), for 14 days in 1 human, adult, 23 years age, male, with infection
from wound.

(AD) Hearing loss confirmed by audiometry.
(AD) Discussion of 10 case reports.   (ENG)

Aminosidine

247

No ototoxic effects due to parenteral, subcutaneous, administration of low
doses used in therapy, 20 mg per kg daily in 2 doses every 12 hours, of
antibiotic, aminosidine (aminosidine sulfate), for 60 days in 20 animals,
guinea pigs, adult, 300 g average weight.
  (CT) Study of 5 guinea pigs, control group.
  (CT) Test for Preyer reflex and vestibular function tests, pretreatment
  and during treatment.
  (AD) Previous studies showed ototoxic effects of high doses of aminosidine
  in animals.
  (AD) Suggested clinical use of aminosidine in low doses for short periods.
  (IT)

251

Damage to organ of Corti and crista ampullaris due to parenteral, subcutaneous, administration of 200 or 400 mg per kg daily in 3 doses every 8
hours of antibiotic, aminosidine (aminosidine sulfate), for 30 days in 2
groups of 16 animals, guinea pigs, 300 g weight.
Less damage to organ of Corti and crista ampullaris due to parenteral, subcutaneous, administration of 50 or 100 mg per kg daily in 3 doses every 8 hours
of antibiotic, aminosidine (aminosidine sulfate), for 30 days in 2 groups of
16 animals, guinea pigs, 300 g weight.
  (CT) Study of 8 guinea pigs, control group.
  (CT) Observation of function of cochlea and vestibular apparatus, pretreatment and during treatment.   (IT)

252

No cochlear impairment or vestibular problems due to parenteral, intramuscular, administration of average daily dose of 16 mg per kg in 2 doses every 12
hours of antibiotic, aminosidine (aminosidine sulfate), for range of 10 to 30
days in 118 humans, adult, male and female, with disorders.
  (CT) Audiometry and vestibular function tests, pretreatment and posttreatment, immediately after cessation of treatment and 1 month later.   (IT)

Ampicillin

384

Usually transient hearing loss and no structural damage to organ of Corti,
stria vascularis, and spiral ganglion due to oral or topical administration
of salicylates in humans.
Hearing loss due to antimalarial, quinine, in humans.
Usually permanent hearing loss due to antimalarial, chloroquine, in humans.
Transient and permanent hearing loss and possible damage to hair cells of
organ of Corti due to diuretic, ethacrynic acid, in humans.
Sensorineural hearing loss due to cardiovascular agent, hexadimethrine
bromide, in humans with kidney disorder.
Sensorineural hearing loss and damage to organ of Corti due to topical ad-
ministration of antineoplastic, nitrogen mustard, in humans.
Sensorineural hearing loss due to high doses of antibiotic, chloramphenicol,
in humans.
Primary vestibular problems due to antibiotic, streptomycin, in humans.
Hearing loss due to high doses usually of antibiotic, streptomycin, in humans.
  (AD) Early detection of hearing loss by audiometry prevents permanent
  damage.
High frequency hearing loss and severe damage to outer hair cells and slight
damage to inner hair cells of organ of Corti due to antibiotic, kanamycin, in
humans.
Sensorineural hearing loss due to parenteral, oral, and topical administration of antibiotic, neomycin, in humans with or without kidney disorders.
Degeneration of hair cells of organ of Corti and of nerve process due to
antibiotics, aminoglycoside, in animals.
  (AD) Literature review of physiological and structural cochleo-vestibulo-

toxic effects of ototoxic drugs.
   (AD) Discussion of suggested mechanism of ototoxicity and routes of drugs
   to inner ear.
Bilateral sensorineural hearing loss due to oral administration of antibiotic, neomycin, in 4 of 8 humans with liver disease.
Bilateral sensorineural hearing loss due to oral administration of range of
doses of antibiotic, neomycin (SM), in 2 of 5 humans with liver disease.
Bilateral sensorineural hearing loss due to diuretics (SM), in 2 of 5 humans
with liver disease.
Transient progression of previous hearing loss due to parenteral, intravenous, administration of diuretic, ethacrynic acid (SM), in 1 injection in 1
of 5 humans with liver disease.
   (CT) Normal cochlear function in 6 humans, control group, with liver
   disease and not treated with neomycin or diuretics.
   (CT) Normal cochlear function in 13 humans, control group, with liver
   disease and treated with diuretics but not with neomycin.
   (AD) Hearing loss confirmed by audiometry.
   (AD) Reported that hearing loss due to neomycin or diuretics in humans
   with liver disease not related to dosage.
   (AD) Clinical study of effects of treatment with neomycin and diuretics in
   humans with liver disease.
Bilateral sensorineural hearing loss and vertigo due to antibiotic, ampicil-
lin, in 1 human, adolescent, 17 years age, female, with tonsillitis.
   (AD) Cited case report.
Severe sensorineural hearing loss and vertigo due to topical administration
in ear drops of antibiotic, framycetin, in 1 human, adult, 42 years age,
male, with previous slight high frequency hearing loss.
   (AD) Cited case report.
Atrophy of hair cells of organ of Corti and hearing loss due to antibiotic,
dihydrostreptomycin, in humans with tuberculous meningitis.
   (AD) Cited study.
Loss of inner hair cells and damage to outer hair cells due to 18 g of anti-
biotic, neomycin, for 18 days in 1 human.
   (AD) Cited case report.   (ENG)

                                                                          457
Tinnitus and progressive sensorineural hearing loss due to parenteral, intramuscular, administration of antibiotic, (SQ) streptomycin, for 10 days in 1
human, adult, 38 years age, female, with infections and later development of
kidney disorder.
Tinnitus and progressive sensorineural hearing loss due to 13.2 g of antibiotic, (SQ) kanamycin, for 11 days in 1 human, adult, 38 years age, female,
with infections and kidney disorder.
Hearing loss due to antimalarial, (SQ) quinine, in 1 human, adult, 20 years
age, male, with various infections and later development of kidney disorder.
Hearing loss due to 400 mg 2 times daily, total dose of 6.5 g, of antibiotic,
(SQ) kanamycin (SM), for 8 days in 1 human, adult, 20 years age, male, with
various infections and later development of kidney disorder.
Hearing loss due to 150 mg 2 times daily, total dose of 2400 mg, of antibiotic, (SQ) colistin (SM), for 8 days in 1 human, adult, 20 years age, male,
with various infections and later development of kidney disorder.
Tinnitus, total bilateral hearing loss, and vestibular problems due to parenteral, intramuscular, administration of 4.0 g daily, total of 21 g, of antibiotic, (SQ) kanamycin (SM), for 5 days in 1 human, adult, 20 years age,
male, with infections and kidney disorder.
Tinnitus, total bilateral hearing loss, and vestibular problems due to 0.6 g
daily, total dose of 1.3 g, of antibiotic, (SQ) colistin (SM), for 2 days in
1 human, adult, 20 years age, male, with infections and kidney disorder.
Tinnitus, total bilateral hearing loss, and vestibular problems due to 2 g
and then 8 g per 24 hours in divided doses, total dose of 26.5 g, of antibiotic, (SQ) chloramphenicol, for 9 days in 1 human, adult, 20 years age, male,
with infections and kidney disorder.
Bilateral hearing loss due to 1 g daily of antibiotic, actinomycin (SM), for
5 days in 1 human, adult, 62 years age, male, with infections and kidney
disorder.
Bilateral hearing loss due to unknown dose of antibiotic, kanamycin (SM), for
5 days in 1 human, adult, 62 years age, male, with infections and kidney
disorder.

Bilateral hearing loss and vestibular problems due to parenteral administration of high doses of antibiotic, (SQ) neomycin, for total of 21 days in 1 human, adult, 25 years age, male, with infection from wound.
Previous administration of unspecified doses of antibiotic, (SQ) streptomycin, in 1 human, adult, 25 years age, male, with infection from wound.
Later administration of antibiotic, (SQ) chloramphenicol, in 1 human, adult, 25 years age, male, with infection from wound.
Tinnitus and rapidly progressive bilateral hearing loss due to parenteral, intramuscular, administration of 0.5 g every 12 hours of antibiotic, (SQ) streptomycin, for 5 days in 1 human, adult, 21 years age, male, with infection from wound.
Tinnitus and rapidly progressive bilateral hearing loss due to parenteral, intramuscular, administration of 200 mg daily, total of 6.8 g, of antibiotic, (SQ) colistin (SM), in 1 human, adult, 21 years age, male, with infection from wound.
Tinnitus and rapidly progressive bilateral hearing loss due to parenteral administration of unspecified doses of antibiotic, (SQ) neomycin (SM), for about 35 days in 1 human, adult, 21 years age, male, with infection from wound.
Tinnitus and progressive bilateral hearing loss due to parenteral administration of 2 l per 24 hours of 1 percent solution of antibiotic, (SQ) neomycin, for 10 days in 1 human, adult, 26 years age, male, with infection from wound.
    (AD) Hearing loss confirmed by audiometry.
Previous administration of 500 mg four times a day of antibiotic, (SQ) ampicillin, in 1 human, adult, 26 years age, male, with infection from wound.
Bilateral sudden deafness due to administration in dialysis fluid of less than 150 mg of antibiotic, neomycin (SM), in 1 human, adult, 44 years age, female, with kidney disorder.
Bilateral sudden deafness due to 50 mg of diuretic, ethacrynic acid (SM), in 1 human, adult, 44 years age, female, with kidney disorder.
    (AD) Hearing loss confirmed by audiology.
Tinnitus and progressive bilateral hearing loss beginning after 8 days of treatment due to parenteral administration of 1 l every 4 hours for 3 days and then every 8 hours for 10 days of 1 percent solution of antibiotic, neomycin, in 1 human, adult, 20 years age, male, with infection from wound.
    (AD) Hearing loss confirmed by audiology.
Tinnitus and bilateral sensorineural hearing loss due to parenteral, intramuscular, administration of 1 g and then 0.5 g every 12 hours of antibiotic, streptomycin (SM), for 15 days in 1 human, adult, 23 years age, male, with infection from wound.
Tinnitus and bilateral sensorineural hearing loss due to topical administration by irrigation of 1 percent solution every 12 hours of antibiotic, neomycin (SM), for 14 days in 1 human, adult, 23 years age, male, with infection from wound.
    (AD) Hearing loss confirmed by audiometry.
    (AD) Discussion of 10 case reports. (ENG)

                         Capreomycin

                                                                  062
High frequency hearing loss and tinnitus due to parenteral, intramuscular, administration of 1 g daily for first 60 days and then 1 g daily for 2 days each week of antibiotic, capreomycin (SM), for 1 year in 7 of 89 humans, range of ages, male and female, with pulmonary tuberculosis.
    (CT) No auditory system problems before treatment.
    (CT) Audiometry 1 time each month for duration of treatment.
    (AD) Previous resistance to primary antituberculous agents reported.
Simultaneous oral administration of 25 mg per kg daily for first 60 days and then 15 mg per kg daily of antituberculous agent, ethambutol (SM), for 1 year in 89 humans, range of ages, male and female, with pulmonary tuberculosis.
No reported ototoxic effects due to oral administration of 300 mg daily of antituberculous agent, isoniazid (SM), for 1 year in 89 humans, range of ages, male and female, with pulmonary tuberculosis.
    (AD) Previous resistance to isoniazid reported. (ENG)

                                                                  068
Hearing loss and tinnitus or hyperacusis due to oral administration of 1 g daily of antibiotic, (SQ) capreomycin, for 2 years in 3 of first group of 34

humans with tuberculosis.
No reported ototoxic effects due to previous unspecified method of administration of unspecified doses of antibiotic, (SQ) streptomycin, in first group
of 34 humans with tuberculosis.
Hearing loss due to previous unspecified method of administration of unspecified doses of antibiotic, (SQ) streptomycin, in 9 of second group of 31
humans with tuberculosis.
More severe hearing loss due to oral administration of 1 g daily of antibiotic, (SQ) capreomycin, for 2 years in 1 of second group of 31 humans with
tuberculosis.   (ENG)

                                                                          075
Hearing loss due to previous administration of antibiotic, (SQ) streptomycin,
in 18 of total of 67 humans with tuberculosis.
More severe hearing loss, tinnitus, or hyperacusis due to unspecified method
of administration of unspecified doses of antibiotic, (SQ) capreomycin, for
long period in 4 of 45 humans with tuberculosis.
No ototoxic effects due to unspecified method of administration of unspecified doses of antibiotic, (SQ) capreomycin, for short period in other 22
humans with tuberculosis.   (ENG)

                                                                          076
Ototoxic effects due to parenteral, intramuscular, administration of 1 g
daily of antibiotic, capreomycin (SM), for 9 months in 4 of 65 humans, adult
and aged, range of 20 to 70 years age, male and female, with pulmonary tuberculosis.
Simultaneous administration of ethambutol (SM) in 65 humans, adult and aged,
range of 20 to 70 years age, male and female, with pulmonary tuberculosis.
Simultaneous administration of antibiotic, rifampicin (SM), in 65 humans,
adult and aged, range of 20 to 70 years age, male and female, with pulmonary
tuberculosis.   (ENG)

                                                                          077
Moderate ototoxic effects due to unspecified method of administration of
range of 25 to 515 g of antibiotic, capreomycin, for long period in 3 of 82
humans with pulmonary tuberculosis.
    (AD) Preliminary study for primary study of kidney function in capreomycin
    treatment.   (ENG)

                                                                          137
Vestibular problems due to 1 g daily of antibiotic, capreomycin (SM), for
long period in 2 of 20 humans with tuberculosis.
Simultaneous administration of 25 mg per kg for first 60 days and then 15 mg
per kg of antituberculous agent, ethambutol (SM), in 20 humans with tuberculosis.
Simultaneous administration of 300 mg twice daily for several months and then
450 mg in 1 dose of antibiotic, rifampicin (SM), in 20 humans with tuberculosis.   (ENG)

                                                                          207
Cochleotoxic effects due to antibiotic, capreomycin, in humans with tuberculosis.
    (AD) Report on new antituberculous agents.
    (AD) Need for careful consideration before use of capreomycin in treatment
    of tuberculosis.   (FR)

                                                                          255
Slight hearing loss and vertigo due to parenteral, intramuscular, administration of 1 g every 24 hours of antibiotic, capreomycin (SM), for range of 5 to
12 months in 4 of 21 humans, adult, with pulmonary tuberculosis and without
pretreatment audiometric changes.
Slight and severe hearing loss and vertigo due to parenteral, intramuscular,
administration of 1 g every 24 hours of antibiotic, capreomycin (SM), for
range of 5 to 12 months in 12 of 40 humans, adult, with pulmonary tuberculosis and without pretreatment audiometric changes.
Simultaneous administration of antituberculous agent, ethambutol (SM), in all
of 61 humans, adult, with pulmonary tuberculosis.
    (AD) Treatment with capreomycin discontinued in 4 humans with severe

ototoxic effects.
  (AD) Audiometry every 4 weeks during treatment. (ENG)

                                                                    297
Possible vestibular problems and hearing loss due to recommended 1 g daily of
antibiotic, capreomycin, in humans with tuberculosis.
  (AD) Ototoxicity due to capreomycin similar to ototoxicity due to streptomycin. (ENG)

                                                                    308
Possible hearing loss due to antibiotic, kanamycin, in humans with tuberculosis.
Possible vestibular problems and cochlear impairment due to antibiotic,
capreomycin, in humans with tuberculosis.
  (AD) Comment on possible cochleo-vestibulotoxic effects of antibiotics
  used in treatment of tuberculosis. (ENG)

                                                                    322
Cochleo-vestibulotoxic effects due to parenteral, intramuscular, administra-
tion of 1 g daily and then 1 g every other day of antibiotic, (SQ) capreomycin (SM), for 6 months in 3 of 36 humans, adult and aged, range of 20 to 80
years age, male and female, with pulmonary tuberculosis.
  (AD) Ototoxic effects confirmed by audiogram.
Simultaneous administration of 600 mg daily of antibiotic, (SQ) rifampicin
(SM), for 6 months in 36 humans, adult and aged, range of 20 to 80 years age,
male and female, with pulmonary tuberculosis.
Simultaneous administration of 25 mg per kg daily and then 15 mg per kg daily
of antituberculous agent, (SQ) ethambutol (SM), for 6 months in 36 humans,
adult and aged, range of 20 to 80 years age, male and female, with pulmonary
tuberculosis.
Cochleo-vestibulotoxic effects due to previous administration of (SQ) antibiotics, aminoglycoside, in 36 humans, adult and aged, range of 20 to 80
years age, male and female, with pulmonary tuberculosis.
  (AD) Therapy with antibiotics not satisfactory. (FR)

                                                                    325
High frequency hearing loss due to parenteral, intramuscular, administration
of total of 15 mg per kg in 2 doses 5 times a week of antibiotic, (SQ) capreomycin (SM), for 37 and 45 days in 2 of 70 humans, adult, 35 and 64 years
age, with pulmonary tuberculosis and with previous treatment with other
ototoxic drugs.
Transient vertigo due to parenteral, intramuscular, administration of total
of 15 mg per kg in 2 doses 5 times a week of antibiotic, (SQ) capreomycin
(SM), for 5, 25, and 94 days in 3 of 70 humans, adult, 39, 61, and 62 years
age, with pulmonary tuberculosis and with previous treatment with streptomycin.
Simultaneous administration of other (SQ) antituberculous agents (SM), in 70
humans, adult, male and female, with pulmonary tuberculosis.
Possible ototoxic effects due to previous administration of antibiotic, (SQ)
streptomycin, in 3 of 70 humans, adult, 39, 61, and 62 years age, with pulmonary tuberculosis. (ENG)

                                                                    326
Hearing loss due to parenteral, intramuscular, administration of 1.0 g daily
of antibiotic, capreomycin (SM), for less than 6 months in 2 of 53 humans
with cavitary pulmonary tuberculosis and no previous chemotherapy.
No reported ototoxic effects due to oral administration of 12.0 g daily in 3
divided doses of antituberculous agent, PAS (SM), for up to 6 months in 53
humans with cavitary pulmonary tuberculosis and no previous chemotherapy.
(ENG)

                                                                    327
More severe hearing loss due to parenteral, intramuscular, administration of
1 g daily of antibiotic, (SQ) capreomycin (SM), for long period in 1 of 32
humans, male, with pulmonary tuberculosis and with previous antibiotic therapy.
Hearing loss before capreomycin treatment due to (SQ) antibiotics, aminoglycoside, in 1 of 32 humans, male, with pulmonary tuberculosis.

(AD) Hearing loss confirmed by audiogram.
Tinnitus due to parenteral, intramuscular, administration of 1 g daily of
antibiotic, (SQ) capreomycin (SM), for long period in 3 of 32 humans with
pulmonary tuberculosis.
Simultaneous administration of other (SQ) antituberculous agents (SM), in 32
humans, adult and aged, 20 to 69 years age, male and female, with pulmonary
tuberculosis.
Previous administration of antituberculous agent, (SQ) PAS, in 32 humans,
adult and aged, 20 to 69 years age, male and female, with pulmonary tuberculosis.   (ENG)

                                                                         328
Moderate hearing loss, subjective, due to total dose of 100 g of antibiotic,
capreomycin (SM), for 31 days or more in 1 of 38 humans, Negro, adult, 63
years age, male, with tuberculosis.
   (CT) Audiometry, pretreatment and during treatment.
   (AD) Audiometry showed possible hearing loss due to capreomycin.
Simultaneous administration of antituberculous agent, ethionamide (SM), in 1
of 38 humans, Negro, adult, 63 years age, male, with tuberculosis.   (ENG)

                                                                         329
Hearing loss or dizziness due to parenteral, intramuscular, administration of
1 g daily, total doses of 20 to 445 g, of antibiotic, (SQ) capreomycin (SM),
for range of 20 days to over 18 months in 5 of 43 humans, adult and aged, 24
to 83 years age, male and female, with pulmonary tuberculosis and with previous treatment with antituberculous agents.
   (CT) Audiometry, pretreatment and during treatment.
Simultaneous administration of 500 to 1000 mg daily in single or divided
doses of antituberculous agent, (SQ) ethionamide (SM), for range of 20 days
to over 18 months in 43 humans, adult and aged, 24 to 83 years age, male and
female, with pulmonary tuberculosis and with previous treatment with antituberculous agents.
Previous administration of other (SQ) antituberculous agents in 43 humans,
adult and aged, 24 to 83 years age, male and female, with pulmonary tuberculosis.   (ENG)

                                                                         330
Hearing loss due to parenteral, intramuscular, administration of 31 mg per kg
or 62 mg per kg daily of antibiotic, capreomycin (capreomycin disulfate), for
more than 1000 days in 4 animals, dogs, male and female.
Hearing loss due to parenteral, subcutaneous, administration of 13 mg per kg
or 130 mg per kg daily of antibiotic, capreomycin (capreomycin tetrahydroch-
loride), for 91 days in 2 animals, cats, male.
   (AD) Hearing loss determined by response of animals to reproducible sound.
   (ENG)

                                                                         331
Possible decr in ototoxicity due to decr dosage, from 1 g daily to 1 g 5 days
a week, of antibiotic, capreomycin, in humans with pulmonary tuberculosis.
(ENG)

                                                                         332
No subjective hearing loss but objective hearing loss over 20 decibels and
tinnitus due to parenteral, intramuscular, administration of 1 g daily for
first 60 days and then 1 g twice a week of antibiotic, capreomycin (SM), for
6 months in 3 of 100 humans treated for pulmonary tuberculosis.
Hearing loss, tinnitus, or dizziness due to parenteral, intramuscular, administration of 1 g daily for first 60 days and then 1 g twice a week of
antibiotic, streptomycin (SM), for 6 months in 8 of 99 humans treated for
pulmonary tuberculosis.
Hearing loss over 20 decibels due to parenteral, intramuscular, administration of 1 g daily for first 60 days and then 1 g twice a week of antibiotic,
streptomycin (SM), for 6 months in 3 of 99 humans treated for pulmonary
tuberculosis.
Simultaneous oral administration of 0.3 g daily in 2 doses of antituberculous
agent, isoniazid (SM), for 6 months in humans treated for pulmonary tuberculosis.
Simultaneous administration of 10 g daily in 3 doses of antituberculous

agent, PAS (SM), for 6 months in humans treated for pulmonary tuberculosis.
   (AD) Report on ototoxic effects of antibiotics used in initial treatment
   of tuberculosis.
High frequency hearing loss, tinnitus, or dizziness due to parenteral, intramuscular, administration of 1 g daily for first 60 days and then 1 g twice a
week of antibiotic, capreomycin (SM), for 6 months in 6 of 66 humans retreated for pulmonary tuberculosis.
No subjective auditory system problems but objective hearing loss over 20
decibels due to parenteral, intramuscular, administration of 1 g 3 times a
week of antibiotic, kanamycin (SM), for 6 months in 4 of 40 humans retreated
for pulmonary tuberculosis.
No subjective auditory system problems but objective hearing loss over 20
decibels due to parenteral, intramuscular, administration of 1 g daily for
first 60 days and then 1 g twice a week of antibiotic, streptomycin (SM), for
6 months in 1 of 13 humans retreated for pulmonary tuberculosis.
Simultaneous oral administration of 0.3 g daily in 2 doses of antituberculous
agent, isoniazid (SM), for 6 months in humans retreated for pulmonary tuberculosis.
   (AD) Report on ototoxic effects of antibiotics used in retreatment of
   tuberculosis.
   (CT) Audiometry, pretreatment and during treatment, 2 times a month in
   first 2 months and then 1 time a month.
   (AD) Comparative study of clinical use and cochleo-vestibulotoxic effects
   of capreomycin and other antibiotics in treatment and retreatment of
   pulmonary tuberculosis. (ENG)

                                                                        342
More severe sensorineural hearing loss of 20 decibels or more due to parenteral administration of total doses of 173 and 172 g of antibiotic, (SQ)
capreomycin, for long period, range of 2 to 18 months, in 2 of 294 humans,
male and female, with pulmonary tuberculosis and with previous hearing loss.
   (CT) Audiometry, pretreatment and during treatment.
   (AD) Suggested that occurrence of auditory system problems due to capreomycin not high.
Sensorineural hearing loss due to previous administration of antibiotic, (SQ)
streptomycin, in 1 of 294 humans with pulmonary tuberculosis. (ENG)

                                                                        343
No hearing loss but decr in vestibular function, asymptomatic except for
dizziness in 1 case, due to 1 g daily of antibiotic, capreomycin (SM), for 4
months or more in 4 of 25 humans, adolescent, adult, and aged, range of 17 to
67 years age, male and female, 80 to 160 lb weight, with pulmonary tuberculosis and with kidney disorder in 2 cases.
Transient dizziness with no objective decr in vestibular function due to 1 g
daily of antibiotic, capreomycin (SM), for 4 months or more in 3 of 25 humans, adolescent, adult, and aged, range of 17 to 67 years age, male and
female, 80 to 160 lb weight, with pulmonary tuberculosis.
Simultaneous administration of 300 mg daily of antituberculous agent, isoniazid (SM), for 4 months or more in 25 humans, adolescent, adult, and aged,
range of 17 to 67 years age, male and female, 80 to 160 lb weight, with
pulmonary tuberculosis.
   (CT) Pure tone audiometry, caloric tests, and cupulometry, pretreatment
   and during treatment with capreomycin.
   (AD) Study of clinical use and cochleo-vestibulotoxic effects of capreomycin.
Hearing loss, asymptomatic in 1 case and symptomatic in 1 case, due to 1 g
daily of antibiotic, viomycin, in 2 of 75 humans with pulmonary tuberculosis.
Objective decr in vestibular function due to 1 g daily of antibiotic, viomycin, in 21 of 75 humans with pulmonary tuberculosis.
Hearing loss, asymptomatic, due to 1 g daily of antibiotic, streptomycin, in
2 of 61 humans with pulmonary tuberculosis.
Objective decr in vestibular function due to 1 g daily of antibiotic, streptomycin, in 8 of 61 humans with pulmonary tuberculosis.
   (CT) Audiometry and vestibular function tests, pretreatment and during
   treatment with viomycin or streptomycin.
   (AD) Results of study on capreomycin comp w results of previous study on
   viomycin and streptomycin. (ENG)

368

Possible vestibular problems and hearing loss due to antibiotic, streptomycin, in humans with tuberculosis.
Permanent hearing loss due to antibiotic, dihydrostreptomycin, in humans with
tuberculosis.
Possible permanent hearing loss due to antibiotic, kanamycin, in humans with
tuberculosis.
Possible vestibular problems and hearing loss due to antibiotic, viomycin, in
humans with tuberculosis.
Possible damage to eighth cranial nerve due to antibiotic, capreomycin, in
humans with tuberculosis.
    (AD) Discussion of primary and secondary drugs used in tuberculosis chemo-
    therapy. (FR)

400

Transient mild cochlear impairment due to parenteral, intramuscular, administration of 1 g daily, maximum dose of 100 g, of antibiotic, capreomycin, in 1
of 21 humans with chronic tuberculosis of genitourinary system.
    (AD) Report on clinical use and toxic effects of new drugs in treatment of
    tuberculosis of genitourinary system.   (GER)

460

No significant decr in cochlear microphonics due to parenteral, subcutaneous,
administration of 100 mg per kg daily for 5 days a week, total dose of 7.5 g
per kg, of antibiotic, streptomycin (streptomycin sulfate), for 75 days in
animals, guinea pigs.
Statistically significant decr in cochlear microphonics at 1 of 18 points
examined, damage to hair cells of organ of Corti, slight damage to stria
vascularis and spiral ganglion, damage to macula utriculi and cristae, slight
damage to macula sacculi, and vestibular problems due to parenteral, subcutaneous, administration of 200 mg per kg daily, then 400 mg per kg, followed
by return to 200 mg per kg, total dose of 15 g per kg, of antibiotic, streptomycin (streptomycin sulfate), for 58 days in animals, guinea pigs.
    (AD) Vestibular problems confirmed by vestibular function tests.
No significant decr in cochlear microphonics due to parenteral, subcutaneous,
administration of 100 mg per kg daily for 5 days a week, total dose of 7.5 g
per kg, of antibiotic, viomycin (viomycin sulfate), for 75 days in animals,
guinea pigs.
Significant decr in cochlear microphonics, damage to hair cells of organ of
Corti and to stria vascularis, slight damage to spiral ganglion, and slight
damage to macula utriculi and crista ampullaris due to parenteral, subcutaneous, administration of 200 mg per kg daily for 5 days a week, then 400 mg
per kg, total dose of 15 g per kg, of antibiotic, viomycin (viomycin sulfate), for total of 67 days in animals, guinea pigs.
    (AD) Most toxicity for cochlear microphonics in guinea pig due to viomy-
    cin.
No significant decr in cochlear microphonics due to parenteral, subcutaneous,
administration of 100 mg per kg daily for 5 days each week, total dose of 7.5
g per kg, of antibiotic, capreomycin (capreomycin sulfate), for 75 days in
animals, guinea pigs.
No significant decr in cochlear microphonics, slight damage to outer hair
cells of organ of Corti and to stria vascularis, and no damage to vestibular
apparatus due to parenteral, subcutaneous, administration of 200 mg per kg
daily for 5 days a week, then 400 mg per kg, total dose of 15 g per kg, of
antibiotic, capreomycin (capreomycin sulfate), for total of 67 days in animals, guinea pigs.
    (CT) Same method using subcutaneous administration of 0.25 cc daily of
    isotonic saline in guinea pigs, control group.
    (AD) Least toxicity for inner ear of guinea pig due to capreomycin.
    (AD) Study of functional and structural cochleo-vestibulotoxic effects of
    streptomycin, viomycin, and capreomycin.
    (AD) Statistical analysis of results.   (ENG)

473

Possible vestibular problems due to antibiotic, viomycin, in humans with
infections.
Possible vestibular problems due to antibiotic, capreomycin, in humans with
infections.

(AD) Experiments to find new derivatives of viomycin and capreomycin with
biological activity but with less toxic effects. (ENG)

501

Ototoxic effects due to antibiotic, capreomycin, in humans treated for tuberculosis.
   (AD) Capreomycin less ototoxic than streptomycin and viomycin. (ENG)

519

Dizziness but no other ototoxic effects due to parenteral, intramuscular,
administration of 1 g daily in single dose of antibiotic, capreomycin (SM),
for long period in 1 of 33 humans, adult and aged, 21 to over 70 years age,
with pulmonary tuberculosis of long duration and with previous treatment with
other drugs.
Simultaneous oral administration of 25 mg per kg during first 60 days and
then 15 mg per kg of antituberculous agent, ethambutol (SM), in 1 of 33
humans, adult and aged, 21 to over 70 years age, with pulmonary tuberculosis
of long duration and with previous treatment with other drugs.
Simultaneous administration of 600 mg of antibiotic, rifampicin (SM), in 1 of
33 humans, adult and aged, 21 to over 70 years age, with pulmonary tuberculosis of long duration and with previous treatment with other drugs.
   (AD) Otoneurology tests every 4 to 8 weeks. (ENG)

555

Cochlear impairment due to parenteral, intramuscular, administration of 100
mg per kg 3 times per week or 25 or 50 mg per kg daily of antibiotic, capreomycin, for 2 years in several animals, dogs.
Vestibular problems due to parenteral, subcutaneous, administration of 125 mg
per kg daily of antibiotic, capreomycin, for 84 days in several animals,
cats.
   (AD) Discussion of chemistry of capreomycin, results of in vitro and in
   vivo studies, and toxicity of capreomycin in animals. (ENG)

556

Moderate lesion of cochlea due to unspecified doses of antibiotic, capreomycin, for long period in 5(12.5 percent) of 40 humans, in treatment or retreatment for pulmonary tuberculosis.
   (AD) Cochlear function monitored by audiometry. (ENG)

557

Ototoxic effects due to previous administration of antibiotic, (SQ) streptomycin, in 8 humans with pulmonary tuberculosis.
No ototoxic effects due to 1.0 g daily of antibiotic, (SQ) capreomycin (SM),
for long period in same 8 of 38 humans with pulmonary tuberculosis.
Simultaneous administration of antituberculous agent, (SQ) ethambutol (SM),
in 38 humans with pulmonary tuberculosis. (ENG)

568

Mild ototoxic effects due to 1 g on 6 days a week or 0.75 g when body weight
below 50 kg, total of 30 to over 330 g, of antibiotic, capreomycin, for long
period in 3 of 82 humans, adult and aged, 21 to 80 years age, male and female, with chronic tuberculosis. (ENG)

569

Slight hearing loss due to 1 g daily in single dose of antibiotic, capreomycin (SM), in 2 of 31 humans with chronic pulmonary tuberculosis.
   (AD) Audiometry and vestibular function tests every 4 weeks and then every
   6 weeks.
   (AD) Cessation of treatment with capreomycin in 4 cases to prevent hearing
   loss.
Simultaneous administration of 25 mg per kg daily in single dose for 12 weeks
and then 15 mg per kg of antituberculous agent, ethambutol (SM), in 31 humans
with chronic pulmonary tuberculosis.
Simultaneous oral administration of 1 other antituberculous agent (SM), in 31
humans with chronic pulmonary tuberculosis. (ENG)

570

Transient slight hearing loss due to parenteral, intramuscular, administra-

tion of 1 g daily, maximum dose of 90 g, of antibiotic, capreomycin (SM), in
1 of 16 humans with chronic tuberculosis of genitourinary system.
Simultaneous administration of 2 other antituberculous agents (SM), in 16
humans with chronic tuberculosis of genitourinary system.
Hearing loss due to 1 g daily average dose of antibiotic, capreomycin (SM),
for long period in 1 of 20 humans, adult, male and female, with chronic
tuberculosis, and 5 also alcoholics.
Simultaneous administration of other antituberculous agents (SM), in 20
humans, adult, male and female, with chronic tuberculosis, and 5 also alcoholics.
    (AD) Discussion of various reports of auditory system problems due to
    capreomycin therapy. (ENG)

590

Ototoxic effects due to antibiotic, capreomycin, in animals.
    (AD) In vivo and in vitro studies of capreomycin. (IT)

591

Hearing loss due to antibiotic, capreomycin, for long period in 2 of 28
humans with tuberculosis.
    (AD) Results of 1 study of effects of capreomycin.
No ototoxic effects due to antibiotic, (SQ) capreomycin, for 1 to 24 months
in 16 humans with tuberculosis.
    (AD) Results of other study of effects of capreomycin.
Vestibular problems due to previous administration of antibiotic, (SQ) streptomycin, in 8 of 16 humans with tuberculosis.
    (AD) Suggested that less ototoxicity due to capreomycin than to streptomy-
    cin. (ENG)

610

Possible ototoxic effects due to antibiotic, capreomycin, in humans with
tuberculosis of genitourinary system.
Possible hearing loss due to antibiotic, kanamycin, in humans with tuberculosis of genitourinary system.
Possible hearing loss and vestibular problems due to antibiotic, viomycin, in
humans with tuberculosis of genitourinary system.
    (AD) Discussion of treatment of tuberculosis of genitourinary system.
    (GER)

641

Possible damage to eighth cranial nerve due to antibiotic, capreomycin, in
humans.
Possible vestibular problems and hearing loss due to antibiotic, gentamicin,
in humans.
Possible delayed transient or permanent hearing loss due to antibiotic,
kanamycin (SM), in humans, in particular with kidney disorders or with simultaneous administration of ethacrynic acid.
Possible delayed transient or permanent hearing loss due to diuretic, ethacrynic acid (SM), in humans.
Possible delayed transient or permanent severe hearing loss due to oral,
parenteral, or topical administration of antibiotic, neomycin, in humans.
Possible damage to eighth cranial nerve, primarily hearing loss, due to
antibiotic, paromomycin, in humans.
Possible hearing loss due to antibiotic, rifampicin, in humans.
High risk of damage to eighth cranial nerve, primarily transient or permanent
vestibular problems but also hearing loss, due to antibiotic, streptomycin,
in humans.
Possible damage to eighth cranial nerve, primarily hearing loss, due to high
doses of antibiotic, vancomycin, for long period of more than 10 days in
humans, in particular with kidney disorders.
Risk of damage to eighth cranial nerve, vestibular problems and hearing loss,
due to high doses of antibiotic, viomycin, for long period of more than 10
days in humans, in particular with kidney disorders.
    (AD) Discussion of toxic effects of antibiotics. (ENG)

656

Possible permanent severe damage to eighth cranial nerve, primarily vestibular problems but also hearing loss, due to parenteral administration of

antibiotic, streptomycin, in humans with tuberculosis, in particular with
concurrent kidney disorder.
Possible permanent severe damage to eighth cranial nerve due to parenteral
administration of antibiotic, viomycin, in humans with tuberculosis.
Possible permanent severe damage to eighth cranial nerve due to parenteral
administration of antibiotic, kanamycin, in humans with tuberculosis.
Possible permanent severe damage to eighth cranial nerve due to parenteral
administration of antibiotic, capreomycin, in humans with tuberculosis.
   (AD) Discussion of primary and secondary drugs used in treatment of tuberculosis. (ENG)

                                                                             711
Vestibular problems due to antibiotic, capreomycin, for more than 3 months in
1 of 35 humans with pulmonary tuberculosis. (POL)

                                                                             715
Loss of outer hair cells of organ of Corti in lower part of first coil of
cochlea due to parenteral, intramuscular, administration of 400 mg per kg of
antibiotic, capreomycin, for 28 days in 40 percent of 10 animals, guinea
pigs, albino, 300 g weight.
Severe loss of outer hair cells of organ of Corti from lower part of basal
coil to upper coil of cochlea due to parenteral, intramuscular, administration of 400 mg per kg of antibiotic, kanamycin, for 28 days in 100 percent of
11 animals, guinea pigs, albino, 300 g weight.
   (CT) Test of Preyer reflex before, during, and after administration of
   antibiotics.
   (AD) Study suggested that capreomycin less ototoxic than kanamycin in
   guinea pigs.
   (AD) No observed damage to vestibular apparatus. (JAP)

                              Cephaloridine

                                                                             520
Decr in time of latency with incr in intensity of acoustic stimuli due to
parenteral, intraperitoneal, administration of 80 mg per kg daily, total of
480 mg, of antibiotic, cephalothin (cephalothin sodium), for 15 days in 10
animals, guinea pigs, albino.
Decr in time of latency with incr in intensity of acoustic stimuli due to
parenteral, intraperitoneal, administration of 20 mg per kg daily, total of
120 mg, of antibiotic, lincomycin (lincomycin chloride), for 15 days in 10
animals, guinea pigs, albino.
Decr in time of latency with incr in intensity of acoustic stimuli due to
parenteral, intraperitoneal, administration of 50 mg per kg daily, total of
300 mg, of antibiotic, cephaloridine, for 15 days in 10 animals, guinea pigs,
albino.
   (CT) Study of guinea pigs, control group, not treated with antibiotics.
   (AD) Study of response of guinea pigs to acoustic stimuli after treatment
   with antibiotics. (IT)

                              Cephalothin

                                                                             520
Decr in time of latency with incr in intensity of acoustic stimuli due to
parenteral, intraperitoneal, administration of 80 mg per kg daily, total of
480 mg, of antibiotic, cephalothin (cephalothin sodium), for 15 days in 10
animals, guinea pigs, albino.
Decr in time of latency with incr in intensity of acoustic stimuli due to
parenteral, intraperitoneal, administration of 20 mg per kg daily, total of
120 mg, of antibiotic, lincomycin (lincomycin chloride), for 15 days in 10
animals, guinea pigs, albino.
Decr in time of latency with incr in intensity of acoustic stimuli due to
parenteral, intraperitoneal, administration of 50 mg per kg daily, total of
300 mg, of antibiotic, cephaloridine, for 15 days in 10 animals, guinea pigs,
albino.
   (CT) Study of guinea pigs, control group, not treated with antibiotics.
   (AD) Study of response of guinea pigs to acoustic stimuli after treatment
   with antibiotics. (IT)

Chloramphenicol

002

Damage to organ of Corti and stria vascularis due to topical administration
to round window of 16 mg of 1.44M solution and 8 mg of 0.72M solution of
antibiotic, chloramphenicol (chloramphenicol succinate), for 30 minutes in 11
animals, guinea pigs, adult, for each solution.
   (CT) Same method using 1.44M solution of sodium (sodium succinate) in 8
   guinea pigs, control group, showed no histological damage. (ENG)

051

Progressive permanent sensorineural hearing loss and tinnitus due to topical
administration to joint of left knee and parenteral, intramuscular, administration of high doses, total of 42.5 g, of antibiotic, (SQ) neomycin, for
long period, 19 days, in 1 human, adult, with infection of left knee.
Previous administration of high doses of antibiotic, (SQ) chloramphenicol,
for unspecified period in 1 human, adult, with infection of left knee.
   (AD) Report of case in court with claim of negligence for administration
   of high doses of neomycin that resulted in hearing loss. (ENG)

069

Progressive decr in cochlear response due to topical administration by insufflation to round window in powder of 8 mg (only 0.5 mg actually fell on round
window) of antibiotic, chloramphenicol, in 1 administration in 8 animals,
guinea pigs, 459 to 996 g weight.
   (CT) Same method using saline in 2 guinea pigs, control group.
   (AD) Measurement of cochlear response at 15 minutes and 1, 5, and 20 hours
   after insufflation. (ENG)

089

Sudden deafness due to parenteral, intravenous, administration of 100 mg, in
100 ml saline solution, of diuretic, (SQ) ethacrynic acid, in 1 injection in
1 human, adult, 42 years age, female, quadriplegic, with kidney disorder.
Previous administration of unspecified dose of antibiotic, (SQ) chloram25pheni-
col, for unspecified period in 1 human, adult, 42 years age, female, quadriplegic, with kidney disorder.
Previous administration of 1 g of antibiotic, (SQ) kanamycin, for unspecified
period in 1 human, adult, 42 years age, female, quadriplegic, with kidney
disorder and genitourinary system infection. (ENG)

170

Sensorineural hearing loss due to topical administration in ear drops of
antibiotic, neomycin, in humans with no other explanation for hearing loss.
Sensorineural hearing loss due to topical administration in ear drops of
antibiotic, chloramphenicol, in humans with no other explanation for hearing
loss.
Sensorineural hearing loss due to topical administration in ear drops of
antibiotic, framycetin, in humans with no other explanation for hearing loss.
   (AD) Comment on topical use of antibiotics and possible risk of cochleotoxic effects. (ENG)

181

Decr in succinic dehydrogenase in outer hair cells of organ of Corti due to
parenteral, intratympanic, administration of 200 mg per ml solution of antibiotic, kanamycin (kanamycin sulfate), in animals, guinea pigs, adult.
Decr in succinic dehydrogenase in outer hair cells of organ of Corti due to
parenteral, intratympanic, administration of 200 mg per ml solution of antibiotic, dihydrostreptomycin (dihydrostreptomycin sulfate), in animals, guinea
pigs, adult.
Decr in succinic dehydrogenase in outer hair cells of organ of Corti due to
parenteral, intratympanic, administration of 200 mg per ml solution of antibiotic, chloramphenicol (chloramphenicol succinate), in animals, guinea pigs,
adult.
   (AD) Same type of damage to organ of Corti due to all 3 antibiotics.
Severe decr in succinic dehydrogenase in organ of Corti, in particular in
outer hair cells, and atrophy of outer hair cells due to saturated solution
of antimalarial, quinine (quinine hydrochloride), in animals, guinea pigs.

Complete degeneration of organ of Corti due to saturated solution of antimalarial, quinine (quinine hydrochloride), in animals, guinea pigs.
   (AD) Damage to organ of Corti more severe due to quinine than to antibiotics.
   (AD) Activity of succinic dehydrogenase often higher in outer hair cells.
   (AD) Possible that damage to outer hair cells due to higher rate of metabolism. (ENG)

183

Inhibition of oxygen consumption of cochlea due to 0.04 mg of antibiotic,
chloramphenicol (chloramphenicol sodium succinate), in animals, guinea pigs,
adult, 300 g weight, with normal Preyer reflex.
More inhibition of oxygen consumption of cochlea due to 0.04 mg of antibiotic, kanamycin (kanamycin sulfate), in animals, guinea pigs, adult, 300 g
weight, with normal Preyer reflex.
   (CT) Study of oxygen consumption in normal cochlea.
   (AD) Measurement of oxygen consumption with differential type of microres-
pirometer.
   (AD) In vitro study.
No detected change in Preyer reflex due to parenteral, intracutaneous, ad-
ministration of 400 mg per kg of antibiotic, chloramphenicol, for 20 days in
animals, guinea pigs.
   (AD) In vivo study.
   (AD) Results with chloramphenicol in vivo not same as results in vitro.
   (ENG)

282

Limited effects on blood vessels of stria vascularis and spiral prominence
due to 300 mg per kg daily of antibiotic, kanamycin, for 4 to 9 days in
animals, guinea pigs.
Limited effects on blood vessels of stria vascularis and spiral prominence
due to 30 mg per kg daily of antibiotic, dihydrostreptomycin, for 4 to 9 days
in animals, guinea pigs.
Limited effects on blood vessels of stria vascularis and spiral prominence
due to 30 mg per kg daily of antibiotic, chloramphenicol, for 4 to 9 days in
animals, guinea pigs.
   (CT) Study of guinea pigs, control group. (JAP)

289

Possible cochlear impairment due to antibiotic, chloramphenicol, in humans.
   (AD) Report on toxic effects of chloramphenicol. (RUM)

314

Loss of enzymes, succinic dehydrogenase and DPN diaphorase, in outer hair
cells of organ of Corti but usually no enzyme loss in inner hair cells due to
topical administration to bulla of 200 mg per ml of antibiotic, kanamycin
(kanamycin sulfate), in 1 injection in animals, guinea pigs.
Loss of enzymes, succinic dehydrogenase and DPN diaphorase, in outer hair
cells of organ of Corti but usually no enzyme loss in inner hair cells due to
topical administration to bulla of 200 mg per ml of antibiotic, dihydrostreptomycin (dihydrostreptomycin sulfate), in 1 injection in animals, guinea
pigs.
Loss of enzymes, succinic dehydrogenase and DPN diaphorase, in outer hair
cells of organ of Corti but usually no enzyme loss in inner hair cells due to
topical administration to bulla of 200 mg per ml of antibiotic, chloramphenicol (chloramphenicol succinate), in 1 injection in animals, guinea pigs.
More severe effects on enzymes, succinic hydrogenase and DPN diaphorase, in
outer hair cells of organ of Corti due to topical administration to bulla of
saturated solution of antimalarial, quinine (quinine hydrochloride), in 1
injection in animals, guinea pigs.
   (CT) Activity of succinic dehydrogenase often higher in outer hair cells
than in inner hair cells of organ of Corti in guinea pigs, control group.
   (AD) Suggested correlation between cochleotoxic effects of drugs and
metabolic activity of hair cells. (ENG)

323

Progressive severe bilateral sensorineural hearing loss and vestibular problems due to parenteral administration of 1 g twice weekly of antibiotic, (SQ)

viomycin (viomycin pantothenate), for total of 10 weeks in 1 human, adult, 59
years age, female, with pulmonary tuberculosis and kidney disorder.
    (AD) Cochleo-vestibulotoxic effects confirmed by audiometry at different
    periods during and after treatment and by caloric test.
Previous administration of antibiotic, (SQ) chloramphenicol, in 1 human,
adult, 59 years age, female, for infection before diagnosis of tuberculosis.
Possible but not reported auditory system problems due to previous parenteral
administration of 0.5 g twice daily of antibiotic, (SQ) streptomycin, for 1
week in 1 human, adult, 59 years age, female, for infection before diagnosis
of tuberculosis.
    (AD) Suggested that possible previous ototoxic effects of streptomycin
    potentiated by viomycin (viomycin pantothenate).
Previous administration of antituberculous agent, (SQ) PAS, in 1 human,
adult, 59 years age, female, with pulmonary tuberculosis and kidney disorder.
(ENG)

                                                                        384
Usually transient hearing loss and no structural damage to organ of Corti,
stria vascularis, and spiral ganglion due to oral or topical administration
of salicylates in humans.
Hearing loss due to antimalarial, quinine, in humans.
Usually permanent hearing loss due to antimalarial, chloroquine, in humans.
Transient and permanent hearing loss and possible damage to hair cells of
organ of Corti due to diuretic, ethacrynic acid, in humans.
Sensorineural hearing loss due to cardiovascular agent, hexadimethrine
bromide, in humans with kidney disorder.
Sensorineural hearing loss and damage to organ of Corti due to topical ad-
ministration of antineoplastic, nitrogen mustard, in humans.
Sensorineural hearing loss due to high doses of antibiotic, chloramphenicol,
in humans.
Primary vestibular problems due to antibiotic, streptomycin, in humans.
Hearing loss due to high doses usually of antibiotic, streptomycin, in humans.
    (AD) Early detection of hearing loss by audiometry prevents permanent
    damage.
High frequency hearing loss and severe damage to outer hair cells and slight
damage to inner hair cells of organ of Corti due to antibiotic, kanamycin, in
humans.
Sensorineural hearing loss due to parenteral, oral, and topical administration of antibiotic, neomycin, in humans with or without kidney disorders.
Degeneration of hair cells of organ of Corti and of nerve process due to
antibiotics, aminoglycoside, in animals.
    (AD) Literature review of physiological and structural cochleo-vestibulo-
    toxic effects of ototoxic drugs.
    (AD) Discussion of suggested mechanism of ototoxicity and routes of drugs
    to inner ear.
Bilateral sensorineural hearing loss due to oral administration of antibiotic, neomycin, in 4 of 8 humans with liver disease.
Bilateral sensorineural hearing loss due to oral administration of range of
doses of antibiotic, neomycin (SM), in 2 of 5 humans with liver disease.
Bilateral sensorineural hearing loss due to diuretics (SM), in 2 of 5 humans
with liver disease.
Transient progression of previous hearing loss due to parenteral, intravenous, administration of diuretic, ethacrynic acid (SM), in 1 injection in 1
of 5 humans with liver disease.
    (CT) Normal cochlear function in 6 humans, control group, with liver
    disease and not treated with neomycin or diuretics.
    (CT) Normal cochlear function in 13 humans, control group, with liver
    disease and treated with diuretics but not with neomycin.
    (AD) Hearing loss confirmed by audiometry.
    (AD) Reported that hearing loss due to neomycin or diuretics in humans
    with liver disease not related to dosage.
    (AD) Clinical study of effects of treatment with neomycin and diuretics in
    humans with liver disease.
Bilateral sensorineural hearing loss and vertigo due to antibiotic, ampicil-
lin, in 1 human, adolescent, 17 years age, female, with tonsillitis.
    (AD) Cited case report.
Severe sensorineural hearing loss and vertigo due to topical administration

in ear drops of antibiotic, framycetin, in 1 human, adult, 42 years age,
male, with previous slight high frequency hearing loss.
    (AD) Cited case report.
Atrophy of hair cells of organ of Corti and hearing loss due to antibiotic,
dihydrostreptomycin, in humans with tuberculous meningitis.
    (AD) Cited study.
Loss of inner hair cells and damage to outer hair cells due to 18 g of antibiotic, neomycin, for 18 days in 1 human.
    (AD) Cited case report.   (ENG)

457

Tinnitus and progressive sensorineural hearing loss due to parenteral, intramuscular, administration of antibiotic, (SQ) streptomycin, for 10 days in 1
human, adult, 38 years age, female, with infections and later development of
kidney disorder.
Tinnitus and progressive sensorineural hearing loss due to 13.2 g of antibiotic, (SQ) kanamycin, for 11 days in 1 human, adult, 38 years age, female,
with infections and kidney disorder.
Hearing loss due to antimalarial, (SQ) quinine, in 1 human, adult, 20 years
age, male, with various infections and later development of kidney disorder.
Hearing loss due to 400 mg 2 times daily, total dose of 6.5 g, of antibiotic,
(SQ) kanamycin (SM), for 8 days in 1 human, adult, 20 years age, male, with
various infections and later development of kidney disorder.
Hearing loss due to 150 mg 2 times daily, total dose of 2400 mg, of antibiotic, (SQ) colistin (SM), for 8 days in 1 human, adult, 20 years age, male,
with various infections and later development of kidney disorder.
Tinnitus, total bilateral hearing loss, and vestibular problems due to parenteral, intramuscular, administration of 4.0 g daily, total of 21 g, of antibiotic, (SQ) kanamycin (SM), for 5 days in 1 human, adult, 20 years age,
male, with infections and kidney disorder.
Tinnitus, total bilateral hearing loss, and vestibular problems due to 0.6 g
daily, total dose of 1.3 g, of antibiotic, (SQ) colistin (SM), for 2 days in
1 human, adult, 20 years age, male, with infections and kidney disorder.
Tinnitus, total bilateral hearing loss, and vestibular problems due to 2 g
and then 8 g per 24 hours in divided doses, total dose of 26.5 g, of antibiotic, (SQ) chloramphenicol, for 9 days in 1 human, adult, 20 years age, male,
with infections and kidney disorder.
Bilateral hearing loss due to 1 g daily of antibiotic, actinomycin (SM), for
5 days in 1 human, adult, 62 years age, male, with infections and kidney
disorder.
Bilateral hearing loss due to unknown dose of antibiotic, kanamycin (SM), for
5 days in 1 human, adult, 62 years age, male, with infections and kidney
disorder.
Bilateral hearing loss and vestibular problems due to parenteral administration of high doses of antibiotic, (SQ) neomycin, for total of 21 days in 1
human, adult, 25 years age, male, with infection from wound.
Previous administration of unspecified doses of antibiotic, (SQ) streptomycin, in 1 human, adult, 25 years age, male, with infection from wound.
Later administration of antibiotic, (SQ) chloramphenicol, in 1 human, adult,
25 years age, male, with infection from wound.
Tinnitus and rapidly progressive bilateral hearing loss due to parenteral,
intramuscular, administration of 0.5 g every 12 hours of antibiotic, (SQ)
streptomycin, for 5 days in 1 human, adult, 21 years age, male, with infection from wound.
Tinnitus and rapidly progressive bilateral hearing loss due to parenteral,
intramuscular, administration of 200 mg daily, total of 6.8 g, of antibiotic,
(SQ) colistin (SM), in 1 human, adult, 21 years age, male, with infection
from wound.
Tinnitus and rapidly progressive bilateral hearing loss due to parenteral
administration of unspecified doses of antibiotic, (SQ) neomycin (SM), for
about 35 days in 1 human, adult, 21 years age, male, with infection from
wound.
Tinnitus and progressive bilateral hearing loss due to parenteral administration of 2 l per 24 hours of 1 percent solution of antibiotic, (SQ) neomycin,
for 10 days in 1 human, adult, 26 years age, male, with infection from wound.
    (AD) Hearing loss confirmed by audiometry.
Previous administration of 500 mg four times a day of antibiotic, (SQ) ampicillin, in 1 human, adult, 26 years age, male, with infection from wound.

Bilateral sudden deafness due to administration in dialysis fluid of less
than 150 mg of antibiotic, neomycin (SM), in 1 human, adult, 44 years age,
female, with kidney disorder.
Bilateral sudden deafness due to 50 mg of diuretic, ethacrynic acid (SM), in
1 human, adult, 44 years age, female, with kidney disorder.
   (AD) Hearing loss confirmed by audiology.
Tinnitus and progressive bilateral hearing loss beginning after 8 days of
treatment due to parenteral administration of 1 l every 4 hours for 3 days
and then every 8 hours for 10 days of 1 percent solution of antibiotic,
neomycin, in 1 human, adult, 20 years age, male, with infection from wound.
   (AD) Hearing loss confirmed by audiology.
Tinnitus and bilateral sensorineural hearing loss due to parenteral, intramuscular, administration of 1 g and then 0.5 g every 12 hours of antibiotic,
streptomycin (SM), for 15 days in 1 human, adult, 23 years age, male, with
infection from wound.
Tinnitus and bilateral sensorineural hearing loss due to topical administration by irrigation of 1 percent solution every 12 hours of antibiotic, neomycin (SM), for 14 days in 1 human, adult, 23 years age, male, with infection
from wound.
   (AD) Hearing loss confirmed by audiometry.
   (AD) Discussion of 10 case reports. (ENG)

                                                                        565

Inhibition of oxygen consumption of cochlea due to 0.04 M of antibiotic,
kanamycin (kanamycin sulfate), in animals, guinea pigs, adult, 300 g weight,
with normal Preyer reflex.
Inhibition of oxygen consumption of cochlea due to 0.04 M of antibiotic,
chloramphenicol (chloramphenicol sodium succinate), in animals, guinea pigs,
adult, 300 g weight, with normal Preyer reflex.
   (AD) Less inhibition of oxygen consumption by chloramphenicol than by
   kanamycin.
Incr inhibition of oxygen consumption of cochlea due to 0.04 M of antibiotic,
kanamycin (SM) (kanamycin sulfate), in animals, guinea pigs, adult, 300 g
weight, with normal Preyer reflex.
Incr inhibition of oxygen consumption of cochlea due to 0.04 M of antibiotic,
chloramphenicol (SM) (chloramphenicol sodium succinate), in animals, guinea
pigs, adult, 300 g weight, with normal Preyer reflex.
   (CT) Measurement of oxygen consumption of normal cochlea without administration of ototoxic drugs.
   (AD) In vitro study using microrespirometer of effect of interaction of
   kanamycin and chloramphenicol on oxygen consumption in guinea pig cochlea.
   (AD) Potentiation of inhibition of oxygen consumption of cochlea with
   simultaneous administration of kanamycin and chloramphenicol.
   (AD) Suggested risk of ototoxicity in clinical use of kanamycin and
   chloramphenicol. (ENG)

                                                                        674

No ototoxic effects due to parenteral, intramuscular, administration of 1 g
twice daily for 1 to 2 days, followed by 1 g daily for 8 to 10 days, with
reduced doses in patients with kidney disorder, of antibiotic, kanamycin
(SM), for total of about 9 to 12 days in 28 humans, adult and aged, 26 to 80
years age, male and female, with severe infections due to gram-negative
bacilli, with bacteremia in 16 cases and kidney disorder in 8 cases.
Simultaneous administration of antibiotic, chloramphenicol (SM), in most of
16 humans with bacteremia.
   (AD) Use of kanamycin without ototoxic effects in patients with kidney
   disorders due to decr in dosage and tests of serum levels of antibiotic.
   (ENG)

                                  Colistin

                                                                        006

Range of degrees of degeneration of endorgan of organ of Corti due to parenteral, intratympanic, administration of range of 1 to 100 mg per ml concentration of antibiotic, neomycin, in 1 injection in animals, guinea pigs,
young, 250 g average weight.
Range of degrees of degeneration of endorgan of organ of Corti due to parenteral, intratympanic, administration of range of 1 to 100 mg per ml concen-

tration of antibiotic, polymyxin B, in 1 injection in animals, guinea pigs,
young, 250 g average weight.
Range of degrees of degeneration of endorgan of organ of Corti due to parenteral, intratympanic, administration of range of 1 to 100 mg per ml concentration of antibiotic, colistin, in 1 injection in animals, guinea pigs,
young, 250 g average weight.
   (CT) Same method using comparable concentration of saline solution or
   solution of glucose or sodium G penicillin in guinea pigs, control group,
   showed no histological damage.
Degeneration of endorgan of organ of Corti due to topical administration to
ear canal of range of 5 to 100 mg per ml 1 time daily of antibiotic, neomycin, for 8 to 25 days in 14 animals, guinea pigs. (ENG)

                                                                         016
Progressive bilateral sensorineural hearing loss and vertigo due to unspecified method of administration of total of 3 g of antibiotic, (SQ) streptomycin (SM), for unspecified period in 1 human, Caucasian, adult, 32 years age,
male, with kidney disorder and on intermittent hemodialysis.
Progressive bilateral sensorineural hearing loss and vertigo due to unspecified method of administration of antibiotic, (SQ) colistin (SM), for unspecified period in 1 human, Caucasian, adult, 32 years age, male, with kidney
disorder and on intermittent hemodialysis.
Permanent sensorineural hearing loss due to parenteral, intravenous, administration of 1.6 mg per kg 2 times daily, total of 500 mg of antibiotic, (SQ)
gentamicin, for unspecified period in 1 human, Caucasian, adult, 32 years
age, male, with kidney disorder and on intermittent hemodialysis.
No definite ototoxic effects reported due to unspecified method of administration of 1 g every 2 weeks, total of 12 g, of antibiotic, (SQ) vancomycin,
for about 6 months in 1 human, Caucasian, adult, 32 years age, male, with
kidney disorder and on intermittent hemodialysis.
   (AD) Hearing loss due to streptomycin and colistin potentiated by gentamicin. (ENG)

                                                                         140
Total bilateral sensorineural hearing loss due to 40 mg daily, total of 1.80
g, of antibiotic, gentamicin, for 45 days in 1 human, aged, 69 years age,
female, with kidney disorder.
   (AD) Hearing loss confirmed by audiogram.
Sensorineural hearing loss due to parenteral administration of 40 mg in 2
injections daily, total of 480 mg, of antibiotic, gentamicin (SM), in 1
human, aged, 65 years age, male.
Simultaneous administration of antibiotic, transcycline (SM), in 1 human,
aged, 65 years age, male.
Simultaneous administration of antibiotic, colistin (SM) (colistimethate), in
1 human, aged, 65 years age, male.
Sensorineural hearing loss due to 40 mg daily, total of 0.84 g, of antibiotic, gentamicin, for 21 days in 1 human, adult, 50 years age, male, with
normal kidney function.
   (AD) Hearing loss confirmed by audiogram.
   (AD) Discussion of 3 case reports of gentamicin ototoxicity. (FR)

                                                                         206
Transient bilateral sensorineural hearing loss due to oral administration of
50 mg every 6 hours of diuretic, ethacrynic acid, for 4 days initially and
then again 2 weeks later for 2 days in 1 human, Negro, adult, 55 years age,
female, with diabetes mellitus and kidney disorder.
   (AD) Hearing loss confirmed by audiogram.
Transient sensorineural hearing loss and tinnitus due to (SQ) oral and parenteral, (SQ) intravenous, administration of 300,300,400, and 500 mg of diuretic, ethacrynic acid, in 4 doses in 1 human, Caucasian, adult, 40 years age,
female, with chronic kidney disorder.
No auditory system problems due to parenteral, intravenous, administration of
(SQ) unspecified doses of diuretic, (SQ) ethacrynic acid, in (SQ) 3 injections in 1 human, Caucasian, adult, 20 years age, female, with kidney disorder.
Transient severe bilateral tinnitus, sensorineural hearing loss, and bilateral nystagmus due to parenteral, intravenous, administration of (SQ) 50 and
100 mg of diuretic, (SQ) ethacrynic acid, in (SQ) 2 injections in 1 human,

Caucasian, adult, 20 years age, female, with kidney disorder.
Previous administration, 2 days before onset of ototoxic effects, of antibiotic, (SQ) colistin (sodium colistimethate), in 1 injection in 1 human, Caucasian, adult, 20 years age, female, with kidney disorder.
Transient sensorineural hearing loss within 12 hours of first dose due to
oral administration of 50 mg of diuretic, ethacrynic acid, in 4 doses in 1
human, Caucasian, aged, 76 years age, male, with kidney disorder and with
previous moderate hearing loss due to otosclerosis.
Severe tinnitus within 1 hour of first dose and sensorineural hearing loss
within 1 half hour of second dose due to parenteral, intravenous, administration of 50 and 100 mg of diuretic, (SQ) ethacrynic acid, in 2 injections in 1
human, Caucasian, adult, 57 years age, female, with leukemia and kidney
disorder.
Administration about 1 week previously of antibiotic, (SQ) streptomycin, in 1
human, Caucasian, adult, 57 years age, female, with leukemia and kidney
disorder, for pneumonitis.
Administration about 1 week previously of antibiotic, (SQ) colistin (sodium
colistimethate), in 1 human, Caucasian, adult, 57 years age, female, with
leukemia and kidney disorder, for pneumonitis.
    (AD) Discussion of 5 case reports of transient hearing loss due to treat-
    ment with ethacrynic acid.   (ENG)

                                                                        213
Dizziness due to antibiotic, polymyxin B (polymyxin B sulfate), in humans.
Dizziness due to antibiotic, colistin (sodium colistimethate), in humans.
Ototoxic effects due to antibiotic, ristocetin, in humans.
Hearing loss due to antibiotic, vancomycin, in humans.
    (AD) Report on pharmacology, clinical use, and toxicity of antibiotics.
    (ENG)

                                                                        316
Possible vestibular problems and cochlear impairment due to more than recommended dose of 15 to 30 mg per kg daily of antibiotic, streptomycin, for long
period in humans.
Hearing loss due to parenteral, intramuscular, administration of total doses
of 5 to 6 g of antibiotic, kanamycin, in humans, adult, with kidney disorder.
Possible hearing loss due to parenteral, topical, or oral administration of
high doses of antibiotic, neomycin, for long period in humans.
Possible hearing loss due to high doses of antibiotic, framycetin, for long
period in humans.
Possible hearing loss due to antibiotic, vancomycin, in humans.
Possible hearing loss and vestibular problems due to antibiotic, viomycin, in
humans.
    (AD) High risk of ototoxicity with simultaneous administration of viomycin
    and streptomycin.
Possible vestibular problems due to antibiotic, gentamicin, in humans.
    (AD) Administration of gentamicin not recommended for newborn infants, for
    humans during pregnancy, and for humans treated with other ototoxic drugs.
Ataxia and hearing loss due to antibiotic, colistin, in humans.
    (AD) Literature review on ototoxic antibiotics.
    (AD) Results of studies on use of pantothenate salt of some antibiotics
    for decr in ototoxicity not clear.
    (AD) Suggested effect of ototoxic antibiotics on breakdown of glucose on
    which hair cells of inner ear depend for energy.   (ENG)

                                                                        412
Damage to organ of Corti and eighth cranial nerve due to parenteral, intramuscular, administration of antibiotic, colistin, in animals, guinea pigs.
    (AD) Study showed individual differences in response to colistin.
    (AD) Administration of colistin to guinea pigs in study of toxic neuritis
    of eighth cranial nerve.   (RUS)

                                                                        420
Acute hearing loss due to 10 mg on first day and then 60 mg daily for 3 days,
total of 220 mg, of antibiotic, (SQ) gentamicin, in total of 4 days in 1
human, adolescent, 16 years age, with kidney disorder.
    (AD) Hearing loss confirmed by audiogram.
Previous administration of antibiotic, (SQ) colistin, in 1 human, adolescent,

16 years age, with kidney disorder.
Vestibular problems due to 40 mg daily, total of 400 mg, of antibiotic,
gentamicin, in total of 10 days in 1 human, aged, 68 years age, with kidney
disorder. (GER)

429

Necrosis of cells of organ of Corti and hearing loss, partial or total, due
to parenteral, intramuscular, administration of high doses, 150,000 units per
kg daily, of antibiotic, colistin (colistin sulfate), for 7 to 21 days in
animals, guinea pigs. (RUS)

430

Permanent hearing loss, partial or total, due to parenteral, intramuscular,
administration of 200,000 units per kg daily of antibiotic, streptomycin, for
30 days in animals, guinea pigs.
Permanent hearing loss, partial or total, due to parenteral, intramuscular,
administration of 150,000 units per kg daily of antibiotic, colistin (colistin sulfate), for 7 to 21 days in animals, guinea pigs. (RUS)

457

Tinnitus and progressive sensorineural hearing loss due to parenteral, intramuscular, administration of antibiotic, (SQ) streptomycin, for 10 days in 1
human, adult, 38 years age, female, with infections and later development of
kidney disorder.
Tinnitus and progressive sensorineural hearing loss due to 13.2 g of antibiotic, (SQ) kanamycin, for 11 days in 1 human, adult, 38 years age, female,
with infections and kidney disorder.
Hearing loss due to antimalarial, (SQ) quinine, in 1 human, adult, 20 years
age, male, with various infections and later development of kidney disorder.
Hearing loss due to 400 mg 2 times daily, total dose of 6.5 g, of antibiotic,
(SQ) kanamycin (SM), for 8 days in 1 human, adult, 20 years age, male, with
various infections and later development of kidney disorder.
Hearing loss due to 150 mg 2 times daily, total dose of 2400 mg, of antibiotic, (SQ) colistin (SM), for 8 days in 1 human, adult, 20 years age, male,
with various infections and later development of kidney disorder.
Tinnitus, total bilateral hearing loss, and vestibular problems due to parenteral, intramuscular, administration of 4.0 g daily, total of 21 g, of antibiotic, (SQ) kanamycin (SM), for 5 days in 1 human, adult, 20 years age,
male, with infections and kidney disorder.
Tinnitus, total bilateral hearing loss, and vestibular problems due to 0.6 g
daily, total dose of 1.3 g, of antibiotic, (SQ) colistin (SM), for 2 days in
1 human, adult, 20 years age, male, with infections and kidney disorder.
Tinnitus, total bilateral hearing loss, and vestibular problems due to 2 g
and then 8 g per 24 hours in divided doses, total dose of 26.5 g, of antibiotic, (SQ) chloramphenicol, for 9 days in 1 human, adult, 20 years age, male,
with infections and kidney disorder.
Bilateral hearing loss due to 1 g daily of antibiotic, actinomycin (SM), for
5 days in 1 human, adult, 62 years age, male, with infections and kidney
disorder.
Bilateral hearing loss due to unknown dose of antibiotic, kanamycin (SM), for
5 days in 1 human, adult, 62 years age, male, with infections and kidney
disorder.
Bilateral hearing loss and vestibular problems due to parenteral administration of high doses of antibiotic, (SQ) neomycin, for total of 21 days in 1
human, adult, 25 years age, male, with infection from wound.
Previous administration of unspecified doses of antibiotic, (SQ) streptomycin, in 1 human, adult, 25 years age, male, with infection from wound.
Later administration of antibiotic, (SQ) chloramphenicol, in 1 human, adult,
25 years age, male, with infection from wound.
Tinnitus and rapidly progressive bilateral hearing loss due to parenteral,
intramuscular, administration of 0.5 g every 12 hours of antibiotic, (SQ)
streptomycin, for 5 days in 1 human, adult, 21 years age, male, with infection from wound.
Tinnitus and rapidly progressive bilateral hearing loss due to parenteral,
intramuscular, administration of 200 mg daily, total of 6.8 g, of antibiotic,
(SQ) colistin (SM), in 1 human, adult, 21 years age, male, with infection
from wound.
Tinnitus and rapidly progressive bilateral hearing loss due to parenteral

administration of unspecified doses of antibiotic, (SQ) neomycin (SM), for
about 35 days in 1 human, adult, 21 years age, male, with infection from
wound.
Tinnitus and progressive bilateral hearing loss due to parenteral administration of 2 l per 24 hours of 1 percent solution of antibiotic, (SQ) neomycin,
for 10 days in 1 human, adult, 26 years age, male, with infection from wound.
   (AD) Hearing loss confirmed by audiometry.
Previous administration of 500 mg four times a day of antibiotic, (SQ) ampicillin, in 1 human, adult, 26 years age, male, with infection from wound.
Bilateral sudden deafness due to administration in dialysis fluid of less
than 150 mg of antibiotic, neomycin (SM), in 1 human, adult, 44 years age,
female, with kidney disorder.
Bilateral sudden deafness due to 50 mg of diuretic, ethacrynic acid (SM), in
1 human, adult, 44 years age, female, with kidney disorder.
   (AD) Hearing loss confirmed by audiology.
Tinnitus and progressive bilateral hearing loss beginning after 8 days of
treatment due to parenteral administration of 1 l every 4 hours for 3 days
and then every 8 hours for 10 days of 1 percent solution of antibiotic,
neomycin, in 1 human, adult, 20 years age, male, with infection from wound.
   (AD) Hearing loss confirmed by audiology.
Tinnitus and bilateral sensorineural hearing loss due to parenteral, intramuscular, administration of 1 g and then 0.5 g every 12 hours of antibiotic,
streptomycin (SM), for 15 days in 1 human, adult, 23 years age, male, with
infection from wound.
Tinnitus and bilateral sensorineural hearing loss due to topical administration by irrigation of 1 percent solution every 12 hours of antibiotic, neomycin (SM), for 14 days in 1 human, adult, 23 years age, male, with infection
from wound.
   (AD) Hearing loss confirmed by audiometry.
   (AD) Discussion of 10 case reports. (ENG)

                                                                      685
Total loss of vestibular function but no hearing loss due to total of 840 mg
of antibiotic, gentamicin (SM), in 47 day period in 1 of 181 humans, aged, 70
years age, female, with kidney disorder.
Total loss of vestibular function but no hearing loss due to 2 g of antibiotic, streptomycin (SM), in 47 day period in 1 of 181 humans, aged, 70 years
age, female, with kidney disorder.
Permanent vestibular problems due to 2.56 g of antibiotic, (SQ) gentamicin,
for 18 days in 1 of 181 humans, adult, 39 years age, female, with kidney
disorder.
Vestibular problems due to previous administration of antibiotic, (SQ) streptomycin, in 1 of 181 humans, adult, 39 years age, female, with kidney disorder.
Permanent vestibular problems, with dizziness, due to antibiotic, gentamicin,
in 1 of 181 humans, adult, 38 years age, female, with kidney disorder.
Transient dizziness after 3 days due to antibiotic, gentamicin, in 1 of 181
humans, adolescent, 16 years age, female, with kidney disorder.
   (AD) Serial vestibular function tests and audiometry not conducted in 181
   patients.
Vestibular problems due to parenteral, intramuscular, administration of 1 g
daily of antibiotic, (SQ) streptomycin (SM), in 1 human, adult, 19 years age,
male, with pseudomonas infection.
   (AD) Vestibular problems due to previous streptomycin therapy.
Simultaneous administration of 300 mg daily of antibiotic, (SQ) colistin (SM)
(colistimethate), for 15 days in 1 human, adult, 19 years age, male, with
pseudomonas infection.
Sequential parenteral, intramuscular, administration of 40 mg 3 times a day
of antibiotic, (SQ) gentamicin, for 36 days in 1 human, adult, 19 years age,
male, with pseudomonas infection.
Dizziness after 4 days due to parenteral, intramuscular, administration of 40
mg 4 times a day, total of 2.56 g, of antibiotic, gentamicin, for 16 days in
1 human, adult, 30 years age, female, with kidney disorder.
   (AD) Discussion of 6 case reports of vestibulotoxic effects of gentamicin.
   (ENG)

Dihydrostreptomycin

009

Delayed permanent sensorineural hearing loss and damage to outer hair cells of basal and middle coils of cochlea due to unspecified doses of antibiotic, dihydrostreptomycin, in humans.
Vertigo and dizziness due to unspecified method of administration of 2 to 3 g daily of antibiotic, streptomycin (streptomycin sulfate), for 30 to 50 days in humans with tuberculosis.
Hearing loss due to unspecified method of administration of high doses of antibiotic, streptomycin (streptomycin sulfate), for long period in humans.
Gradual high frequency hearing loss and tinnitus and degeneration of hair cells of organ of Corti in basal coil of cochlea due to unspecified doses of antibiotic, kanamycin, in humans.
Delayed severe high frequency hearing loss due to parenteral, oral, or topical administration by inhalation of unspecified doses of antibiotic, neomycin, for unspecified period in humans with kidney disorder.
Complete degeneration of inner hair cells due to unspecified method of administration of 18 g of antibiotic, neomycin, for unspecified period in humans with bacterial endocarditis.
Lesions in organ of Corti due to parenteral administration of unspecified doses of antibiotic, polymyxin B, for unspecified period in animals, guinea pigs.
Sensorineural hearing loss due to parenteral, intravenous, administration of 80 to 95 mg per ml of antibiotic, vancomycin, for unspecified period in humans with kidney disorder.
  (AD) Sensorineural hearing loss and vestibular problems due to 6 antibiotics in humans and animals, guinea pigs.
  (AD) Literature review of ototoxic effects of antibiotics. (ENG)

019

Progressive severe sensorineural hearing loss and tinnitus due to unspecified method of administration of 0.5 g twice daily, total of 16 g, of antibiotic, kanamycin, for 16 days in 1 human, Caucasian, adult, 25 years age, male, with kidney disorder and treated with peritoneal dialysis.
  (AD) Audiograms showed hearing loss and recruitment test showed reversed recruitment.
Severe sensorineural hearing loss due to unspecified method of administration of 0.5 g daily for 40 days and then 0.5 g 3 times a week for 3 weeks of antibiotic, streptomycin, for total period of about 9 weeks in 1 human, Negro, child, 9 years age, male, with pulmonary tuberculosis and kidney disorder.
  (AD) No record of hearing loss before treatment with streptomycin.
Delayed severe bilateral high frequency hearing loss due to unspecified method of administration of 0.5 g daily for 8 months and then 0.5 g every 3 days for 4 months, followed by a break of 3.5 months, and then 0.5 g every 3 days for 1.5 months, total of 153 g of antibiotic, dihydrostreptomycin, for total period of about 13.5 months in 1 human, Negro, infant, 16 months age, female, with tuberculosis.
  (AD) Hearing loss detected at 13 years age.
Hearing loss and tinnitus due to unspecified method of administration of 1 g daily of antibiotic, streptomycin, for 10 weeks and possibly for a longer period after discharge in 1 human, Negro, adult, 23 years age, male, treated for infection in tuberculosis hospital.
  (AD) Hearing loss detected 1 month after treatment with streptomycin.
Progressive severe sensorineural hearing loss due to unspecified method of administration of 0.5 g 3 times a week, total of 61 g of antibiotic, streptomycin, for about 10 months in 1 human, Negro, child, 9 years age, female, with pulmonary tuberculosis.
  (AD) Discussion of 5 case reports. (ENG)

044

Change in cochlear response and damage to hair cells of organ of Corti due to 100 mg per kg daily of antibiotic, dihydrostreptomycin, in animals, rabbits.
Change in cochlear response and damage to stria vascularis due to 250 mg per kg daily and 500 mg per kg daily of antibiotic, dihydrostreptomycin, in 2 other groups of animals, rabbits. (JAP)

045
Progressive degeneration of endorgan of cochlea due to low doses of antibiotic, dihydrostreptomycin, in animals, guinea pigs.
Progressive degeneration of endorgan of cochlea due to low doses of antibiotic, neomycin, in animals, guinea pigs.   (JAP)

050
Higher concentrations of dihydrostreptomycin in perilymph than in endolymph
due to parenteral, intraperitoneal, administration of 20 to 30 mc per kg
concentration, tritium-labelled, of antibiotic, dihydrostreptomycin (dihydrostreptomycin sulfate), in 1 injection in 8 animals, guinea pigs, albino, 200
to 250 g weight.
    (CT) Control group of 3 guinea pigs used.
    (AD) Study showed that dihydrostreptomycin carried by blood stream to
    spiral ligament earlier than to stria vascularis.   (ENG)

056
Range of degree of hearing loss due to range of 40 to 300 g of antibiotic,
(SQ) streptomycin, in 59 of 338 humans, male and female, with no previous
treatment with streptomycin.
    (AD) No auditory system problems before treatment.
    (AD) Hearing loss often detected in alcoholics in group.
Range of degree of hearing loss due to range of 40 to 100 g of antibiotic,
(SQ) streptomycin, in 8 of 32 humans with previous treatment with streptomy-
cin.
    (AD) No reported auditory system problems before treatment.
    (AD) More severe hearing loss with administration of 100 g or more of
    streptomycin in both groups.
    (AD) More severe hearing loss in group with previous streptomycin treat-
    ment.
No reported ototoxic effects due to high doses of antibiotic, (SQ) dihydros-
treptomycin, in some of total of 370 humans treated with streptomycin.   (SER)

057
No ototoxic effects within 2 months due to antibiotic, dihydrostreptomycin
(dihydrostreptomycin ascorbinate), in humans with pulmonary tuberculosis.
    (AD) Audiometry used to determine ototoxic effects.
Tinnitus and vertigo due to antibiotic, streptomycin (streptomycin sulfate),
in humans with pulmonary tuberculosis.
    (AD) Comparative study of effects of 2 antibiotics used in treatment of
    pulmonary tuberculosis.   (RUS)

073
Permanent hearing loss due to 10 to 35 mg per kg daily or twice daily of
antibiotic, dihydrostreptomycin, in 23(26.4 percent) of 87 humans, child,
with pulmonary and meningeal tuberculosis.
Permanent hearing loss due to 15 to 35 mg per kg daily or twice daily of
antibiotic, streptomycin, in 1(5.2 percent)of 19 humans, child, with pulmonary and meningeal tuberculosis.
    (AD) More ototoxic effects with 1 dose per day than with 2 doses per day.
Permanent hearing loss due to 15 to 20 mg per kg daily or twice daily of
antibiotic, dihydrostreptomycin (CB), in 4(18.6 percent) of 46 humans, child,
with pulmonary and meningeal tuberculosis.
Permanent hearing loss due to 15 to 20 mg per kg daily or twice daily of
antibiotic, streptomycin (CB), in 4(18.6 percent) of 46 humans, child, with
pulmonary and meningeal tuberculosis.
    (CT) No hearing loss in 14 children, control group, treated with PAS and
    isoniazid.
    (AD) Need to confirm hearing loss with audiometry discussed.   (SER)

080
Hearing loss and vertigo due to parenteral administration of antibiotic,
streptomycin, in humans, child and adult, with normal kidney function and
with kidney disorder.
    (AD) Suggested use for severe infections only.
Delayed permanent hearing loss due to antibiotic, dihydrostreptomycin, in
humans.
    (AD) High risk of ototoxic effects with clinical use.

Hearing loss due to oral administration of antibiotic, paromomycin, in humans.
Progressive permanent hearing loss and tinnitus due to parenteral administration of antibiotic, kanamycin, in humans.
Progressive permanent hearing loss and tinnitus due to parenteral and topical
administration of antibiotic, neomycin, in humans.
  (AD) Need for careful consideration in use of paromomycin, kanamycin, and
  neomycin due to potential ototoxicity.
  (AD) Discussion of ototoxic effects of 5 antibiotics. (ENG)

088

Ototoxic effects in fetus due to unspecified method of administration of
unspecified doses of antibiotic, streptomycin, for long period in humans,
female, treated for tuberculosis during pregnancy.
Ototoxic effects in fetus due to unspecified method of administration of
unspecified doses of antibiotic, dihydrostreptomycin, for long period in
humans, female, treated for tuberculosis during pregnancy. (ENG)

091

Ototoxic effects due to antibiotic, streptomycin (streptomycin sulfate), in
humans with pulmonary tuberculosis.
Ototoxic effects due to antibiotic, dihydrostreptomycin, in humans with
pulmonary tuberculosis.
Ototoxic effects due to antibiotic, florimycin, in humans with pulmonary
tuberculosis.
Ototoxic effects due to antibiotic, kanamycin, in humans with pulmonary
tuberculosis.
  (AD) Comparative study of ototoxicity of different derivatives of antibiotics. (RUS)

106

Severe sensorineural hearing loss due to antibiotic, dihydrostreptomycin, in
humans.
  (AD) Comment on risk of ototoxic effects with clinical use of dihydrostreptomycin. (NOR)

116

Moderate unilateral sensorineural hearing loss in 1 of 36 fetuses due to
total of 13 g of antibiotic, dihydrostreptomycin, in 33 humans, female,
treated during pregnancy for tuberculosis.
  (AD) Child not treated with dihydrostreptomycin or streptomycin.
Sensorineural hearing loss due to 1 g daily for the first 30 days and then 1
g twice a week of antibiotic, dihydrostreptomycin (CB), in 8(24 percent)of 33
humans, female, treated during pregnancy for tuberculosis.
Sensorineural hearing loss due to 1 g daily for the first 30 days and then 1
g twice a week of antibiotic, streptomycin (CB), in 8(24 percent)of 33 humans, female, treated during pregnancy for tuberculosis.
Vestibular problems due to antibiotic, (SQ) dihydrostreptomycin, in 1 of 33
humans, female, treated during pregnancy for tuberculosis and chronic pyelonephritis.
Vestibular problems due to antibiotic, (SQ) streptomycin, in 1 of 33 humans,
female, treated during pregnancy for tuberculosis and chronic pyelonephritis.
  (AD) Case histories, audiometry, and vestibular function tests for children and adults. (ENG)

142

No toxic effects on eighth cranial nerve due to antibiotic, modified dihydrostreptomycin, in animals, guinea pigs and mice.
  (AD) Decr in antibiotic action and toxicity due to modification of quanidine group of dihydrostreptomycin molecule.
  (AD) Study of effect of chemical modification of dihydrostreptomycin
  molecule on biological activity and toxic effects of antibiotic. (RUS)

181

Decr in succinic dehydrogenase in outer hair cells of organ of Corti due to
parenteral, intratympanic, administration of 200 mg per ml solution of antibiotic, kanamycin (kanamycin sulfate), in animals, guinea pigs, adult.
Decr in succinic dehydrogenase in outer hair cells of organ of Corti due to

parenteral, intratympanic, administration of 200 mg per ml solution of antibiotic, dihydrostreptomycin (dihydrostreptomycin sulfate), in animals, guinea
pigs, adult.
Decr in succinic dehydrogenase in outer hair cells of organ of Corti due to
parenteral, intratympanic, administration of 200 mg per ml solution of antibiotic, chloramphenicol (chloramphenicol succinate), in animals, guinea pigs,
adult.
   (AD) Same type of damage to organ of Corti due to all 3 antibiotics.
Severe decr in succinic dehydrogenase in organ of Corti, in particular in
outer hair cells, and atrophy of outer hair cells due to saturated solution
of antimalarial, quinine (quinine hydrochloride), in animals, guinea pigs.
Complete degeneration of organ of Corti due to saturated solution of antimalarial, quinine (quinine hydrochloride), in animals, guinea pigs.
   (AD) Damage to organ of Corti more severe due to quinine than to antibiotics.
   (AD) Activity of succinic dehydrogenase often higher in outer hair cells.
   (AD) Possible that damage to outer hair cells due to higher rate of metabolism. (ENG)

                                                                          184
Incr in ATP hydrolyzing system in stria vascularis and spiral ligament and
incr in ATP activity in membranous labyrinth due to parenteral, intraperitoneal, administration of 400 mg per kg 5 days a week of antibiotic, kanamycin (kanamycin sulfate), for 20 days in animals, guinea pigs, adult, with
normal pinna reflex.
Incr in ATP hydrolyzing system in stria vascularis and spiral ligament due to
parenteral, intraperitoneal, administration of 400 mg per kg 5 days a week of
antibiotic, streptomycin (streptomycin sulfate), for 20 days in animals,
guinea pigs, adult, with normal pinna reflex.
Decr in ATP hydrolyzing system in stria vascularis and spiral ligament and
decr in ATP activity in membranous labyrinth due to parenteral, intraperitoneal, administration of 400 mg per kg 5 days a week of antibiotic, dihydrostreptomycin (dihydrostreptomycin sulfate), for 20 days in animals, guinea
pigs, adult, with normal pinna reflex.
   (CT) Study of normal activity of ATP hydrolyzing system. (ENG)

                                                                          187
Unspecified ototoxic effects due to parenteral, intravenous, intramuscular,
and intraperitoneal, administration of 0.9 percent sodium chloride solution
of antibiotics, aminoglycoside, in animals, mice, albino, adult, male and
female, 15 to 30 g weight.
   (CT) Same method using 0.9 percent sodium chloride solution in mice,
   control group.
   (AD) Comment on relationship of study to ototoxicity of antibiotics.
Risk of ototoxic effects due to antibiotic, dihydrostreptomycin, in chronic
intoxication in humans. (ENG)

                                                                          197
Progressive degeneration of organ of Corti beginning at base of cochlea due
to antibiotic, neomycin, in animals, guinea pigs.
Progressive degeneration of organ of Corti beginning at base of cochlea due
to antibiotic, kanamycin, in animals, guinea pigs.
Progressive degeneration of organ of Corti beginning at base of cochlea due
to antibiotic, framycetin, in animals, guinea pigs.
No damage to hair cells of organ of Corti due to parenteral administration of
high doses of antibiotic, dihydrostreptomycin, for long periods in animals,
guinea pigs.
   (AD) Surface specimen technique used in study of organ of Corti.
   (AD) Damage to organ of Corti due to ototoxic drugs different from that
   due to noise. (ENG)

                                                                          245
Degeneration of outer hair cells of organ of Corti and changes in supporting
cells due to 400 mg per kg daily of antibiotic, kanamycin, for 14 days in
animals, guinea pigs.
Degeneration of organ of Corti due to 400 mg per kg daily of antibiotic,
dihydrostreptomycin, for 14 days in animals, guinea pigs.
   (AD) Comparative study of cochleotoxic effects of kanamycin and dihydros-

treptomycin.   (FR)

250

Damage to vestibular apparatus due to more than 1 g daily of antibiotic,
streptomycin, for 60 to 120 days in 25 percent of humans.
Dizziness 5 days after cessation of treatment due to parenteral, intramuscular, administration of 1 g every 12 hours of antibiotic, streptomycin (SM),
for 9 days in 1 human, adult, 44 years age, female, with peritonitis.
Simultaneous parenteral, intravenous, administration of 600 mg every 18 hours
of antibiotic, lincomycin (SM), for 9 days in 1 human, adult, 44 years age,
female, with peritonitis.
   (AD) Case report of vestibular problem due to streptomycin.
Damage to cochlea due to antibiotic, dihydrostreptomycin, for more than 1
week in 4 to 15 percent of humans.
Sensorineural hearing loss and damage to organ of Corti due to antibiotic,
kanamycin, in humans.
Sensorineural hearing loss and damage to organ of Corti due to antibiotic,
vancomycin, in humans.
   (AD) Discussion of cochleo-vestibulotoxic effects due to antibiotic therapy in surgery.   (ENG)

282

Limited effects on blood vessels of stria vascularis and spiral prominence
due to 300 mg per kg daily of antibiotic, kanamycin, for 4 to 9 days in
animals, guinea pigs.
Limited effects on blood vessels of stria vascularis and spiral prominence
due to 30 mg per kg daily of antibiotic, dihydrostreptomycin, for 4 to 9 days
in animals, guinea pigs.
Limited effects on blood vessels of stria vascularis and spiral prominence
due to 30 mg per kg daily of antibiotic, chloramphenicol, for 4 to 9 days in
animals, guinea pigs.
   (CT) Study of guinea pigs, control group.   (JAP)

285

Transient inhibition of endorgan of ampulla due to range of doses of antibiotic, streptomycin (streptomycin sulfate), in animals, frogs.
Transient inhibition of endorgan of ampulla due to range of doses of antibio-
tic, dihydrostreptomycin (dihydrostreptomycin sulfate), in animals, frogs.
Transient inhibition of endorgan of ampulla due to range of doses of antibiotic, neomycin (neomycin sulfate), in animals, frogs.
Transient inhibition of endorgan of ampulla due to range of doses of antibiotic, kanamycin (kanamycin sulfate), in animals, frogs.
   (CT) Study of frogs, control group.
   (AD) More inhibition of endorgan of ampulla with streptomycin than with
   other aminoglycoside antibiotics.
   (AD) Agreement between in vivo and in vitro observations of intensity of
   action on endorgans of vestibular apparatus.   (ENG)

290

Vestibular problems, sensorineural hearing loss, and tinnitus due to total
doses of 12 to 63 g of antibiotic, streptomycin, in 24 humans with tuberculosis.
   (AD) Subjects tested after streptomycin intoxication with audiology and
   cupulometry.
   (AD) Individual responses to streptomycin observed.
Changes in cupulometric curves for postrotatory nystagmus, showing changes in
vestibular apparatus, due to 0.5 g daily, total doses of 30 to 100 g, of
antibiotic, streptomycin (SM) (streptomycin sulfate), in 23 humans with
various infections.
Simultaneous administration of 0.5 g of antibiotic, dihydrostreptomycin (SM),
in 23 humans with various infections.
Simultaneous administration of antituberculous agent, PAS (SM), in 23 humans
with various infections.
   (CT) Pretreatment vestibular function normal.
   (CT) Subjects tested with audiology and cupulometry before and during
   treatment with streptomycin.
   (AD) Hearing loss in 1 subject in group with cupulometry during treatment
   but in 5 subjects in other group with cupulometry only after treatment.

(AD) Suggested use of cupulometry for possible prevention of streptomycin intoxication. (ENG)

311

Vertigo or hearing loss of 10 to 20 decibels due to antibiotic, streptomycin, in 14 of 67 humans with pulmonary tuberculosis.
Vertigo or hearing loss of 30 to 40 decibels due to antibiotic, streptomycin (CB), in 12 of 59 humans with pulmonary tuberculosis.
Vertigo or hearing loss of 30 to 40 decibels due to antibiotic, dihydrostreptomycin (CB), in 12 of 59 humans with pulmonary tuberculosis.
    (AD) Hearing loss confirmed by audiometry. (DUT)

314

Loss of enzymes, succinic dehydrogenase and DPN diaphorase, in outer hair cells of organ of Corti but usually no enzyme loss in inner hair cells due to topical administration to bulla of 200 mg per ml of antibiotic, kanamycin (kanamycin sulfate), in 1 injection in animals, guinea pigs.
Loss of enzymes, succinic dehydrogenase and DPN diaphorase, in outer hair cells of organ of Corti but usually no enzyme loss in inner hair cells due to topical administration to bulla of 200 mg per ml of antibiotic, dihydrostreptomycin (dihydrostreptomycin sulfate), in 1 injection in animals, guinea pigs.
Loss of enzymes, succinic dehydrogenase and DPN diaphorase, in outer hair cells of organ of Corti but usually no enzyme loss in inner hair cells due to topical administration to bulla of 200 mg per ml of antibiotic, chloramphenicol (chloramphenicol succinate), in 1 injection in animals, guinea pigs.
More severe effects on enzymes, succinic hydrogenase and DPN diaphorase, in outer hair cells of organ of Corti due to topical administration to bulla of saturated solution of antimalarial, quinine (quinine hydrochloride), in 1 injection in animals, guinea pigs.
    (CT) Activity of succinic dehydrogenase often higher in outer hair cells than in inner hair cells of organ of Corti in guinea pigs, control group.
    (AD) Suggested correlation between cochleotoxic effects of drugs and metabolic activity of hair cells. (ENG)

317

Possible decr in ototoxic effects due to antibiotic, dihydrostreptomycin (IB), in humans, with administration of pantothenate salt.
    (AD) Discussion of clinical use of dihydrostreptomycin and possible decr in ototoxicity with use of pantothenate salt of antibiotic. (GER)

318

High risk of ototoxic effects due to antibiotic, dihydrostreptomycin, in humans with bacterial infections.
Risk of ototoxic effects due to antibiotic, streptomycin, in humans with bacterial infections, with administration of pantothenic acid.
    (AD) Literature review on clinical use and ototoxicity of streptomycin.
    (AD) Recommended use of streptomycin only for tuberculosis due to high risk of ototoxic effects. (GER)

333

Vestibular problems due to antibiotic, streptomycin, in humans.
Severe cochlear impairment due to antibiotic, dihydrostreptomycin, in humans.
Loss of hair cells in organ of Corti and hearing loss due to antibiotics, aminoglycoside, in humans.
Hearing loss in fetus due to antimalarial, quinine, in humans, female, treated during pregnancy.
Transient hearing loss due to high doses of salicylate, aspirin, for long period in humans.
    (AD) Discussion of possible cochleo-vestibulotoxic effects of ototoxic drugs.
    (AD) Ototoxic effects related to concurrent disorders, dosage, duration of treatment, and age of individuals. (ENG)

334

Effect on organ of Corti of fetuses due to parenteral, intraperitoneal, administration of daily doses of antibiotic, streptomycin, in animals, rats, female, during pregnancy.

Effect on organ of Corti of fetuses due to parenteral, intraperitoneal,
administration of daily doses of antibiotic, dihydrostreptomycin, in animals,
rats, female, during pregnancy.
   (AD) Determined concentration of antibiotic in blood of fetus.   (GER)

335

Vestibular problems due to antibiotic, streptomycin, in humans.
Severe cochlear impairment due to antibiotic, dihydrostreptomycin, in humans.
Cochlear impairment due to parenteral, oral, and topical administration of
antibiotic, neomycin, in humans.
Tinnitus and hearing loss due to antibiotic, kanamycin, in humans.
Vestibular problems and hearing loss due to antibiotic, gentamicin, in hu-
mans.
   (AD) Discussion of clinical use and possible cochleo-vestibulotoxic ef-
   fects of aminoglycoside antibiotics.   (SP)

338

No loss of pinna reflex and no significant histological changes due to parenteral, subcutaneous, administration of 400 mg per kg daily in 1 injection of
antibiotic, dihydrostreptomycin, for 8 to 37 injections in 8 animals, guinea
pigs, young, 200 to 290 g weight.
Hearing loss after 64 injections and moderate damage to hair cells of cochlea
due to parenteral, subcutaneous, administration of 600 mg per kg daily, total
dose of 38.4 g, of antibiotic, dihydrostreptomycin, for 9 to 64 injections in
1 of 5 animals, guinea pigs, young, 200 to 290 g weight.
No loss of pinna reflex and no significant histological changes due to 50 mg
per kg daily of antibiotic, kanamycin, for 64 injections in 10 animals,
guinea pigs.
   (CT) Test of pinna reflex, pretreatment and daily during treatment with
   antibiotics.
   (AD) Suggested relationship between degree of kanamycin damage to cochlea
   and daily dose rather than total dose.   (ENG)

368

Possible vestibular problems and hearing loss due to antibiotic, streptomycin, in humans with tuberculosis.
Permanent hearing loss due to antibiotic, dihydrostreptomycin, in humans with
tuberculosis.
Possible permanent hearing loss due to antibiotic, kanamycin, in humans with
tuberculosis.
Possible vestibular problems and hearing loss due to antibiotic, viomycin, in
humans with tuberculosis.
Possible damage to eighth cranial nerve due to antibiotic, capreomycin, in
humans with tuberculosis.
   (AD) Discussion of primary and secondary drugs used in tuberculosis chemotherapy.   (FR)

382

Damage to hair cells of organ of Corti and nervous tissue of osseous spiral
lamina due to topical administration to inner ear of 9.8 percent tritium-
labelled solution, in same amount of Ringer's solution, of antibiotic, dihydrostreptomycin, in animals, guinea pigs, 250 to 450 g weight.
   (AD) Autoradiographical study of distribution of dihydrostreptomycin in
   cochlear duct.
   (AD) Suggested that ototoxicity of dihydrostreptomycin due to retention of
   drug for long period in perilymph and specific accumulation of drug in
   hair cells and nervous tissue of organ of Corti.   (ENG)

384

Usually transient hearing loss and no structural damage to organ of Corti,
stria vascularis, and spiral ganglion due to oral or topical administration
of salicylates in humans.
Hearing loss due to antimalarial, quinine, in humans.
Usually permanent hearing loss due to antimalarial, chloroquine, in humans.
Transient and permanent hearing loss and possible damage to hair cells of
organ of Corti due to diuretic, ethacrynic acid, in humans.
Sensorineural hearing loss due to cardiovascular agent, hexadimethrine
bromide, in humans with kidney disorder.

Sensorineural hearing loss and damage to organ of Corti due to topical administration of antineoplastic, nitrogen mustard, in humans.
Sensorineural hearing loss due to high doses of antibiotic, chloramphenicol,
in humans.
Primary vestibular problems due to antibiotic, streptomycin, in humans.
Hearing loss due to high doses usually of antibiotic, streptomycin, in humans.
   (AD) Early detection of hearing loss by audiometry prevents permanent
   damage.
High frequency hearing loss and severe damage to outer hair cells and slight
damage to inner hair cells of organ of Corti due to antibiotic, kanamycin, in
humans.
Sensorineural hearing loss due to parenteral, oral, and topical administration of antibiotic, neomycin, in humans with or without kidney disorders.
Degeneration of hair cells of organ of Corti and of nerve process due to
antibiotics, aminoglycoside, in animals.
   (AD) Literature review of physiological and structural cochleo-vestibulotoxic effects of ototoxic drugs.
   (AD) Discussion of suggested mechanism of ototoxicity and routes of drugs
   to inner ear.
Bilateral sensorineural hearing loss due to oral administration of antibiotic, neomycin, in 4 of 8 humans with liver disease.
Bilateral sensorineural hearing loss due to oral administration of range of
doses of antibiotic, neomycin (SM), in 2 of 5 humans with liver disease.
Bilateral sensorineural hearing loss due to diuretics (SM), in 2 of 5 humans
with liver disease.
Transient progression of previous hearing loss due to parenteral, intravenous, administration of diuretic, ethacrynic acid (SM), in 1 injection in 1
of 5 humans with liver disease.
   (CT) Normal cochlear function in 6 humans, control group, with liver
   disease and not treated with neomycin or diuretics.
   (CT) Normal cochlear function in 13 humans, control group, with liver
   disease and treated with diuretics but not with neomycin.
   (AD) Hearing loss confirmed by audiometry.
   (AD) Reported that hearing loss due to neomycin or diuretics in humans
   with liver disease not related to dosage.
   (AD) Clinical study of effects of treatment with neomycin and diuretics in
   humans with liver disease.
Bilateral sensorineural hearing loss and vertigo due to antibiotic, ampicil-
lin, in 1 human, adolescent, 17 years age, female, with tonsillitis.
   (AD) Cited case report.
Severe sensorineural hearing loss and vertigo due to topical administration
in ear drops of antibiotic, framycetin, in 1 human, adult, 42 years age,
male, with previous slight high frequency hearing loss.
   (AD) Cited case report.
Atrophy of hair cells of organ of Corti and hearing loss due to antibiotic,
dihydrostreptomycin, in humans with tuberculous meningitis.
   (AD) Cited study.
Loss of inner hair cells and damage to outer hair cells due to 18 g of anti-
biotic, neomycin, for 18 days in 1 human.
   (AD) Cited case report. (ENG)

                                                                      434
Slight ototoxic effects due to range of doses of antibiotic, streptomycin, in
8 of 40 humans, female, treated for tuberculosis during pregnancy.
Slight ototoxic effects due to range of doses of antibiotic, dihydrostreptomycin, in 2 of 40 humans, female, treated for tuberculosis during pregnancy.
Vestibular problems and sensorineural hearing loss in mother and vestibular
problems in fetus due to total of 27 g of antibiotic, streptomycin (CB), for
2.5 months in 1 human, adult, 28 years age, female, treated for pulmonary
tuberculosis at end of pregnancy.
Vestibular problems and sensorineural hearing loss in mother and vestibular
problems in fetus due to total of 27 g of antibiotic, dihydrostreptomycin
(CB), for 2.5 months in 1 human, adult, 28 years age, female, treated for
pulmonary tuberculosis at end of pregnancy.
   (AD) Pure tone audiometry and vestibular function tests in child, female,
   at 10 years age.

Mixed hearing loss in mother and severe sensorineural hearing loss and vestibular problems in fetus due to total of 28 g of antibiotic, (SQ) dihydrostreptomycin, for 2.5 months in 1 human, adult, 22 years age, female, treated for
tuberculosis at beginning of pregnancy.
Mixed hearing loss in mother and severe sensorineural hearing loss and vestibular problems in fetus due to total of 28 g of antibiotic, (SQ) streptomycin, for 2.5 months in 1 human, adult, 22 years age, female, treated for
tuberculosis at beginning of pregnancy.
    (AD) Pure tone audiometry and vestibular function tests in child, female,
    at 10 years age.   (ENG)

464

Possible decr in damage to organ of Corti and eighth cranial nerve due to
antibiotic, dihydrostreptomycin (IB), in animals, guinea pigs, with administration of citrobioflavonoid complex.   (IT)

468

Complete inhibition of acetylcholine induced decr in cochlear potential due
to parenteral, intravenous, administration of 1.0 mg of antibiotic, streptomycin (streptomycin sulfate), in 1 injection in 5 animals, cats, male and
female, 1.5 to 2.8 kg weight, with injection of acetylcholine.
Minimum inhibition of acetylcholine induced decr in cochlear potential due to
parenteral, intravenous, administration of 1.0 mg of antibiotic, dihydrostreptomycin (dihydrostreptomycin sulfate), in 1 injection in 5 animals, cats,
male and female, 1.5 to 2.8 kg weight, with injection of acetylcholine.
Complete inhibition of acetylcholine induced decr in cochlear potential due
to parenteral, intravenous, administration of 1.0 mg of antibiotic, kanamycin
(kanamycin sulfate), in 1 injection in 5 animals, cats, male and female, 1.5
to 2.8 kg weight, with injection of acetylcholine.
Complete inhibition of acetylcholine induced decr in cochlear potential due
to parenteral, intravenous, administration of 1.0 mg of antibiotic, neomycin
(neomycin sulfate), in 1 injection in 5 animals, cats, male and female, 1.5
to 2.8 kg weight, with injection of acetylcholine.
Acute inhibition of acetylcholine induced decr in cochlear potential due to
parenteral, intravenous, administration of 1.0 mg of antimalarial, quinine
(quinine hydrochloride), in 1 injection in 5 animals, cats, male and female,
1.5 to 2.8 kg weight, with injection of acetylcholine.
    (CT) Injections of 0.1 ml isotonic saline in cats, control group.
Inhibition of acetylcholine induced decr in cochlear potential due to parenteral, subcutaneous, administration of 300 mg per kg daily of antibiotic,
streptomycin, for 7 to 9 days in 10 animals, cats.
Inhibition of acetylcholine induced decr in cochlear potential due to parenteral, subcutaneous, administration of 100 mg per kg daily of antibiotic,
neomycin, for 7 to 9 days in 10 animals, cats.
    (CT) Study of 7 cats, control group, not treated with antibiotics.
    (AD) Study of effect of acetylcholine on cochlear potential after acute
    and chronic administration of ototoxic drugs.
    (AD) Suggested relationship between change in acetylcholine activity and
    ototoxic drugs.
    (AD) Suggested that ototoxicity partially due to disruption of efferent
    effect on cochlea.   (ENG)

477

Significant decr in oxygen consumption of cochlea due to high doses of antibiotic, kanamycin, in animals, guinea pigs.
Significant decr in oxygen consumption of cochlea due to high doses of antibiotic, streptomycin, in animals, guinea pigs.
Incr followed by significant decr in oxygen consumption of cochlea due to
high doses of antibiotic, dihydrostreptomycin, in animals, guinea pigs.
    (CT) Determination of oxygen consumption of guinea pigs, control group,
    not treated with ototoxic drugs.
    (AD) Suggested that ototoxicity of aminoglycoside antibiotics due to
    inhibition of respiratory enzymes of cells of inner ear.   (ENG)

478

Nystagmus due to parenteral, intramuscular, administration of 0.5 g daily,
total dose of 50 g, of antibiotic, dihydrostreptomycin, in 6 humans with
pulmonary tuberculosis.

Nystagmus due to parenteral, intramuscular, administration of total doses of
105 to 300 g of antibiotic, dihydrostreptomycin, in 10 humans with pulmonary
tuberculosis.
    (AD) Case report included.
    (AD) Study using cupulometry of vestibular problems due to dihydrostrep-
    tomycin therapy.   (GER)

482

Decr in cochlear function and vestibular function due to parenteral, intramuscular, administration of 50 to 100 mg per kg of antibiotic, streptomycin
(streptomycin sulfate), for 35 days in animals, guinea pigs, pigmented, 400
to 500 g weight.
    (AD) More ototoxic effects with higher dosage.
Decr in cochlear function with both doses but decr in vestibular function
with only higher dose due to parenteral, intramuscular, administration of 50
to 100 mg per kg of antibiotic, dihydrostreptomycin (dihydrostreptomycin
sulfate), for 35 days in animals, guinea pigs, pigmented, 400 to 500 g
weight.
    (AD) More decr in cochlear function with higher dosage.
Decr in cochlear function in all animals but decr in vestibular function in 2
groups only due to parenteral, intramuscular, administration of 50 to 100 mg
per kg of antibiotic, kanamycin, for 35 days in animals, guinea pigs, pigmented, 400 to 500 g weight.
    (AD) More decr in cochlear function with higher dosage.
Decr in cochlear function due to parenteral, intramuscular, administration of
20 mg per kg of diuretic, ethacrynic acid, for 35 days in animals, guinea
pigs, pigmented, 400 to 500 g weight.
    (CT) Study of guinea pigs, control group, not treated with ototoxic drugs.
Decr in ototoxic effects due to parenteral, intramuscular, administration of
100 mg per kg of antibiotic, streptomycin (IB) (streptomycin sulfate), for 35
days in animals, guinea pigs, pigmented, 400 to 500 g weight, with administration of 1 mg per kg of various inhibitors.
Decr in ototoxic effects due to parenteral, intramuscular, administration of
100 mg per kg of antibiotic, dihydrostreptomycin (IB) (dihydrostreptomycin
sulfate), for 35 days in animals, guinea pigs, pigmented, 400 to 500 g
weight, with administration of 1 mg per kg of various inhibitors.
Decr in ototoxic effects due to parenteral, intramuscular, administration of
100 mg per kg of antibiotic, kanamycin (IB), for 35 days in animals, guinea
pigs, pigmented, 400 to 500 g weight, with administration of 1 mg per kg of
various inhibitors.
Decr in ototoxic effects due to parenteral, intramuscular, administration of
20 mg per kg of diuretic, ethacrynic acid (IB), for 35 days in animals,
guinea pigs, pigmented, 400 to 500 g weight, with administration of 1 mg per
kg of various inhibitors.
    (AD) Measurement of Preyer reflex and vestibular function tests.
Ototoxic effects, functional and structural, due to parenteral, intraperitoneal, administration of 100 mg per kg of antibiotic, streptomycin (streptomycin sulfate), for 50 days in animals, mice, male, 18 to 22 g weight.
No ototoxic effects due to parenteral, intraperitoneal, administration of 100
mg per kg of antibiotic, dihydrostreptomycin (dihydrostreptomycin sulfate),
for 50 days in animals, mice, male, 18 to 22 g weight.
Ototoxic effects, functional and structural, due to parenteral, intraperitoneal, administration of 100 mg per kg of antibiotic, kanamycin, for 50 days
in animals, mice, male, 18 to 22 g weight.
    (CT) Study of mice, control group, not treated with ototoxic drugs.
No ototoxic effects due to parenteral, intraperitoneal, administration of 100
mg per kg of antibiotic, streptomycin (IB) (streptomycin sulfate), for 50
days in animals, mice, male, 18 to 22 g weight, with administration of 1 mg
per kg of vitamin B.
No ototoxic effects due to parenteral, intraperitoneal, administration of 100
mg per kg of antibiotic, dihydrostreptomycin (IB) (dihydrostreptomycin sulfate), for 50 days in animals, mice, male, 18 to 22 g weight, with administration of 1 mg per kg of vitamin B.
No ototoxic effects due to parenteral, intraperitoneal, administration of 100
mg per kg of antibiotic, kanamycin (IB), for 50 days in animals, mice, male,
18 to 22 g weight, with administration of vitamin B.
    (AD) More ototoxic effects of aminoglycoside antibiotics in guinea pigs
    than in mice.

(AD) Ototoxic effects of diuretic in guinea pigs.   (IT)

485

High concentration in fluids of inner ear and ototoxic effects due to 250 mg
per kg of antibiotic, streptomycin, in animals, guinea pigs.
High concentration in fluids of inner ear and ototoxic effects due to 250 mg
per kg of antibiotic, kanamycin, in animals, guinea pigs.
Higher concentration in fluids of inner ear and more severe ototoxic effects
due to 250 mg per kg of antibiotic, dihydrostreptomycin, in animals, guinea
pigs.
Higher concentration in fluids of inner ear and more severe ototoxic effects
due to 100 mg per kg of antibiotic, neomycin, in animals, guinea pigs.
    (AD) High concentration of aminoglycoside antibiotics in fluids of inner
    ear due to low doses as well as high doses.
    (AD) Ototoxic effect of aminoglycoside antibiotics due to retention of
    high concentrations in inner ear for long period and slow elimination of
    drugs.
Significant decr in concentration in fluids of inner ear and in serum and
decr in ototoxicity due to 250 mg per kg or 100 mg per kg of antibiotics
(IB), aminoglycoside, in animals, guinea pigs, with administration of ozothin.
Decr in concentration in fluids of inner ear and decr in ototoxicity due to
250 mg per kg or 100 mg per kg of antibiotics (IB), aminoglycoside, in animals, guinea pigs, with administration of pantothenic acid.   (GER)

486

Incr in ATP activity of stria vascularis and spiral ligament but no pattern
of enzyme changes observed in membranous labyrinth due to 400 mg per kg daily
of antibiotic, kanamycin, for 3 weeks in animals, guinea pigs.
Incr in ATP activity of stria vascularis and spiral ligament but no pattern
of enzyme changes observed in membranous labyrinth due to 400 mg per kg daily
of antibiotic, streptomycin, for 3 weeks in animals, guinea pigs.
Decr in ATP activity of stria vascularis and spiral ligament but no pattern
of enzyme changes observed in membranous labyrinth due to 400 mg per kg daily
of antibiotic, dihydrostreptomycin, for 3 weeks in animals, guinea pigs.
    (CT) Study of guinea pigs, control group, not treated with aminoglycoside
    antibiotics.
    (AD) Study of effects of ototoxic drugs on ATP activity of inner ear of
    guinea pigs.   (JAP)

529

Total loss of Preyer reflex within several days but no vestibular problems
due to parenteral, subcutaneous, administration of range of high doses to
more than 1000 mg per kg daily of antibiotic, kanamycin (kanamycin sulfate),
in animals, rats, Wistar, albino, female, 50 g weight.
    (AD) Linear relationship between hearing loss and kanamycin dosage.
Loss of Preyer reflex but no vestibular problems due to parenteral, subcutaneous, administration of range of high doses to more than 600 mg per kg
daily of antibiotic, neomycin, in animals, rats, Wistar, albino, female, 50 g
weight.
    (AD) Linear relationship between hearing loss and neomycin dosage.
    (AD) Hearing loss observed with lower doses of neomycin than kanamycin.
Moderate to severe vestibular problems but cochlear impairment in only 1 case
due to parenteral, subcutaneous, administration of high doses, 471, 583, 720,
887, and 1089 mg per kg daily, of antibiotic, streptomycin (streptomycin
sulfate), in animals, rats, Wistar, albino, female, 50 g weight.
    (AD) Linear realtionship between vestibular problems and streptomycin
    dosage.
Transient moderate to severe vestibular problems but cochlear impairment in
only 1 case due to parenteral, subcutaneous, administration of high doses,
765, 940, 1151, and 1377 mg per kg daily, of antibiotic, dihydrostreptomycin
(dihydrostreptomycin sulfate), in 40 animals, rats, Wistar, albino, female,
50 g weight.
    (CT) Same method using saline in 30 rats, control group, showed no coch-
    leo-vestibulotoxic effects.
Hearing loss due to parenteral, subcutaneous, administration of 500 mg per kg
daily of antibiotic, kanamycin (SM), in animals, rats, Wistar, albino, female, 50 g weight.

Hearing loss due to parenteral, subcutaneous, administration of range of
doses of antibiotic, neomycin (SM), in animals, rats, Wistar, albino, female,
50 g weight.
   (AD) Incr in ototoxicity of neomycin due to kanamycin.
Hearing loss but no vestibular problems due to parenteral, subcutaneous,
administration of 500 mg per kg of antibiotic, kanamycin (SM), in animals,
rats, Wistar, albino, female, 50 g weight.
Hearing loss but no vestibular problems due to parenteral, subcutaneous,
administration of 200, 270, 364.5, and 492 mg per kg daily of antibiotic,
streptomycin (SM), in animals, rats, Wistar, albino, female, 50 g weight.
Hearing loss but no vestibular problems due to parenteral, subcutaneous,
administration of 500 mg per kg daily of antibiotic, kanamycin (SM), in
animals, rats, Wistar, albino, female, 50 g weight.
Hearing loss but no vestibular problems due to parenteral, subcutaneous,
administration of 350, 472.5, 637.9, and 861.1 mg per kg daily of antibiotic,
dihydrostreptomycin (SM), in animals, rats, Wistar, albino, female, 50 g
weight.
   (AD) Tests of cochlear function and vestibular function, pretreatment and
   daily during treatment.
   (AD) Comparative study of ototoxic effects of aminoglycoside antibiotics
   in Wistar rats.
   (AD) Report of hearing loss in 321 (43.4 percent) of total of 740 rats in
   study.
   (AD) Suggested that ototoxic effects of kanamycin and neomycin due to
   different mechanisms of action than ototoxic effects of streptomycin and
   dihydrostreptomycin.   (ENG)

                                                                         551
Sensorineural hearing loss due to parenteral administration of range of
doses, 3, 15, 25, and 40 g, of antibiotic, dihydrostreptomycin, in humans,
adult and child, range of ages, male and female, in 4 families.
   (AD) Study of familial incidence of dihydrostreptomycin hearing loss and
   hereditary susceptibility of cochlea.
   (AD) Suggested that administration of dihydrostreptomycin in humans with
   hereditary susceptibility of cochlea results in hearing loss.   (ENG)

                                                                         602
Effect on eighth cranial nerve due to antibiotic, streptomycin, in humans.
Effect on eighth cranial nerve due to antibiotic, dihydrostreptomycin, in
humans.
   (AD) Comparative study of effect of 2 antibiotics on eighth cranial nerve.
   (ENG)

                                                                         621
Primarily vestibular problems due to antibiotic, streptomycin, in humans.
Primarily hearing loss but also vestibular problems due to antibiotic, dihy-
drostreptomycin, in humans.
Primarily hearing loss but also vestibular problems due to antibiotic, kana-
mycin, in humans.
Primarily hearing loss but also vestibular problems due to antibiotic, neomy-
cin, in humans.
Primarily hearing loss but also vestibular problems due to antibiotic, genta-
micin, in humans.
Vertigo and ataxia due to antituberculous agent, isoniazid, in humans.
Hearing loss due to salicylate, aspirin, in humans.
Hearing loss and vertigo due to antimalarial, quinine, in humans.
Nystagmus due to barbiturates in humans.
Vestibular problems due to analgesic, morphine, in humans.
Nystagmus due to sedative, alcohol, in humans.
Nystagmus and hearing loss due to chemical agent, carbon monoxide, in humans.
Ototoxic effects due to antineoplastic, nitrogen mustard, in humans.
Ototoxic effects due to chemical agent, aniline, in humans.
Ototoxic effects due to chemical agent, tobacco, in humans.
Nystagmus due to chemical agent, nicotine, in humans.
Vestibular problems due to anticonvulsants in humans.
Vestibular problems due to anesthetics in humans.
Vestibular problems due to diuretics in humans.
   (AD) Inclusion of comprehensive list of ototoxic agents.   (SP)

645

Permanent severe hearing loss due to antibiotic, dihydrostreptomycin, in
humans.
  (AD) Suggested that no preparations of dihydrostreptomycin be used in
  therapy. (ENG)

670

Possible vestibular problems due to parenteral administration of antibiotic,
gentamicin, in humans.
Damage to eighth cranial nerve, primarily hearing loss, usually permanent,
due to parenteral administration of high doses of antibiotic, kanamycin, for
more than 10 days in humans, in particular with kidney disorders.
Damage to eighth cranial nerve, primarily hearing loss, usually permanent,
due to parenteral administration of high doses of antibiotic, neomycin, for
more than 10 days in humans, in particular with kidney disorders.
Possible damage to eighth cranial nerve, primarily hearing loss, due to
parenteral administration of antibiotic, paromomycin, in humans.
Transient or permanent vestibular problems due to parenteral administration
of antibiotic, streptomycin, in humans.
Permanent severe hearing loss due to parenteral administration of antibiotic,
dihydrostreptomycin, in humans.
Damage to eighth cranial nerve, primarily hearing loss, due to parenteral
administration of high doses of antibiotic, vancomycin, for more than 10 days
in humans, in particular with kidney disorders.
Damage to eighth cranial nerve, vestibular problems and hearing loss, due to
parenteral administration of high doses of antibiotic, viomycin, for more
than 10 days in humans, in particular with kidney disorders.
  (AD) Discussion of toxic effects of antibiotics. (ENG)

676

Vestibular problems due to antibiotic, streptomycin, in humans.
  (AD) Ototoxic effects of streptomycin particularly with high doses, long
  period of treatment, concurrent kidney disorders, and in older patients.
Hearing loss due to antibiotic, dihydrostreptomycin, in humans.
Hearing loss due to antibiotic, viomycin, in humans.
  (AD) Discussion of toxic effects of various antibiotics.
  (AD) Comment that effect of some inhibitors on ototoxicity not known
  definitely. (FR)

681

Degrees of inhibition of potential of endorgan of ampulla of posterior semicircular canal due to 50, 200, 300, and 500 mcg per cc, in Tyrode solution,
of antibiotic, streptomycin (streptomycin sulfate), in animals, frogs.
Degrees of inhibition of potential of endorgan of ampulla of posterior semicircular canal due to 100, 200, and 500 mcg per cc, in Tyrode solution, of
antibiotic, dihydrostreptomycin, in animals, frogs.
  (AD) Recovery of potential after cessation of administration of antibiotics. (IT)

726

Effect on concentration of cytoplasmic RNS in organ of Corti due to parenteral, intramuscular, administration of 100 mg per kg of antibiotic, dihydrostreptomycin, for 20 days in 5 animals, guinea pigs.
  (AD) Study of effect of dihydrostreptomycin on concentration of cytoplasmic RNS in inner ear of guinea pigs. (GER)

Florimycin

091

Ototoxic effects due to antibiotic, streptomycin (streptomycin sulfate), in
humans with pulmonary tuberculosis.
Ototoxic effects due to antibiotic, dihydrostreptomycin, in humans with
pulmonary tuberculosis.
Ototoxic effects due to antibiotic, florimycin, in humans with pulmonary
tuberculosis.
Ototoxic effects due to antibiotic, kanamycin, in humans with pulmonary
tuberculosis.
  (AD) Comparative study of ototoxicity of different derivatives of antibio-

tics. (RUS)

522
Hearing loss due to antibiotic, kanamycin, for 2 to 10 months in 30.4 percent
of 56 humans with chronic pulmonary tuberculosis and treated previously with
other drugs.
No significant ototoxic effects due to antibiotic, florimycin, for 2 to 10
months in 50 humans with chronic pulmonary tuberculosis and treated previously with other drugs.
  (AD) Study of effects of kanamycin and florimycin in treatment of pulmonary tuberculosis. (RUS)

Framycetin

170
Sensorineural hearing loss due to topical administration in ear drops of
antibiotic, neomycin, in humans with no other explanation for hearing loss.
Sensorineural hearing loss due to topical administration in ear drops of
antibiotic, chloramphenicol, in humans with no other explanation for hearing
loss.
Sensorineural hearing loss due to topical administration in ear drops of
antibiotic, framycetin, in humans with no other explanation for hearing loss.
  (AD) Comment on topical use of antibiotics and possible risk of cochleotoxic effects. (ENG)

197
Progressive degeneration of organ of Corti beginning at base of cochlea due
to antibiotic, neomycin, in animals, guinea pigs.
Progressive degeneration of organ of Corti beginning at base of cochlea due
to antibiotic, kanamycin, in animals, guinea pigs.
Progressive degeneration of organ of Corti beginning at base of cochlea due
to antibiotic, framycetin, in animals, guinea pigs.
No damage to hair cells of organ of Corti due to parenteral administration of
high doses of antibiotic, dihydrostreptomycin, for long periods in animals,
guinea pigs.
  (AD) Surface specimen technique used in study of organ of Corti.
  (AD) Damage to organ of Corti due to ototoxic drugs different from that
  due to noise. (ENG)

316
Possible vestibular problems and cochlear impairment due to more than recommended dose of 15 to 30 mg per kg daily of antibiotic, streptomycin, for long
period in humans.
Hearing loss due to parenteral, intramuscular, administration of total doses
of 5 to 6 g of antibiotic, kanamycin, in humans, adult, with kidney disorder.
Possible hearing loss due to parenteral, topical, or oral administration of
high doses of antibiotic, neomycin, for long period in humans.
Possible hearing loss due to high doses of antibiotic, framycetin, for long
period in humans.
Possible hearing loss due to antibiotic, vancomycin, in humans.
Possible hearing loss and vestibular problems due to antibiotic, viomycin, in
humans.
  (AD) High risk of ototoxicity with simultaneous administration of viomycin
  and streptomycin.
Possible vestibular problems due to antibiotic, gentamicin, in humans.
  (AD) Administration of gentamicin not recommended for newborn infants, for
  humans during pregnancy, and for humans treated with other ototoxic drugs.
Ataxia and hearing loss due to antibiotic, colistin, in humans.
  (AD) Literature review on ototoxic antibiotics.
  (AD) Results of studies on use of pantothenate salt of some antibiotics
  for decr in ototoxicity not clear.
  (AD) Suggested effect of ototoxic antibiotics on breakdown of glucose on
  which hair cells of inner ear depend for energy. (ENG)

384
Usually transient hearing loss and no structural damage to organ of Corti,
stria vascularis, and spiral ganglion due to oral or topical administration
of salicylates in humans.

Hearing loss due to antimalarial, quinine, in humans.
Usually permanent hearing loss due to antimalarial, chloroquine, in humans.
Transient and permanent hearing loss and possible damage to hair cells of
organ of Corti due to diuretic, ethacrynic acid, in humans.
Sensorineural hearing loss due to cardiovascular agent, hexadimethrine
bromide, in humans with kidney disorder.
Sensorineural hearing loss and damage to organ of Corti due to topical ad-
ministration of antineoplastic, nitrogen mustard, in humans.
Sensorineural hearing loss due to high doses of antibiotic, chloramphenicol,
in humans.
Primary vestibular problems due to antibiotic, streptomycin, in humans.
Hearing loss due to high doses usually of antibiotic, streptomycin, in humans.
   (AD) Early detection of hearing loss by audiometry prevents permanent
   damage.
High frequency hearing loss and severe damage to outer hair cells and slight
damage to inner hair cells of organ of Corti due to antibiotic, kanamycin, in
humans.
Sensorineural hearing loss due to parenteral, oral, and topical administration of antibiotic, neomycin, in humans with or without kidney disorders.
Degeneration of hair cells of organ of Corti and of nerve process due to
antibiotics, aminoglycoside, in animals.
   (AD) Literature review of physiological and structural cochleo-vestibulotoxic effects of ototoxic drugs.
   (AD) Discussion of suggested mechanism of ototoxicity and routes of drugs
   to inner ear.
Bilateral sensorineural hearing loss due to oral administration of antibiotic, neomycin, in 4 of 8 humans with liver disease.
Bilateral sensorineural hearing loss due to oral administration of range of
doses of antibiotic, neomycin (SM), in 2 of 5 humans with liver disease.
Bilateral sensorineural hearing loss due to diuretics (SM), in 2 of 5 humans
with liver disease.
Transient progression of previous hearing loss due to parenteral, intravenous, administration of diuretic, ethacrynic acid (SM), in 1 injection in 1
of 5 humans with liver disease.
   (CT) Normal cochlear function in 6 humans, control group, with liver
   disease and not treated with neomycin or diuretics.
   (CT) Normal cochlear function in 13 humans, control group, with liver
   disease and treated with diuretics but not with neomycin.
   (AD) Hearing loss confirmed by audiometry.
   (AD) Reported that hearing loss due to neomycin or diuretics in humans
   with liver disease not related to dosage.
   (AD) Clinical study of effects of treatment with neomycin and diuretics in
   humans with liver disease.
Bilateral sensorineural hearing loss and vertigo due to antibiotic, ampicil-
lin, in 1 human, adolescent, 17 years age, female, with tonsillitis.
   (AD) Cited case report.
Severe sensorineural hearing loss and vertigo due to topical administration
in ear drops of antibiotic, framycetin, in 1 human, adult, 42 years age,
male, with previous slight high frequency hearing loss.
   (AD) Cited case report.
Atrophy of hair cells of organ of Corti and hearing loss due to antibiotic,
dihydrostreptomycin, in humans with tuberculous meningitis.
   (AD) Cited study.
Loss of inner hair cells and damage to outer hair cells due to 18 g of anti-
biotic, neomycin, for 18 days in 1 human.
   (AD) Cited case report.   (ENG)

                           Gentamicin

                                                                    008
Severe vestibular problems and bilateral sensorineural hearing loss due to
unspecified method of administration of more than 1 mg per kg recommended
daily dosage of antibiotic, gentamicin (gentamicin sulfate), for unspecified
period in 5 humans with kidney disorder.
   (AD) No pretreatment tests conducted.
Severe vestibular problems and unilateral sensorineural hearing loss due to
unspecified method of administration of more than 1 mg per kg recommended

daily dosage of antibiotic, gentamicin (gentamicin sulfate), for unspecified
period in 3 humans with kidney disorder.
  (CT) Pretreatment vestibular function tests and audiometry showed normal
  vestibular function and normal hearing.
Transient vestibular problems only due to unspecified method of administration of more than 1 mg per kg recommended daily dosage of antibiotic, gentamicin (gentamicin sulfate), for unspecified period in 2 humans with normal
kidney function.
  (CT) Pretreatment vestibular function tests showed normal vestibular
  function. (ENG)

                                                                        016
Progressive bilateral sensorineural hearing loss and vertigo due to unspecified method of administration of total of 3 g of antibiotic, (SQ) streptomycin (SM), for unspecified period in 1 human, Caucasian, adult, 32 years age,
male, with kidney disorder and on intermittent hemodialysis.
Progressive bilateral sensorineural hearing loss and vertigo due to unspecified method of administration of antibiotic, (SQ) colistin (SM), for unspecified period in 1 human, Caucasian, adult, 32 years age, male, with kidney
disorder and on intermittent hemodialysis.
Permanent sensorineural hearing loss due to parenteral, intravenous, administration of 1.6 mg per kg 2 times daily, total of 500 mg of antibiotic, (SQ)
gentamicin, for unspecified period in 1 human, Caucasian, adult, 32 years
age, male, with kidney disorder and on intermittent hemodialysis.
No definite ototoxic effects reported due to unspecified method of administration of 1 g every 2 weeks, total of 12 g, of antibiotic, (SQ) vancomycin,
for about 6 months in 1 human, Caucasian, adult, 32 years age, male, with
kidney disorder and on intermittent hemodialysis.
  (AD) Hearing loss due to streptomycin and colistin potentiated by gentamicin. (ENG)

                                                                        020
Effect on function of inner ear due to parenteral, subcutaneous, administration of high doses, range of 30 to 75 mg per kg of antibiotic, gentamicin,
for about 8 to 20 days in 11 animals, cats.
  (AD) Preliminary study of dosage levels.
Damage to semicircular canal, membranous labyrinth, and outer hair cells and
inner hair cells of the cochlea due to parenteral, subcutaneous, administration of high doses, range of 30 to 75 mg per kg of antibiotic, gentamicin,
for about 8 to 20 days in 11 animals, cats, with kidney damage resulting from
gentamicin.
  (AD) Preliminary study of dosage levels.
Partial hearing loss due to parenteral, subcutaneous, administration of 20 mg
per kg of antibiotic, gentamicin, for 14 days in 1 out of 15 animals, cats.
Complete degeneration of outer hair cells of organ of Corti due to parenteral, subcutaneous, administration of 20 mg per kg of antibiotic, gentamicin, for 14 days in 1 out of 15 animals, cats.
Range of degree of damage, transient and permanent, to vestibular apparatus
due to parenteral, subcutaneous, administration of 20 mg per kg of antibiotic, gentamicin, for 14 days in 15 animals, cats.
Complete damage to vestibular apparatus due to parenteral, subcutaneous,
administration of 200 mg per kg of antibiotic, streptomycin, for 9 days in
animals, cats.
Higher incidence and earlier symptoms of ototoxic effects due to parenteral,
subcutaneous, administration of 20 mg per kg of antibiotic, gentamicin, for
14 days in 66.6 percent of 15 animals, cats, with kidney damage than in cats
with normal kidney function.
  (AD) Study of correlation of functional and histological effects of gentamicin.
  (AD) Comparative study of effect on vestibular apparatus of gentamicin and
  streptomycin. (ENG)

                                                                        022
Progressive degeneration of hair cells of organ of Corti and membranous
labyrinth due to topical administration to middle ear of 0.2 ml 1 time daily
of 50 percent saline solution of antibiotic, gentamicin, for 1 to 4 days in
animals, guinea pigs.
Severe damage to sensory epithelia of vestibular apparatus and degeneration

of hair cells of cochlea due to topical administration to middle ear of 0.2
ml of 0.3 percent solution of antibiotic, gentamicin, for 13 days in animals,
guinea pigs.
 (AD) Degeneration due to topical administration of low concentration of
 gentamicin for long period similar to degeneration due to intramuscular
 injections of high doses of gentamicin for long period in other studies.
 (AD) Study includes literature review of clinical and experimental ototoxicity. (ENG)

                                                                          036
Damage to vestibular apparatus due to parenteral or topical administration of
antibiotic, gentamicin (gentamicin sulfate), in humans. (ENG)

                                                                          042
Transient bilateral sensorineural hearing loss due to parenteral, intravenous, administration of 50 mg of diuretic, (SQ) ethacrynic acid, in 1
injection in 1 human, adult, 45 years age, female, with lymphosarcoma and
with normal kidney function.
 (AD) Hearing loss reported 15 minutes after treatment with ethacrynic
 acid.
Previous parenteral, intramuscular, administration of 60 mg every 6 hours of
antibiotic, (SQ) gentamicin (gentamicin sulfate), for unspecified period in 1
human, adult, 45 years age, female, with lymphosarcoma and with normal kidney
function.
Bilateral sensorineural hearing loss due to parenteral, intravenous, administration of 100 mg of diuretic, (SQ) ethacrynic acid, in 2 injections of 50 mg
each 6 hours apart in 1 human, adult, 64 years age, female, with acute leukemia and with normal kidney function.
 (AD) Histological study after death showed no damage to inner ear.
Previous unspecified method of administration of unspecified dose of antibiotic, (SQ) polymyxin B (polymyxin B sulfate), in 1 human, adult, 64 years age,
female, with acute leukemia and with normal kidney function.
Previous parenteral, intramuscular, administration of 0.5 g every 12 hours of
antibiotic, (SQ) kanamycin (kanamycin sulfate), for unspecified period in 1
human, adult, 64 years age, female, with acute leukemia and with normal
kidney function.
 (AD) Suggested that hearing loss due to combined action of ethacrynic acid
 and antibiotics. (ENG)

                                                                          079
Hearing loss and range of degree of damage to hair cells of organ of Corti
due to parenteral, intramuscular, administration of 50, 80, 110, and 140 mg
per kg daily of antibiotic, gentamicin (gentamicin sulfate), for 7 to 28 days
in 4 groups of 12 animals, guinea pigs, adult, 250 to 500 g weight.
 (AD) Comparative study showed that degree of damage determined by dosage.
 (AD) Hearing loss determined by Preyer reflex. (ENG)

                                                                          081
Dizziness, tinnitus, and high frequency hearing loss due to parenteral,
intramuscular, administration of 40 mg daily, total of 1470 mg intermittently, of antibiotic, gentamicin, in 74 days in 1 human, adolescent, 15 years
age, male, with kidney disorder.
 (AD) Hearing loss confirmed by audiogram.
 (AD) Loss of hair and visual perception defect due to gentamicin treatment. (ENG)

                                                                          093
Cochleo-vestibulotoxic effects due to parenteral administration of 50 to 100
mg per kg daily of antibiotic, gentamicin (gentamicin sulfate), for 20 days
in humans and animals, cats and guinea pigs.
 (AD) Literature review showed ototoxic effects of gentamicin in 2.8 percent of cases reported. (ENG)

                                                                          101
Primary damage to vestibular apparatus but also cochlear impairment due to
parenteral, intramuscular, administration of 40 mg every 8 hours and 80 mg
every 8 hours of antibiotic, gentamicin, in 7 of 16 (2 groups of 8) humans,
adult, male and female, with normal kidney function.

Primary damage to vestibular apparatus but also cochlear impairment due to
parenteral, intramuscular, administration of 40 mg daily of antibiotic,
gentamicin, in 7 of 8 humans, adult, male and female, with kidney disorder.
Primary damage to vestibular apparatus but also cochlear impairment due to
parenteral, intravenous, administration of 80 mg of antibiotic, gentamicin,
in 6 of 7 humans, adult, male and female, with chronic kidney disorder and
treated with hemodialysis.
   (AD) Comparative study of humans with normal kidney function and with
   kidney disorder.
   (AD) Higher incidence of ototoxic effects due to gentamicin in humans with
   kidney disorder.
   (AD) Cochleo-vestibulotoxic effects confirmed by audiometry and vestibular
   function tests.   (FR)

                                                                          117
Transient sensorineural hearing loss due to parenteral, intramuscular, administration of 80 mg daily, total of 320 mg, of antibiotic, gentamicin, for
1 to 4 days in 1 of 339 humans, adult, female, with chronic pyelonephritis.
Transient sensorineural hearing loss due to parenteral, intramuscular, administration of 80 mg daily, total of 1200 mg, of antibiotic, gentamicin, for
1 to 15 days in 1 of 339 humans, adult, female.
Transient vestibular problem due to 80 mg daily, total of 560 mg, of antibiotic, gentamicin, for 7 days in 1 of 339 humans, adult, female, with kidney
disorder.
   (AD) Need for vestibular function tests with use of gentamicin in humans
   with kidney disorder.
   (AD) Report of results of 33 investigations.   (ENG)

                                                                          119
Damage to hair cells of organ of Corti and change in action potential due to
parenteral, intramuscular, administration of 20 mg per kg and 150 mg per kg
of antibiotic, gentamicin (gentamicin sulfate), in 2 groups of 59 animals,
guinea pigs.
   (CT) Control group of 26 guinea pigs used.
   (AD) More severe damage due to 150 mg per kg of gentamicin than due to 20
   mg per kg.   (GER)

                                                                          140
Total bilateral sensorineural hearing loss due to 40 mg daily, total of 1.80
g, of antibiotic, gentamicin, for 45 days in 1 human, aged, 69 years age,
female, with kidney disorder.
   (AD) Hearing loss confirmed by audiogram.
Sensorineural hearing loss due to parenteral administration of 40 mg in 2
injections daily, total of 480 mg, of antibiotic, gentamicin (SM), in 1
human, aged, 65 years age, male.
Simultaneous administration of antibiotic, transcycline (SM), in 1 human,
aged, 65 years age, male.
Simultaneous administration of antibiotic, colistin (SM) (colistimethate), in
1 human, aged, 65 years age, male.
Sensorineural hearing loss due to 40 mg daily, total of 0.84 g, of antibiotic, gentamicin, for 21 days in 1 human, adult, 50 years age, male, with
normal kidney function.
   (AD) Hearing loss confirmed by audiogram.
   (AD) Discussion of 3 case reports of gentamicin ototoxicity.   (FR)

                                                                          141
Total bilateral sensorineural hearing loss, tinnitus, and vestibular problems
due to 120 mg daily, total of 1.2 g, of antibiotic, gentamicin (SM), for 10
days in 1 human, adult, 22 years age, female, 46 kg weight, with purulent
pleurisy after surgery.
Total bilateral sensorineural hearing loss, tinnitus, and vestibular problems
due to 1 g every 2 days, total of 9 g, of antibiotic, kanamycin (SM), for 18
days in 1 human, adult, 22 years age, female, 46 kg weight, with purulent
pleurisy after surgery.
Total bilateral sensorineural hearing loss and vestibular problems due to
high doses, 160 mg daily, of antibiotic, gentamicin, for long period, 47
days, in 1 human, adult, 35 years age, with pleurisy.
Total bilateral sensorineural hearing loss and vestibular problems due to 1 g

every 2 days of antibiotic, kanamycin, for 26 days in 1 human, adult, 35
years age, with pleurisy.
Total bilateral sensorineural hearing loss and vestibular problems due to 160
mg daily of antibiotic, gentamicin (SM), for 12 days in 1 human, adult, 35
years age, with pleurisy.
Total bilateral sensorineural hearing loss and vestibular problems due to 1 g
every 2 days of antibiotic, kanamycin (SM), for 12 days in 1 human, adult, 35
years age, with pleurisy.
   (AD) Hearing loss confirmed by audiogram.
   (AD) Discussion of 2 case reports of gentamicin ototoxicity.   (FR)

164

Ototoxic effects not determined due to parenteral, intramuscular and intrathecal, administration of 1.5 mg per kg every 8 to 12 hours, to produce peak
serum levels of 2.5 to 5.0 mcg per ml, of antibiotic, (SQ) gentamicin, for 9
to 13 days in 5 humans, newborn infant, with infections.
Ototoxic effects not determined due to parenteral, intramuscular, administration of 7.5 mg per kg every 12 hours of antibiotic, (SQ) kanamycin, for 7 to
17 days in 3 of 5 humans, newborn infant, with infections.
   (AD) No follow up studies of gentamicin over long period to determine
   ototoxic effects.
   (AD) Need for audiometry and vestibular function tests after several
   months to determine ototoxic effects.
   (AD) Study of clinical pharmacology of gentamicin.   (ENG)

185

Ataxia, damage to hair cells of macula, and damage to hair cells of organ of
Corti due to parenteral, subcutaneous, administration of 10 to 80 mg per kg
daily of antibiotic, gentamicin (gentamicin sulfate), for 19 to 120 days in
animals, cats.
Ataxia due to 100 and 200 mg per kg daily of antibiotic, streptomycin (streptomycin sulfate), for 8 to 40 days in animals, cats.
Loss of Preyer reflex, decr in cochlear potential and eighth cranial nerve
action potential, and loss of outer hair cells of organ of Corti due to 80 to
200 mg per kg daily of antibiotic, gentamicin (gentamicin sulfate), in animals, guinea pigs.
Damage to cochlea due to 100 and 200 mg per kg of antibiotic, kanamycin
(kanamycin sulfate), in animals, guinea pigs.
   (AD) Comparative study of ototoxicity of gentamicin and other aminoglycoside antibiotics.
   (AD) Study suggested low risk of ototoxicity when gentamicin used in
   recommended clinical dose of 1 to 3 mg per kg.   (ENG)

195

Damage to vestibular nerve and cochlear nerve due to antibiotic, gentamicin,
in humans.
   (AD) Comment on use in therapy and cochleo-vestibulotoxic effects of
   gentamicin.   (ENG)

218

Transient vertigo due to parenteral, intramuscular, administration of 2 x 40
mg of antibiotic, gentamicin, for 15 days in 1 human, adult, 39 years age, 72
kg weight, with diabetes mellitus and chronic pyelonephritis.   (GER)

225

Vestibular problems, in particular dizziness, due to antibiotic, gentamicin,
in 19 of 1327 humans, range of ages, with normal kidney function and with
kidney disorder.
Vestibular problems and high frequency hearing loss due to antibiotic, gentamicin, in 8 of 1327 humans, range of ages, with normal kidney function and
with kidney disorder.
High frequency hearing loss due to antibiotic, gentamicin, in 4 of 1327
humans, range of ages, with normal kidney function and with kidney disorder.
   (AD) Kidney disorders in 33.3 percent of patients, previous or simultaneous treatment with other ototoxic drugs in 50 percent, and 50 years or
   more age in about 50 percent.
   (AD) Comparison of incidence of ototoxicity due to gentamicin and other
   aminoglycoside antibiotics.   (ENG)

256

Loss of outer hair cells of organ of Corti in basal coil of cochlea due to
parenteral, intramuscular, administration of 110 mg per kg daily of antibiotic, gentamicin, for 28 days in animals, guinea pigs.
Less damage to hair cells of organ of Corti in second and third coils of
cochlea due to parenteral, intramuscular, administration of 110 mg per kg
daily of antibiotic, gentamicin, for 19 days in animals, guinea pigs.
   (AD) Suggested relationship between duration of administration of gentamicin and degree of damage to inner ear.   (ENG)

277

Sensorineural hearing loss due to parenteral administration of total doses of
160 mg to more than 4000 mg of antibiotic, gentamicin, in 52 humans.
Vestibular problems due to parenteral administration of total doses of 160 mg
to more than 4000 mg of antibiotic, gentamicin, in 34 humans.
   (CT) Audiometry and vestibular function tests before and after treatment
   with gentamicin.   (GER)

298

Possible vestibular problems and high frequency hearing loss due to more than
225 mg daily of antibiotic, gentamicin, in humans.
   (AD) Report on chemistry, pharmacology, clinical use, and cochleo-vestibulotoxic effects of gentamicin.
   (AD) More risk of ototoxicity with gentamicin, dose for dose, than with
   other aminoglycoside antibiotics.
Range of degrees of vestibular problems 1 to 14 days after cessation of
treatment due to total doses of 0.74 to 3.15 g of antibiotic, gentamicin, in
5 of 57 humans with kidney disorder.
   (AD) Report of cases in previous study.   (ENG)

300

Possible vestibular problems due to more than recommended 240 mg daily of
antibiotic, gentamicin, in humans, in particular with kidney disorder or 40
years or over age.
   (AD) More risk of ototoxicity with gentamicin than with other aminoglycoside antibiotics.
   (AD) Need for study of relationship between vestibular problems and dosage
   and duration of therapy.   (ENG)

301

Severe vertigo 2 days after cessation of treatment due to topical (SM) administration of 0.1 percent solution of antibiotic, gentamicin, for 4 weeks
in 1 human, aged, 65 years age, male, with mild kidney disorder.
Severe vertigo 2 days after cessation of treatment due to parenteral (SM)
administration of 40 mg every 6 hours of antibiotic, gentamicin (gentamicin
sulfate), for 4 weeks in 1 human, aged, 65 years age, male, with mild kidney
disorder.
   (CT) Study of gentamicin serum levels in normal subjects and humans
   treated for pseudomonas infections with recommended dose of gentamicin.
   (AD) Case report of vestibulotoxic effect of gentamicin.   (ENG)

302

Transient dizziness due to parenteral, intramuscular, administration of 120
mg 2 or 3 times daily of antibiotic, gentamicin, for several weeks in 4 of 23
humans, adult and aged, range of 50 to over 70 years age, male, with bronchial infections and with normal kidney function.
   (AD) Vestibulotoxic effect confirmed by caloric tests.   (ENG)

306

Vestibular problems due to unspecified dose of antibiotic, gentamicin, for 10
days in 1 human.
Significant vestibular problems and hearing loss due to antibiotic, gentamicin, in 14 of 27 humans, some with kidney disorders, with previous treatment
with ototoxic drugs, or over 40 years age.
   (AD) Vestibular problems confirmed by vestibular function tests.
   (AD) Report on clinical pharmacology, clinical use, and cochleo-vestibulotoxic effects of gentamicin.
   (AD) Reported 2.5 percent incidence in USA of vestibular problems due to

gentamicin.
(AD) Suggested that otqtoxicity of gentamicin is dose related.   (ENG)

316

Possible vestibular problems and cochlear impairment due to more than recommended dose of 15 to 30 mg per kg daily of antibiotic, streptomycin, for long
period in humans.
Hearing loss due to parenteral, intramuscular, administration of total doses
of 5 to 6 g of antibiotic, kanamycin, in humans, adult, with kidney disorder.
Possible hearing loss due to parenteral, topical, or oral administration of
high doses of antibiotic, neomycin, for long period in humans.
Possible hearing loss due to high doses of antibiotic, framycetin, for long
period in humans.
Possible hearing loss due to antibiotic, vancomycin, in humans.
Possible hearing loss and vestibular problems due to antibiotic, viomycin, in
humans.
(AD) High risk of ototoxicity with simultaneous administration of viomycin
    and streptomycin.
Possible vestibular problems due to antibiotic, gentamicin, in humans.
(AD) Administration of gentamicin not recommended for newborn infants, for
    humans during pregnancy, and for humans treated with other ototoxic drugs.
Ataxia and hearing loss due to antibiotic, colistin, in humans.
(AD) Literature review on ototoxic antibiotics.
(AD) Results of studies on use of pantothenate salt of some antibiotics
    for decr in ototoxicity not clear.
(AD) Suggested effect of ototoxic antibiotics on breakdown of glucose on
    which hair cells of inner ear depend for energy.   (ENG)

324

Ataxia, vestibular problems with improvement in some, and damage to hair
cells of vestibular apparatus due to parenteral, subcutaneous, administration
of 20 mg per kg of antibiotic, gentamicin (gentamicin sulfate), for 19 days
maximum for acute intoxication and 14 days for chronic intoxication in 15
animals, cats.
Hearing loss and damage to hair cells of cochlea due to parenteral, subcutaneous, administration of 20 mg per kg of antibiotic, gentamicin (gentamicin
sulfate), for 19 days maximum for acute intoxication and 14 days for chronic
intoxication in 1 of 15 animals, cats.
(AD) Preliminary study to determine minimum toxic level of gentamicin by
    parenteral route made previously.
(AD) Cochleo-vestibulotoxic effects determined by audiometry and vestibu-
    lar function tests.
Permanent severe vestibular problems and damage to hair cells of vestibular
apparatus due to parenteral, subcutaneous, administration of 200 mg per kg of
antibiotic, streptomycin (streptomycin sulfate), in 3 animals, cats.
Hearing loss and damage to hair cells of cochlea due to parenteral, subcutaneous, administration of 200 mg per kg of antibiotic, streptomycin (streptomycin sulfate), in 2 of 3 animals, cats.
Ataxia, vestibular problems, and damage to hair cells of vestibular apparatus
due to topical administration to bulla in solution of 6 percent concentration
in water of antibiotic, gentamicin (gentamicin sulfate), for 19 days in 1
animal, cat.
Ataxia, vestibular problems, and more severe damage to hair cells of vestibular apparatus due to topical administration to bulla in solution of 6 percent
concentration in Monex of antibiotic, gentamicin (gentamicin sulfate), for 5
days in 3 animals, cats.
(CT) Same method using water or Monex without gentamicin in 11 cats,
    control group, showed no ototoxic effects.
(AD) Preliminary study to determine concentration of gentamicin for topi-
    cal route made previously.
Vestibular problems due to topical administration to bulla in solution of 6
percent concentration in water of antibiotic, neomycin, for 31 days in 2
animals, cats.
(AD) Comparative study of effects of gentamicin and other aminoglycoside
    antibiotics.
(AD) Ototoxicity of gentamicin dose related.   (ENG)

335

Vestibular problems due to antibiotic, streptomycin, in humans.
Severe cochlear impairment due to antibiotic, dihydrostreptomycin, in humans.
Cochlear impairment due to parenteral, oral, and topical administration of
antibiotic, neomycin, in humans.
Tinnitus and hearing loss due to antibiotic, kanamycin, in humans.
Vestibular problems and hearing loss due to antibiotic, gentamicin, in hu-
mans.
   (AD) Discussion of clinical use and possible cochleo-vestibulotoxic ef-
   fects of aminoglycoside antibiotics.   (SP)

369

Rapid loss of Preyer reflex and more gradual changes in vestibular function
due to parenteral, intramuscular, administration of 100 mg per kg daily in 2
doses of antibiotic, gentamicin, for 6 to 49 days in 8 animals, guinea pigs.
Loss of Preyer reflex and changes in vestibular function due to parenteral,
intramuscular, administration of 75 mg per kg daily in 2 doses of antibiotic,
gentamicin, for 15 to 52 days in 8 animals, guinea pigs.
Less effect on Preyer reflex and vestibular function due to parenteral,
intramuscular, administration of 50 mg per kg daily in 2 doses of antibiotic,
gentamicin, for 35 to 53 days in 8 animals, guinea pigs.
   (CT) Use of 6 guinea pigs, control group.
   (CT) Determination of Preyer reflex and vestibular function, pretreatment
   and during treatment with audiometry and vestibular function tests.
   (AD) Relationship but not precise correlation between cochleo-vestibuloto-
   xic effects of gentamicin and daily dosage and duration of treatment.
   (IT)

370

Severe damage to hair cells of organ of Corti, supporting cells, stria vascularis, Reissner's membrane, spiral ganglion, crista ampullaris, and semicircular canal due to parenteral, intramuscular, administration of 100 mg per kg
daily of antibiotic, gentamicin, for 28, 35, or 49 days in 4 animals, guinea
pigs.
Damage to hair cells of organ of Corti in basal coil of cochlea, supporting
cells, and spiral ganglion, and severe damage to crista ampullaris and semicircular canal due to parenteral, intramuscular, administration of 75 mg per
kg daily of antibiotic, gentamicin, for 35, 42, or 49 days in 3 animals,
guinea pigs.
Moderate damage to hair cells of organ of Corti in basal coil of cochlea,
supporting cells, spiral ganglion, crista ampullaris, and semicircular canal
due to parenteral, intramuscular, administration of 50 mg per kg daily of
antibiotic, gentamicin, for 38 or 46 days in 2 animals, guinea pigs.
   (CT) Normal function of cochlea and vestibular apparatus in 3 guinea pigs,
   control group, not treated with gentamicin.
   (AD) Relationship but not precise correlation between cochleo-vestibulotoxic effects of gentamicin and dosage and duration of treatment.
   (AD) Individual differences in response to same doses of gentamicin for
   same period.
   (AD) Not precise correlation between results of histological study and
   results of previous functional study.   (IT)

409

Primary damage to hair cells of organ of Corti, hearing loss, and possible
vestibular problems due to antibiotic, viomycin, in humans.
Damage to hair cells of organ of Corti and hearing loss due to antibiotic,
neomycin, in humans.
Damage to hair cells of organ of Corti and hearing loss due to antibiotic,
kanamycin, in humans.
Primary damage to vestibular apparatus, vestibular problems, and possible
hearing loss due to antibiotic, streptomycin, in humans.
Primary damage to vestibular apparatus, vestibular problems, and possible
hearing loss due to antibiotic, gentamicin, in humans.
   (AD) Need for audiometry and vestibular function tests, pretreatment and
   during treatment, with clinical use of aminoglycoside antibiotics.
   (AD) Incr in blood levels and ototoxicity of antibiotics in humans with
   kidney disorders.   (ENG)

420

Acute hearing loss due to 10 mg on first day and then 60 mg daily for 3 days,
total of 220 mg, of antibiotic, (SQ) gentamicin, in total of 4 days in 1
human, adolescent, 16 years age, with kidney disorder.
  (AD) Hearing loss confirmed by audiogram.
Previous administration of antibiotic, (SQ) colistin, in 1 human, adolescent,
16 years age, with kidney disorder.
Vestibular problems due to 40 mg daily, total of 400 mg, of antibiotic,
gentamicin, in total of 10 days in 1 human, aged, 68 years age, with kidney
disorder.   (GER)

426

Damage to vestibular function due to sufficient doses to produce blood level
of over 10 mcg per ml of antibiotic, gentamicin, in humans with or without
kidney disorders.
  (AD) High blood levels due to kidney disorders or due to high doses or
  long period of treatment in humans with normal kidney function.
  (AD) Comment on study that reported vestibulotoxic effects of gentamicin
  with blood levels lower than 10 mcg per ml.   (ENG)

427

Damage to vestibular function due to high doses of antibiotic, gentamicin, in
humans with normal kidney function.
Damage to vestibular function due to antibiotic, gentamicin, in humans with
kidney disorder.
  (AD) Risk of gentamicin ototoxicity with blood levels of over 10 mcg per
  ml.
  (AD) Suggested that gentamicin ototoxicity is dose related.
  (AD) Comment on study that reported vestibulotoxic effects of gentamicin
  with blood levels lower than 10 mcg per ml.   (ENG)

428

Possible damage to eighth cranial nerve due to high blood level of over 10
mcg per ml of antibiotic, gentamicin, in humans.
  (AD) Need for serum assays and other tests in clinical use of gentamicin.
  (AD) Comment on study that reported vestibulotoxic effects of gentamicin
  with blood levels lower than 10 mcg per ml.   (ENG)

431

No vestibular problems or hearing loss due to parenteral, intravenous, administration for 30 to 45 minutes of high doses, 4 to 5 mg per kg daily,
diluted in 30 to 50 cc of sterile water, to produce blood levels of 6.25 mcg
per ml or less, of antibiotic, gentamicin (gentamicin sulfate), for total of
20 days in 1 human, adolescent, 13 years age, with cystic fibrosis.
No vestibular problems or hearing loss due to parenteral, intravenous, administration for 30 to 45 minutes of high doses, 4 to 5 mg per kg daily,
diluted in 30 to 50 cc of sterile water, to produce blood levels of 6.25 mcg
per ml or less of antibiotic, gentamicin (SM) (gentamicin sulfate), for range
of 2 to 13 days in 4 humans, adolescent and child, 2 to 13 years age, with
cystic fibrosis.
Simultaneous parenteral, intravenous, administration of high doses, 100 to
600 mg per kg every 4 hours, of antibiotic, carbenicillin (SM) (disodium
carbenicillin), for range of 2 to 19 days in 4 humans, adolescent and child,
2 to 13 years age, with cystic fibrosis.
  (CT) Audiograms and vestibular function tests before and after treatment
  with gentamicin.
  (AD) Comment on high doses of gentamicin without toxicity.   (ENG)

451

No eighth cranial nerve toxicity due to 80 mg every 6 or 8 hours, and lower
dosage in humans with kidney disorder, to produce serum levels of 5 to 8 mcg
per ml of antibiotic, gentamicin, in 104 humans, adult, aged, and child, 2 to
80 years age, with various infections.
  (AD) Suggested that prevention of ototoxicity due to daily assays of serum
  levels.   (ENG)

454

Damage to vestibular apparatus due to high doses of antibiotic, gentamicin,
in animals, guinea pigs.

Damage to vestibular apparatus due to low doses of antibiotic, gentamicin, in humans with disorders. (GER)

                                                                              471
Damage to vestibular apparatus due to antibiotic, gentamicin, in humans with genitourinary system infections.
   (AD) Comment on risk of vestibulotoxic effects in clinical use of gentami-
   cin. (GER)

                                                                              474
Transient dizziness due to parenteral, intramuscular, administration of 80 mg, to produce serum level of 12 mcg per ml, of antibiotic, gentamicin, in 1 injection in 1 human, adult, 62 years age, female, 46.5 kg weight. (ENG)

                                                                              475
Possible damage to eighth cranial nerve with vestibular problems due to parenteral administration of low doses to produce recommended serum levels of antibiotic, gentamicin, in humans with genitourinary system infections. (ENG)

                                                                              483
Possible damage to vestibular nerve and cochlear nerve due to antibiotic, streptomycin, in humans with or without kidney disorder.
Possible damage to vestibular nerve and cochlear nerve due to antibiotic, gentamicin, in humans with or without kidney disorder.
Possible damage to vestibular nerve and cochlear nerve due to antibiotic, kanamycin, in humans with or without kidney disorder.
Possible damage to vestibular nerve and cochlear nerve due to antibiotic, neomycin, in humans with or without kidney disorder.
   (AD) Incidence of effects on vestibular function highest in streptomycin, followed by gentamicin, kanamycin, and neomycin.
   (AD) Incidence of effects on cochlear function highest in neomycin, fol-
   lowed by kanamycin, gentamicin, and streptomycin.
   (AD) Need for careful consideration in clinical use of aminoglycoside antibiotics.
Possible cochlear impairment and vestibular problems due to antibiotic, paromomycin, in humans.
Possible dizziness and ataxia due to antibiotic, polymyxin B, in humans.
Possible but rare dizziness and vertigo due to antibiotic, nalidixic acid, in humans. (ENG)

                                                                              528
No reported ototoxic effects due to parenteral, intravenous or intramuscular, administration of 40 mg every 8 hours in 1 injection, to produce blood level of 20 mcg per ml in 1 case, of antibiotic, (SQ) gentamicin (SM), for 3 to 10 days in 25 humans with pseudomonas infection.
Parenteral, intravenous, administration of 1 dose of 2 g and then 1 g every 2 hours for 12 hours, followed by 1 g every 3 hours for 3 to 7 days of antibio-
tic, (SQ) carbenicillin (SM), in 25 humans with pseudomonas infection.
   (AD) Study of treatment of pseudomonas infection with gentamicin and carbenicillin.
   (AD) Decr in blood level of gentamicin when used simultaneously with carbenicillin. (ENG)

                                                                              539
Transient unilateral or bilateral ototoxic effects, vestibular problems in 66.6 percent of cases, due to antibiotic, gentamicin, in 14 humans.
   (AD) Literature review showed small number of cases of gentamicin ototoxi-
   city reported in Germany.
   (AD) Primary factor in gentamicin ototoxicity is kidney disorder.
   (AD) Other factors in gentamicin ototoxicity include dosage and simul-
   taneous administration of other ototoxic drugs.
Hearing loss due to diuretic, ethacrynic acid, in humans with kidney disor-
der. (GER)

                                                                              546
Degeneration and fusion of hair cells of crista ampullaris, first in central part and later in peripheral parts, due to topical administration to bulla of

0.2 ml in 1 injection daily of 0.3 percent solution of antibiotic, gentamicin (gentamicin sulfate), for total of 7 injections in animals, guinea pigs.
  (AD) Electron microscopic study of effects of gentamicin on vestibular apparatus.
  (AD) Study showed more damage to type 1 hair cells than to type 2 hair cells. (ENG)

548
Transient vestibular problems due to parenteral administration of antibiotic, gentamicin, in humans. (GER)

573
Bilateral vestibular problems, ataxia, and damage to hair cells of organ of Corti in basal coil of cochlea and of cristae and maculae due to parenteral, intramuscular, administration of 80 or 50 mg per kg on 5 days a week of antibiotic, gentamicin, in 5 animals, squirrel monkeys, Saimiri sciureus, about 2 years age, male and female.
Loss of equilibrium, ataxia, damage to hair cells of cristae and maculae, and some degeneration of nerve process near hair cells due to parenteral, subcutaneous, administration of 60, 30, or 20 mg per kg on 7 days a week of antibiotic, gentamicin, in 7 animals, squirrel monkeys, Saimiri sciureus, about 2 years age, male and female.
  (AD) Type 1 hair cells of cristae and maculae more vulnerable to gentamicin than type 2 hair cells.
  (CT) Squirrel monkey rail method and test of nystagmus, pretreatment and posttreatment.
  (AD) Earlier onset of equilibrium disorders with high daily doses than with low daily doses.
  (AD) Total doses before onset of ataxia slightly more in group with high daily doses.
  (AD) Less ototoxic effects and slower onset with administration of gentamicin 5 days a week than 7 days a week.
  (AD) Lower doses in group with injections 7 days a week resulted in more severe and earlier onset of loss of equilibrium.
  (AD) Damage to vestibular apparatus slightly more severe in animals with higher daily doses.
  (AD) Correlation between equilibrium test and electron microscopic findings. (ENG)

574
Ataxia due to parenteral, subcutaneous, administration of 20, 40, or 60 mg per kg daily, dissolved in distilled water in volume of 0.5 ml per kg, of antibiotic, gentamicin (gentamicin sulfate), for 10 to 70 days in animals, cats, male, 2.5 to 5.0 kg weight.
  (AD) Tests to determine ataxia conducted.
  (AD) Relationship between onset of ataxia and dosage.
Permanent ataxia due to parenteral, subcutaneous, administration of 40 mg per kg daily of antibiotic, gentamicin (gentamicin sulfate), for 16, 18, or 19 days, followed by a rest for 29 to 32 days, and then 19 to 20 days more in 3 animals, cats.
  (AD) Ataxia persisted during period without gentamicin treatment.
Ataxia due to parenteral, subcutaneous, administration of 20, 40, or 60 mg per kg daily, total doses of 600 to about 900 mg per kg, of antibiotic, gentamicin (gentamicin sulfate), in animals, cats.
  (AD) Occurrence of ataxia after smaller average total dose at lower dosage levels than at higher levels.
  (AD) Inverse relationship between onset of ataxia and total dosage suggests that duration of treatment possibly significant factor at dosage levels studied.
Ataxia after 25 days due to parenteral, subcutaneous, administration of 40 mg per kg daily of antibiotic, gentamicin (gentamicin sulfate), for 5 days in 5 animals, cats.
Ataxia after 18 days due to parenteral, subcutaneous, administration of 40 mg per kg daily of antibiotic, gentamicin (gentamicin sulfate), for 7 days in 5 animals, cats.
  (AD) Results of experiment suggest significance of total dosage and duration of treatment.
Ataxia after 17 days due to parenteral, subcutaneous, administration of 40 mg

per kg 1 time daily, average total of 680 mg per kg, of antibiotic, gentamicin (gentamicin sulfate), in 6 animals, cats.
Ataxia after 19.4 days due to parenteral, subcutaneous, administration of 20
mg per kg twice daily, average total of 776 mg per kg of antibiotic, gentamicin (gentamicin sulfate), in 5 animals, cats.
  (AD) Average total dose to produce ataxia higher with 2 doses daily than
  with single daily dose.
Ataxia after 16 days due to parenteral, (SQ) subcutaneous, administration of
40 mg per kg daily, to produce blood levels of 100 mcg per ml 30 minutes
after treatment, of antibiotic, gentamicin (gentamicin sulfate), in 1 dose in
2 animals, cats.
  (AD) Rapid decr in blood levels 24 hours after treatment.
Ataxia after 16 days due to parenteral, (SQ) intraarterial, administration of
40 mg per kg daily of antibiotic, gentamicin (gentamicin sulfate), in 2
animals, cats.
  (AD) Blood levels monitored daily.
  (AD) Peak blood levels with intraarterial administration 2 to 6 times as
  high as with subcutaneous route and decr rapidly to less than 1 mcg per ml
  24 hours after treatment.
  (AD) Decr in kidney function at time of occurrence of ataxia.
  (AD) Report on various experiments in study of factors in effect of gentamicin on vestibular function in cats.
  (AD) Suggested that total dosage and duration of treatment possibly more
  significant factors than peak blood levels with reference to time of onset
  of ataxia at dosage levels studied.   (ENG)

575

Transient and permanent vestibular problems only in 29 cases, hearing loss
only in 7 cases, and vestibular problems and hearing loss in 8 cases, beginning less than 10 to 14 days after treatment, due to antibiotic, gentamicin,
in 44 humans, with kidney disorder in 64 percent of cases.
  (AD) Survey of clinical experience in USA with gentamicin ototoxicity.
  (AD) Statistical analysis of administration of gentamicin with and without
  ototoxic effects to determine significant factors in ototoxicity.
  (AD) Reported 2 percent incidence of ototoxicity due to gentamicin.
  (AD) Kidney disorders in patients and size of daily dose, mg per kg,
  reported most significant factors in gentamicin ototoxicity.
  (AD) Relationship between daily dose and ototoxicity suggests that blood
  level of gentamicin possibly significant factor in ototoxicity.
  (AD) Previous therapy with gentamicin or other ototoxic drugs, total dose,
  mg and mg per kg, and duration of therapy reported significant factors in
  gentamicin ototoxicity in patients with kidney disorder.
  (AD) Occurrence of gentamicin ototoxicity in patients with kidney disorders at younger age than in patients with normal kidney function.
  (AD) Suggested highest risk of gentamicin ototoxicity in younger patients
  with kidney disorder.   (ENG)

576

Progressive ataxia beginning after 4 days of treatment due to topical administration to bulla of 0.4 ml daily of aqueous solution of 10 percent concentration, to produce blood level of 7 mcg per ml, of antibiotic, gentamicin,
for 19 days maximum in 1 of 2 animals, cats.
Minimal transient ataxia beginning after 10 to 18 days of treatment and
moderate damage to cristae and maculae but normal cochlea due to topical
administration to bulla of 0.4 ml daily of aqueous solution of 3 percent
concentration, to produce blood levels of less than 0.5 mcg per ml, of antibiotic, gentamicin, for 19 days maximum in 1 of 3 animals, cats.
  (AD) Preliminary studies of topical gentamicin in cats.
  (AD) Not possible to obtain audiograms due to administration of gentamicin
  in middle ear so evaluation of cochlear function depended on histological
  study of cochlea.
  (AD) Evaluation of vestibular function with vestibular function tests.
Ataxia beginning after 12 days of treatment, decr in duration of rotatory
nystagmus, change in ENG, and loss of hair cells of cristae and of organ of
Corti in basal coil of cochlea due to topical administration to bulla of 0.4
ml daily of aqueous solution of 6 percent concentration of antibiotic, gentamicin, for 19 days maximum in 4 animals, cats.
No clinical vestibular problems and no significant change in duration of

rotatory nystagmus and in ENG but degeneration of cochlea and spiral ganglion
and changes in saccule due to topical administration to bulla of 0.4 ml daily
of aqueous solution of 3 percent concentration of antibiotic, gentamicin, for
30 days maximum in 5 animals, cats.
  (AD) Direct relationship between onset of ataxia and concentration of
    gentamicin solution.
  (AD) Correlation between duration of rotatory nystagmus and ataxia.
  (AD) Topical gentamicin most toxic to cochlea and saccule.
  (AD) Need to monitor clinical use of gentamicin with audiology.
No clinical vestibular problems, transient decr in duration of rotatory
nystagmus, transient bilateral decr in ENG, and loss of hair cells of organ
of Corti in basal coil of cochlea but normal vestibular apparatus due to
topical administration to bulla of 0.4 ml daily of solution of 6 percent
concentration of antibiotic, neomycin, for 30 days maximum in 2 animals,
cats.
  (AD) Comparative study of effects of topical gentamicin and neomycin.
  (CT) Same methods using 0.4 ml distilled water for 30 days in 7 cats,
    control group, showed no clinical vestibular problems and no histological
    changes. (ENG)

                                                                      577

No ototoxic effects due to parenteral, intramuscular, administration of 3 to
5 mg per kg daily in 3 or 4 divided doses, average total dose of 3.0 g, of
antibiotic, gentamicin, for 12.7 days average in 41 humans, adolescent,
adult, and aged, 14 to 87 years age, male and female, with genitourinary
system infections primarily and with kidney disorder in 13 cases.
No ototoxic effects due to parenteral, intramuscular, administration of 15 mg
per kg daily in 2 or 3 divided doses, average total dose of 6.6 g, of antibiotic, kanamycin (SM), for 8 days average in 34 humans, adult and aged, 40
to 81 years age, male and female, with genitourinary system infection and
with kidney disorder in 8 cases.
No ototoxic effects due to parenteral, intramuscular or intravenous administration of 1.5 to 2.5 mg per kg daily in 2 to 4 divided doses, average total
dose of 1.0 g, of antibiotic, polymyxin B (SM), for 6 days average in 34
humans, adult and aged, 40 to 81 years age, male and female, with genitourinary system infection and with kidney disorder in 8 cases.
  (AD) Comparative study of effects of 3 antibiotics on infections due to
    gram-negative bacilli. (ENG)

                                                                      578

No clinical evidence of ototoxic effects due to high doses, 3 to 6 mg per kg
daily, of antibiotic, gentamicin, in 53 humans, child, adolescent, adult, and
aged, 10 to 84 years age, male and female, with bacteremia due to gram-negative bacilli and with kidney disorder in 14 cases.
  (AD) Monitored for clinical symptoms of ototoxic effects.
  (AD) No audiology or vestibular function tests to determine ototoxic
    effects. (ENG)

                                                                      579

No clinical evidence of ototoxic effects due to parenteral, intravenous,
administration of 1.5 to 6 mg per kg daily, average of 3 mg per kg daily, of
antibiotic, gentamicin, for as long as 36 days in 25 humans, child and adolescent, 2.5 to 15 years age, with acute leukemia and infections.
  (AD) No audiology or vestibular function tests used to determine ototoxic
    effects. (ENG)

                                                                      580

No observed ototoxic effects in follow up study of 10 months due to parenteral, intramuscular, administration of 4 or 5 mg per kg daily in 2 equal
doses at 12 hour intervals, to produce blood levels of 4.9 mcg per ml or
less, of antibiotic, gentamicin, for 1 to 31 days in 16 humans, newborn
infant, 0 to 22 days age, less than 2500 g weight in 8 patients, with infections.
No observed ototoxic effects due to parenteral, intravenous and intraventricular, administration of 1.6 mg per kg of antibiotic, gentamicin, in 1 human,
newborn infant, low birth weight, with infection.
  (AD) Responses of newborn infants to sound monitored. (ENG)

581
No hearing loss detected due to parenteral, intrathecal (SM), administration
of 1 mg daily of antibiotic, gentamicin, in 13 humans, infant.
No hearing loss detected due to parenteral, intramuscular (SM), administration of 2 mg per kg daily of antibiotic, gentamicin, in 13 humans, infant.
  (AD) Evaluation of cochlear function difficult in infants but no hearing
  loss detected after gentamicin therapy. (ENG)

582
No observed ototoxic effects due to 2 mg per kg daily of antibiotic, gentamicin, for 5 to 10 days in over 100 humans, child, with genitourinary system
infections.
  (AD) Patients observed for evidence of ototoxicity. (ENG)

583
No observed ototoxic effects but possible damage to inner ear due to parenteral, intramuscular, administration of 3.0 or 5.0 mg per kg daily, to produce serum levels as high as 7.8 mcg per ml, of antibiotic, gentamicin, for 6
to 7 days in 45 humans, newborn infant, 1.4 to 21 days average age, low birth
weight, with infections.
  (AD) Measurement of blood levels at 0.5, 1, 4, 8, and 12 hours after first
  injection and on third day.
  (AD) Follow up studies with audiology planned to determine if ototoxic
  effects resulted from gentamicin therapy. (ENG)

584
No observed ototoxic effects due to parenteral, intramuscular, administration
of 2.5 mg per kg every 12 hours or 1.7 mg per kg every 8 hours, daily total
of 5 mg per kg, to produce blood levels of 6 mcg per ml or less, of antibiotic, gentamicin, for 10 days in 60 humans, infant, male and female, with
genitourinary system infections.
  (AD) Determination of blood levels at 1, 2, 4, and 8 hours after first
  injection and at 12 hours in group with administration of gentamicin every
  12 hours.
  (AD) Blood levels higher and for longer duration in group with administration every 12 hours.
  (AD) Follow up studies with audiograms planned to determine if ototoxic
  effects resulted from gentamicin therapy. (ENG)

585
High frequency hearing loss due to parenteral, intramuscular, administration
of 3.0 mg per kg daily or less of antibiotic, (SQ) gentamicin (gentamicin
sulfate), for several days in 1 of 215 humans, child, with genitourinary
system infection.
High frequency hearing loss due to previous administration of (SQ) other
antibiotics in 1 of 215 humans, child, with genitourinary system infection.
  (AD) Clinical evaluation of effect of gentamicin on eighth cranial nerve
  in patients and audiometry and vestibular function tests when indicated.
  (ENG)

586
Mild sensorineural hearing loss due to parenteral administration of 4 mg per
kg every 24 hours in 4 divided doses, total doses of 1000 and 7788 mg, of
antibiotic, gentamicin (gentamicin sulfate), for 25 to 138 days in 1 of 10
humans with infection secondary to burns.
  (AD) Audiology in 10 patients with therapy of long duration confirmed
  hearing loss in 1 patient.
No reported ototoxic effects due to parenteral (SM) administration of 4 mg
per kg every 24 hours in 4 divided doses of antibiotic, gentamicin (gentamicin sulfate), for several days to over 30 days in other 85 humans, newborn
infant, infant, child, and adolescent, 0 to 16 years age, with infection
secondary to burns.
Simultaneous topical, direct site (SM), administration in cream of 0.1 percent of antibiotic, gentamicin (gentamicin sulfate), in some of 95 humans,
newborn infant, infant, child, and adolescent, 0 to 16 years age, with infection secondary to burns. (ENG)

No ototoxic effects due to parenteral (SM) administration of 3 mg per kg
every 24 hours of antibiotic, gentamicin (SM), for 5 to 132 days in 99 humans
with burns and with infection secondary to burns.
Simultaneous parenteral administration of other antibiotics (SM) in 99 humans
with burns and with infection secondary to burns.
No ototoxic effects due to topical, direct site (SM), administration in cream
or ointment of 0.1 percent of antibiotic, gentamicin, in 50 humans with burns
and with infection secondary to burns.
   (AD) No topical gentamicin therapy in 2 patients.   (ENG)

588

No observed ototoxic effects due to parenteral, intramuscular, administration
of range of 1.36 to 7.00 mg per kg daily, in 6 dosage regimens, to produce
blood levels of 10.5 to 18.5 mcg per ml in 8 patients tested, of antibiotic,
gentamicin, for short period in 160 humans, Filipino, adolescent and adult,
15 to 62 years age, male, 78 to 168 lb weight, with venereal disease.
   (AD) Clinical evaluation of vestibular function and cochlear function
   after gentamicin therapy.   (ENG)

589

Dizziness during or after 5 or 6 injections but no evidence of hearing loss
due to parenteral, intramuscular and then intravenous (SM), administration of
7 mg per kg total daily, not exceeding 180 mg total dose every 24 hours, of
antibiotic, (SQ) gentamicin, for as long as 30 days in 5 of 80 humans, infant, child, and adult, 8 months to 36 years age, with cystic fibrosis and
severe pulmonary infection.
   (AD) Audiology in 40 of 80 patients showed no evidence of hearing loss.
   (AD) Dizziness possibly due to rapid administration of gentamicin.
High frequency hearing loss before gentamicin therapy possibly due to previous administration of (SQ) ototoxic drugs in some of 80 humans, infant,
child, and adult, 8 months to 36 years age, with cystic fibrosis and severe
pulmonary infection.
Dizziness due to topical administration by inhalation (SM) of 16 to 20 mg up
to 4 times a day, in 2 ml of 0.125 percent phenylephrine hydrochloride and
propylene glycol, of antibiotic, (SQ) gentamicin (CB), in some of 80 humans,
infant, child, and adult, 8 months to 36 years age, with cystic fibrosis and
severe pulmonary infection.
Dizziness due to topical administration by inhalation (SM) of 16 to 20 mg up
to 4 times a day, in 2 ml of 0.125 percent phenylephrine hydrochloride and
propylene glycol, of antibiotic, (SQ) neomycin (CB), in some of 80 humans,
infant, child, and adult, 8 months to 36 years age, with cystic fibrosis and
severe pulmonary infection.   (ENG)

595

Bilateral hearing loss due to parenteral, intramuscular, administration of 80
mg daily of antibiotic, gentamicin, in 1 human, adult, 38 years age, male,
with pulmonary infection.
   (AD) Hearing loss confirmed by audiogram.   (FR)

599

Unspecified ototoxic effects due to parenteral, intramuscular, administration
of 40 mg, to produce blood levels of 3.7 mcg per ml 1 hour after treatment to
less than 0.1 and 0.2 mcg per ml after 8 hours, of antibiotic, gentamicin
(gentamicin sulfate), in 1 dose in 10 humans, male and female, 59 to 87 kg
weight.
   (AD) Risk of ototoxic effects with gentamicin.
   (AD) Study in unpaid subjects of pharmacology and clinical use of gentamicin.   (GER)

600

No ototoxic effects due to parenteral, intramuscular or intravenous, administration of 40 or 80 mg daily of antibiotic, gentamicin, in humans with pseudomonas infection.
No ototoxic effects due to topical, direct site, administration in cream of
0.3 percent daily of antibiotic, gentamicin, in humans with pseudomonas
infection.   (GER)

605

Decr in ototoxic effects due to parenteral, subcutaneous, administration of high doses of antibiotic, gentamicin (IB) (gentamicin sulfate), in acute intoxication in 20 animals, mice, male, 20 g weight, with simultaneous subcutaneous administration of calcium chloride.
   (CT) Same method using 8 mg of calcium chloride in mice, control group, showed no ototoxic effects.
   (CT) Same method using 12.5 mg of gentamicin (gentamicin sulfate) in mice, control group, showed ototoxic effects.
Decr in ototoxic effects due to parenteral, subcutaneous or intravenous, administration of 25 mg per ml solution of antibiotic, gentamicin (IB) (gentamicin sulfate), in acute intoxication in animals, mice, male, 20 g weight, with combined administration of 1, 2, 4, 8, 16, or 32 mg per ml concentrations of calcium chloride.
Decr in ototoxic effects due to parenteral, subcutaneous, administration of antibiotic, gentamicin (IB) (gentamicin hydrochloride), in acute intoxication in animals, mice, male, 20 g weight, with combined administration of complex of calcium chloride.
   (AD) Decr in ototoxic effects in mice to less than 0.2 of effects of gentamicin (gentamicin hydrochloride) and to less than 0.5 of effects of gentamicin (gentamicin sulfate) due to calcium chloride.
Ataxia and equilibrium disorder due to parenteral, subcutaneous, administration of 60 and 120 mg per kg 1 time daily of antibiotic, gentamicin (gentamicin sulfate), in chronic intoxication in 20 animals, cats, male and female.
   (CT) Same method using saline in cats, control group.
Ataxia and equilibrium disorder due to parenteral, subcutaneous, administration of 60 and 120 mg per kg 1 time daily of antibiotic, gentamicin (IB) (gentamicin hydrochloride), in chronic intoxication in 20 animals, cats, male and female, with administration of complex of calcium chloride.
   (AD) No decr in ototoxicity due to calcium chloride in cats.   (ENG)

606

Transient vertigo after 7 days due to doses to produce blood level of 20 mcg per ml of antibiotic, gentamicin, in 1 human, adult, 53 years age, male, with kidney disorder and with previous hearing loss due to other aminoglycoside antibiotics.
Transient vertigo after 5 days due to doses to produce blood level of 10 mcg per ml of antibiotic, gentamicin, in 1 human, adult, 32 years age, female, with chronic pyelonephritis.
Transient vertigo and hearing loss after 6 days due to high doses to produce blood level of 40 mcg per ml of antibiotic, gentamicin, in 1 human, adult, 20 years age, male, with kidney disorder and severe pseudomonas infection.
   (CT) Audiometry and vestibular function tests, pretreatment and posttreatment.
   (AD) Ototoxic effects in 3 of 58 patients in study.
Unilateral vestibular problem with dizziness due to high daily doses and high total doses to produce blood levels of 4 to 32 mcg per ml of antibiotic, gentamicin, in 10 of 40 humans, 7 with kidney disorders.
   (CT) Audiometry and vestibular function tests, pretreatment and posttreatment in 5 patients.
   (AD) Ototoxic effects in 10 of 40 patients in study.
   (AD) Bilateral high frequency hearing loss in 2 patients without pretreatment audiograms possibly not due to gentamicin.
Unilateral tinnitus possibly due to topical, (SQ) direct site, administration of 40 mg of antibiotic, gentamicin, in 1 human with previous noise induced hearing loss.
Unilateral tinnitus possibly due to parenteral, (SQ) intramuscular, administration of total of 160 mg of antibiotic, gentamicin, in 1 human with previous noise induced hearing loss.
   (AD) Tinnitus, as well as hearing loss, possibly present before administration of gentamicin.
Incr vertigo due to 120 mg daily of antibiotic, gentamicin, in 1 human, adult, 36 years age, male, with previous vertigo.
   (CT) Audiometry and vestibular function tests, pretreatment and posttreatment.
   (AD) Ototoxic effects in possibly 2 of 148 patients in study treated with topical or parenteral gentamicin.
   (AD) Discussion of 3 studies of ototoxic effects of gentamicin.   (ENG)

616

Range of degrees of damage to hair cells of organ of Corti due to parenteral,
intramuscular, administration of 50 to 140 mg per kg daily of antibiotic,
gentamicin, for 7 to 20 days in 4 groups of animals, guinea pigs.
    (AD) Relationship between hair cell damage and dosage of gentamicin.
    (ENG)

621

Primarily vestibular problems due to antibiotic, streptomycin, in humans.
Primarily hearing loss but also vestibular problems due to antibiotic, dihy-
drostreptomycin, in humans.
Primarily hearing loss but also vestibular problems due to antibiotic, kana-
mycin, in humans.
Primarily hearing loss but also vestibular problems due to antibiotic, neomy-
cin, in humans.
Primarily hearing loss but also vestibular problems due to antibiotic, genta-
micin, in humans.
Vertigo and ataxia due to antituberculous agent, isoniazid, in humans.
Hearing loss due to salicylate, aspirin, in humans.
Hearing loss and vertigo due to antimalarial, quinine, in humans.
Nystagmus due to barbiturates in humans.
Vestibular problems due to analgesic, morphine, in humans.
Nystagmus due to sedative, alcohol, in humans.
Nystagmus and hearing loss due to chemical agent, carbon monoxide, in humans.
Ototoxic effects due to antineoplastic, nitrogen mustard, in humans.
Ototoxic effects due to chemical agent, aniline, in humans.
Ototoxic effects due to chemical agent, tobacco, in humans.
Nystagmus due to chemical agent, nicotine, in humans.
Vestibular problems due to anticonvulsants in humans.
Vestibular problems due to anesthetics in humans.
Vestibular problems due to diuretics in humans.
    (AD) Inclusion of comprehensive list of ototoxic agents.   (SP)

624

Possible ototoxic effects due to antibiotic, gentamicin, in humans with
pseudomonas infections.   (ENG)

628

Hearing loss due to parenteral, intravenous, administration of 1 mg per kg
initial dose and then 0.75 mg per kg every 6 hours, dissolved in 200 ml of 5
percent glucose solution, of antibiotic, (SQ) gentamicin (gentamicin sulfate), in 4 of 60 humans, child, adolescent, adult, and aged, 6 to 76 years
age, with carcinoma, lymphoma, or leukemia and with azotemia in 3 of 4 and
previous hearing loss in 1 of 4.
Hearing loss due to previous administration of diuretic, (SQ) ethacrynic
acid, in 1 of 4 humans with gentamicin hearing loss.
    (AD) Suggested that hearing loss in 1 patient due to both gentamicin and
    ethacrynic acid.   (ENG)

629

Hearing loss and vestibular problems due to antibiotic, (SQ) gentamicin
(gentamicin sulfate), in 16(2.8 percent) of 565 humans, with kidney disorder
in 10 cases and with previous treatment with ototoxic drugs in 7 cases.
Possible ototoxic effects due to previous administration of other (SQ) ototoxic drugs in 7 of 16 humans.
Hearing loss and vestibular problems due to antibiotic, gentamicin, in 23(2
percent) of 1152 humans.
    (AD) Discussion of incidence of ototoxicity due to gentamicin reported in
    2 studies.   (ENG)

632

Ototoxic effects due to antibiotic, gentamicin, in humans with infections.
    (AD) Suggested dosage of 1 to maximum of 1.5 mg per kg of gentamicin in
    therapy.   (GER)

639

Hearing loss in 6 cases and vestibular problems in 17 cases due to parenteral
administration of antibiotic, gentamicin, in 23(2 percent) of 1152 humans.
(ENG)

641

Possible damage to eighth cranial nerve due to antibiotic, capreomycin, in humans.
Possible vestibular problems and hearing loss due to antibiotic, gentamicin, in humans.
Possible delayed transient or permanent hearing loss due to antibiotic, kanamycin (SM), in humans, in particular with kidney disorders or with simultaneous administration of ethacrynic acid.
Possible delayed transient or permanent hearing loss due to diuretic, ethacrynic acid (SM), in humans.
Possible delayed transient or permanent severe hearing loss due to oral, parenteral, or topical administration of antibiotic, neomycin, in humans.
Possible damage to eighth cranial nerve, primarily hearing loss, due to antibiotic, paromomycin, in humans.
Possible hearing loss due to antibiotic, rifampicin, in humans.
High risk of damage to eighth cranial nerve, primarily transient or permanent vestibular problems but also hearing loss, due to antibiotic, streptomycin, in humans.
Possible damage to eighth cranial nerve, primarily hearing loss, due to high doses of antibiotic, vancomycin, for long period of more than 10 days in humans, in particular with kidney disorders.
Risk of damage to eighth cranial nerve, vestibular problems and hearing loss, due to high doses of antibiotic, viomycin, for long period of more than 10 days in humans, in particular with kidney disorders.
   (AD) Discussion of toxic effects of antibiotics. (ENG)

642

Possible transient or permanent damage to eighth cranial nerve, primarily vestibular problems, due to parenteral, intramuscular, administration of high doses of antibiotic, gentamicin (gentamicin sulfate), for long period in humans, in particular with kidney disorders.
   (AD) Need to monitor vestibular function and cochlear function with doses over 3 mg per kg daily or with administration of gentamicin for more than 10 days.
   (AD) Recommended that serum concentrations of gentamicin not be higher than 10 mcg per ml.
   (AD) Dizziness possibly early symptom of ototoxicity. (ENG)

650

Transient bilateral hearing loss and moderate dizziness after 6 days due to 0.8 mg per kg daily of antibiotic, gentamicin, in 1 of 44 humans with various infections and with normal kidney function.
   (CT) Vestibular function tests and audiometry, before, during, and after gentamicin treatment. (ENG)

651

No vestibular problems due to 4 to 6 mg per kg daily of antibiotic, gentamicin, in 100 humans, infant, 3 to 12 months age, with various severe infections.
   (AD) Vestibular function tests used to determine vestibulotoxic effects. (ENG)

652

No vestibular problems or hearing loss observed due to parenteral, intravenous, administration of 1 mg per kg initial dose, and then 0.75 mg per kg every 6 hours, in 200 ml dextrose solution over 2 hour period, of antibiotic, gentamicin (SM), for 2 weeks minimum or for 5 days after cessation of fever, whichever longer, in 23 humans, adolescent, adult, and aged, 13 to 68 years age, with acute leukemia or metastatic cancer and with previous treatment with other antibiotics in some.
   (AD) No vestibular function tests or audiometry used to determine if ototoxic effects.
Simultaneous parenteral, intravenous, administration of 4 g every 4 hours of antibiotic, carbenicillin (SM), for 2 weeks minimum or for 5 days after cessation of fever, whichever longer, in 23 humans, adolescent, adult, and aged, 13 to 68 years age, with acute leukemia or metastatic cancer and with

previous treatment with other antibiotics in some.   (ENG)

653

Possible ototoxic effects due to antibiotic, kanamycin, in humans with acute
genitourinary system infections.
Possible ototoxic effects due to antibiotic, gentamicin, in humans with acute
genitourinary system infections.
   (AD) Need for careful consideration in use of kanamycin and gentamicin in
   therapy, in particular in patients with kidney disorders.   (ENG)

670

Possible vestibular problems due to parenteral administration of antibiotic,
gentamicin, in humans.
Damage to eighth cranial nerve, primarily hearing loss, usually permanent,
due to parenteral administration of high doses of antibiotic, kanamycin, for
more than 10 days in humans, in particular with kidney disorders.
Damage to eighth cranial nerve, primarily hearing loss, usually permanent,
due to parenteral administration of high doses of antibiotic, neomycin, for
more than 10 days in humans, in particular with kidney disorders.
Possible damage to eighth cranial nerve, primarily hearing loss, due to
parenteral administration of antibiotic, paromomycin, in humans.
Transient or permanent vestibular problems due to parenteral administration
of antibiotic, streptomycin, in humans.
Permanent severe hearing loss due to parenteral administration of antibiotic,
dihydrostreptomycin, in humans.
Damage to eighth cranial nerve, primarily hearing loss, due to parenteral
administration of high doses of antibiotic, vancomycin, for more than 10 days
in humans, in particular with kidney disorders.
Damage to eighth cranial nerve, vestibular problems and hearing loss, due to
parenteral administration of high doses of antibiotic, viomycin, for more
than 10 days in humans, in particular with kidney disorders.
   (AD) Discussion of toxic effects of antibiotics.   (ENG)

672

Possible sensorineural hearing loss due to parenteral administration of
antibiotic, kanamycin, in humans with kidney disorders.
   (AD) Need for decr in dosage and 3 to 4 days interval between doses in
   patients with kidney disorders.
Possible vestibular problems and hearing loss due to parenteral administration of antibiotic, streptomycin, in humans with kidney disorders.
   (AD) Need for decr in dosage and 3 to 4 days interval between doses in
   patients with kidney disorders.
Possible vestibular problems due to parenteral administration of antibiotic,
gentamicin, in humans with kidney disorders.
   (AD) Need for decr in dosage and unknown period between doses in patients
   with kidney disorders.
Possible hearing loss due to parenteral administration of antibiotic, van-
comycin, in humans with kidney disorders.
   (AD) Need for decr in dosage and 9 days interval between doses in patients
   with kidney disorders.
   (AD) Report on use of antibiotics in patients with kidney disorders.
   (AD) Need for total initial dose followed by 50 percent of initial dose at
   recommended intervals.
   (AD) Change in dosage based on serum half-life of antibiotic.
   (AD) Literature review of effect of antibiotics in patients with kidney
   disorders.   (ENG)

677

Transient or permanent, bilateral or unilateral, vestibular problems primarily but also possible high frequency hearing loss due to parenteral administration of high doses to produce serum levels over 10 mcg per ml of antibiotic, gentamicin, in humans, in particular with kidney disorders.
   (AD) Gentamicin ototoxicity also in patients with previous treatment with
   ototoxic drugs or with previous auditory system problems.
   (AD) Reported 2 to 2.5 percent incidence of vestibular problems due to
   parenteral gentamicin.
   (AD) Literature review of mechanism of action, pharmacology, dosage,
   clinical use, and toxic effects of gentamicin.   (ENG)

678

Primarily transient but also permanent severe vestibular problems due to
doses to produce serum levels over 12 mcg per ml of antibiotic, gentamicin,
in humans.
   (AD) Study of in vitro activity of gentamicin only or gentamicin combined
   with other antibiotics.   (ENG)

679

Damage to eighth cranial nerve due to antibiotic, gentamicin, in humans.
   (AD) Factors in gentamicin ototoxicity include concurrent kidney disorders, total doses over 1 g, serum levels over 12 mcg per ml, 60 years or
   more age, and previous administration of ototoxic drugs, antibiotics.
   (ENG)

680

Damage to vestibular apparatus and cochlea due to high doses of antibiotic,
gentamicin, for several weeks in animals, guinea pigs.
   (AD) Electron microscopical study of effects of gentamicin on inner ear of
   guinea pig.   (ENG)

683

Primarily transient or permanent, unilateral or bilateral, vestibular problems but also high frequency hearing loss due to parenteral administration of
high doses to produce blood levels over 10 mcg per ml of antibiotic, gentamicin, in humans, in particular with kidney disorders or with previous treatment with ototoxic drugs, or with previous auditory system problems.
   (AD) Discussion of chemical structure, antibiotic activity, clinical
   pharmacology, use in therapy, and toxic effects.
   (AD) Reported 2 to 2.5 percent incidence of vestibular problems due to
   parenteral gentamicin.
   (AD) Unilateral vestibular problems in 50 percent of patients tested.
   (ENG)

684

Possible permanent severe vestibular problems and some hearing loss due to
antibiotic, gentamicin, in humans.
   (AD) Possible to use potential ototoxic drugs with minimum risk of permanent ototoxic effects by regulation of dosage and cessation of therapy
   at first symptom of ototoxicity.   (ENG)

685

Total loss of vestibular function but no hearing loss due to total of 840 mg
of antibiotic, gentamicin (SM), in 47 day period in 1 of 181 humans, aged, 70
years age, female, with kidney disorder.
Total loss of vestibular function but no hearing loss due to 2 g of antibiotic, streptomycin (SM), in 47 day period in 1 of 181 humans, aged, 70 years
age, female, with kidney disorder.
Permanent vestibular problems due to 2.56 g of antibiotic, (SQ) gentamicin,
for 18 days in 1 of 181 humans, adult, 39 years age, female, with kidney
disorder.
Vestibular problems due to previous administration of antibiotic, (SQ) streptomycin, in 1 of 181 humans, adult, 39 years age, female, with kidney disorder.
Permanent vestibular problems, with dizziness, due to antibiotic, gentamicin,
in 1 of 181 humans, adult, 38 years age, female, with kidney disorder.
Transient dizziness after 3 days due to antibiotic, gentamicin, in 1 of 181
humans, adolescent, 16 years age, female, with kidney disorder.
   (AD) Serial vestibular function tests and audiometry not conducted in 181
   patients.
Vestibular problems due to parenteral, intramuscular, administration of 1 g
daily of antibiotic, (SQ) streptomycin (SM), in 1 human, adult, 19 years age,
male, with pseudomonas infection.
   (AD) Vestibular problems due to previous streptomycin therapy.
Simultaneous administration of 300 mg daily of antibiotic, (SQ) colistin (SM)
(colistimethate), for 15 days in 1 human, adult, 19 years age, male, with
pseudomonas infection.
Sequential parenteral, intramuscular, administration of 40 mg 3 times a day
of antibiotic, (SQ) gentamicin, for 36 days in 1 human, adult, 19 years age,

male, with pseudomonas infection.
Dizziness after 4 days due to parenteral, intramuscular, administration of 40
mg 4 times a day, total of 2.56 g, of antibiotic, gentamicin, for 16 days in
1 human, adult, 30 years age, female, with kidney disorder.
  (AD) Discussion of 6 case reports of vestibulotoxic effects of gentamicin.
  (ENG)

702

Permanent total bilateral sensorineural hearing loss 5 days after cessation
of treatment but no vestibular problems due to parenteral, intramuscular,
administration of total dose of 0.32 g of antibiotic, gentamicin, in 16
single injections in 1 human, adult, 27 years age, male, with severe bilateral kidney disorder.
  (AD) Hearing loss confirmed by audiology.   (GER)

725

Damage to eighth cranial nerve due to 20, 40, or 150 mg per kg of antibiotic,
gentamicin (gentamicin sulfate), in 10 injections in animals, guinea pigs.
  (CT) Study of normal guinea pigs, control group.   (GER)

729

No hearing loss or vestibular problems due to parenteral, intramuscular,
administration of total dose of 160 to more than 4000 mg of antibiotic,
gentamicin, for 2 to 40 days in 72 humans with various infections.
No hearing loss or vestibular problems due to topical administration in
solution or ointment of antibiotic, gentamicin, for 2 to 40 days in 55 humans
with various infections or in surgery.   (GER)

731

Possible damage to eighth cranial nerve, vestibular problems, due to antibiotic, streptomycin, in humans with gram-negative bacilli.
Possible damage to eighth cranial nerve, hearing loss, due to antibiotic,
kanamycin, in humans with gram-negative bacilli.
Possible damage to eighth cranial nerve, hearing loss, due to antibiotic,
neomycin, in humans with gram-negative bacilli.
Possible damage to eighth cranial nerve, vestibular problems, due to antibio-
tic, gentamicin, in humans with gram-negative bacilli.
Possible ototoxic effects due to antibiotic, vancomycin, in humans with gram-
positive cocci.
  (AD) Need to decr dosage of antibiotics in patients with kidney disorders.
  (AD) Discussion of possible toxic effects of antibiotics used in surgery.
  (ENG)

Kanamycin

009

Delayed permanent sensorineural hearing loss and damage to outer hair cells
of basal and middle coils of cochlea due to unspecified doses of antibiotic,
dihydrostreptomycin, in humans.
Vertigo and dizziness due to unspecified method of administration of 2 to 3 g
daily of antibiotic, streptomycin (streptomycin sulfate), for 30 to 50 days
in humans with tuberculosis.
Hearing loss due to unspecified method of administration of high doses of
antibiotic, streptomycin (streptomycin sulfate), for long period in humans.
Gradual high frequency hearing loss and tinnitus and degeneration of hair
cells of organ of Corti in basal coil of cochlea due to unspecified doses of
antibiotic, kanamycin, in humans.
Delayed severe high frequency hearing loss due to parenteral, oral, or topical administration by inhalation of unspecified doses of antibiotic, neomycin, for unspecified period in humans with kidney disorder.
Complete degeneration of inner hair cells due to unspecified method of administration of 18 g of antibiotic, neomycin, for unspecified period in
humans with bacterial endocarditis.
Lesions in organ of Corti due to parenteral administration of unspecified
doses of antibiotic, polymyxin B, for unspecified period in animals, guinea
pigs.
Sensorineural hearing loss due to parenteral, intravenous, administration of
80 to 95 mg per ml of antibiotic, vancomycin, for unspecified period in

humans with kidney disorder.
  (AD) Sensorineural hearing loss and vestibular problems due to 6 antibio-
  tics in humans and animals, guinea pigs.
  (AD) Literature review of ototoxic effects of antibiotics. (ENG)

010

Permanent sensorineural hearing loss due to parenteral, intramuscular, administration of low doses, less than 2 g, of antibiotic, (SQ) kanamycin
(kanamycin sulfate), for short period in 5 humans, adult, range of 33 to 47
years age, range of 90 to 177 lb weight, with kidney disorder.
Permanent sensorineural hearing loss due to parenteral, intramuscular, administration of low doses, less than 2 g, of antibiotic, (SQ) streptomycin,
for short period in 5 humans, adult, range of 33 to 47 years age, range of 90
to 177 lb weight, with kidney disorder.
Permanent sensorineural hearing loss due to parenteral, intramuscular, administration of low doses, less than 2 g, of antibiotic, (SQ) neomycin, for
short period in 5 humans, adult, range of 33 to 47 years age, range of 90 to
177 lb weight, with kidney disorder.
Permanent sensorineural hearing loss due to parenteral, intramuscular, administration of low doses, less than 2 g, of diuretic, (SQ) ethacrynic acid,
for short period in 5 humans, adult, range of 33 to 47 years age, range of 90
to 177 lb weight, with kidney disorder.
  (AD) Study of cochleotoxic effects of kanamycin with other antibiotics and
  with ethacrynic acid. (ENG)

011

Transient cochleo-vestibulotoxic effects due to topical administration by
inhalation and parenteral, intramuscular, administration of 0.5 g twice a day
for 6 days, followed by a 1-day break, of antibiotic, (SQ) kanamycin (kanamycin sulfate), for 1 to 3 months in 2 of 17 humans treated for tuberculosis.
  (CT) Pretreatment audiometry and vestibular function tests conducted.
Ototoxic effects due to previous administration of antibiotic, (SQ) streptomycin, in 2 of 17 humans with tuberculosis. (RUS)

012

Permanent sensorineural hearing loss due to parenteral, intramuscular, administration of high doses, about 100 mg per kg daily, total of more than 6 g
of antibiotic, (SQ) neomycin (neomycin sulfate), for 7 days in 1 human,
Caucasian, infant, 13 months age.
Unspecified effects due to parenteral, intramuscular, administration of about
12 mg per kg daily recommended dosage, total of 20 mg, of antibiotic, (SQ)
kanamycin (kanamycin sulfate), for less than 24 hours in 1 human, Caucasian,
infant, 13 months age.
  (CT) Normal response to acoustic stimulus before administration of antibiotics.
  (AD) Suggested that ototoxicity of neomycin not potentiated by administration of kanamycin in this case. (ENG)

019

Progressive severe sensorineural hearing loss and tinnitus due to unspecified
method of administration of 0.5 g twice daily, total of 16 g, of antibiotic,
kanamycin, for 16 days in 1 human, Caucasian, adult, 25 years age, male, with
kidney disorder and treated with peritoneal dialysis.
  (AD) Audiograms showed hearing loss and recruitment test showed reversed
  recruitment.
Severe sensorineural hearing loss due to unspecified method of administration
of 0.5 g daily for 40 days and then 0.5 g 3 times a week for 3 weeks of
antibiotic, streptomycin, for total period of about 9 weeks in 1 human,
Negro, child, 9 years age, male, with pulmonary tuberculosis and kidney
disorder.
  (AD) No record of hearing loss before treatment with streptomycin.
Delayed severe bilateral high frequency hearing loss due to unspecified
method of administration of 0.5 g daily for 8 months and then 0.5 g every 3
days for 4 months, followed by a break of 3.5 months, and then 0.5 g every 3
days for 1.5 months, total of 153 g of antibiotic, dihydrostreptomycin, for
total period of about 13.5 months in 1 human, Negro, infant, 16 months age,
female, with tuberculosis.
  (AD) Hearing loss detected at 13 years age.

Hearing loss and tinnitus due to unspecified method of administration of 1 g
daily of antibiotic, streptomycin, for 10 weeks and possibly for a longer
period after discharge in 1 human, Negro, adult, 23 years age, male, treated
for infection in tuberculosis hospital.
(AD) Hearing loss detected 1 month after treatment with streptomycin.
Progressive severe sensorineural hearing loss due to unspecified method of
administration of 0.5 g 3 times a week, total of 61 g of antibiotic, streptomycin, for about 10 months in 1 human, Negro, child, 9 years age, female,
with pulmonary tuberculosis.
(AD) Discussion of 5 case reports.   (ENG)

042

Transient bilateral sensorineural hearing loss due to parenteral, intravenous, administration of 50 mg of diuretic, (SQ) ethacrynic acid, in 1
injection in 1 human, adult, 45 years age, female, with lymphosarcoma and
with normal kidney function.
(AD) Hearing loss reported 15 minutes after treatment with ethacrynic
  acid.
Previous parenteral, intramuscular, administration of 60 mg every 6 hours of
antibiotic, (SQ) gentamicin (gentamicin sulfate), for unspecified period in 1
human, adult, 45 years age, female, with lymphosarcoma and with normal kidney
function.
Bilateral sensorineural hearing loss due to parenteral, intravenous, administration of 100 mg of diuretic, (SQ) ethacrynic acid, in 2 injections of 50 mg
each 6 hours apart in 1 human, adult, 64 years age, female, with acute leukemia and with normal kidney function.
(AD) Histological study after death showed no damage to inner ear.
Previous unspecified method of administration of unspecified dose of antibiotic, (SQ) polymyxin B (polymyxin B sulfate), in 1 human, adult, 64 years age,
female, with acute leukemia and with normal kidney function.
Previous parenteral, intramuscular, administration of 0.5 g every 12 hours of
antibiotic, (SQ) kanamycin (kanamycin sulfate), for unspecified period in 1
human, adult, 64 years age, female, with acute leukemia and with normal
kidney function.
(AD) Suggested that hearing loss due to combined action of ethacrynic acid
  and antibiotics.   (ENG)

043

Histochemical and electron microscopic changes in Reissner's membrane due to
parenteral, intramuscular, administration of 400 mg per kg daily of antibiotic, kanamycin, for 15 days in 10 animals, guinea pigs, 300 to 400 g weight.
(ENG)

046

Concentration of kanamycin in perilymph for more than 24 hours due to parenteral administration of 400 mg per kg of antibiotic, kanamycin, in 1 injection in animals, guinea pigs.
(AD) Study of kanamycin levels in blood, cerebrospinal fluid, perilymph,
  and endolymph.   (JAP)

058

Ototoxic effects due to parenteral, subcutaneous, administration of 250 mg
per kg daily of antibiotic, kanamycin (kanamycin sulfate), for 10 days in 60
animals, guinea pigs, 250 g average weight.
(AD) Tests made 30, 60, and 120 minutes after last injection.
Ototoxic effects due to parenteral, subcutaneous, administration of 250 mg
per kg daily of antibiotic, kanamycin (kanamycin sulfate), for 11 days in 20
animals, guinea pigs.
(AD) Tests made 5 or 12 hours after last injection.
(AD) High concentration of kanamycin in perilymph and, in particular,
  endolymph.
(AD) High concentration and long period of action of kanamycin in inner
  ear causes ototoxic effects.   (GER)

074

Decr in cochlear microphonic due to topical administration to round window of
range of 210 to 680 g of antibiotic, streptomycin, in animals, guinea pigs.
Decr in cochlear microphonic due to topical administration to round window of

range of 210 to 680 g of antibiotic, kanamycin, in animals, guinea pigs.
No decr in cochlear microphonic due to topical administration to round window
of range of 210 to 680 g of antibiotic, neomycin, in animals, guinea pigs.
(POL)

080

Hearing loss and vertigo due to parenteral administration of antibiotic,
streptomycin, in humans, child and adult, with normal kidney function and
with kidney disorder.
    (AD) Suggested use for severe infections only.
Delayed permanent hearing loss due to antibiotic, dihydrostreptomycin, in
humans.
    (AD) High risk of ototoxic effects with clinical use.
Hearing loss due to oral administration of antibiotic, paromomycin, in humans.
Progressive permanent hearing loss and tinnitus due to parenteral administration of antibiotic, kanamycin, in humans.
Progressive permanent hearing loss and tinnitus due to parenteral and topical
administration of antibiotic, neomycin, in humans.
    (AD) Need for careful consideration in use of paromomycin, kanamycin, and
    neomycin due to potential ototoxicity.
    (AD) Discussion of ototoxic effects of 5 antibiotics.   (ENG)

084

Decr in damage to organ of Corti due to topical administration of antibiotic,
kanamycin (IB), in animals, guinea pigs, 300 to 500 g weight, with intravenous administration of cytochrome C.
Decr in damage to organ of Corti due to topical administration of antibiotic,
streptomycin (IB) (streptomycin sulfate), in animals, guinea pigs, 300 to 500
g weight, with intravenous administration of cytochrome C.   (POL)

085

Hearing loss due to antibiotic, viomycin, in 17.7 percent of 152 humans with
tuberculosis.
    (CT) Systematic controls with audiology.
Hearing loss due to antibiotic, viomycin (IB), in only 5.3 percent of 36
humans with previous hearing loss with administration of nialamid.
Hearing loss due to antibiotic, kanamycin, in 20 percent of 55 humans with
tuberculosis.
Hearing loss due to antibiotic, kanamycin (IB), in 0 of 25 humans with previous hearing loss with administration of nialamid.
Lesion of inner ear due to antibiotic, neomycin (IB), in only 1 human with
previous hearing loss with administration of nialamid.   (GER)

086

Damage to organ of Corti due to parenteral, subcutaneous, administration of
150 mg per kg and 250 mg per kg of antibiotic, kanamycin, in 10 days in
animals, cats.
    (AD) Comparative study of ototoxicity of 4 compounds of kanamycin.   (GER)

089

Sudden deafness due to parenteral, intravenous, administration of 100 mg, in
100 ml saline solution, of diuretic, (SQ) ethacrynic acid, in 1 injection in
1 human, adult, 42 years age, female, quadriplegic, with kidney disorder.
Previous administration of unspecified dose of antibiotic, (SQ) chloramphenicol, for unspecified period in 1 human, adult, 42 years age, female, quadriplegic, with kidney disorder.
Previous administration of 1 g of antibiotic, (SQ) kanamycin, for unspecified
period in 1 human, adult, 42 years age, female, quadriplegic, with kidney
disorder and genitourinary system infection.   (ENG)

091

Ototoxic effects due to antibiotic, streptomycin (streptomycin sulfate), in
humans with pulmonary tuberculosis.
Ototoxic effects due to antibiotic, dihydrostreptomycin, in humans with
pulmonary tuberculosis.
Ototoxic effects due to antibiotic, florimycin, in humans with pulmonary
tuberculosis.

Ototoxic effects due to antibiotic, kanamycin, in humans with pulmonary
tuberculosis.
    (AD) Comparative study of ototoxicity of different derivatives of antibio-
    tics. (RUS)

                                                            094
Inhibition of RNA metabolism in cells of Reissner's membrane due to unspecified method of administration of 400 mg per kg daily of antibiotic, kanamycin
(kanamycin sulfate), for 14 days in 15 animals, guinea pigs, albino, 300 g
weight. (ENG)

                                                            096
Loss of outer hair cells and inner hair cells and damage to reticular membrane of organ of Corti due to parenteral, intraperitoneal (SM), administration of 400 mg per kg (SM) of antibiotic, kanamycin (kanamycin sulfate), in 5
days in animals, 15 cats, adult, 2.5 kg weight, and 30 guinea pigs, young,
300 g weight.
Simultaneous topical (SM) administration to middle ear cavity of 0.6 ml of 20
percent solution (SM) of antibiotic, kanamycin (kanamycin sulfate), for 1 day
in animals, 15 cats, adult, 2.5 kg weight, and 30 guinea pigs, young, 300 g
weight.
    (AD) Study of repair pattern in reticular membrane after loss of hair
    cells. (ENG)

                                                            107
Vertigo and nystagmus due to antibiotic, kanamycin, in humans, male and
female.
Vertigo and nystagmus due to antibiotic, streptomycin, in humans, male and
female.
    (AD) Preclinical detection of vestibular problems by ENG. (FR)

                                                            108
Degeneration of outer hair cells of organ of Corti due to parenteral, intramuscular, administration of 400 mg per kg daily of antibiotic, kanamycin, for
14 days in animals, guinea pigs.
Degeneration of outer hair cells of organ of Corti due to parenteral, intramuscular, administration of 400 mg per kg daily of antibiotic, kanamycin, in
animals, guinea pigs, after acoustic trauma.
More severe damage to outer hair cells and inner hair cells of organ of Corti
due to parenteral, intramuscular, administration of 400 mg per kg daily of
antibiotic, kanamycin, in animals, guinea pigs, before acoustic trauma.
    (AD) More severe cochleotoxic effects due to treatment with kanamycin
    before acoustic trauma. (FR)

                                                            109
Damage to hair cells in organ of Corti due to topical administration of 300
mg per kg of antibiotic, kanamycin, in 14 injections in animals, guinea pigs.
Severe degeneration of hair cells of organ of Corti and membranous labyrinth
due to topical administration to middle ear of low doses of antibiotics in
animals, guinea pigs.
    (AD) Report on studies of several years on cochleo-vestibulotoxic effects
    due to antibiotics. (ENG)

                                                            121
Tinnitus and high frequency hearing loss and damage to organ of Corti due to
antibiotic, kanamycin, in humans.
    (AD) Literature review of kanamycin, use in therapy and toxic effects.
    (AD) Suggested clinical procedures for use of kanamycin with minimum risk
    of ototoxicity. (ENG)

                                                            126
Decr in acid mucopolysaccharides in stria vascularis and spiral ligament due
to parenteral, subcutaneous, administration of 400 mg per kg daily for 5 days
a week of antibiotic, kanamycin (kanamycin sulfate), for 10 days in 60 animals, guinea pigs, pigmented, 250 to 350 g weight, with normal pinna reflex.
    (CT) Control group of 8 guinea pigs used.
    (AD) Study of role of mucopolysaccharides in hearing. (ENG)

129

Incr in sodium in perilymph but no significant change in potassium due to
parenteral, intraperitoneal, administration of 20 mg per kg and 200 mg per kg
of antibiotic, kanamycin (kanamycin sulfate), for about 5 days in animals,
guinea pigs, 400 to 600 g weight.
    (CT) Control group of 5 guinea pigs used.   (SP)

131

Severe sensorineural hearing loss due to antibiotic, kanamycin, in humans,
adult and child, female and male.
    (AD) Hearing loss confirmed by audiometry.   (JAP)

139

Cochleotoxic effects due to antibiotic, kanamycin, in humans and animals,
guinea pigs.
Cochleotoxic effects due to antibiotic, streptomycin, in humans and animals,
guinea pigs.
    (AD) Literature review of mechanism of action of ototoxic antibiotics.
    (POL)

141

Total bilateral sensorineural hearing loss, tinnitus, and vestibular problems
due to 120 mg daily, total of 1.2 g, of antibiotic, gentamicin (SM), for 10
days in 1 human, adult, 22 years age, female, 46 kg weight, with purulent
pleurisy after surgery.
Total bilateral sensorineural hearing loss, tinnitus, and vestibular problems
due to 1 g every 2 days, total of 9 g, of antibiotic, kanamycin (SM), for 18
days in 1 human, adult, 22 years age, female, 46 kg weight, with purulent
pleurisy after surgery.
Total bilateral sensorineural hearing loss and vestibular problems due to
high doses, 160 mg daily, of antibiotic, gentamicin, for long period, 47
days, in 1 human, adult, 35 years age, with pleurisy.
Total bilateral sensorineural hearing loss and vestibular problems due to 1 g
every 2 days of antibiotic, kanamycin, for 26 days in 1 human, adult, 35
years age, with pleurisy.
Total bilateral sensorineural hearing loss and vestibular problems due to 160
mg daily of antibiotic, gentamicin (SM), for 12 days in 1 human, adult, 35
years age, with pleurisy.
Total bilateral sensorineural hearing loss and vestibular problems due to 1 g
every 2 days of antibiotic, kanamycin (SM), for 12 days in 1 human, adult, 35
years age, with pleurisy.
    (AD) Hearing loss confirmed by audiogram.
    (AD) Discussion of 2 case reports of gentamicin ototoxicity.   (FR)

145

Decr of only 33.3 percent in cells of spiral ganglion due to 12 g of antibiotic, kanamycin, for 8 days in 1 human with kidney disorder.
    (AD) Temporal bone study of number of cells of spiral ganglion after
    treatment with kanamycin.
    (AD) Near normal number of spiral ganglion cells after treatment with
    ototoxic drug.   (ENG)

146

Cochleotoxic effects due to antibiotic, kanamycin, in chronic intoxication in
animals, rabbits.
    (AD) Electrophysiological study of ototoxicity of kanamycin.   (JAP)

147

Protection from ototoxic effects on inner ear due to antibiotic, kanamycin
(IB), in animals, cats, with administration of vitamin B.
    (AD) Preliminary study.   (SP)

159

Hearing loss due to antibiotic, kanamycin, in humans with infections.   (JAP)

161

No reported ototoxic effects due to parenteral, intramuscular, administration
of 2 g of antibiotic, kanamycin, in 1 injection in 4 humans, adult, 27 to 36

years age, with rectal gonorrhea.
  (AD) Audiogram after treatment with kanamycin within normal range. (ENG)

164

Ototoxic effects not determined due to parenteral, intramuscular and intrathecal, administration of 1.5 mg per kg every 8 to 12 hours, to produce peak
serum levels of 2.5 to 5.0 mcg per ml, of antibiotic, (SQ) gentamicin, for 9
to 13 days in 5 humans, newborn infant, with infections.
Ototoxic effects not determined due to parenteral, intramuscular, administration of 7.5 mg per kg every 12 hours of antibiotic (SQ) kanamycin, for 7 to
17 days in 3 of 5 humans, newborn infant, with infections.
  (AD) No follow up studies of gentamicin over long period to determine
  ototoxic effects.
  (AD) Need for audiometry and vestibular function tests after several
  months to determine ototoxic effects.
  (AD) Study of clinical pharmacology of gentamicin. (ENG)

165

Hearing loss, tinnitus, or vertigo due to parenteral administration of 36.0
mg per kg daily, total of 46.7 g, of antibiotic, kanamycin, for 20.3 average
days in 22 of 106 humans, adult, 50.8 years average age.
  (AD) Report on case study from previous study.
  (AD) Literature review of clinical and experimental studies. (ENG)

169

Progressive sensorineural hearing loss, complete range of degrees of damage
to organ of Corti, and degeneration in cochlear nuclei due to parenteral,
intramuscular, administration of 15 to 100 mg per kg daily of antibiotic,
kanamycin (kanamycin sulfate), for 28 to 180 days in 3 animals, monkeys,
young, 2 to 6 years age, male and female, 3 to 9 kg weight, conditioned.
High frequency hearing loss and damage to organ of Corti due to parenteral,
intramuscular, administration of 100 mg per kg daily of antibiotic, neomycin
(neomycin sulfate), for 5 days in 1 animal, monkey, young, conditioned.
Delayed severe sensorineural hearing loss after 2 months and severe damage to
organ of Corti due to parenteral, intramuscular, administration of 50 mg per
kg of antibiotic, neomycin (neomycin sulfate), for 15 days in 1 animal,
monkey, young, conditioned.
  (CT) Pretreatment hearing baseline determined.
  (AD) Study showed correlation of measurement of hearing loss and histopathology of cochlea in same subject.
  (AD) Cochleograms made to show patterns of cell loss.
  (AD) Reported that neomycin more ototoxic than kanamycin. (ENG)

173

Decr in oxygen consumption of cochlea due to parenteral, intraperitoneal,
administration of 400 mg per kg daily of antibiotic, kanamycin (kanamycin
sulfate), for 5,10, and 20 days in 3 groups of 22 animals, guinea pigs,
white, 300 to 400 g weight.
  (CT) Study of oxygen consumption in 35 guinea pigs, control group, not
  treated with kanamycin.
  (AD) Measurement of oxygen consumption with differential type of microrespirometer. (ENG)

176

Possible ototoxic effects due to low doses of antibiotic, kanamycin, in
humans.
  (AD) Literature review of infections with report on toxic effects of
  antibiotic therapy. (ENG)

179

Progressive high frequency hearing loss and tinnitus due to 1 g daily of
antibiotic, kanamycin, in 3 humans, adolescent and adult, male, with tuberculosis and with previous treatment with ototoxic drugs but with no report of
toxic effects.
Less severe sensorineural hearing loss and no tinnitus due to 1 g 5 times a
week of antibiotic, kanamycin, in 1 human, male, with tuberculosis and with
previous treatment with ototoxic drugs.
Sensorineural hearing loss and tinnitus due to 6 g of antibiotic, kanamycin

(SM), in 1 human, male, with tuberculosis and with previous treatment with
ototoxic drugs.
Sensorineural hearing loss and tinnitus due to parenteral administration of
1000 mg per day of antibiotic, streptomycin (SM), in 1 human, male, with
tuberculosis and with previous treatment with ototoxic drugs.
No high frequency hearing loss due to parenteral administration of 1 g daily
of antibiotic, streptomycin, in 1 human, female, with tuberculosis and with
previous treatment with ototoxic drugs.
High frequency hearing loss but no tinnitus due to 750 mg daily of antibiotic, streptomycin, in 1 human, female, with tuberculosis and with previous
treatment with ototoxic drugs.
Simultaneous administration of range of doses of other antituberculous agents
(SM) in total of 7 humans, adolescent and adult, 13 to 49 years age, male and
female, with tuberculosis and with previous treatment with ototoxic drugs.
   (AD) Study using high frequency audiometry and conventional audiometry.
   (CT) Pretreatment audiograms obtained.   (ENG)

                                                                         181
Decr in succinic dehydrogenase in outer hair cells of organ of Corti due to
parenteral, intratympanic, administration of 200 mg per ml solution of antibiotic, kanamycin (kanamycin sulfate), in animals, guinea pigs, adult.
Decr in succinic dehydrogenase in outer hair cells of organ of Corti due to
parenteral, intratympanic, administration of 200 mg per ml solution of antibiotic, dihydrostreptomycin (dihydrostreptomycin sulfate), in animals, guinea
pigs, adult.
Decr in succinic dehydrogenase in outer hair cells of organ of Corti due to
parenteral, intratympanic, administration of 200 mg per ml solution of antibiotic, chloramphenicol (chloramphenicol succinate), in animals, guinea pigs,
adult.
   (AD) Same type of damage to organ of Corti due to all 3 antibiotics.
Severe decr in succinic dehydrogenase in organ of Corti, in particular in
outer hair cells, and atrophy of outer hair cells due to saturated solution
of antimalarial, quinine (quinine hydrochloride), in animals, guinea pigs.
Complete degeneration of organ of Corti due to saturated solution of antimalarial, quinine (quinine hydrochloride), in animals, guinea pigs.
   (AD) Damage to organ of Corti more severe due to quinine than to antibiotics.
   (AD) Activity of succinic dehydrogenase often higher in outer hair cells.
   (AD) Possible that damage to outer hair cells due to higher rate of metabolism.   (ENG)

                                                                         183
Inhibition of oxygen consumption of cochlea due to 0.04 mg of antibiotic,
chloramphenicol (chloramphenicol sodium succinate), in animals, guinea pigs,
adult, 300 g weight, with normal Preyer reflex.
More inhibition of oxygen consumption of cochlea due to 0.04 mg of antibio-
tic, kanamycin (kanamycin sulfate), in animals, guinea pigs, adult, 300 g
weight, with normal Preyer reflex.
   (CT) Study of oxygen consumption in normal cochlea.
   (AD) Measurement of oxygen consumption with differential type of microres-
   pirometer.
   (AD) In vitro study.
No detected change in Preyer reflex due to parenteral, intracutaneous, ad-
ministration of 400 mg per kg of antibiotic, chloramphenicol, for 20 days in
animals, guinea pigs.
   (AD) In vivo study.
   (AD) Results with chloramphenicol in vivo not same as results in vitro.
   (ENG)

                                                                         184
Incr in ATP hydrolyzing system in stria vascularis and spiral ligament and
incr in ATP activity in membranous labyrinth due to parenteral, intraperitoneal, administration of 400 mg per kg 5 days a week of antibiotic, kanamycin (kanamycin sulfate), for 20 days in animals, guinea pigs, adult, with
normal pinna reflex.
Incr in ATP hydrolyzing system in stria vascularis and spiral ligament due to
parenteral, intraperitoneal, administration of 400 mg per kg 5 days a week of
antibiotic, streptomycin (streptomycin sulfate), for 20 days in animals,

quinea pigs, adult, with normal pinna reflex.
Decr in ATP hydrolyzing system in stria vascularis and spiral ligament and
decr in ATP activity in membranous labyrinth due to parenteral, intraperitoneal, administration of 400 mg per kg 5 days a week of antibiotic, dihydrostreptomycin (dihydrostreptomycin sulfate), for 20 days in animals, guinea
pigs, adult, with normal pinna reflex.
   (CT) Study of normal activity of ATP hydrolyzing system. (ENG)

                                                                             185
Ataxia, damage to hair cells of macula, and damage to hair cells of organ of
Corti due to parenteral, subcutaneous, administration of 10 to 80 mg per kg
daily of antibiotic, gentamicin (gentamicin sulfate), for 19 to 120 days in
animals, cats.
Ataxia due to 100 and 200 mg per kg daily of antibiotic, streptomycin (streptomycin sulfate), for 8 to 40 days in animals, cats.
Loss of Preyer reflex, decr in cochlear potential and eighth cranial nerve
action potential, and loss of outer hair cells of organ of Corti due to 80 to
200 mg per kg daily of antibiotic, gentamicin (gentamicin sulfate), in animals, guinea pigs.
Damage to cochlea due to 100 and 200 mg per kg of antibiotic, kanamycin
(kanamycin sulfate), in animals, guinea pigs.
   (AD) Comparative study of ototoxicity of gentamicin and other aminoglycoside antibiotics.
   (AD) Study suggested low risk of ototoxicity when gentamicin used in
   recommended clinical dose of 1 to 3 mg per kg. (ENG)

                                                                             196
Sensorineural hearing loss due to unspecified doses of antibiotic, streptomycin, in 8.9 percent of 2917 humans, child, adolescent, and adult, 10 to 34
years age, with pulmonary tuberculosis.
Sensorineural hearing loss due to unspecified doses of antibiotic, streptomy-
cin (SM), in high percent of 608 humans, child, adolescent, and adult, 10 to
34 years age, with pulmonary tuberculosis.
Sensorineural hearing loss due to unspecified doses of antibiotic, kanamycin
(SM), in high percent of 608 humans, child, adolescent, and adult, 10 to 34
years age, with pulmonary tuberculosis.
   (CT) Study of 314 humans, control group, without pulmonary tuberculosis.
   (CT) No subjective hearing loss before treatment with antibiotics.
   (CT) Hearing loss after antibiotic treatment confirmed by audiometry.
   (AD) Statistical analysis of 3525 cases with antibiotic therapy.
   (AD) Highest incidence of hearing loss in 30 to 34 years age group.
   (AD) Higher incidence of severe hearing loss in group treated with two
   antibiotics than in group treated with streptomycin only. (ENG)

                                                                             197
Progressive degeneration of organ of Corti beginning at base of cochlea due
to antibiotic, neomycin, in animals, guinea pigs.
Progressive degeneration of organ of Corti beginning at base of cochlea due
to antibiotic, kanamycin, in animals, guinea pigs.
Progressive degeneration of organ of Corti beginning at base of cochlea due
to antibiotic, framycetin, in animals, guinea pigs.
No damage to hair cells of organ of Corti due to parenteral administration of
high doses of antibiotic, dihydrostreptomycin, for long periods in animals,
guinea pigs.
   (AD) Surface specimen technique used in study of organ of Corti.
   (AD) Damage to organ of Corti due to ototoxic drugs different from that
   due to noise. (ENG)

                                                                             199
Progressive high frequency hearing loss due to parenteral, intramuscular,
administration of 500 mg twice a day of antibiotic, kanamycin, in 1 human,
aged, male, with diabetes mellitus, vascular disorder, and osteomyelitis.
   (AD) Hearing loss confirmed by audiogram.
   (AD) Report on clinical use and toxicity of antibiotics. (ENG)

                                                                             203
Permanent high frequency hearing loss due to range of less than 30 g to more
than 180 g of antibiotic, kanamycin, for long period in 55.6 percent of 72

humans with tuberculosis.
   (AD) Need for audiometry during treatment with kanamycin for prevention of
   more severe hearing loss. (GER)

204

Incr then decr in activity of 3 lysosomal enzymes in gradual permanent degeneration of hair cells of organ of Corti due to parenteral, intraperitoneal, administration of 250 mg per kg daily, total doses of 1750 to 10500
mg per kg, of antibiotic, kanamycin (kanamycin sulfate), for 1 to 6 weeks in
36 animals, guinea pigs, 250 to 300 g weight, with normal pinna reflex and no
middle ear infection.
Transient incr then decr in activity of 3 lysosomal enzymes in spiral ganglion due to parenteral, intraperitoneal, administration of 250 mg per kg
daily, total doses of 1750 to 10500 mg per kg, of antibiotic, kanamycin
(kanamycin sulfate), for 1 to 6 weeks in 36 animals, guinea pigs, 250 to 300
g weight, with normal pinna reflex and no middle ear infection.
   (CT) Study of 9 guinea pigs, control group, not treated with kanamycin.
   (AD) Suggested that histochemical changes in spiral ganglion independent
   of damage to organ of Corti. (ENG)

223

Sensorineural hearing loss due to antibiotic, kanamycin, in 1 human, adult,
female.
   (AD) Claim of negligence in treatment with kanamycin. (JAP)

226

Changes in hair cells of inner ear but no damage to stria vascularis due to
parenteral, intramuscular, administration of 300 mg per kg of antibiotic,
streptomycin (streptomycin sulfate), in animals, guinea pigs.
Damage to hair cells, then complete degeneration of organ of Corti, and
degeneration of spiral ganglion due to parenteral, intramuscular, administration of 200 or 300 mg per kg daily of antibiotic, kanamycin (kanamycin sulfate), for range of 7 to 29 injections in 28 animals, guinea pigs.
   (AD) Studies using electron microscopy and light microscopy.
   (AD) Study of transport in cochlea.
   (AD) Suggested that debris from degeneration in cochlea removed by Claudius cells and Reissner's membrane. (ENG)

229

Auditory system problems due to parenteral, intramuscular, administration of
high doses of antibiotic, kanamycin, for long period in humans, infant, for
infections.
   (AD) Recommended kanamycin dosage for infants of 7.5 mg per kg daily in
   divided doses every 12 hours by intramuscular administration for 12 days
   at most. (ENG)

232

Degeneration of hair cells of vestibular apparatus due to parenteral administration of antibiotic, kanamycin, in animals, guinea pigs.
Degeneration of hair cells of vestibular apparatus due to administration to
middle ear of antibiotic, streptomycin, in animals, guinea pigs.
   (AD) Study using surface specimen technique. (ENG)

236

Bilateral high frequency hearing loss due to parenteral, intramuscular,
administration of high dose, 90 mg per kg daily, total of 99.2 g, of antibiotic, kanamycin, for 62 days in 1 human, child, with miliary tuberculosis.
High frequency hearing loss due to parenteral, intramuscular, administration
of high dose, 25 mg per kg daily, total of 22.2 g, of antibiotic, kanamycin,
for 148 days in 1 human, child, with miliary tuberculosis.
Permanent severe sensorineural hearing loss due to parenteral, intramuscular,
administration of high doses of antibiotic, kanamycin, in 1 human, child,
with multiple infections.
Progressive sensorineural hearing loss due to oral administration of antibiotic, neomycin, for 11 months in 1 human, child, 11.5 years age, male, with
severe ulcerative ileocolitis.
   (AD) Hearing loss confirmed by audiogram.
   (AD) Discussion of 4 case reports of ototoxic effects due to kanamycin or

neomycin.
(AD) Suggested that risk of kanamycin ototoxicity less in children than in adults.
Sensorineural hearing loss due to 10 to 100 mg per kg daily of antibiotic, kanamycin, for 5 to 95 days in 5 of 30 humans, child and infant, with infections.
(CT) Study of 30 children and infants, control group, not treated with kanamycin.
(AD) Suggested that cochleotoxic effects related to total dose of kanamycin.
(AD) Report on studies made during 8 years of clinical use of kanamycin. (ENG)

237

Hearing loss due to parenteral, intramuscular, administration of 15 mg per kg daily of antibiotic, kanamycin, for 6 to 10 days in 5.1 percent of 143 humans, child, treated when newborn infant for infection.
Hearing loss due to parenteral, intramuscular, administration of 40 mg per kg daily of antibiotic, streptomycin, for 6 to 12 days in 5.6 percent of 93 humans, child, treated when newborn infant for infection.
(CT) Hearing loss in 4.4 percent of 170 children, control group, without antibiotic therapy.
(AD) Hearing loss confirmed by audiogram.
(AD) Suggested low kanamycin ototoxicity in newborn infants with use of recommended dosage. (ENG)

241

Risk of damage to organ of Corti and hearing loss due to antibiotic, kanamycin, in humans, infant.
(AD) Study of dose response relationships.
(AD) Recommended dose of 15 mg per kg daily every 12 hours for infants. (ENG)

242

Variations in decr in cochlear microphonic due to parenteral, intraperitoneal, administration of 100 mg per kg of antibiotic, kanamycin, for period until measurement of cochlear microphonic not possible in 12 animals, rabbits, adult, normal.
Changes in outer hair cells and supporting cells, in particular in basal coil of cochlea, and slight damage to inner hair cells of organ of Corti due to parenteral, intraperitoneal, administration of 100 mg per kg of antibiotic, kanamycin, for period until measurement of cochlear microphonic not possible in 12 animals, rabbits, adult, normal.
(AD) Serial observations on beginning and progression of cochleotoxic effects of kanamycin by daily measurement of cochlear microphonic and study of correlations between electrophysiological and histopathological changes.
(AD) Variations in response of cochlea to kanamycin but correlation between electrophysiological and histopathological changes. (ENG)

245

Degeneration of outer hair cells of organ of Corti and changes in supporting cells due to 400 mg per kg daily of antibiotic, kanamycin, for 14 days in animals, guinea pigs.
Degeneration of organ of Corti due to 400 mg per kg daily of antibiotic, dihydrostreptomycin, for 14 days in animals, guinea pigs.
(AD) Comparative study of cochleotoxic effects of kanamycin and dihydrostreptomycin. (FR)

250

Damage to vestibular apparatus due to more than 1 g daily of antibiotic, streptomycin, for 60 to 120 days in 25 percent of humans.
Dizziness 5 days after cessation of treatment due to parenteral, intramuscular, administration of 1 g every 12 hours of antibiotic, streptomycin (SM), for 9 days in 1 human, adult, 44 years age, female, with peritonitis.
Simultaneous parenteral, intravenous, administration of 600 mg every 18 hours of antibiotic, lincomycin (SM), for 9 days in 1 human, adult, 44 years age, female, with peritonitis.

(AD) Case report of vestibular problem due to streptomycin.
Damage to cochlea due to antibiotic, dihydrostreptomycin, for more than 1
week in 4 to 15 percent of humans.
Sensorineural hearing loss and damage to organ of Corti due to antibiotic,
kanamycin, in humans.
Sensorineural hearing loss and damage to organ of Corti due to antibiotic,
vancomycin, in humans.
  (AD) Discussion of cochleo-vestibulotoxic effects due to antibiotic therapy in surgery. (ENG)

                                                                      261
Nystagmus, ataxia, and loss of pinna reflex after 4 to 5 hours due to parenteral, intratympanic, administration of 5 to 20 mg, in 0.1 ml Ringer's solution, of antibiotic, streptomycin (streptomycin sulfate), in 1 ear of 15
animals, guinea pigs, pigmented, 250 to 350 g weight, with normal pinna
reflex.
  (CT) Use of other ear of 15 guinea pigs, control group.
No detected vestibular problems due to parenteral administration of 300 mg
per kg daily of antibiotic, kanamycin (kanamycin sulfate), for 8 to 15 days
in 5 animals, guinea pigs, pigmented, 250 to 350 g weight, with normal pinna
reflex.
Degeneration of hair cells of vestibular apparatus and organ of Corti due to
parenteral, intratympanic, administration of 5 to 20 mg, in 0.1 ml Ringer's
solution, of antibiotic, streptomycin (streptomycin sulfate), in all 15
animals, guinea pigs, pigmented, 250 to 350 g weight, with normal pinna
reflex.
  (AD) Suggested relationship between histological changes and streptomycin
  dosage.
Degeneration of hair cells of vestibular apparatus and organ of Corti due to
parenteral administration of 300 mg per kg daily of antibiotic, kanamycin
(kanamycin sulfate), for 8 to 15 days in 4 out of 5 animals, guinea pigs,
pigmented, 250 to 350 g weight, with normal pinna reflex.
  (AD) Same pattern of degeneration in vestibular apparatus due to streptomycin and kanamycin.
  (AD) Hair cells of vestibular apparatus more sensitive to streptomycin and
  hair cells of organ of Corti more sensitive to kanamycin. (ENG)

                                                                      267
Degeneration of outer hair cells of organ of Corti and damage to spiral
ganglion due to 400 mg per kg daily of antibiotic, kanamycin, for 14 days in
animals, guinea pigs.
Permanent histological changes in cochlea due to 100 mg per kg of antibiotic,
kanamycin, in animals, guinea pigs.
Damage to organ of Corti of fetuses due to 200 mg per kg of antibiotic,
kanamycin, in animals, guinea pigs, treated during pregnancy.
  (AD) Report on previous results of experimentation.
Cochleotoxic effects due to antibiotic, kanamycin, in average of 30 percent
of more than 1000 humans, adult.
  (AD) Discussion of relationship between kanamycin ototoxicity and dosage,
  duration of treatment, age, previous auditory system problems, administration of other ototoxic drugs, kidney function, and individual responses to
  drug. (ENG)

                                                                      268
Hearing loss due to antibiotic, kanamycin, in humans, adult.
  (AD) Discussion on incidence of hearing loss due to kanamycin, correlation
  between blood levels and ototoxicity, and relationship between kidney
  function and cochleotoxic effects. (ENG)

                                                                      270
Damage to organ of Corti due to antibiotic, kanamycin, in animals, guinea
pigs. (JAP)

                                                                      274
Degrees of damage, from loss of hair cells to complete destruction of organ
of Corti, but with partial replacement of organ of Corti by other structures
due to parenteral, intraperitoneal, administration of 200 mg per kg 5 days a
week of antibiotic, kanamycin (kanamycin sulfate), for 10, 15, and 20 days in

3 groups of 30 animals, guinea pigs, pigmented, young, 300 g weight.
   (AD) Report on degeneration and regeneration processes of organ of Corti.
   (AD) Study of patterns of replacement structure of reticular membrane.
   (ENG)

                                                                  275
Loss of some hair cells of crista ampullaris with replacement by supporting
cells due to parenteral, intraperitoneal, administration of 250 mg per kg
every other day of antibiotic, streptomycin (streptomycin sulfate), for 8
weeks in 1 group of 48 animals, guinea pigs, pigmented, young, 300 g average
weight.
Loss of some hair cells of crista ampullaris with replacement by supporting
cells due to parenteral, intraperitoneal, administration of 250 mg per kg
every other day of antibiotic, kanamycin (kanamycin sulfate), for 8 weeks in
1 group of 48 animals, guinea pigs, pigmented, young, 300 g average weight.
Loss of some hair cells of crista ampullaris with replacement by supporting
cells due to topical administration to middle ear of 0.6 ml of 250 mg per kg
of antibiotic, streptomycin (streptomycin sulfate), for 3 times with interval
of 1 week in 1 group of 48 animals, guinea pigs, pigmented, young, 300 g
average weight.
Loss of some hair cells of crista ampullaris with replacement by supporting
cells due to topical administration to middle ear of 0.6 ml of 250 mg per kg
of antibiotic, kanamycin (kanamycin sulfate), for 3 times with interval of 1
week in 1 group of 48 animals, guinea pigs, pigmented, young, 300 g average
weight.
   (AD) Degeneration of hair cells of crista ampullaris most severe in group
   with topical administration of streptomycin to middle ear.
   (AD) Degeneration of hair cells of crista ampullaris least severe in group
   with intraperitoneal administration of kanamycin. (ENG)

                                                                  282
Limited effects on blood vessels of stria vascularis and spiral prominence
due to 300 mg per kg daily of antibiotic, kanamycin, for 4 to 9 days in
animals, guinea pigs.
Limited effects on blood vessels of stria vascularis and spiral prominence
due to 30 mg per kg daily of antibiotic, dihydrostreptomycin, for 4 to 9 days
in animals, guinea pigs.
Limited effects on blood vessels of stria vascularis and spiral prominence
due to 30 mg per kg daily of antibiotic, chloramphenicol, for 4 to 9 days in
animals, guinea pigs.
   (CT) Study of guinea pigs, control group. (JAP)

                                                                  283
Effect on action potentials and cochlear microphonic and on vestibular apparatus due to range of doses of antibiotic, streptomycin, for range of
periods in animals, cats.
Effect on action potentials and cochlear microphonic and on vestibular apparatus due to range of doses of antibiotic, kanamycin, for range of periods
in animals, cats. (IT)

                                                                  285
Transient inhibition of endorgan of ampulla due to range of doses of antibio-
tic, streptomycin (streptomycin sulfate), in animals, frogs.
Transient inhibition of endorgan of ampulla due to range of doses of antibio-
tic, dihydrostreptomycin (dihydrostreptomycin sulfate), in animals, frogs.
Transient inhibition of endorgan of ampulla due to range of doses of antibio-
tic, neomycin (neomycin sulfate), in animals, frogs.
Transient inhibition of endorgan of ampulla due to range of doses of antibiotic, kanamycin (kanamycin sulfate), in animals, frogs.
   (CT) Study of frogs, control group.
   (AD) More inhibition of endorgan of ampulla with streptomycin than with
   other aminoglycoside antibiotics.
   (AD) Agreement between in vivo and in vitro observations of intensity of
   action on endorgans of vestibular apparatus. (ENG)

                                                                  286
Decr in cochlear microphonic due to antibiotic, kanamycin (kanamycin sulfate), in animals, guinea pigs.

Minimum effect on cochlear microphonic due to antibiotic, kanamycin (IB)
(kanamycin sulfate), in animals, guinea pigs, with administration of pantothenic acid.   (GER)

287

Cochlear impairment in fetus due to antibiotic, kanamycin, in humans, female,
treated during pregnancy.
   (AD) Discussion of cochleotoxic effects of kanamycin in newborn infants
   and infants.   (JAP)

288

Changes in cochlear microphonic due to parenteral, intramuscular, administration of 300 mg per kg daily of antibiotic, kanamycin, in animals, cats.
Changes in cochlear microphonic due to parenteral, intramuscular, administration of 200 and 100 mg per kg daily of antibiotic, streptomycin, in animals,
cats.
Hearing loss due to 300 mg per kg daily of antibiotic, kanamycin, in humans.
Hearing loss due to range of 50 to 200 mg per kg daily of antibiotic, streptomycin, in humans.
   (CT) Study of subjects, control group, not treated with aminoglycoside
   antibiotics.
   (AD) Hearing loss confirmed by audiogram.   (JAP)

307

No sensorineural hearing loss due to unspecified method of administration of
5 to 21 mg per kg daily, total doses of 30 to 450 mg, of antibiotic, kanamycin, for 3 to 11 days in 20 humans, infant and child, 1 to 4 years age,
treated when newborn infant for various infections.
   (CT) Study of 7 children, control group, treated with other antibiotics
   during neonatal period for similar infections.
   (AD) Use of pure tone audiometry or clinical evaluation only to determine
   hearing loss.
   (AD) Study to determine cochleotoxic effects of kanamycin when used in
   treatment of newborn infants.   (ENG)

308

Possible hearing loss due to antibiotic, kanamycin, in humans with tuberculosis.
Possible vestibular problems and cochlear impairment due to antibiotic,
capreomycin, in humans with tuberculosis.
   (AD) Comment on possible cochleo-vestibulotoxic effects of antibiotics
   used in treatment of tuberculosis.   (ENG)

309

Bilateral sensorineural hearing loss and tinnitus, tinnitus only, or vertigo
due to parenteral, intramuscular, administration of 1 g daily in 2 doses or
15 mg per kg, total doses of 6 to 9 g, of antibiotic, kanamycin, for 6 to 9
days in 5 of 17 humans, adult and aged, female and male, with genitourinary
system infections and normal kidney function.
Bilateral sensorineural hearing loss, tinnitus, and vertigo due to parenteral, intramuscular, administration of less than normal dosage of antibiotic, kanamycin, for 6 to 9 days in 2 of 17 humans, adult, male and female,
with genitourinary system infections and kidney disorder.
   (CT) Pure tone audiometry, pretreatment, during treatment, and posttreatment.
   (AD) Discussion of case reports.
   (AD) Prospective study to determine clinical effectiveness of kanamycin in
   genitourinary system infections.   (ENG)

314

Loss of enzymes, succinic dehydrogenase and DPN diaphorase, in outer hair
cells of organ of Corti but usually no enzyme loss in inner hair cells due to
topical administration to bulla of 200 mg per ml of antibiotic, kanamycin
(kanamycin sulfate), in 1 injection in animals, guinea pigs.
Loss of enzymes, succinic dehydrogenase and DPN diaphorase, in outer hair
cells of organ of Corti but usually no enzyme loss in inner hair cells due to
topical administration to bulla of 200 mg per ml of antibiotic, dihydrostreptomycin (dihydrostreptomycin sulfate), in 1 injection in animals, guinea

pigs.
Loss of enzymes, succinic dehydrogenase and DPN diaphorase, in outer hair
cells of organ of Corti but usually no enzyme loss in inner hair cells due to
topical administration to bulla of 200 mg per ml of antibiotic, chloramphenicol (chloramphenicol succinate), in 1 injection in animals, guinea pigs.
More severe effects on enzymes, succinic hydrogenase and DPN diaphorase, in
outer hair cells of organ of Corti due to topical administration to bulla of
saturated solution of antimalarial, quinine (quinine hydrochloride), in 1
injection in animals, guinea pigs.
  (CT) Activity of succinic dehydrogenase often higher in outer hair cells
  than in inner hair cells of organ of Corti in guinea pigs, control group.
  (AD) Suggested correlation between cochleotoxic effects of drugs and
  metabolic activity of hair cells. (ENG)

316
Possible vestibular problems and cochlear impairment due to more than recommended dose of 15 to 30 mg per kg daily of antibiotic, streptomycin, for long
period in humans.
Hearing loss due to parenteral, intramuscular, administration of total doses
of 5 to 6 g of antibiotic, kanamycin, in humans, adult, with kidney disorder.
Possible hearing loss due to parenteral, topical, or oral administration of
high doses of antibiotic, neomycin, for long period in humans.
Possible hearing loss due to high doses of antibiotic, framycetin, for long
period in humans.
Possible hearing loss due to antibiotic, vancomycin, in humans.
Possible hearing loss and vestibular problems due to antibiotic, viomycin, in
humans.
  (AD) High risk of ototoxicity with simultaneous administration of viomycin
  and streptomycin.
Possible vestibular problems due to antibiotic, gentamicin, in humans.
  (AD) Administration of gentamicin not recommended for newborn infants, for
  humans during pregnancy, and for humans treated with other ototoxic drugs.
Ataxia and hearing loss due to antibiotic, colistin, in humans.
  (AD) Literature review on ototoxic antibiotics.
  (AD) Results of studies on use of pantothenate salt of some antibiotics
  for decr in ototoxicity not clear.
  (AD) Suggested effect of ototoxic antibiotics on breakdown of glucose on
  which hair cells of inner ear depend for energy. (ENG)

332
No subjective hearing loss but objective hearing loss over 20 decibels and
tinnitus due to parenteral, intramuscular, administration of 1 g daily for
first 60 days and then 1 g twice a week of antibiotic, capreomycin (SM), for
6 months in 3 of 100 humans treated for pulmonary tuberculosis.
Hearing loss, tinnitus, or dizziness due to parenteral, intramuscular, administration of 1 g daily for first 60 days and then 1 g twice a week of
antibiotic, streptomycin (SM), for 6 months in 8 of 99 humans treated for
pulmonary tuberculosis.
Hearing loss over 20 decibels due to parenteral, intramuscular, administration of 1 g daily for first 60 days and then 1 g twice a week of antibiotic,
streptomycin (SM), for 6 months in 3 of 99 humans treated for pulmonary
tuberculosis.
Simultaneous oral administration of 0.3 g daily in 2 doses of antituberculous
agent, isoniazid (SM), for 6 months in humans treated for pulmonary tuberculosis.
Simultaneous administration of 10 g daily in 3 doses of antituberculous
agent, PAS (SM), for 6 months in humans treated for pulmonary tuberculosis.
  (AD) Report on ototoxic effects of antibiotics used in initial treatment
  of tuberculosis.
High frequency hearing loss, tinnitus, or dizziness due to parenteral, intramuscular, administration of 1 g daily for first 60 days and then 1 g twice a
week of antibiotic, capreomycin (SM), for 6 months in 6 of 66 humans retreated for pulmonary tuberculosis.
No subjective auditory system problems but objective hearing loss over 20
decibels due to parenteral, intramuscular, administration of 1 g 3 times a
week of antibiotic, kanamycin (SM), for 6 months in 4 of 40 humans retreated
for pulmonary tuberculosis.
No subjective auditory system problems but objective hearing loss over 20

decibels due to parenteral, intramuscular, administration of 1 g daily for
first 60 days and then 1 g twice a week of antibiotic, streptomycin (SM), for
6 months in 1 of 13 humans retreated for pulmonary tuberculosis.
Simultaneous oral administration of 0.3 g daily in 2 doses of antituberculous
agent, isoniazid (SM), for 6 months in humans retreated for pulmonary tuberculosis.
   (AD) Report on ototoxic effects of antibiotics used in retreatment of
   tuberculosis.
   (CT) Audiometry, pretreatment and during treatment, 2 times a month in
   first 2 months and then 1 time a month.
   (AD) Comparative study of clinical use and cochleo-vestibulotoxic effects
   of capreomycin and other antibiotics in treatment and retreatment of
   pulmonary tuberculosis.   (ENG)

                                                                        335
Vestibular problems due to antibiotic, streptomycin, in humans.
Severe cochlear impairment due to antibiotic, dihydrostreptomycin, in humans.
Cochlear impairment due to parenteral, oral, and topical administration of
antibiotic, neomycin, in humans.
Tinnitus and hearing loss due to antibiotic, kanamycin, in humans.
Vestibular problems and hearing loss due to antibiotic, gentamicin, in hu-
mans.
   (AD) Discussion of clinical use and possible cochleo-vestibulotoxic ef-
   fects of aminoglycoside antibiotics.   (SP)

                                                                        337
Shifts in cochlear microphonic and action potential thresholds and loss of
Preyer reflex due to parenteral, subcutaneous, administration of 400 mg per
kg daily of antibiotic, kanamycin, for 10, 14, or 20 days in 3 groups of
animals, guinea pigs, adult, male.
   (CT) Study of guinea pigs, control group.
   (AD) Correlation between duration of dosage and decr in function.
   (AD) Study of guinea pigs showed individual responses to kanamycin.
Shifts in cochlear microphonic and action potential thresholds and loss of
Preyer reflex due to parenteral, subcutaneous, administration of 400 mg per
kg daily of antibiotic, kanamycin, for 10, 14, or 20 days in 3 groups of
animals, rats, adult, male.
   (CT) Study of rats, control group.
   (AD) Results of study of rats showed high degree of individual response to
   kanamycin or technical difficulty in recording from round window of rat.
Shifts in cochlear microphonic and action potential thresholds and loss of
Preyer reflex due to parenteral, subcutaneous, administration of 400 mg per
kg daily of antibiotic, kanamycin, for 10, 14, or 20 days in 3 groups of
animals, rabbits, adult, male.
   (CT) Study of rabbits, control group.
   (AD) Similarity between cochlear impairment of rabbit and hearing loss in
   humans due to kanamycin.
Destruction of hair cells of organ of Corti in all coils of cochlea and
damage to stria vascularis and spiral ganglion due to unspecified method of
administration of 200 mg per kg of antibiotic, kanamycin, for 20 days in
animals, guinea pigs.
   (AD) Difference in pattern and degree of cochlear impairment in different
   species of animals.
   (AD) Suggested that physiological changes precede histological changes and
   so show more clearly the ototoxic effects of the drug.   (ENG)

                                                                        338
No loss of pinna reflex and no significant histological changes due to parenteral, subcutaneous, administration of 400 mg per kg daily in 1 injection of
antibiotic, dihydrostreptomycin, for 8 to 37 injections in 8 animals, guinea
pigs, young, 200 to 290 g weight.
Hearing loss after 64 injections and moderate damage to hair cells of cochlea
due to parenteral, subcutaneous, administration of 600 mg per kg daily, total
dose of 38.4 g, of antibiotic, dihydrostreptomycin, for 9 to 64 injections in
1 of 5 animals, guinea pigs, young, 200 to 290 g weight.
No loss of pinna reflex and no significant histological changes due to 50 mg
per kg daily of antibiotic, kanamycin, for 64 injections in 10 animals,
guinea pigs.

(CT) Test of pinna reflex, pretreatment and daily during treatment with
antibiotics.
(AD) Suggested relationship between degree of kanamycin damage to cochlea
and daily dose rather than total dose.   (ENG)

349

Effect on hearing loss due to antibiotic, kanamycin (IB), in animals, rabbits, with administration of vitamin B derivatives.
(AD) Study of effects of vitamin B derivatives on cochleotoxic effects of
kanamycin.   (JAP)

350

Cochleotoxic effects due to 0.75 or 1 g daily, total doses of 30.0 to 116.75
g, of antibiotic, streptomycin, in 9(7.2 percent)of 125 humans with disorders.
Cochleotoxic effects due to 1 g daily, total of less than 30 to over 180 g,
of antibiotic, kanamycin, in 40 (55.6 percent) of 72 humans with disorders.
   (AD) Comparative study of ototoxic effects of 2 aminoglycoside antibiotics.   (GER)

368

Possible vestibular problems and hearing loss due to antibiotic, streptomycin, in humans with tuberculosis.
Permanent hearing loss due to antibiotic, dihydrostreptomycin, in humans with
tuberculosis.
Possible permanent hearing loss due to antibiotic, kanamycin, in humans with
tuberculosis.
Possible vestibular problems and hearing loss due to antibiotic, viomycin, in
humans with tuberculosis.
Possible damage to eighth cranial nerve due to antibiotic, capreomycin, in
humans with tuberculosis.
   (AD) Discussion of primary and secondary drugs used in tuberculosis chemotherapy.   (FR)

371

Damage to hair cells of organ of Corti due to parenteral administration of
150 mg per kg of antibiotic, kanamycin (kanamycin sulfate), for 20 and 30
injections in animals, guinea pigs.
Decr in damage to hair cells of organ of Corti due to parenteral administration of 150 mg per kg of antibiotic, kanamycin (IB), for 20 and 30 injections
in animals, guinea pigs, with administration of pantothenic acid.
Slight decr in damage to hair cells of organ of Corti due to parenteral
administration of 150 mg per kg of antibiotic, kanamycin (IB) (kanamycin
sulfate), for 20 injections in animals, guinea pigs, with administration of
ozothin.
Slight decr in damage to hair cells of organ of Corti due to parenteral
administration of 150 mg per kg of antibiotic, kanamycin (IB), for 20 injections in animals, guinea pigs, with administration of pantothenic acid and
ozothin.
   (AD) Study of cochleotoxic effects of kanamycin without and with pantothenic acid and ozothin.   (GER)

373

Possible progressive sensorineural hearing loss due to antibiotics, aminogly-
coside, in humans.
Possible transient hearing loss due to high doses of salicylate, aspirin, in
humans.
Possible transient hearing loss due to high doses of antimalarial, quinine,
in humans.
Possible hearing loss due to diuretic, ethacrynic acid, in humans.
Bilateral sudden deafness due to antibiotic, kanamycin, in 4 humans, adult,
34 years average age, male and female.
   (AD) Hearing loss due to ototoxic drugs usually progressive.
   (AD) Sudden deafness due to ototoxic drugs possible in some cases, as in
   humans with kidney disorder.
   (AD) Literature review on etiology of sudden deafness.   (ENG)

Usually transient hearing loss and no structural damage to organ of Corti,
stria vascularis, and spiral ganglion due to oral or topical administration
of salicylates in humans.
Hearing loss due to antimalarial, quinine, in humans.
Usually permanent hearing loss due to antimalarial, chloroquine, in humans.
Transient and permanent hearing loss and possible damage to hair cells of
organ of Corti due to diuretic, ethacrynic acid, in humans.
Sensorineural hearing loss due to cardiovascular agent, hexadimethrine
bromide, in humans with kidney disorder.
Sensorineural hearing loss and damage to organ of Corti due to topical ad-
ministration of antineoplastic, nitrogen mustard, in humans.
Sensorineural hearing loss due to high doses of antibiotic, chloramphenicol,
in humans.
Primary vestibular problems due to antibiotic, streptomycin, in humans.
Hearing loss due to high doses usually of antibiotic, streptomycin, in humans.
    (AD) Early detection of hearing loss by audiometry prevents permanent
    damage.
High frequency hearing loss and severe damage to outer hair cells and slight
damage to inner hair cells of organ of Corti due to antibiotic, kanamycin, in
humans.
Sensorineural hearing loss due to parenteral, oral, and topical administration of antibiotic, neomycin, in humans with or without kidney disorders.
Degeneration of hair cells of organ of Corti and of nerve process due to
antibiotics, aminoglycoside, in animals.
    (AD) Literature review of physiological and structural cochleo-vestibulo-
    toxic effects of ototoxic drugs.
    (AD) Discussion of suggested mechanism of ototoxicity and routes of drugs
    to inner ear.
Bilateral sensorineural hearing loss due to oral administration of antibiotic, neomycin, in 4 of 8 humans with liver disease.
Bilateral sensorineural hearing loss due to oral administration of range of
doses of antibiotic, neomycin (SM), in 2 of 5 humans with liver disease.
Bilateral sensorineural hearing loss due to diuretics (SM), in 2 of 5 humans
with liver disease.
Transient progression of previous hearing loss due to parenteral, intravenous, administration of diuretic, ethacrynic acid (SM), in 1 injection in 1
of 5 humans with liver disease.
    (CT) Normal cochlear function in 6 humans, control group, with liver
    disease and not treated with neomycin or diuretics.
    (CT) Normal cochlear function in 13 humans, control group, with liver
    disease and treated with diuretics but not with neomycin.
    (AD) Hearing loss confirmed by audiometry.
    (AD) Reported that hearing loss due to neomycin or diuretics in humans
    with liver disease not related to dosage.
    (AD) Clinical study of effects of treatment with neomycin and diuretics in
    humans with liver disease.
Bilateral sensorineural hearing loss and vertigo due to antibiotic, ampicillin, in 1 human, adolescent, 17 years age, female, with tonsillitis.
    (AD) Cited case report.
Severe sensorineural hearing loss and vertigo due to topical administration
in ear drops of antibiotic, framycetin, in 1 human, adult, 42 years age,
male, with previous slight high frequency hearing loss.
    (AD) Cited case report.
Atrophy of hair cells of organ of Corti and hearing loss due to antibiotic,
dihydrostreptomycin, in humans with tuberculous meningitis.
    (AD) Cited study.
Loss of inner hair cells and damage to outer hair cells due to 18 g of antibiotic, neomycin, for 18 days in 1 human.
    (AD) Cited case report.   (ENG)

                                                                    391
Hearing loss in 15 fetuses due to parenteral, intramuscular, administration
of 200 mg per kg daily of antibiotic, kanamycin, for 15 days in animals,
rats, Wistar strain, female, about 150 g weight, during pregnancy.
    (AD) Test of Preyer reflex of rats, newborn infant, 30 days after birth.
No hearing loss due to 20 mg per kg daily of antibiotic, kanamycin, for 1 to
5 days in 15 humans, newborn infant.

(CT) EEG in newborn infants, before and about 1 month after kanamycin administration.
No hearing loss in fetuses due to antibiotic, kanamycin, in humans, female, treated for pulmonary tuberculosis during pregnancy.
(AD) Follow up study for 3 years after birth showed no hearing loss in children.
(AD) Discussion of clinical and experimental studies on effects of kanamycin.
Hearing loss due to range of 30 to 100 mg per kg daily of antibiotic, kanamycin, for range of 3 to 46 days in 9 of 391 humans, newborn infant.
No hearing loss due to less than 60 mg per kg daily of antibiotic, kanamycin, for less than 11 days in 382 humans, newborn infant.
(AD) Discussion of reports from 100 hospitals in Japan on effects of kanamycin in newborn infants.
(AD) Relationship between cochleotoxic effects of kanamycin and daily dosage and duration of treatment.   (ENG)

                                                                    392
No hearing loss but tinnitus due to parenteral, intramuscular, administration of range of 0.05 to 1.0 g daily according to age of antibiotic, kanamycin, for short period in 4 of 125 humans, infant, child, and adult, with acute otorhinolaryngological infections.
(AD) Audiograms showed no hearing loss.
Hearing loss, subjective in 1 case and latent in others, but no vestibular problems due to 1.0 g daily 2 times a week of antibiotic, (SQ) kanamycin, for long period in 15 of 66 humans, adolescent and adult, 15 to 55 years age, with pulmonary tuberculosis and with previous streptomycin treatment.
(CT) Audiogram before and during treatment with kanamycin.
Hearing loss due to previous administration of antibiotic, (SQ) streptomycin, in 31 of 272 humans.
Sensorineural hearing loss due to previous administration of total of 600 g of antibiotic, (SQ) streptomycin, in 1 human, adult, 27 years age.
More severe sensorineural hearing loss, subjective, due to total of 136 g of antibiotic, (SQ) kanamycin, in 1 human, adult, 27 years age.
(AD) Case report of hearing loss due to streptomycin potentiated by treatment with kanamycin.
Hearing loss, latent, and tinnitus, but no vestibular problems due to total of over 20 g to over 300 g of antibiotic, kanamycin, for long period in 10 of 70 humans with pulmonary tuberculosis and no previous chemotherapy.
(CT) Audiogram before and during treatment with kanamycin.
(AD) Clinical studies of effects of treatment with kanamycin for short and long periods.
Vestibular problems after 10 to 12 days due to parenteral administration of 100 mg per kg daily of antibiotic, streptomycin, in 3 animals, cats, 2 kg weight.
Slight vestibular problems after 30 days due to 300 mg per kg daily of antibiotic, kanamycin, in 3 animals, cats, 2 kg weight.
Decr in cochlear microphonic due to 200 mg per kg daily of antibiotic, streptomycin, in 11 injections in animals, cats.
Slight decr in cochlear microphonic due to 300 mg per kg daily of antibiotic, kanamycin, in 11 to 60 injections in animals, cats.
(AD) Comparative experimental studies of cochleo-vestibulotoxic effects of kanamycin and streptomycin in cats.
(AD) Different effects of 2 aminoglycoside antibiotics on vestibular function but similar effects on cochlear function.   (ENG)

                                                                    393
Severe hearing loss due to parenteral administration of 1 to 2 g daily, total doses of 30, 40, 21, and 4 g, of antibiotic, kanamycin, in 4 humans, adult, 53, 20, 32, and 37 years age, female and male, with kidney disorders.
(AD) Case reports of cochleotoxic effects of kanamycin in humans with kidney disorders.   (ENG)

                                                                    394
Tinnitus and hearing loss due to total of 50 to 100 g, in some cases, of antibiotic, (SQ) kanamycin, in 176 (9 percent) of 2054 humans with surgery for pulmonary tuberculosis.
(AD) Improvement in hearing in only 30 percent of humans.

Possible hearing loss due to previous administration of antibiotic, (SQ)
streptomycin, for long period in 176 of 2054 humans before surgery for pulmonary tuberculosis. (ENG)

409

Primary damage to hair cells of organ of Corti, hearing loss, and possible
vestibular problems due to antibiotic, viomycin, in humans.
Damage to hair cells of organ of Corti and hearing loss due to antibiotic,
neomycin, in humans.
Damage to hair cells of organ of Corti and hearing loss due to antibiotic,
kanamycin, in humans.
Primary damage to vestibular apparatus, vestibular problems, and possible
hearing loss due to antibiotic, streptomycin, in humans.
Primary damage to vestibular apparatus, vestibular problems, and possible
hearing loss due to antibiotic, gentamicin, in humans.
  (AD) Need for audiometry and vestibular function tests, pretreatment and
  during treatment, with clinical use of aminoglycoside antibiotics.
  (AD) Incr in blood levels and ototoxicity of antibiotics in humans with
  kidney disorders. (ENG)

432

Damage to sensory epithelia of macula utriculi and macula sacculi due to
parenteral, intraperitoneal, administration of 250 mg per kg every other day
of antibiotic, streptomycin (streptomycin sulfate), for 8 weeks in 12 animals, guinea pigs, pigmented, young, about 300 g weight.
Least severe damage to sensory epithelia of macula utriculi and macula sacculi due to parenteral, intraperitoneal, administration of 250 mg per kg every
day of antibiotic, kanamycin (kanamycin sulfate), for 8 weeks in 12 animals,
guinea pigs, pigmented, young, about 300 g weight.
Most severe damage to sensory epithelia of macula utriculi and macula sacculi
due to topical administration to middle ear cavity through tympanic membrane
of about 0.6 ml of concentration of 250 mg per kg of antibiotic, streptomycin
(streptomycin sulfate), in 8 injections, with interval of 1 week between
injections, in 12 animals, guinea pigs, pigmented, young, about 300 g weight.
Damage to sensory epithelia of macula utriculi and macula sacculi due to
topical administration to middle ear cavity through tympanic membrane of
about 0.6 ml of concentration of 250 mg per kg of antibiotic, kanamycin
(kanamycin sulfate), in 8 injections, with interval of 1 week between injections, in 12 animals, guinea pigs, pigmented, young, about 300 g weight.
  (AD) More damage to vestibular apparatus due to topical administration
  than due to parenteral administration of antibiotics.
  (AD) More loss of hair cells in sensory epithelium of macula utriculi than
  in that of macula sacculi.
  (AD) Type 1 hair cells more vulnerable to aminoglycoside antibiotics than
  type 2 hair cells.
  (AD) Comment on morphological and phylogenetical vulnerability of hair
  cells.
  (AD) Replacement of hair cells of vestibular apparatus by supporting
  cells. (ENG)

435

Decr in cochlear microphonic, summating potential, and eighth nerve action
potential due to parenteral, subcutaneous, administration of 800 mg per kg
daily of antibiotic, kanamycin, for 5 to 7 days in 8 animals, guinea pigs.
Slow decr of endocochlear potential in cochlear duct and low maximum negative
value of endocochlear potential due to parenteral, subcutaneous, administration of 800 mg per kg daily of antibiotic, kanamycin, for 5 to 7 days in 8
animals, guinea pigs, with anoxia.
  (AD) Longer survival time of endocochlear potential with severe decr in
  cochlear microphonic.
  (AD) Study of negative potential in cochlear duct of guinea pig during
  anoxia. (ENG)

438

Suppression of microphonic potentials of saccule due to topical, intraluminal, administration of antibiotic, streptomycin, in animals, goldfish.
Suppression of microphonic potentials of saccule due to topical, intraluminal, administration of antibiotic, kanamycin, in animals, goldfish.

Suppression of microphonic potentials of saccule due to topical, intraluminal
or extraluminal, administration of 0.5 mg of chemical agent, cyanide, in
animals, goldfish.
Suppression of microphonic potentials of saccule due to topical, intraluminal
or extraluminal, administration of 0.1 mg of antimalarial, quinine, in animals, goldfish.
Suppression of microphonic potentials of saccule due to topical, intraluminal
or extraluminal, administration of 2 mg of anesthetic, procaine, in animals,
goldfish.
No effect on microphonic potentials of saccule due to topical administration
of salicylates in animals, goldfish.   (ENG)

439

Decr in cochlear potentials due to parenteral, intramuscular, administration
of 400 mg per kg of antibiotic, kanamycin, for 10 days in 8 animals, guinea
pigs.   (FR)

440

Possible damage to organ of Corti in fetuses due to antibiotic, kanamycin, in
animals, guinea pigs, adult, during pregnancy.
   (AD) Study of transmission of drugs from mother to fetus.
   (AD) Serum levels of kanamycin in fetus about 7 percent of serum levels in
   mother and not related to variations in dosage.
   (AD) Slow elimination of kanamycin from fetus.   (ENG)

455

Damage to sensory epithelia of vestibular apparatus due to 250 mg per kg of
antibiotic, streptomycin, in animals.
Damage to sensory epithelia of vestibular apparatus due to 250 mg per kg of
antibiotic, kanamycin, in animals.   (JAP)

457

Tinnitus and progressive sensorineural hearing loss due to parenteral, intramuscular, administration of antibiotic, (SQ) streptomycin, for 10 days in 1
human, adult, 38 years age, female, with infections and later development of
kidney disorder.
Tinnitus and progressive sensorineural hearing loss due to 13.2 g of antibiotic, (SQ) kanamycin, for 11 days in 1 human, adult, 38 years age, female,
with infections and kidney disorder.
Hearing loss due to antimalarial, (SQ) quinine, in 1 human, adult, 20 years
age, male, with various infections and later development of kidney disorder.
Hearing loss due to 400 mg 2 times daily, total dose of 6.5 g, of antibiotic,
(SQ) kanamycin (SM), for 8 days in 1 human, adult, 20 years age, male, with
various infections and later development of kidney disorder.
Hearing loss due to 150 mg 2 times daily, total dose of 2400 mg, of antibiotic, (SQ) colistin (SM), for 8 days in 1 human, adult, 20 years age, male,
with various infections and later development of kidney disorder.
Tinnitus, total bilateral hearing loss, and vestibular problems due to parenteral, intramuscular, administration of 4.0 g daily, total of 21 g, of antibiotic, (SQ) kanamycin (SM), for 5 days in 1 human, adult, 20 years age,
male, with infections and kidney disorder.
Tinnitus, total bilateral hearing loss, and vestibular problems due to 0.6 g
daily, total dose of 1.3 g, of antibiotic, (SQ) colistin (SM), for 2 days in
1 human, adult, 20 years age, male, with infections and kidney disorder.
Tinnitus, total bilateral hearing loss, and vestibular problems due to 2 g
and then 8 g per 24 hours in divided doses, total dose of 26.5 g, of antibiotic, (SQ) chloramphenicol, for 9 days in 1 human, adult, 20 years age, male,
with infections and kidney disorder.
Bilateral hearing loss due to 1 g daily of antibiotic, actinomycin (SM), for
5 days in 1 human, adult, 62 years age, male, with infections and kidney
disorder.
Bilateral hearing loss due to unknown dose of antibiotic, kanamycin (SM), for
5 days in 1 human, adult, 62 years age, male, with infections and kidney
disorder.
Bilateral hearing loss and vestibular problems due to parenteral administration of high doses of antibiotic, (SQ) neomycin, for total of 21 days in 1
human, adult, 25 years age, male, with infection from wound.
Previous administration of unspecified doses of antibiotic, (SQ) streptomy-

cin, in 1 human, adult, 25 years age, male, with infection from wound.
Later administration of antibiotic, (SQ) chloramphenicol, in 1 human, adult,
25 years age, male, with infection from wound.
Tinnitus and rapidly progressive bilateral hearing loss due to parenteral,
intramuscular, administration of 0.5 g every 12 hours of antibiotic, (SQ)
streptomycin, for 5 days in 1 human, adult, 21 years age, male, with infection from wound.
Tinnitus and rapidly progressive bilateral hearing loss due to parenteral,
intramuscular, administration of 200 mg daily, total of 6.8 g, of antibiotic,
(SQ) colistin (SM), in 1 human, adult, 21 years age, male, with infection
from wound.
Tinnitus and rapidly progressive bilateral hearing loss due to parenteral
administration of unspecified doses of antibiotic, (SQ) neomycin (SM), for
about 35 days in 1 human, adult, 21 years age, male, with infection from
wound.
Tinnitus and progressive bilateral hearing loss due to parenteral administration of 2 l per 24 hours of 1 percent solution of antibiotic, (SQ) neomycin,
for 10 days in 1 human, adult, 26 years age, male, with infection from wound.
    (AD) Hearing loss confirmed by audiometry.
Previous administration of 500 mg four times a day of antibiotic, (SQ) ampicillin, in 1 human, adult, 26 years age, male, with infection from wound.
Bilateral sudden deafness due to administration in dialysis fluid of less
than 150 mg of antibiotic, neomycin (SM), in 1 human, adult, 44 years age,
female, with kidney disorder.
Bilateral sudden deafness due to 50 mg of diuretic, ethacrynic acid (SM), in
1 human, adult, 44 years age, female, with kidney disorder.
    (AD) Hearing loss confirmed by audiology.
Tinnitus and progressive bilateral hearing loss beginning after 8 days of
treatment due to parenteral administration of 1 l every 4 hours for 3 days
and then every 8 hours for 10 days of 1 percent solution of antibiotic,
neomycin, in 1 human, adult, 20 years age, male, with infection from wound.
    (AD) Hearing loss confirmed by audiology.
Tinnitus and bilateral sensorineural hearing loss due to parenteral, intramuscular, administration of 1 g and then 0.5 g every 12 hours of antibiotic,
streptomycin (SM), for 15 days in 1 human, adult, 23 years age, male, with
infection from wound.
Tinnitus and bilateral sensorineural hearing loss due to topical administration by irrigation of 1 percent solution every 12 hours of antibiotic, neomycin (SM), for 14 days in 1 human, adult, 23 years age, male, with infection
from wound.
    (AD) Hearing loss confirmed by audiometry.
    (AD) Discussion of 10 case reports. (ENG)

                                                                        459
No significant decr in cochlear microphonic due to parenteral, subcutaneous,
administration of 100 mg per kg daily for 5 days a week, total dose of 3 g
per kg, of antibiotic, kanamycin (kanamycin sulfate), for 30 days in animals,
guinea pigs.
Decr in cochlear microphonics in 14 of 15 ears, damage to hair cells of organ
of Corti and to stria vascularis, slight to severe damage to spiral ganglion,
damage to macula utriculi, and slight damage to crista ampullaris and macula
sacculi due to parenteral, subcutaneous, administration of 250 mg per kg
daily for 5 days a week, total dose of 5 g per kg, of antibiotic, kanamycin
(kanamycin sulfate), for 20 days in animals, guinea pigs.
Significant decr in cochlear microphonics in all ears, damage to outer hair
cells of organ of Corti and to stria vascularis, and slight damage to spiral
ganglion due to parenteral, subcutaneous, administration of 200 mg per kg
daily for 5 days a week, total dose of 6 g per kg, of antibiotic, kanamycin
(kanamycin sulfate), for 30 days in animals, guinea pigs.
Significant decr in cochlear microphonics due to parenteral, subcutaneous,
administration of 200 mg per kg daily for 5 days a week, total dose of 6 g
per kg, of antibiotic, kanamycin (IB) (kanamycin sulfate), for 30 days in
animals, guinea pigs, with subcutaneous administration of 1.5 mg per kg of
nialamide.
Significant decr in cochlear microphonics, damage to hair cells of organ of
Corti and to stria vascularis, and slight damage to spiral ganglion due to
parenteral, subcutaneous, administration of 200 mg per kg daily for 5 days a
week, total dose of 6 g per kg, of antibiotic, kanamycin (IB) (kanamycin

sulfate), for 30 days in animals, guinea pigs, with subcutaneous administration of 8 mg per kg of nialamide.
Significant decr in cochlear microphonics, damage to hair cells of organ of Corti and to stria vascularis, slight to severe damage to spiral ganglion, slight damage to limbus, and slight damage to macula utriculi and cristae due to parenteral, subcutaneous, administration of 200 mg per kg daily for 5 days a week, total dose of 6 g per kg, of antibiotic, kanamycin (IB) (kanamycin sulfate), for 30 days in animals, guinea pigs, with subcutaneous administration of 15 mg per kg of nialamide.
  (AD) No prevention of kanamycin effects on cochlear microphonics with administration of nialamide.
Less decr in cochlear microphonics in 6, 10, and 11 of 3 groups of 15 ears, damage to hair cells of organ of Corti and to stria vascularis, slight damage to spiral ganglion and to limbus, damage to macula utriculi, and slight damage to crista ampullaris due to parenteral, subcutaneous, administration of 250 mg per kg daily for 5 days a week, total dose of 5 g per kg, of antibiotic, kanamycin (IB), for 20 days in 3 groups of animals, guinea pigs, with pantothenic acid.
  (CT) Same method using daily subcutaneous administration of 0.25 cc of isotonic saline in guinea pigs, control group.
  (AD) Decr in kanamycin effects on cochlear microphonics with pantothenic acid.
  (AD) Study of functional and structural cochleo-vestibulotoxic effects of kanamycin with and without inhibitors.
  (AD) Statistical analysis of results. (ENG)

                                                                     466
Possible decr in damage to organ of Corti due to antibiotic, kanamycin (IB), in animals, guinea pigs, with administration of vitamin B, nialamide, dexamethasone, or glutathione. (FR)

                                                                     468
Complete inhibition of acetylcholine induced decr in cochlear potential due to parenteral, intravenous, administration of 1.0 mg of antibiotic, streptomycin (streptomycin sulfate), in 1 injection in 5 animals, cats, male and female, 1.5 to 2.8 kg weight, with injection of acetylcholine.
Minimum inhibition of acetylcholine induced decr in cochlear potential due to parenteral, intravenous, administration of 1.0 mg of antibiotic, dihydrostreptomycin (dihydrostreptomycin sulfate), in 1 injection in 5 animals, cats, male and female, 1.5 to 2.8 kg weight, with injection of acetylcholine.
Complete inhibition of acetylcholine induced decr in cochlear potential due to parenteral, intravenous, administration of 1.0 mg of antibiotic, kanamycin (kanamycin sulfate), in 1 injection in 5 animals, cats, male and female, 1.5 to 2.8 kg weight, with injection of acetylcholine.
Complete inhibition of acetylcholine induced decr in cochlear potential due to parenteral, intravenous, administration of 1.0 mg of antibiotic, neomycin (neomycin sulfate), in 1 injection in 5 animals, cats, male and female, 1.5 to 2.8 kg weight, with injection of acetylcholine.
Acute inhibition of acetylcholine induced decr in cochlear potential due to parenteral, intravenous, administration of 1.0 mg of antimalarial, quinine (quinine hydrochloride), in 1 injection in 5 animals, cats, male and female, 1.5 to 2.8 kg weight, with injection of acetylcholine.
  (CT) Injections of 0.1 ml isotonic saline in cats, control group.
Inhibition of acetylcholine induced decr in cochlear potential due to parenteral, subcutaneous, administration of 300 mg per kg daily of antibiotic, streptomycin, for 7 to 9 days in 10 animals, cats.
Inhibition of acetylcholine induced decr in cochlear potential due to parenteral, subcutaneous, administration of 100 mg per kg daily of antibiotic, neomycin, for 7 to 9 days in 10 animals, cats.
  (CT) Study of 7 cats, control group, not treated with antibiotics.
  (AD) Study of effect of acetylcholine on cochlear potential after acute and chronic administration of ototoxic drugs.
  (AD) Suggested relationship between change in acetylcholine activity and ototoxic drugs.
  (AD) Suggested that ototoxicity partially due to disruption of efferent effect on cochlea. (ENG)

Significant decr in oxygen consumption of cochlea due to high doses of antibiotic, kanamycin, in animals, guinea pigs.
Significant decr in oxygen consumption of cochlea due to high doses of antibiotic, streptomycin, in animals, guinea pigs.
Incr followed by significant decr in oxygen consumption of cochlea due to
high doses of antibiotic, dihydrostreptomycin, in animals, guinea pigs.
   (CT) Determination of oxygen consumption of guinea pigs, control group,
   not treated with ototoxic drugs.
   (AD) Suggested that ototoxicity of aminoglycoside antibiotics due to
   inhibition of respiratory enzymes of cells of inner ear. (ENG)

Decr in cochlear function and vestibular function due to parenteral, intramuscular, administration of 50 to 100 mg per kg of antibiotic, streptomycin
(streptomycin sulfate), for 35 days in animals, guinea pigs, pigmented, 400
to 500 g weight.
   (AD) More ototoxic effects with higher dosage.
Decr in cochlear function with both doses but decr in vestibular function
with only higher dose due to parenteral, intramuscular, administration of 50
to 100 mg per kg of antibiotic, dihydrostreptomycin (dihydrostreptomycin
sulfate), for 35 days in animals, guinea pigs, pigmented, 400 to 500 g
weight.
   (AD) More decr in cochlear function with higher dosage.
Decr in cochlear function in all animals but decr in vestibular function in 2
groups only due to parenteral, intramuscular, administration of 50 to 100 mg
per kg of antibiotic, kanamycin, for 35 days in animals, guinea pigs, pigmented, 400 to 500 g weight.
   (AD) More decr in cochlear function with higher dosage.
Decr in cochlear function due to parenteral, intramuscular, administration of
20 mg per kg of diuretic, ethacrynic acid, for 35 days in animals, guinea
pigs, pigmented, 400 to 500 g weight.
   (CT) Study of guinea pigs, control group, not treated with ototoxic drugs.
Decr in ototoxic effects due to parenteral, intramuscular, administration of
100 mg per kg of antibiotic, streptomycin (IB) (streptomycin sulfate), for 35
days in animals, guinea pigs, pigmented, 400 to 500 g weight, with administration of 1 mg per kg of various inhibitors.
Decr in ototoxic effects due to parenteral, intramuscular, administration of
100 mg per kg of antibiotic, dihydrostreptomycin (IB) (dihydrostreptomycin
sulfate), for 35 days in animals, guinea pigs, pigmented, 400 to 500 g
weight, with administration of 1 mg per kg of various inhibitors.
Decr in ototoxic effects due to parenteral, intramuscular, administration of
100 mg per kg of antibiotic, kanamycin (IB), for 35 days in animals, guinea
pigs, pigmented, 400 to 500 g weight, with administration of 1 mg per kg of
various inhibitors.
Decr in ototoxic effects due to parenteral, intramuscular, administration of
20 mg per kg of diuretic, ethacrynic acid (IB), for 35 days in animals,
guinea pigs, pigmented, 400 to 500 g weight, with administration of 1 mg per
kg of various inhibitors.
   (AD) Measurement of Preyer reflex and vestibular function tests.
Ototoxic effects, functional and structural, due to parenteral, intraperitoneal, administration of 100 mg per kg of antibiotic, streptomycin (streptomycin sulfate), for 50 days in animals, mice, male, 18 to 22 g weight.
No ototoxic effects due to parenteral, intraperitoneal, administration of 100
mg per kg of antibiotic, dihydrostreptomycin (dihydrostreptomycin sulfate),
for 50 days in animals, mice, male, 18 to 22 g weight.
Ototoxic effects, functional and structural, due to parenteral, intraperitoneal, administration of 100 mg per kg of antibiotic, kanamycin, for 50 days
in animals, mice, male, 18 to 22 g weight.
   (CT) Study of mice, control group, not treated with ototoxic drugs.
No ototoxic effects due to parenteral, intraperitoneal, administration of 100
mg per kg of antibiotic, streptomycin (IB) (streptomycin sulfate), for 50
days in animals, mice, male, 18 to 22 g weight, with administration of 1 mg
per kg of vitamin B.
No ototoxic effects due to parenteral, intraperitoneal, administration of 100
mg per kg of antibiotic, dihydrostreptomycin (IB) (dihydrostreptomycin sulfate), for 50 days in animals, mice, male, 18 to 22 g weight, with administration of 1 mg per kg of vitamin B.
No ototoxic effects due to parenteral, intraperitoneal, administration of 100

mg per kg of antibiotic, kanamycin (IB), for 50 days in animals, mice, male,
18 to 22 g weight, with administration of vitamin B.
   (AD) More ototoxic effects of aminoglycoside antibiotics in guinea pigs
   than in mice.
   (AD) Ototoxic effects of diuretic in guinea pigs.   (IT)

                                                                            483

Possible damage to vestibular nerve and cochlear nerve due to antibiotic,
streptomycin, in humans with or without kidney disorder.
Possible damage to vestibular nerve and cochlear nerve due to antibiotic,
gentamicin, in humans with or without kidney disorder.
Possible damage to vestibular nerve and cochlear nerve due to antibiotic,
kanamycin, in humans with or without kidney disorder.
Possible damage to vestibular nerve and cochlear nerve due to antibiotic,
neomycin, in humans with or without kidney disorder.
   (AD) Incidence of effects on vestibular function highest in streptomycin,
   followed by gentamicin, kanamycin, and neomycin.
   (AD) Incidence of effects on cochlear function highest in neomycin, fol-
   lowed by kanamycin, gentamicin, and streptomycin.
   (AD) Need for careful consideration in clinical use of aminoglycoside
   antibiotics.
Possible cochlear impairment and vestibular problems due to antibiotic,
paromomycin, in humans.
Possible dizziness and ataxia due to antibiotic, polymyxin B, in humans.
Possible but rare dizziness and vertigo due to antibiotic, nalidixic acid, in
humans.   (ENG)

                                                                            485
High concentration in fluids of inner ear and ototoxic effects due to 250 mg
per kg of antibiotic, streptomycin, in animals, guinea pigs.
High concentration in fluids of inner ear and ototoxic effects due to 250 mg
per kg of antibiotic, kanamycin, in animals, guinea pigs.
Higher concentration in fluids of inner ear and more severe ototoxic effects
due to 250 mg per kg of antibiotic, dihydrostreptomycin, in animals, guinea
pigs.
Higher concentration in fluids of inner ear and more severe ototoxic effects
due to 100 mg per kg of antibiotic, neomycin, in animals, guinea pigs.
   (AD) High concentration of aminoglycoside antibiotics in fluids of inner
   ear due to low doses as well as high doses.
   (AD) Ototoxic effect of aminoglycoside antibiotics due to retention of
   high concentrations in inner ear for long period and slow elimination of
   drugs.
Significant decr in concentration in fluids of inner ear and in serum and
decr in ototoxicity due to 250 mg per kg or 100 mg per kg of antibiotics
(IB), aminoglycoside, in animals, guinea pigs, with administration of ozothin.
Decr in concentration in fluids of inner ear and decr in ototoxicity due to
250 mg per kg or 100 mg per kg of antibiotics (IB), aminoglycoside, in animals, guinea pigs, with administration of pantothenic acid.   (GER)

                                                                            486
Incr in ATP activity of stria vascularis and spiral ligament but no pattern
of enzyme changes observed in membranous labyrinth due to 400 mg per kg daily
of antibiotic, kanamycin, for 3 weeks in animals, guinea pigs.
Incr in ATP activity of stria vascularis and spiral ligament but no pattern
of enzyme changes observed in membranous labyrinth due to 400 mg per kg daily
of antibiotic, streptomycin, for 3 weeks in animals, guinea pigs.
Decr in ATP activity of stria vascularis and spiral ligament but no pattern
of enzyme changes observed in membranous labyrinth due to 400 mg per kg daily
of antibiotic, dihydrostreptomycin, for 3 weeks in animals, guinea pigs.
   (CT) Study of guinea pigs, control group, not treated with aminoglycoside
   antibiotics.
   (AD) Study of effects of ototoxic drugs on ATP activity of inner ear of
   guinea pigs.   (JAP)

                                                                            489
Loss of Preyer reflex and progressive damage to hair cells of organ of Corti
beginning with basal coil of cochlea due to 400 mg per kg of antibiotic,

kanamycin (kanamycin sulfate), in 3 to 18 injections in 25 animals, guinea
pigs, adult, 250 to 350 g weight, with normal Preyer reflex.
  (CT) Daily administration of Ringer's solution in 4 guinea pigs, control
  group.
  (AD) Discussion of difference between ototoxic effects of kanamycin and
  streptomycin on organ of Corti.   (ENG)

                                                                      491
Changes in sensory epithelium of otocyst due to antibiotic, streptomycin, in
animals, chickens, embryo.
Changes in sensory epithelium of otocyst due to antibiotic, neomycin, in
animals, chickens, embryo.
Changes in sensory epithelium of otocyst due to antibiotic, kanamycin, in
animals, chickens, embryo.
  (CT) Study of otocysts of chickens, control group, not treated with aminoglycoside antibiotics.
  (AD) Neomycin and kanamycin more toxic to otocysts of chickens than streptomycin.   (CZ)

                                                                      492
Damage to hair cells of organ of Corti due to 400, 200, or 100 mg per kg
daily of antibiotic, kanamycin, for 14 days in animals, guinea pigs.
  (CT) Study of normal guinea pigs, control group, not treated with aminoglycoside antibiotic.
Possible protection of organ of Corti from damage due to antibiotic, kanamycin (IB), in animals, guinea pigs with administration of inhibitor.
  (AD) Electrophysiological and histological study of effect of ototoxic
  drug on cochlea of guinea pigs.   (FR)

                                                                      493
Decr in cochlear microphonics due to parenteral, intramuscular, administration of 400 or 200 mg per kg daily of antibiotic, kanamycin, in animals,
guinea pigs.
Decr in cochlear microphonics due to parenteral, intravenous, administration
of 100 mg per kg daily of antibiotic, kanamycin, for 3 to 10 days in animals,
guinea pigs.
No ototoxic effect in fetuses due to antibiotic, kanamycin, in animals,
guinea pigs, female, treated during pregnancy.
  (AD) More rapid and severe ototoxic effect with intravenous administration
  than with intramuscular administration.   (ENG)

                                                                      494
Accumulation in fluids of inner ear due to antibiotic, kanamycin, in animals,
guinea pigs.
  (AD) Suggested that route of kanamycin to inner ear is through stria
  vascularis, plexus cochlearis, and round window.   (JAP)

                                                                      496
Perilymph level of 2.5 mcg per ml and blood level of 36 mcg per ml due to
parenteral, subcutaneous, administration of 25 mg per kg of antibiotic,
kanamycin (kanamycin sulfate), in 1 injection in animals, guinea pigs.
Incr of 10 times of perilymph level and incr in blood level due to parenteral, subcutaneous, administration of 50 mg per kg of antibiotic, kanamycin
(kanamycin sulfate), in 1 injection in animals, guinea pigs.
No incr in perilymph level but incr in blood level due to parenteral, subcutaneous, administration of 250 mg per kg of antibiotic, kanamycin (kanamycin
sulfate), in 1 injection in animals, guinea pigs.
Some incr in inner ear level due to parenteral, subcutaneous, administration
of 250 mg per kg daily, total of 2500 mg per kg, of antibiotic, kanamycin
(kanamycin sulfate), for 10 days in animals, guinea pigs.
More incr in inner ear level due to parenteral, subcutaneous, administration
of total of 5000 mg per kg of antibiotic, kanamycin (kanamycin sulfate), for
20 days in animals, guinea pigs.
  (AD) Continuous accumulation of kanamycin in inner ear due to treatment
  with daily injections of long duration.
  (AD) High concentration of kanamycin in fluids of inner ear and slow
  elimination of more than 25 hours.
  (AD) Results of study showed direct linear relationship between dosage of

kanamycin and concentration in blood.
(AD) Results of study showed initial rapid accumulation with 25 and 50 mg
per kg doses in single injections and later lack of accumulation of kanamycin in perilymph.
(AD) Rapid incr in kanamycin level of inner ear with small incr in dosage
significant for clinical use of drug.
(AD) Accumulation of kanamycin in inner ear due to membrane sealing effect
of antibiotic.   (ENG)

515

Bilateral hearing loss due to oral (SM) administration of 480 mg daily of
diuretic, furosemide (SM), for 10 days in 1 human with kidney disorder.
Bilateral hearing loss due to parenteral, intravenous (SM), administration of
600 mg daily of diuretic, furosemide (SM), for 10 days in 1 human with kidney
disorder.
Bilateral hearing loss due to 500 mg of antibiotic, kanamycin (SM) (kanamycin
sulfate), in 2 doses in 1 human with kidney disorder.
(AD) No pretreatment audiogram.
(AD) Posttreatment audiogram confirmed hearing loss.
(AD) Suggested audiometry, pretreatment and during treatment, for humans,
in particular with kidney disorder, treated with high doses of intravenous
furosemide.   (ENG)

522

Hearing loss due to antibiotic, kanamycin, for 2 to 10 months in 30.4 percent
of 56 humans with chronic pulmonary tuberculosis and treated previously with
other drugs.
No significant ototoxic effects due to antibiotic, florimycin, for 2 to 10
months in 50 humans with chronic pulmonary tuberculosis and treated previously with other drugs.
(AD) Study of effects of kanamycin and florimycin in treatment of pulmonary tuberculosis.   (RUS)

529

Total loss of Preyer reflex within several days but no vestibular problems
due to parenteral, subcutaneous, administration of range of high doses to
more than 1000 mg per kg daily of antibiotic, kanamycin (kanamycin sulfate),
in animals, rats, Wistar, albino, female, 50 g weight.
(AD) Linear relationship between hearing loss and kanamycin dosage.
Loss of Preyer reflex but no vestibular problems due to parenteral, subcutaneous, administration of range of high doses to more than 600 mg per kg
daily of antibiotic, neomycin, in animals, rats, Wistar, albino, female, 50 g
weight.
(AD) Linear relationship between hearing loss and neomycin dosage.
(AD) Hearing loss observed with lower doses of neomycin than kanamycin.
Moderate to severe vestibular problems but cochlear impairment in only 1 case
due to parenteral, subcutaneous, administration of high doses, 471, 583, 720,
887, and 1089 mg per kg daily, of antibiotic, streptomycin (streptomycin
sulfate), in animals, rats, Wistar, albino, female, 50 g weight.
(AD) Linear realtionship between vestibular problems and streptomycin
dosage.
Transient moderate to severe vestibular problems but cochlear impairment in
only 1 case due to parenteral, subcutaneous, administration of high doses,
765, 940, 1151, and 1377 mg per kg daily, of antibiotic, dihydrostreptomycin
(dihydrostreptomycin sulfate), in 40 animals, rats, Wistar, albino, female,
50 g weight.
(CT) Same method using saline in 30 rats, control group, showed no cochleo-vestibulotoxic effects.
Hearing loss due to parenteral, subcutaneous, administration of 500 mg per kg
daily of antibiotic, kanamycin (SM), in animals, rats, Wistar, albino, female, 50 g weight.
Hearing loss due to parenteral, subcutaneous, administration of range of
doses of antibiotic, neomycin (SM), in animals, rats, Wistar, albino, female,
50 g weight.
(AD) Incr in ototoxicity of neomycin due to kanamycin.
Hearing loss but no vestibular problems due to parenteral, subcutaneous,
administration of 500 mg per kg of antibiotic, kanamycin (SM), in animals,
rats, Wistar, albino, female, 50 g weight.

Hearing loss but no vestibular problems due to parenteral, subcutaneous,
administration of 200, 270, 364.5, and 492 mg per kg daily of antibiotic,
streptomycin (SM), in animals, rats, Wistar, albino, female, 50 g weight.
Hearing loss but no vestibular problems due to parenteral, subcutaneous,
administration of 500 mg per kg daily of antibiotic, kanamycin (SM), in
animals, rats, Wistar, albino, female, 50 g weight.
Hearing loss but no vestibular problems due to parenteral, subcutaneous,
administration of 350, 472.5, 637.9, and 861.1 mg per kg daily of antibiotic,
dihydrostreptomycin (SM), in animals, rats, Wistar, albino, female, 50 g
weight.
  (AD) Tests of cochlear function and vestibular function, pretreatment and
  daily during treatment.
  (AD) Comparative study of ototoxic effects of aminoglycoside antibiotics
  in Wistar rats.
  (AD) Report of hearing loss in 321 (43.4 percent) of total of 740 rats in
  study.
  (AD) Suggested that ototoxic effects of kanamycin and neomycin due to
  different mechanisms of action than ototoxic effects of streptomycin and
  dihydrostreptomycin.   (ENG)

                                                                        558
Severe hearing loss due to antibiotic, kanamycin (SM), in 1 human, adult, 44
years age, female, with basilar meningitis.
Simultaneous administration of 1 g daily of antituberculous agent, ethambutol
(SM), in 1 human, adult, 44 years age, female, with basilar meningitis.
(ENG)

                                                                        560
Ototoxic effects due to antibiotic, streptomycin, in humans with tuberculo-
sis.
Ototoxic effects due to antibiotic, kanamycin, in humans with tuberculosis.
  (AD) Reported 4 to 5 percent incidence in audiometry of ototoxicity from
  streptomycin and kanamycin.
  (AD) Decr in ototoxicity with administration of streptomycin or kanamycin
  in evening before sleeping.   (JAP)

                                                                        562
Decr in microphonic potential of saccule due to topical, intraluminal, administration of antibiotic, streptomycin, in animals, goldfish.
Decr in microphonic potential of saccule due to topical, intraluminal, administration of antibiotic, kanamycin, in animals, goldfish.
Permanent decr in microphonic potential of saccule due to topical, intraluminal or extraluminal, administration of 0.5 mg per ml of chemical agent,
cyanide, in animals, goldfish.
Permanent decr in microphonic potential of saccule due to topical, intraluminal or extraluminal, administration of 0.1 mg per ml of antimalarial,
quinine, in animals, goldfish.
No effect on microphonic potential of saccule due to salicylate, aspirin, in
animals, goldfish.
Some decr in microphonic potential of saccule due to 2 mg per ml of anesthetic, procaine, in animals, goldfish.
  (AD) Study of effects of various agents on microphonic potential of saccule of goldfish.   (JAP)

                                                                        564
Hearing loss due to antibiotic, kanamycin (SM), for long period in 3 of 4
humans, adult, range of ages, male and female, during retreatment for pulmonary tuberculosis.
Simultaneous administration of 25 mg per kg for 2 months and then 15 mg per
kg of antituberculous agent, ethambutol (SM), in 4 humans, adult, range of
ages, male and female, during retreatment for pulmonary tuberculosis.
  (CT) Treatment with ethambutol and 2 other antituberculous agents in
  humans, control group.   (ENG)

                                                                        565
Inhibition of oxygen consumption of cochlea due to 0.04 M of antibiotic,
kanamycin (kanamycin sulfate), in animals, guinea pigs, adult, 300 g weight,
with normal Preyer reflex.

Inhibition of oxygen consumption of cochlea due to 0.04 M of antibiotic,
chloramphenicol (chloramphenicol sodium succinate), in animals, guinea pigs,
adult, 300 g weight, with normal Preyer reflex.
    (AD) Less inhibition of oxygen consumption by chloramphenicol than by
    kanamycin.
Incr inhibition of oxygen consumption of cochlea due to 0.04 M of antibiotic,
kanamycin (SM) (kanamycin sulfate), in animals, guinea pigs, adult, 300 g
weight, with normal Preyer reflex.
Incr inhibition of oxygen consumption of cochlea due to 0.04 M of antibiotic,
chloramphenicol (SM) (chloramphenicol sodium succinate), in animals, guinea
pigs, adult, 300 g weight, with normal Preyer reflex.
    (CT) Measurement of oxygen consumption of normal cochlea without adminis-
    tration of ototoxic drugs.
    (AD) In vitro study using microrespirometer of effect of interaction of
    kanamycin and chloramphenicol on oxygen consumption in guinea pig cochlea.
    (AD) Potentiation of inhibition of oxygen consumption of cochlea with
    simultaneous administration of kanamycin and chloramphenicol.
    (AD) Suggested risk of ototoxicity in clinical use of kanamycin and
    chloramphenicol.   (ENG)

577

No ototoxic effects due to parenteral, intramuscular, administration of 3 to
5 mg per kg daily in 3 or 4 divided doses, average total dose of 3.0 g, of
antibiotic, gentamicin, for 12.7 days average in 41 humans, adolescent,
adult, and aged, 14 to 87 years age, male and female, with genitourinary
system infections primarily and with kidney disorder in 13 cases.
No ototoxic effects due to parenteral, intramuscular, administration of 15 mg
per kg daily in 2 or 3 divided doses, average total dose of 6.6 g, of antibiotic, kanamycin (SM), for 8 days average in 34 humans, adult and aged, 40
to 81 years age, male and female, with genitourinary system infection and
with kidney disorder in 8 cases.
No ototoxic effects due to parenteral, intramuscular or intravenous administration of 1.5 to 2.5 mg per kg daily in 2 to 4 divided doses, average total
dose of 1.0 g, of antibiotic, polymyxin B (SM), for 6 days average in 34
humans, adult and aged, 40 to 81 years age, male and female, with genitourinary system infection and with kidney disorder in 8 cases.
    (AD) Comparative study of effects of 3 antibiotics on infections due to
    gram-negative bacilli.   (ENG)

601

Effect on eighth cranial nerve due to antibiotic, kanamycin, in humans with
infections and with or without kidney disorder.
    (AD) Study of use of kanamycin for therapy of various infections.   (ENG)

610

Possible ototoxic effects due to antibiotic, capreomycin, in humans with
tuberculosis of genitourinary system.
Possible hearing loss due to antibiotic, kanamycin, in humans with tuberculosis of genitourinary system.
Possible hearing loss and vestibular problems due to antibiotic, viomycin, in
humans with tuberculosis of genitourinary system.
    (AD) Discussion of treatment of tuberculosis of genitourinary system.
    (GER)

617

Hearing loss observed after several years possibly due to high doses, 125 mg
per kg daily, total of 10.75 g, of antibiotic, kanamycin, for total of 43
days in 1 human, child, treated after surgery for congenital intestinal
atresia when newborn infant.
    (AD) Hearing loss possibly congenital and not due to kanamycin therapy.
Bilateral hearing loss detected after 8 to 10 years but no subjective symptoms due to 100 mg per kg daily of antibiotic, kanamycin, for 8 to 14 days in
1 of 51 humans, child, treated for disorder when infant.
    (AD) Study with audiometry of effects of kanamycin used in treatment of 51
    newborn infants and infants.
    (CT) Study of 43 children, control group, without kanamycin therapy.
    (AD) Suggested that high doses of kanamycin not be used.
    (AD) Suggested that less ototoxic effects due to kanamycin in infants and

children than in adults.   (ENG)

618

Hearing loss due to parenteral, intramuscular, administration of 2 g in 2
doses, twice weekly, of antibiotic, kanamycin, in 7(1.1 percent) of 608
humans with pulmonary tuberculosis.
    (AD) Relationship between hearing loss and total dosage of kanamycin.
No hearing loss due to parenteral, intravenous, administration of 1 g twice
weekly, dissolved in 300 ml of saline solution, of antibiotic, kanamycin, for
long period in 1 human, adult, 40 years age, male, with pulmonary tuberculosis.
    (AD) Cochlear function monitored by audiometry during therapy.
    (AD) Higher blood levels of kanamycin with intravenous route than with
    intramuscular route.   (ENG)

621

Primarily vestibular problems due to antibiotic, streptomycin, in humans.
Primarily hearing loss but also vestibular problems due to antibiotic, dihy-
drostreptomycin, in humans.
Primarily hearing loss but also vestibular problems due to antibiotic, kana-
mycin, in humans.
Primarily hearing loss but also vestibular problems due to antibiotic, neomy-
cin, in humans.
Primarily hearing loss but also vestibular problems due to antibiotic, genta-
micin, in humans.
Vertigo and ataxia due to antituberculous agent, isoniazid, in humans.
Hearing loss due to salicylate, aspirin, in humans.
Hearing loss and vertigo due to antimalarial, quinine, in humans.
Nystagmus due to barbiturates in humans.
Vestibular problems due to analgesic, morphine, in humans.
Nystagmus due to sedative, alcohol, in humans.
Nystagmus and hearing loss due to chemical agent, carbon monoxide, in humans.
Ototoxic effects due to antineoplastic, nitrogen mustard, in humans.
Ototoxic effects due to chemical agent, aniline, in humans.
Ototoxic effects due to chemical agent, tobacco, in humans.
Nystagmus due to chemical agent, nicotine, in humans.
Vestibular problems due to anticonvulsants in humans.
Vestibular problems due to anesthetics in humans.
Vestibular problems due to diuretics in humans.
    (AD) Inclusion of comprehensive list of ototoxic agents.   (SP)

633

Cochlear impairment due to antibiotic, kanamycin, in humans, female, treated
for gynecologic infections.   (FR)

635

Effect on cochlear impairment due to antibiotic, kanamycin (IB), in animals,
rabbits, with administration of derivative of thiamine.   (JAP)

641

Possible damage to eighth cranial nerve due to antibiotic, capreomycin, in
humans.
Possible vestibular problems and hearing loss due to antibiotic, gentamicin,
in humans.
Possible delayed transient or permanent hearing loss due to antibiotic,
kanamycin (SM), in humans, in particular with kidney disorders or with simultaneous administration of ethacrynic acid.
Possible delayed transient or permanent hearing loss due to diuretic, ethacrynic acid (SM), in humans.
Possible delayed transient or permanent severe hearing loss due to oral,
parenteral, or topical administration of antibiotic, neomycin, in humans.
Possible damage to eighth cranial nerve, primarily hearing loss, due to
antibiotic, paromomycin, in humans.
Possible hearing loss due to antibiotic, rifampicin, in humans.
High risk of damage to eighth cranial nerve, primarily transient or permanent
vestibular problems but also hearing loss, due to antibiotic, streptomycin,
in humans.
Possible damage to eighth cranial nerve, primarily hearing loss, due to high

doses of antibiotic, vancomycin, for long period of more than 10 days in
humans, in particular with kidney disorders.
Risk of damage to eighth cranial nerve, vestibular problems and hearing loss,
due to high doses of antibiotic, viomycin, for long period of more than 10
days in humans, in particular with kidney disorders.
   (AD) Discussion of toxic effects of antibiotics.   (ENG)

653

Possible ototoxic effects due to antibiotic, kanamycin, in humans with acute
genitourinary system infections.
Possible ototoxic effects due to antibiotic, gentamicin, in humans with acute
genitourinary system infections.
   (AD) Need for careful consideration in use of kanamycin and gentamicin in
   therapy, in particular in patients with kidney disorders.   (ENG)

656

Possible permanent severe damage to eighth cranial nerve, primarily vestibular problems but also hearing loss, due to parenteral administration of
antibiotic, streptomycin, in humans with tuberculosis, in particular with
concurrent kidney disorder.
Possible permanent severe damage to eighth cranial nerve due to parenteral
administration of antibiotic, viomycin, in humans with tuberculosis.
Possible permanent severe damage to eighth cranial nerve due to parenteral
administration of antibiotic, kanamycin, in humans with tuberculosis.
Possible permanent severe damage to eighth cranial nerve due to parenteral
administration of antibiotic, capreomycin, in humans with tuberculosis.
   (AD) Discussion of primary and secondary drugs used in treatment of tuberculosis.   (ENG)

657

Possible ototoxic effects due to parenteral, intramuscular, administration of
2 g of antibiotic, kanamycin, in humans with gonorrhea, in particular with
concurrent kidney disorders.   (ENG)

662

Hearing loss due to 250 mg of antibiotic, kanamycin (kanamycin sulfate), for
8 days in animals, guinea pigs, 200 to 300 g weight with exposure to noise.
   (CT) Same method using 0.9 percent sodium chloride in guinea pigs, control
   group.
   (AD) Study of ototoxic effects of kanamycin when administered to guinea
   pigs with exposure to noise.   (GER)

666

Permanent severe and possibly delayed and progressive hearing loss and vestibular problems due to parenteral administration of antibiotic, kanamycin, in
humans, in particular with severe kidney disorders.
Permanent severe and possibly delayed and progressive hearing loss and vestibular problems due to parenteral administration of antibiotic, neomycin, in
humans, in particular with severe kidney disorders.
   (AD) Cochleo-vestibulotoxic effects of kanamycin and neomycin usually dose
   related but occur also after low doses.
   (AD) Higher risk of ototoxic effects due to kanamycin and neomycin in
   older patients.
   (AD) Need for audiometry 2 times a week with administration of antibiotics
   for more than 7 days.
   (AD) Recommended adult dose of 1.5 g daily for not more than 1 week and
   lower doses in patients with kidney disorder and dehydration.
   (AD) Suggested use of kanamycin and neomycin for only severe infections.
   (AD) Kanamycin reported less toxic than neomycin.
Hearing loss due to oral administration of antibiotic, neomycin, in humans.
 (ENG)

670

Possible vestibular problems due to parenteral administration of antibiotic,
gentamicin, in humans.
Damage to eighth cranial nerve, primarily hearing loss, usually permanent,
due to parenteral administration of high doses of antibiotic, kanamycin, for
more than 10 days in humans, in particular with kidney disorders.

Damage to eighth cranial nerve, primarily hearing loss, usually permanent, due to parenteral administration of high doses of antibiotic, neomycin, for more than 10 days in humans, in particular with kidney disorders.
Possible damage to eighth cranial nerve, primarily hearing loss, due to parenteral administration of antibiotic, paromomycin, in humans.
Transient or permanent vestibular problems due to parenteral administration of antibiotic, streptomycin, in humans.
Permanent severe hearing loss due to parenteral administration of antibiotic, dihydrostreptomycin, in humans.
Damage to eighth cranial nerve, primarily hearing loss, due to parenteral administration of high doses of antibiotic, vancomycin, for more than 10 days in humans, in particular with kidney disorders.
Damage to eighth cranial nerve, vestibular problems and hearing loss, due to parenteral administration of high doses of antibiotic, viomycin, for more than 10 days in humans, in particular with kidney disorders.
   (AD) Discussion of toxic effects of antibiotics. (ENG)

672

Possible sensorineural hearing loss due to parenteral administration of antibiotic, kanamycin, in humans with kidney disorders.
   (AD) Need for decr in dosage and 3 to 4 days interval between doses in patients with kidney disorders.
Possible vestibular problems and hearing loss due to parenteral administration of antibiotic, streptomycin, in humans with kidney disorders.
   (AD) Need for decr in dosage and 3 to 4 days interval between doses in patients with kidney disorders.
Possible vestibular problems due to parenteral administration of antibiotic, gentamicin, in humans with kidney disorders.
   (AD) Need for decr in dosage and unknown period between doses in patients with kidney disorders.
Possible hearing loss due to parenteral administration of antibiotic, vancomycin, in humans with kidney disorders.
   (AD) Need for decr in dosage and 9 days interval between doses in patients with kidney disorders.
   (AD) Report on use of antibiotics in patients with kidney disorders.
   (AD) Need for total initial dose followed by 50 percent of initial dose at recommended intervals.
   (AD) Change in dosage based on serum half-life of antibiotic.
   (AD) Literature review of effect of antibiotics in patients with kidney disorders. (ENG)

674

No ototoxic effects due to parenteral, intramuscular, administration of 1 g twice daily for 1 to 2 days, followed by 1 g daily for 8 to 10 days, with reduced doses in patients with kidney disorder, of antibiotic, kanamycin (SM), for total of about 9 to 12 days in 28 humans, adult and aged, 26 to 80 years age, male and female, with severe infections due to gram-negative bacilli, with bacteremia in 16 cases and kidney disorder in 8 cases. Simultaneous administration of antibiotic, chloramphenicol (SM), in most of 16 humans with bacteremia.
   (AD) Use of kanamycin without ototoxic effects in patients with kidney disorders due to decr in dosage and tests of serum levels of antibiotic. (ENG)

675

Possible total hearing loss due to parenteral administration of antibiotic, kanamycin (kanamycin sulfate), in humans with genitourinary system infections and with concurrent kidney disorder. (ENG)

688

Hearing loss due to antibiotic, kanamycin, in 2 (8 percent) of 26 humans after 3 months and in 1 (5 percent) of 21 humans after 6 months of retreatment for pulmonary tuberculosis.
   (CT) Audiograms, pretreatment and posttreatment.
Hearing loss due to antibiotic, kanamycin, for 6 months in 14.9 percent of humans during retreatment for pulmonary tuberculosis.
   (AD) Hearing loss confirmed by audiograms. (ENG)

692

Bilateral sensorineural hearing loss possibly due to topical, direct site,
administration in vertebral canal of 500 mg, in 2 cc water, of antibiotic,
kanamycin (kanamycin sulfate), in 1 dose in 1 human, aged, 67 years age,
male, with previous hearing loss, during surgery for lumbar disc.
   (AD) Case report of hearing loss possibly due to kanamycin.
   (AD) Hearing loss confirmed by audiometry.
   (AD) Neurotoxic effects resulted from kanamycin administration.   (ENG)

698

Hearing loss, after 3 months in most cases, due to parenteral administration
of 0.5 g twice daily for 7 days a week of antibiotic, kanamycin, in 29 (39
percent) of 75 humans with pulmonary tuberculosis.
Damage to eighth cranial nerve due to parenteral administration of 1 g twice
daily for 2 days a week of antibiotic, kanamycin, for more than 12 months in
5 (7 percent) of 64 humans with pulmonary tuberculosis.
   (AD) Low incidence of ototoxic effects reported in study possibly due to
   administration of kanamycin only 2 days a week.
Damage to eighth cranial nerve due to parenteral administration of 15 mg per
kg daily of antibiotic, kanamycin, in 4 (6 percent) of 65 humans with pulmonary tuberculosis and with previous hearing loss.
Hearing loss due to parenteral administration of 15 to 20 mg per kg for 5
days a week of antibiotic, (SQ) kanamycin, in 19 (22 percent) of 82 humans
with pulmonary tuberculosis and with previous hearing loss in 10 cases.
   (AD) Hearing loss confirmed by audiometry.
   (AD) Ototoxic effects in patients 50 years or over age in 15 of 19 cases.
Previous administration of antibiotic, (SQ) streptomycin, for long period in
82 humans with pulmonary tuberculosis.
Previous administration of antibiotic, (SQ) viomycin, in 10 of 82 humans with
pulmonary tuberculosis.
   (AD) Discussion of ototoxic effects of kanamycin reported in 4 studies.
   (AD) Significant factors in kanamycin ototoxicity reported to be age over
   50 years, high daily dose of more than 20 mg per kg, high serum level of
   more than 25 mcg per ml, concurrent kidney disorders, and previous hearing
   loss.   (ENG)

699

Permanent hearing loss due to parenteral, intramuscular, administration of
0.5 g at 6-hour intervals for 48 hours and then at 12-hour intervals for 5
days, total dose of more than 12 g, to produce peak serum levels of 10 to 30
mcg per ml after 12 hours, of antibiotic, kanamycin, for about 7 days in 2 of
about 300 humans with various infections.
   (AD) Higher risk of kanamycin ototoxicity in patients with dehydration or
   kidney disorder or with total doses of about 20 g.
   (AD) Prevention or decr in ototoxic effects with regulation of daily dose
   and duration of therapy and with tests of kidney function.   (ENG)

701

Hearing loss due to antibiotic, kanamycin, in humans.
   (AD) Study of clinical use of vitamin K-1 in hearing loss due to kanamycin.   (JAP)

705

No significant loss of hair cells of organ of Corti due to 15, 50, or 100 mg
per kg daily of antibiotic, kanamycin, for 3 or 5 weeks in animals, guinea
pigs.
No significant loss of hair cells of organ of Corti due to 15 or 50 mg per kg
daily of antibiotic, kanamycin, for 3 weeks in animals, guinea pigs, with
exposure to low level noise, 68 to 72 decibels at 125 Hz.
Damage to outer hair cells primarily in apical coil of cochlea due to 15 or
50 mg per kg daily of antibiotic, kanamycin, for 5 weeks in animals, guinea
pigs, with exposure to low level noise, 68 to 72 decibels at 125 Hz.
Damage to outer hair cells primarily in apical coil of cochlea due to 100 mg
per kg daily of antibiotic, kanamycin, for 3 weeks in animals, guinea pigs,
with exposure to low level noise, 68 to 72 decibels at 125 Hz.
   (AD) Earlier occurrence of hair cell damage with incr in dosage of kanamycin in guinea pigs with exposure to low level noise.
   (AD) Study of sensitization by low level noise of hair cells of cochlea to

damage by low doses of kanamycin. (ENG)

715

Loss of outer hair cells of organ of Corti in lower part of first coil of
cochlea due to parenteral, intramuscular, administration of 400 mg per kg of
antibiotic, capreomycin, for 28 days in 40 percent of 10 animals, guinea
pigs, albino, 300 g weight.
Severe loss of outer hair cells of organ of Corti from lower part of basal
coil to upper coil of cochlea due to parenteral, intramuscular, administration of 400 mg per kg of antibiotic, kanamycin, for 28 days in 100 percent of
11 animals, guinea pigs, albino, 300 g weight.
   (CT) Test of Preyer reflex before, during, and after administration of
   antibiotics.
   (AD) Study suggested that capreomycin less ototoxic than kanamycin in
   guinea pigs.
   (AD) No observed damage to vestibular apparatus. (JAP)

724

Hearing loss due to antibiotic, kanamycin, in humans in dental treatment.
(ENG)

727

Decr in cochleotoxic effects due to parenteral, subcutaneous, administration
of antibiotic, kanamycin (IB), in animals, cats, with administration of
pantothenic acid.
   (AD) Electrophysiological study of effect of pantothenic acid on kanamycin
   ototoxicity in cats. (GER)

731

Possible damage to eighth cranial nerve, vestibular problems, due to antibiotic, streptomycin, in humans with gram-negative bacilli.
Possible damage to eighth cranial nerve, hearing loss, due to antibiotic,
kanamycin, in humans with gram-negative bacilli.
Possible damage to eighth cranial nerve, hearing loss, due to antibiotic,
neomycin, in humans with gram-negative bacilli.
Possible damage to eighth cranial nerve, vestibular problems, due to antibio-
tic, gentamicin, in humans with gram-negative bacilli.
Possible ototoxic effects due to antibiotic, vancomycin, in humans with gram-
positive cocci.
   (AD) Need to decr dosage of antibiotics in patients with kidney disorders.
   (AD) Discussion of possible toxic effects of antibiotics used in surgery.
   (ENG)

                              Lincomycin

250

Damage to vestibular apparatus due to more than 1 g daily of antibiotic,
streptomycin, for 60 to 120 days in 25 percent of humans.
Dizziness 5 days after cessation of treatment due to parenteral, intramuscular, administration of 1 g every 12 hours of antibiotic, streptomycin (SM),
for 9 days in 1 human, adult, 44 years age, female, with peritonitis.
Simultaneous parenteral, intravenous, administration of 600 mg every 18 hours
of antibiotic, lincomycin (SM), for 9 days in 1 human, adult, 44 years age,
female, with peritonitis.
   (AD) Case report of vestibular problem due to streptomycin.
Damage to cochlea due to antibiotic, dihydrostreptomycin, for more than 1
week in 4 to 15 percent of humans.
Sensorineural hearing loss and damage to organ of Corti due to antibiotic,
kanamycin, in humans.
Sensorineural hearing loss and damage to organ of Corti due to antibiotic,
vancomycin, in humans.
   (AD) Discussion of cochleo-vestibulotoxic effects due to antibiotic therapy in surgery. (ENG)

520

Decr in time of latency with incr in intensity of acoustic stimuli due to
parenteral, intraperitoneal, administration of 80 mg per kg daily, total of
480 mg, of antibiotic, cephalothin (cephalothin sodium), for 15 days in 10

animals, guinea pigs, albino.
Decr in time of latency with incr in intensity of acoustic stimuli due to
parenteral, intraperitoneal, administration of 20 mg per kg daily, total of
120 mg, of antibiotic, lincomycin (lincomycin chloride), for 15 days in 10
animals, guinea pigs, albino.
Decr in time of latency with incr in intensity of acoustic stimuli due to
parenteral, intraperitoneal, administration of 50 mg per kg daily, total of
300 mg, of antibiotic, cephaloridine, for 15 days in 10 animals, guinea pigs,
albino.
  (CT) Study of guinea pigs, control group, not treated with antibiotics.
  (AD) Study of response of guinea pigs to acoustic stimuli after treatment
  with antibiotics.   (IT)

531

Hearing loss due to antibiotic, lincomycin, in 1 human treated with hemodialysis after bilateral nephrectomy for kidney disorder.
  (AD) Hearing loss confirmed by audiogram.   (CZ)

Nalidixic acid

414

Transient hearing loss in short time after injection due to parenteral,
intravenous, administration of (SQ) high doses, 500 mg each dose, of diuretic, (SQ) furosemide, in (SQ) total of 2 doses, each for duration of 3
minutes, on consecutive days in 1 human, adult, 49 years age, female, with
chronic kidney disorder.
  (AD) No observed hearing loss before treatment with furosemide.
  (AD) Normal hearing within 4 hours.
No hearing loss due to parenteral, intravenous, administration of (SQ) 240 mg
of diuretic, (SQ) furosemide, in (SQ) 1 dose for duration of 5 minutes in 1
human, adult, 49 years age, female, with chronic kidney disorder.
  (AD) Suggested that cochleotoxic effect of furosemide is dose related.
  (AD) Different individual responses to furosemide suggest other factors in
  ototoxic effects.
Previous administration of antibiotic, (SQ) nalidixic acid, in 1 human,
adult, 49 years age, female, with chronic kidney disorder.   (ENG)

483

Possible damage to vestibular nerve and cochlear nerve due to antibiotic,
streptomycin, in humans with or without kidney disorder.
Possible damage to vestibular nerve and cochlear nerve due to antibiotic,
gentamicin, in humans with or without kidney disorder.
Possible damage to vestibular nerve and cochlear nerve due to antibiotic,
kanamycin, in humans with or without kidney disorder.
Possible damage to vestibular nerve and cochlear nerve due to antibiotic,
neomycin, in humans with or without kidney disorder.
  (AD) Incidence of effects on vestibular function highest in streptomycin,
  followed by gentamicin, kanamycin, and neomycin.
  (AD) Incidence of effects on cochlear function highest in neomycin, fol-
  lowed by kanamycin, gentamicin, and streptomycin.
  (AD) Need for careful consideration in clinical use of aminoglycoside
  antibiotics.
Possible cochlear impairment and vestibular problems due to antibiotic,
paromomycin, in humans.
Possible dizziness and ataxia due to antibiotic, polymyxin B, in humans.
Possible but rare dizziness and vertigo due to antibiotic, nalidixic acid, in
humans.   (ENG)

623

Vertigo due to oral administration of antibiotic, nalidixic acid, in humans.
  (ENG)

Neomycin

001

Permanent bilateral high frequency hearing loss due to topical administration
by irrigation of joint cavity of left knee with 50 cc of 10 percent solution
of antibiotic, neomycin, for every 3 hours for 3 days and every 6 hours for 5

days in 1 human, child, 6 years age, male, 56 lb weight.
   (CT) Pretreatment audiogram showed normal bilateral hearing sensitivity.
   (ENG)

004

Bilateral sensorineural hearing loss due to oral administration of total of
600 g of antibiotic, neomycin, in 300 days in 1 human, child, 11 years age,
male, with chronic colitis.
   (AD) Literature review showed 4 other case reports of hearing loss due to
   oral administration of neomycin. (ENG)

006

Range of degrees of degeneration of endorgan of organ of Corti due to parenteral, intratympanic, administration of range of 1 to 100 mg per ml concentration of antibiotic, neomycin, in 1 injection in animals, guinea pigs,
young, 250 g average weight.
Range of degrees of degeneration of endorgan of organ of Corti due to parenteral, intratympanic, administration of range of 1 to 100 mg per ml concentration of antibiotic, polymyxin B, in 1 injection in animals, guinea pigs,
young, 250 g average weight.
Range of degrees of degeneration of endorgan of organ of Corti due to parenteral, intratympanic, administration of range of 1 to 100 mg per ml concentration of antibiotic, colistin, in 1 injection in animals, guinea pigs,
young, 250 g average weight.
   (CT) Same method using comparable concentration of saline solution or
   solution of glucose or sodium G penicillin in guinea pigs, control group,
   showed no histological damage.
Degeneration of endorgan of organ of Corti due to topical administration to
ear canal of range of 5 to 100 mg per ml 1 time daily of antibiotic, neomycin, for 8 to 25 days in 14 animals, guinea pigs. (ENG)

009

Delayed permanent sensorineural hearing loss and damage to outer hair cells
of basal and middle coils of cochlea due to unspecified doses of antibiotic,
dihydrostreptomycin, in humans.
Vertigo and dizziness due to unspecified method of administration of 2 to 3 g
daily of antibiotic, streptomycin (streptomycin sulfate), for 30 to 50 days
in humans with tuberculosis.
Hearing loss due to unspecified method of administration of high doses of
antibiotic, streptomycin (streptomycin sulfate), for long period in humans.
Gradual high frequency hearing loss and tinnitus and degeneration of hair
cells of organ of Corti in basal coil of cochlea due to unspecified doses of
antibiotic, kanamycin, in humans.
Delayed severe high frequency hearing loss due to parenteral, oral, or topical administration by inhalation of unspecified doses of antibiotic, neomycin, for unspecified period in humans with kidney disorder.
Complete degeneration of inner hair cells due to unspecified method of administration of 18 g of antibiotic, neomycin, for unspecified period in
humans with bacterial endocarditis.
Lesions in organ of Corti due to parenteral administration of unspecified
doses of antibiotic, polymyxin B, for unspecified period in animals, guinea
pigs.
Sensorineural hearing loss due to parenteral, intravenous, administration of
80 to 95 mg per ml of antibiotic, vancomycin, for unspecified period in
humans with kidney disorder.
   (AD) Sensorineural hearing loss and vestibular problems due to 6 antibiotics in humans and animals, guinea pigs.
   (AD) Literature review of ototoxic effects of antibiotics. (ENG)

010

Permanent sensorineural hearing loss due to parenteral, intramuscular, administration of low doses, less than 2 g, of antibiotic, (SQ) kanamycin
(kanamycin sulfate), for short period in 5 humans, adult, range of 33 to 47
years age, range of 90 to 177 lb weight, with kidney disorder.
Permanent sensorineural hearing loss due to parenteral, intramuscular, administration of low doses, less than 2 g, of antibiotic, (SQ) streptomycin,
for short period in 5 humans, adult, range of 33 to 47 years age, range of 90
to 177 lb weight, with kidney disorder.

Permanent sensorineural hearing loss due to parenteral, intramuscular, administration of low doses, less than 2 g, of antibiotic, (SQ) neomycin, for
short period in 5 humans, adult, range of 33 to 47 years age, range of 90 to
177 lb weight, with kidney disorder.
Permanent sensorineural hearing loss due to parenteral, intramuscular, administration of low doses, less than 2 g, of diuretic, (SQ) ethacrynic acid,
for short period in 5 humans, adult, range of 33 to 47 years age, range of 90
to 177 lb weight, with kidney disorder.
   (AD) Study of cochleotoxic effects of kanamycin with other antibiotics and
   with ethacrynic acid.   (ENG)

                                                                     012

Permanent sensorineural hearing loss due to parenteral, intramuscular, administration of high doses, about 100 mg per kg daily, total of more than 6 g
of antibiotic, (SQ) neomycin (neomycin sulfate), for 7 days in 1 human,
Caucasian, infant, 13 months age.
Unspecified effects due to parenteral, intramuscular, administration of about
12 mg per kg daily recommended dosage, total of 20 mg, of antibiotic, (SQ)
kanamycin (kanamycin sulfate), for less than 24 hours in 1 human, Caucasian,
infant, 13 months age.
   (CT) Normal response to acoustic stimulus before administration of antibiotics.
   (AD) Suggested that ototoxicity of neomycin not potentiated by administration of kanamycin in this case.   (ENG)

                                                                     013

No reported ototoxic effects due to antibiotic, neomycin (CB), in 26 humans
with inflammation of external auditory meatus.
No reported ototoxic effects due to antibiotic, polymyxin B (CB), in 26
humans with inflammation of external auditory meatus.
   (AD) Study of use of neomycin, polymyxin B, and fluocinolone acetonide in
   treatment of inflammation of external auditory meatus.   (FR)

                                                                     025

Effect on electrical response of cochlea due to 300 mg per kg and 50 mg per
kg of antibiotic, neomycin, for 6 days and 10 days respectively in 2 groups
of animals, guinea pigs.
Decr in cochleotoxic effect due to antibiotic, neomycin (IB), in animals,
guinea pigs, with administration of ATP.   (GER)

                                                                     027

Progressive bilateral high frequency hearing loss and tinnitus due to topical
administration by irrigation of wound with 80 ml every 4 hours for 2 weeks
and then 40 ml every 4 hours of 0.5 percent solution of antibiotic, (SQ)
neomycin (SM), in 1 human, adult, 24 years age, male, paraplegic, with infection of ulcer of left hip.
Progressive bilateral high frequency hearing loss and tinnitus due to topical
administration by irrigation of wound with 80 ml every 4 hours for 2 weeks
and then 40 ml every 4 hours of 0.1 percent solution of antibiotic, (SQ)
polymyxin B (SM), in 1 human, adult, 24 years age, male, paraplegic, with
infection of ulcer of left hip.
No reported ototoxic effects due to unspecified method of administration of 1
g daily of antibiotic, (SQ) streptomycin, for 5 days in 1 human, adult, 24
years age, male, paraplegic, with infection of ulcer of left hip.   (ENG)

                                                                     045

Progressive degeneration of endorgan of cochlea due to low doses of antibiotic, dihydrostreptomycin, in animals, guinea pigs.
Progressive degeneration of endorgan of cochlea due to low doses of antibiotic, neomycin, in animals, guinea pigs.   (JAP)

                                                                     051

Progressive permanent sensorineural hearing loss and tinnitus due to topical
administration to joint of left knee and parenteral, intramuscular, administration of high doses, total of 42.5 g, of antibiotic, (SQ) neomycin, for
long period, 19 days, in 1 human, adult, with infection of left knee.
Previous administration of high doses of antibiotic, (SQ) chloramphenicol,
for unspecified period in 1 human, adult, with infection of left knee.

(AD) Report of case in court with claim of negligence for administration
of high doses of neomycin that resulted in hearing loss. (ENG)

                                                                    052
Ototoxic effects due to parenteral, oral, and topical administration of
antibiotic, neomycin, in humans.
    (AD) Discussion of neomycin ototoxicity due to all usual administration
    routes. (ENG)

                                                                    053
Ototoxic effects due to topical administration of high doses of antibiotic,
neomycin, in humans.
    (AD) Need for careful consideration of dosage of neomycin used in topical
    administration. (ENG)

                                                                    059
Bilateral sensorineural hearing loss due to oral administration of 0 to 12 g
daily, total of 2500 g, of antibiotic, neomycin, for 16 months in 1 human,
Caucasian, adult, 49 years age, female, chronic alcoholic, with hepatic
encephalopathy and normal kidney function.
Bilateral sensorineural hearing loss due to oral administration of 0 to 4 g
daily, total of 800 g, of antibiotic, (SQ) neomycin, for 21 months in 1
human, Caucasian, adult, 47 years age, female, chronic alcoholic, with hepatic encephalopathy and normal kidney function.
More severe sensorineural hearing loss due to oral administration of 6 g
daily, total of 111 g, of antibiotic, (SQ) paromomycin, for 9 months in 1
human, Caucasian, adult, 47 years age, female, chronic alcoholic, with hepatic encephalopathy and normal kidney function.
Sensorineural hearing loss due to oral administration of 0 to 12 g daily,
total of 1500 g, of antibiotic, neomycin, for 11 months in 1 human, Caucasian, adult, 39 years age, female, chronic alcoholic, with hepatic encephalopathy and some kidney disorder.
Sensorineural hearing loss in right ear due to oral administration of 3 to 4
g daily, total of 500 g, of antibiotic, (SQ) neomycin, for 8 months in 1
human, Caucasian, aged, 66 years age, female, with hepatic encephalopathy and
kidney disorder.
    (AD) Tinnitus and sudden deafness in left ear 27 years earlier.
Sensorineural hearing loss in right ear due to oral administration of total
of 240 g of antibiotic, (SQ) paromomycin, for long period in 1 human, Caucasian, aged, 66 years age, female, with hepatic encephalopathy and kidney
disorder.
Sequential administration of unspecified doses of diuretic, (SQ) furosemide,
for unspecified period in 1 human, Caucasian, aged, 66 years age, female,
with hepatic encephalopathy and kidney disorder.
Bilateral sensorineural hearing loss due to oral administration of 0 to 12 g
daily, total of 1000 to 1500 g, of antibiotic, (SQ) neomycin, for 28 months
in 1 human, Caucasian, adult, 60 years age, male, chronic alcoholic, with
hepatic encephalopathy and kidney disorder.
Bilateral sensorineural hearing loss due to oral administration of total of
300 g of antibiotic, (SQ) paromomycin, for long period in 1 human, Caucasian,
adult, 60 years age, male, chronic alcoholic, with hepatic encephalopathy and
kidney disorder.
Sequential administration of unspecified doses of (SQ) diuretics for unspecified period in 1 human, Caucasian, adult, 60 years age, male, chronic alcoholic, with hepatic encephalopathy and kidney disorder.
    (AD) Discussion of 5 case reports of hearing loss due to antibiotic thera-
    py.
    (AD) Audiograms confirmed hearing loss in all cases. (ENG)

                                                                    063
Progressive permanent bilateral sensorineural hearing loss due to topical
administration by irrigation of wound with 1000 ml of 1 percent solution (6.5
g) of antibiotic, neomycin (CB) (neomycin sulfate), in 1 administration in 1
human, Caucasian, adolescent, 18 years age, male, with gunshot wound of
abdomen.
    (AD) Hearing loss reported 21 days after treatment.
Progressive permanent bilateral sensorineural hearing loss due to topical
administration by irrigation of wound with 1000 ml of 0.1 percent solution

(650 mg) of antibiotic, polymyxin B (CB) (polymyxin B sulfate), in 1 administration in 1 human, Caucasian, adolescent, 18 years age, male, with gunshot wound of abdomen.

(AD) Study reported that ototoxic effects only due to neomycin.

(AD) Hemodialysis 24 hours after treatment for prevention of hearing loss not satisfactory.

Progressive permanent bilateral sensorineural hearing loss due to topical administration by irrigation of wound with high doses of 1 percent solution of antibiotic, (SQ) neomycin, for 22 days in 1 human, Caucasian, adult, 20 years age, male, with gunshot wounds.

(AD) Hearing loss reported after 19 days of treatment.

Previous administration of unspecified dose of antibiotic, (SQ) streptomycin, for 6 days in 1 human, Caucasian, adult, 20 years age, male, with gunshot wounds.

Progressive permanent bilateral sensorineural hearing loss due to topical administration by irrigation of wound with total of 4000 ml of 1 percent solution of antibiotic, neomycin (CB) (neomycin sulfate), in 4 days in 1 human, Caucasian, adult, 39 years age, male, with wounds.

(AD) Hearing loss reported within 5 days.

Progressive permanent bilateral sensorineural hearing loss due to topical administration by irrigation of wound with total of 4000 ml of 0.1 percent solution of antibiotic, polymyxin B (CB) (polymyxin B sulfate), in 4 days in 1 human, Caucasian, adult, 39 years age, male, with wounds.

(AD) Discussion of 3 case reports of hearing loss due to topical administration of antibiotics. (ENG)

064

Risk of hearing loss due to topical administration of more than 1 g of antibiotic, neomycin, in more than 7 days in humans.

(AD) Comment on risk of hearing loss with topical administration of neomycin. (ENG)

074

Decr in cochlear microphonic due to topical administration to round window of range of 210 to 680 g of antibiotic, streptomycin, in animals, guinea pigs.
Decr in cochlear microphonic due to topical administration to round window of range of 210 to 680 g of antibiotic, kanamycin, in animals, guinea pigs.
No decr in cochlear microphonic due to topical administration to round window of range of 210 to 680 g of antibiotic, neomycin, in animals, guinea pigs.
(POL)

080

Hearing loss and vertigo due to parenteral administration of antibiotic, streptomycin, in humans, child and adult, with normal kidney function and with kidney disorder.

(AD) Suggested use for severe infections only.

Delayed permanent hearing loss due to antibiotic, dihydrostreptomycin, in humans.

(AD) High risk of ototoxic effects with clinical use.

Hearing loss due to oral administration of antibiotic, paromomycin, in humans.

Progressive permanent hearing loss and tinnitus due to parenteral administration of antibiotic, kanamycin, in humans.

Progressive permanent hearing loss and tinnitus due to parenteral and topical administration of antibiotic, neomycin, in humans.

(AD) Need for careful consideration in use of paromomycin, kanamycin, and neomycin due to potential ototoxicity.

(AD) Discussion of ototoxic effects of 5 antibiotics. (ENG)

085

Hearing loss due to antibiotic, viomycin, in 17.7 percent of 152 humans with tuberculosis.

(CT) Systematic controls with audiology.

Hearing loss due to antibiotic, viomycin (IB), in only 5.3 percent of 36 humans with previous hearing loss with administration of nialamid.

Hearing loss due to antibiotic, kanamycin, in 20 percent of 55 humans with tuberculosis.

Hearing loss due to antibiotic, kanamycin (IB), in 0 of 25 humans with pre-

vious hearing loss with administration of nialamid.
Lesion of inner ear due to antibiotic, neomycin (IB), in only 1 human with
previous hearing loss with administration of nialamid.   (GER)

104

Hearing loss due to 1.5 g daily, total of 12 g, of antibiotic, neomycin, in 1
human, aged, 90 years age.
  (AD) Cochleotoxic effect due to negligence of physician.   (SW)

150

Total sensorineural hearing loss due to topical administration by irrigation
of mediastinum with 2400 ml per 24 hours, total of 72 g, of 0.3 percent
solution of antibiotic, neomycin, for 11 days in 1 human, adult, 60 years
age, male, with purulent mediastinitis.
  (AD) High serum neomycin concentrations decr by hemodialysis.   (ENG)

157

Damage to hair cells of organ of Corti and membranous labyrinth and to
neurons of spiral ganglion due to parenteral, subcutaneous, administration of
100 mg per kg, in physiological saline, of antibiotic, neomycin (neomycin
sulfate), in 5 and 7 doses in 21 animals, guinea pigs, albino, 250 to 700 g
weight.
Moderate damage to organ of Corti, less degeneration of hair cells of membranous labyrinth, and decr in number of neurons of spiral ganglion due to
parenteral, subcutaneous, administration of 100 mg per kg of antibiotic,
neomycin (neomycin sulfate), in 10,12,14,15, and 20 doses in 33 animals,
guinea pigs, albino, 250 to 700 g weight.
Range of degrees of degeneration up to complete destruction of organ of Corti
and disappearance of most of neurons of spiral ganglion due to parenteral,
subcutaneous, administration of 100 mg per kg of antibiotic, neomycin (neomycin sulfate), in 30 doses in 6 animals, guinea pigs, albino, 250 to 700 g
weight.
Range of degrees of degeneration up to complete destruction of organ of Corti
and disappearance of most of neurons of spiral ganglion due to parenteral,
subcutaneous, administration of 150 mg per kg of antibiotic, neomycin (neomycin sulfate), in 10 and 20 doses in 4 animals, guinea pigs, albino, 250 to
700 g weight.
  (CT) Study of 19 guinea pigs, control group.
  (AD) Damage due to high doses for shorter period similar to damage due to
  low doses for longer period.   (ENG)

158

No reported ototoxic effects due to 5 g of antibiotic, (SQ) streptomycin, in
1 human, adult, 63 years age, male, with bronchopleural fistula and staphylococcal empyema.
Progressive total bilateral sensorineural hearing loss due to topical administration by irrigation of empyema cavity with (SQ) 1200 ml of 1 percent
solution of antibiotic, (SQ) neomycin, for 10 days, total of 33 irrigations,
in 1 human, adult, 63 years age, male, with bronchopleural fistula and staphylococcal empyema.
Progressive total bilateral sensorineural hearing loss due to topical administration by irrigation of empyema cavity with (SQ) 700 ml of 1 percent solution, total of 403 g in all, of antibiotic, (SQ) neomycin, in 1 administration in 1 human, adult, 63 years age, male, at time of surgery to close
cavity.
Sequential parenteral, intramuscular, administration of total of 4 g of
antibiotic, (SQ) streptomycin (streptomycin sulfate), for 4 to 5 days in 1
human, adult, 63 years age, male, after closure of empyema cavity.
  (AD) No hearing loss before closure of cavity.
  (AD) Hearing loss confirmed by audiogram but no vestibular problems detected by vestibular function tests.
  (AD) Suggested that hearing loss due to neomycin only and not to streptomycin.   (ENG)

169

Progressive sensorineural hearing loss, complete range of degrees of damage
to organ of Corti, and degeneration in cochlear nuclei due to parenteral,
intramuscular, administration of 15 to 100 mg per kg daily of antibiotic,

kanamycin (kanamycin sulfate), for 28 to 180 days in 3 animals, monkeys,
young, 2 to 6 years age, male and female, 3 to 9 kg weight, conditioned.
High frequency hearing loss and damage to organ of Corti due to parenteral,
intramuscular, administration of 100 mg per kg daily of antibiotic, neomycin
(neomycin sulfate), for 5 days in 1 animal, monkey, young, conditioned.
Delayed severe sensorineural hearing loss after 2 months and severe damage to
organ of Corti due to parenteral, intramuscular, administration of 50 mg per
kg of antibiotic, neomycin (neomycin sulfate), for 15 days in 1 animal,
monkey, young, conditioned.
   (CT) Pretreatment hearing baseline determined.
   (AD) Study showed correlation of measurement of hearing loss and histopathology of cochlea in same subject.
   (AD) Cochleograms made to show patterns of cell loss.
   (AD) Reported that neomycin more ototoxic than kanamycin.   (ENG)

                                                                      170

Sensorineural hearing loss due to topical administration in ear drops of
antibiotic, neomycin, in humans with no other explanation for hearing loss.
Sensorineural hearing loss due to topical administration in ear drops of
antibiotic, chloramphenicol, in humans with no other explanation for hearing
loss.
Sensorineural hearing loss due to topical administration in ear drops of
antibiotic, framycetin, in humans with no other explanation for hearing loss.
   (AD) Comment on topical use of antibiotics and possible risk of cochleotoxic effects.   (ENG)

                                                                      192

Sensorineural hearing loss, dizziness, vertigo, and nystagmus due to topical,
cutaneous, administration in ointment of 0.3 percent concentration of antibiotic, (SQ) neomycin, for 5 months in 1 human, Caucasian, child, 9 years
age, with dermatomyositis.
Sensorineural hearing loss, dizziness, vertigo, and nystagmus due to topical,
cutaneous, administration in ointment of 1 percent concentration of antibiotic, (SQ) neomycin (CB), for 2 months in 1 human, Caucasian, child, 9 years
age, with dermatomyositis.
Sensorineural hearing loss, dizziness, vertigo, and nystagmus due to topical,
cutaneous, administration in ointment of 11 percent concentration of chemical
agent, (SQ) dimethyl sulfoxide (CB), for 2 months in 1 human, Caucasian,
child, 9 years age, with dermatomyositis.
   (AD) Potentiation of cochleo-vestibulotoxic effects of neomycin as result
   of incr cutaneous absorption due to dimethyl sulfoxide.
   (AD) Hearing loss confirmed by audiogram.   (ENG)

                                                                      197

Progressive degeneration of organ of Corti beginning at base of cochlea due
to antibiotic, neomycin, in animals, guinea pigs.
Progressive degeneration of organ of Corti beginning at base of cochlea due
to antibiotic, kanamycin, in animals, guinea pigs.
Progressive degeneration of organ of Corti beginning at base of cochlea due
to antibiotic, framycetin, in animals, guinea pigs.
No damage to hair cells of organ of Corti due to parenteral administration of
high doses of antibiotic, dihydrostreptomycin, for long periods in animals,
guinea pigs.
   (AD) Surface specimen technique used in study of organ of Corti.
   (AD) Damage to organ of Corti due to ototoxic drugs different from that
   due to noise.   (ENG)

                                                                      231

No hearing loss due to 8 g and then 12 g daily of antibiotic, neomycin
(neomycin sulfate), for total of 19 months in 1 human, adult, 48 years age,
male, chronic alcoholic, treated for infections.   (ENG)

                                                                      236

Bilateral high frequency hearing loss due to parenteral, intramuscular,
administration of high dose, 90 mg per kg daily, total of 99.2 g, of antibiotic, kanamycin, for 62 days in 1 human, child, with miliary tuberculosis.
High frequency hearing loss due to parenteral, intramuscular, administration
of high dose, 25 mg per kg daily, total of 22.2 g, of antibiotic, kanamycin,

for 148 days in 1 human, child, with miliary tuberculosis.
Permanent severe sensorineural hearing loss due to parenteral, intramuscular,
administration of high doses of antibiotic, kanamycin, in 1 human, child,
with multiple infections.
Progressive sensorineural hearing loss due to oral administration of antibiotic, neomycin, for 11 months in 1 human, child, 11.5 years age, male, with
severe ulcerative ileocolitis.
  (AD) Hearing loss confirmed by audiogram.
  (AD) Discussion of 4 case reports of ototoxic effects due to kanamycin or
  neomycin.
  (AD) Suggested that risk of kanamycin ototoxicity less in children than in
  adults.
Sensorineural hearing loss due to 10 to 100 mg per kg daily of antibiotic,
kanamycin, for 5 to 95 days in 5 of 30 humans, child and infant, with infections.
  (CT) Study of 30 children and infants, control group, not treated with
  kanamycin.
  (AD) Suggested that cochleotoxic effects related to total dose of kanamy-
  cin.
  (AD) Report on studies made during 8 years of clinical use of kanamycin.
  (ENG)

                                                                        238
Sensorineural hearing loss due to oral administration of 50 to 100 mg per kg
of antibiotic, neomycin, in 9 of 17 humans, child, 2.5 to 7 years age, with
dyspepsia.
  (AD) Hearing loss determined by audiometry. (FR)

                                                                        254
Hearing loss due to antibiotic, neomycin, in humans, infant.
  (AD) Routine use of neomycin for gastroenteritis in infants not recom-
  mended. (ENG)

                                                                        257
Degeneration of hair cells of organ of Corti due to parenteral, intramuscular, administration of 200 mg per kg of antibiotic, neomycin (neomycin sulfate), for 6 days in 15 animals, guinea pigs, albino.
  (CT) Study of 7 guinea pigs, control group.
  (AD) Use of surface specimen technique in study of cochleotoxic effects of
  neomycin. (ENG)

                                                                        273
Vertigo and hearing loss due to topical administration in ear drops of
500,000 ED in distilled water, in 6 to 8 ear drops daily, of antibiotic,
neomycin, for 8 days in 1 human with suppuration from right ear.
  (AD) Hearing loss confirmed by audiometry. (RUS)

                                                                        285
Transient inhibition of endorgan of ampulla due to range of doses of antibio-
tic, streptomycin (streptomycin sulfate), in animals, frogs.
Transient inhibition of endorgan of ampulla due to range of doses of antibio-
tic, dihydrostreptomycin (dihydrostreptomycin sulfate), in animals, frogs.
Transient inhibition of endorgan of ampulla due to range of doses of antibio-
tic, neomycin (neomycin sulfate), in animals, frogs.
Transient inhibition of endorgan of ampulla due to range of doses of antibiotic, kanamycin (kanamycin sulfate), in animals, frogs.
  (CT) Study of frogs, control group.
  (AD) More inhibition of endorgan of ampulla with streptomycin than with
  other aminoglycoside antibiotics.
  (AD) Agreement between in vivo and in vitro observations of intensity of
  action on endorgans of vestibular apparatus. (ENG)

                                                                        316
Possible vestibular problems and cochlear impairment due to more than recommended dose of 15 to 30 mg per kg daily of antibiotic, streptomycin, for long
period in humans.
Hearing loss due to parenteral, intramuscular, administration of total doses
of 5 to 6 g of antibiotic, kanamycin, in humans, adult, with kidney disorder.

Possible hearing loss due to parenteral, topical, or oral administration of
high doses of antibiotic, neomycin, for long period in humans.
Possible hearing loss due to high doses of antibiotic, framycetin, for long
period in humans.
Possible hearing loss due to antibiotic, vancomycin, in humans.
Possible hearing loss and vestibular problems due to antibiotic, viomycin, in
humans.
    (AD) High risk of ototoxicity with simultaneous administration of viomycin
    and streptomycin.
Possible vestibular problems due to antibiotic, gentamicin, in humans.
    (AD) Administration of gentamicin not recommended for newborn infants, for
    humans during pregnancy, and for humans treated with other ototoxic drugs.
Ataxia and hearing loss due to antibiotic, colistin, in humans.
    (AD) Literature review on ototoxic antibiotics.
    (AD) Results of studies on use of pantothenate salt of some antibiotics
    for decr in ototoxicity not clear.
    (AD) Suggested effect of ototoxic antibiotics on breakdown of glucose on
    which hair cells of inner ear depend for energy.   (ENG)

                                                                      324
Ataxia, vestibular problems with improvement in some, and damage to hair
cells of vestibular apparatus due to parenteral, subcutaneous, administration
of 20 mg per kg of antibiotic, gentamicin (gentamicin sulfate), for 19 days
maximum for acute intoxication and 14 days for chronic intoxication in 15
animals, cats.
Hearing loss and damage to hair cells of cochlea due to parenteral, subcutaneous, administration of 20 mg per kg of antibiotic, gentamicin (gentamicin
sulfate), for 19 days maximum for acute intoxication and 14 days for chronic
intoxication in 1 of 15 animals, cats.
    (AD) Preliminary study to determine minimum toxic level of gentamicin by
    parenteral route made previously.
    (AD) Cochleo-vestibulotoxic effects determined by audiometry and vestibu-
    lar function tests.
Permanent severe vestibular problems and damage to hair cells of vestibular
apparatus due to parenteral, subcutaneous, administration of 200 mg per kg of
antibiotic, streptomycin (streptomycin sulfate), in 3 animals, cats.
Hearing loss and damage to hair cells of cochlea due to parenteral, subcutaneous, administration of 200 mg per kg of antibiotic, streptomycin (streptomycin sulfate), in 2 of 3 animals, cats.
Ataxia, vestibular problems, and damage to hair cells of vestibular apparatus
due to topical administration to bulla in solution of 6 percent concentration
in water of antibiotic, gentamicin (gentamicin sulfate), for 19 days in 1
animal, cat.
Ataxia, vestibular problems, and more severe damage to hair cells of vestibular apparatus due to topical administration to bulla in solution of 6 percent
concentration in Monex of antibiotic, gentamicin (gentamicin sulfate), for 5
days in 3 animals, cats.
    (CT) Same method using water or Monex without gentamicin in 11 cats,
    control group, showed no ototoxic effects.
    (AD) Preliminary study to determine concentration of gentamicin for topi-
    cal route made previously.
Vestibular problems due to topical administration to bulla in solution of 6
percent concentration in water of antibiotic, neomycin, for 31 days in 2
animals, cats.
    (AD) Comparative study of effects of gentamicin and other aminoglycoside
    antibiotics.
    (AD) Ototoxicity of gentamicin dose related.   (ENG)

                                                                      335
Vestibular problems due to antibiotic, streptomycin, in humans.
Severe cochlear impairment due to antibiotic, dihydrostreptomycin, in humans.
Cochlear impairment due to parenteral, oral, and topical administration of
antibiotic, neomycin, in humans.
Tinnitus and hearing loss due to antibiotic, kanamycin, in humans.
Vestibular problems and hearing loss due to antibiotic, gentamicin, in hu-
mans.
    (AD) Discussion of clinical use and possible cochleo-vestibulotoxic ef-
    fects of aminoglycoside antibiotics.   (SP)

348

No ototoxic effects due to topical administration in ear drops of 3 to 4 ear
drops 3 times daily of fluocinolone acetonide (CB), for 5 to 10 days in 54
humans, child, adolescent, adult, and aged, male and female, with infections
of middle ear and external ear.
No ototoxic effects due to topical administration in ear drops of 3 to 4 ear
drops 3 times daily of antibiotic, polymyxin B (CB), for 5 to 10 days in 54
humans, child, adolescent, adult, and aged, male and female, with infections
of middle ear and external ear.
No ototoxic effects due to topical administration in ear drops of 3 to 4 ear
drops 3 times daily of antibiotic, neomycin (CB) (neomycin sulfate), for 5 to
10 days in 54 humans, child, adolescent, adult, and aged, male and female,
with infections of middle ear and external ear.   (IT)

356

Hearing loss due to antibiotic, streptomycin, in 120 of 150 humans, child, 2
to 4 years age, most treated when newborn infant or infant for different
disorders.
Hearing loss due to antibiotic, streptomycin (SM), in 30 of 150 humans,
child, 2 to 4 years age, most treated when newborn infant or infant for
different disorders.
Hearing loss due to antibiotic, neomycin (SM), in 30 of 150 humans, child, 2
to 4 years age, most treated when newborn infant or infant for different
disorders.
Hearing loss due to other antibiotics (SM) in 30 of 150 humans, child, 2 to 4
years age, most treated when newborn infant or infant for different disorders.
   (AD) Hearing loss determined by play audiometry.
   (AD) No relationship between hearing loss and dosage or duration of treatment with antibiotics.
   (AD) No improvement in hearing after 1 to 2 years. (RUS)

358

Severe to total hearing loss due to antibiotic, paromomycin, in most of
humans treated.
Severe to total hearing loss due to antibiotic, streptomycin, in most of
humans treated.
Severe to total hearing loss due to antibiotic, neomycin, in most of humans
treated.
Objective but no subjective vestibular problems due to antibiotic, streptomycin, in 2 humans. (RUS)

362

Hearing loss due to high and low doses of antibiotic, streptomycin, in humans, child and adult, with different disorders and with previous hearing
loss in 2 humans.
Hearing loss due to high doses of antibiotic, neomycin, in humans, child and
adult, with different disorders.
   (AD) Need for daily audiometry and vestibular function tests with administration of aminoglycoside antibiotics.
   (AD) If ototoxic effect observed, need to withdraw ototoxic drug or ad-
   minister vitamins, glucose, dimedrol, calcium chloride, or electrophoresis
   with potassium iodide. (RUS)

376

High concentration of drug in fluids of ear for long period due to parenteral, intravenous, administration of 15000 units per kg of antibiotic,
neomycin, in 22 animals, cats.
   (AD) Comparative study of neomycin level in fluids of ear and in other
   biological fluids. (RUS)

381

Degeneration of organ of Corti and hearing loss due to various methods of
administration of antibiotic, neomycin, in humans.
   (AD) Literature review of toxic effects of new antibiotics. (GER)

384

Usually transient hearing loss and no structural damage to organ of Corti,

stria vascularis, and spiral ganglion due to oral or topical administration
of salicylates in humans.
Hearing loss due to antimalarial, quinine, in humans.
Usually permanent hearing loss due to antimalarial, chloroquine, in humans.
Transient and permanent hearing loss and possible damage to hair cells of
organ of Corti due to diuretic, ethacrynic acid, in humans.
Sensorineural hearing loss due to cardiovascular agent, hexadimethrine
bromide, in humans with kidney disorder.
Sensorineural hearing loss and damage to organ of Corti due to topical ad-
ministration of antineoplastic, nitrogen mustard, in humans.
Sensorineural hearing loss due to high doses of antibiotic, chloramphenicol,
in humans.
Primary vestibular problems due to antibiotic, streptomycin, in humans.
Hearing loss due to high doses usually of antibiotic, streptomycin, in humans.
    (AD) Early detection of hearing loss by audiometry prevents permanent
    damage.
High frequency hearing loss and severe damage to outer hair cells and slight
damage to inner hair cells of organ of Corti due to antibiotic, kanamycin, in
humans.
Sensorineural hearing loss due to parenteral, oral, and topical administration of antibiotic, neomycin, in humans with or without kidney disorders.
Degeneration of hair cells of organ of Corti and of nerve process due to
antibiotics, aminoglycoside, in animals.
    (AD) Literature review of physiological and structural cochleo-vestibulo-
    toxic effects of ototoxic drugs.
    (AD) Discussion of suggested mechanism of ototoxicity and routes of drugs
    to inner ear.
Bilateral sensorineural hearing loss due to oral administration of antibiotic, neomycin, in 4 of 8 humans with liver disease.
Bilateral sensorineural hearing loss due to oral administration of range of
doses of antibiotic, neomycin (SM), in 2 of 5 humans with liver disease.
Bilateral sensorineural hearing loss due to diuretics (SM), in 2 of 5 humans
with liver disease.
Transient progression of previous hearing loss due to parenteral, intravenous, administration of diuretic, ethacrynic acid (SM), in 1 injection in 1
of 5 humans with liver disease.
    (CT) Normal cochlear function in 6 humans, control group, with liver
    disease and not treated with neomycin or diuretics.
    (CT) Normal cochlear function in 13 humans, control group, with liver
    disease and treated with diuretics but not with neomycin.
    (AD) Hearing loss confirmed by audiometry.
    (AD) Reported that hearing loss due to neomycin or diuretics in humans
    with liver disease not related to dosage.
    (AD) Clinical study of effects of treatment with neomycin and diuretics in
    humans with liver disease.
Bilateral sensorineural hearing loss and vertigo due to antibiotic, ampicillin, in 1 human, adolescent, 17 years age, female, with tonsillitis.
    (AD) Cited case report.
Severe sensorineural hearing loss and vertigo due to topical administration
in ear drops of antibiotic, framycetin, in 1 human, adult, 42 years age,
male, with previous slight high frequency hearing loss.
    (AD) Cited case report.
Atrophy of hair cells of organ of Corti and hearing loss due to antibiotic,
dihydrostreptomycin, in humans with tuberculous meningitis.
    (AD) Cited study.
Loss of inner hair cells and damage to outer hair cells due to 18 g of antibiotic, neomycin, for 18 days in 1 human.
    (AD) Cited case report.   (ENG)

                                                                   385
Possible hearing loss due to oral administration of antibiotic, neomycin, in
humans, infant, with enteritis.
    (AD) Literature review of possible toxic effects of antibiotics in treat-
    ment of enteritis.   (GER)

                                                                   387
Risk of hearing loss due to parenteral and oral administration of antibiotic,

neomycin, in humans.
Possible hearing loss due to topical, rectal, administration of antibiotic,
neomycin, in humans.
  (AD) Study of rectal administration as possible route for neomycin therapy. (ENG)

                                                                          409
Primary damage to hair cells of organ of Corti, hearing loss, and possible
vestibular problems due to antibiotic, viomycin, in humans.
Damage to hair cells of organ of Corti and hearing loss due to antibiotic,
neomycin, in humans.
Damage to hair cells of organ of Corti and hearing loss due to antibiotic,
kanamycin, in humans.
Primary damage to vestibular apparatus, vestibular problems, and possible
hearing loss due to antibiotic, streptomycin, in humans.
Primary damage to vestibular apparatus, vestibular problems, and possible
hearing loss due to antibiotic, gentamicin, in humans.
  (AD) Need for audiometry and vestibular function tests, pretreatment and
  during treatment, with clinical use of aminoglycoside antibiotics.
  (AD) Incr in blood levels and ototoxicity of antibiotics in humans with
  kidney disorders. (ENG)

                                                                          424
Effect on muscles of middle ear due to antibiotic, neomycin, in animals,
guinea pigs. (CZ)

                                                                          437
Hearing loss and damage to cochlea due to antibiotic, neomycin, in animals,
guinea pigs and monkeys, and humans.
Hearing loss and damage to cochlea due to antibiotic, streptomycin, in animals, guinea pigs and monkeys, and humans.
  (AD) Discussion of findings on decr of ototoxicity of aminoglycoside
  antibiotics. (GER)

                                                                          457
Tinnitus and progressive sensorineural hearing loss due to parenteral, intramuscular, administration of antibiotic, (SQ) streptomycin, for 10 days in 1
human, adult, 38 years age, female, with infections and later development of
kidney disorder.
Tinnitus and progressive sensorineural hearing loss due to 13.2 g of antibiotic, (SQ) kanamycin, for 11 days in 1 human, adult, 38 years age, female,
with infections and kidney disorder.
Hearing loss due to antimalarial, (SQ) quinine, in 1 human, adult, 20 years
age, male, with various infections and later development of kidney disorder.
Hearing loss due to 400 mg 2 times daily, total dose of 6.5 g, of antibiotic,
(SQ) kanamycin (SM), for 8 days in 1 human, adult, 20 years age, male, with
various infections and later development of kidney disorder.
Hearing loss due to 150 mg 2 times daily, total dose of 2400 mg, of antibiotic, (SQ) colistin (SM), for 8 days in 1 human, adult, 20 years age, male,
with various infections and later development of kidney disorder.
Tinnitus, total bilateral hearing loss, and vestibular problems due to parenteral, intramuscular, administration of 4.0 g daily, total of 21 g, of antibiotic, (SQ) kanamycin (SM), for 5 days in 1 human, adult, 20 years age,
male, with infections and kidney disorder.
Tinnitus, total bilateral hearing loss, and vestibular problems due to 0.6 g
daily, total dose of 1.3 g, of antibiotic, (SQ) colistin (SM), for 2 days in
1 human, adult, 20 years age, male, with infections and kidney disorder.
Tinnitus, total bilateral hearing loss, and vestibular problems due to 2 g
and then 8 g per 24 hours in divided doses, total dose of 26.5 g, of antibiotic, (SQ) chloramphenicol, for 9 days in 1 human, adult, 20 years age, male,
with infections and kidney disorder.
Bilateral hearing loss due to 1 g daily of antibiotic, actinomycin (SM), for
5 days in 1 human, adult, 62 years age, male, with infections and kidney
disorder.
Bilateral hearing loss due to unknown dose of antibiotic, kanamycin (SM), for
5 days in 1 human, adult, 62 years age, male, with infections and kidney
disorder.
Bilateral hearing loss and vestibular problems due to parenteral administra-

tion of high doses of antibiotic, (SQ) neomycin, for total of 21 days in 1
human, adult, 25 years age, male, with infection from wound.
Previous administration of unspecified doses of antibiotic, (SQ) streptomycin, in 1 human, adult, 25 years age, male, with infection from wound.
Later administration of antibiotic, (SQ) chloramphenicol, in 1 human, adult,
25 years age, male, with infection from wound.
Tinnitus and rapidly progressive bilateral hearing loss due to parenteral,
intramuscular, administration of 0.5 g every 12 hours of antibiotic, (SQ)
streptomycin, for 5 days in 1 human, adult, 21 years age, male, with infection from wound.
Tinnitus and rapidly progressive bilateral hearing loss due to parenteral,
intramuscular, administration of 200 mg daily, total of 6.8 g, of antibiotic,
(SQ) colistin (SM), in 1 human, adult, 21 years age, male, with infection
from wound.
Tinnitus and rapidly progressive bilateral hearing loss due to parenteral
administration of unspecified doses of antibiotic, (SQ) neomycin (SM), for
about 35 days in 1 human, adult, 21 years age, male, with infection from
wound.
Tinnitus and progressive bilateral hearing loss due to parenteral administration of 2 l per 24 hours of 1 percent solution of antibiotic, (SQ) neomycin,
for 10 days in 1 human, adult, 26 years age, male, with infection from wound.
    (AD) Hearing loss confirmed by audiometry.
Previous administration of 500 mg four times a day of antibiotic, (SQ) ampicillin, in 1 human, adult, 26 years age, male, with infection from wound.
Bilateral sudden deafness due to administration in dialysis fluid of less
than 150 mg of antibiotic, neomycin (SM), in 1 human, adult, 44 years age,
female, with kidney disorder.
Bilateral sudden deafness due to 50 mg of diuretic, ethacrynic acid (SM), in
1 human, adult, 44 years age, female, with kidney disorder.
    (AD) Hearing loss confirmed by audiology.
Tinnitus and progressive bilateral hearing loss beginning after 8 days of
treatment due to parenteral administration of 1 l every 4 hours for 3 days
and then every 8 hours for 10 days of 1 percent solution of antibiotic,
neomycin, in 1 human, adult, 20 years age, male, with infection from wound.
    (AD) Hearing loss confirmed by audiology.
Tinnitus and bilateral sensorineural hearing loss due to parenteral, intramuscular, administration of 1 g and then 0.5 g every 12 hours of antibiotic,
streptomycin (SM), for 15 days in 1 human, adult, 23 years age, male, with
infection from wound.
Tinnitus and bilateral sensorineural hearing loss due to topical administration by irrigation of 1 percent solution every 12 hours of antibiotic, neomycin (SM), for 14 days in 1 human, adult, 23 years age, male, with infection
from wound.
    (AD) Hearing loss confirmed by audiometry.
    (AD) Discussion of 10 case reports. (ENG)

461

Destruction of cochlear microphonics, destruction of hair cells of organ of
Corti in basal coil of cochlea, severe damage to stria vascularis, damage to
nuclei of limbus, and slight damage to macula utriculi due to parenteral,
subcutaneous, administration of 100 mg per kg daily for 5 days a week, total
dose of 3 g per kg, of antibiotic, neomycin (neomycin sulfate), for 30 days
in animals, guinea pigs.
No damage to cochlear microphonics and no structural damage to cochlea or
vestibular apparatus due to parenteral, subcutaneous, administration of 100
mg per kg daily for 5 days a week, total dose of 3 g per kg, of antibiotic,
neomycin (methylneomycin), for 30 days in animals, guinea pigs.
Decr in cochlear microphonics due to parenteral, subcutaneous, administration
of 100 mg per kg daily for 5 days a week, total dose of 1.5 g per kg, of
antibiotic, neomycin (neomycin sulfate), for 15 days in animals, guinea pigs.
Decr in cochlear microphonics due to parenteral, subcutaneous, administration
of 200 mg per kg daily for 5 days a week, total dose of 2 g per kg, of antibiotic, neomycin (neomycin sulfate), for 10 days in animals, guinea pigs.
Decr in cochlear microphonics due to parenteral, subcutaneous, administration
of 200 mg per kg daily for 5 days a week, total dose of 2 g per kg, of antibiotic, neomycin (IB) (neomycin sulfate), for 10 days in animals, guinea
pigs, with administration of vitamin B.
    (CT) Same method with daily subcutaneous administration of 0.25 cc iso-

tonic saline in guinea pigs, control group.
(AD) No decr in ototoxic effects of neomycin on cochlear microphonics with administration of vitamin B.
(AD) Study of functional and structural cochleo-vestibulotoxic effects of neomycin.
(AD) Statistical analysis of results.   (ENG)

468

Complete inhibition of acetylcholine induced decr in cochlear potential due to parenteral, intravenous, administration of 1.0 mg of antibiotic, streptomycin (streptomycin sulfate), in 1 injection in 5 animals, cats, male and female, 1.5 to 2.8 kg weight, with injection of acetylcholine.
Minimum inhibition of acetylcholine induced decr in cochlear potential due to parenteral, intravenous, administration of 1.0 mg of antibiotic, dihydrostreptomycin (dihydrostreptomycin sulfate), in 1 injection in 5 animals, cats, male and female, 1.5 to 2.8 kg weight, with injection of acetylcholine.
Complete inhibition of acetylcholine induced decr in cochlear potential due to parenteral, intravenous, administration of 1.0 mg of antibiotic, kanamycin (kanamycin sulfate), in 1 injection in 5 animals, cats, male and female, 1.5 to 2.8 kg weight, with injection of acetylcholine.
Complete inhibition of acetylcholine induced decr in cochlear potential due to parenteral, intravenous, administration of 1.0 mg of antibiotic, neomycin (neomycin sulfate), in 1 injection in 5 animals, cats, male and female, 1.5 to 2.8 kg weight, with injection of acetylcholine.
Acute inhibition of acetylcholine induced decr in cochlear potential due to parenteral, intravenous, administration of 1.0 mg of antimalarial, quinine (quinine hydrochloride), in 1 injection in 5 animals, cats, male and female, 1.5 to 2.8 kg weight, with injection of acetylcholine.
(CT) Injections of 0.1 ml isotonic saline in cats, control group.
Inhibition of acetylcholine induced decr in cochlear potential due to parenteral, subcutaneous, administration of 300 mg per kg daily of antibiotic, streptomycin, for 7 to 9 days in 10 animals, cats.
Inhibition of acetylcholine induced decr in cochlear potential due to parenteral, subcutaneous, administration of 100 mg per kg daily of antibiotic, neomycin, for 7 to 9 days in 10 animals, cats.
(CT) Study of 7 cats, control group, not treated with antibiotics.
(AD) Study of effect of acetylcholine on cochlear potential after acute and chronic administration of ototoxic drugs.
(AD) Suggested relationship between change in acetylcholine activity and ototoxic drugs.
(AD) Suggested that ototoxicity partially due to disruption of efferent effect on cochlea.   (ENG)

469

Hearing loss due to parenteral administration of antibiotic, neomycin, in humans.   (FR)

483

Possible damage to vestibular nerve and cochlear nerve due to antibiotic, streptomycin, in humans with or without kidney disorder.
Possible damage to vestibular nerve and cochlear nerve due to antibiotic, gentamicin, in humans with or without kidney disorder.
Possible damage to vestibular nerve and cochlear nerve due to antibiotic, kanamycin, in humans with or without kidney disorder.
Possible damage to vestibular nerve and cochlear nerve due to antibiotic, neomycin, in humans with or without kidney disorder.
(AD) Incidence of effects on vestibular function highest in streptomycin, followed by gentamicin, kanamycin, and neomycin.
(AD) Incidence of effects on cochlear function highest in neomycin, followed by kanamycin, gentamicin, and streptomycin.
(AD) Need for careful consideration in clinical use of aminoglycoside antibiotics.
Possible cochlear impairment and vestibular problems due to antibiotic, paromomycin, in humans.
Possible dizziness and ataxia due to antibiotic, polymyxin B, in humans.
Possible but rare dizziness and vertigo due to antibiotic, nalidixic acid, in humans.   (ENG)

485

High concentration in fluids of inner ear and ototoxic effects due to 250 mg
per kg of antibiotic, streptomycin, in animals, guinea pigs.
High concentration in fluids of inner ear and ototoxic effects due to 250 mg
per kg of antibiotic, kanamycin, in animals, guinea pigs.
Higher concentration in fluids of inner ear and more severe ototoxic effects
due to 250 mg per kg of antibiotic, dihydrostreptomycin, in animals, guinea
pigs.
Higher concentration in fluids of inner ear and more severe ototoxic effects
due to 100 mg per kg of antibiotic, neomycin, in animals, guinea pigs.
   (AD) High concentration of aminoglycoside antibiotics in fluids of inner
   ear due to low doses as well as high doses.
   (AD) Ototoxic effect of aminoglycoside antibiotics due to retention of
   high concentrations in inner ear for long period and slow elimination of
   drugs.
Significant decr in concentration in fluids of inner ear and in serum and
decr in ototoxicity due to 250 mg per kg or 100 mg per kg of antibiotics
(IB), aminoglycoside, in animals, guinea pigs, with administration of ozothin.
Decr in concentration in fluids of inner ear and decr in ototoxicity due to
250 mg per kg or 100 mg per kg of antibiotics (IB), aminoglycoside, in animals, guinea pigs, with administration of pantothenic acid.   (GER)

491

Changes in sensory epithelium of otocyst due to antibiotic, streptomycin, in
animals, chickens, embryo.
Changes in sensory epithelium of otocyst due to antibiotic, neomycin, in
animals, chickens, embryo.
Changes in sensory epithelium of otocyst due to antibiotic, kanamycin, in
animals, chickens, embryo.
   (CT) Study of otocysts of chickens, control group, not treated with aminoglycoside antibiotics.
   (AD) Neomycin and kanamycin more toxic to otocysts of chickens than streptomycin.   (CZ)

495

Ototoxic effects due to parenteral, intramuscular, administration of 100 mg
per kg of antibiotic, neomycin (neomycin sulfate), in 10 injections in 10
animals, guinea pigs.
Significant decr in ototoxic effects due to parenteral, intramuscular, administration of 100 mg per kg of antibiotic, neomycin (IB) (neomycin sulfate), in 10 injections in 10 animals, guinea pigs, with combined administration of 1.2 ml per kg of ozothin.
Ototoxic effects due to parenteral, intramuscular, administration of 250 mg
per kg of antibiotic, streptomycin (streptomycin sulfate), in 10 injections
in animals, guinea pigs.
Decr in ototoxic effects due to parenteral, intramuscular, administration of
250 mg per kg of antibiotic, streptomycin (IB) (streptomycin sulfate), in 10
injections in 15 animals, guinea pigs, with combined administration of 1.2 ml
per kg of ozothin.
No ototoxic effects due to parenteral, intramuscular, administration of 250
mg per kg of antibiotic, streptomycin (IB) (streptomycin sulfate), in 10
injections in 6 animals, guinea pigs, with previous intramuscular administration of 1.2 ml per kg of ozothin.
   (CT) Study of 12 guinea pigs, control group.
   (AD) Electrophysiological study of effects of ozothin on ototoxicity of
   aminoglycoside antibiotics.   (GER)

498

Severe hearing loss 8 days after first dose due to oral administration of 7 g
on first day followed by 4 g on second day, total dose of 11 g, of antibiotic, neomycin, for total of 2 days in 1 human, adult, 45 years age, female,
treated before surgery.
   (AD) Case report of severe hearing loss due to neomycin therapy.
   (AD) Hearing clinically normal before neomycin treatment.
   (AD) Audiometry 1.5 years later confirmed auditory system problem.   (ENG)

518

Hearing loss and damage to hair cells of organ of Corti but no histological changes in vascular strip of spiral fissure due to antibiotic, neomycin, in animals, guinea pigs.
   (CT) Study of guinea pigs, control group, not treated with neomycin.
   (RUS)

529

Total loss of Preyer reflex within several days but no vestibular problems due to parenteral, subcutaneous, administration of range of high doses to more than 1000 mg per kg daily of antibiotic, kanamycin (kanamycin sulfate), in animals, rats, Wistar, albino, female, 50 g weight.
   (AD) Linear relationship between hearing loss and kanamycin dosage.
Loss of Preyer reflex but no vestibular problems due to parenteral, subcutaneous, administration of range of high doses to more than 600 mg per kg daily of antibiotic, neomycin, in animals, rats, Wistar, albino, female, 50 g weight.
   (AD) Linear relationship between hearing loss and neomycin dosage.
   (AD) Hearing loss observed with lower doses of neomycin than kanamycin.
Moderate to severe vestibular problems but cochlear impairment in only 1 case due to parenteral, subcutaneous, administration of high doses, 471, 583, 720, 887, and 1089 mg per kg daily, of antibiotic, streptomycin (streptomycin sulfate), in animals, rats, Wistar, albino, female, 50 g weight.
   (AD) Linear realtionship between vestibular problems and streptomycin
   dosage.
Transient moderate to severe vestibular problems but cochlear impairment in only 1 case due to parenteral, subcutaneous, administration of high doses, 765, 940, 1151, and 1377 mg per kg daily, of antibiotic, dihydrostreptomycin (dihydrostreptomycin sulfate), in 40 animals, rats, Wistar, albino, female, 50 g weight.
   (CT) Same method using saline in 30 rats, control group, showed no coch-
   leo-vestibulotoxic effects.
Hearing loss due to parenteral, subcutaneous, administration of 500 mg per kg daily of antibiotic, kanamycin (SM), in animals, rats, Wistar, albino, female, 50 g weight.
Hearing loss due to parenteral, subcutaneous, administration of range of doses of antibiotic, neomycin (SM), in animals, rats, Wistar, albino, female, 50 g weight.
   (AD) Incr in ototoxicity of neomycin due to kanamycin.
Hearing loss but no vestibular problems due to parenteral, subcutaneous, administration of 500 mg per kg of antibiotic, kanamycin (SM), in animals, rats, Wistar, albino, female, 50 g weight.
Hearing loss but no vestibular problems due to parenteral, subcutaneous, administration of 200, 270, 364.5, and 492 mg per kg daily of antibiotic, streptomycin (SM), in animals, rats, Wistar, albino, female, 50 g weight.
Hearing loss but no vestibular problems due to parenteral, subcutaneous, administration of 500 mg per kg daily of antibiotic, kanamycin (SM), in animals, rats, Wistar, albino, female, 50 g weight.
Hearing loss but no vestibular problems due to parenteral, subcutaneous, administration of 350, 472.5, 637.9, and 861.1 mg per kg daily of antibiotic, dihydrostreptomycin (SM), in animals, rats, Wistar, albino, female, 50 g weight.
   (AD) Tests of cochlear function and vestibular function, pretreatment and
   daily during treatment.
   (AD) Comparative study of ototoxic effects of aminoglycoside antibiotics
   in Wistar rats.
   (AD) Report of hearing loss in 321 (43.4 percent) of total of 740 rats in
   study.
   (AD) Suggested that ototoxic effects of kanamycin and neomycin due to
   different mechanisms of action than ototoxic effects of streptomycin and
   dihydrostreptomycin.   (ENG)

547

Bilateral sensorineural hearing loss within 20 minutes but normal vestibular function due to parenteral, intravenous, administration of 50 mg of diuretic, ethacrynic acid (SM), in 1 injection in 1 human, adult, 53 years age, female, with kidney disorder.
   (AD) Hearing loss confirmed by audiogram.
   (AD) Vestibular function tests showed normal vestibular function.

Simultaneous oral administration of 18 g of antibiotic, neomycin (SM), in 7
days in 1 human, adult, 53 years age, female, with kidney disorder.
Severe destruction of outer hair cells of organ of Corti in basal coil of
cochlea due to parenteral, intravenous, administration of 50 mg of diuretic,
ethacrynic acid (SM), in 1 injection in 1 human, adult, 53 years age, female,
with kidney disorder.
  (AD) Suggested that damage to hair cells possibly due to neomycin also.
  (AD) Suggested possible permanent hearing loss as result of ethacrynic
  acid treatment in patients with kidney disorders.
Transient and permanent total hearing loss within 15 minutes due to parenteral administration of diuretic, ethacrynic acid, in animals, cats. (ENG)

576

Progressive ataxia beginning after 4 days of treatment due to topical administration to bulla of 0.4 ml daily of aqueous solution of 10 percent concentration, to produce blood level of 7 mcg per ml, of antibiotic, gentamicin,
for 19 days maximum in 1 of 2 animals, cats.
Minimal transient ataxia beginning after 10 to 18 days of treatment and
moderate damage to cristae and maculae but normal cochlea due to topical
administration to bulla of 0.4 ml daily of aqueous solution of 3 percent
concentration, to produce blood levels of less than 0.5 mcg per ml, of antibiotic, gentamicin, for 19 days maximum in 1 of 3 animals, cats.
  (AD) Preliminary studies of topical gentamicin in cats.
  (AD) Not possible to obtain audiograms due to administration of gentamicin
  in middle ear so evaluation of cochlear function depended on histological
  study of cochlea.
  (AD) Evaluation of vestibular function with vestibular function tests.
Ataxia beginning after 12 days of treatment, decr in duration of rotatory
nystagmus, change in ENG, and loss of hair cells of cristae and of organ of
Corti in basal coil of cochlea due to topical administration to bulla of 0.4
ml daily of aqueous solution of 6 percent concentration of antibiotic, gentamicin, for 19 days maximum in 4 animals, cats.
No clinical vestibular problems and no significant change in duration of
rotatory nystagmus and in ENG but degeneration of cochlea and spiral ganglion
and changes in saccule due to topical administration to bulla of 0.4 ml daily
of aqueous solution of 3 percent concentration of antibiotic, gentamicin, for
30 days maximum in 5 animals, cats.
  (AD) Direct relationship between onset of ataxia and concentration of
  gentamicin solution.
  (AD) Correlation between duration of rotatory nystagmus and ataxia.
  (AD) Topical gentamicin most toxic to cochlea and saccule.
  (AD) Need to monitor clinical use of gentamicin with audiology.
No clinical vestibular problems, transient decr in duration of rotatory
nystagmus, transient bilateral decr in ENG, and loss of hair cells of organ
of Corti in basal coil of cochlea but normal vestibular apparatus due to
topical administration to bulla of 0.4 ml daily of solution of 6 percent
concentration of antibiotic, neomycin, for 30 days maximum in 2 animals,
cats.
  (AD) Comparative study of effects of topical gentamicin and neomycin.
  (CT) Same methods using 0.4 ml distilled water for 30 days in 7 cats,
  control group, showed no clinical vestibular problems and no histological
  changes. (ENG)

589

Dizziness during or after 5 or 6 injections but no evidence of hearing loss
due to parenteral, intramuscular and then intravenous (SM), administration of
7 mg per kg total daily, not exceeding 180 mg total dose every 24 hours, of
antibiotic, (SQ) gentamicin, for as long as 30 days in 5 of 80 humans, infant, child, and adult, 8 months to 36 years age, with cystic fibrosis and
severe pulmonary infection.
  (AD) Audiology in 40 of 80 patients showed no evidence of hearing loss.
  (AD) Dizziness possibly due to rapid administration of gentamicin.
High frequency hearing loss before gentamicin therapy possibly due to previous administration of (SQ) ototoxic drugs in some of 80 humans, infant,
child, and adult, 8 months to 36 years age, with cystic fibrosis and severe
pulmonary infection.
Dizziness due to topical administration by inhalation (SM) of 16 to 20 mg up
to 4 times a day, in 2 ml of 0.125 percent phenylephrine hydrochloride and

propylene glycol, of antibiotic, (SQ) gentamicin (CB), in some of 80 humans,
infant, child, and adult, 8 months to 36 years age, with cystic fibrosis and
severe pulmonary infection.
Dizziness due to topical administration by inhalation (SM) of 16 to 20 mg up
to 4 times a day, in 2 ml of 0.125 percent phenylephrine hydrochloride and
propylene glycol, of antibiotic, (SQ) neomycin (CB), in some of 80 humans,
infant, child, and adult, 8 months to 36 years age, with cystic fibrosis and
severe pulmonary infection.   (ENG)

                                                                          611
Hearing loss due to range of 0.8 to 15 g of antibiotic, neomycin (SM), in 9
humans, child, adult, and aged, 4 or less to 65 years age, with various
infections.
Simultaneous administration of antibiotic, streptomycin (SM), in 6 humans,
child, adult, and aged, 4 or less to 65 years age, with various infections.
Simultaneous administration of antibiotic, polymyxin (SM), in 1 human, child,
less than 4 years age, with various infections.
   (AD) Hearing loss confirmed by audiograms.
   (AD) Discussion of 9 case reports.   (HUN)

                                                                          621
Primarily vestibular problems due to antibiotic, streptomycin, in humans.
Primarily hearing loss but also vestibular problems due to antibiotic, dihy-
drostreptomycin, in humans.
Primarily hearing loss but also vestibular problems due to antibiotic, kana-
mycin, in humans.
Primarily hearing loss but also vestibular problems due to antibiotic, neomy-
cin, in humans.
Primarily hearing loss but also vestibular problems due to antibiotic, genta-
micin, in humans.
Vertigo and ataxia due to antituberculous agent, isoniazid, in humans.
Hearing loss due to salicylate, aspirin, in humans.
Hearing loss and vertigo due to antimalarial, quinine, in humans.
Nystagmus due to barbiturates in humans.
Vestibular problems due to analgesic, morphine, in humans.
Nystagmus due to sedative, alcohol, in humans.
Nystagmus and hearing loss due to chemical agent, carbon monoxide, in humans.
Ototoxic effects due to antineoplastic, nitrogen mustard, in humans.
Ototoxic effects due to chemical agent, aniline, in humans.
Ototoxic effects due to chemical agent, tobacco, in humans.
Nystagmus due to chemical agent, nicotine, in humans.
Vestibular problems due to anticonvulsants in humans.
Vestibular problems due to anesthetics in humans.
Vestibular problems due to diuretics in humans.
   (AD) Inclusion of comprehensive list of ototoxic agents.   (SP)

                                                                          627
Sensorineural hearing loss and vestibular problems due to parenteral, oral,
and topical administration of antibiotics in humans with and without kidney
disorder.
Degeneration of cochlea due to parenteral, intratympanic, administration of
antibiotic, neomycin, in animals, guinea pigs.
Transient sensorineural hearing loss due to high doses of salicylates in
humans.
Sensorineural hearing loss due to antimalarial, quinine, in humans.
Sensorineural hearing loss due to chemical agent, tobacco, in humans.
Sensorineural hearing loss due to sedative, alcohol, in humans.
   (AD) Discussion of ototoxicity of various drugs as 1 etiology of sen-
   sorineural hearing loss in adults.   (ENG)

                                                                          641
Possible damage to eighth cranial nerve due to antibiotic, capreomycin, in
humans.
Possible vestibular problems and hearing loss due to antibiotic, gentamicin,
in humans.
Possible delayed transient or permanent hearing loss due to antibiotic,
kanamycin (SM), in humans, in particular with kidney disorders or with simultaneous administration of ethacrynic acid.

Possible delayed transient or permanent hearing loss due to diuretic, ethacrynic acid (SM), in humans.
Possible delayed transient or permanent severe hearing loss due to oral,
parenteral, or topical administration of antibiotic, neomycin, in humans.
Possible damage to eighth cranial nerve, primarily hearing loss, due to
antibiotic, paromomycin, in humans.
Possible hearing loss due to antibiotic, rifampicin, in humans.
High risk of damage to eighth cranial nerve, primarily transient or permanent
vestibular problems but also hearing loss, due to antibiotic, streptomycin,
in humans.
Possible damage to eighth cranial nerve, primarily hearing loss, due to high
doses of antibiotic, vancomycin, for long period of more than 10 days in
humans, in particular with kidney disorders.
Risk of damage to eighth cranial nerve, vestibular problems and hearing loss,
due to high doses of antibiotic, viomycin, for long period of more than 10
days in humans, in particular with kidney disorders.
   (AD) Discussion of toxic effects of antibiotics.   (ENG)

666

Permanent severe and possibly delayed and progressive hearing loss and vestibular problems due to parenteral administration of antibiotic, kanamycin, in
humans, in particular with severe kidney disorders.
Permanent severe and possibly delayed and progressive hearing loss and vestibular problems due to parenteral administration of antibiotic, neomycin, in
humans, in particular with severe kidney disorders.
   (AD) Cochleo-vestibulotoxic effects of kanamycin and neomycin usually dose
   related but occur also after low doses.
   (AD) Higher risk of ototoxic effects due to kanamycin and neomycin in
   older patients.
   (AD) Need for audiometry 2 times a week with administration of antibiotics
   for more than 7 days.
   (AD) Recommended adult dose of 1.5 g daily for not more than 1 week and
   lower doses in patients with kidney disorder and dehydration.
   (AD) Suggested use of kanamycin and neomycin for only severe infections.
   (AD) Kanamycin reported less toxic than neomycin.
Hearing loss due to oral administration of antibiotic, neomycin, in humans.
   (ENG)

670

Possible vestibular problems due to parenteral administration of antibiotic,
gentamicin, in humans.
Damage to eighth cranial nerve, primarily hearing loss, usually permanent,
due to parenteral administration of high doses of antibiotic, kanamycin, for
more than 10 days in humans, in particular with kidney disorders.
Damage to eighth cranial nerve, primarily hearing loss, usually permanent,
due to parenteral administration of high doses of antibiotic, neomycin, for
more than 10 days in humans, in particular with kidney disorders.
Possible damage to eighth cranial nerve, primarily hearing loss, due to
parenteral administration of antibiotic, paromomycin, in humans.
Transient or permanent vestibular problems due to parenteral administration
of antibiotic, streptomycin, in humans.
Permanent severe hearing loss due to parenteral administration of antibiotic,
dihydrostreptomycin, in humans.
Damage to eighth cranial nerve, primarily hearing loss, due to parenteral
administration of high doses of antibiotic, vancomycin, for more than 10 days
in humans, in particular with kidney disorders.
Damage to eighth cranial nerve, vestibular problems and hearing loss, due to
parenteral administration of high doses of antibiotic, viomycin, for more
than 10 days in humans, in particular with kidney disorders.
   (AD) Discussion of toxic effects of antibiotics.   (ENG)

731

Possible damage to eighth cranial nerve, vestibular problems, due to antibiotic, streptomycin, in humans with gram-negative bacilli.
Possible damage to eighth cranial nerve, hearing loss, due to antibiotic,
kanamycin, in humans with gram-negative bacilli.
Possible damage to eighth cranial nerve, hearing loss, due to antibiotic,
neomycin, in humans with gram-negative bacilli.

Possible damage to eighth cranial nerve, vestibular problems, due to antibio-
tic, gentamicin, in humans with gram-negative bacilli.
Possible ototoxic effects due to antibiotic, vancomycin, in humans with gram-
positive cocci.
   (AD) Need to decr dosage of antibiotics in patients with kidney disorders.
   (AD) Discussion of possible toxic effects of antibiotics used in surgery.
   (ENG)

                              Paromomycin

                                                                       059
Bilateral sensorineural hearing loss due to oral administration of 0 to 12 g
daily, total of 2500 g, of antibiotic, neomycin, for 16 months in 1 human,
Caucasian, adult, 49 years age, female, chronic alcoholic, with hepatic
encephalopathy and normal kidney function.
Bilateral sensorineural hearing loss due to oral administration of 0 to 4 g
daily, total of 800 g, of antibiotic, (SQ) neomycin, for 21 months in 1
human, Caucasian, adult, 47 years age, female, chronic alcoholic, with hepatic encephalopathy and normal kidney function.
More severe sensorineural hearing loss due to oral administration of 6 g
daily, total of 111 g, of antibiotic, (SQ) paromomycin, for 9 months in 1
human, Caucasian, adult, 47 years age, female, chronic alcoholic, with hepatic encephalopathy and normal kidney function.
Sensorineural hearing loss due to oral administration of 0 to 12 g daily,
total of 1500 g, of antibiotic, neomycin, for 11 months in 1 human, Caucasian, adult, 39 years age, female, chronic alcoholic, with hepatic encephalopathy and some kidney disorder.
Sensorineural hearing loss in right ear due to oral administration of 3 to 4
g daily, total of 500 g, of antibiotic, (SQ) neomycin, for 8 months in 1
human, Caucasian, aged, 66 years age, female, with hepatic encephalopathy and
kidney disorder.
   (AD) Tinnitus and sudden deafness in left ear 27 years earlier.
Sensorineural hearing loss in right ear due to oral administration of total
of 240 g of antibiotic, (SQ) paromomycin, for long period in 1 human, Caucasian, aged, 66 years age, female, with hepatic encephalopathy and kidney
disorder.
Sequential administration of unspecified doses of diuretic, (SQ) furosemide,
for unspecified period in 1 human, Caucasian, aged, 66 years age, female,
with hepatic encephalopathy and kidney disorder.
Bilateral sensorineural hearing loss due to oral administration of 0 to 12 g
daily, total of 1000 to 1500 g, of antibiotic, (SQ) neomycin, for 28 months
in 1 human, Caucasian, adult, 60 years age, male, chronic alcoholic, with
hepatic encephalopathy and kidney disorder.
Bilateral sensorineural hearing loss due to oral administration of total of
300 g of antibiotic, (SQ) paromomycin, for long period in 1 human, Caucasian,
adult, 60 years age, male, chronic alcoholic, with hepatic encephalopathy and
kidney disorder.
Sequential administration of unspecified doses of (SQ) diuretics for unspecified period in 1 human, Caucasian, adult, 60 years age, male, chronic alcoholic, with hepatic encephalopathy and kidney disorder.
   (AD) Discussion of 5 case reports of hearing loss due to antibiotic therapy.
   (AD) Audiograms confirmed hearing loss in all cases.   (ENG)

                                                                       080
Hearing loss and vertigo due to parenteral administration of antibiotic,
streptomycin, in humans, child and adult, with normal kidney function and
with kidney disorder.
   (AD) Suggested use for severe infections only.
Delayed permanent hearing loss due to antibiotic, dihydrostreptomycin, in
humans.
   (AD) High risk of ototoxic effects with clinical use.
Hearing loss due to oral administration of antibiotic, paromomycin, in hu-
mans.
Progressive permanent hearing loss and tinnitus due to parenteral administration of antibiotic, kanamycin, in humans.
Progressive permanent hearing loss and tinnitus due to parenteral and topical
administration of antibiotic, neomycin, in humans.

(AD) Need for careful consideration in use of paromomycin, kanamycin, and neomycin due to potential ototoxicity.
(AD) Discussion of ototoxic effects of 5 antibiotics. (ENG)

358

Severe to total hearing loss due to antibiotic, paromomycin, in most of humans treated.
Severe to total hearing loss due to antibiotic, streptomycin, in most of humans treated.
Severe to total hearing loss due to antibiotic, neomycin, in most of humans treated.
Objective but no subjective vestibular problems due to antibiotic, streptomycin, in 2 humans. (RUS)

483

Possible damage to vestibular nerve and cochlear nerve due to antibiotic, streptomycin, in humans with or without kidney disorder.
Possible damage to vestibular nerve and cochlear nerve due to antibiotic, gentamicin, in humans with or without kidney disorder.
Possible damage to vestibular nerve and cochlear nerve due to antibiotic, kanamycin, in humans with or without kidney disorder.
Possible damage to vestibular nerve and cochlear nerve due to antibiotic, neomycin, in humans with or without kidney disorder.
    (AD) Incidence of effects on vestibular function highest in streptomycin, followed by gentamicin, kanamycin, and neomycin.
    (AD) Incidence of effects on cochlear function highest in neomycin, followed by kanamycin, gentamicin, and streptomycin.
    (AD) Need for careful consideration in clinical use of aminoglycoside antibiotics.
Possible cochlear impairment and vestibular problems due to antibiotic, paromomycin, in humans.
Possible dizziness and ataxia due to antibiotic, polymyxin B, in humans.
Possible but rare dizziness and vertigo due to antibiotic, nalidixic acid, in humans. (ENG)

641

Possible damage to eighth cranial nerve due to antibiotic, capreomycin, in humans.
Possible vestibular problems and hearing loss due to antibiotic, gentamicin, in humans.
Possible delayed transient or permanent hearing loss due to antibiotic, kanamycin (SM), in humans, in particular with kidney disorders or with simultaneous administration of ethacrynic acid.
Possible delayed transient or permanent hearing loss due to diuretic, ethacrynic acid (SM), in humans.
Possible delayed transient or permanent severe hearing loss due to oral, parenteral, or topical administration of antibiotic, neomycin, in humans.
Possible damage to eighth cranial nerve, primarily hearing loss, due to antibiotic, paromomycin, in humans.
Possible hearing loss due to antibiotic, rifampicin, in humans.
High risk of damage to eighth cranial nerve, primarily transient or permanent vestibular problems but also hearing loss, due to antibiotic, streptomycin, in humans.
Possible damage to eighth cranial nerve, primarily hearing loss, due to high doses of antibiotic, vancomycin, for long period of more than 10 days in humans, in particular with kidney disorders.
Risk of damage to eighth cranial nerve, vestibular problems and hearing loss, due to high doses of antibiotic, viomycin, for long period of more than 10 days in humans, in particular with kidney disorders.
    (AD) Discussion of toxic effects of antibiotics. (ENG)

670

Possible vestibular problems due to parenteral administration of antibiotic, gentamicin, in humans.
Damage to eighth cranial nerve, primarily hearing loss, usually permanent, due to parenteral administration of high doses of antibiotic, kanamycin, for more than 10 days in humans, in particular with kidney disorders.
Damage to eighth cranial nerve, primarily hearing loss, usually permanent,

due to parenteral administration of high doses of antibiotic, neomycin, for
more than 10 days in humans, in particular with kidney disorders.
Possible damage to eighth cranial nerve, primarily hearing loss, due to
parenteral administration of antibiotic, paromomycin, in humans.
Transient or permanent vestibular problems due to parenteral administration
of antibiotic, streptomycin, in humans.
Permanent severe hearing loss due to parenteral administration of antibiotic,
dihydrostreptomycin, in humans.
Damage to eighth cranial nerve, primarily hearing loss, due to parenteral
administration of high doses of antibiotic, vancomycin, for more than 10 days
in humans, in particular with kidney disorders.
Damage to eighth cranial nerve, vestibular problems and hearing loss, due to
parenteral administration of high doses of antibiotic, viomycin, for more
than 10 days in humans, in particular with kidney disorders.
    (AD) Discussion of toxic effects of antibiotics.   (ENG)

Penicillin

292

Cochlear impairment due to parenteral, intramuscular, administration of 1.2,
10, or 1 ml of antibiotic, penicillin (procaine penicillin G), in humans,
adult, with various infections.
    (AD) Discussion of 3 case reports.   (SL)

614

Vertigo due to parenteral administration of 0.5 g twice daily of antibiotic,
streptomycin (SM), for 7 days in 3 of 59 humans, aged, 70 years or over age,
with chronic bronchitis.
Simultaneous administration of 3,000,000 units twice daily of antibiotic,
penicillin (SM), for 14 days in 3 of 59 humans, aged, 70 years or over age,
with chronic bronchitis.   (ENG)

637

Ototoxic effects due to antibiotic, streptomycin (CB), in humans.
Ototoxic effects due to antibiotic, penicillin (CB), in humans.   (GER)

Polymyxin B

006

Range of degrees of degeneration of endorgan of organ of Corti due to parenteral, intratympanic, administration of range of 1 to 100 mg per ml concentration of antibiotic, neomycin, in 1 injection in animals, guinea pigs,
young, 250 g average weight.
Range of degrees of degeneration of endorgan of organ of Corti due to parenteral, intratympanic, administration of range of 1 to 100 mg per ml concentration of antibiotic, polymyxin B, in 1 injection in animals, guinea pigs,
young, 250 g average weight.
Range of degrees of degeneration of endorgan of organ of Corti due to parenteral, intratympanic, administration of range of 1 to 100 mg per ml concentration of antibiotic, colistin, in 1 injection in animals, guinea pigs,
young, 250 g average weight.
    (CT) Same method using comparable concentration of saline solution or
    solution of glucose or sodium G penicillin in guinea pigs, control group,
    showed no histological damage.
Degeneration of endorgan of organ of Corti due to topical administration to
ear canal of range of 5 to 100 mg per ml 1 time daily of antibiotic, neomycin, for 8 to 25 days in 14 animals, guinea pigs.   (ENG)

009

Delayed permanent sensorineural hearing loss and damage to outer hair cells
of basal and middle coils of cochlea due to unspecified doses of antibiotic,
dihydrostreptomycin, in humans.
Vertigo and dizziness due to unspecified method of administration of 2 to 3 g
daily of antibiotic, streptomycin (streptomycin sulfate), for 30 to 50 days
in humans with tuberculosis.
Hearing loss due to unspecified method of administration of high doses of
antibiotic, streptomycin (streptomycin sulfate), for long period in humans.
Gradual high frequency hearing loss and tinnitus and degeneration of hair

cells of organ of Corti in basal coil of cochlea due to unspecified doses of
antibiotic, kanamycin, in humans.
Delayed severe high frequency hearing loss due to parenteral, oral, or topical administration by inhalation of unspecified doses of antibiotic, neomycin, for unspecified period in humans with kidney disorder.
Complete degeneration of inner hair cells due to unspecified method of administration of 18 g of antibiotic, neomycin, for unspecified period in
humans with bacterial endocarditis.
Lesions in organ of Corti due to parenteral administration of unspecified
doses of antibiotic, polymyxin B, for unspecified period in animals, guinea
pigs.
Sensorineural hearing loss due to parenteral, intravenous, administration of
80 to 95 mg per ml of antibiotic, vancomycin, for unspecified period in
humans with kidney disorder.
    (AD) Sensorineural hearing loss and vestibular problems due to 6 antibio-
    tics in humans and animals, guinea pigs.
    (AD) Literature review of ototoxic effects of antibiotics. (ENG)

013

No reported ototoxic effects due to antibiotic, neomycin (CB), in 26 humans
with inflammation of external auditory meatus.
No reported ototoxic effects due to antibiotic, polymyxin B (CB), in 26
humans with inflammation of external auditory meatus.
    (AD) Study of use of neomycin, polymyxin B, and fluocinolone acetonide in
    treatment of inflammation of external auditory meatus. (FR)

027

Progressive bilateral high frequency hearing loss and tinnitus due to topical
administration by irrigation of wound with 80 ml every 4 hours for 2 weeks
and then 40 ml every 4 hours of 0.5 percent solution of antibiotic, (SQ)
neomycin (SM), in 1 human, adult, 24 years age, male, paraplegic, with infection of ulcer of left hip.
Progressive bilateral high frequency hearing loss and tinnitus due to topical
administration by irrigation of wound with 80 ml every 4 hours for 2 weeks
and then 40 ml every 4 hours of 0.1 percent solution of antibiotic, (SQ)
polymyxin B (SM), in 1 human, adult, 24 years age, male, paraplegic, with
infection of ulcer of left hip.
No reported ototoxic effects due to unspecified method of administration of 1
g daily of antibiotic, (SQ) streptomycin, for 5 days in 1 human, adult, 24
years age, male, paraplegic, with infection of ulcer of left hip. (ENG)

042

Transient bilateral sensorineural hearing loss due to parenteral, intravenous, administration of 50 mg of diuretic, (SQ) ethacrynic acid, in 1
injection in 1 human, adult, 45 years age, female, with lymphosarcoma and
with normal kidney function.
    (AD) Hearing loss reported 15 minutes after treatment with ethacrynic
    acid.
Previous parenteral, intramuscular, administration of 60 mg every 6 hours of
antibiotic, (SQ) gentamicin (gentamicin sulfate), for unspecified period in 1
human, adult, 45 years age, female, with lymphosarcoma and with normal kidney
function.
Bilateral sensorineural hearing loss due to parenteral, intravenous, administration of 100 mg of diuretic, (SQ) ethacrynic acid, in 2 injections of 50 mg
each 6 hours apart in 1 human, adult, 64 years age, female, with acute leukemia and with normal kidney function.
    (AD) Histological study after death showed no damage to inner ear.
Previous unspecified method of administration of unspecified dose of antibiotic, (SQ) polymyxin B (polymyxin B sulfate), in 1 human, adult, 64 years age,
female, with acute leukemia and with normal kidney function.
Previous parenteral, intramuscular, administration of 0.5 g every 12 hours of
antibiotic, (SQ) kanamycin (kanamycin sulfate), for unspecified period in 1
human, adult, 64 years age, female, with acute leukemia and with normal
kidney function.
    (AD) Suggested that hearing loss due to combined action of ethacrynic acid
    and antibiotics. (ENG)

Progressive permanent bilateral sensorineural hearing loss due to topical
administration by irrigation of wound with 1000 ml of 1 percent solution (6.5
g) of antibiotic, neomycin (CB) (neomycin sulfate), in 1 administration in 1
human, Caucasian, adolescent, 18 years age, male, with gunshot wound^of
abdomen.
   (AD) Hearing loss reported 21 days after treatment.
Progressive permanent bilateral sensorineural hearing loss due to topical
administration by irrigation of wound with 1000 ml of 0.1 percent solution
(650 mg) of antibiotic, polymyxin B (CB) (polymyxin B sulfate), in 1 administration in 1 human, Caucasian, adolescent, 18 years age, male, with gunshot
wound of abdomen.
   (AD) Study reported that ototoxic effects only due to neomycin.
   (AD) Hemodialysis 24 hours after treatment for prevention of hearing loss
   not satisfactory.
Progressive permanent bilateral sensorineural hearing loss due to topical
administration by irrigation of wound with high doses of 1 percent solution
of antibiotic, (SQ) neomycin, for 22 days in 1 human, Caucasian, adult, 20
years age, male, with gunshot wounds.
   (AD) Hearing loss reported after 19 days of treatment.
Previous administration of unspecified dose of antibiotic, (SQ) streptomycin,
for 6 days in 1 human, Caucasian, adult, 20 years age, male, with gunshot
wounds.
Progressive permanent bilateral sensorineural hearing loss due to topical
administration by irrigation of wound with total of 4000 ml of 1 percent
solution of antibiotic, neomycin (CB) (neomycin sulfate), in 4 days in 1
human, Caucasian, adult, 39 years age, male, with wounds.
   (AD) Hearing loss reported within 5 days.
Progressive permanent bilateral sensorineural hearing loss due to topical
administration by irrigation of wound with total of 4000 ml of 0.1 percent
solution of antibiotic, polymyxin B (CB) (polymyxin B sulfate), in 4 days in
1 human, Caucasian, adult, 39 years age, male, with wounds.
   (AD) Discussion of 3 case reports of hearing loss due to topical administration of antibiotics.   (ENG)

213
Dizziness due to antibiotic, polymyxin B (polymyxin B sulfate), in humans.
Dizziness due to antibiotic, colistin (sodium colistimethate), in humans.
Ototoxic effects due to antibiotic, ristocetin, in humans.
Hearing loss due to antibiotic, vancomycin, in humans.
   (AD) Report on pharmacology, clinical use, and toxicity of antibiotics.
   (ENG)

348
No ototoxic effects due to topical administration in ear drops of 3 to 4 ear
drops 3 times daily of fluocinolone acetonide (CB), for 5 to 10 days in 54
humans, child, adolescent, adult, and aged, male and female, with infections
of middle ear and external ear.
No ototoxic effects due to topical administration in ear drops of 3 to 4 ear
drops 3 times daily of antibiotic, polymyxin B (CB), for 5 to 10 days in 54
humans, child, adolescent, adult, and aged, male and female, with infections
of middle ear and external ear.
No ototoxic effects due to topical administration in ear drops of 3 to 4 ear
drops 3 times daily of antibiotic, neomycin (CB) (neomycin sulfate), for 5 to
10 days in 54 humans, child, adolescent, adult, and aged, male and female,
with infections of middle ear and external ear.   (IT)

483
Possible damage to vestibular nerve and cochlear nerve due to antibiotic,
streptomycin, in humans with or without kidney disorder.
Possible damage to vestibular nerve and cochlear nerve due to antibiotic,
gentamicin, in humans with or without kidney disorder.
Possible damage to vestibular nerve and cochlear nerve due to antibiotic,
kanamycin, in humans with or without kidney disorder.
Possible damage to vestibular nerve and cochlear nerve due to antibiotic,
neomycin, in humans with or without kidney disorder.
   (AD) Incidence of effects on vestibular function highest in streptomycin,
   followed by gentamicin, kanamycin, and neomycin.
   (AD) Incidence of effects on cochlear function highest in neomycin, fol-

lowed by kanamycin, gentamicin, and streptomycin.
   (AD) Need for careful consideration in clinical use of aminoglycoside
   antibiotics.
Possible cochlear impairment and vestibular problems due to antibiotic,
paromomycin, in humans.
Possible dizziness and ataxia due to antibiotic, polymyxin B, in humans.
Possible but rare dizziness and vertigo due to antibiotic, nalidixic acid, in
humans. (ENG)

577

No ototoxic effects due to parenteral, intramuscular, administration of 3 to
5 mg per kg daily in 3 or 4 divided doses, average total dose of 3.0 g, of
antibiotic, gentamicin, for 12.7 days average in 41 humans, adolescent,
adult, and aged, 14 to 87 years age, male and female, with genitourinary
system infections primarily and with kidney disorder in 13 cases.
No ototoxic effects due to parenteral, intramuscular, administration of 15 mg
per kg daily in 2 or 3 divided doses, average total dose of 6.6 g, of antibiotic, kanamycin (SM), for 8 days average in 34 humans, adult and aged, 40
to 81 years age, male and female, with genitourinary system infection and
with kidney disorder in 8 cases.
No ototoxic effects due to parenteral, intramuscular or intravenous administration of 1.5 to 2.5 mg per kg daily in 2 to 4 divided doses, average total
dose of 1.0 g, of antibiotic, polymyxin B (SM), for 6 days average in 34
humans, adult and aged, 40 to 81 years age, male and female, with genitourinary system infection and with kidney disorder in 8 cases.
   (AD) Comparative study of effects of 3 antibiotics on infections due to
   gram-negative bacilli. (ENG)

682

Possible dizziness and ataxia due to high blood levels of over 5 mcg per ml
of antibiotic, polymyxin B, in humans, adult.
   (AD) Discussion of clinical pharmacology, dosage, toxic effects, and use
   in therapy of polymyxins. (ENG)

Rifampicin

076

Ototoxic effects due to parenteral, intramuscular, administration of 1 g
daily of antibiotic, capreomycin (SM), for 9 months in 4 of 65 humans, adult
and aged, range of 20 to 70 years age, male and female, with pulmonary tuberculosis.
Simultaneous administration of ethambutol (SM) in 65 humans, adult and aged,
range of 20 to 70 years age, male and female, with pulmonary tuberculosis.
Simultaneous administration of antibiotic, rifampicin (SM), in 65 humans,
adult and aged, range of 20 to 70 years age, male and female, with pulmonary
tuberculosis. (ENG)

137

Vestibular problems due to 1 g daily of antibiotic, capreomycin (SM), for
long period in 2 of 20 humans with tuberculosis.
Simultaneous administration of 25 mg per kg for first 60 days and then 15 mg
per kg of antituberculous agent, ethambutol (SM), in 20 humans with tuberculosis.
Simultaneous administration of 300 mg twice daily for several months and then
450 mg in 1 dose of antibiotic, rifampicin (SM), in 20 humans with tuberculosis. (ENG)

322

Cochleo-vestibulotoxic effects due to parenteral, intramuscular, administration of 1 g daily and then 1 g every other day of antibiotic, (SQ) capreomycin (SM), for 6 months in 3 of 36 humans, adult and aged, range of 20 to 80
years age, male and female, with pulmonary tuberculosis.
   (AD) Ototoxic effects confirmed by audiogram.
Simultaneous administration of 600 mg daily of antibiotic, (SQ) rifampicin
(SM), for 6 months in 36 humans, adult and aged, range of 20 to 80 years age,
male and female, with pulmonary tuberculosis.
Simultaneous administration of 25 mg per kg daily and then 15 mg per kg daily
of antituberculous agent, (SQ) ethambutol (SM), for 6 months in 36 humans,

adult and aged, range of 20 to 80 years age, male and female, with pulmonary
tuberculosis.
Cochleo-vestibulotoxic effects due to previous administration of (SQ) antibiotics, aminoglycoside, in 36 humans, adult and aged, range of 20 to 80
years age, male and female, with pulmonary tuberculosis.
   (AD) Therapy with antibiotics not satisfactory.   (FR)

                                                                           346
Temporary inhibition of oxygen consumption at level of mitochondria of cen-
tral vestibular nuclei due to antibiotic, streptomycin, in animals.
Temporary inhibition of oxygen consumption at level of mitochondria of cen-
tral vestibular nuclei due to antibiotic, rifampicin, in animals.
   (AD) Discussion of chronic and acute vestibular toxicity.   (ENG)

                                                                           502
Possible transient hearing loss or dizziness due to antibiotic, rifampicin,
in humans treated for tuberculosis or other infections.
   (AD) Literature review of clinical use, pharmacology, toxicity, and other
   aspects of rifampicin.   (ENG)

                                                                           519
Dizziness but no other ototoxic effects due to parenteral, intramuscular,
administration of 1 g daily in single dose of antibiotic, capreomycin (SM),
for long period in 1 of 33 humans, adult and aged, 21 to over 70 years age,
with pulmonary tuberculosis of long duration and with previous treatment with
other drugs.
Simultaneous oral administration of 25 mg per kg during first 60 days and
then 15 mg per kg of antituberculous agent, ethambutol (SM), in 1 of 33
humans, adult and aged, 21 to over 70 years age, with pulmonary tuberculosis
of long duration and with previous treatment with other drugs.
Simultaneous administration of 600 mg of antibiotic, rifampicin (SM), in 1 of
33 humans, adult and aged, 21 to over 70 years age, with pulmonary tuberculosis of long duration and with previous treatment with other drugs.
   (AD) Otoneurology tests every 4 to 8 weeks.   (ENG)

                                                                           538
Dizziness due to parenteral administration of 1 g daily for first 8 weeks and
then 1 g twice weekly for 12 weeks of antibiotic, streptomycin (SM), for
total of 20 weeks in 5 of 77 humans with pulmonary tuberculosis.
Simultaneous administration of 300 mg daily in single dose of antituberculous
agent, isoniazid (SM), in 77 humans with pulmonary tuberculosis.
Simultaneous administration of 15 mg per kg daily of antituberculous agent,
ethambutol (SM), in 77 humans with pulmonary tuberculosis.
No reported ototoxic effects due to 600 mg daily in single dose of antibiotic, rifampicin, in 157 humans with pulmonary tuberculosis.   (ENG)

                                                                           571
No significant effect on vestibular apparatus due to oral administration of
50 or 150 mg per kg daily, total of 1.55 and 4.65 g per kg, of antibiotic,
rifampicin, for 5 weeks in 2 groups of 7 animals, rabbits, male.
   (CT) Same method using 1 percent carboxymethyl-cellulose in rabbits,
   control group.
   (AD) Measurement of horizontal nystagmus 2, 3, 4, and 5 weeks after beginning of treatment.
No accumulation in perilymph due to oral administration of 100 mg per kg of
antibiotic, rifampicin, for 1 dose in animals, guinea pigs.
   (AD) Determination of rifampicin concentration in perilymph and blood
   after 2, 6, and 24 hours.
   (AD) Study of vestibulotoxic effects and retention in inner ear of rifampicin.   (ENG)

                                                                           622
Possible transient hearing loss due to antibiotic, rifampicin, in humans.
(ENG)

                                                                           626
Transient hearing loss during therapy due to 300 mg 3 times a day of antibiotic, rifampicin, for 14 days in 2 of 27 humans, adult and aged, 20 to 79

years age, female and male, with genitourinary system infections. (ENG)

641

Possible damage to eighth cranial nerve due to antibiotic, capreomycin, in
humans.
Possible vestibular problems and hearing loss due to antibiotic, gentamicin,
in humans.
Possible delayed transient or permanent hearing loss due to antibiotic,
kanamycin (SM), in humans, in particular with kidney disorders or with simultaneous administration of ethacrynic acid.
Possible delayed transient or permanent hearing loss due to diuretic, ethacrynic acid (SM), in humans.
Possible delayed transient or permanent severe hearing loss due to oral,
parenteral, or topical administration of antibiotic, neomycin, in humans.
Possible damage to eighth cranial nerve, primarily hearing loss, due to
antibiotic, paromomycin, in humans.
Possible hearing loss due to antibiotic, rifampicin, in humans.
High risk of damage to eighth cranial nerve, primarily transient or permanent
vestibular problems but also hearing loss, due to antibiotic, streptomycin,
in humans.
Possible damage to eighth cranial nerve, primarily hearing loss, due to high
doses of antibiotic, vancomycin, for long period of more than 10 days in
humans, in particular with kidney disorders.
Risk of damage to eighth cranial nerve, vestibular problems and hearing loss,
due to high doses of antibiotic, viomycin, for long period of more than 10
days in humans, in particular with kidney disorders.
   (AD) Discussion of toxic effects of antibiotics. (ENG)

Ristocetin

213

Dizziness due to antibiotic, polymyxin B (polymyxin B sulfate), in humans.
Dizziness due to antibiotic, colistin (sodium colistimethate), in humans.
Ototoxic effects due to antibiotic, ristocetin, in humans.
Hearing loss due to antibiotic, vancomycin, in humans.
   (AD) Report on pharmacology, clinical use, and toxicity of antibiotics.
   (ENG)

Spectinomycin

647

No damage to eighth cranial nerve observed but possible dizziness due to
parenteral administration of antibiotic, spectinomycin, in humans with gonorrhea.
   (AD) New antibiotic for treatment of gonorrhea.
   (AD) Spectinomycin chemically related to ototoxic drugs as streptomycin
   and kanamycin. (ENG)

Streptomycin

009

Delayed permanent sensorineural hearing loss and damage to outer hair cells
of basal and middle coils of cochlea due to unspecified doses of antibiotic,
dihydrostreptomycin, in humans.
Vertigo and dizziness due to unspecified method of administration of 2 to 3 g
daily of antibiotic, streptomycin (streptomycin sulfate), for 30 to 50 days
in humans with tuberculosis.
Hearing loss due to unspecified method of administration of high doses of
antibiotic, streptomycin (streptomycin sulfate), for long period in humans.
Gradual high frequency hearing loss and tinnitus and degeneration of hair
cells of organ of Corti in basal coil of cochlea due to unspecified doses of
antibiotic, kanamycin, in humans.
Delayed severe high frequency hearing loss due to parenteral, oral, or topical administration by inhalation of unspecified doses of antibiotic, neomycin, for unspecified period in humans with kidney disorder.
Complete degeneration of inner hair cells due to unspecified method of administration of 18 g of antibiotic, neomycin, for unspecified period in
humans with bacterial endocarditis.

Lesions in organ of Corti due to parenteral administration of unspecified
doses of antibiotic, polymyxin B, for unspecified period in animals, guinea
pigs.
Sensorineural hearing loss due to parenteral, intravenous, administration of
80 to 95 mg per ml of antibiotic, vancomycin, for unspecified period in
humans with kidney disorder.
   (AD) Sensorineural hearing loss and vestibular problems due to 6 antibiotics in humans and animals, guinea pigs.
   (AD) Literature review of ototoxic effects of antibiotics.   (ENG)

                                                                      010

Permanent sensorineural hearing loss due to parenteral, intramuscular, administration of low doses, less than 2 g, of antibiotic, (SQ) kanamycin
(kanamycin sulfate), for short period in 5 humans, adult, range of 33 to 47
years age, range of 90 to 177 lb weight, with kidney disorder.
Permanent sensorineural hearing loss due to parenteral, intramuscular, administration of low doses, less than 2 g, of antibiotic, (SQ) streptomycin,
for short period in 5 humans, adult, range of 33 to 47 years age, range of 90
to 177 lb weight, with kidney disorder.
Permanent sensorineural hearing loss due to parenteral, intramuscular, administration of low doses, less than 2 g, of antibiotic, (SQ) neomycin, for
short period in 5 humans, adult, range of 33 to 47 years age, range of 90 to
177 lb weight, with kidney disorder.
Permanent sensorineural hearing loss due to parenteral, intramuscular, administration of low doses, less than 2 g, of diuretic, (SQ) ethacrynic acid,
for short period in 5 humans, adult, range of 33 to 47 years age, range of 90
to 177 lb weight, with kidney disorder.
   (AD) Study of cochleotoxic effects of kanamycin with other antibiotics and
   with ethacrynic acid.   (ENG)

                                                                      011

Transient cochleo-vestibulotoxic effects due to topical administration by
inhalation and parenteral, intramuscular, administration of 0.5 g twice a day
for 6 days, followed by a 1-day break, of antibiotic, (SQ) kanamycin (kanamycin sulfate), for 1 to 3 months in 2 of 17 humans treated for tuberculosis.
   (CT) Pretreatment audiometry and vestibular function tests conducted.
Ototoxic effects due to previous administration of antibiotic, (SQ) streptomycin, in 2 of 17 humans with tuberculosis.   (RUS)

                                                                      014

No permanent sensorineural hearing loss or damage to cochlea or vestibular
apparatus due to 20 to 30 mg per kg daily, total of 2 to 39 g, of antibiotic,
streptomycin, for 6 months to 5 years in 205 humans, child and adolescent,
range of 6 to 14 years age, with various disorders.   (POL)

                                                                      016

Progressive bilateral sensorineural hearing loss and vertigo due to unspecified method of administration of total of 3 g of antibiotic, (SQ) streptomycin (SM), for unspecified period in 1 human, Caucasian, adult, 32 years age,
male, with kidney disorder and on intermittent hemodialysis.
Progressive bilateral sensorineural hearing loss and vertigo due to unspecified method of administration of antibiotic, (SQ) colistin (SM), for unspecified period in 1 human, Caucasian, adult, 32 years age, male, with kidney
disorder and on intermittent hemodialysis.
Permanent sensorineural hearing loss due to parenteral, intravenous, administration of 1.6 mg per kg 2 times daily, total of 500 mg of antibiotic, (SQ)
gentamicin, for unspecified period in 1 human, Caucasian, adult, 32 years
age, male, with kidney disorder and on intermittent hemodialysis.
No definite ototoxic effects reported due to unspecified method of administration of 1 g every 2 weeks, total of 12 g, of antibiotic, (SQ) vancomycin,
for about 6 months in 1 human, Caucasian, adult, 32 years age, male, with
kidney disorder and on intermittent hemodialysis.
   (AD) Hearing loss due to streptomycin and colistin potentiated by gentamicin.   (ENG)

                                                                      017

Ototoxic effects, vestibular problems and cochlear impairment in 78 percent,
vestibular problems only in 14 percent, and cochlear impairment only in 8

percent due to unspecified method of administration of unspecified doses of
antibiotic, streptomycin (streptomycin sulfate), for unspecified period in
100 humans with tuberculosis and other infections.
  (CT) No symptoms of damage to cochlea or vestibular apparatus before
  treatment with streptomycin.
  (AD) Recommendation of audiometry and vestibular function test, pretreatment and during treatment, for early detection of ototoxic effects. (ENG)

018

Hearing loss due to parenteral administration of low doses, 1 g daily, of
antibiotic, (SQ) streptomycin, in 3 injections in 1 human, adult, 22 years
age, male, with pulmonary tuberculosis.
Unspecified effects due to previous administration of 3 unspecified doses of
antimalarial, (SQ) quinine, in 1 human, adult, 22 years age, male, with
pulmonary tuberculosis. (ENG)

019

Progressive severe sensorineural hearing loss and tinnitus due to unspecified
method of administration of 0.5 g twice daily, total of 16 g, of antibiotic,
kanamycin, for 16 days in 1 human, Caucasian, adult, 25 years age, male, with
kidney disorder and treated with peritoneal dialysis.
  (AD) Audiograms showed hearing loss and recruitment test showed reversed
  recruitment.
Severe sensorineural hearing loss due to unspecified method of administration
of 0.5 g daily for 40 days and then 0.5 g 3 times a week for 3 weeks of
antibiotic, streptomycin, for total period of about 9 weeks in 1 human,
Negro, child, 9 years age, male, with pulmonary tuberculosis and kidney
disorder.
  (AD) No record of hearing loss before treatment with streptomycin.
Delayed severe bilateral high frequency hearing loss due to unspecified
method of administration of 0.5 g daily for 8 months and then 0.5 g every 3
days for 4 months, followed by a break of 3.5 months, and then 0.5 g every 3
days for 1.5 months, total of 153 g of antibiotic, dihydrostreptomycin, for
total period of about 13.5 months in 1 human, Negro, infant, 16 months age,
female, with tuberculosis.
  (AD) Hearing loss detected at 13 years age.
Hearing loss and tinnitus due to unspecified method of administration of 1 g
daily of antibiotic, streptomycin, for 10 weeks and possibly for a longer
period after discharge in 1 human, Negro, adult, 23 years age, male, treated
for infection in tuberculosis hospital.
  (AD) Hearing loss detected 1 month after treatment with streptomycin.
Progressive severe sensorineural hearing loss due to unspecified method of
administration of 0.5 g 3 times a week, total of 61 g of antibiotic, streptomycin, for about 10 months in 1 human, Negro, child, 9 years age, female,
with pulmonary tuberculosis.
  (AD) Discussion of 5 case reports. (ENG)

020

Effect on function of inner ear due to parenteral, subcutaneous, administration of high doses, range of 30 to 75 mg per kg of antibiotic, gentamicin,
for about 8 to 20 days in 11 animals, cats.
  (AD) Preliminary study of dosage levels.
Damage to semicircular canal, membranous labyrinth, and outer hair cells and
inner hair cells of the cochlea due to parenteral, subcutaneous, administration of high doses, range of 30 to 75 mg per kg of antibiotic, gentamicin,
for about 8 to 20 days in 11 animals, cats, with kidney damage resulting from
gentamicin.
  (AD) Preliminary study of dosage levels.
Partial hearing loss due to parenteral, subcutaneous, administration of 20 mg
per kg of antibiotic, gentamicin, for 14 days in 1 out of 15 animals, cats.
Complete degeneration of outer hair cells of organ of Corti due to parenteral, subcutaneous, administration of 20 mg per kg of antibiotic, gentamicin, for 14 days in 1 out of 15 animals, cats.
Range of degree of damage, transient and permanent, to vestibular apparatus
due to parenteral, subcutaneous, administration of 20 mg per kg of antibiotic, gentamicin, for 14 days in 15 animals, cats.
Complete damage to vestibular apparatus due to parenteral, subcutaneous,
administration of 200 mg per kg of antibiotic, streptomycin, for 9 days in

animals, cats.
Higher incidence and earlier symptoms of ototoxic effects due to parenteral,
subcutaneous, administration of 20 mg per kg of antibiotic, gentamicin, for
14 days in 66.6 percent of 15 animals, cats, with kidney damage than in cats
with normal kidney function.
   (AD) Study of correlation of functional and histological effects of gentamicin.
   (AD) Comparative study of effect on vestibular apparatus of gentamicin and
   streptomycin. (ENG)

                                                                         023
No degeneration in inner hair cells and outer hair cells of organ of Corti
due to parenteral, intramuscular, administration of 200 mg per kg daily of
antibiotic, streptomycin (streptomycin sulfate), for 10 days in 15 animals,
guinea pigs, 150 to 200 g weight.
   (CT) Study of 5 guinea pigs, control group.
Changes in succinic dehydrogenase activity in hair cells of organ of Corti
due to parenteral, intramuscular, administration of 200 mg per kg daily of
antibiotic, streptomycin (streptomycin sulfate), for 10 days in 15 animals,
guinea pigs, 150 to 200 g weight.
   (CT) Study of 10 guinea pigs, control group.
   (AD) Difference between inner hair cells and outer hair cells discussed.
   (ENG)

                                                                         024
Suppression of semicircular canal function due to parenteral administration
of range of 22.5 to 54 g, total doses, of antibiotic, streptomycin (streptomycin sulfate), for range of 7.5 to 26 days in 4 humans, adult, male and
female, treated for Meniere's disease.
   (AD) Use of ototoxic effect of streptomycin in treatment of Meniere's
   disease. (ENG)

                                                                         027
Progressive bilateral high frequency hearing loss and tinnitus due to topical
administration by irrigation of wound with 80 ml every 4 hours for 2 weeks
and then 40 ml every 4 hours of 0.5 percent solution of antibiotic, (SQ)
neomycin (SM), in 1 human, adult, 24 years age, male, paraplegic, with infection of ulcer of left hip.
Progressive bilateral high frequency hearing loss and tinnitus due to topical
administration by irrigation of wound with 80 ml every 4 hours for 2 weeks
and then 40 ml every 4 hours of 0.1 percent solution of antibiotic, (SQ)
polymyxin B (SM), in 1 human, adult, 24 years age, male, paraplegic, with
infection of ulcer of left hip.
No reported ototoxic effects due to unspecified method of administration of 1
g daily of antibiotic, (SQ) streptomycin, for 5 days in 1 human, adult, 24
years age, male, paraplegic, with infection of ulcer of left hip. (ENG)

                                                                         028
Bilateral sensorineural hearing loss and tinnitus due to parenteral, intravenous, administration of 100 mg of diuretic, ethacrynic acid (SM), in 2
doses in 1 human, adult, 24 years age, male, with kidney disorder.
Bilateral sensorineural hearing loss and tinnitus due to parenteral, intravenous, administration of 4 g of antibiotic, streptomycin (SM), for 5 days in
1 human, adult, 24 years age, male, with kidney disorder.
Bilateral sensorineural hearing loss due to parenteral, intravenous, administration of 500 mg of diuretic, ethacrynic acid (SM), for 4 days in 1 human,
adult, 35 years age, female, with kidney disorder.
Bilateral sensorineural hearing loss due to parenteral, intravenous, administration of 1.5 g of antibiotic, streptomycin (SM), for 4 days in 1 human,
adult, 35 years age, female, with kidney disorder.
Permanent hearing loss due to parenteral, intravenous, administration of 200
mg of diuretic, ethacrynic acid, in humans. (ENG)

                                                                         029
Concentration of streptomycin in blood and perilymph due to 250, 50, 25, and
15 mg per kg of antibiotic, streptomycin (streptomycin sulfate), in 4 injections in 325 animals, guinea pigs.
Concentration of streptomycin in blood and perilymph due to 250, 50, 25, and

15 mg per kg of antibiotic, streptomycin (IB) (streptomycin sulfate), in 4
injections in 325 animals, guinea pigs, with administration of ozothin.
   (AD) Protective action of ozothin not dependable. (GER)

031

Damage to cochlea due to antibiotic, streptomycin, in animals, guinea pigs.
   (AD) Study of RNA and protein in cochlea for evaluation of streptomycin
   ototoxicity. (GER)

037

Progressive hearing loss due to 0.75 to 1 g daily of antibiotic, streptomycin, for long period in 7.2 percent of 125 humans. (GER)

040

Sensorineural hearing loss due to parenteral, intramuscular, administration
of 1 g twice a week of antibiotic, streptomycin (streptomycin sulfate), for
335 days in 1 human, adult, 63 years age, male, with bone tuberculosis.
   (AD) Pretreatment hearing loss reported.
Sensorineural hearing loss due to parenteral, intramuscular, administration
of 0.5 g twice a week of antibiotic, streptomycin (streptomycin sulfate), for
333 days in 1 human, child, 3 years age, with bone tuberculosis. (ENG)

041

Cochleo-vestibulotoxic effects due to unspecified method of administration of
300 mg daily of antituberculous agent, isoniazid, for 6 to 18 months in 12.9
percent of 70 humans with tuberculosis.
Cochleo-vestibulotoxic effects due to unspecified method of administration of
300 mg of antituberculous agent, isoniazid (SM), for 6 to 18 months in 22
percent of 297 humans with tuberculosis.
Cochleo-vestibulotoxic effects due to unspecified method of administration of
150 mg of antituberculous agent, thiacetazone (SM), for 6 to 18 months in 22
percent of 297 humans with tuberculosis.
Cochleo-vestibulotoxic effects due to unspecified method of administration of
antituberculous agent, isoniazid (SM), for 6 to 18 months in 82.9 percent of
82 humans with tuberculosis.
Cochleo-vestibulotoxic effects due to unspecified method of administration of
antituberculous agent, thiacetazone (SM), for 6 to 8 months in 82.9 percent
of 82 humans with tuberculosis.
Cochleo-vestibulotoxic effects due to unspecified method of administration of
1 g of antibiotic, streptomycin (SM), for 6 to 18 months in 82.9 percent of
82 humans with tuberculosis.
Cochleo-vestibulotoxic effects due to unspecified method of administration of
300 mg of antituberculous agent, isoniazid (SM), for 6 to 18 months in 25
percent of 20 humans with tuberculosis.
Cochleo-vestibulotoxic effects due to unspecified method of administration of
1 g of antibiotic, streptomycin (SM), for 6 to 18 months in 25 percent of 20
humans with tuberculosis.
   (AD) Potentiation by thiacetazone of cochleo-vestibulotoxic effects of
   streptomycin suggested.
   (AD) Audiometry and vestibular function tests every 2 weeks for 6 to 18
   months in total of 469 humans with tuberculosis. (ENG)

056

Range of degree of hearing loss due to range of 40 to 300 g of antibiotic,
(SQ) streptomycin, in 59 of 338 humans, male and female, with no previous
treatment with streptomycin.
   (AD) No auditory system problems before treatment.
   (AD) Hearing loss often detected in alcoholics in group.
Range of degree of hearing loss due to range of 40 to 100 g of antibiotic,
(SQ) streptomycin, in 8 of 32 humans with previous treatment with streptomy-
cin.
   (AD) No reported auditory system problems before treatment.
   (AD) More severe hearing loss with administration of 100 g or more of
   streptomycin in both groups.
   (AD) More severe hearing loss in group with previous streptomycin treat-
   ment.
No reported ototoxic effects due to high doses of antibiotic, (SQ) dihydros-
treptomycin, in some of total of 370 humans treated with streptomycin. (SER)

057

No ototoxic effects within 2 months due to antibiotic, dihydrostreptomycin
(dihydrostreptomycin ascorbinate), in humans with pulmonary tuberculosis.
    (AD) Audiometry used to determine ototoxic effects.
Tinnitus and vertigo due to antibiotic, streptomycin (streptomycin sulfate),
in humans with pulmonary tuberculosis.
    (AD) Comparative study of effects of 2 antibiotics used in treatment of
    pulmonary tuberculosis.   (RUS)

063

Progressive permanent bilateral sensorineural hearing loss due to topical
administration by irrigation of wound with 1000 ml of 1 percent solution (6.5
g) of antibiotic, neomycin (CB) (neomycin sulfate), in 1 administration in 1
human, Caucasian, adolescent, 18 years age, male, with gunshot wound of
abdomen.
    (AD) Hearing loss reported 21 days after treatment.
Progressive permanent bilateral sensorineural hearing loss due to topical
administration by irrigation of wound with 1000 ml of 0.1 percent solution
(650 mg) of antibiotic, polymyxin B (CB) (polymyxin B sulfate), in 1 administration in 1 human, Caucasian, adolescent, 18 years age, male, with gunshot
wound of abdomen.
    (AD) Study reported that ototoxic effects only due to neomycin.
    (AD) Hemodialysis 24 hours after treatment for prevention of hearing loss
    not satisfactory.
Progressive permanent bilateral sensorineural hearing loss due to topical
administration by irrigation of wound with high doses of 1 percent solution
of antibiotic, (SQ) neomycin, for 22 days in 1 human, Caucasian, adult, 20
years age, male, with gunshot wounds.
    (AD) Hearing loss reported after 19 days of treatment.
Previous administration of unspecified dose of antibiotic, (SQ) streptomycin,
for 6 days in 1 human, Caucasian, adult, 20 years age, male, with gunshot
wounds.
Progressive permanent bilateral sensorineural hearing loss due to topical
administration by irrigation of wound with total of 4000 ml of 1 percent
solution of antibiotic, neomycin (CB) (neomycin sulfate), in 4 days in 1
human, Caucasian, adult, 39 years age, male, with wounds.
    (AD) Hearing loss reported within 5 days.
Progressive permanent bilateral sensorineural hearing loss due to topical
administration by irrigation of wound with total of 4000 ml of 0.1 percent
solution of antibiotic, polymyxin B (CB) (polymyxin B sulfate), in 4 days in
1 human, Caucasian, adult, 39 years age, male, with wounds.
    (AD) Discussion of 3 case reports of hearing loss due to topical adminis-
    tration of antibiotics. (ENG)

067

High frequency hearing loss in 11.4 percent of fetuses due to 10 g to more
than 100 g of antibiotic, streptomycin, in 44 humans, female, treated for
tuberculosis during pregnancy.
    (AD) Hearing loss confirmed by audiogram.
    (AD) Damage most often due to streptomycin treatment during first trimes-
    ter. (GER)

068

Hearing loss and tinnitus or hyperacusis due to oral administration of 1 g
daily of antibiotic, (SQ) capreomycin, for 2 years in 3 of first group of 34
humans with tuberculosis.
No reported ototoxic effects due to previous unspecified method of administration of unspecified doses of antibiotic, (SQ) streptomycin, in first group
of 34 humans with tuberculosis.
Hearing loss due to previous unspecified method of administration of unspecified doses of antibiotic, (SQ) streptomycin, in 9 of second group of 31
humans with tuberculosis.
More severe hearing loss due to oral administration of 1 g daily of antibiotic, (SQ) capreomycin, for 2 years in 1 of second group of 31 humans with
tuberculosis.   (ENG)

070

Cochleo-vestibulotoxic effects due to range of less than 50 g to more than

200 g of antibiotic, streptomycin, in 127 humans with pulmonary tuberculosis
and 1 human with croupous pneumonia.
>   (AD) Statistical analysis showed correlation between ototoxic effects and
>   dosage.
>   (AD) Vestibular problems detected earlier than hearing loss.
>   (AD) Suggested use of audiometry before streptomycin treatment and every
>   10 to 15 days during treatment.   (RUS)

                                                                          071

Cochleo-vestibulotoxic effects due to antibiotic, streptomycin (SM) (streptomycin sulfate), in 65.5 percent of 553 humans, child and adolescent, 3 to
15 years age, with pulmonary tuberculosis.
Simultaneous administration of other unspecified antituberculous agents (SM)
in 553 humans, child and adolescent, 3 to 15 years age, with pulmonary tuberculosis.
>   (CT) No cochleo-vestibulotoxic effects in 113 humans, child and adoles-
>   cent, control group, not treated with streptomycin.
>   (AD) Analysis by audiometry of ototoxic effects of streptomycin in chil-
>   dren and adolescents.   (SER)

                                                                          073

Permanent hearing loss due to 10 to 35 mg per kg daily or twice daily of
antibiotic, dihydrostreptomycin, in 23(26.4 percent) of 87 humans, child,
with pulmonary and meningeal tuberculosis.
Permanent hearing loss due to 15 to 35 mg per kg daily or twice daily of
antibiotic, streptomycin, in 1(5.2 percent)of 19 humans, child, with pulmonary and meningeal tuberculosis.
>   (AD) More ototoxic effects with 1 dose per day than with 2 doses per day.
Permanent hearing loss due to 15 to 20 mg per kg daily or twice daily of
antibiotic, dihydrostreptomycin (CB), in 4(18.6 percent) of 46 humans, child,
with pulmonary and meningeal tuberculosis.
Permanent hearing loss due to 15 to 20 mg per kg daily or twice daily of
antibiotic, streptomycin (CB), in 4(18.6 percent) of 46 humans, child, with
pulmonary and meningeal tuberculosis.
>   (CT) No hearing loss in 14 children, control group, treated with PAS and
>   isoniazid.
>   (AD) Need to confirm hearing loss with audiometry discussed.   (SER)

                                                                          074

Decr in cochlear microphonic due to topical administration to round window of
range of 210 to 680 g of antibiotic, streptomycin, in animals, guinea pigs.
Decr in cochlear microphonic due to topical administration to round window of
range of 210 to 680 g of antibiotic, kanamycin, in animals, guinea pigs.
No decr in cochlear microphonic due to topical administration to round window
of range of 210 to 680 g of antibiotic, neomycin, in animals, guinea pigs.
(POL)

                                                                          075

Hearing loss due to previous administration of antibiotic, (SQ) streptomycin,
in 18 of total of 67 humans with tuberculosis.
More severe hearing loss, tinnitus, or hyperacusis due to unspecified method
of administration of unspecified doses of antibiotic, (SQ) capreomycin, for
long period in 4 of 45 humans with tuberculosis.
No ototoxic effects due to unspecified method of administration of unspecified doses of antibiotic, (SQ) capreomycin, for short period in other 22
humans with tuberculosis.   (ENG)

                                                                          080

Hearing loss and vertigo due to parenteral administration of antibiotic,
streptomycin, in humans, child and adult, with normal kidney function and
with kidney disorder.
>   (AD) Suggested use for severe infections only.
Delayed permanent hearing loss due to antibiotic, dihydrostreptomycin, in
humans.
>   (AD) High risk of ototoxic effects with clinical use.
Hearing loss due to oral administration of antibiotic, paromomycin, in humans.
Progressive permanent hearing loss and tinnitus due to parenteral administra-

tion of antibiotic, kanamycin, in humans.
Progressive permanent hearing loss and tinnitus due to parenteral and topical
administration of antibiotic, neomycin, in humans.
  (AD) Need for careful consideration in use of paromomycin, kanamycin, and
  neomycin due to potential ototoxicity.
  (AD) Discussion of ototoxic effects of 5 antibiotics.   (ENG)

                                                  084
Decr in damage to organ of Corti due to topical administration of antibiotic,
kanamycin (IB), in animals, guinea pigs, 300 to 500 g weight, with intravenous administration of cytochrome C.
Decr in damage to organ of Corti due to topical administration of antibiotic,
streptomycin (IB) (streptomycin sulfate), in animals, guinea pigs, 300 to 500
g weight, with intravenous administration of cytochrome C.   (POL)

                                                  087
High frequency hearing loss and tinnitus due to antibiotics in humans, parti-
cularly infant and aged, and humans with kidney disorder.
Degeneration in hair cells of organ of Corti due to antibiotics in humans.
Vertigo and unsteady gait due to antibiotic, streptomycin, in humans.
Bilateral damage to vestibular apparatus due to antibiotic, streptomycin, in
humans.
  (AD) Literature review of physiological and structural cochleo-vestibulo-
  toxic effects of antibiotics.
  (AD) Degree of damage determined by dosage and duration of dosage of
  antibiotics.   (ENG)

                                                  088
Ototoxic effects in fetus due to unspecified method of administration of
unspecified doses of antibiotic, streptomycin, for long period in humans,
female, treated for tuberculosis during pregnancy.
Ototoxic effects in fetus due to unspecified method of administration of
unspecified doses of antibiotic, dihydrostreptomycin, for long period in
humans, female, treated for tuberculosis during pregnancy.   (ENG)

                                                090
Tinnitus and vertigo due to unspecified method of administration of 0.75 g
daily of antibiotic, (SQ) streptomycin (SM), for 5 weeks in 1 human, adult,
38 years age, female, with pulmonary tuberculosis.
Simultaneous administration of antituberculous agent, (SQ) PAS (SM), in 1
human, adult, 38 years age, female, with pulmonary tuberculosis.
Simultaneous administration of antituberculous agent, (SQ) isoniazid (SM), in
1 human, adult, 38 years age, female, with pulmonary tuberculosis.
No reported ototoxic effects due to unspecified method of administration of
150 mg daily of antituberculous agent, (SQ) thiacetazone, for 11 months in 1
human, adult, 38 years age, female, with pulmonary tuberculosis.
  (AD) Hemolytic disease due to treatment with thiacetazone.   (ENG)

                                                091
Ototoxic effects due to antibiotic, streptomycin (streptomycin sulfate), in
humans with pulmonary tuberculosis.
Ototoxic effects due to antibiotic, dihydrostreptomycin, in humans with
pulmonary tuberculosis.
Ototoxic effects due to antibiotic, florimycin, in humans with pulmonary
tuberculosis.
Ototoxic effects due to antibiotic, kanamycin, in humans with pulmonary
tuberculosis.
  (AD) Comparative study of ototoxicity of different derivatives of antibiotics.   (RUS)

                                                092
Decr of enzyme activity in vestibular apparatus due to topical administration
to bulla of 0.2 cc of 50 percent solution of antibiotic, streptomycin, in 10
animals, guinea pigs.   (GER)

                                                095
Ototoxic effects due to unspecified method of administration of (SQ) 0.75 g
daily of antibiotic, streptomycin (SM), for (SQ) 3 months initial treatment

in 6 of 140 humans with tuberculosis.
Simultaneous unspecified method of administration of (SQ) 300 mg of antituberculous agent, isoniazid (SM), in 140 humans with tuberculosis.
Ototoxic effects due to unspecified method of administration of (SQ) 1 g 3
days a week of antibiotic, streptomycin (SM), for (SQ) 18 months following
initial treatment in 24 of 140 humans with tuberculosis.
Dizziness due to simultaneous unspecified method of administration of (SQ)
600 mg of antituberculous agent, isoniazid (SM), in unspecified number of
humans with tuberculosis and with other toxic effects due to isoniazid.
(ENG)

                                                                              100
Hearing loss due to antibiotic, streptomycin, in human, male.
   (AD) Court case on ototoxic effects due to streptomycin.   (GER)

                                                                              103
Cochleo-vestibulotoxic effects due to range of less than 50 g to 300 g of
antibiotic, streptomycin (SM) (streptomycin sulfate), for 6 to 8 months in
humans, adult, with tuberculous meningitis.
Simultaneous administration of antituberculous agent, PAS (SM), in humans,
adult, with tuberculous meningitis.
Simultaneous administration of antituberculous agent, isoniazid (SM), in
humans, adult, with tuberculous meningitis.
   (AD) Follow up study after average of 7 years.   (GER)

                                                                              107
Vertigo and nystagmus due to antibiotic, kanamycin, in humans, male and
female.
Vertigo and nystagmus due to antibiotic, streptomycin, in humans, male and
female.
   (AD) Preclinical detection of vestibular problems by ENG.   (FR)

                                                                              110
Nystagmus and other vestibular problems due to topical administration to
bulla of 0.5 g of antibiotic, streptomycin, in 1 injection in cats.
   (AD) Suggested route of streptomycin in cat from bulla by way of large
   membrane of round window to inner ear.
Changes in chromatin in hair cells, type 1, of maculae due to topical administration to bulla of 0.5 g of antibiotic, streptomycin, in 1 injection in
cats.
   (AD) Suggested that destruction of hair cells due to changes in protein
   metabolism as result of action of streptomycin.   (ENG)

                                                                              111
Damage to organ ofCorti and vestibular apparatus due to antibiotic, streptomycin, in humans and animals, guinea pigs.
   (AD) Comparative study of ototoxic effects of streptomycin in humans and
   animals.   (GER)

                                                                              112
Permanent inhibition of cochlear microphonic due to parenteral administration
of high doses of antibiotic, streptomycin, in animals, guinea pigs and rabbits.
Rapid decr in cochlear potentials due to lower doses of antibiotic, streptomycin, in animals, guinea pigs and rabbits, sensitized with horse serum.
   (AD) Study to show pathogenesis of cochlear neuritis in association with
   streptomycin treatment.   (RUS)

                                                                              116
Moderate unilateral sensorineural hearing loss in 1 of 36 fetuses due to
total of 13 g of antibiotic, dihydrostreptomycin, in 33 humans, female,
treated during pregnancy for tuberculosis.
   (AD) Child not treated with dihydrostreptomycin or streptomycin.
Sensorineural hearing loss due to 1 g daily for the first 30 days and then 1
g twice a week of antibiotic, dihydrostreptomycin (CB), in 8(24 percent)of 33
humans, female, treated during pregnancy for tuberculosis.
Sensorineural hearing loss due to 1 g daily for the first 30 days and then 1
g twice a week of antibiotic, streptomycin (CB), in 8(24 percent)of 33 hu-

mans, female, treated during pregnancy for tuberculosis.
Vestibular problems due to antibiotic, (SQ) dihydrostreptomycin, in 1 of 33
humans, female, treated during pregnancy for tuberculosis and chronic pyelonephritis.
Vestibular problems due to antibiotic, (SQ) streptomycin, in 1 of 33 humans,
female, treated during pregnancy for tuberculosis and chronic pyelonephritis.
   (AD) Case histories, audiometry, and vestibular function tests for children and adults.   (ENG)

                                                                      133
Sensorineural hearing loss due to antibiotic, streptomycin, in 6 of 420
humans, child, with suppurative meningitis.   (RUS)

                                                                      139
Cochleotoxic effects due to antibiotic, kanamycin, in humans and animals,
guinea pigs.
Cochleotoxic effects due to antibiotic, streptomycin, in humans and animals,
guinea pigs.
   (AD) Literature review of mechanism of action of ototoxic antibiotics.
   (POL)

                                                                      155
Suppression of function of semicircular canal due to parenteral, intramuscular, administration of range of 1100 to 4600 mg total doses of antibiotic,
streptomycin (streptomycin sulfate), for 16 to 23 doses in 8 animals, squirrel monkeys, with normal semicircular canal function.
   (CT) Vestibular function tests used to confirm pretreatment normal function of semicircular canal.
Moderate to severe damage to hair cells of cristae and organ of Corti and
some changes in spiral ganglion and maculae due to parenteral, intramuscular,
administration of range of 1100 to 4600 mg total doses of antibiotic, streptomycin (streptomycin sulfate), for 16 to 23 doses in 8 animals, squirrel
monkeys, with normal semicircular canal function.
   (AD) Report on 8 case studies to show clinical and pathological correlations.   (ENG)

                                                                      156
Sensorineural hearing loss due to unspecified method of administration of
high doses of antibiotic, streptomycin (SM), in 7 humans, infant and child,
with tuberculous meningitis.
Simultaneous administration of unspecified doses of antituberculous agent,
PAS (SM), in 7 humans, infant and child, with tuberculous meningitis.
Simultaneous administration of unspecified doses of antituberculous agent,
isoniazid (SM), in 7 humans, infant and child, with tuberculous meningitis.
Sensorineural hearing loss due to unspecified method of administration of
high doses of antibiotic, viomycin, in 7 humans, infant and child, with
tuberculous meningitis.
   (AD) Cochleotoxic effect due to antibiotic therapy or infection.   (ENG)

                                                                      158
No reported ototoxic effects due to 5 g of antibiotic, (SQ) streptomycin, in
1 human, adult, 63 years age, male, with bronchopleural fistula and staphylococcal empyema.
Progressive total bilateral sensorineural hearing loss due to topical administration by irrigation of empyema cavity with (SQ) 1200 ml of 1 percent
solution of antibiotic, (SQ) neomycin, for 10 days, total of 33 irrigations,
in 1 human, adult, 63 years age, male, with bronchopleural fistula and staphylococcal empyema.
Progressive total bilateral sensorineural hearing loss due to topical administration by irrigation of empyema cavity with (SQ) 700 ml of 1 percent solution, total of 403 g in all, of antibiotic, (SQ) neomycin, in 1 administration in 1 human, adult, 63 years age, male, at time of surgery to close
cavity.
Sequential parenteral, intramuscular, administration of total of 4 g of
antibiotic, (SQ) streptomycin (streptomycin sulfate), for 4 to 5 days in 1
human, adult, 63 years age, male, after closure of empyema cavity.
   (AD) No hearing loss before closure of cavity.
   (AD) Hearing loss confirmed by audiogram but no vestibular problems de-

tected by vestibular function tests.
(AD) Suggested that hearing loss due to neomycin only and not to streptomycin. (ENG)

172

Vertigo due to sedative, alcohol, ethyl, in humans.
Vertigo due to antibiotic, streptomycin, in humans.
(AD) Report on etiology of vertigo. (GER)

179

Progressive high frequency hearing loss and tinnitus due to 1 g daily of
antibiotic, kanamycin, in 3 humans, adolescent and adult, male, with tuberculosis and with previous treatment with ototoxic drugs but with no report of
toxic effects.
Less severe sensorineural hearing loss and no tinnitus due to 1 g 5 times a
week of antibiotic, kanamycin, in 1 human, male, with tuberculosis and with
previous treatment with ototoxic drugs.
Sensorineural hearing loss and tinnitus due to 6 g of antibiotic, kanamycin
(SM), in 1 human, male, with tuberculosis and with previous treatment with
ototoxic drugs.
Sensorineural hearing loss and tinnitus due to parenteral administration of
1000 mg per day of antibiotic, streptomycin (SM), in 1 human, male, with
tuberculosis and with previous treatment with ototoxic drugs.
No high frequency hearing loss due to parenteral administration of 1 g daily
of antibiotic, streptomycin, in 1 human, female, with tuberculosis and with
previous treatment with ototoxic drugs.
High frequency hearing loss but no tinnitus due to 750 mg daily of antibiotic, streptomycin, in 1 human, female, with tuberculosis and with previous
treatment with ototoxic drugs.
Simultaneous administration of range of doses of other antituberculous agents
(SM) in total of 7 humans, adolescent and adult, 13 to 49 years age, male and
female, with tuberculosis and with previous treatment with ototoxic drugs.
   (AD) Study using high frequency audiometry and conventional audiometry.
   (CT) Pretreatment audiograms obtained. (ENG)

184

Incr in ATP hydrolyzing system in stria vascularis and spiral ligament and
incr in ATP activity in membranous labyrinth due to parenteral, intraperitoneal, administration of 400 mg per kg 5 days a week of antibiotic, kanamycin (kanamycin sulfate), for 20 days in animals, guinea pigs, adult, with
normal pinna reflex.
Incr in ATP hydrolyzing system in stria vascularis and spiral ligament due to
parenteral, intraperitoneal, administration of 400 mg per kg 5 days a week of
antibiotic, streptomycin (streptomycin sulfate), for 20 days in animals,
guinea pigs, adult, with normal pinna reflex.
Decr in ATP hydrolyzing system in stria vascularis and spiral ligament and
decr in ATP activity in membranous labyrinth due to parenteral, intraperitoneal, administration of 400 mg per kg 5 days a week of antibiotic, dihydrostreptomycin (dihydrostreptomycin sulfate), for 20 days in animals, guinea
pigs, adult, with normal pinna reflex.
   (CT) Study of normal activity of ATP hydrolyzing system. (ENG)

185

Ataxia, damage to hair cells of macula, and damage to hair cells of organ of
Corti due to parenteral, subcutaneous, administration of 10 to 80 mg per kg
daily of antibiotic, gentamicin (gentamicin sulfate), for 19 to 120 days in
animals, cats.
Ataxia due to 100 and 200 mg per kg daily of antibiotic, streptomycin (streptomycin sulfate), for 8 to 40 days in animals, cats.
Loss of Preyer reflex, decr in cochlear potential and eighth cranial nerve
action potential, and loss of outer hair cells of organ of Corti due to 80 to
200 mg per kg daily of antibiotic, gentamicin (gentamicin sulfate), in animals, guinea pigs.
Damage to cochlea due to 100 and 200 mg per kg of antibiotic, kanamycin
(kanamycin sulfate), in animals, guinea pigs.
   (AD) Comparative study of ototoxicity of gentamicin and other aminoglycoside antibiotics.
   (AD) Study suggested low risk of ototoxicity when gentamicin used in

recommended clinical dose of 1 to 3 mg per kg. (ENG)

191

Vestibular problems due to unspecified method of administration of unspecified doses of antibiotic, streptomycin, for long period in 9 of 155 humans
with tuberculosis.
Cochlear impairment due to unspecified method of administration of unspecified doses of antibiotic, streptomycin, for long period in 4 of 155 humans
with tuberculosis.
Vestibular problems and cochlear impairment due to unspecified method of
administration of unspecified doses of antibiotic, streptomycin, for long
period in 1 of 155 humans with tuberculosis. (ENG)

196

Sensorineural hearing loss due to unspecified doses of antibiotic, streptomycin, in 8.9 percent of 2917 humans, child, adolescent, and adult, 10 to 34
years age, with pulmonary tuberculosis.
Sensorineural hearing loss due to unspecified doses of antibiotic, streptomy-
cin (SM), in high percent of 608 humans, child, adolescent, and adult, 10 to
34 years age, with pulmonary tuberculosis.
Sensorineural hearing loss due to unspecified doses of antibiotic, kanamycin
(SM), in high percent of 608 humans, child, adolescent, and adult, 10 to 34
years age, with pulmonary tuberculosis.
   (CT) Study of 314 humans, control group, without pulmonary tuberculosis.
   (CT) No subjective hearing loss before treatment with antibiotics.
   (CT) Hearing loss after antibiotic treatment confirmed by audiometry.
   (AD) Statistical analysis of 3525 cases with antibiotic therapy.
   (AD) Highest incidence of hearing loss in 30 to 34 years age group.
   (AD) Higher incidence of severe hearing loss in group treated with two
   antibiotics than in group treated with streptomycin only. (ENG)

198

Severe vertigo due to parenteral, intramuscular, administration of 1 g daily
in single dose of antibiotic, streptomycin (SM) (streptomycin sulfate), for 6
months in 2 of 41 humans, 108.2 lb average weight, with pulmonary tuberculosis and with previous streptomycin therapy in some.
Simultaneous oral administration of 15 g daily in single dose of antituberculous agent, PAS (SM) (sodium PAS), for 6 months in 2 of 41 humans, 108.2 lb
average weight, with pulmonary tuberculosis and with previous streptomycin
therapy in some.
No vestibulotoxic effects due to parenteral, intramuscular, administration of
1 g daily in single dose of antibiotic, streptomycin (SM) (streptomycin
sulfate), for 6 months in 41 humans, 113.5 lb average weight, with pulmonary
tuberculosis and with previous streptomycin therapy in some.
Simultaneous oral administration of 15 g daily in 2 doses of antituberculous
agent, PAS (SM) (sodium PAS), for 6 months in 41 humans, 113.5 lb average
weight, with pulmonary tuberculosis and with previous streptomycin therapy in
some.
   (AD) Study of retreatment of pulmonary tuberculosis in humans with no
   response to previous chemotherapy. (ENG)

200

Moderate to profound sensorineural hearing loss, possibly due to 25 mg per kg
every 12 hours of antibiotic, streptomycin (streptomycin sulfate), in 8 doses
in 16 of 17 humans, child, about 4 years age, treated in neonatal period for
hemolytic disease or hyperbilirubinemia.
   (AD) Hearing loss determined by pure tone audiometry using play audiometry
   methods.
   (AD) Reported that not possible to determine role of streptomycin independent of high bilirubin level in hearing loss of 16 children. (ENG)

206

Transient bilateral sensorineural hearing loss due to oral administration of
50 mg every 6 hours of diuretic, ethacrynic acid, for 4 days initially and
then again 2 weeks later for 2 days in 1 human, Negro, adult, 55 years age,
female, with diabetes mellitus and kidney disorder.
   (AD) Hearing loss confirmed by audiogram.
Transient sensorineural hearing loss and tinnitus due to (SQ) oral and paren-

teral, (SQ) intravenous, administration of 300,300,400, and 500 mg of diuretic, ethacrynic acid, in 4 doses in 1 human, Caucasian, adult, 40 years age,
female, with chronic kidney disorder.
No auditory system problems due to parenteral, intravenous, administration of
(SQ) unspecified doses of diuretic, (SQ) ethacrynic acid, in (SQ) 3 injections in 1 human, Caucasian, adult, 20 years age, female, with kidney disorder.
Transient severe bilateral tinnitus, sensorineural hearing loss, and bilateral nystagmus due to parenteral, intravenous, administration of (SQ) 50 and
100 mg of diuretic, (SQ) ethacrynic acid, in (SQ) 2 injections in 1 human,
Caucasian, adult, 20 years age, female, with kidney disorder.
Previous administration, 2 days before onset of ototoxic effects, of antibiotic, (SQ) colistin (sodium colistimethate), in 1 injection in 1 human, Caucasian, adult, 20 years age, female, with kidney disorder.
Transient sensorineural hearing loss within 12 hours of first dose due to
oral administration of 50 mg of diuretic, ethacrynic acid, in 4 doses in 1
human, Caucasian, aged, 76 years age, male, with kidney disorder and with
previous moderate hearing loss due to otosclerosis.
Severe tinnitus within 1 hour of first dose and sensorineural hearing loss
within 1 half hour of second dose due to parenteral, intravenous, administration of 50 and 100 mg of diuretic, (SQ) ethacrynic acid, in 2 injections in 1
human, Caucasian, adult, 57 years age, female, with leukemia and kidney
disorder.
Administration about 1 week previously of antibiotic, (SQ) streptomycin, in 1
human, Caucasian, adult, 57 years age, female, with leukemia and kidney
disorder, for pneumonitis.
Administration about 1 week previously of antibiotic, (SQ) colistin (sodium
colistimethate), in 1 human, Caucasian, adult, 57 years age, female, with
leukemia and kidney disorder, for pneumonitis.
   (AD) Discussion of 5 case reports of transient hearing loss due to treatment with ethacrynic acid.   (ENG)

                                                                         211
Severe and slight vertigo due to total of 29 to 57 g of antibiotic, streptomycin, for long period in 14 of 180 humans, adult, 50 years or less age,
male, with pneumoconiosis.   (ENG)

                                                                         212
Changes in hair cells of vestibular apparatus due to 250 mg per kg daily of
antibiotic, streptomycin (streptomycin sulfate), for 10 or 20 days in 9
animals, guinea pigs, 140 to 300 g weight.
Decr in damage to cochlea due to 250 mg per kg daily of antibiotic, streptomycin (IB) (streptomycin sulfate), for 10 or 15 days in 10 animals, guinea
pigs, 140 to 300 g weight, with intramuscular administration of 1.25 ml per
kg daily of ozothin.
   (CT) Study of 10 guinea pigs, control group, 5 normal and 5 with parenteral administration of 2.5 ml per kg daily of ozothin for 10 days.
   (AD) Study not show decr in streptomycin damage to vestibular apparatus
   with administration of ozothin.   (GER)

                                                                         215
Primary damage to vestibular function but also cochlear impairment due to
blood levels over 25 mcg per ml of antibiotic, streptomycin, in humans.
   (AD) Report on dosage, clinical use, and toxicity of streptomycin.
   (AD) Relationship between cochleo-vestibulotoxic effects and daily dosage
   and duration of treatment.
   (AD) Need for audiometry and vestibular function tests during treatment
   and for 6 months after treatment with streptomycin.   (ENG)

                                                                         216
Damage to hair cells and decr in excitation of vestibular apparatus due to
parenteral, intramuscular, administration of 250 mg per kg of antibiotic,
streptomycin (streptomycin sulfate), for 10 and 30 days in animals, guinea
pigs.
Damage to hair cells and decr in excitation of vestibular apparatus due to
parenteral, intramuscular, administration of 250 mg per kg of antibiotic,
streptomycin (IB) (streptomycin sulfate), for 10 and 30 days in animals,
guinea pigs, with intramuscular administration of 1.25 ml per kg of ozothin.

(CT) Study of 14 guinea pigs, control group, with 1.25 ml per kg or 2.5 ml per kg daily of ozothin.
(AD) No decr in streptomycin damage to hair cells of vestibular apparatus with administration of ozothin.
(AD) Evaluation of damage with cytovestibulogram and caloric test.
(AD) Vestibulotoxic effects depend on total dosage of streptomycin used.
(GER)

217

Sensorineural hearing loss due to antibiotic, streptomycin, in humans.
(AD) Comment on ototoxic effects of drugs.   (FIN)

226

Changes in hair cells of inner ear but no damage to stria vascularis due to parenteral, intramuscular, administration of 300 mg per kg of antibiotic, streptomycin (streptomycin sulfate), in animals, guinea pigs.
Damage to hair cells, then complete degeneration of organ of Corti, and degeneration of spiral ganglion due to parenteral, intramuscular, administration of 200 or 300 mg per kg daily of antibiotic, kanamycin (kanamycin sulfate), for range of 7 to 29 injections in 28 animals, guinea pigs.
(AD) Studies using electron microscopy and light microscopy.
(AD) Study of transport in cochlea.
(AD) Suggested that debris from degeneration in cochlea removed by Claudius cells and Reissner's membrane.   (ENG)

232

Degeneration of hair cells of vestibular apparatus due to parenteral administration of antibiotic, kanamycin, in animals, guinea pigs.
Degeneration of hair cells of vestibular apparatus due to administration to middle ear of antibiotic, streptomycin, in animals, guinea pigs.
(AD) Study using surface specimen technique.   (ENG)

237

Hearing loss due to parenteral, intramuscular, administration of 15 mg per kg daily of antibiotic, kanamycin, for 6 to 10 days in 5.1 percent of 143 humans, child, treated when newborn infant for infection.
Hearing loss due to parenteral, intramuscular, administration of 40 mg per kg daily of antibiotic, streptomycin, for 6 to 12 days in 5.6 percent of 93 humans, child, treated when newborn infant for infection.
(CT) Hearing loss in 4.4 percent of 170 children, control group, without antibiotic therapy.
(AD) Hearing loss confirmed by audiogram.
(AD) Suggested low kanamycin ototoxicity in newborn infants with use of recommended dosage.   (ENG)

243

Hearing loss and vestibular problems due to 1.5 g of antibiotic, streptomycin (streptomycin pantothenate), in 1 human, child, male.
(AD) Literature review of pharmacology and toxicology of aminoglycoside antibiotics, streptomycin, dihydrostreptomycin, kanamycin, and neomycin.
(GER)

250

Damage to vestibular apparatus due to more than 1 g daily of antibiotic, streptomycin, for 60 to 120 days in 25 percent of humans.
Dizziness 5 days after cessation of treatment due to parenteral, intramuscular, administration of 1 g every 12 hours of antibiotic, streptomycin (SM), for 9 days in 1 human, adult, 44 years age, female, with peritonitis.
Simultaneous parenteral, intravenous, administration of 600 mg every 18 hours of antibiotic, lincomycin (SM), for 9 days in 1 human, adult, 44 years age, female, with peritonitis.
(AD) Case report of vestibular problem due to streptomycin.
Damage to cochlea due to antibiotic, dihydrostreptomycin, for more than 1 week in 4 to 15 percent of humans.
Sensorineural hearing loss and damage to organ of Corti due to antibiotic, kanamycin, in humans.
Sensorineural hearing loss and damage to organ of Corti due to antibiotic, vancomycin, in humans.

(AD) Discussion of cochleo-vestibulotoxic effects due to antibiotic therapy in surgery. (ENG)

253

Severe vestibular problems, as nystagmus, after 3 to 6 hours due to topical
administration to middle ear and parenteral administration of high doses of
antibiotic, streptomycin, for range of 1 to 7 days in 28 animals, cats.
Decr in ribosomes of cytoplasm of type 1 hair cells of vestibular apparatus
due to topical administration to middle ear and parenteral administration of
high doses of antibiotic, streptomycin, for range of 1 to 7 days in 28 animals, cats.
   (CT) Study of cats, control group.
   (AD) Suggested that primary location of action of streptomycin is protein
   synthesis of cells. (GER)

259

Damage to hair cells of organ of Corti and decr in action potentials due to
parenteral, intramuscular, administration of 250 mg per kg, in distilled
water, of antibiotic, streptomycin (streptomycin sulfate), in 10 doses in 1
group of total of over 100 animals, guinea pigs, 200 g average weight.
Normal hair cells of organ of Corti and no decr in action potentials due to
parenteral, intramuscular, administration of 250 mg per kg of antibiotic,
streptomycin (IB) (streptomycin sulfate), in 10 doses in 1 group of total of
over 100 animals, guinea pigs, 200 g average weight, with administration of
1.2 ml of ozothin.
   (CT) Study of guinea pigs, control group.
   (AD) Significant decr in ototoxicity of streptomycin due to administration
   of ozothin. (ENG)

261

Nystagmus, ataxia, and loss of pinna reflex after 4 to 5 hours due to parenteral, intratympanic, administration of 5 to 20 mg, in 0.1 ml Ringer's solution, of antibiotic, streptomycin (streptomycin sulfate), in 1 ear of 15
animals, guinea pigs, pigmented, 250 to 350 g weight, with normal pinna
reflex.
   (CT) Use of other ear of 15 guinea pigs, control group.
No detected vestibular problems due to parenteral administration of 300 mg
per kg daily of antibiotic, kanamycin (kanamycin sulfate), for 8 to 15 days
in 5 animals, guinea pigs, pigmented, 250 to 350 g weight, with normal pinna
reflex.
Degeneration of hair cells of vestibular apparatus and organ of Corti due to
parenteral, intratympanic, administration of 5 to 20 mg, in 0.1 ml Ringer's
solution, of antibiotic, streptomycin (streptomycin sulfate), in all 15
animals, guinea pigs, pigmented, 250 to 350 g weight, with normal pinna
reflex.
   (AD) Suggested relationship between histological changes and streptomycin
   dosage.
Degeneration of hair cells of vestibular apparatus and organ of Corti due to
parenteral administration of 300 mg per kg daily of antibiotic, kanamycin
(kanamycin sulfate), for 8 to 15 days in 4 out of 5 animals, guinea pigs,
pigmented, 250 to 350 g weight, with normal pinna reflex.
   (AD) Same pattern of degeneration in vestibular apparatus due to streptomycin and kanamycin.
   (AD) Hair cells of vestibular apparatus more sensitive to streptomycin and
   hair cells of organ of Corti more sensitive to kanamycin. (ENG)

271

Sensorineural hearing loss due to antibiotic, streptomycin, in humans, child.
   (AD) Statistical analysis of etiology and occurrence of sensorineural
   hearing loss in children. (JAP)

275

Loss of some hair cells of crista ampullaris with replacement by supporting
cells due to parenteral, intraperitoneal, administration of 250 mg per kg
every other day of antibiotic, streptomycin (streptomycin sulfate), for 8
weeks in 1 group of 48 animals, guinea pigs, pigmented, young, 300 g average
weight.
Loss of some hair cells of crista ampullaris with replacement by supporting

cells due to parenteral, intraperitoneal, administration of 250 mg per kg
every other day of antibiotic, kanamycin (kanamycin sulfate), for 8 weeks in
1 group of 48 animals, guinea pigs, pigmented, young, 300 g average weight.
Loss of some hair cells of crista ampullaris with replacement by supporting
cells due to topical administration to middle ear of 0.6 ml of 250 mg per kg
of antibiotic, streptomycin (streptomycin sulfate), for 3 times with interval
of 1 week in 1 group of 48 animals, guinea pigs, pigmented, young, 300 g
average weight.
Loss of some hair cells of crista ampullaris with replacement by supporting
cells due to topical administration to middle ear of 0.6 ml of 250 mg per kg
of antibiotic, kanamycin (kanamycin sulfate), for 3 times with interval of 1
week in 1 group of 48 animals, guinea pigs, pigmented, young, 300 g average
weight.
   (AD) Degeneration of hair cells of crista ampullaris most severe in group
   with topical administration of streptomycin to middle ear.
   (AD) Degeneration of hair cells of crista ampullaris least severe in group
   with intraperitoneal administration of kanamycin. (ENG)

276

Decr in vestibular responses due to parenteral, intramuscular, administration
of 250 mg per kg of antibiotic, streptomycin (streptomycin sulfate), in 10 or
25 injections in 13 animals, guinea pigs, 250 to 300 g weight.
Decr in vestibular responses for several hours due to parenteral, intraperitoneal, administration of 1.5, 3.0, or 4.5 mg of analeptic, dimorpholamine,
in 17 animals, guinea pigs, 250 to 300 g weight. (GER)

283

Effect on action potentials and cochlear microphonic and on vestibular apparatus due to range of doses of antibiotic, streptomycin, for range of
periods in animals, cats.
Effect on action potentials and cochlear microphonic and on vestibular apparatus due to range of doses of antibiotic, kanamycin, for range of periods
in animals, cats. (IT)

285

Transient inhibition of endorgan of ampulla due to range of doses of antibiotic, streptomycin (streptomycin sulfate), in animals, frogs.
Transient inhibition of endorgan of ampulla due to range of doses of antibio-
tic, dihydrostreptomycin (dihydrostreptomycin sulfate), in animals, frogs.
Transient inhibition of endorgan of ampulla due to range of doses of antibiotic, neomycin (neomycin sulfate), in animals, frogs.
Transient inhibition of endorgan of ampulla due to range of doses of antibiotic, kanamycin (kanamycin sulfate), in animals, frogs.
   (CT) Study of frogs, control group.
   (AD) More inhibition of endorgan of ampulla with streptomycin than with
   other aminoglycoside antibiotics.
   (AD) Agreement between in vivo and in vitro observations of intensity of
   action on endorgans of vestibular apparatus. (ENG)

288

Changes in cochlear microphonic due to parenteral, intramuscular, administration of 300 mg per kg daily of antibiotic, kanamycin, in animals, cats.
Changes in cochlear microphonic due to parenteral, intramuscular, administration of 200 and 100 mg per kg daily of antibiotic, streptomycin, in animals,
cats.
Hearing loss due to 300 mg per kg daily of antibiotic, kanamycin, in humans.
Hearing loss due to range of 50 to 200 mg per kg daily of antibiotic, streptomycin, in humans.
   (CT) Study of subjects, control group, not treated with aminoglycoside
   antibiotics.
   (AD) Hearing loss confirmed by audiogram. (JAP)

290

Vestibular problems, sensorineural hearing loss, and tinnitus due to total
doses of 12 to 63 g of antibiotic, streptomycin, in 24 humans with tuberculosis.
   (AD) Subjects tested after streptomycin intoxication with audiology and
   cupulometry.

(AD) Individual responses to streptomycin observed.
Changes in cupulometric curves for postrotatory nystagmus, showing changes in
vestibular apparatus, due to 0.5 g daily, total doses of 30 to 100 g, of
antibiotic, streptomycin (SM) (streptomycin sulfate), in 23 humans with
various infections.
Simultaneous administration of 0.5 g of antibiotic, dihydrostreptomycin (SM),
in 23 humans with various infections.
Simultaneous administration of antituberculous agent, PAS (SM), in 23 humans
with various infections.
   (CT) Pretreatment vestibular function normal.
   (CT) Subjects tested with audiology and cupulometry before and during
   treatment with streptomycin.
   (AD) Hearing loss in 1 subject in group with cupulometry during treatment
   but in 5 subjects in other group with cupulometry only after treatment.
   (AD) Suggested use of cupulometry for possible prevention of streptomycin
   intoxication. (ENG)

                                                                      293
Cochleo-vestibulotoxic effects due to antibiotic, streptomycin (SM), in
humans, range of ages, with pulmonary tuberculosis.
Simultaneous administration of other antituberculous agents (SM) in humans,
range of ages, with pulmonary tuberculosis.
   (AD) Report on toxic effects due to simultaneous treatment with various
   antituberculous agents.   (BUL)

                                                                      296
Ototoxic effects due to antibiotic, streptomycin, in large number of humans.
(BUL)

                                                                      311
Vertigo or hearing loss of 10 to 20 decibels due to antibiotic, streptomycin,
in 14 of 67 humans with pulmonary tuberculosis.
Vertigo or hearing loss of 30 to 40 decibels due to antibiotic, streptomycin
(CB), in 12 of 59 humans with pulmonary tuberculosis.
Vertigo or hearing loss of 30 to 40 decibels due to antibiotic, dihydrostrep-
tomycin (CB), in 12 of 59 humans with pulmonary tuberculosis.
   (AD) Hearing loss confirmed by audiometry.   (DUT)

                                                                      316
Possible vestibular problems and cochlear impairment due to more than recommended dose of 15 to 30 mg per kg daily of antibiotic, streptomycin, for long
period in humans.
Hearing loss due to parenteral, intramuscular, administration of total doses
of 5 to 6 g of antibiotic, kanamycin, in humans, adult, with kidney disorder.
Possible hearing loss due to parenteral, topical, or oral administration of
high doses of antibiotic, neomycin, for long period in humans.
Possible hearing loss due to high doses of antibiotic, framycetin, for long
period in humans.
Possible hearing loss due to antibiotic, vancomycin, in humans.
Possible hearing loss and vestibular problems due to antibiotic, viomycin, in
humans.
   (AD) High risk of ototoxicity with simultaneous administration of viomycin
   and streptomycin.
Possible vestibular problems due to antibiotic, gentamicin, in humans.
   (AD) Administration of gentamicin not recommended for newborn infants, for
   humans during pregnancy, and for humans treated with other ototoxic drugs.
Ataxia and hearing loss due to antibiotic, colistin, in humans.
   (AD) Literature review on ototoxic antibiotics.
   (AD) Results of studies on use of pantothenate salt of some antibiotics
   for decr in ototoxicity not clear.
   (AD) Suggested effect of ototoxic antibiotics on breakdown of glucose on
   which hair cells of inner ear depend for energy.   (ENG)

                                                                      318
High risk of ototoxic effects due to antibiotic, dihydrostreptomycin, in
humans with bacterial infections.
Risk of ototoxic effects due to antibiotic, streptomycin, in humans with
bacterial infections, with administration of pantothenic acid.

(AD) Literature review on clinical use and ototoxicity of streptomycin.
(AD) Recommended use of streptomycin only for tuberculosis due to high
risk of ototoxic effects. (GER)

                                                                        319
Ototoxic effects due to antibiotic, streptomycin, in humans with infections
of ear.
(AD) Literature review of clinical use and ototoxicity of streptomycin.
(GER)

                                                                        321
Vestibular problems due to antibiotic, streptomycin, in humans.
(AD) Use of ENG to determine extent of vestibular problems due to strep-
tomycin.   (RUM)

                                                                        323
Progressive severe bilateral sensorineural hearing loss and vestibular problems due to parenteral administration of 1 g twice weekly of antibiotic, (SQ)
viomycin (viomycin pantothenate), for total of 10 weeks in 1 human, adult, 59
years age, female, with pulmonary tuberculosis and kidney disorder.
(AD) Cochleo-vestibulotoxic effects confirmed by audiometry at different
periods during and after treatment and by caloric test.
Previous administration of antibiotic, (SQ) chloramphenicol, in 1 human,
adult, 59 years age, female, for infection before diagnosis of tuberculosis.
Possible but not reported auditory system problems due to previous parenteral
administration of 0.5 g twice daily of antibiotic, (SQ) streptomycin, for 1
week in 1 human, adult, 59 years age, female, for infection before diagnosis
of tuberculosis.
(AD) Suggested that possible previous ototoxic effects of streptomycin
potentiated by viomycin (viomycin pantothenate).
Previous administration of antituberculous agent, (SQ) PAS, in 1 human,
adult, 59 years age, female, with pulmonary tuberculosis and kidney disorder.
(ENG)

                                                                        324
Ataxia, vestibular problems with improvement in some, and damage to hair
cells of vestibular apparatus due to parenteral, subcutaneous, administration
of 20 mg per kg of antibiotic, gentamicin (gentamicin sulfate), for 19 days
maximum for acute intoxication and 14 days for chronic intoxication in 15
animals, cats.
Hearing loss and damage to hair cells of cochlea due to parenteral, subcutaneous, administration of 20 mg per kg of antibiotic, gentamicin (gentamicin
sulfate), for 19 days maximum for acute intoxication and 14 days for chronic
intoxication in 1 of 15 animals, cats.
(AD) Preliminary study to determine minimum toxic level of gentamicin by
parenteral route made previously.
(AD) Cochleo-vestibulotoxic effects determined by audiometry and vestibular function tests.
Permanent severe vestibular problems and damage to hair cells of vestibular
apparatus due to parenteral, subcutaneous, administration of 200 mg per kg of
antibiotic, streptomycin (streptomycin sulfate), in 3 animals, cats.
Hearing loss and damage to hair cells of cochlea due to parenteral, subcutaneous, administration of 200 mg per kg of antibiotic, streptomycin (streptomycin sulfate), in 2 of 3 animals, cats.
Ataxia, vestibular problems, and damage to hair cells of vestibular apparatus
due to topical administration to bulla in solution of 6 percent concentration
in water of antibiotic, gentamicin (gentamicin sulfate), for 19 days in 1
animal, cat.
Ataxia, vestibular problems, and more severe damage to hair cells of vestibular apparatus due to topical administration to bulla in solution of 6 percent
concentration in Monex of antibiotic, gentamicin (gentamicin sulfate), for 5
days in 3 animals, cats.
(CT) Same method using water or Monex without gentamicin in 11 cats,
control group, showed no ototoxic effects.
(AD) Preliminary study to determine concentration of gentamicin for topical route made previously.
Vestibular problems due to topical administration to bulla in solution of 6
percent concentration in water of antibiotic, neomycin, for 31 days in 2

animals, cats.
   (AD) Comparative study of effects of gentamicin and other aminoglycoside
   antibiotics.
   (AD) Ototoxicity of gentamicin dose related.   (ENG)

                                                                        325
High frequency hearing loss due to parenteral, intramuscular, administration
of total of 15 mg per kg in 2 doses 5 times a week of antibiotic, (SQ) capreomycin (SM), for 37 and 45 days in 2 of 70 humans, adult, 35 and 64 years
age, with pulmonary tuberculosis and with previous treatment with other
ototoxic drugs.
Transient vertigo due to parenteral, intramuscular, administration of total
of 15 mg per kg in 2 doses 5 times a week of antibiotic, (SQ) capreomycin
(SM), for 5, 25, and 94 days in 3 of 70 humans, adult, 39, 61, and 62 years
age, with pulmonary tuberculosis and with previous treatment with streptomycin.
Simultaneous administration of other (SQ) antituberculous agents (SM), in 70
humans, adult, male and female, with pulmonary tuberculosis.
Possible ototoxic effects due to previous administration of antibiotic, (SQ)
streptomycin, in 3 of 70 humans, adult, 39, 61, and 62 years age, with pulmonary tuberculosis.   (ENG)

                                                                        332
No subjective hearing loss but objective hearing loss over 20 decibels and
tinnitus due to parenteral, intramuscular, administration of 1 g daily for
first 60 days and then 1 g twice a week of antibiotic, capreomycin (SM), for
6 months in 3 of 100 humans treated for pulmonary tuberculosis.
Hearing loss, tinnitus, or dizziness due to parenteral, intramuscular, administration of 1 g daily for first 60 days and then 1 g twice a week of
antibiotic, streptomycin (SM), for 6 months in 8 of 99 humans treated for
pulmonary tuberculosis.
Hearing loss over 20 decibels due to parenteral, intramuscular, administration of 1 g daily for first 60 days and then 1 g twice a week of antibiotic,
streptomycin (SM), for 6 months in 3 of 99 humans treated for pulmonary
tuberculosis.
Simultaneous oral administration of 0.3 g daily in 2 doses of antituberculous
agent, isoniazid (SM), for 6 months in humans treated for pulmonary tuberculosis.
Simultaneous administration of 10 g daily in 3 doses of antituberculous
agent, PAS (SM), for 6 months in humans treated for pulmonary tuberculosis.
   (AD) Report on ototoxic effects of antibiotics used in initial treatment
   of tuberculosis.
High frequency hearing loss, tinnitus, or dizziness due to parenteral, intramuscular, administration of 1 g daily for first 60 days and then 1 g twice a
week of antibiotic, capreomycin (SM), for 6 months in 6 of 66 humans retreated for pulmonary tuberculosis.
No subjective auditory system problems but objective hearing loss over 20
decibels due to parenteral, intramuscular, administration of 1 g 3 times a
week of antibiotic, kanamycin (SM), for 6 months in 4 of 40 humans retreated
for pulmonary tuberculosis.
No subjective auditory system problems but objective hearing loss over 20
decibels due to parenteral, intramuscular, administration of 1 g daily for
first 60 days and then 1 g twice a week of antibiotic, streptomycin (SM), for
6 months in 1 of 13 humans retreated for pulmonary tuberculosis.
Simultaneous oral administration of 0.3 g daily in 2 doses of antituberculous
agent, isoniazid (SM), for 6 months in humans retreated for pulmonary tuberculosis.
   (AD) Report on ototoxic effects of antibiotics used in retreatment of
   tuberculosis.
   (CT) Audiometry, pretreatment and during treatment, 2 times a month in
   first 2 months and then 1 time a month.
   (AD) Comparative study of clinical use and cochleo-vestibulotoxic effects
   of capreomycin and other antibiotics in treatment and retreatment of
   pulmonary tuberculosis.   (ENG)

                                                                        333
Vestibular problems due to antibiotic, streptomycin, in humans.
Severe cochlear impairment due to antibiotic, dihydrostreptomycin, in humans.

Loss of hair cells in organ of Corti and hearing loss due to antibiotics,
aminoglycoside, in humans.
Hearing loss in fetus due to antimalarial, quinine, in humans, female,
treated during pregnancy.
Transient hearing loss due to high doses of salicylate, aspirin, for long
period in humans.
   (AD) Discussion of possible cochleo-vestibulotoxic effects of ototoxic
   drugs.
   (AD) Ototoxic effects related to concurrent disorders, dosage, duration of
   treatment, and age of individuals. (ENG)

                                                                        334
Effect on organ of Corti of fetuses due to parenteral, intraperitoneal,
administration of daily doses of antibiotic, streptomycin, in animals, rats,
female, during pregnancy.
Effect on organ of Corti of fetuses due to parenteral, intraperitoneal,
administration of daily doses of antibiotic, dihydrostreptomycin, in animals,
rats, female, during pregnancy.
   (AD) Determined concentration of antibiotic in blood of fetus.   (GER)

                                                                        335
Vestibular problems due to antibiotic, streptomycin, in humans.
Severe cochlear impairment due to antibiotic, dihydrostreptomycin, in humans.
Cochlear impairment due to parenteral, oral, and topical administration of
antibiotic, neomycin, in humans.
Tinnitus and hearing loss due to antibiotic, kanamycin, in humans.
Vestibular problems and hearing loss due to antibiotic, gentamicin, in hu-
mans.
   (AD) Discussion of clinical use and possible cochleo-vestibulotoxic ef-
   fects of aminoglycoside antibiotics. (SP)

                                                                        336
Damage to type 1 hair cells of vestibular apparatus and vestibular problems
due to topical administration to middle ear of antibiotic, streptomycin, in 1
injection in animals.
   (AD) Destruction of hair cells and ototoxicity result of effect of streptomycin on protein synthesis of cells. (FR)

                                                                        340
Vestibular problems due to 150 mg daily of antituberculous agent, thiaceta-
zone (SM), in 15 of 75 humans with pulmonary tuberculosis.
Vestibular problems due to 0.75 to 1 g daily of antibiotic, streptomycin (SM)
(streptomycin sulfate), in 15 of 75 humans with pulmonary tuberculosis.
Vestibular problems due to 300 mg daily of antituberculous agent, isoniazid
(SM), in 15 of 75 humans with pulmonary tuberculosis.
   (AD) Vestibulotoxic effects confirmed by vestibular function tests.
   (AD) Statistical analysis showed higher occurrence of vestibular problems
   in humans with thiacetazone in drug regimen than without thiacetazone.
   (SL)

                                                                        341
Transient vestibular problems due to 1.0 g daily of antibiotic, streptomycin
(streptomycin sulfate), for short period, 1 or 2 months, in 32 of 84 humans
with tuberculosis.
   (AD) Vestibulotoxic effects determined by ENG.
   (AD) Slight vestibular problem in only 2 humans 1 year after cessation of
   treatment. (POL)

                                                                        342
More severe sensorineural hearing loss of 20 decibels or more due to parenteral administration of total doses of 173 and 172 g of antibiotic, (SQ)
capreomycin, for long period, range of 2 to 18 months, in 2 of 294 humans,
male and female, with pulmonary tuberculosis and with previous hearing loss.
   (CT) Audiometry, pretreatment and during treatment.
   (AD) Suggested that occurrence of auditory system problems due to capreomycin not high.
Sensorineural hearing loss due to previous administration of antibiotic, (SQ)
streptomycin, in 1 of 294 humans with pulmonary tuberculosis. (ENG)

343

No hearing loss but decr in vestibular function, asymptomatic except for
dizziness in 1 case, due to 1 g daily of antibiotic, capreomycin (SM), for 4
months or more in 4 of 25 humans, adolescent, adult, and aged, range of 17 to
67 years age, male and female, 80 to 160 lb weight, with pulmonary tuberculosis and with kidney disorder in 2 cases.
Transient dizziness with no objective decr in vestibular function due to 1 g
daily of antibiotic, capreomycin (SM), for 4 months or more in 3 of 25 humans, adolescent, adult, and aged, range of 17 to 67 years age, male and
female, 80 to 160 lb weight, with pulmonary tuberculosis.
Simultaneous administration of 300 mg daily of antituberculous agent, isoniazid (SM), for 4 months or more in 25 humans, adolescent, adult, and aged,
range of 17 to 67 years age, male and female, 80 to 160 lb weight, with
pulmonary tuberculosis.
   (CT) Pure tone audiometry, caloric tests, and cupulometry, pretreatment
   and during treatment with capreomycin.
   (AD) Study of clinical use and cochleo-vestibulotoxic effects of capreomycin.
Hearing loss, asymptomatic in 1 case and symptomatic in 1 case, due to 1 g
daily of antibiotic, viomycin, in 2 of 75 humans with pulmonary tuberculosis.
Objective decr in vestibular function due to 1 g daily of antibiotic, viomycin, in 21 of 75 humans with pulmonary tuberculosis.
Hearing loss, asymptomatic, due to 1 g daily of antibiotic, streptomycin, in
2 of 61 humans with pulmonary tuberculosis.
Objective decr in vestibular function due to 1 g daily of antibiotic, streptomycin, in 8 of 61 humans with pulmonary tuberculosis.
   (CT) Audiometry and vestibular function tests, pretreatment and during
   treatment with viomycin or streptomycin.
   (AD) Results of study on capreomycin comp w results of previous study on
   viomycin and streptomycin. (ENG)

346

Temporary inhibition of oxygen consumption at level of mitochondria of central vestibular nuclei due to antibiotic, streptomycin, in animals.
Temporary inhibition of oxygen consumption at level of mitochondria of central vestibular nuclei due to antibiotic, rifampicin, in animals.
   (AD) Discussion of chronic and acute vestibular toxicity. (ENG)

347

Delayed hearing loss at 2 different times due to 15 g each time of antibiotic, streptomycin, in 1 human, child, male, treated at 8 years age for rheumatism and at 13 years age for pneumonia.
   (AD) Similar audiograms after 2 periods of treatment.
Delayed hearing loss due to 6 and 8 g of antibiotic, streptomycin, in 2
humans, adult and child, female, mother and daughter.
Delayed hearing loss due to 6 and 5 g of antibiotic, streptomycin, in 2
humans, adult, 34 and 36 years age, female, sisters.
Delayed hearing loss due to 10 and 8 g of antibiotic, streptomycin, in 2
humans, adult, 23 and 24 years age, female, sisters.
Sensorineural hearing loss due to 10 and 4 g of antibiotic, streptomycin, in
3 humans, female, sisters.
Delayed hearing loss due to low doses of antibiotic, streptomycin, in 3
humans, adult and child, 50, 26, and 8 years age, female, mother, daughter,
and granddaughter.
   (AD) Suggested familial and constitutional predisposition in streptomycin
   ototoxicity. (FR)

350

Cochleotoxic effects due to 0.75 or 1 g daily, total doses of 30.0 to 116.75
g, of antibiotic, streptomycin, in 9(7.2 percent)of 125 humans with disorders.
Cochleotoxic effects due to 1 g daily, total of less than 30 to over 180 g,
of antibiotic, kanamycin, in 40 (55.6 percent) of 72 humans with disorders.
   (AD) Comparative study of ototoxic effects of 2 aminoglycoside antibiotics. (GER)

354

Vestibular problems due to 1 g daily, total doses of 1 to 115 g before onset

of ototoxicity, of antibiotic, streptomycin (SM), for several days to 9
months in 56 of 364 humans, adolescent and adult, 16 to 64 years age, female,
with tuberculosis of genitourinary system.
No specified ototoxic effects due to range of doses of antituberculous agent,
PAS (SM), for several days to 9 months in 13 of 369 humans, adolescent and
adult, 16 to 64 years age, female, with tuberculosis of genitourinary system.
Simultaneous administration of antituberculous agent, isoniazid (SM), in 274
humans, adolescent and adult, 16 to 64 years age, female, with tuberculosis
of genitourinary system.   (ENG)

356

Hearing loss due to antibiotic, streptomycin, in 120 of 150 humans, child, 2
to 4 years age, most treated when newborn infant or infant for different
disorders.
Hearing loss due to antibiotic, streptomycin (SM), in 30 of 150 humans,
child, 2 to 4 years age, most treated when newborn infant or infant for
different disorders.
Hearing loss due to antibiotic, neomycin (SM), in 30 of 150 humans, child, 2
to 4 years age, most treated when newborn infant or infant for different
disorders.
Hearing loss due to other antibiotics (SM) in 30 of 150 humans, child, 2 to 4
years age, most treated when newborn infant or infant for different disorders.
   (AD) Hearing loss determined by play audiometry.
   (AD) No relationship between hearing loss and dosage or duration of treatment with antibiotics.
   (AD) No improvement in hearing after 1 to 2 years.   (RUS)

358

Severe to total hearing loss due to antibiotic, paromomycin, in most of
humans treated.
Severe to total hearing loss due to antibiotic, streptomycin, in most of
humans treated.
Severe to total hearing loss due to antibiotic, neomycin, in most of humans
treated.
Objective but no subjective vestibular problems due to antibiotic, streptomycin, in 2 humans.   (RUS)

362

Hearing loss due to high and low doses of antibiotic, streptomycin, in humans, child and adult, with different disorders and with previous hearing
loss in 2 humans.
Hearing loss due to high doses of antibiotic, neomycin, in humans, child and
adult, with different disorders.
   (AD) Need for daily audiometry and vestibular function tests with administration of aminoglycoside antibiotics.
   (AD) If ototoxic effect observed, need to withdraw ototoxic drug or ad-
   minister vitamins, glucose, dimedrol, calcium chloride, or electrophoresis
   with potassium iodide.   (RUS)

363

Decr in hearing loss due to antibiotic, streptomycin (IB), in 9 of 40 humans
with administration of ATP, vitamin A, vitamin E, ascorbic acid, or nicotinic
acid.
Decr in hearing loss due to other antibiotics (IB) in 9 of 40 humans with
administration of ATP, vitamin A, vitamin E, ascorbic acid, or nicotinic
acid.
   (CT) Audiology before and 5 to 6 days after administration of inhibitors.
   (AD) Study of effectiveness of treatment of auditory system problems due
   to ototoxic drugs.   (RUS)

364

Damage to organ of Corti, spiral ganglion, and cochlear nuclei of medulla
oblongata 15 days after beginning of treatment due to 100 mg per kg of antibiotic, streptomycin, in 38 animals, guinea pigs.
Decr in damage to spiral ganglion and cochlear nuclei of medulla oblongata
due to 100 mg per kg of antibiotic, streptomycin (IB), in 8 of 18 animals,
guinea pigs, with simultaneous administration of 2 ml of 5 percent unitiol

for 30 to 60 days.
Decr in hearing loss due to ototoxic drugs (IB) in 3 of 25 humans with ad-
ministration of unitiol.
No hearing loss due to antibiotic, streptomycin (IB), in 25 humans with
pulmonary tuberculosis with administration of unitiol.
   (AD) Study of effect of inhibitor, unitiol, on streptomycin ototoxicity.
   (RUS)

367

Auditory system problems due to oral administration of 150 mg daily of antituberculous agent, thiacetazone (CB), for 12 weeks in 47 of 581 humans,
adolescent and adult, 15 years or over age, male and female, with pulmonary
tuberculosis.
Auditory system problems due to oral administration of 150 mg daily of antituberculous agent, thiacetazone (CB) (IB), for 12 weeks in 39 of 584 humans,
adolescent and adult, 15 years or over age, male and female, with pulmonary
tuberculosis, with administration of vitamins and antihistamine.
Combined oral administration of 300 mg daily of antituberculous agent, i-
soniazid (CB), for 12 weeks in humans, adolescent and adult, 15 years or over
age, male and female, with pulmonary tuberculosis.
   (AD) Study of effect of inhibitors on toxicity of drugs in 1 group with
   drug regimen of thiacetazone and isoniazid in combination.
Auditory system problems due to parenteral administration of 1 g daily of
antibiotic, streptomycin (SM), for 12 weeks in 227 of 689 humans, adolescent
and adult, 15 years or over age, male and female, with pulmonary tuberculosis.
Auditory system problems due to parenteral administration of 1 g daily of
antibiotic, streptomycin (SM) (IB), for 12 weeks in 218 of 707 humans, adolescent and adult, 15 years or over age, male and female, with pulmonary tuberculosis, with administration of vitamins and antihistamine.
Auditory system problems due to simultaneous oral administration of 150 mg
daily of antituberculous agent, thiacetazone (SM), for 12 weeks in humans,
adolescent and adult, 15 years or over age, male and female, with pulmonary
tuberculosis.
Simultaneous oral administration of 300 mg daily of antituberculous agent,
isoniazid (SM), for 12 weeks in humans, adolescent and adult, 15 years or
over age, male and female, with pulmonary tuberculosis.
   (AD) Study of effect of inhibitors on toxicity of drugs in 1 group with
   drug regimen of streptomycin, thiacetazone, and isoniazid.
Auditory system problems due to parenteral administration of 1 g daily of
antibiotic, streptomycin (SM), for 12 weeks in 109 of 711 humans, adolescent
and adult, 15 years or over age, male and female, with pulmonary tuberculosis.
Auditory system problems due to parenteral administration of 1 g daily of
antibiotic, streptomycin (SM) (IB), for 12 weeks in 111 of 696 humans, adolescent and adult, 15 years or over age, male and female, with pulmonary tuberculosis, with administration of vitamins and antihistamine.
Simultaneous oral administration of 300 mg daily of antituberculous agent,
isoniazid (SM), for 12 weeks in humans, adolescent and adult, 15 years or
over age, male and female, with pulmonary tuberculosis.
   (AD) Study of effect of inhibitors on toxicity of drugs in 1 group with
   drug regimen of streptomycin and isoniazid.
   (AD) Study of effectiveness of inhibitors in prevention of toxic effects
   of thiacetazone and streptomycin.
   (AD) Study suggested that vitamins and antihistamine not effective in
   prevention of toxicity. (ENG)

368

Possible vestibular problems and hearing loss due to antibiotic, streptomycin, in humans with tuberculosis.
Permanent hearing loss due to antibiotic, dihydrostreptomycin, in humans with
tuberculosis.
Possible permanent hearing loss due to antibiotic, kanamycin, in humans with
tuberculosis.
Possible vestibular problems and hearing loss due to antibiotic, viomycin, in
humans with tuberculosis.
Possible damage to eighth cranial nerve due to antibiotic, capreomycin, in
humans with tuberculosis.

(AD) Discussion of primary and secondary drugs used in tuberculosis chemotherapy. (FR)

375

Possible hearing loss due to antibiotic, streptomycin, in humans.
(AD) Discussion of value of experimentation with animals to determine use
and effects of drugs in humans.
(AD) Possible to determine total hearing loss due to drugs in dogs and
monkeys but more difficult to determine partial hearing loss in animals.
(AD) Possible that high doses of drugs used in experimentation help to
determine effects in therapeutic doses. (ENG)

377

Lesion of vestibular apparatus due to about 22 g of antibiotic, streptomycin
(SM), in human with pulmonary tuberculosis.
(AD) Lesion of vestibular apparatus confirmed by vestibular function test.
Simultaneous administration of 185 g of antituberculous agent, PAS (SM), in
human with pulmonary tuberculosis.
Simultaneous administration of 16.5 g of antituberculous agent, isoniazid
(SM), in human with pulmonary tuberculosis. (POL)

380

Unilateral loss of vestibular function and no ataxia due to parenteral administration, infusion into carotid artery, of 150 cc in Ringer's Lactate
every 24 hours, total dose of 0.84 to 1.5 g per kg, of antibiotic, streptomycin (streptomycin sulfate), for 3 to 10 days in 5 animals, cat s, adult, 1.9
to 3.1 kg weight.
Bilateral loss of vestibular function with ataxia and destruction of hair
cells of crista ampullaris and semicircular canal due to parenteral administration, infusion into carotid artery, of 150 cc in Ringer's Lactate every 24
hours, total dose of 1.2 to 2.5 g per kg, of antibiotic, streptomycin (streptomycin sulfate), for 6 to 12 days in 5 animals, cats, adult, 2.3 to 5.1 kg
weight.
No hearing loss and no damage to hair cells of organ of Corti due to parenteral administration, infusion into carotid artery, of 150 cc in Ringer's
Lactate every 24 hours, total dose of 0.84 to 2.5 g per kg, of antibiotic,
streptomycin (streptomycin sulfate), for 3 to 12 days in 10 animals, cats,
adult, 1.9 to 5.1 kg weight.
Decr in cochlear microphonic but no damage to hair cells of organ of Corti
due to parenteral administration, infusion into carotid artery, of 150 cc in
Ringer's Lactate every 24 hours, total dose of 1.0 g per kg, of antibiotic,
streptomycin (streptomycin sulfate), for 4 days in 1 animal, cat, adult, 3.0
kg weight.
(CT) Measurement of cochlear function and vestibular function before and
after infusion of streptomycin.
(AD) Type of loss of vestibular function due to total dosage of streptomycin and duration of administration.
(AD) Unilateral destruction of vestibular function without cochlear impairment is goal in treatment of Meniere's disease. (ENG)

384

Usually transient hearing loss and no structural damage to organ of Corti,
stria vascularis, and spiral ganglion due to oral or topical administration
of salicylates in humans.
Hearing loss due to antimalarial, quinine, in humans.
Usually permanent hearing loss due to antimalarial, chloroquine, in humans.
Transient and permanent hearing loss and possible damage to hair cells of
organ of Corti due to diuretic, ethacrynic acid, in humans.
Sensorineural hearing loss due to cardiovascular agent, hexadimethrine
bromide, in humans with kidney disorder.
Sensorineural hearing loss and damage to organ of Corti due to topical ad-
ministration of antineoplastic, nitrogen mustard, in humans.
Sensorineural hearing loss due to high doses of antibiotic, chloramphenicol,
in humans.
Primary vestibular problems due to antibiotic, streptomycin, in humans.
Hearing loss due to high doses usually of antibiotic, streptomycin, in hu-
mans.
(AD) Early detection of hearing loss by audiometry prevents permanent

damage.
High frequency hearing loss and severe damage to outer hair cells and slight
damage to inner hair cells of organ of Corti due to antibiotic, kanamycin, in
humans.
Sensorineural hearing loss due to parenteral, oral, and topical administration of antibiotic, neomycin, in humans with or without kidney disorders.
Degeneration of hair cells of organ of Corti and of nerve process due to
antibiotics, aminoglycoside, in animals.
    (AD) Literature review of physiological and structural cochleo-vestibulo-
    toxic effects of ototoxic drugs.
    (AD) Discussion of suggested mechanism of ototoxicity and routes of drugs
    to inner ear.
Bilateral sensorineural hearing loss due to oral administration of antibiotic, neomycin, in 4 of 8 humans with liver disease.
Bilateral sensorineural hearing loss due to oral administration of range of
doses of antibiotic, neomycin (SM), in 2 of 5 humans with liver disease.
Bilateral sensorineural hearing loss due to diuretics (SM), in 2 of 5 humans
with liver disease.
Transient progression of previous hearing loss due to parenteral, intravenous, administration of diuretic, ethacrynic acid (SM), in 1 injection in 1
of 5 humans with liver disease.
    (CT) Normal cochlear function in 6 humans, control group, with liver
    disease and not treated with neomycin or diuretics.
    (CT) Normal cochlear function in 13 humans, control group, with liver
    disease and treated with diuretics but not with neomycin.
    (AD) Hearing loss confirmed by audiometry.
    (AD) Reported that hearing loss due to neomycin or diuretics in humans
    with liver disease not related to dosage.
    (AD) Clinical study of effects of treatment with neomycin and diuretics in
    humans with liver disease.
Bilateral sensorineural hearing loss and vertigo due to antibiotic, ampicillin, in 1 human, adolescent, 17 years age, female, with tonsillitis.
    (AD) Cited case report.
Severe sensorineural hearing loss and vertigo due to topical administration
in ear drops of antibiotic, framycetin, in 1 human, adult, 42 years age,
male, with previous slight high frequency hearing loss.
    (AD) Cited case report.
Atrophy of hair cells of organ of Corti and hearing loss due to antibiotic,
dihydrostreptomycin, in humans with tuberculous meningitis.
    (AD) Cited study.
Loss of inner hair cells and damage to outer hair cells due to 18 g of antibiotic, neomycin, for 18 days in 1 human.
    (AD) Cited case report. (ENG)

                                                                        390
Sensorineural hearing loss due to antibiotic, streptomycin, in 2.2 percent of
3250 humans with pulmonary tuberculosis.
    (AD) Symptoms of cochlear impairment more delayed than symptoms of disor-
    der of vestibular function. (RUS)

                                                                        392
No hearing loss but tinnitus due to parenteral, intramuscular, administration
of range of 0.05 to 1.0 g daily according to age of antibiotic, kanamycin,
for short period in 4 of 125 humans, infant, child, and adult, with acute
otorhinolaryngological infections.
    (AD) Audiograms showed no hearing loss.
Hearing loss, subjective in 1 case and latent in others, but no vestibular
problems due to 1.0 g daily 2 times a week of antibiotic, (SQ) kanamycin, for
long period in 15 of 66 humans, adolescent and adult, 15 to 55 years age,
with pulmonary tuberculosis and with previous streptomycin treatment.
    (CT) Audiogram before and during treatment with kanamycin.
Hearing loss due to previous administration of antibiotic, (SQ) streptomycin,
in 31 of 272 humans.
Sensorineural hearing loss due to previous administration of total of 600 g
of antibiotic, (SQ) streptomycin, in 1 human, adult, 27 years age.
More severe sensorineural hearing loss, subjective, due to total of 136 g of
antibiotic, (SQ) kanamycin, in 1 human, adult, 27 years age.
    (AD) Case report of hearing loss due to streptomycin potentiated by treat-

ment with kanamycin.
Hearing loss, latent, and tinnitus, but no vestibular problems due to total
of over 20 g to over 300 g of antibiotic, kanamycin, for long period in 10 of
70 humans with pulmonary tuberculosis and no previous chemotherapy.
  (CT) Audiogram before and during treatment with kanamycin.
  (AD) Clinical studies of effects of treatment with kanamycin for short and
  long periods.
Vestibular problems after 10 to 12 days due to parenteral administration of
100 mg per kg daily of antibiotic, streptomycin, in 3 animals, cats, 2 kg
weight.
Slight vestibular problems after 30 days due to 300 mg per kg daily of antibiotic, kanamycin, in 3 animals, cats, 2 kg weight.
Decr in cochlear microphonic due to 200 mg per kg daily of antibiotic, streptomycin, in 11 injections in animals, cats.
Slight decr in cochlear microphonic due to 300 mg per kg daily of antibiotic,
kanamycin, in 11 to 60 injections in animals, cats.
  (AD) Comparative experimental studies of cochleo-vestibulotoxic effects of
  kanamycin and streptomycin in cats.
  (AD) Different effects of 2 aminoglycoside antibiotics on vestibular
  function but similar effects on cochlear function. (ENG)

394

Tinnitus and hearing loss due to total of 50 to 100 g, in some cases, of
antibiotic, (SQ) kanamycin, in 176(9 percent) of 2054 humans with surgery for
pulmonary tuberculosis.
  (AD) Improvement in hearing in only 30 percent of humans.
Possible hearing loss due to previous administration of antibiotic, (SQ)
streptomycin, for long period in 176 of 2054 humans before surgery for pulmonary tuberculosis. (ENG)

395

Damage first to outer hair cells of organ of Corti in basal coil of cochlea
due to high doses of antibiotics, aminoglycoside, in animals, guinea pigs.
  (AD) Same damage due to x-ray radiation.
Primary damage to central areas of crista ampullaris, crista neglecta, and
macula due to antibiotics, aminoglycoside, in animals, guinea pigs.
  (AD) Damage to peripheral areas of crista ampullaris, crista neglecta, and
  macula due to x-ray radiation.
Disturbance of protein synthesis due to topical administration to bulla of
antibiotic, streptomycin, in animals, guinea pigs.
  (AD) Similar electron microscopy findings for streptomycin administration
  to bulla and for x-ray radiation.
  (AD) Cochleo-vestibulotoxic effects due to x-ray radiation comp w effects
  due to antibiotics. (ENG)

399

Risk of vestibular problems due to antibiotic, streptomycin, in humans,
adult, with tuberculous meningitis.
  (AD) Report on treatment of meningitis and possible toxic effects of drugs
  used. (GER)

403

Risk of damage to function of eighth cranial nerve due to antibiotic, streptomycin, for long period in humans, adult and child, with tuberculous meningitis.
  (AD) Need for tests of function of eighth cranial nerve with clinical use
  of streptomycin.
  (AD) Literature review of treatment of infections of CNS. (ENG)

408

Ototoxic effects due to antibiotic, streptomycin, in humans.
  (AD) Discussion of streptomycin ototoxicity, 1 of topics at conference on
  various aspects of the ear and hearing. (FR)

409

Primary damage to hair cells of organ of Corti, hearing loss, and possible
vestibular problems due to antibiotic, viomycin, in humans.
Damage to hair cells of organ of Corti and hearing loss due to antibiotic,

neomycin, in humans.
Damage to hair cells of organ of Corti and hearing loss due to antibiotic,
kanamycin, in humans.
Primary damage to vestibular apparatus, vestibular problems, and possible
hearing loss due to antibiotic, streptomycin, in humans.
Primary damage to vestibular apparatus, vestibular problems, and possible
hearing loss due to antibiotic, gentamicin, in humans.
  (AD) Need for audiometry and vestibular function tests, pretreatment and
  during treatment, with clinical use of aminoglycoside antibiotics.
  (AD) Incr in blood levels and ototoxicity of antibiotics in humans with
  kidney disorders. (ENG)

419

Hearing loss and vestibular problems due to antibiotic, streptomycin, in
humans with various disorders.
Hearing loss and vestibular problems due to other ototoxic drugs in humans
with various disorders.
  (AD) Discussion of cochleo-vestibulotoxic effects of ototoxic drugs used
  in therapy for various disorders. (GER)

421

Damage to cochlear function and vestibular function due to antibiotic, streptomycin, in humans, adult, with tuberculosis. (RUS)

425

Decr in ototoxic effect on organ of Corti and crista ampullaris due to topical administration to bulla of 0.2 ccm of 50 percent solution of antibiotic,
streptomycin (IB) (streptomycin sulfate), in 10 animals, guinea pigs with
intramuscular administration of 1 ml per 100 g ozothin.
  (AD) Histochemical study of effect of ozothin on ototoxicity of streptomycin in guinea pigs. (GER)

430

Permanent hearing loss, partial or total, due to parenteral, intramuscular,
administration of 200,000 units per kg daily of antibiotic, streptomycin, for
30 days in animals, guinea pigs.
Permanent hearing loss, partial or total, due to parenteral, intramuscular,
administration of 150,000 units per kg daily of antibiotic, colistin (colistin sulfate), for 7 to 21 days in animals, guinea pigs. (RUS)

432

Damage to sensory epithelia of macula utriculi and macula sacculi due to
parenteral, intraperitoneal, administration of 250 mg per kg every other day
of antibiotic, streptomycin (streptomycin sulfate), for 8 weeks in 12 animals, guinea pigs, pigmented, young, about 300 g weight.
Least severe damage to sensory epithelia of macula utriculi and macula sacculi due to parenteral, intraperitoneal, administration of 250 mg per kg every
day of antibiotic, kanamycin (kanamycin sulfate), for 8 weeks in 12 animals,
guinea pigs, pigmented, young, about 300 g weight.
Most severe damage to sensory epithelia of macula utriculi and macula sacculi
due to topical administration to middle ear cavity through tympanic membrane
of about 0.6 ml of concentration of 250 mg per kg of antibiotic, streptomycin
(streptomycin sulfate), in 8 injections, with interval of 1 week between
injections, in 12 animals, guinea pigs, pigmented, young, about 300 g weight.
Damage to sensory epithelia of macula utriculi and macula sacculi due to
topical administration to middle ear cavity through tympanic membrane of
about 0.6 ml of concentration of 250 mg per kg of antibiotic, kanamycin
(kanamycin sulfate), in 8 injections, with interval of 1 week between injections, in 12 animals, guinea pigs, pigmented, young, about 300 g weight.
  (AD) More damage to vestibular apparatus due to topical administration
  than due to parenteral administration of antibiotics.
  (AD) More loss of hair cells in sensory epithelium of macula utriculi than
  in that of macula sacculi.
  (AD) Type 1 hair cells more vulnerable to aminoglycoside antibiotics than
  type 2 hair cells.
  (AD) Comment on morphological and phylogenetical vulnerability of hair
  cells.
  (AD) Replacement of hair cells of vestibular apparatus by supporting

cells.   (ENG)

Dizziness due to 1 g daily of antibiotic, streptomycin (SM), for 6 months in
32 percent of 114 humans with pulmonary tuberculosis.
Dizziness due to 300 mg daily of antituberculous agent, isoniazid (SM), for 6
months with streptomycin and then 6 months alone in 32 percent of 114 humans
with pulmonary tuberculosis.
   (AD) Regimen of simultaneous administration of streptomycin and isoniazid
   for 6 months followed by administration of isoniazid only for 6 months.
Dizziness due to 1 g daily of antibiotic, streptomycin (SM), for 6 months in
54 percent of 94 humans with pulmonary tuberculosis.
Dizziness due to 150 mg daily of antituberculous agent, thiacetazone (SM),
for 6 months with streptomycin and isoniazid and then 6 months with isoniazid
in 54 percent of 94 humans with pulmonary tuberculosis.
Dizziness due to 300 mg daily of antituberculous agent, isoniazid (SM), for 6
months with streptomycin and thiacetazone and then 6 months with thiacetazone
in 54 percent of 94 humans with pulmonary tuberculosis.
   (AD) Regimen of simultaneous administration of streptomycin, thiacetazone,
   and isoniazid for 6 months followed by administration of thiacetazone and
   isoniazid for 6 months.
Dizziness due to 150 mg daily of antituberculous agent, thiacetazone (SM),
for 1 year in 13 percent of 78 humans with pulmonary tuberculosis.
Dizziness due to 300 mg daily of antituberculous agent, isoniazid (SM), for 1
year in 13 percent of 78 humans with pulmonary tuberculosis.
   (AD) Regimen of simultaneous administration of thiacetazone and isoniazid
   for 1 year.
   (AD) Study of role of drug regimens with thiacetazone in treatment of
   pulmonary tuberculosis.   (ENG)

Slight ototoxic effects due to range of doses of antibiotic, streptomycin, in
8 of 40 humans, female, treated for tuberculosis during pregnancy.
Slight ototoxic effects due to range of doses of antibiotic, dihydrostreptomycin, in 2 of 40 humans, female, treated for tuberculosis during pregnancy.
Vestibular problems and sensorineural hearing loss in mother and vestibular
problems in fetus due to total of 27 g of antibiotic, streptomycin (CB), for
2.5 months in 1 human, adult, 28 years age, female, treated for pulmonary
tuberculosis at end of pregnancy.
Vestibular problems and sensorineural hearing loss in mother and vestibular
problems in fetus due to total of 27 g of antibiotic, dihydrostreptomycin
(CB), for 2.5 months in 1 human, adult, 28 years age, female, treated for
pulmonary tuberculosis at end of pregnancy.
   (AD) Pure tone audiometry and vestibular function tests in child, female,
   at 10 years age.
Mixed hearing loss in mother and severe sensorineural hearing loss and vestibular problems in fetus due to total of 28 g of antibiotic, (SQ) dihydrostreptomycin, for 2.5 months in 1 human, adult, 22 years age, female, treated for
tuberculosis at beginning of pregnancy.
Mixed hearing loss in mother and severe sensorineural hearing loss and vestibular problems in fetus due to total of 28 g of antibiotic, (SQ) streptomycin, for 2.5 months in 1 human, adult, 22 years age, female, treated for
tuberculosis at beginning of pregnancy.
   (AD) Pure tone audiometry and vestibular function tests in child, female,
   at 10 years age.   (ENG)

Hearing loss and damage to cochlea due to antibiotic, neomycin, in animals,
guinea pigs and monkeys, and humans.
Hearing loss and damage to cochlea due to antibiotic, streptomycin, in animals, guinea pigs and monkeys, and humans.
   (AD) Discussion of findings on decr of ototoxicity of aminoglycoside
   antibiotics.   (GER)

Suppression of microphonic potentials of saccule due to topical, intraluminal, administration of antibiotic, streptomycin, in animals, goldfish.

Suppression of microphonic potentials of saccule due to topical, intraluminal, administration of antibiotic, kanamycin, in animals, goldfish.
Suppression of microphonic potentials of saccule due to topical, intraluminal
or extraluminal, administration of 0.5 mg of chemical agent, cyanide, in
animals, goldfish.
Suppression of microphonic potentials of saccule due to topical, intraluminal
or extraluminal, administration of 0.1 mg of antimalarial, quinine, in animals, goldfish.
Suppression of microphonic potentials of saccule due to topical, intraluminal
or extraluminal, administration of 2 mg of anesthetic, procaine, in animals,
goldfish.
No effect on microphonic potentials of saccule due to topical administration
of salicylates in animals, goldfish.   (ENG)

446

Vestibular problems only in 5 and dizziness, tinnitus, and hearing loss in 1
due to parenteral, intramuscular, administration of 1 g daily in single
injection of antibiotic, streptomycin (SM) (streptomycin sulfate), for 6
months only in 6 (6 percent) of 65 humans, Negro, adolescent and adult, 15 to
over 55 years age, male and female, 80 to over 140 lb weight, for retreatment
of pulmonary tuberculosis.
Simultaneous oral administration of 15 g of antituberculous agent, PAS (SM)
(sodium PAS), for 1 year in 65 humans, Negro, adolescent and adult, 15 to
over 55 years age, male and female, 80 to over 140 lb weight, for retreatment
of pulmonary tuberculosis.
   (AD) Study of value of regimen of streptomycin, PAS, and pyrazinamide in
   retreatment of pulmonary tuberculosis.   (ENG)

449

Vertigo due to antibiotic, streptomycin, in 1 human, adult, female.   (JAP)

452

Hearing loss due to 0.5 g daily, total of 30 to 50 g, of antibiotic, streptomycin, in some of 187 humans, child, adolescent, and adult, 12 to 20 years
age, with tuberculosis.
   (AD) Audiogram confirmed hearing loss.
   (AD) Inclusion of 3 case reports.   (HUN)

453

Damage to vestibular function due to antibiotic, streptomycin, in 2 humans,
adult, 20 and 60 years age, male, with tuberculosis.
   (AD) Vestibular problem confirmed by vestibular function tests.
   (AD) Discussion of restoration of vestibular function after damage due to
   streptomycin therapy.   (GER)

455

Damage to sensory epithelia of vestibular apparatus due to 250 mg per kg of
antibiotic, streptomycin, in animals.
Damage to sensory epithelia of vestibular apparatus due to 250 mg per kg of
antibiotic, kanamycin, in animals.   (JAP)

456

Damage to type 1 hair cells of cristae and macula utriculi, no significant
changes in macula sacculi, and no changes in type 2 hair cells of vestibular
apparatus due to parenteral, intramuscular, administration of 200 mg per kg
daily, total doses of 1600 to 3800 mg per kg, of antibiotic, streptomycin
(streptomycin sulfate), for range of 10 to 26 days, until decline in caloric
threshold values of 2 to 10 degrees C, in 4 animals, squirrel monkeys, 500 to
600 g weight.
Severe damage to type 1 and 2 hair cells of cristae, loss of type 1 hair
cells of macula utriculi, and slight changes in macula sacculi due to parenteral, intramuscular, administration of 200 mg per kg daily, total doses of
2000 and 2600 mg per kg, of antibiotic, streptomycin (streptomycin sulfate),
for 14 and 18 days, until complete suppression of vestibular function, in 2
animals, squirrel monkeys, 500 to 600 g weight.
   (AD) Damage to vestibular function determined by vestibular function
   tests.
   (AD) Relative mild damage in early period of intoxication result of low

concentration of streptomycin in endolymph due to intramuscular route.
(AD) Suggested mechanism of streptomycin action is damage to enzyme system, damage to cytoplasmic membrane, and inhibition of protein synthesis
and ribosome function.   (ENG)

457

Tinnitus and progressive sensorineural hearing loss due to parenteral, intramuscular, administration of antibiotic, (SQ) streptomycin, for 10 days in 1
human, adult, 38 years age, female, with infections and later development of
kidney disorder.
Tinnitus and progressive sensorineural hearing loss due to 13.2 g of antibiotic, (SQ) kanamycin, for 11 days in 1 human, adult, 38 years age, female,
with infections and kidney disorder.
Hearing loss due to antimalarial, (SQ) quinine, in 1 human, adult, 20 years
age, male, with various infections and later development of kidney disorder.
Hearing loss due to 400 mg 2 times daily, total dose of 6.5 g, of antibiotic,
(SQ) kanamycin (SM), for 8 days in 1 human, adult, 20 years age, male, with
various infections and later development of kidney disorder.
Hearing loss due to 150 mg 2 times daily, total dose of 2400 mg, of antibiotic, (SQ) colistin (SM), for 8 days in 1 human, adult, 20 years age, male,
with various infections and later development of kidney disorder.
Tinnitus, total bilateral hearing loss, and vestibular problems due to parenteral, intramuscular, administration of 4.0 g daily, total of 21 g, of antibiotic, (SQ) kanamycin (SM), for 5 days in 1 human, adult, 20 years age,
male, with infections and kidney disorder.
Tinnitus, total bilateral hearing loss, and vestibular problems due to 0.6 g
daily, total dose of 1.3 g, of antibiotic, (SQ) colistin (SM), for 2 days in
1 human, adult, 20 years age, male, with infections and kidney disorder.
Tinnitus, total bilateral hearing loss, and vestibular problems due to 2 g
and then 8 g per 24 hours in divided doses, total dose of 26.5 g, of antibiotic, (SQ) chloramphenicol, for 9 days in 1 human, adult, 20 years age, male,
with infections and kidney disorder.
Bilateral hearing loss due to 1 g daily of antibiotic, actinomycin (SM), for
5 days in 1 human, adult, 62 years age, male, with infections and kidney
disorder.
Bilateral hearing loss due to unknown dose of antibiotic, kanamycin (SM), for
5 days in 1 human, adult, 62 years age, male, with infections and kidney
disorder.
Bilateral hearing loss and vestibular problems due to parenteral administration of high doses of antibiotic, (SQ) neomycin, for total of 21 days in 1
human, adult, 25 years age, male, with infection from wound.
Previous administration of unspecified doses of antibiotic, (SQ) streptomycin, in 1 human, adult, 25 years age, male, with infection from wound.
Later administration of antibiotic, (SQ) chloramphenicol, in 1 human, adult,
25 years age, male, with infection from wound.
Tinnitus and rapidly progressive bilateral hearing loss due to parenteral,
intramuscular, administration of 0.5 g every 12 hours of antibiotic, (SQ)
streptomycin, for 5 days in 1 human, adult, 21 years age, male, with infection from wound.
Tinnitus and rapidly progressive bilateral hearing loss due to parenteral,
intramuscular, administration of 200 mg daily, total of 6.8 g, of antibiotic,
(SQ) colistin (SM), in 1 human, adult, 21 years age, male, with infection
from wound.
Tinnitus and rapidly progressive bilateral hearing loss due to parenteral
administration of unspecified doses of antibiotic, (SQ) neomycin (SM), for
about 35 days in 1 human, adult, 21 years age, male, with infection from
wound.
Tinnitus and progressive bilateral hearing loss due to parenteral administration of 2 l per 24 hours of 1 percent solution of antibiotic, (SQ) neomycin,
for 10 days in 1 human, adult, 26 years age, male, with infection from wound.
    (AD) Hearing loss confirmed by audiometry.
Previous administration of 500 mg four times a day of antibiotic, (SQ) ampicillin, in 1 human, adult, 26 years age, male, with infection from wound.
Bilateral sudden deafness due to administration in dialysis fluid of less
than 150 mg of antibiotic, neomycin (SM), in 1 human, adult, 44 years age,
female, with kidney disorder.
Bilateral sudden deafness due to 50 mg of diuretic, ethacrynic acid (SM), in
1 human, adult, 44 years age, female, with kidney disorder.

(AD) Hearing loss confirmed by audiology.
Tinnitus and progressive bilateral hearing loss beginning after 8 days of treatment due to parenteral administration of 1 l every 4 hours for 3 days and then every 8 hours for 10 days of 1 percent solution of antibiotic, neomycin, in 1 human, adult, 20 years age, male, with infection from wound.
(AD) Hearing loss confirmed by audiology.
Tinnitus and bilateral sensorineural hearing loss due to parenteral, intramuscular, administration of 1 g and then 0.5 g every 12 hours of antibiotic, streptomycin (SM), for 15 days in 1 human, adult, 23 years age, male, with infection from wound.
Tinnitus and bilateral sensorineural hearing loss due to topical administration by irrigation of 1 percent solution every 12 hours of antibiotic, neomycin (SM), for 14 days in 1 human, adult, 23 years age, male, with infection from wound.
(AD) Hearing loss confirmed by audiometry.
(AD) Discussion of 10 case reports.   (ENG)

460

No significant decr in cochlear microphonics due to parenteral, subcutaneous, administration of 100 mg per kg daily for 5 days a week, total dose of 7.5 g per kg, of antibiotic, streptomycin (streptomycin sulfate), for 75 days in animals, guinea pigs.
Statistically significant decr in cochlear microphonics at 1 of 18 points examined, damage to hair cells of organ of Corti, slight damage to stria vascularis and spiral ganglion, damage to macula utriculi and cristae, slight damage to macula sacculi, and vestibular problems due to parenteral, subcutaneous, administration of 200 mg per kg daily, then 400 mg per kg, followed by return to 200 mg per kg, total dose of 15 g per kg, of antibiotic, streptomycin (streptomycin sulfate), for 58 days in animals, guinea pigs.
(AD) Vestibular problems confirmed by vestibular function tests.
No significant decr in cochlear microphonics due to parenteral, subcutaneous, administration of 100 mg per kg daily for 5 days a week, total dose of 7.5 g per kg, of antibiotic, viomycin (viomycin sulfate), for 75 days in animals, guinea pigs.
Significant decr in cochlear microphonics, damage to hair cells of organ of Corti and to stria vascularis, slight damage to spiral ganglion, and slight damage to macula utriculi and crista ampullaris due to parenteral, subcutaneous, administration of 200 mg per kg daily for 5 days a week, then 400 mg per kg, total dose of 15 g per kg, of antibiotic, viomycin (viomycin sulfate), for total of 67 days in animals, guinea pigs.
(AD) Most toxicity for cochlear microphonics in guinea pig due to viomycin.
No significant decr in cochlear microphonics due to parenteral, subcutaneous, administration of 100 mg per kg daily for 5 days each week, total dose of 7.5 g per kg, of antibiotic, capreomycin (capreomycin sulfate), for 75 days in animals, guinea pigs.
No significant decr in cochlear microphonics, slight damage to outer hair cells of organ of Corti and to stria vascularis, and no damage to vestibular apparatus due to parenteral, subcutaneous, administration of 200 mg per kg daily for 5 days a week, then 400 mg per kg, total dose of 15 g per kg, of antibiotic, capreomycin (capreomycin sulfate), for total of 67 days in animals, guinea pigs.
(CT) Same method using subcutaneous administration of 0.25 cc daily of isotonic saline in guinea pigs, control group.
(AD) Least toxicity for inner ear of guinea pig due to capreomycin.
(AD) Study of functional and structural cochleo-vestibulotoxic effects of streptomycin, viomycin, and capreomycin.
(AD) Statistical analysis of results.   (ENG)

468

Complete inhibition of acetylcholine induced decr in cochlear potential due to parenteral, intravenous, administration of 1.0 mg of antibiotic, streptomycin (streptomycin sulfate), in 1 injection in 5 animals, cats, male and female, 1.5 to 2.8 kg weight, with injection of acetylcholine.
Minimum inhibition of acetylcholine induced decr in cochlear potential due to parenteral, intravenous, administration of 1.0 mg of antibiotic, dihydrostreptomycin (dihydrostreptomycin sulfate), in 1 injection in 5 animals, cats, male and female, 1.5 to 2.8 kg weight, with injection of acetylcholine.

168Streptomycin

Complete inhibition of acetylcholine induced decr in cochlear potential due
to parenteral, intravenous, administration of 1.0 mg of antibiotic, kanamycin
(kanamycin sulfate), in 1 injection in 5 animals, cats, male and female, 1.5
to 2.8 kg weight, with injection of acetylcholine.
Complete inhibition of acetylcholine induced decr in cochlear potential due
to parenteral, intravenous, administration of 1.0 mg of antibiotic, neomycin
(neomycin sulfate), in 1 injection in 5 animals, cats, male and female, 1.5
to 2.8 kg weight, with injection of acetylcholine.
Acute inhibition of acetylcholine induced decr in cochlear potential due to
parenteral, intravenous, administration of 1.0 mg of antimalarial, quinine
(quinine hydrochloride), in 1 injection in 5 animals, cats, male and female,
1.5 to 2.8 kg weight, with injection of acetylcholine.
  (CT) Injections of 0.1 ml isotonic saline in cats, control group.
Inhibition of acetylcholine induced decr in cochlear potential due to parenteral, subcutaneous, administration of 300 mg per kg daily of antibiotic,
streptomycin, for 7 to 9 days in 10 animals, cats.
Inhibition of acetylcholine induced decr in cochlear potential due to parenteral, subcutaneous, administration of 100 mg per kg daily of antibiotic,
neomycin, for 7 to 9 days in 10 animals, cats.
  (CT) Study of 7 cats, control group, not treated with antibiotics.
  (AD) Study of effect of acetylcholine on cochlear potential after acute
  and chronic administration of ototoxic drugs.
  (AD) Suggested relationship between change in acetylcholine activity and
  ototoxic drugs.
  (AD) Suggested that ototoxicity partially due to disruption of efferent
  effect on cochlea. (ENG)

470
Damage to vestibular apparatus due to antibiotic, streptomycin, in humans.
  (AD) Study of effect of drugs on kidney function and vestibular function.
  (FR)

476
Vestibulotoxic effects due to 100 mg per kg of antibiotic, streptomycin, in
animals, pigeons.
Some decr in vestibulotoxic effects due to 100 mg per kg of antibiotic,
streptomycin (IB), for 30 days in animals, pigeons, with administration of
25000 units of vitamin A.
  (AD) Structural damage similar in both groups of pigeons. (POL)

477
Significant decr in oxygen consumption of cochlea due to high doses of antibiotic, kanamycin, in animals, guinea pigs.
Significant decr in oxygen consumption of cochlea due to high doses of antibiotic, streptomycin, in animals, guinea pigs.
Incr followed by significant decr in oxygen consumption of cochlea due to
high doses of antibiotic, dihydrostreptomycin, in animals, guinea pigs.
  (CT) Determination of oxygen consumption of guinea pigs, control group,
  not treated with ototoxic drugs.
  (AD) Suggested that ototoxicity of aminoglycoside antibiotics due to
  inhibition of respiratory enzymes of cells of inner ear. (ENG)

480
Changes in acid phosphatase activity of vestibular apparatus due to antibiotic, streptomycin (streptomycin sulfate), in animals.
  (AD) Study using electron microscopy of acid phosphatase activity of
  vestibular apparatus. (JAP)

481
Damage to vestibular apparatus due to 1 g daily or twice daily of antibiotic,
streptomycin (SM), for maximum of 3 months in 9 of 108 humans, range of 2 to
86 years age, male and female, with pulmonary tuberculosis.
Simultaneous administration of 12 g daily of antituberculous agent, PAS (SM),
for 12 to 18 months in 108 humans, range of 2 to 86 years age, male and
female, with pulmonary tuberculosis.
Simultaneous administration of 300 mg daily of antituberculous agent, isoniazid (SM), for 12 to 18 months in 108 humans, range of 2 to 86 years age, male
and female, with pulmonary tuberculosis. (ENG)

482

Decr in cochlear function and vestibular function due to parenteral, intramuscular, administration of 50 to 100 mg per kg of antibiotic, streptomycin
(streptomycin sulfate), for 35 days in animals, guinea pigs, pigmented, 400
to 500 g weight.
  (AD) More ototoxic effects with higher dosage.
Decr in cochlear function with both doses but decr in vestibular function
with only higher dose due to parenteral, intramuscular, administration of 50
to 100 mg per kg of antibiotic, dihydrostreptomycin (dihydrostreptomycin
sulfate), for 35 days in animals, guinea pigs, pigmented, 400 to 500 g
weight.
  (AD) More decr in cochlear function with higher dosage.
Decr in cochlear function in all animals but decr in vestibular function in 2
groups only due to parenteral, intramuscular, administration of 50 to 100 mg
per kg of antibiotic, kanamycin, for 35 days in animals, guinea pigs, pigmented, 400 to 500 g weight.
  (AD) More decr in cochlear function with higher dosage.
Decr in cochlear function due to parenteral, intramuscular, administration of
20 mg per kg of diuretic, ethacrynic acid, for 35 days in animals, guinea
pigs, pigmented, 400 to 500 g weight.
  (CT) Study of guinea pigs, control group, not treated with ototoxic drugs.
Decr in ototoxic effects due to parenteral, intramuscular, administration of
100 mg per kg of antibiotic, streptomycin (IB) (streptomycin sulfate), for 35
days in animals, guinea pigs, pigmented, 400 to 500 g weight, with administration of 1 mg per kg of various inhibitors.
Decr in ototoxic effects due to parenteral, intramuscular, administration of
100 mg per kg of antibiotic, dihydrostreptomycin (IB) (dihydrostreptomycin
sulfate), for 35 days in animals, guinea pigs, pigmented, 400 to 500 g
weight, with administration of 1 mg per kg of various inhibitors.
Decr in ototoxic effects due to parenteral, intramuscular, administration of
100 mg per kg of antibiotic, kanamycin (IB), for 35 days in animals, guinea
pigs, pigmented, 400 to 500 g weight, with administration of 1 mg per kg of
various inhibitors.
Decr in ototoxic effects due to parenteral, intramuscular, administration of
20 mg per kg of diuretic, ethacrynic acid (IB), for 35 days in animals,
guinea pigs, pigmented, 400 to 500 g weight, with administration of 1 mg per
kg of various inhibitors.
  (AD) Measurement of Preyer reflex and vestibular function tests.
Ototoxic effects, functional and structural, due to parenteral, intraperitoneal, administration of 100 mg per kg of antibiotic, streptomycin (streptomycin sulfate), for 50 days in animals, mice, male, 18 to 22 g weight.
No ototoxic effects due to parenteral, intraperitoneal, administration of 100
mg per kg of antibiotic, dihydrostreptomycin (dihydrostreptomycin sulfate),
for 50 days in animals, mice, male, 18 to 22 g weight.
Ototoxic effects, functional and structural, due to parenteral, intraperitoneal, administration of 100 mg per kg of antibiotic, kanamycin, for 50 days
in animals, mice, male, 18 to 22 g weight.
  (CT) Study of mice, control group, not treated with ototoxic drugs.
No ototoxic effects due to parenteral, intraperitoneal, administration of 100
mg per kg of antibiotic, streptomycin (IB) (streptomycin sulfate), for 50
days in animals, mice, male, 18 to 22 g weight, with administration of 1 mg
per kg of vitamin B.
No ototoxic effects due to parenteral, intraperitoneal, administration of 100
mg per kg of antibiotic, dihydrostreptomycin (IB) (dihydrostreptomycin sulfate), for 50 days in animals, mice, male, 18 to 22 g weight, with administration of 1 mg per kg of vitamin B.
No ototoxic effects due to parenteral, intraperitoneal, administration of 100
mg per kg of antibiotic, kanamycin (IB), for 50 days in animals, mice, male,
18 to 22 g weight, with administration of vitamin B.
  (AD) More ototoxic effects of aminoglycoside antibiotics in guinea pigs
  than in mice.
  (AD) Ototoxic effects of diuretic in guinea pigs.   (IT)

483

Possible damage to vestibular nerve and cochlear nerve due to antibiotic,
streptomycin, in humans with or without kidney disorder.
Possible damage to vestibular nerve and cochlear nerve due to antibiotic,
gentamicin, in humans with or without kidney disorder.

Possible damage to vestibular nerve and cochlear nerve due to antibiotic, kanamycin, in humans with or without kidney disorder.
Possible damage to vestibular nerve and cochlear nerve due to antibiotic, neomycin, in humans with or without kidney disorder.
  (AD) Incidence of effects on vestibular function highest in streptomycin, followed by gentamicin, kanamycin, and neomycin.
  (AD) Incidence of effects on cochlear function highest in neomycin, followed by kanamycin, gentamicin, and streptomycin.
  (AD) Need for careful consideration in clinical use of aminoglycoside antibiotics.
Possible cochlear impairment and vestibular problems due to antibiotic, paromomycin, in humans.
Possible dizziness and ataxia due to antibiotic, polymyxin B, in humans.
Possible but rare dizziness and vertigo due to antibiotic, nalidixic acid, in humans. (ENG)

                                                                        485
High concentration in fluids of inner ear and ototoxic effects due to 250 mg per kg of antibiotic, streptomycin, in animals, guinea pigs.
High concentration in fluids of inner ear and ototoxic effects due to 250 mg per kg of antibiotic, kanamycin, in animals, guinea pigs.
Higher concentration in fluids of inner ear and more severe ototoxic effects due to 250 mg per kg of antibiotic, dihydrostreptomycin, in animals, guinea pigs.
Higher concentration in fluids of inner ear and more severe ototoxic effects due to 100 mg per kg of antibiotic, neomycin, in animals, guinea pigs.
  (AD) High concentration of aminoglycoside antibiotics in fluids of inner ear due to low doses as well as high doses.
  (AD) Ototoxic effect of aminoglycoside antibiotics due to retention of high concentrations in inner ear for long period and slow elimination of drugs.
Significant decr in concentration in fluids of inner ear and in serum and decr in ototoxicity due to 250 mg per kg or 100 mg per kg of antibiotics (IB), aminoglycoside, in animals, guinea pigs, with administration of ozothin.
Decr in concentration in fluids of inner ear and decr in ototoxicity due to 250 mg per kg or 100 mg per kg of antibiotics (IB), aminoglycoside, in animals, guinea pigs, with administration of pantothenic acid. (GER)

                                                                        486
Incr in ATP activity of stria vascularis and spiral ligament but no pattern of enzyme changes observed in membranous labyrinth due to 400 mg per kg daily of antibiotic, kanamycin, for 3 weeks in animals, guinea pigs.
Incr in ATP activity of stria vascularis and spiral ligament but no pattern of enzyme changes observed in membranous labyrinth due to 400 mg per kg daily of antibiotic, streptomycin, for 3 weeks in animals, guinea pigs.
Decr in ATP activity of stria vascularis and spiral ligament but no pattern of enzyme changes observed in membranous labyrinth due to 400 mg per kg daily of antibiotic, dihydrostreptomycin, for 3 weeks in animals, guinea pigs.
  (CT) Study of guinea pigs, control group, not treated with aminoglycoside antibiotics.
  (AD) Study of effects of ototoxic drugs on ATP activity of inner ear of guinea pigs. (JAP)

                                                                        487
Severe vestibular problems due to parenteral, intramuscular, administration of antibiotic, streptomycin (streptomycin sulfate), for long period in 8 percent of 600 humans with tuberculosis and with previous hearing loss in some cases.
Transient hearing loss in most cases due to parenteral, intramuscular, administration of antibiotic, streptomycin (streptomycin sulfate), for long period in some of 600 humans with tuberculosis and with previous hearing loss in some cases.
  (CT) Audiometry and vestibular function tests before, during, and after streptomycin treatment.
  (AD) Improvement in vestibular function after cessation of streptomycin treatment.
  (AD) Transient hearing loss in most cases due to early detection with

audiology.   (GER)

488
Permanent cochleo-vestibulotoxic effects due to range of doses of antibiotic,
streptomycin (streptomycin sulfate), in some of 1198 humans treated for
tuberculosis and other disorders.
    (AD) Auditory system problems detected by audiology.
    (AD) Comment on differences in individual responses to streptomycin.
    (SER)

490
No hearing loss due to average dose of 36.8 mg per kg daily, average total
dose of 118.9 mg per kg, of antibiotic, streptomycin (streptomycin sulfate),
for short period, average of 3.2 days, in 98 humans, child, 7 and 8 years
age, female and male, treated when newborn infants.
    (AD) Follow up study with audiometry of children treated in neonatal
    period with streptomycin.
    (CT) Study of 102 children, control group, not treated in neonatal period
    with ototoxic drugs.
    (AD) Sensorineural hearing loss detected in 3 of 98 children treated with
    streptomycin not attributed to antibiotic.   (ENG)

491
Changes in sensory epithelium of otocyst due to antibiotic, streptomycin, in
animals, chickens, embryo.
Changes in sensory epithelium of otocyst due to antibiotic, neomycin, in
animals, chickens, embryo.
Changes in sensory epithelium of otocyst due to antibiotic, kanamycin, in
animals, chickens, embryo.
    (CT) Study of otocysts of chickens, control group, not treated with amino-
    glycoside antibiotics.
    (AD) Neomycin and kanamycin more toxic to otocysts of chickens than strep-
    tomycin.   (CZ)

495
Ototoxic effects due to parenteral, intramuscular, administration of 100 mg
per kg of antibiotic, neomycin (neomycin sulfate), in 10 injections in 10
animals, guinea pigs.
Significant decr in ototoxic effects due to parenteral, intramuscular, administration of 100 mg per kg of antibiotic, neomycin (IB) (neomycin sulfate), in 10 injections in 10 animals, guinea pigs, with combined administration of 1.2 ml per kg of ozothin.
Ototoxic effects due to parenteral, intramuscular, administration of 250 mg
per kg of antibiotic, streptomycin (streptomycin sulfate), in 10 injections
in animals, guinea pigs.
Decr in ototoxic effects due to parenteral, intramuscular, administration of
250 mg per kg of antibiotic, streptomycin (IB) (streptomycin sulfate), in 10
injections in 15 animals, guinea pigs, with combined administration of 1.2 ml
per kg of ozothin.
No ototoxic effects due to parenteral, intramuscular, administration of 250
mg per kg of antibiotic, streptomycin (IB) (streptomycin sulfate), in 10
injections in 6 animals, guinea pigs, with previous intramuscular administration of 1.2 ml per kg of ozothin.
    (CT) Study of 12 guinea pigs, control group.
    (AD) Electrophysiological study of effects of ozothin on ototoxicity of
    aminoglycoside antibiotics.   (GER)

500
Sensorineural hearing loss due to antibiotic, streptomycin, in humans, newborn infant.
    (AD) Discussion of etiology of hearing loss in children.   (ENG)

509
Hearing loss due to high doses of antibiotic, streptomycin, for long period
in humans.   (POL)

524
Damage to eighth cranial nerve due to antibiotics in 8 of 103 humans with

172   Streptomycin

kidney disorder.
Hearing loss due to antibiotic, streptomycin, in 6 of 103 humans with kidney
disorder.
   (AD) Study of effects of ototoxic drugs in humans with kidney disorder.
   (ENG)

                                                                        529
Total loss of Preyer reflex within several days but no vestibular problems
due to parenteral, subcutaneous, administration of range of high doses to
more than 1000 mg per kg daily of antibiotic, kanamycin (kanamycin sulfate),
in animals, rats, Wistar, albino, female, 50 g weight.
   (AD) Linear relationship between hearing loss and kanamycin dosage.
Loss of Preyer reflex but no vestibular problems due to parenteral, subcutaneous, administration of range of high doses to more than 600 mg per kg
daily of antibiotic, neomycin, in animals, rats, Wistar, albino, female, 50 g
weight.
   (AD) Linear relationship between hearing loss and neomycin dosage.
   (AD) Hearing loss observed with lower doses of neomycin than kanamycin.
Moderate to severe vestibular problems but cochlear impairment in only 1 case
due to parenteral, subcutaneous, administration of high doses, 471, 583, 720,
887, and 1089 mg per kg daily, of antibiotic, streptomycin (streptomycin
sulfate), in animals, rats, Wistar, albino, female, 50 g weight.
   (AD) Linear realtionship between vestibular problems and streptomycin
   dosage.
Transient moderate to severe vestibular problems but cochlear impairment in
only 1 case due to parenteral, subcutaneous, administration of high doses,
765, 940, 1151, and 1377 mg per kg daily, of antibiotic, dihydrostreptomycin
(dihydrostreptomycin sulfate), in 40 animals, rats, Wistar, albino, female,
50 g weight.
   (CT) Same method using saline in 30 rats, control group, showed no cochleo-vestibulotoxic effects.
Hearing loss due to parenteral, subcutaneous, administration of 500 mg per kg
daily of antibiotic, kanamycin (SM), in animals, rats, Wistar, albino, female, 50 g weight.
Hearing loss due to parenteral, subcutaneous, administration of range of
doses of antibiotic, neomycin (SM), in animals, rats, Wistar, albino, female,
50 g weight.
   (AD) Incr in ototoxicity of neomycin due to kanamycin.
Hearing loss but no vestibular problems due to parenteral, subcutaneous,
administration of 500 mg per kg of antibiotic, kanamycin (SM), in animals,
rats, Wistar, albino, female, 50 g weight.
Hearing loss but no vestibular problems due to parenteral, subcutaneous,
administration of 200, 270, 364.5, and 492 mg per kg daily of antibiotic,
streptomycin (SM), in animals, rats, Wistar, albino, female, 50 g weight.
Hearing loss but no vestibular problems due to parenteral, subcutaneous,
administration of 500 mg per kg daily of antibiotic, kanamycin (SM), in
animals, rats, Wistar, albino, female, 50 g weight.
Hearing loss but no vestibular problems due to parenteral, subcutaneous,
administration of 350, 472.5, 637.9, and 861.1 mg per kg daily of antibiotic,
dihydrostreptomycin (SM), in animals, rats, Wistar, albino, female, 50 g
weight.
   (AD) Tests of cochlear function and vestibular function, pretreatment and
   daily during treatment.
   (AD) Comparative study of ototoxic effects of aminoglycoside antibiotics
   in Wistar rats.
   (AD) Report of hearing loss in 321 (43.4 percent) of total of 740 rats in
   study.
   (AD) Suggested that ototoxic effects of kanamycin and neomycin due to
   different mechanisms of action than ototoxic effects of streptomycin and
   dihydrostreptomycin.   (ENG)

                                                                        534
Dizziness within 6 weeks due to parenteral, intramuscular, administration of
0.75 g daily of antibiotic, streptomycin, in 8 (31 percent) of 27 humans,
child, adult, and aged, 12 to 76 years age, female and male, 34 to 89 kg
weight, with tuberculosis.
   (AD) Use of vestibular function tests in patients reporting dizziness.
   (AD) Study showed significant relationship between higher 24 hour serum

levels and dizziness.
(AD) Suggested decr in dosage when serum streptomycin more than 3 mcg per
ml at 24 hours.
(AD) More risk of vestibulotoxic effects due to streptomycin in patients
over 45 years age.   (ENG)

535

Dizziness due to parenteral administration of 0.75 g on 6 days a week for 3
months and then 1 g on 2 days a week with intervals of 2 to 3 days for 15
months of antibiotic, streptomycin (SM), for total of 18 months in 2 of 80
humans, adult, range of ages, female and male, 16 to 92 kg weight, with
pulmonary tuberculosis.
Dizziness due to 300 mg on 6 days a week for 3 months and then 600 mg on 2
days a week with intervals of 2 to 3 days for 15 months of antituberculous
agent, isoniazid (SM), for total of 18 months in 1 of 80 humans, adult, range
of ages, female and male, 16 to 92 kg weight, with pulmonary tuberculosis.
Simultaneous administration of 12 g on 6 days a week of antituberculous
agent, PAS (SM), for 3 months in 80 humans, adult, range of ages, female and
male, 16 to 92 kg weight, with pulmonary tuberculosis.   (ENG)

536

Damage to eighth cranial nerve and vertigo due to 1 g or 0.75 g daily of
antibiotic, streptomycin (SM), for about 3 months usually in less than 55 of
181 humans, adult and aged, primarily 50 years or over age, male and female,
with pulmonary tuberculosis.
Simultaneous administration of 300 mg daily of antituberculous agent, isoniazid (SM), for 18 months to 2 years usually in 181 humans, adult and aged,
primarily 50 years or over age, male and female, with pulmonary tuberculosis.
Simultaneous administration of 12 g daily of antituberculous agent, PAS (SM),
for 18 months to 2 years usually in 181 humans, adult and aged, primarily 50
years or over age, male and female, with pulmonary tuberculosis.   (ENG)

537

Dizziness due to oral administration in tablet of 150 mg daily of antituberculous agent, thiacetazone (CB) (SM), in 1 of 147 humans, African, adolescent
and adult, 15 years or more age, with pulmonary tuberculosis and without
previous treatment.
Dizziness due to oral administration in tablet of 300 mg daily of antituberculous agent, isoniazid (CB) (SM), in 1 of 147 humans, African, adolescent
and adult, 15 years or more age, with pulmonary tuberculosis and without
previous treatment.
   (AD) Dizziness in 1 patient due to combined treatment with thiacetazone
   and isoniazid only.
Dizziness due to parenteral, intramuscular, administration of 1 g daily of
antibiotic, streptomycin (SM) (streptomycin sulfate), for first 2 weeks in 1
of 161 humans, African, adolescent and adult, 15 years or more age, with
pulmonary tuberculosis and without previous treatment.
   (AD) Dizziness in 1 patient due to simultaneous treatment with thiacetazone and isoniazid in 1 tablet and intramuscular streptomycin for 2 weeks.
Dizziness due to parenteral, intramuscular, administration of 1 g daily of
antibiotic, streptomycin (SM) (streptomycin sulfate), for first 8 weeks in 10
of 162 humans, African, adolescent and adult, 15 years or more age, with
pulmonary tuberculosis and without previous treatment.
   (AD) Dizziness in 10 patients due to simultaneous treatment with thiacetazone and isoniazid in 1 tablet and intramuscular streptomycin for 8 weeks.
   (AD) Study showed vestibulotoxic effects in total of 12 of 818 patients
   treated for pulmonary tuberculosis.   (ENG)

538

Dizziness due to parenteral administration of 1 g daily for first 8 weeks and
then 1 g twice weekly for 12 weeks of antibiotic, streptomycin (SM), for
total of 20 weeks in 5 of 77 humans with pulmonary tuberculosis.
Simultaneous administration of 300 mg daily in single dose of antituberculous
agent, isoniazid (SM), in 77 humans with pulmonary tuberculosis.
Simultaneous administration of 15 mg per kg daily of antituberculous agent,
ethambutol (SM), in 77 humans with pulmonary tuberculosis.
No reported ototoxic effects due to 600 mg daily in single dose of antibiotic, rifampicin, in 157 humans with pulmonary tuberculosis.   (ENG)

542

Deaf-mutism in fetus due to antibiotic, streptomycin, in human, female,
treated during pregnancy.
   (AD) Case report of congenital hearing loss due to streptomycin therapy in
   mother during pregnancy.   (ENG)

557

Ototoxic effects due to previous administration of antibiotic, (SQ) streptomycin, in 8 humans with pulmonary tuberculosis.
No ototoxic effects due to 1.0 g daily of antibiotic, (SQ) capreomycin (SM),
for long period in same 8 of 38 humans with pulmonary tuberculosis.
Simultaneous administration of antituberculous agent, (SQ) ethambutol (SM),
in 38 humans with pulmonary tuberculosis.   (ENG)

560

Ototoxic effects due to antibiotic, streptomycin, in humans with tuberculosis.
Ototoxic effects due to antibiotic, kanamycin, in humans with tuberculosis.
   (AD) Reported 4 to 5 percent incidence in audiometry of ototoxicity from
   streptomycin and kanamycin.
   (AD) Decr in ototoxicity with administration of streptomycin or kanamycin
   in evening before sleeping.   (JAP)

561

Sensorineural hearing loss due to antibiotic, streptomycin, in humans.
   (AD) Study of incidence of various types of hearing loss.
   (AD) Reported that some cases of sensorineural hearing loss of unknown
   etiology possibly due to streptomycin therapy.   (JAP)

562

Decr in microphonic potential of saccule due to topical, intraluminal, administration of antibiotic, streptomycin, in animals, goldfish.
Decr in microphonic potential of saccule due to topical, intraluminal, administration of antibiotic, kanamycin, in animals, goldfish.
Permanent decr in microphonic potential of saccule due to topical, intraluminal or extraluminal, administration of 0.5 mg per ml of chemical agent,
cyanide, in animals, goldfish.
Permanent decr in microphonic potential of saccule due to topical, intraluminal or extraluminal, administration of 0.1 mg per ml of antimalarial,
quinine, in animals, goldfish.
No effect on microphonic potential of saccule due to salicylate, aspirin, in
animals, goldfish.
Some decr in microphonic potential of saccule due to 2 mg per ml of anesthetic, procaine, in animals, goldfish.
   (AD) Study of effects of various agents on microphonic potential of saccule of goldfish.   (JAP)

591

Hearing loss due to antibiotic, capreomycin, for long period in 2 of 28
humans with tuberculosis.
   (AD) Results of 1 study of effects of capreomycin.
No ototoxic effects due to antibiotic, (SQ) capreomycin, for 1 to 24 months
in 16 humans with tuberculosis.
   (AD) Results of other study of effects of capreomycin.
Vestibular problems due to previous administration of antibiotic, (SQ) strep-
tomycin, in 8 of 16 humans with tuberculosis.
   (AD) Suggested that less ototoxicity due to capreomycin than to streptomy-
   cin.   (ENG)

593

Vestibular problems due to 1 g in 24 hours of antibiotic, (SQ) streptomycin
(SM), in 1 human, adult, 32 years age, female, with tuberculosis.
Vestibular problems due to 450 mg of antituberculous agent, (SQ) isoniazid
(SM), in 1 human, adult, 32 years age, female, with tuberculosis.
Vestibular problems due to oral administration in tablets of 0.10 g of anti-
convulsant, (SQ) diphenylhydantoin, in 1 human, adult, 32 years age, female,
with tuberculosis.
Vestibular problems due to oral administration in tablets of 3 tablets of

0.10 g each daily of anticonvulsant, (SQ) diphenylhydantoin (SM), in 1 human,
adult, 49 years age, female, with tuberculosis.
Vestibular problems due to 300 mg of antituberculous agent, (SQ) isoniazid
(SM), in 1 human, adult, 49 years age, female, with tuberculosis.
Simultaneous administration of 500 cm of antituberculous agent, (SQ) PAS
(SM), in 1 human, adult, 49 years age, female, with tuberculosis.
    (AD) Report of vestibulotoxic effects in 2 patients due to diphenylhydan-
    toin with isoniazid or streptomycin.   (FR)

                                                                              597
Hearing loss due to salicylates in humans.
Hearing loss due to antimalarial, quinine, in humans.
Hearing loss due to antibiotic, streptomycin, in humans.
Tinnitus due to chemical agent, camphor, in humans.
Tinnitus due to chemical agent, tobacco, in humans.
Tinnitus due to cardiovascular agent, quinidine, in humans.
Tinnitus due to chemical agent, ergot, in humans.
Tinnitus due to chemical agent, alcohol, methyl, in humans.
    (AD) Discussion of toxic effects of drugs.   (ENG)

                                                                              602
Effect on eighth cranial nerve due to antibiotic, streptomycin, in humans.
Effect on eighth cranial nerve due to antibiotic, dihydrostreptomycin, in
humans.
    (AD) Comparative study of effect of 2 antibiotics on eighth cranial nerve.
    (ENG)

                                                                              611
Hearing loss due to range of 0.8 to 15 g of antibiotic, neomycin (SM), in 9
humans, child, adult, and aged, 4 or less to 65 years age, with various
infections.
Simultaneous administration of antibiotic, streptomycin (SM), in 6 humans,
child, adult, and aged, 4 or less to 65 years age, with various infections.
Simultaneous administration of antibiotic, polymyxin (SM), in 1 human, child,
less than 4 years age, with various infections.
    (AD) Hearing loss confirmed by audiograms.
    (AD) Discussion of 9 case reports.   (HUN)

                                                                              612
Hearing loss due to parenteral administration of antibiotic, streptomycin, in
humans.
    (AD) Literature review of ototoxic effects of streptomycin.
    (AD) Ototoxic effects of neomycin and kanamycin comp w effects of strep-
    tomycin and dihydrostreptomycin.   (SP)

                                                                              614
Vertigo due to parenteral administration of 0.5 g twice daily of antibiotic,
streptomycin (SM), for 7 days in 3 of 59 humans, aged, 70 years or over age,
with chronic bronchitis.
Simultaneous administration of 3,000,000 units twice daily of antibiotic,
penicillin (SM), for 14 days in 3 of 59 humans, aged, 70 years or over age,
with chronic bronchitis.   (ENG)

                                                                              615
Tinnitus, hearing loss, vertigo, and dizziness due to oral administration in
tablet of 150 mg daily of antituberculous agent, thiacetazone (CB) (SM), in
some of 1002 humans with tuberculosis.
Tinnitus, hearing loss, vertigo, and dizziness due to oral administration in
tablet of 300 mg daily of antituberculous agent, isoniazid (CB) (SM), in some
of 1002 humans with tuberculosis.
Tinnitus, hearing loss, vertigo, and dizziness due to parenteral administration of 1 g daily of antibiotic, streptomycin (SM), in some of 1002 humans
with tuberculosis.
    (AD) Reported 21.4 percent incidence of toxic effects in regimen of thia-
    cetazone, isoniazid, and streptomycin.
    (AD) Suggested that effects of streptomycin potentiated by thiacetazone.
Unspecified ototoxic effects due to oral administration of 300 mg daily of
antituberculous agent, isoniazid (SM), in 987 humans with tuberculosis.

Unspecified ototoxic effects due to parenteral administration of 1 g daily of antibiotic, streptomycin (SM), in 987 humans with tuberculosis.
   (AD) Reported 7.8 percent incidence of toxic effects in regimen of isoniazid and streptomycin without thiacetazone.   (ENG)

                                                                          619

Tinnitus in 7 cases and vertigo in 2 cases due to 1 g twice weekly of antibiotic, streptomycin (SM), in total of 9 of 190 humans, Japanese, adult, 20 to 61 years age, male and female, with pulmonary tuberculosis and without previous chemotherapy.
Tinnitus in 7 cases and vertigo in 2 cases due to about 7.5 mg per kg in single dose daily of antituberculous agent, isoniazid (SM), in total of 9 of 190 humans, Japanese, adult, 20 to 61 years age, male and female, with pulmonary tuberculosis and without previous chemotherapy.
Simultaneous administration of 10 g daily in 3 divided doses of antituberculous agent, PAS (SM), in 190 humans, Japanese, adult, 20 to 61 years age, male and female, with pulmonary tuberculosis and without previous chemotherapy.
Tinnitus in 3 cases and hearing loss in 2 cases due to 1 g twice weekly of antibiotic, streptomycin (SM), in total of 5 of 160 humans, Japanese, adult, 20 to 61 years age, male and female, with pulmonary tuberculosis and without previous chemotherapy.
Tinnitus in 3 cases and hearing loss in 2 cases due to 18 mg per kg in 3 divided doses of antituberculous agent, isoniazid (SM), in total of 5 of 160 humans, Japanese, adult, 20 to 61 years age, male and female, with pulmonary tuberculosis and without previous chemotherapy.
Simultaneous administration of 10 g daily in 3 divided doses of antituberculous agent, PAS (SM), in 160 humans, Japanese, adult, 20 to 61 years age, male and female, with pulmonary tuberculosis and without previous chemotherapy.
   (AD) Similar ototoxic effects in both drug regimens.   (ENG)

                                                                          620

Changes of various degrees of intensity in cerebellar vermis, including Purkinje's cell, due to 30 mg per kg, total doses of 600 mg and 1200 mg, of antibiotic, streptomycin, in 2 groups of 24 animals, pigeons.   (POL)

                                                                          621

Primarily vestibular problems due to antibiotic, streptomycin, in humans.
Primarily hearing loss but also vestibular problems due to antibiotic, dihydrostreptomycin, in humans.
Primarily hearing loss but also vestibular problems due to antibiotic, kanamycin, in humans.
Primarily hearing loss but also vestibular problems due to antibiotic, neomycin, in humans.
Primarily hearing loss but also vestibular problems due to antibiotic, gentamicin, in humans.
Vertigo and ataxia due to antituberculous agent, isoniazid, in humans.
Hearing loss due to salicylate, aspirin, in humans.
Hearing loss and vertigo due to antimalarial, quinine, in humans.
Nystagmus due to barbiturates in humans.
Vestibular problems due to analgesic, morphine, in humans.
Nystagmus due to sedative, alcohol, in humans.
Nystagmus and hearing loss due to chemical agent, carbon monoxide, in humans.
Ototoxic effects due to antineoplastic, nitrogen mustard, in humans.
Ototoxic effects due to chemical agent, aniline, in humans.
Ototoxic effects due to chemical agent, tobacco, in humans.
Nystagmus due to chemical agent, nicotine, in humans.
Vestibular problems due to anticonvulsants in humans.
Vestibular problems due to anesthetics in humans.
Vestibular problems due to diuretics in humans.
   (AD) Inclusion of comprehensive list of ototoxic agents.   (SP)

                                                                          631

Ototoxic effects due to antibiotic, streptomycin, in humans with pulmonary tuberculosis.   (BUL)

637
Ototoxic effects due to antibiotic, streptomycin (CB), in humans.
Ototoxic effects due to antibiotic, penicillin (CB), in humans. (GER)

641
Possible damage to eighth cranial nerve due to antibiotic, capreomycin, in
humans.
Possible vestibular problems and hearing loss due to antibiotic, gentamicin,
in humans.
Possible delayed transient or permanent hearing loss due to antibiotic,
kanamycin (SM), in humans, in particular with kidney disorders or with simul-
taneous administration of ethacrynic acid.
Possible delayed transient or permanent hearing loss due to diuretic, ethacrynic acid (SM), in humans.
Possible delayed transient or permanent severe hearing loss due to oral,
parenteral, or topical administration of antibiotic, neomycin, in humans.
Possible damage to eighth cranial nerve, primarily hearing loss, due to
antibiotic, paromomycin, in humans.
Possible hearing loss due to antibiotic, rifampicin, in humans.
High risk of damage to eighth cranial nerve, primarily transient or permanent
vestibular problems but also hearing loss, due to antibiotic, streptomycin,
in humans.
Possible damage to eighth cranial nerve, primarily hearing loss, due to high
doses of antibiotic, vancomycin, for long period of more than 10 days in
humans, in particular with kidney disorders.
Risk of damage to eighth cranial nerve, vestibular problems and hearing loss,
due to high doses of antibiotic, viomycin, for long period of more than 10
days in humans, in particular with kidney disorders.
    (AD) Discussion of toxic effects of antibiotics. (ENG)

643
Possible transient or permanent damage to eighth cranial nerve, vestibular
problems and hearing loss, due to antibiotic, streptomycin, in humans with
tuberculosis and in particular with concurrent kidney disorders.
    (AD) Need for careful consideration in use of streptomycin in therapy.
    (ENG)

648
Vertigo due to antibiotic, streptomycin, in 3 humans with tuberculosis.
    (AD) Report on testing with ENG of 191 patients with vertigo of various
    etiologies. (ENG)

656
Possible permanent severe damage to eighth cranial nerve, primarily vestibular problems but also hearing loss, due to parenteral administration of
antibiotic, streptomycin, in humans with tuberculosis, in particular with
concurrent kidney disorder.
Possible permanent severe damage to eighth cranial nerve due to parenteral
administration of antibiotic, viomycin, in humans with tuberculosis.
Possible permanent severe damage to eighth cranial nerve due to parenteral
administration of antibiotic, kanamycin, in humans with tuberculosis.
Possible permanent severe damage to eighth cranial nerve due to parenteral
administration of antibiotic, capreomycin, in humans with tuberculosis.
    (AD) Discussion of primary and secondary drugs used in treatment of tuber-
    culosis. (ENG)

663
Vertigo due to antibiotic, streptomycin, in 2 humans.
Tinnitus and sensorineural hearing loss but no vertigo due to antibiotic,
streptomycin, in 3 humans.
    (AD) Treatment with dogmatil of vestibular problems and hearing loss due
    to streptomycin. (FR)

670
Possible vestibular problems due to parenteral administration of antibiotic,
gentamicin, in humans.
Damage to eighth cranial nerve, primarily hearing loss, usually permanent,
due to parenteral administration of high doses of antibiotic, kanamycin, for
more than 10 days in humans, in particular with kidney disorders.

Damage to eighth cranial nerve, primarily hearing loss, usually permanent,
due to parenteral administration of high doses of antibiotic, neomycin, for
more than 10 days in humans, in particular with kidney disorders.
Possible damage to eighth cranial nerve, primarily hearing loss, due to
parenteral administration of antibiotic, paromomycin, in humans.
Transient or permanent vestibular problems due to parenteral administration
of antibiotic, streptomycin, in humans.
Permanent severe hearing loss due to parenteral administration of antibiotic,
dihydrostreptomycin, in humans.
Damage to eighth cranial nerve, primarily hearing loss, due to parenteral
administration of high doses of antibiotic, vancomycin, for more than 10 days
in humans, in particular with kidney disorders.
Damage to eighth cranial nerve, vestibular problems and hearing loss, due to
parenteral administration of high doses of antibiotic, viomycin, for more
than 10 days in humans, in particular with kidney disorders.
    (AD) Discussion of toxic effects of antibiotics. (ENG)

                                                                          672
Possible sensorineural hearing loss due to parenteral administration of
antibiotic, kanamycin, in humans with kidney disorders.
    (AD) Need for decr in dosage and 3 to 4 days interval between doses in
    patients with kidney disorders.
Possible vestibular problems and hearing loss due to parenteral administration of antibiotic, streptomycin, in humans with kidney disorders.
    (AD) Need for decr in dosage and 3 to 4 days interval between doses in
    patients with kidney disorders.
Possible vestibular problems due to parenteral administration of antibiotic,
gentamicin, in humans with kidney disorders.
    (AD) Need for decr in dosage and unknown period between doses in patients
    with kidney disorders.
Possible hearing loss due to parenteral administration of antibiotic, vancomycin, in humans with kidney disorders.
    (AD) Need for decr in dosage and 9 days interval between doses in patients
    with kidney disorders.
    (AD) Report on use of antibiotics in patients with kidney disorders.
    (AD) Need for total initial dose followed by 50 percent of initial dose at
    recommended intervals.
    (AD) Change in dosage based on serum half-life of antibiotic.
    (AD) Literature review of effect of antibiotics in patients with kidney
    disorders. (ENG)

                                                                          676
Vestibular problems due to antibiotic, streptomycin, in humans.
    (AD) Ototoxic effects of streptomycin particularly with high doses, long
    period of treatment, concurrent kidney disorders, and in older patients.
Hearing loss due to antibiotic, dihydrostreptomycin, in humans.
Hearing loss due to antibiotic, viomycin, in humans.
    (AD) Discussion of toxic effects of various antibiotics.
    (AD) Comment that effect of some inhibitors on ototoxicity not known
    definitely. (FR)

                                                                          681
Degrees of inhibition of potential of endorgan of ampulla of posterior semicircular canal due to 50, 200, 300, and 500 mcg per cc, in Tyrode solution,
of antibiotic, streptomycin (streptomycin sulfate), in animals, frogs.
Degrees of inhibition of potential of endorgan of ampulla of posterior semicircular canal due to 100, 200, and 500 mcg per cc, in Tyrode solution, of
antibiotic, dihydrostreptomycin, in animals, frogs.
    (AD) Recovery of potential after cessation of administration of antibio-
    tics. (IT)

                                                                          685
Total loss of vestibular function but no hearing loss due to total of 840 mg
of antibiotic, gentamicin (SM), in 47 day period in 1 of 181 humans, aged, 70
years age, female, with kidney disorder.
Total loss of vestibular function but no hearing loss due to 2 g of antibiotic, streptomycin (SM), in 47 day period in 1 of 181 humans, aged, 70 years
age, female, with kidney disorder.

Permanent vestibular problems due to 2.56 g of antibiotic, (SQ) gentamicin,
for 18 days in 1 of 181 humans, adult, 39 years age, female, with kidney
disorder.
Vestibular problems due to previous administration of antibiotic, (SQ) streptomycin, in 1 of 181 humans, adult, 39 years age, female, with kidney disorder.
Permanent vestibular problems, with dizziness, due to antibiotic, gentamicin,
in 1 of 181 humans, adult, 38 years age, female, with kidney disorder.
Transient dizziness after 3 days due to antibiotic, gentamicin, in 1 of 181
humans, adolescent, 16 years age, female, with kidney disorder.
   (AD) Serial vestibular function tests and audiometry not conducted in 181
   patients.
Vestibular problems due to parenteral, intramuscular, administration of 1 g
daily of antibiotic, (SQ) streptomycin (SM), in 1 human, adult, 19 years age,
male, with pseudomonas infection.
   (AD) Vestibular problems due to previous streptomycin therapy.
Simultaneous administration of 300 mg daily of antibiotic, (SQ) colistin (SM)
(colistimethate), for 15 days in 1 human, adult, 19 years age, male, with
pseudomonas infection.
Sequential parenteral, intramuscular, administration of 40 mg 3 times a day
of antibiotic, (SQ) gentamicin, for 36 days in 1 human, adult, 19 years age,
male, with pseudomonas infection.
Dizziness after 4 days due to parenteral, intramuscular, administration of 40
mg 4 times a day, total of 2.56 g, of antibiotic, gentamicin, for 16 days in
1 human, adult, 30 years age, female, with kidney disorder.
   (AD) Discussion of 6 case reports of vestibulotoxic effects of gentamicin.
   (ENG)

                                                                          687
Vestibular problems and hearing loss due to high doses of antibiotic, strep-
tomycin, in humans.
   (AD) Discussion of toxic effects of drugs.   (GER)

                                                                          698
Hearing loss, after 3 months in most cases, due to parenteral administration
of 0.5 g twice daily for 7 days a week of antibiotic, kanamycin, in 29 (39
percent) of 75 humans with pulmonary tuberculosis.
Damage to eighth cranial nerve due to parenteral administration of 1 g twice
daily for 2 days a week of antibiotic, kanamycin, for more than 12 months in
5 (7 percent) of 64 humans with pulmonary tuberculosis.
   (AD) Low incidence of ototoxic effects reported in study possibly due to
   administration of kanamycin only 2 days a week.
Damage to eighth cranial nerve due to parenteral administration of 15 mg per
kg daily of antibiotic, kanamycin, in 4 (6 percent) of 65 humans with pulmonary tuberculosis and with previous hearing loss.
Hearing loss due to parenteral administration of 15 to 20 mg per kg for 5
days a week of antibiotic, (SQ) kanamycin, in 19 (22 percent) of 82 humans
with pulmonary tuberculosis and with previous hearing loss in 10 cases.
   (AD) Hearing loss confirmed by audiometry.
   (AD) Ototoxic effects in patients 50 years or over age in 15 of 19 cases.
Previous administration of antibiotic, (SQ) streptomycin, for long period in
82 humans with pulmonary tuberculosis.
Previous administration of antibiotic, (SQ) viomycin, in 10 of 82 humans with
pulmonary tuberculosis.
   (AD) Discussion of ototoxic effects of kanamycin reported in 4 studies.
   (AD) Significant factors in kanamycin ototoxicity reported to be age over
   50 years, high daily dose of more than 20 mg per kg, high serum level of
   more than 25 mcg per ml, concurrent kidney disorders, and previous hearing
   loss.   (ENG)

                                                                          700
Dizziness or vertigo, during first 3 months in 7 cases and after 3 to 6
months in 5 cases, due to 1 g daily for first 3 months, and then 1 g 3 times
a week for second 3 months in patients 50 years age or less, or 1 g 3 times a
week for 6 months in patients over 50 years age, of antibiotic, streptomycin
(SM) (streptomycin sulfate), for 6 months in 12 (20 percent) of 59 humans,
adult and aged, 55 years or more age in most cases, male, with chronic pulmonary tuberculosis and pneumoconiosis.

(AD) Reported 20 percent incidence of streptomycin ototoxicity in first
   year of therapy.
Incr hearing loss reported after 6 months due to 1 g daily for first 3
months, and then 1 g 3 times a week for second 3 months in patients 50 years
age or less, or 1 g 3 times a week for 6 months in patients over 50 years
age, of antibiotic, streptomycin (SM) (streptomycin sulfate), for 6 months in
1 of 59 humans, adult and aged, 55 years or more age in most cases, male,
with chronic pulmonary tuberculosis and pneumoconiosis and with previous
hearing loss.
   (AD) Reported 1 case of hearing loss due to streptomycin in first year of
   therapy.
Dizziness and tinnitus after 14 months due to 1 g daily for first 3 months,
and then 1 g 3 times a week for second 3 months in patients 50 years age or
less, or 1 g 3 times a week for 6 months in patients over 50 years age, of
antibiotic, streptomycin (SM) (streptomycin sulfate), for 6 months in 1 of 31
humans, male, with chronic pulmonary tuberculosis and pneumoconiosis.
   (AD) Reported 1 case with ototoxic effects within 18 months of therapy.
Simultaneous oral administration in cachets of 333 mg daily of antituberculous agent, isoniazid (SM) (CB), for 18 months or more in 59 humans, male,
with chronic pulmonary tuberculosis and pneumoconiosis.
Simultaneous oral administration in cachets of 15 g daily of antituberculous
agent, PAS (SM) (CB) (sodium PAS), for 18 months or more in 59 humans, male,
with chronic pulmonary tuberculosis and pneumoconiosis.   (ENG)

                                                                         723
Possible sensorineural hearing loss and vestibular problems due to antibio-
tic, streptomycin, in humans treated for tuberculosis during pregnancy.
(GER)

                                                                         731
Possible damage to eighth cranial nerve, vestibular problems, due to antibio-
tic, streptomycin, in humans with gram-negative bacilli.
Possible damage to eighth cranial nerve, hearing loss, due to antibiotic,
kanamycin, in humans with gram-negative bacilli.
Possible damage to eighth cranial nerve, hearing loss, due to antibiotic,
neomycin, in humans with gram-negative bacilli.
Possible damage to eighth cranial nerve, vestibular problems, due to antibio-
tic, gentamicin, in humans with gram-negative bacilli.
Possible ototoxic effects due to antibiotic, vancomycin, in humans with gram-
positive cocci.
   (AD) Need to decr dosage of antibiotics in patients with kidney disorders.
   (AD) Discussion of possible toxic effects of antibiotics used in surgery.
   (ENG)

                                   Tobramycin

                                                                         049
Hearing loss and damage to hair cells of organ of Corti due to parenteral,
(SQ) intraperitoneal, administration of 200 mg per kg daily of antibiotic,
tobramycin (nebramycin (factor 6)), for 6 days in 13 animals, guinea pigs,
220 to 260 g weight.
Hearing loss and damage to hair cells of organ of Corti due to parenteral,
(SQ) subcutaneous, administration of 150 mg per kg daily of antibiotic,
tobramycin (nebramycin (factor 6)), for 6 weeks in 13 animals, guinea pigs,
220 to 260 g weight.
   (CT) Control group of 5 guinea pigs used.
   (AD) Loss of Preyer reflex showed hearing loss.   (ENG)

                                   Vancomycin

                                                                         009
Delayed permanent sensorineural hearing loss and damage to outer hair cells
of basal and middle coils of cochlea due to unspecified doses of antibiotic,
dihydrostreptomycin, in humans.
Vertigo and dizziness due to unspecified method of administration of 2 to 3 g
daily of antibiotic, streptomycin (streptomycin sulfate), for 30 to 50 days
in humans with tuberculosis.
Hearing loss due to unspecified method of administration of high doses of

antibiotic, streptomycin (streptomycin sulfate), for long period in humans.
Gradual high frequency hearing loss and tinnitus and degeneration of hair
cells of organ of Corti in basal coil of cochlea due to unspecified doses of
antibiotic, kanamycin, in humans.
Delayed severe high frequency hearing loss due to parenteral, oral, or topical administration by inhalation of unspecified doses of antibiotic, neomycin, for unspecified period in humans with kidney disorder.
Complete degeneration of inner hair cells due to unspecified method of administration of 18 g of antibiotic, neomycin, for unspecified period in
humans with bacterial endocarditis.
Lesions in organ of Corti due to parenteral administration of unspecified
doses of antibiotic, polymyxin B, for unspecified period in animals, guinea
pigs.
Sensorineural hearing loss due to parenteral, intravenous, administration of
80 to 95 mg per ml of antibiotic, vancomycin, for unspecified period in
humans with kidney disorder.
    (AD) Sensorineural hearing loss and vestibular problems due to 6 antibio-
    tics in humans and animals, guinea pigs.
    (AD) Literature review of ototoxic effects of antibiotics. (ENG)

                                                                 016
Progressive bilateral sensorineural hearing loss and vertigo due to unspecified method of administration of total of 3 g of antibiotic, (SQ) streptomycin (SM), for unspecified period in 1 human, Caucasian, adult, 32 years age,
male, with kidney disorder and on intermittent hemodialysis.
Progressive bilateral sensorineural hearing loss and vertigo due to unspecified method of administration of antibiotic, (SQ) colistin (SM), for unspecified period in 1 human, Caucasian, adult, 32 years age, male, with kidney
disorder and on intermittent hemodialysis.
Permanent sensorineural hearing loss due to parenteral, intravenous, administration of 1.6 mg per kg 2 times daily, total of 500 mg of antibiotic, (SQ)
gentamicin, for unspecified period in 1 human, Caucasian, adult, 32 years
age, male, with kidney disorder and on intermittent hemodialysis.
No definite ototoxic effects reported due to unspecified method of administration of 1 g every 2 weeks, total of 12 g, of antibiotic, (SQ) vancomycin,
for about 6 months in 1 human, Caucasian, adult, 32 years age, male, with
kidney disorder and on intermittent hemodialysis.
    (AD) Hearing loss due to streptomycin and colistin potentiated by gentami-
    cin. (ENG)

                                                                 213
Dizziness due to antibiotic, polymyxin B (polymyxin B sulfate), in humans.
Dizziness due to antibiotic, colistin (sodium colistimethate), in humans.
Ototoxic effects due to antibiotic, ristocetin, in humans.
Hearing loss due to antibiotic, vancomycin, in humans.
    (AD) Report on pharmacology, clinical use, and toxicity of antibiotics.
    (ENG)

                                                                 214
Hearing loss due to high blood levels of 90 mcg per ml or more of antibiotic,
vancomycin, in humans.
    (AD) Report on chemical composition, mechanism of action, clinical use,
    and toxicity of vancomycin. (ENG)

                                                                 250
Damage to vestibular apparatus due to more than 1 g daily of antibiotic,
streptomycin, for 60 to 120 days in 25 percent of humans.
Dizziness 5 days after cessation of treatment due to parenteral, intramuscular, administration of 1 g every 12 hours of antibiotic, streptomycin (SM),
for 9 days in 1 human, adult, 44 years age, female, with peritonitis.
Simultaneous parenteral, intravenous, administration of 600 mg every 18 hours
of antibiotic, lincomycin (SM), for 9 days in 1 human, adult, 44 years age,
female, with peritonitis.
    (AD) Case report of vestibular problem due to streptomycin.
Damage to cochlea due to antibiotic, dihydrostreptomycin, for more than 1
week in 4 to 15 percent of humans.
Sensorineural hearing loss and damage to organ of Corti due to antibiotic,
kanamycin, in humans.

Sensorineural hearing loss and damage to organ of Corti due to antibiotic,
vancomycin, in humans.
   (AD) Discussion of cochleo-vestibulotoxic effects due to antibiotic therapy in surgery. (ENG)

316

Possible vestibular problems and cochlear impairment due to more than recommended dose of 15 to 30 mg per kg daily of antibiotic, streptomycin, for long
period in humans.
Hearing loss due to parenteral, intramuscular, administration of total doses
of 5 to 6 g of antibiotic, kanamycin, in humans, adult, with kidney disorder.
Possible hearing loss due to parenteral, topical, or oral administration of
high doses of antibiotic, neomycin, for long period in humans.
Possible hearing loss due to high doses of antibiotic, framycetin, for long
period in humans.
Possible hearing loss due to antibiotic, vancomycin, in humans.
Possible hearing loss and vestibular problems due to antibiotic, viomycin, in
humans.
   (AD) High risk of ototoxicity with simultaneous administration of viomycin
   and streptomycin.
Possible vestibular problems due to antibiotic, gentamicin, in humans.
   (AD) Administration of gentamicin not recommended for newborn infants, for
   humans during pregnancy, and for humans treated with other ototoxic drugs.
Ataxia and hearing loss due to antibiotic, colistin, in humans.
   (AD) Literature review on ototoxic antibiotics.
   (AD) Results of studies on use of pantothenate salt of some antibiotics
   for decr in ototoxicity not clear.
   (AD) Suggested effect of ototoxic antibiotics on breakdown of glucose on
   which hair cells of inner ear depend for energy. (ENG)

404

No cochleo-vestibulotoxic effects due to parenteral, intravenous, administration of 1 g, dissolved in 250 ml isotonic saline, of antibiotic, vancomycin,
for every 14 days for long period, more than 60 days, in 25 humans with
chronic kidney disorder and treated with intermittent hemodialysis.
   (AD) Audiometry every 12 weeks.
   (AD) Previous reports of severe ototoxicity due to vancomycin.
   (AD) Previous report suggested occurrence of ototoxicity with vancomycin
   serum levels over 80 mcg per ml.
   (AD) Suggested that vancomycin ototoxicity not related to total dosage or
   duration of treatment. (ENG)

641

Possible damage to eighth cranial nerve due to antibiotic, capreomycin, in
humans.
Possible vestibular problems and hearing loss due to antibiotic, gentamicin,
in humans.
Possible delayed transient or permanent hearing loss due to antibiotic,
kanamycin (SM), in humans, in particular with kidney disorders or with simultaneous administration of ethacrynic acid.
Possible delayed transient or permanent hearing loss due to diuretic, ethacrynic acid (SM), in humans.
Possible delayed transient or permanent severe hearing loss due to oral,
parenteral, or topical administration of antibiotic, neomycin, in humans.
Possible damage to eighth cranial nerve, primarily hearing loss, due to
antibiotic, paromomycin, in humans.
Possible hearing loss due to antibiotic, rifampicin, in humans.
High risk of damage to eighth cranial nerve, primarily transient or permanent
vestibular problems but also hearing loss, due to antibiotic, streptomycin,
in humans.
Possible damage to eighth cranial nerve, primarily hearing loss, due to high
doses of antibiotic, vancomycin, for long period of more than 10 days in
humans in particular with kidney disorders.
Risk of damage to eighth cranial nerve, vestibular problems and hearing loss,
due to high doses of antibiotic, viomycin, for long period of more than 10
days in humans, in particular with kidney disorders.
   (AD) Discussion of toxic effects of antibiotics. (ENG)

670

Possible vestibular problems due to parenteral administration of antibiotic, gentamicin, in humans.
Damage to eighth cranial nerve, primarily hearing loss, usually permanent, due to parenteral administration of high doses of antibiotic, kanamycin, for more than 10 days in humans, in particular with kidney disorders.
Damage to eighth cranial nerve, primarily hearing loss, usually permanent, due to parenteral administration of high doses of antibiotic, neomycin, for more than 10 days in humans, in particular with kidney disorders.
Possible damage to eighth cranial nerve, primarily hearing loss, due to parenteral administration of antibiotic, paromomycin, in humans.
Transient or permanent vestibular problems due to parenteral administration of antibiotic, streptomycin, in humans.
Permanent severe hearing loss due to parenteral administration of antibiotic, dihydrostreptomycin, in humans.
Damage to eighth cranial nerve, primarily hearing loss, due to parenteral administration of high doses of antibiotic, vancomycin, for more than 10 days in humans, in particular with kidney disorders.
Damage to eighth cranial nerve, vestibular problems and hearing loss, due to parenteral administration of high doses of antibiotic, viomycin, for more than 10 days in humans, in particular with kidney disorders.
    (AD) Discussion of toxic effects of antibiotics. (ENG)

672

Possible sensorineural hearing loss due to parenteral administration of antibiotic, kanamycin, in humans with kidney disorders.
    (AD) Need for decr in dosage and 3 to 4 days interval between doses in patients with kidney disorders.
Possible vestibular problems and hearing loss due to parenteral administration of antibiotic, streptomycin, in humans with kidney disorders.
    (AD) Need for decr in dosage and 3 to 4 days interval between doses in patients with kidney disorders.
Possible vestibular problems due to parenteral administration of antibiotic, gentamicin, in humans with kidney disorders.
    (AD) Need for decr in dosage and unknown period between doses in patients with kidney disorders.
Possible hearing loss due to parenteral administration of antibiotic, vancomycin, in humans with kidney disorders.
    (AD) Need for decr in dosage and 9 days interval between doses in patients with kidney disorders.
    (AD) Report on use of antibiotics in patients with kidney disorders.
    (AD) Need for total initial dose followed by 50 percent of initial dose at recommended intervals.
    (AD) Change in dosage based on serum half-life of antibiotic.
    (AD) Literature review of effect of antibiotics in patients with kidney disorders. (ENG)

731

Possible damage to eighth cranial nerve, vestibular problems, due to antibiotic, streptomycin, in humans with gram-negative bacilli.
Possible damage to eighth cranial nerve, hearing loss, due to antibiotic, kanamycin, in humans with gram-negative bacilli.
Possible damage to eighth cranial nerve, hearing loss, due to antibiotic, neomycin, in humans with gram-negative bacilli.
Possible damage to eighth cranial nerve, vestibular problems, due to antibiotic, gentamicin, in humans with gram-negative bacilli.
Possible ototoxic effects due to antibiotic, vancomycin, in humans with gram-positive cocci.
    (AD) Need to decr dosage of antibiotics in patients with kidney disorders.
    (AD) Discussion of possible toxic effects of antibiotics used in surgery.
    (ENG)

Viomycin

015

Damage to cells of ampulla due to range of doses of antibiotic, viomycin, in animals.
    (AD) Electron microscopic study of effects of viomycin on vestibular

apparatus.   (JAP)

047

Range of degree of damage to crista ampullaris and macula due to parenteral,
intramuscular, administration of 150 mg per kg daily of antibiotic, viomycin
(viomycin sulfate), for about 2 to 3 weeks in 3 animals, squirrel monkeys.
Range of degree of damage to crista ampullaris and macula due to parenteral,
intramuscular, administration of 200 to 300 mg per kg daily of antibiotic,
viomycin (viomycin sulfate), for about 2 to 3 weeks in 3 animals, cats.
More severe damage to crista ampullaris and macula due to topical administration in solution of range of 113 mg per ml to 500 mg per ml solution of
antibiotic, viomycin (viomycin sulfate), in 1 or 2 doses in 9 animals, cats.
   (CT) Control group of 2 monkeys and 2 cats used.   (ENG)

085

Hearing loss due to antibiotic, viomycin, in 17.7 percent of 152 humans with
tuberculosis.
   (CT) Systematic controls with audiology.
Hearing loss due to antibiotic, viomycin (IB), in only 5.3 percent of 36
humans with previous hearing loss with administration of nialamid.
Hearing loss due to antibiotic, kanamycin, in 20 percent of 55 humans with
tuberculosis.
Hearing loss due to antibiotic, kanamycin (IB), in 0 of 25 humans with previous hearing loss with administration of nialamid.
Lesion of inner ear due to antibiotic, neomycin (IB), in only 1 human with
previous hearing loss with administration of nialamid.   (GER)

120

Sensorineural hearing loss and damage to eighth cranial nerve due to parenteral, intramuscular, administration of 1 g daily of antibiotic, viomycin
(IB), for 1 month or more in 5 percent of 60 humans with pulmonary tuberculosis and treated with vitamin B.
   (AD) Need for audiometry with clinical use of viomycin.   (POL)

122

Damage to eighth cranial nerve and sensorineural hearing loss and vestibular
problems due to unspecified doses of antibiotic, viomycin, for long period in
humans.
   (AD) Literature review of viomycin, use in therapy and toxic effects.
   (AD) Recommended intramuscular administration of 1 to 2 g daily dose of
   viomycin for 2 to 3 weeks for minimum risk of ototoxicity.   (ENG)

156

Sensorineural hearing loss due to unspecified method of administration of
high doses of antibiotic, streptomycin (SM), in 7 humans, infant and child,
with tuberculous meningitis.
Simultaneous administration of unspecified doses of antituberculous agent,
PAS (SM), in 7 humans, infant and child, with tuberculous meningitis.
Simultaneous administration of unspecified doses of antituberculous agent,
isoniazid (SM), in 7 humans, infant and child, with tuberculous meningitis.
Sensorineural hearing loss due to unspecified method of administration of
high doses of antibiotic, viomycin, in 7 humans, infant and child, with
tuberculous meningitis.
   (AD) Cochleotoxic effect due to antibiotic therapy or infection.   (ENG)

316

Possible vestibular problems and cochlear impairment due to more than recommended dose of 15 to 30 mg per kg daily of antibiotic, streptomycin, for long
period in humans.
Hearing loss due to parenteral, intramuscular, administration of total doses
of 5 to 6 g of antibiotic, kanamycin, in humans, adult, with kidney disorder.
Possible hearing loss due to parenteral, topical, or oral administration of
high doses of antibiotic, neomycin, for long period in humans.
Possible hearing loss due to high doses of antibiotic, framycetin, for long
period in humans.
Possible hearing loss due to antibiotic, vancomycin, in humans.
Possible hearing loss and vestibular problems due to antibiotic, viomycin, in
humans.

(AD) High risk of ototoxicity with simultaneous administration of viomycin and streptomycin.
Possible vestibular problems due to antibiotic, gentamicin, in humans.
(AD) Administration of gentamicin not recommended for newborn infants, for humans during pregnancy, and for humans treated with other ototoxic drugs.
Ataxia and hearing loss due to antibiotic, colistin, in humans.
(AD) Literature review on ototoxic antibiotics.
(AD) Results of studies on use of pantothenate salt of some antibiotics for decr in ototoxicity not clear.
(AD) Suggested effect of ototoxic antibiotics on breakdown of glucose on which hair cells of inner ear depend for energy.   (ENG)

323

Progressive severe bilateral sensorineural hearing loss and vestibular problems due to parenteral administration of 1 g twice weekly of antibiotic, (SQ) viomycin (viomycin pantothenate), for total of 10 weeks in 1 human, adult, 59 years age, female, with pulmonary tuberculosis and kidney disorder.
(AD) Cochleo-vestibulotoxic effects confirmed by audiometry at different periods during and after treatment and by caloric test.
Previous administration of antibiotic, (SQ) chloramphenicol, in 1 human, adult, 59 years age, female, for infection before diagnosis of tuberculosis.
Possible but not reported auditory system problems due to previous parenteral administration of 0.5 g twice daily of antibiotic, (SQ) streptomycin, for 1 week in 1 human, adult, 59 years age, female, for infection before diagnosis of tuberculosis.
(AD) Suggested that possible previous ototoxic effects of streptomycin potentiated by viomycin (viomycin pantothenate).
Previous administration of antituberculous agent, (SQ) PAS, in 1 human, adult, 59 years age, female, with pulmonary tuberculosis and kidney disorder. (ENG)

343

No hearing loss but decr in vestibular function, asymptomatic except for dizziness in 1 case, due to 1 g daily of antibiotic, capreomycin (SM), for 4 months or more in 4 of 25 humans, adolescent, adult, and aged, range of 17 to 67 years age, male and female, 80 to 160 lb weight, with pulmonary tuberculosis and with kidney disorder in 2 cases.
Transient dizziness with no objective decr in vestibular function due to 1 g daily of antibiotic, capreomycin (SM), for 4 months or more in 3 of 25 humans, adolescent, adult, and aged, range of 17 to 67 years age, male and female, 80 to 160 lb weight, with pulmonary tuberculosis.
Simultaneous administration of 300 mg daily of antituberculous agent, isoniazid (SM), for 4 months or more in 25 humans, adolescent, adult, and aged, range of 17 to 67 years age, male and female, 80 to 160 lb weight, with pulmonary tuberculosis.
(CT) Pure tone audiometry, caloric tests, and cupulometry, pretreatment and during treatment with capreomycin.
(AD) Study of clinical use and cochleo-vestibulotoxic effects of capreomycin.
Hearing loss, asymptomatic in 1 case and symptomatic in 1 case, due to 1 g daily of antibiotic, viomycin, in 2 of 75 humans with pulmonary tuberculosis.
Objective decr in vestibular function due to 1 g daily of antibiotic, viomycin, in 21 of 75 humans with pulmonary tuberculosis.
Hearing loss, asymptomatic, due to 1 g daily of antibiotic, streptomycin, in 2 of 61 humans with pulmonary tuberculosis.
Objective decr in vestibular function due to 1 g daily of antibiotic, streptomycin, in 8 of 61 humans with pulmonary tuberculosis.
(CT) Audiometry and vestibular function tests, pretreatment and during treatment with viomycin or streptomycin.
(AD) Results of study on capreomycin comp w results of previous study on viomycin and streptomycin.   (ENG)

368

Possible vestibular problems and hearing loss due to antibiotic, streptomycin, in humans with tuberculosis.
Permanent hearing loss due to antibiotic, dihydrostreptomycin, in humans with tuberculosis.
Possible permanent hearing loss due to antibiotic, kanamycin, in humans with

tuberculosis.
Possible vestibular problems and hearing loss due to antibiotic, viomycin, in
humans with tuberculosis.
Possible damage to eighth cranial nerve due to antibiotic, capreomycin, in
humans with tuberculosis.
    (AD) Discussion of primary and secondary drugs used in tuberculosis chemo-
    therapy.   (FR)

                                                                        409
Primary damage to hair cells of organ of Corti, hearing loss, and possible
vestibular problems due to antibiotic, viomycin, in humans.
Damage to hair cells of organ of Corti and hearing loss due to antibiotic,
neomycin, in humans.
Damage to hair cells of organ of Corti and hearing loss due to antibiotic,
kanamycin, in humans.
Primary damage to vestibular apparatus, vestibular problems, and possible
hearing loss due to antibiotic, streptomycin, in humans.
Primary damage to vestibular apparatus, vestibular problems, and possible
hearing loss due to antibiotic, gentamicin, in humans.
    (AD) Need for audiometry and vestibular function tests, pretreatment and
    during treatment, with clinical use of aminoglycoside antibiotics.
    (AD) Incr in blood levels and ototoxicity of antibiotics in humans with
    kidney disorders.   (ENG)

                                                                        460
No significant decr in cochlear microphonics due to parenteral, subcutaneous,
administration of 100 mg per kg daily for 5 days a week, total dose of 7.5 g
per kg, of antibiotic, streptomycin (streptomycin sulfate), for 75 days in
animals, guinea pigs.
Statistically significant decr in cochlear microphonics at 1 of 18 points
examined, damage to hair cells of organ of Corti, slight damage to stria
vascularis and spiral ganglion, damage to macula utriculi and cristae, slight
damage to macula sacculi, and vestibular problems due to parenteral, subcutaneous, administration of 200 mg per kg daily, then 400 mg per kg, followed
by return to 200 mg per kg, total dose of 15 g per kg, of antibiotic, streptomycin (streptomycin sulfate), for 58 days in animals, guinea pigs.
    (AD) Vestibular problems confirmed by vestibular function tests.
No significant decr in cochlear microphonics due to parenteral, subcutaneous,
administration of 100 mg per kg daily for 5 days a week, total dose of 7.5 g
per kg, of antibiotic, viomycin (viomycin sulfate), for 75 days in animals,
guinea pigs.
Significant decr in cochlear microphonics, damage to hair cells of organ of
Corti and to stria vascularis, slight damage to spiral ganglion, and slight
damage to macula utriculi and crista ampullaris due to parenteral, subcutaneous, administration of 200 mg per kg daily for 5 days a week, then 400 mg
per kg, total dose of 15 g per kg, of antibiotic, viomycin (viomycin sulfate), for total of 67 days in animals, guinea pigs.
    (AD) Most toxicity for cochlear microphonics in guinea pig due to viomy-
    cin.
No significant decr in cochlear microphonics due to parenteral, subcutaneous,
administration of 100 mg per kg daily for 5 days each week, total dose of 7.5
g per kg, of antibiotic, capreomycin (capreomycin sulfate), for 75 days in
animals, guinea pigs.
No significant decr in cochlear microphonics, slight damage to outer hair
cells of organ of Corti and to stria vascularis, and no damage to vestibular
apparatus due to parenteral, subcutaneous, administration of 200 mg per kg
daily for 5 days a week, then 400 mg per kg, total dose of 15 g per kg, of
antibiotic, capreomycin (capreomycin sulfate), for total of 67 days in animals, guinea pigs.
    (CT) Same method using subcutaneous administration of 0.25 cc daily of
    isotonic saline in guinea pigs, control group.
    (AD) Least toxicity for inner ear of guinea pig due to capreomycin.
    (AD) Study of functional and structural cochleo-vestibulotoxic effects of
    streptomycin, viomycin, and capreomycin.
    (AD) Statistical analysis of results.   (ENG)

                                                                        473
Possible vestibular problems due to antibiotic, viomycin, in humans with

infections.
Possible vestibular problems due to antibiotic, capreomycin, in humans with
infections.
   (AD) Experiments to find new derivatives of viomycin and capreomycin with
   biological activity but with less toxic effects.   (ENG)

                                                                        610
Possible ototoxic effects due to antibiotic, capreomycin, in humans with
tuberculosis of genitourinary system.
Possible hearing loss due to antibiotic, kanamycin, in humans with tuberculo-
sis of genitourinary system.
Possible hearing loss and vestibular problems due to antibiotic, viomycin, in
humans with tuberculosis of genitourinary system.
   (AD) Discussion of treatment of tuberculosis of genitourinary system.
   (GER)

                                                                        641
Possible damage to eighth cranial nerve due to antibiotic, capreomycin, in
humans.
Possible vestibular problems and hearing loss due to antibiotic, gentamicin,
in humans.
Possible delayed transient or permanent hearing loss due to antibiotic,
kanamycin (SM), in humans, in particular with kidney disorders or with simul-
taneous administration of ethacrynic acid.
Possible delayed transient or permanent hearing loss due to diuretic, ethacrynic acid (SM), in humans.
Possible delayed transient or permanent severe hearing loss due to oral,
parenteral, or topical administration of antibiotic, neomycin, in humans.
Possible damage to eighth cranial nerve, primarily hearing loss, due to
antibiotic, paromomycin, in humans.
Possible hearing loss due to antibiotic, rifampicin, in humans.
High risk of damage to eighth cranial nerve, primarily transient or permanent
vestibular problems but also hearing loss, due to antibiotic, streptomycin,
in humans.
Possible damage to eighth cranial nerve, primarily hearing loss, due to high
doses of antibiotic, vancomycin, for long period of more than 10 days in
humans, in particular with kidney disorders.
Risk of damage to eighth cranial nerve, vestibular problems and hearing loss,
due to high doses of antibiotic, viomycin, for long period of more than 10
days in humans, in particular with kidney disorders.
   (AD) Discussion of toxic effects of antibiotics.   (ENG)

                                                                        656
Possible permanent severe damage to eighth cranial nerve, primarily vestibular problems but also hearing loss, due to parenteral administration of
antibiotic, streptomycin, in humans with tuberculosis, in particular with
concurrent kidney disorder.
Possible permanent severe damage to eighth cranial nerve due to parenteral
administration of antibiotic, viomycin, in humans with tuberculosis.
Possible permanent severe damage to eighth cranial nerve due to parenteral
administration of antibiotic, kanamycin, in humans with tuberculosis.
Possible permanent severe damage to eighth cranial nerve due to parenteral
administration of antibiotic, capreomycin, in humans with tuberculosis.
   (AD) Discussion of primary and secondary drugs used in treatment of tuberculosis.   (ENG)

                                                                        670
Possible vestibular problems due to parenteral administration of antibiotic,
gentamicin, in humans.
Damage to eighth cranial nerve, primarily hearing loss, usually permanent,
due to parenteral administration of high doses of antibiotic, kanamycin, for
more than 10 days in humans, in particular with kidney disorders.
Damage to eighth cranial nerve, primarily hearing loss, usually permanent,
due to parenteral administration of high doses of antibiotic, neomycin, for
more than 10 days in humans, in particular with kidney disorders.
Possible damage to eighth cranial nerve, primarily hearing loss, due to
parenteral administration of antibiotic, paromomycin, in humans.
Transient or permanent vestibular problems due to parenteral administration

of antibiotic, streptomycin, in humans.
Permanent severe hearing loss due to parenteral administration of antibiotic,
dihydrostreptomycin, in humans.
Damage to eighth cranial nerve, primarily hearing loss, due to parenteral
administration of high doses of antibiotic, vancomycin, for more than 10 days
in humans, in particular with kidney disorders.
Damage to eighth cranial nerve, vestibular problems and hearing loss, due to
parenteral administration of high doses of antibiotic, viomycin, for more
than 10 days in humans, in particular with kidney disorders.
    (AD) Discussion of toxic effects of antibiotics. (ENG)

676

Vestibular problems due to antibiotic, streptomycin, in humans.
    (AD) Ototoxic effects of streptomycin particularly with high doses, long
    period of treatment, concurrent kidney disorders, and in older patients.
Hearing loss due to antibiotic, dihydrostreptomycin, in humans.
Hearing loss due to antibiotic, viomycin, in humans.
    (AD) Discussion of toxic effects of various antibiotics.
    (AD) Comment that effect of some inhibitors on ototoxicity not known
    definitely. (FR)

698

Hearing loss, after 3 months in most cases, due to parenteral administration
of 0.5 g twice daily for 7 days a week of antibiotic, kanamycin, in 29 (39
percent) of 75 humans with pulmonary tuberculosis.
Damage to eighth cranial nerve due to parenteral administration of 1 g twice
daily for 2 days a week of antibiotic, kanamycin, for more than 12 months in
5 (7 percent) of 64 humans with pulmonary tuberculosis.
    (AD) Low incidence of ototoxic effects reported in study possibly due to
    administration of kanamycin only 2 days a week.
Damage to eighth cranial nerve due to parenteral administration of 15 mg per
kg daily of antibiotic, kanamycin, in 4 (6 percent) of 65 humans with pulmonary tuberculosis and with previous hearing loss.
Hearing loss due to parenteral administration of 15 to 20 mg per kg for 5
days a week of antibiotic, (SQ) kanamycin, in 19 (22 percent) of 82 humans
with pulmonary tuberculosis and with previous hearing loss in 10 cases.
    (AD) Hearing loss confirmed by audiometry.
    (AD) Ototoxic effects in patients 50 years or over age in 15 of 19 cases.
Previous administration of antibiotic, (SQ) streptomycin, for long period in
82 humans with pulmonary tuberculosis.
Previous administration of antibiotic, (SQ) viomycin, in 10 of 82 humans with
pulmonary tuberculosis.
    (AD) Discussion of ototoxic effects of kanamycin reported in 4 studies.
    (AD) Significant factors in kanamycin ototoxicity reported to be age over
    50 years, high daily dose of more than 20 mg per kg, high serum level of
    more than 25 mcg per ml, concurrent kidney disorders, and previous hearing
    loss. (ENG)

ANTICONVULSANTS

621

Primarily vestibular problems due to antibiotic, streptomycin, in humans.
Primarily hearing loss but also vestibular problems due to antibiotic, dihy-
drostreptomycin, in humans.
Primarily hearing loss but also vestibular problems due to antibiotic, kana-
mycin, in humans.
Primarily hearing loss but also vestibular problems due to antibiotic, neomy-
cin, in humans.
Primarily hearing loss but also vestibular problems due to antibiotic, genta-
micin, in humans.
Vertigo and ataxia due to antituberculous agent, isoniazid, in humans.
Hearing loss due to salicylate, aspirin, in humans.
Hearing loss and vertigo due to antimalarial, quinine, in humans.
Nystagmus due to barbiturates in humans.
Vestibular problems due to analgesic, morphine, in humans.
Nystagmus due to sedative, alcohol, in humans.
Nystagmus and hearing loss due to chemical agent, carbon monoxide, in humans.
Ototoxic effects due to antineoplastic, nitrogen mustard, in humans.

Ototoxic effects due to chemical agent, aniline, in humans.
Ototoxic effects due to chemical agent, tobacco, in humans.
Nystagmus due to chemical agent, nicotine, in humans.
Vestibular problems due to anticonvulsants in humans.
Vestibular problems due to anesthetics in humans.
Vestibular problems due to diuretics in humans.
   (AD) Inclusion of comprehensive list of ototoxic agents. (SP)

Amino-oxyacetic acid

721

Decr in eighth cranial nerve action potential and change in Preyer reflex
threshold due to parenteral, subcutaneous, administration of 2 or 3 to 20 mg
per kg of anticonvulsant, amino-oxyacetic acid, in animals, guinea pigs.
   (CT) Same method using saline in guinea pigs, control group, showed no
   change in reflex threshold.
   (AD) Changes in Preyer reflex threshold in part due to effects on auditory
   pathway. (ENG)

Carbamazepine

541

Vertigo due to anticonvulsant, carbamazepine, in 58(11.4 percent) of humans
treated for paroxysmal trigeminal neuralgia.
Tinnitus due to anticonvulsant, carbamazepine, in 1(0.2 percent)of humans
treated for paroxysmal trigeminal neuralgia.
   (AD) Need to monitor use of carbamazepine in therapy. (ENG)

665

Transient slight dizziness and equilibrium disorder due to oral administration in tablets of range of less than 600 mg to 1200 mg daily, of anticonvulsant, carbamazepine, for long period in large group of humans, adult and
aged, 30 to over 80 years age, male and female, with facial pain.
Severe dizziness due to oral administration in tablets of range of less than
600 mg to 1200 mg daily, of anticonvulsant, carbamazepine, for long period in
2 of 71 humans, adult and aged, 30 to over 80 years age, male and female,
with facial pain and with concurrent multiple sclerosis in 1 and cerebral
arteriosclerosis in other. (ENG)

669

Possible transient dizziness due to anticonvulsant, carbamazepine, in humans
with trigeminal neuralgia. (ENG)

Diphenylhydantoin

160

Tinnitus due to unspecified method of administration of 300 mg daily of
anticonvulsant, diphenylhydantoin (diphenylhydantoin sodium), for 2 years in
1 human, aged, 77 years age, female, for dizziness.
   (AD) No tinnitus after cessation of treatment with diphenylhydantoin
   (diphenylhydantoin sodium). (ENG)

383

Nystagmus and cochlear impairment due to high doses of anticonvulsant, di-
phenylhydantoin, in humans, infant and child.
   (AD) Literature review of toxic risks of antibiotics and other drugs.
   (GER)

593

Vestibular problems due to 1 g in 24 hours of antibiotic, (SQ) streptomycin
(SM), in 1 human, adult, 32 years age, female, with tuberculosis.
Vestibular problems due to 450 mg of antituberculous agent, (SQ) isoniazid
(SM), in 1 human, adult, 32 years age, female, with tuberculosis.
Vestibular problems due to oral administration in tablets of 0.10 g of anti-
convulsant, (SQ) diphenylhydantoin, in 1 human, adult, 32 years age, female,
with tuberculosis.
Vestibular problems due to oral administration in tablets of 3 tablets of
0.10 g each daily of anticonvulsant, (SQ) diphenylhydantoin (SM), in 1 human,

adult, 49 years age, female, with tuberculosis.
Vestibular problems due to 300 mg of antituberculous agent, (SQ) isoniazid
(SM), in 1 human, adult, 49 years age, female, with tuberculosis.
Simultaneous administration of 500 cm of antituberculous agent, (SQ) PAS
(SM), in 1 human, adult, 49 years age, female, with tuberculosis.
   (AD) Report of vestibulotoxic effects in 2 patients due to diphenylhydan-
   toin with isoniazid or streptomycin.   (FR)

654

Possible ataxia due to high doses to produce blood level of 3 mg per 100 ml
or more of anticonvulsant, diphenylhydantoin, in humans, child and adult,
with epilepsy.
Possible nystagmus due to doses to produce blood level of more than 2 mg per
100 ml of anticonvulsant, diphenylhydantoin, in humans, child and adult, with
epilepsy.   (ENG)

655

Possible ataxia and nystagmus due to anticonvulsant, diphenylhydantoin, in
humans with convulsive disorders.   (ENG)

658

Vertigo due to parenteral, intravenous, administration of 250 mg of anticonvulsant, diphenylhydantoin, in some of 123 humans, adult and aged, male and
female, with heart disorders.   (GER)

664

Nystagmus due to parenteral, intramuscular or intravenous, administration of
1000 to 1500 mg on first day, and then 400 to 1500 mg on second day, followed
by 400 to 600 mg, to produce blood levels of 8.6 to 35.0 mcg per ml, of
anticonvulsant, diphenylhydantoin, in 8 of 10 humans, adult and aged, 40 to
65 years age, male and female, 50-94 kg weight, with heart disorders.   (ENG)

671

Nystagmus due to anticonvulsant, diphenylhydantoin, in humans, child and
adult, male and female, with epilepsy.   (FIN)

ANTIDEPRESSANTS

Imipramine hydrochloride

396

No hearing loss but decr in vestibular function due to parenteral, intramuscular, administration of 25 mg of antidepressant, imipramine hydrochloride,
in 20 humans.   (IT)

ANTIDIABETICS

Insulin

397

Sensorineural hearing loss possibly due to antidiabetic, insulin, in humans
treated for diabetes.
   (AD) Reported that hearing loss in many humans treated with insulin for
   diabetes.
   (AD) Hearing loss confirmed by audiometry.   (ENG)

R 94

174

Transient high frequency hearing loss and tinnitus after 4 hours due to oral
administration of 1 g daily of antidiabetic, (SQ) R 94, for 28 days at most
in 26 humans, adolescent and adult, 15 to 55 years age, male, with moderate
to severe diabetes.
Incr in high frequency hearing loss due to oral administration of 1 g of
antidiabetic, (SQ) R 94, for 7 days after onset of hearing loss in 9 of 26
humans, adolescent and adult, 15 to 55 years age, male, with moderate to
severe diabetes.
Decr and complete reversal of hearing loss due to oral administration of 1 g

of antidiabetic, (SQ) R 94 (IB), in 15 of 26 humans, adolescent and adult, 15
to 55 years age, male, with moderate to severe diabetes, with administration
of 100 and 200 mg of nicotinic acid.
  (AD) Reversal of hearing loss after cessation of treatment with R 94 or
  with administration of nicotinic acid.
  (CT) Use of subjects with no recent treatment with ototoxic drugs.
  (CT) Audiometry, pretreatment and 4 hours after every daily dose.
  (AD) Vestibular function tests normal. (ENG)

ANTIHISTAMINES

Dimenhydrinate

118

Nystagmus and unsteady gait due to unspecified doses of antibiotics (SM) in 1
human, adult, 47 years age, male, with epilepsy.
Simultaneous administration of anticonvulsant, primidone (SM), in 1 human,
adult, 47 years age, male, with epilepsy.
Simultaneous administration of antihistamine, dimenhydrinate (SM), in 1
human, adult, 47 years age, male, with epilepsy. (ENG)

344

No significant change in perrotatory neuronal response of medial vestibular
nucleus due to parenteral, intravenous, administration of 2, 8, or 20 mg per
kg of antihistamine, dimenhydrinate, in animals, cats, adult, 2.5 kg average
weight.
Significant decr in perrotatory neuronal response of medial vestibular nucleus due to parenteral, intravenous, administration of 0.4 mg per kg of
diazepan in animals, cat s, adult, 2.5 kg average weight.
  (CT) Same method using 1 ml Ringer's solution in cats, control group,
  showed no significant changes.
  (AD) Possible peripheral or central location, or both, of action of dimenhydrinate.
  (AD) Study to determine if changes in perrotatory response of medial
  vestibular nucleus is result of action on vestibular apparatus.
  (AD) Suggest that endorgan not location of action of dimenhydrinate.
  (ENG)

ANTI-INFLAMMATORY AGENTS

Chymotrypsin

714

Decr in cochlear microphonics due to topical administration to bulla of
concentrations of 1, 3, and 6 units, in 0.1 ml, of anti-inflammatory agent,
chymotrypsin, in 40 animals, guinea pigs.
  (CT) Same method using physiological sodium chloride solution in guinea
  pigs, control group.
  (AD) Electrophysiological study showed more decr in cochlear potentials
  with incr in concentration of chymotrypsin.
  (AD) Suggested careful consideration in clinical use of chymotrypsin in
  treatment of adhesive otitis media. (GER)

Fluorometholone

603

Tinnitus due to oral administration of 25 mg twice a day, total of 50 mg per
kg, of anti-inflammatory agent, fluorometholone (NSC-33001), for 8 weeks in 1
of 112 humans, adult, 25 years average age, with tumors. (ENG)

Ibuprofen

263

Possible dizziness, tinnitus, and hearing loss due to anti-inflammatory
agent, ibuprofen, in humans. (ENG)

355

Tinnitus and hearing loss due to previous oral administration of (SQ) 4.5 g

daily of salicylate, (SQ) aspirin, in 4 of 6 humans with rheumatoid arthritis.
Tinnitus and hearing loss due to oral administration of (SQ) 3.6 g daily of
salicylate, (SQ) aspirin, for short period, 2 weeks, in 1 of 6 humans with
rheumatoid arthritis.
No ototoxic effects due to oral administration of 0.3, 0.6, and 0.9 g daily
of anti-inflammatory agent, (SQ) ibuprofen, for short period, 2 weeks, in 6
humans with rheumatoid arthritis.
No ototoxic effects due to range of 200 to 1200 mg daily, average of 600 mg
daily, of anti-inflammatory agent, ibuprofen, for long period, 3 months to
over 12 months, in 27 humans, adult, 60.6 years average age, male and female,
with rheumatoid arthritis.
    (AD) Comparative study of effectiveness of aspirin and ibuprofen in treat-
    ment of rheumatoid arthritis.   (ENG)

                                                                         359
Hearing loss due to oral administration of 400, 600, or 800 mg of anti-inflammatory agent, ibuprofen, for 2 weeks in 2 of 30 humans, adult and aged, 30
to 79 years age, female and male, with rheumatoid arthritis.
Unspecified ototoxic effects due to oral administration of 2.4, 3.6, or 4.8 g
daily of salicylate, aspirin, for 2 weeks in 18 of 30 humans, adult and aged,
30 to 79 years age, female and male, with rheumatoid arthritis.
    (AD) Comparative study of ibuprofen, aspirin, and placebo in treatment of
    rheumatoid arthritis.   (ENG)

                                                                         360
Transient dizziness due to 0.9 or 0.6 g daily of anti-inflammatory agent,
ibuprofen, for 7 or 14 days in 1 of 39 humans, adult, range of ages, male and
female, with arthritis.
    (AD) Comparative study of ibuprofen and placebo in treatment of arthritis.
    (ENG)

                                                                         361
Transient dizziness and tinnitus due to oral administration of 750 mg daily
of anti-inflammatory agent, ibuprofen, for 5 days in 1 of 9 humans, adult and
aged, 37 to 67 years age, male and female, with rheumatoid arthritis.
    (AD) Ibuprofen therapy discontinued after 5 days.
Hearing loss and tinnitus due to oral administration of 5 g daily of salicylate, aspirin, for 1 week in 3 of 9 humans, adult and aged, 37 to 67 years
age, male and female, with rheumatoid arthritis.
    (AD) Comparative study of ibuprofen, aspirin, and prednisolone in treat-
    ment of rheumatoid arthritis.   (ENG)

                             Indomethacin

                                                                         305
Dizziness, vertigo, tinnitus, and hearing loss due to oral administration of
50, 100, 150, and then 200 mg, incr daily doses each week, of anti-inflammatory agent, indomethacin, for 4 weeks in 7 of 24 humans, adult and aged,
range of 23 to 69 years age, male and female, with rheumatoid arthritis.
Dizziness, vertigo, tinnitus, and hearing loss due to oral administration of
1.6, 3.2, 4.8, and then 6.4 g, incr daily doses each week, of salicylate,
acetylsalicylic acid, for 4 weeks in 18 of 24 humans, adult and aged, range
of 23 to 69 years age, male and female, with rheumatoid arthritis.
    (AD) Comparative study of effectiveness of indomethacin and acetylsalicy-
    lic acid in treatment of rheumatoid arthritis.   (ENG)

                                                                         659
Possible dizziness due to anti-inflammatory agent, indomethacin, in humans.
(ENG)

                                                                         668
Possible vertigo due to anti-inflammatory agent, indomethacin, in humans,
adult.
    (AD) High incidence of vertigo due to indomethacin reported in studies.
    (AD) Incidence and degree of effect usually dose related.   (ENG)

693
Tinnitus due to oral administration in capsules of 75 mg daily of anti-inflammatory agent, indomethacin, for 4 weeks in 1 of 14 humans, male and female, with rheumatoid arthritis.
Dizziness due to oral administration in capsules of 75 mg daily of anti-
inflammatory agent, indomethacin, for 4 weeks in 1 of 14 humans, male and
female, with rheumatoid arthritis.   (ENG)

697
Dizziness in 12 cases and hearing loss in 1 case due to oral (SM) administration in capsules of 25 mg twice a day for 2 days and then 4 times a day for 2
days, followed by 50 mg 3 times a day for 2 days and then 4 times a day, of
anti-inflammatory agent, indomethacin, for 12 weeks in 12 (40 percent) of 30
humans with bone and joint disorder.
Dizziness in 12 cases and hearing loss in 1 case due to topical, rectal (SM),
administration in suppositories of 100 mg daily of anti-inflammatory agent,
indomethacin, for first 6 days in 12(40 percent) of 30 humans with bone and
joint disorder.   (ENG)

707
Dizziness due to 75 mg daily of anti-inflammatory agent, indomethacin, in 1
of 24 humans with bone and joint disorder.   (CZ)

708
Vertigo due to oral administration in capsules of 75 mg in 2 capsules 3 times
daily of anti-inflammatory agent, indomethacin, in 2 of 18 humans during
treatment for arthritis.
Vertigo due to oral administration in capsules of 75 mg in 2 capsules 3 times
daily of anti-inflammatory agent, indomethacin, for 4 weeks in 1 of 7 humans
after treatment for arthritis.
Vertigo due to oral administration in capsules of 1500 mg daily in 2 capsules
3 times daily of anti-inflammatory agent, mefenamic acid, for 4 weeks in 1 of
39 humans after treatment for arthritis.   (ENG)

Mefenamic acid

708
Vertigo due to oral administration in capsules of 75 mg in 2 capsules 3 times
daily of anti-inflammatory agent, indomethacin, in 2 of 18 humans during
treatment for arthritis.
Vertigo due to oral administration in capsules of 75 mg in 2 capsules 3 times
daily of anti-inflammatory agent, indomethacin, for 4 weeks in 1 of 7 humans
after treatment for arthritis.
Vertigo due to oral administration in capsules of 1500 mg daily in 2 capsules
3 times daily of anti-inflammatory agent, mefenamic acid, for 4 weeks in 1 of
39 humans after treatment for arthritis.   (ENG)

Monophenylbutazone

694
Vertigo and tinnitus due to oral administration in 3 tablets of 750 mg daily
of anti-inflammatory agent, (SQ) monophenylbutazone, for 5 days in 1 of 10
humans, male, with rheumatoid arthritis.
Previous oral administration in 3 tablets of 840 mg daily of salicylate, (SQ)
acetylsalicylic acid, for 2 weeks in 1 of 10 humans, male, with rheumatoid
arthritis.   (ENG)

ANTIMALARIALS
Chloroquine

219
Cochleo-vestibulotoxic effects due to antibiotics in humans.
Transient and permanent sensorineural hearing loss due to diuretic, etha-
crynic acid, in humans.
Transient sensorineural hearing loss, tinnitus, and vertigo due to salicy-
late, aspirin, in humans.
Transient and permanent sensorineural hearing loss and dizziness due to
antimalarial, quinine, in humans.

Sensorineural hearing loss due to antimalarial, chloroquine, in humans.
Sensorineural hearing loss, tinnitus, and vertigo due to chemical agents in
humans.
   (AD) Literature review of ototoxic drugs with clinical and histopathologi-
     cal correlations.
   (AD) Comment on ototoxicity of some chemical agents.
   (AD) Review of theories of mechanism of action of ototoxic drugs.   (ENG)

                                                          365
Possible vertigo and tinnitus due to high doses, 300 mg daily, of antimalarial, chloroquine (chloroquine sulfate), in humans with tuberculoid lepro-
sy.   (FR)

                                                          384
Usually transient hearing loss and no structural damage to organ of Corti,
stria vascularis, and spiral ganglion due to oral or topical administration
of salicylates in humans.
Hearing loss due to antimalarial, quinine, in humans.
Usually permanent hearing loss due to antimalarial, chloroquine, in humans.
Transient and permanent hearing loss and possible damage to hair cells of
organ of Corti due to diuretic, ethacrynic acid, in humans.
Sensorineural hearing loss due to cardiovascular agent, hexadimethrine
bromide, in humans with kidney disorder.
Sensorineural hearing loss and damage to organ of Corti due to topical ad-
ministration of antineoplastic, nitrogen mustard, in humans.
Sensorineural hearing loss due to high doses of antibiotic, chloramphenicol,
in humans.
Primary vestibular problems due to antibiotic, streptomycin, in humans.
Hearing loss due to high doses usually of antibiotic, streptomycin, in hu-
mans.
   (AD) Early detection of hearing loss by audiometry prevents permanent
     damage.
High frequency hearing loss and severe damage to outer hair cells and slight
damage to inner hair cells of organ of Corti due to antibiotic, kanamycin, in
humans.
Sensorineural hearing loss due to parenteral, oral, and topical administra-
tion of antibiotic, neomycin, in humans with or without kidney disorders.
Degeneration of hair cells of organ of Corti and of nerve process due to
antibiotics, aminoglycoside, in animals.
   (AD) Literature review of physiological and structural cochleo-vestibulo-
     toxic effects of ototoxic drugs.
   (AD) Discussion of suggested mechanism of ototoxicity and routes of drugs
     to inner ear.
Bilateral sensorineural hearing loss due to oral administration of antibio-
tic, neomycin, in 4 of 8 humans with liver disease.
Bilateral sensorineural hearing loss due to oral administration of range of
doses of antibiotic, neomycin (SM), in 2 of 5 humans with liver disease.
Bilateral sensorineural hearing loss due to diuretics (SM), in 2 of 5 humans
with liver disease.
Transient progression of previous hearing loss due to parenteral, intra-
venous, administration of diuretic, ethacrynic acid (SM), in 1 injection in 1
of 5 humans with liver disease.
   (CT) Normal cochlear function in 6 humans, control group, with liver
     disease and not treated with neomycin or diuretics.
   (CT) Normal cochlear function in 13 humans, control group, with liver
     disease and treated with diuretics but not with neomycin.
   (AD) Hearing loss confirmed by audiometry.
   (AD) Reported that hearing loss due to neomycin or diuretics in humans
     with liver disease not related to dosage.
   (AD) Clinical study of effects of treatment with neomycin and diuretics in
     humans with liver disease.
Bilateral sensorineural hearing loss and vertigo due to antibiotic, ampicil-
lin, in 1 human, adolescent, 17 years age, female, with tonsillitis.
   (AD) Cited case report.
Severe sensorineural hearing loss and vertigo due to topical administration
in ear drops of antibiotic, framycetin, in 1 human, adult, 42 years age,
male, with previous slight high frequency hearing loss.
   (AD) Cited case report.

Atrophy of hair cells of organ of Corti and hearing loss due to antibiotic,
dihydrostreptomycin, in humans with tuberculous meningitis.
   (AD) Cited study.
Loss of inner hair cells and damage to outer hair cells due to 18 g of anti-
biotic, neomycin, for 18 days in 1 human.
   (AD) Cited case report. (ENG)

644

Possible vertigo due to antimalarial, amodiaquine (amodiaquine dihydrochloride), in humans with parasitic infections.
Possible sensorineural hearing loss due to antimalarial, chloroquine (chloroquine hydrochloride) (chloroquine phosphate), in humans with parasitic infections.
Possible vertigo and ataxia due to antiparasitic, metronidazole, in humans
with parasitic infections.
Dizziness due to antiparasitic, quinacrine (quinacrine hydrochloride), in
humans with parasitic infections.
Tinnitus due to antimalarial, quinine (quinine dihydrochloride) (quinine
sulfate), in humans with parasitic infections.
Possible vertigo and tinnitus due to antiparasitic, thiabendazole, in humans
with parasitic infections.
Possible tinnitus due to antiparasitic, tryparsamide, in humans with parasitic infections.
   (AD) Discussion of clinical use and toxic effects of drugs used for parasitic infections. (ENG)

732

Hearing loss and total degeneration of organ of Corti and moderate degeneration of spiral ganglion and nerve process in fetus due to oral ingestion of
250 mg daily of antimalarial, chloroquine (chloroquine phosphate), in humans,
female, during pregnancy.
   (AD) Histopathological study of inner ear after death. (ENG)

Quinine

018

Hearing loss due to parenteral administration of low doses, 1 g daily, of
antibiotic, (SQ) streptomycin, in 3 injections in 1 human, adult, 22 years
age, male, with pulmonary tuberculosis.
Unspecified effects due to previous administration of 3 unspecified doses of
antimalarial, (SQ) quinine, in 1 human, adult, 22 years age, male, with
pulmonary tuberculosis. (ENG)

115

Permanent cochleo-vestibulotoxic effects due to antibiotics, aminoglycoside,
in humans.
Transient cochlear impairment due to salicylates in humans.
Ototoxic effects due to antimalarial, quinine, in humans.
Ototoxic effects due to chemical agent, nicotine, in humans.
   (AD) Report on ototoxic effects of various drugs.
   (AD) Need for audiometry and vestibular function tests with clinical use
   of ototoxic drugs. (FR)

181

Decr in succinic dehydrogenase in outer hair cells of organ of Corti due to
parenteral, intratympanic, administration of 200 mg per ml solution of antibiotic, kanamycin (kanamycin sulfate), in animals, guinea pigs, adult.
Decr in succinic dehydrogenase in outer hair cells of organ of Corti due to
parenteral, intratympanic, administration of 200 mg per ml solution of antibiotic, dihydrostreptomycin (dihydrostreptomycin sulfate), in animals, guinea
pigs, adult.
Decr in succinic dehydrogenase in outer hair cells of organ of Corti due to
parenteral, intratympanic, administration of 200 mg per ml solution of antibiotic, chloramphenicol (chloramphenicol succinate), in animals, guinea pigs,
adult.
   (AD) Same type of damage to organ of Corti due to all 3 antibiotics.
Severe decr in succinic dehydrogenase in organ of Corti, in particular in
outer hair cells, and atrophy of outer hair cells due to saturated solution

of antimalarial, quinine (quinine hydrochloride), in animals, guinea pigs.
Complete degeneration of organ of Corti due to saturated solution of antimalarial, quinine (quinine hydrochloride), in animals, guinea pigs.
    (AD) Damage to organ of Corti more severe due to quinine than to antibio-
    tics.
    (AD) Activity of succinic dehydrogenase often higher in outer hair cells.
    (AD) Possible that damage to outer hair cells due to higher rate of meta-
    bolism. (ENG)

                                                                         186
Diplacusis due to antibiotics, aminoglycoside, in humans.
Diplacusis due to antimalarial, quinine, in humans.
Diplacusis due to salicylate, aspirin, in humans.
Diplacusis due to chemical agent, carbon monoxide, in humans.
    (AD) Report on etiology of diplacusis with comment on ototoxic drugs.
    (ENG)

                                                                         219
Cochleo-vestibulotoxic effects due to antibiotics in humans.
Transient and permanent sensorineural hearing loss due to diuretic, etha-
crynic acid, in humans.
Transient sensorineural hearing loss, tinnitus, and vertigo due to salicy-
late, aspirin, in humans.
Transient and permanent sensorineural hearing loss and dizziness due to
antimalarial, quinine, in humans.
Sensorineural hearing loss due to antimalarial, chloroquine, in humans.
Sensorineural hearing loss, tinnitus, and vertigo due to chemical agents in
humans.
    (AD) Literature review of ototoxic drugs with clinical and histopathologi-
    cal correlations.
    (AD) Comment on ototoxicity of some chemical agents.
    (AD) Review of theories of mechanism of action of ototoxic drugs. (ENG)

                                                                         239
Transient sensorineural hearing loss due to oral ingestion in tablets of 3 to
5 g (10 to 15 tablets) of antimalarial, quinine, in 1 human, adult, 26 years
age, male, with alcohol intoxication.
    (AD) Case of attempted suicide.
    (AD) Hearing loss confirmed by audiogram. (GER)

                                                                         249
Cochleo-vestibulotoxic effects due to antibiotics, aminoglycoside, in humans.
Cochlear impairment due to antimalarial, quinine, in humans.
Transient cochlear impairment and vestibular problems due to salicylates in
humans.
    (AD) Occurrence of ototoxic effects with different dosages due to indivi-
    dual responses to drugs.
    (AD) Need for observation and tests with clinical use of ototoxic drugs.
    (FR)

                                                                         258
Cessation of blood flow in some capillaries of basilar membrane due to parenteral, intraperitoneal, administration of 125 mg of antimalarial, quinine
(quinine dihydrochloride), in 1 dose in animals, guinea pigs, 500 g weight.
Transient cessation of blood flow in some capillaries of basilar membrane due
to parenteral, intraperitoneal, administration of 62.5 mg per dose, total of
125 mg, of antimalarial, quinine (quinine dihydrochloride), in gradual doses
in animals, guinea pigs, 500 g weight.
    (CT) Study of guinea pigs, control group.
    (AD) Transient hearing loss due to quinine (quinine dihydrochloride) known
    from previous studies.
    (AD) Drugs known to produce hearing loss also produce cessation of blood
    flow in capillaries of basilar membrane. (ENG)

                                                                         284
Hearing loss due to antibiotics, aminoglycoside, in humans.
Hearing loss due to salicylate, sodium salicylate, in humans.
Hearing loss due to antimalarial, quinine, in humans.

(AD) Discussion of clinical use and cochleotoxic effects of ototoxic drugs
in humans. (FR)

291

Cochlear impairment due to 5.0 g of antimalarial, quinine (quinine hydroch-
loride), in humans.
Cochlear impairment due to antimalarial, quinine (quinine hydrochloride), in
animals, cats and rabbits.
   (AD) Comparative animal studies and clinical case reports.
   (AD) Study of ocular toxicity with comment on ototoxicity. (GER)

314

Loss of enzymes, succinic dehydrogenase and DPN diaphorase, in outer hair
cells of organ of Corti but usually no enzyme loss in inner hair cells due to
topical administration to bulla of 200 mg per ml of antibiotic, kanamycin
(kanamycin sulfate), in 1 injection in animals, guinea pigs.
Loss of enzymes, succinic dehydrogenase and DPN diaphorase, in outer hair
cells of organ of Corti but usually no enzyme loss in inner hair cells due to
topical administration to bulla of 200 mg per ml of antibiotic, dihydrostreptomycin (dihydrostreptomycin sulfate), in 1 injection in animals, guinea
pigs.
Loss of enzymes, succinic dehydrogenase and DPN diaphorase, in outer hair
cells of organ of Corti but usually no enzyme loss in inner hair cells due to
topical administration to bulla of 200 mg per ml of antibiotic, chloramphenicol (chloramphenicol succinate), in 1 injection in animals, guinea pigs.
More severe effects on enzymes, succinic hydrogenase and DPN diaphorase, in
outer hair cells of organ of Corti due to topical administration to bulla of
saturated solution of antimalarial, quinine (quinine hydrochloride), in 1
injection in animals, guinea pigs.
   (CT) Activity of succinic dehydrogenase often higher in outer hair cells
   than in inner hair cells of organ of Corti in guinea pigs, control group.
   (AD) Suggested correlation between cochleotoxic effects of drugs and
   metabolic activity of hair cells. (ENG)

333

Vestibular problems due to antibiotic, streptomycin, in humans.
Severe cochlear impairment due to antibiotic, dihydrostreptomycin, in humans.
Loss of hair cells in organ of Corti and hearing loss due to antibiotics,
aminoglycoside, in humans.
Hearing loss in fetus due to antimalarial, quinine, in humans, female,
treated during pregnancy.
Transient hearing loss due to high doses of salicylate, aspirin, for long
period in humans.
   (AD) Discussion of possible cochleo-vestibulotoxic effects of ototoxic
   drugs.
   (AD) Ototoxic effects related to concurrent disorders, dosage, duration of
   treatment, and age of individuals. (ENG)

373

Possible progressive sensorineural hearing loss due to antibiotics, aminogly-
coside, in humans.
Possible transient hearing loss due to high doses of salicylate, aspirin, in
humans.
Possible transient hearing loss due to high doses of antimalarial, quinine,
in humans.
Possible hearing loss due to diuretic, ethacrynic acid, in humans.
Bilateral sudden deafness due to antibiotic, kanamycin, in 4 humans, adult,
34 years average age, male and female.
   (AD) Hearing loss due to ototoxic drugs usually progressive.
   (AD) Sudden deafness due to ototoxic drugs possible in some cases, as in
   humans with kidney disorder.
   (AD) Literature review on etiology of sudden deafness. (ENG)

384

Usually transient hearing loss and no structural damage to organ of Corti,
stria vascularis, and spiral ganglion due to oral or topical administration
of salicylates in humans.
Hearing loss due to antimalarial, quinine, in humans.

Usually permanent hearing loss due to antimalarial, chloroquine, in humans.
Transient and permanent hearing loss and possible damage to hair cells of
organ of Corti due to diuretic, ethacrynic acid, in humans.
Sensorineural hearing loss due to cardiovascular agent, hexadimethrine
bromide, in humans with kidney disorder.
Sensorineural hearing loss and damage to organ of Corti due to topical ad-
ministration of antineoplastic, nitrogen mustard, in humans.
Sensorineural hearing loss due to high doses of antibiotic, chloramphenicol,
in humans.
Primary vestibular problems due to antibiotic, streptomycin, in humans.
Hearing loss due to high doses usually of antibiotic, streptomycin, in humans.
    (AD) Early detection of hearing loss by audiometry prevents permanent
    damage.
High frequency hearing loss and severe damage to outer hair cells and slight
damage to inner hair cells of organ of Corti due to antibiotic, kanamycin, in
humans.
Sensorineural hearing loss due to parenteral, oral, and topical administration of antibiotic, neomycin, in humans with or without kidney disorders.
Degeneration of hair cells of organ of Corti and of nerve process due to
antibiotics, aminoglycoside, in animals.
    (AD) Literature review of physiological and structural cochleo-vestibulo-
    toxic effects of ototoxic drugs.
    (AD) Discussion of suggested mechanism of ototoxicity and routes of drugs
    to inner ear.
Bilateral sensorineural hearing loss due to oral administration of antibiotic, neomycin, in 4 of 8 humans with liver disease.
Bilateral sensorineural hearing loss due to oral administration of range of
doses of antibiotic, neomycin (SM), in 2 of 5 humans with liver disease.
Bilateral sensorineural hearing loss due to diuretics (SM), in 2 of 5 humans
with liver disease.
Transient progression of previous hearing loss due to parenteral, intravenous, administration of diuretic, ethacrynic acid (SM), in 1 injection in 1
of 5 humans with liver disease.
    (CT) Normal cochlear function in 6 humans, control group, with liver
    disease and not treated with neomycin or diuretics.
    (CT) Normal cochlear function in 13 humans, control group, with liver
    disease and treated with diuretics but not with neomycin.
    (AD) Hearing loss confirmed by audiometry.
    (AD) Reported that hearing loss due to neomycin or diuretics in humans
    with liver disease not related to dosage.
    (AD) Clinical study of effects of treatment with neomycin and diuretics in
    humans with liver disease.
Bilateral sensorineural hearing loss and vertigo due to antibiotic, ampicillin, in 1 human, adolescent, 17 years age, female, with tonsillitis.
    (AD) Cited case report.
Severe sensorineural hearing loss and vertigo due to topical administration
in ear drops of antibiotic, framycetin, in 1 human, adult, 42 years age,
male, with previous slight high frequency hearing loss.
    (AD) Cited case report.
Atrophy of hair cells of organ of Corti and hearing loss due to antibiotic,
dihydrostreptomycin, in humans with tuberculous meningitis.
    (AD) Cited study.
Loss of inner hair cells and damage to outer hair cells due to 18 g of antibiotic, neomycin, for 18 days in 1 human.
    (AD) Cited case report.   (ENG)

                                                                          388
Hearing loss in 2 fetuses, twin, male, due to oral ingestion of high doses of
antimalarial, quinine, for unspecified period in 1 human, female, at end of
first trimester of pregnancy to induce abortion.
    (AD) No visual perception defect in twins due to ingestion of quinine by
    mother during pregnancy.
    (AD) Suggested vascular or neural mechanism of ototoxic effects of
    quinine.   (ENG)

                                                                          423
More severe and more rapid progression of presbycusis due to antimalarial,

quinine, in humans, adult and aged.
More severe and more rapid progression of presbycusis due to antibiotics,
aminoglycoside, in humans, adult and aged.
More severe and more rapid progression of presbycusis due to salicylate,
aspirin, in humans, adult and aged.
More severe and more rapid progression of presbycusis due to chemical agent,
carbon monoxide, in humans, adult and aged.
    (AD) Discussion of factors resulting in more severe and more rapid pro-
    gression of presbycusis. (FR)

438

Suppression of microphonic potentials of saccule due to topical, intraluminal, administration of antibiotic, streptomycin, in animals, goldfish.
Suppression of microphonic potentials of saccule due to topical, intraluminal, administration of antibiotic, kanamycin, in animals, goldfish.
Suppression of microphonic potentials of saccule due to topical, intraluminal
or extraluminal, administration of 0.5 mg of chemical agent, cyanide, in
animals, goldfish.
Suppression of microphonic potentials of saccule due to topical, intraluminal
or extraluminal, administration of 0.1 mg of antimalarial, quinine, in animals, goldfish.
Suppression of microphonic potentials of saccule due to topical, intraluminal
or extraluminal, administration of 2 mg of anesthetic, procaine, in animals,
goldfish.
No effect on microphonic potentials of saccule due to topical administration
of salicylates in animals, goldfish. (ENG)

450

Hearing loss and vertigo due to high doses of antimalarial, quinine, in
humans, adult, female and male, in suicide attempt.
    (AD) Study with EEG of acute quinine ototoxicity. (IT)

457

Tinnitus and progressive sensorineural hearing loss due to parenteral, intramuscular, administration of antibiotic, (SQ) streptomycin, for 10 days in 1
human, adult, 38 years age, female, with infections and later development of
kidney disorder.
Tinnitus and progressive sensorineural hearing loss due to 13.2 g of antibiotic, (SQ) kanamycin, for 11 days in 1 human, adult, 38 years age, female,
with infections and kidney disorder.
Hearing loss due to antimalarial, (SQ) quinine, in 1 human, adult, 20 years
age, male, with various infections and later development of kidney disorder.
Hearing loss due to 400 mg 2 times daily, total dose of 6.5 g, of antibiotic,
(SQ) kanamycin (SM), for 8 days in 1 human, adult, 20 years age, male, with
various infections and later development of kidney disorder.
Hearing loss due to 150 mg 2 times daily, total dose of 2400 mg, of antibiotic, (SQ) colistin (SM), for 8 days in 1 human, adult, 20 years age, male,
with various infections and later development of kidney disorder.
Tinnitus, total bilateral hearing loss, and vestibular problems due to parenteral, intramuscular, administration of 4.0 g daily, total of 21 g, of antibiotic, (SQ) kanamycin (SM), for 5 days in 1 human, adult, 20 years age,
male, with infections and kidney disorder.
Tinnitus, total bilateral hearing loss, and vestibular problems due to 0.6 g
daily, total dose of 1.3 g, of antibiotic, (SQ) colistin (SM), for 2 days in
1 human, adult, 20 years age, male, with infections and kidney disorder.
Tinnitus, total bilateral hearing loss, and vestibular problems due to 2 g
and then 8 g per 24 hours in divided doses, total dose of 26.5 g, of antibiotic, (SQ) chloramphenicol, for 9 days in 1 human, adult, 20 years age, male,
with infections and kidney disorder.
Bilateral hearing loss due to 1 g daily of antibiotic, actinomycin (SM), for
5 days in 1 human, adult, 62 years age, male, with infections and kidney
disorder.
Bilateral hearing loss due to unknown dose of antibiotic, kanamycin (SM), for
5 days in 1 human, adult, 62 years age, male, with infections and kidney
disorder.
Bilateral hearing loss and vestibular problems due to parenteral administration of high doses of antibiotic, (SQ) neomycin, for total of 21 days in 1
human, adult, 25 years age, male, with infection from wound.

Previous administration of unspecified doses of antibiotic, (SQ) streptomycin, in 1 human, adult, 25 years age, male, with infection from wound.
Later administration of antibiotic, (SQ) chloramphenicol, in 1 human, adult,
25 years age, male, with infection from wound.
Tinnitus and rapidly progressive bilateral hearing loss due to parenteral,
intramuscular, administration of 0.5 g every 12 hours of antibiotic, (SQ)
streptomycin, for 5 days in 1 human, adult, 21 years age, male, with infection from wound.
Tinnitus and rapidly progressive bilateral hearing loss due to parenteral,
intramuscular, administration of 200 mg daily, total of 6.8 g, of antibiotic,
(SQ) colistin (SM), in 1 human, adult, 21 years age, male, with infection
from wound.
Tinnitus and rapidly progressive bilateral hearing loss due to parenteral
administration of unspecified doses of antibiotic, (SQ) neomycin (SM), for
about 35 days in 1 human, adult, 21 years age, male, with infection from
wound.
Tinnitus and progressive bilateral hearing loss due to parenteral administration of 2 l per 24 hours of 1 percent solution of antibiotic, (SQ) neomycin,
for 10 days in 1 human, adult, 26 years age, male, with infection from wound.
    (AD) Hearing loss confirmed by audiometry.
Previous administration of 500 mg four times a day of antibiotic, (SQ) ampicillin, in 1 human, adult, 26 years age, male, with infection from wound.
Bilateral sudden deafness due to administration in dialysis fluid of less
than 150 mg of antibiotic, neomycin (SM), in 1 human, adult, 44 years age,
female, with kidney disorder.
Bilateral sudden deafness due to 50 mg of diuretic, ethacrynic acid (SM), in
1 human, adult, 44 years age, female, with kidney disorder.
    (AD) Hearing loss confirmed by audiology.
Tinnitus and progressive bilateral hearing loss beginning after 8 days of
treatment due to parenteral administration of 1 l every 4 hours for 3 days
and then every 8 hours for 10 days of 1 percent solution of antibiotic,
neomycin, in 1 human, adult, 20 years age, male, with infection from wound.
    (AD) Hearing loss confirmed by audiology.
Tinnitus and bilateral sensorineural hearing loss due to parenteral, intramuscular, administration of 1 g and then 0.5 g every 12 hours of antibiotic,
streptomycin (SM), for 15 days in 1 human, adult, 23 years age, male, with
infection from wound.
Tinnitus and bilateral sensorineural hearing loss due to topical administration by irrigation of 1 percent solution every 12 hours of antibiotic, neomycin (SM), for 14 days in 1 human, adult, 23 years age, male, with infection
from wound.
    (AD) Hearing loss confirmed by audiometry.
    (AD) Discussion of 10 case reports.   (ENG)

                                                                    468
Complete inhibition of acetylcholine induced decr in cochlear potential due
to parenteral, intravenous, administration of 1.0 mg of antibiotic, streptomycin (streptomycin sulfate), in 1 injection in 5 animals, cats, male and
female, 1.5 to 2.8 kg weight, with injection of acetylcholine.
Minimum inhibition of acetylcholine induced decr in cochlear potential due to
parenteral, intravenous, administration of 1.0 mg of antibiotic, dihydrostreptomycin (dihydrostreptomycin sulfate), in 1 injection in 5 animals, cats,
male and female, 1.5 to 2.8 kg weight, with injection of acetylcholine.
Complete inhibition of acetylcholine induced decr in cochlear potential due
to parenteral, intravenous, administration of 1.0 mg of antibiotic, kanamycin
(kanamycin sulfate), in 1 injection in 5 animals, cats, male and female, 1.5
to 2.8 kg weight, with injection of acetylcholine.
Complete inhibition of acetylcholine induced decr in cochlear potential due
to parenteral, intravenous, administration of 1.0 mg of antibiotic, neomycin
(neomycin sulfate), in 1 injection in 5 animals, cats, male and female, 1.5
to 2.8 kg weight, with injection of acetylcholine.
Acute inhibition of acetylcholine induced decr in cochlear potential due to
parenteral, intravenous, administration of 1.0 mg of antimalarial, quinine
(quinine hydrochloride), in 1 injection in 5 animals, cats, male and female,
1.5 to 2.8 kg weight, with injection of acetylcholine.
    (CT) Injections of 0.1 ml isotonic saline in cats, control group.
Inhibition of acetylcholine induced decr in cochlear potential due to parenteral, subcutaneous, administration of 300 mg per kg daily of antibiotic,

streptomycin, for 7 to 9 days in 10 animals, cats.
Inhibition of acetylcholine induced decr in cochlear potential due to parenteral, subcutaneous, administration of 100 mg per kg daily of antibiotic,
neomycin, for 7 to 9 days in 10 animals, cats.
   (CT) Study of 7 cats, control group, not treated with antibiotics.
   (AD) Study of effect of acetylcholine on cochlear potential after acute
   and chronic administration of ototoxic drugs.
   (AD) Suggested relationship between change in acetylcholine activity and
   ototoxic drugs.
   (AD) Suggested that ototoxicity partially due to disruption of efferent
   effect on cochlea. (ENG)

                                                                        484
No observed ototoxic effects in fetuses due to parenteral, intramuscular,
administration of 15, 30, or 50 mg per kg in 1 injection daily of antimalarial, quinine, for 30 days in 3 groups of 12 animals, dogs, during pregnancy.
   (CT) Study of 7 dogs, control group, not treated with quinine.
   (AD) Study of effects of quinine on fetuses of animals. (FR)

                                                                        562
Decr in microphonic potential of saccule due to topical, intraluminal, administration of antibiotic, streptomycin, in animals, goldfish.
Decr in microphonic potential of saccule due to topical, intraluminal, administration of antibiotic, kanamycin, in animals, goldfish.
Permanent decr in microphonic potential of saccule due to topical, intraluminal or extraluminal, administration of 0.5 mg per ml of chemical agent,
cyanide, in animals, goldfish.
Permanent decr in microphonic potential of saccule due to topical, intraluminal or extraluminal, administration of 0.1 mg per ml of antimalarial,
quinine, in animals, goldfish.
No effect on microphonic potential of saccule due to salicylate, aspirin, in
animals, goldfish.
Some decr in microphonic potential of saccule due to 2 mg per ml of anesthetic, procaine, in animals, goldfish.
   (AD) Study of effects of various agents on microphonic potential of saccule of goldfish. (JAP)

                                                                        597
Hearing loss due to salicylates in humans.
Hearing loss due to antimalarial, quinine, in humans.
Hearing loss due to antibiotic, streptomycin, in humans.
Tinnitus due to chemical agent, camphor, in humans.
Tinnitus due to chemical agent, tobacco, in humans.
Tinnitus due to cardiovascular agent, quinidine, in humans.
Tinnitus due to chemical agent, ergot, in humans.
Tinnitus due to chemical agent, alcohol, methyl, in humans.
   (AD) Discussion of toxic effects of drugs. (ENG)

                                                                        607
Transient tinnitus and hearing loss after 2 hours due to oral ingestion of 6
g of antimalarial, quinine (quinine sulfate), in 1 dose in 1 human, adult, 26
years age, female, in suicide attempt.
Transient tinnitus and sensorineural hearing loss within 5 hours due to oral
ingestion of 12 g, to produce serum level of 9.2 mg per l, of antimalarial,
quinine (quinine sulfate), in 1 human, adult, 24 years age, female, during
pregnancy in attempt to induce abortion. (ENG)

                                                                        621
Primarily vestibular problems due to antibiotic, streptomycin, in humans.
Primarily hearing loss but also vestibular problems due to antibiotic, dihy-
drostreptomycin, in humans.
Primarily hearing loss but also vestibular problems due to antibiotic, kana-
mycin, in humans.
Primarily hearing loss but also vestibular problems due to antibiotic, neomy-
cin, in humans.
Primarily hearing loss but also vestibular problems due to antibiotic, genta-
micin, in humans.

Vertigo and ataxia due to antituberculous agent, isoniazid, in humans.
Hearing loss due to salicylate, aspirin, in humans.
Hearing loss and vertigo due to antimalarial, quinine, in humans.
Nystagmus due to barbiturates in humans.
Vestibular problems due to analgesic, morphine, in humans.
Nystagmus due to sedative, alcohol, in humans.
Nystagmus and hearing loss due to chemical agent, carbon monoxide, in humans.
Ototoxic effects due to antineoplastic, nitrogen mustard, in humans.
Ototoxic effects due to chemical agent, aniline, in humans.
Ototoxic effects due to chemical agent, tobacco, in humans.
Nystagmus due to chemical agent, nicotine, in humans.
Vestibular problems due to anticonvulsants in humans.
Vestibular problems due to anesthetics in humans.
Vestibular problems due to diuretics in humans.
    (AD) Inclusion of comprehensive list of ototoxic agents. (SP)

627

Sensorineural hearing loss and vestibular problems due to parenteral, oral,
and topical administration of antibiotics in humans with and without kidney
disorder.
Degeneration of cochlea due to parenteral, intratympanic, administration of
antibiotic, neomycin, in animals, guinea pigs.
Transient sensorineural hearing loss due to high doses of salicylates in
humans.
Sensorineural hearing loss due to antimalarial, quinine, in humans.
Sensorineural hearing loss due to chemical agent, tobacco, in humans.
Sensorineural hearing loss due to sedative, alcohol, in humans.
    (AD) Discussion of ototoxicity of various drugs as 1 etiology of sen-
    sorineural hearing loss in adults. (ENG)

636

Inhibition of potentials of endorgan of ampulla of posterior semicircular
canal due to 2.5, 10, or 20 mcg per ml, in Tyrode solution, of antimalarial,
quinine (quinine hydrochloride), in animals, frogs.
    (CT) Study of effect on potentials of Tyrode solution without quinine.
    (AD) Electrophysiological study of effect of quinine on potentials of
    endorgan of ampulla of posterior semicircular canal.
    (AD) Some recovery of potentials after cessation of quinine administra-
    tion.
    (AD) Suggested that toxic effects on endorgan of semicircular canal result
    from administration of quinine. (ENG)

644

Possible vertigo due to antimalarial, amodiaquine (amodiaquine dihydrochloride), in humans with parasitic infections.
Possible sensorineural hearing loss due to antimalarial, chloroquine (chloroquine hydrochloride) (chloroquine phosphate), in humans with parasitic infections.
Possible vertigo and ataxia due to antiparasitic, metronidazole, in humans
with parasitic infections.
Dizziness due to antiparasitic, quinacrine (quinacrine hydrochloride), in
humans with parasitic infections.
Tinnitus due to antimalarial, quinine (quinine dihydrochloride) (quinine
sulfate), in humans with parasitic infections.
Possible vertigo and tinnitus due to antiparasitic, thiabendazole, in humans
with parasitic infections.
Possible tinnitus due to antiparasitic, tryparsamide, in humans with parasitic infections.
    (AD) Discussion of clinical use and toxic effects of drugs used for para-
    sitic infections. (ENG)

706

Ototoxic effects due to chemical agents and heavy metals in humans.
    (AD) Literature review of ototoxic effects of nicotine, carbon monoxide,
    carbon tetrachloride, mercury, arsenic, and lead.
Cochleo-vestibulotoxic effects, functional and structural, due to antibiotics
in humans.
    (AD) Literature review of ototoxicity of streptomycin, dihydrostreptomy-

cin, neomycin, kanamycin, gentamicin, capreomycin, rifampicin, viomycin,
   isoniazid, aminosidine, and framycetin.
Hearing loss due to salicylates in humans.
Hearing loss due to antimalarial, quinine, in humans.
Hearing loss due to diuretic, ethacrynic acid, in humans.
   (AD) Literature review of effects of various ototoxic agents.   (IT)

                              16-126 RP

                                                                      598
Vertigo or tinnitus due to oral administration in tablets of 1 to 3 tablets
of 200 mg each, total of 200 to 600 mg, of antimalarial, 16-126 RP, in 1 dose
in 3 of 20 humans, African, child, 4 or less to over 9 years age, with malaria.
Vertigo due to oral administration in tablets of 2 to 6 tablets of 200 mg
each, total of 400 to 1200 mg, of antimalarial, 16-126 RP, for 2 days in 1 of
15 humans, African, child, 4 or less to over 9 years age, with malaria. (FR)

                          ANTINEOPLASTICS

                          Mechlorethamine

                                                                      525
No loss of Preyer reflex and no structural changes in organ of Corti and
stria vascularis due to parenteral, intraperitoneal, administration of 3 to 5
mg per kg, in aqueous solution, of antineoplastic, mechlorethamine, for 5
days to 5 weeks in animals, 8 guinea pigs, adult, 300 to 400 g weight, and 6
mice, adult, 25 to 35 g weight, with normal Preyer reflex.
Loss of Preyer reflex and severe destruction of outer hair cells of organ of
Corti in basal and middle coils of cochlea but little or no change in stria
vascularis, spiral ganglion, and cochlear nerve due to parenteral, intraperitoneal, administration of 10 to 30 mg per kg, in aqueous solution, of antineoplastic, mechlorethamine, for 1 day to 5 weeks in animals, 7 guinea
pigs, adult, 300 to 400 g weight, and 19 mice, adult, 25 to 35 g weight, with
normal Preyer reflex.
   (CT) Same method using same volume of Ringer's solution in 5 animals,
   control group.
   (AD) Electron microscopic study of degeneration of cochlea in mechlorethamine intoxicated animals and in animals with congenital hearing loss to
   determine the mechanism of degeneration.
   (AD) Suggested possible effect on protein synthesis in hair cells of organ
   of Corti in early stages of mechlorethamine ototoxicity. (ENG)

                          Nitrogen mustard

                                                                      048
Severe sensorineural hearing loss and loss of hair cells of organ of Corti in
basal and middle coils of cochlea due to parenteral, intravenous, administration of high doses, 1.0 mg per kg, of antineoplastic, nitrogen mustard, in 1
injection in animals, cats, conditioned. (ENG)

                                                                      194
Vestibular problems, primary effect, and bilateral sensorineural hearing loss
due to antineoplastic, nitrogen mustard, for long periods in 24 humans with
malignant tumors and lupus erythematosus.
   (AD) Auditory system problems confirmed by audiometry and vestibular
   function tests.
   (AD) Cochleo-vestibulotoxic effects after treatment with nitrogen mustard
   due to dosage, duration of treatment, and route of administration. (SP)

                                                                      384
Usually transient hearing loss and no structural damage to organ of Corti,
stria vascularis, and spiral ganglion due to oral or topical administration
of salicylates in humans.
Hearing loss due to antimalarial, quinine, in humans.
Usually permanent hearing loss due to antimalarial, chloroquine, in humans.
Transient and permanent hearing loss and possible damage to hair cells of
organ of Corti due to diuretic, ethacrynic acid, in humans.

Sensorineural hearing loss due to cardiovascular agent, hexadimethrine bromide, in humans with kidney disorder.
Sensorineural hearing loss and damage to organ of Corti due to topical administration of antineoplastic, nitrogen mustard, in humans.
Sensorineural hearing loss due to high doses of antibiotic, chloramphenicol, in humans.
Primary vestibular problems due to antibiotic, streptomycin, in humans.
Hearing loss due to high doses usually of antibiotic, streptomycin, in humans.
   (AD) Early detection of hearing loss by audiometry prevents permanent damage.
High frequency hearing loss and severe damage to outer hair cells and slight damage to inner hair cells of organ of Corti due to antibiotic, kanamycin, in humans.
Sensorineural hearing loss due to parenteral, oral, and topical administration of antibiotic, neomycin, in humans with or without kidney disorders.
Degeneration of hair cells of organ of Corti and of nerve process due to antibiotics, aminoglycoside, in animals.
   (AD) Literature review of physiological and structural cochleo-vestibulotoxic effects of ototoxic drugs.
   (AD) Discussion of suggested mechanism of ototoxicity and routes of drugs to inner ear.
Bilateral sensorineural hearing loss due to oral administration of antibiotic, neomycin, in 4 of 8 humans with liver disease.
Bilateral sensorineural hearing loss due to oral administration of range of doses of antibiotic, neomycin (SM), in 2 of 5 humans with liver disease.
Bilateral sensorineural hearing loss due to diuretics (SM), in 2 of 5 humans with liver disease.
Transient progression of previous hearing loss due to parenteral, intravenous, administration of diuretic, ethacrynic acid (SM), in 1 injection in 1 of 5 humans with liver disease.
   (CT) Normal cochlear function in 6 humans, control group, with liver disease and not treated with neomycin or diuretics.
   (CT) Normal cochlear function in 13 humans, control group, with liver disease and treated with diuretics but not with neomycin.
   (AD) Hearing loss confirmed by audiometry.
   (AD) Reported that hearing loss due to neomycin or diuretics in humans with liver disease not related to dosage.
   (AD) Clinical study of effects of treatment with neomycin and diuretics in humans with liver disease.
Bilateral sensorineural hearing loss and vertigo due to antibiotic, ampicillin, in 1 human, adolescent, 17 years age, female, with tonsillitis.
   (AD) Cited case report.
Severe sensorineural hearing loss and vertigo due to topical administration in ear drops of antibiotic, framycetin, in 1 human, adult, 42 years age, male, with previous slight high frequency hearing loss.
   (AD) Cited case report.
Atrophy of hair cells of organ of Corti and hearing loss due to antibiotic, dihydrostreptomycin, in humans with tuberculous meningitis.
   (AD) Cited study.
Loss of inner hair cells and damage to outer hair cells due to 18 g of antibiotic, neomycin, for 18 days in 1 human.
   (AD) Cited case report.   (ENG)

540
Effect on cells of cochlea due to antineoplastic, nitrogen mustard, in animals.   (JAP)

621
Primarily vestibular problems due to antibiotic, streptomycin, in humans.
Primarily hearing loss but also vestibular problems due to antibiotic, dihydrostreptomycin, in humans.
Primarily hearing loss but also vestibular problems due to antibiotic, kanamycin, in humans.
Primarily hearing loss but also vestibular problems due to antibiotic, neomycin, in humans.
Primarily hearing loss but also vestibular problems due to antibiotic, gentamicin, in humans.

Vertigo and ataxia due to antituberculous agent, isoniazid, in humans.
Hearing loss due to salicylate, aspirin, in humans.
Hearing loss and vertigo due to antimalarial, quinine, in humans.
Nystagmus due to barbiturates in humans.
Vestibular problems due to analgesic, morphine, in humans.
Nystagmus due to sedative, alcohol, in humans.
Nystagmus and hearing loss due to chemical agent, carbon monoxide, in humans.
Ototoxic effects due to antineoplastic, nitrogen mustard, in humans.
Ototoxic effects due to chemical agent, aniline, in humans.
Ototoxic effects due to chemical agent, tobacco, in humans.
Nystagmus due to chemical agent, nicotine, in humans.
Vestibular problems due to anticonvulsants in humans.
Vestibular problems due to anesthetics in humans.
Vestibular problems due to diuretics in humans.
   (AD) Inclusion of comprehensive list of ototoxic agents.   (SP)

ANTIPARASITICS

A-16612

594

Transient severe vertigo due to oral administration in tablets of 50 mg per
kg of 500 mg tablets of antiparasitic, A-16612, for 2 days in 1 human, adult,
with schistosomiasis.
Auditory hallucination due to 100 mg per kg daily of antiparasitic, A-16612,
for 3 days in 1 human, adult, with schistosomiasis.
   (AD) Study of chemotherapy of schistosomiasis with new antiparasitic
   agent, A-16612.   (ENG)

Oil of chenopodium

138

Sensorineural hearing loss due to antiparasitic, oil of chenopodium, in 1
human, adult, 56 years age, male.
   (AD) Hearing loss confirmed by audiograms.   (POL)

709

Possible hearing loss and vertigo after 10 to 48 hours due to antiparasitic,
oil of chenopodium, in humans.   (FR)

Quinacrine

644

Possible vertigo due to antimalarial, amodiaquine (amodiaquine dihydrochloride), in humans with parasitic infections.
Possible sensorineural hearing loss due to antimalarial, chloroquine (chloroquine hydrochloride) (chloroquine phosphate), in humans with parasitic infections.
Possible vertigo and ataxia due to antiparasitic, metronidazole, in humans
with parasitic infections.
Dizziness due to antiparasitic, quinacrine (quinacrine hydrochloride), in
humans with parasitic infections.
Tinnitus due to antimalarial, quinine (quinine dihydrochloride) (quinine
sulfate), in humans with parasitic infections.
Possible vertigo and tinnitus due to antiparasitic, thiabendazole, in humans
with parasitic infections.
Possible tinnitus due to antiparasitic, tryparsamide, in humans with parasitic infections.
   (AD) Discussion of clinical use and toxic effects of drugs used for parasitic infections.   (ENG)

Thiabendazole

644

Possible vertigo due to antimalarial, amodiaquine (amodiaquine dihydrochloride), in humans with parasitic infections.
Possible sensorineural hearing loss due to antimalarial, chloroquine (chloroquine hydrochloride) (chloroquine phosphate), in humans with parasitic infec-

tions.
Possible vertigo and ataxia due to antiparasitic, metronidazole, in humans
with parasitic infections.
Dizziness due to antiparasitic, quinacrine (quinacrine hydrochloride), in
humans with parasitic infections.
Tinnitus due to antimalarial, quinine (quinine dihydrochloride) (quinine
sulfate), in humans with parasitic infections.
Possible vertigo and tinnitus due to antiparasitic, thiabendazole, in humans
with parasitic infections.
Possible tinnitus due to antiparasitic, tryparsamide, in humans with parasitic infections.
   (AD) Discussion of clinical use and toxic effects of drugs used for parasitic infections. (ENG)

                                                                        667
Possible vertigo due to antiparasitic, thiabendazole, in humans with parasitic disorder. (ENG)

                           ANTITUBERCULOUS AGENTS

                                                                        154
Ototoxic effects due to antibiotics in humans with tuberculosis.
   (AD) Literature review of some new antituberculous agents of 1968. (GER)

                                                                        179
Progressive high frequency hearing loss and tinnitus due to 1 g daily of
antibiotic, kanamycin, in 3 humans, adolescent and adult, male, with tuberculosis and with previous treatment with ototoxic drugs but with no report of
toxic effects.
Less severe sensorineural hearing loss and no tinnitus due to 1 g 5 times a
week of antibiotic, kanamycin, in 1 human, male, with tuberculosis and with
previous treatment with ototoxic drugs.
Sensorineural hearing loss and tinnitus due to 6 g of antibiotic, kanamycin
(SM), in 1 human, male, with tuberculosis and with previous treatment with
ototoxic drugs.
Sensorineural hearing loss and tinnitus due to parenteral administration of
1000 mg per day of antibiotic, streptomycin (SM), in 1 human, male, with
tuberculosis and with previous treatment with ototoxic drugs.
No high frequency hearing loss due to parenteral administration of 1 g daily
of antibiotic, streptomycin, in 1 human, female, with tuberculosis and with
previous treatment with ototoxic drugs.
High frequency hearing loss but no tinnitus due to 750 mg daily of antibiotic, streptomycin, in 1 human, female, with tuberculosis and with previous
treatment with ototoxic drugs.
Simultaneous administration of range of doses of other antituberculous agents
(SM) in total of 7 humans, adolescent and adult, 13 to 49 years age, male and
female, with tuberculosis and with previous treatment with ototoxic drugs.
   (AD) Study using high frequency audiometry and conventional audiometry.
   (CT) Pretreatment audiograms obtained. (ENG)

                                                                        293
Cochleo-vestibulotoxic effects due to antibiotic, streptomycin (SM), in
humans, range of ages, with pulmonary tuberculosis.
Simultaneous administration of other antituberculous agents (SM) in humans,
range of ages, with pulmonary tuberculosis.
   (AD) Report on toxic effects due to simultaneous treatment with various
   antituberculous agents. (BUL)

                                                                        325
High frequency hearing loss due to parenteral, intramuscular, administration
of total of 15 mg per kg in 2 doses 5 times a week of antibiotic, (SQ) capreomycin (SM), for 37 and 45 days in 2 of 70 humans, adult, 35 and 64 years
age, with pulmonary tuberculosis and with previous treatment with other
ototoxic drugs.
Transient vertigo due to parenteral, intramuscular, administration of total
of 15 mg per kg in 2 doses 5 times a week of antibiotic, (SQ) capreomycin
(SM), for 5, 25, and 94 days in 3 of 70 humans, adult, 39, 61, and 62 years
age, with pulmonary tuberculosis and with previous treatment with streptomy-

cin.
Simultaneous administration of other (SQ) antituberculous agents (SM), in 70
humans, adult, male and female, with pulmonary tuberculosis.
Possible ototoxic effects due to previous administration of antibiotic, (SQ)
streptomycin, in 3 of 70 humans, adult, 39, 61, and 62 years age, with pulmonary tuberculosis.   (ENG)

                                                                        570
Transient slight hearing loss due to parenteral, intramuscular, administration of 1 g daily, maximum dose of 90 g, of antibiotic, capreomycin (SM), in
1 of 16 humans with chronic tuberculosis of genitourinary system.
Simultaneous administration of 2 other antituberculous agents (SM), in 16
humans with chronic tuberculosis of genitourinary system.
Hearing loss due to 1 g daily average dose of antibiotic, capreomycin (SM),
for long period in 1 of 20 humans, adult, male and female, with chronic
tuberculosis, and 5 also alcoholics.
Simultaneous administration of other antituberculous agents (SM), in 20
humans, adult, male and female, with chronic tuberculosis, and 5 also alcoholics.
    (AD) Discussion of various reports of auditory system problems due to
    capreomycin therapy.   (ENG)

                                                                        690
Ototoxic effects due to antituberculous agents in humans with tuberculosis.
(JAP)

                              Ethambutol

                                                                        062
High frequency hearing loss and tinnitus due to parenteral, intramuscular,
administration of 1 g daily for first 60 days and then 1 g daily for 2 days
each week of antibiotic, capreomycin (SM), for 1 year in 7 of 89 humans,
range of ages, male and female, with pulmonary tuberculosis.
    (CT) No auditory system problems before treatment.
    (CT) Audiometry 1 time each month for duration of treatment.
    (AD) Previous resistance to primary antituberculous agents reported.
Simultaneous oral administration of 25 mg per kg daily for first 60 days and
then 15 mg per kg daily of antituberculous agent, ethambutol (SM), for 1 year
in 89 humans, range of ages, male and female, with pulmonary tuberculosis.
No reported ototoxic effects due to oral administration of 300 mg daily of
antituberculous agent, isoniazid (SM), for 1 year in 89 humans, range of
ages, male and female, with pulmonary tuberculosis.
    (AD) Previous resistance to isoniazid reported.   (ENG)

                                                                        076
Ototoxic effects due to parenteral, intramuscular, administration of 1 g
daily of antibiotic, capreomycin (SM), for 9 months in 4 of 65 humans, adult
and aged, range of 20 to 70 years age, male and female, with pulmonary tuberculosis.
Simultaneous administration of ethambutol (SM) in 65 humans, adult and aged,
range of 20 to 70 years age, male and female, with pulmonary tuberculosis.
Simultaneous administration of antibiotic, rifampicin (SM), in 65 humans,
adult and aged, range of 20 to 70 years age, male and female, with pulmonary
tuberculosis.   (ENG)

                                                                        137
Vestibular problems due to 1 g daily of antibiotic, capreomycin (SM), for
long period in 2 of 20 humans with tuberculosis.
Simultaneous administration of 25 mg per kg for first 60 days and then 15 mg
per kg of antituberculous agent, ethambutol (SM), in 20 humans with tuberculosis.
Simultaneous administration of 300 mg twice daily for several months and then
450 mg in 1 dose of antibiotic, rifampicin (SM), in 20 humans with tuberculosis.   (ENG)

                                                                        255
Slight hearing loss and vertigo due to parenteral, intramuscular, administration of 1 g every 24 hours of antibiotic, capreomycin (SM), for range of 5 to

12 months in 4 of 21 humans, adult, with pulmonary tuberculosis and without
pretreatment audiometric changes.
Slight and severe hearing loss and vertigo due to parenteral, intramuscular,
administration of 1 g every 24 hours of antibiotic, capreomycin (SM), for
range of 5 to 12 months in 12 of 40 humans, adult, with pulmonary tuberculosis and with pretreatment audiometric changes.
Simultaneous administration of antituberculous agent, ethambutol (SM), in all
of 61 humans, adult, with pulmonary tuberculosis.
   (AD) Treatment with capreomycin discontinued in 4 humans with severe
   ototoxic effects.
   (AD) Audiometry every 4 weeks during treatment.   (ENG)

                                                                       322
Cochleo-vestibulotoxic effects due to parenteral, intramuscular, administra-
tion of 1 g daily and then 1 g every other day of antibiotic, (SQ) capreomycin (SM), for 6 months in 3 of 36 humans, adult and aged, range of 20 to 80
years age, male and female, with pulmonary tuberculosis.
   (AD) Ototoxic effects confirmed by audiogram.
Simultaneous administration of 600 mg daily of antibiotic, (SQ) rifampicin
(SM), for 6 months in 36 humans, adult and aged, range of 20 to 80 years age,
male and female, with pulmonary tuberculosis.
Simultaneous administration of 25 mg per kg daily and then 15 mg per kg daily
of antituberculous agent, (SQ) ethambutol (SM), for 6 months in 36 humans,
adult and aged, range of 20 to 80 years age, male and female, with pulmonary
tuberculosis.
Cochleo-vestibulotoxic effects due to previous administration of (SQ) antibiotics, aminoglycoside, in 36 humans, adult and aged, range of 20 to 80
years age, male and female, with pulmonary tuberculosis.
   (AD) Therapy with antibiotics not satisfactory.   (FR)

                                                                       519
Dizziness but no other ototoxic effects due to parenteral, intramuscular,
administration of 1 g daily in single dose of antibiotic, capreomycin (SM),
for long period in 1 of 33 humans, adult and aged, 21 to over 70 years age,
with pulmonary tuberculosis of long duration and with previous treatment with
other drugs.
Simultaneous oral administration of 25 mg per kg during first 60 days and
then 15 mg per kg of antituberculous agent, ethambutol (SM), in 1 of 33
humans, adult and aged, 21 to over 70 years age, with pulmonary tuberculosis
of long duration and with previous treatment with other drugs.
Simultaneous administration of 600 mg of antibiotic, rifampicin (SM), in 1 of
33 humans, adult and aged, 21 to over 70 years age, with pulmonary tuberculosis of long duration and with previous treatment with other drugs.
   (AD) Otoneurology tests every 4 to 8 weeks.   (ENG)

                                                                       538
Dizziness due to parenteral administration of 1 g daily for first 8 weeks and
then 1 g twice weekly for 12 weeks of antibiotic, streptomycin (SM), for
total of 20 weeks in 5 of 77 humans with pulmonary tuberculosis.
Simultaneous administration of 300 mg daily in single dose of antituberculous
agent, isoniazid (SM), in 77 humans with pulmonary tuberculosis.
Simultaneous administration of 15 mg per kg daily of antituberculous agent,
ethambutol (SM), in 77 humans with pulmonary tuberculosis.
No reported ototoxic effects due to 600 mg daily in single dose of antibiotic, rifampicin, in 157 humans with pulmonary tuberculosis.   (ENG)

                                                                       544
Vertigo due to antituberculous agent, ethambutol, in 2 of 187 humans treated
for pulmonary tuberculosis.
   (AD) Literature review showed report of 2 cases of vertigo due to ethambutol.   (FR)

                                                                       557
Ototoxic effects due to previous administration of antibiotic, (SQ) strep-
tomycin, in 8 humans with pulmonary tuberculosis.
No ototoxic effects due to 1.0 g daily of antibiotic, (SQ) capreomycin (SM),
for long period in same 8 of 38 humans with pulmonary tuberculosis.
Simultaneous administration of antituberculous agent, (SQ) ethambutol (SM),

in 38 humans with pulmonary tuberculosis.   (ENG)

558
Severe hearing loss due to antibiotic, kanamycin (SM), in 1 human, adult, 44
years age, female, with basilar meningitis.
Simultaneous administration of 1 g daily of antituberculous agent, ethambutol
(SM), in 1 human, adult, 44 years age, female, with basilar meningitis.
(ENG)

564
Hearing loss due to antibiotic, kanamycin (SM), for long period in 3 of 4
humans, adult, range of ages, male and female, during retreatment for pulmonary tuberculosis.
Simultaneous administration of 25 mg per kg for 2 months and then 15 mg per
kg of antituberculous agent, ethambutol (SM), in 4 humans, adult, range of
ages, male and female, during retreatment for pulmonary tuberculosis.
   (CT) Treatment with ethambutol and 2 other antituberculous agents in
   humans, control group.   (ENG)

569
Slight hearing loss due to 1 g daily in single dose of antibiotic, capreomycin (SM), in 2 of 31 humans with chronic pulmonary tuberculosis.
   (AD) Audiometry and vestibular function tests every 4 weeks and then every
   6 weeks.
   (AD) Cessation of treatment with capreomycin in 4 cases to prevent hearing
   loss.
Simultaneous administration of 25 mg per kg daily in single dose for 12 weeks
and then 15 mg per kg of antituberculous agent, ethambutol (SM), in 31 humans
with chronic pulmonary tuberculosis.
Simultaneous oral administration of 1 other antituberculous agent (SM), in 31
humans with chronic pulmonary tuberculosis.   (ENG)

Isoniazid

041
Cochleo-vestibulotoxic effects due to unspecified method of administration of
300 mg daily of antituberculous agent, isoniazid, for 6 to 18 months in 12.9
percent of 70 humans with tuberculosis.
Cochleo-vestibulotoxic effects due to unspecified method of administration of
300 mg of antituberculous agent, isoniazid (SM), for 6 to 18 months in 22
percent of 297 humans with tuberculosis.
Cochleo-vestibulotoxic effects due to unspecified method of administration of
150 mg of antituberculous agent, thiacetazone (SM), for 6 to 18 months in 22
percent of 297 humans with tuberculosis.
Cochleo-vestibulotoxic effects due to unspecified method of administration of
antituberculous agent, isoniazid (SM), for 6 to 18 months in 82.9 percent of
82 humans with tuberculosis.
Cochleo-vestibulotoxic effects due to unspecified method of administration of
antituberculous agent, thiacetazone (SM), for 6 to 8 months in 82.9 percent
of 82 humans with tuberculosis.
Cochleo-vestibulotoxic effects due to unspecified method of administration of
1 g of antibiotic, streptomycin (SM), for 6 to 18 months in 82.9 percent of
82 humans with tuberculosis.
Cochleo-vestibulotoxic effects due to unspecified method of administration of
300 mg of antituberculous agent, isoniazid (SM), for 6 to 18 months in 25
percent of 20 humans with tuberculosis.
Cochleo-vestibulotoxic effects due to unspecified method of administration of
1 g of antibiotic, streptomycin (SM), for 6 to 18 months in 25 percent of 20
humans with tuberculosis.
   (AD) Potentiation by thiacetazone of cochleo-vestibulotoxic effects of
   streptomycin suggested.
   (AD) Audiometry and vestibular function tests every 2 weeks for 6 to 18
   months in total of 469 humans with tuberculosis.   (ENG)

062
High frequency hearing loss and tinnitus due to parenteral, intramuscular,
administration of 1 g daily for first 60 days and then 1 g daily for 2 days
each week of antibiotic, capreomycin (SM), for 1 year in 7 of 89 humans,

range of ages, male and female, with pulmonary tuberculosis.
    (CT) No auditory system problems before treatment.
    (CT) Audiometry 1 time each month for duration of treatment.
    (AD) Previous resistance to primary antituberculous agents reported.
Simultaneous oral administration of 25 mg per kg daily for first 60 days and
then 15 mg per kg daily of antituberculous agent, ethambutol (SM), for 1 year
in 89 humans, range of ages, male and female, with pulmonary tuberculosis.
No reported ototoxic effects due to oral administration of 300 mg daily of
antituberculous agent, isoniazid (SM), for 1 year in 89 humans, range of
ages, male and female, with pulmonary tuberculosis.
    (AD) Previous resistance to isoniazid reported.   (ENG)

                                                                      090
Tinnitus and vertigo due to unspecified method of administration of 0.75 g
daily of antibiotic, (SQ) streptomycin (SM), for 5 weeks in 1 human, adult,
38 years age, female, with pulmonary tuberculosis.
Simultaneous administration of antituberculous agent, (SQ) PAS (SM), in 1
human, adult, 38 years age, female, with pulmonary tuberculosis.
Simultaneous administration of antituberculous agent, (SQ) isoniazid (SM), in
1 human, adult, 38 years age, female, with pulmonary tuberculosis.
No reported ototoxic effects due to unspecified method of administration of
150 mg daily of antituberculous agent, (SQ) thiacetazone, for 11 months in 1
human, adult, 38 years age, female, with pulmonary tuberculosis.
    (AD) Hemolytic disease due to treatment with thiacetazone.   (ENG)

                                                                      095
Ototoxic effects due to unspecified method of administration of (SQ) 0.75 g
daily of antibiotic, streptomycin (SM), for (SQ) 3 months initial treatment
in 6 of 140 humans with tuberculosis.
Simultaneous unspecified method of administration of (SQ) 300 mg of antituberculous agent, isoniazid (SM), in 140 humans with tuberculosis.
Ototoxic effects due to unspecified method of administration of (SQ) 1 g 3
days a week of antibiotic, streptomycin (SM), for (SQ) 18 months following
initial treatment in 24 of 140 humans with tuberculosis.
Dizziness due to simultaneous unspecified method of administration of (SQ)
600 mg of antituberculous agent, isoniazid (SM), in unspecified number of
humans with tuberculosis and with other toxic effects due to isoniazid.
    (ENG)

                                                                      103
Cochleo-vestibulotoxic effects due to range of less than 50 g to 300 g of
antibiotic, streptomycin (SM) (streptomycin sulfate), for 6 to 8 months in
humans, adult, with tuberculous meningitis.
Simultaneous administration of antituberculous agent, PAS (SM), in humans,
adult, with tuberculous meningitis.
Simultaneous administration of antituberculous agent, isoniazid (SM), in
humans, adult, with tuberculous meningitis.
    (AD) Follow up study after average of 7 years.   (GER)

                                                                      136
Vestibular problems due to oral administration of 150 mg daily of antituberculous agent, thiacetazone (CB), for 12 months in 4 of 150 humans with pulmonary tuberculosis and without previous treatment.
Combined oral administration of 30 mg daily of antituberculous agent, isoniazid (CB), for 12 months in 150 humans with pulmonary tuberculosis and without
previous treatment.
No vestibular problems due to 10 g daily in 2 doses of antituberculous agent,
PAS (CB) (sodium PAS), for 12 months in 100 humans with pulmonary tuberculosis and without previous treatment.
Combined administration of 200 mg daily in 2 doses of antituberculous agent,
isoniazid (CB), for 12 months in 100 humans with pulmonary tuberculosis and
without previous treatment.
    (AD) Comparative study of effects of thiacetazone and PAS with isoniazid
    in treatment of tuberculosis.   (ENG)

                                                                      156
Sensorineural hearing loss due to unspecified method of administration of
high doses of antibiotic, streptomycin (SM), in 7 humans, infant and child,

Isoniazid 211

with tuberculous meningitis.
Simultaneous administration of unspecified doses of antituberculous agent, PAS (SM), in 7 humans, infant and child, with tuberculous meningitis.
Simultaneous administration of unspecified doses of antituberculous agent, isoniazid (SM), in 7 humans, infant and child, with tuberculous meningitis.
Sensorineural hearing loss due to unspecified method of administration of high doses of antibiotic, viomycin, in 7 humans, infant and child, with tuberculous meningitis.
(AD) Cochleotoxic effect due to antibiotic therapy or infection. (ENG)

227

Bilateral tinnitus and sudden deafness possibly due to cardiovascular agent, (SQ) hexadimethrine bromide, in 1 human, adult, 32 years age, female, with chronic nephritis and treated with hemodialysis.
Previous administration of antituberculous agent, (SQ) PAS, in 1 human, adult, 32 years age, female, with chronic nephritis and treated with hemodialysis.
Previous administration of antituberculous agent, (SQ) isoniazid, in 1 human, adult, 32 years age, female, with chronic nephritis and treated with hemodialysis.
Damage to Reissner's membrane, degeneration of organ of Corti, stria vascularis, and spiral ganglion, and slight changes in vestibular apparatus possibly due to cardiovascular agent, (SQ) hexadimethrine bromide, in 1 human, adult, 32 years age, female, with chronic nephritis and treated with hemodialysis.
Progressive severe sensorineural hearing loss possibly due to cardiovascular agent, hexadimethrine bromide, in 4 humans, adolescent and adult, 17 to 40 years age, with kidney disorders and treated with hemodialysis.
(AD) Association of hexadimethrine bromide with hearing loss only when used with hemodialysis in treatment of kidney disorder.
(AD) No hearing loss in group treated with hemodialysis without hexadimethrine bromide. (ENG)

332

No subjective hearing loss but objective hearing loss over 20 decibels and tinnitus due to parenteral, intramuscular, administration of 1 g daily for first 60 days and then 1 g twice a week of antibiotic, capreomycin (SM), for 6 months in 3 of 100 humans treated for pulmonary tuberculosis.
Hearing loss, tinnitus, or dizziness due to parenteral, intramuscular, administration of 1 g daily for first 60 days and then 1 g twice a week of antibiotic, streptomycin (SM), for 6 months in 8 of 99 humans treated for pulmonary tuberculosis.
Hearing loss over 20 decibels due to parenteral, intramuscular, administration of 1 g daily for first 60 days and then 1 g twice a week of antibiotic, streptomycin (SM), for 6 months in 3 of 99 humans treated for pulmonary tuberculosis.
Simultaneous oral administration of 0.3 g daily in 2 doses of antituberculous agent, isoniazid (SM), for 6 months in humans treated for pulmonary tuberculosis.
Simultaneous administration of 10 g daily in 3 doses of antituberculous agent, PAS (SM), for 6 months in humans treated for pulmonary tuberculosis.
(AD) Report on ototoxic effects of antibiotics used in initial treatment of tuberculosis.
High frequency hearing loss, tinnitus, or dizziness due to parenteral, intramuscular, administration of 1 g daily for first 60 days and then 1 g twice a week of antibiotic, capreomycin (SM), for 6 months in 6 of 66 humans retreated for pulmonary tuberculosis.
No subjective auditory system problems but objective hearing loss over 20 decibels due to parenteral, intramuscular, administration of 1 g 3 times a week of antibiotic, kanamycin (SM), for 6 months in 4 of 40 humans retreated for pulmonary tuberculosis.
No subjective auditory system problems but objective hearing loss over 20 decibels due to parenteral, intramuscular, administration of 1 g daily for first 60 days and then 1 g twice a week of antibiotic, streptomycin (SM), for 6 months in 1 of 13 humans retreated for pulmonary tuberculosis.
Simultaneous oral administration of 0.3 g daily in 2 doses of antituberculous agent, isoniazid (SM), for 6 months in humans retreated for pulmonary tuberculosis.

(AD) Report on ototoxic effects of antibiotics used in retreatment of
tuberculosis.
(CT) Audiometry, pretreatment and during treatment, 2 times a month in
first 2 months and then 1 time a month.
(AD) Comparative study of clinical use and cochleo-vestibulotoxic effects
of capreomycin and other antibiotics in treatment and retreatment of
pulmonary tuberculosis.   (ENG)

338

No loss of pinna reflex and no significant histological changes due to parenteral, subcutaneous, administration of 400 mg per kg daily in 1 injection of
antibiotic, dihydrostreptomycin, for 8 to 37 injections in 8 animals, guinea
pigs, young, 200 to 290 g weight.
Hearing loss after 64 injections and moderate damage to hair cells of cochlea
due to parenteral, subcutaneous, administration of 600 mg per kg daily, total
dose of 38.4 g, of antibiotic, dihydrostreptomycin, for 9 to 64 injections in
1 of 5 animals, guinea pigs, young, 200 to 290 g weight.
No loss of pinna reflex and no significant histological changes due to 50 mg
per kg daily of antibiotic, kanamycin, for 64 injections in 10 animals,
guinea pigs.
(CT) Test of pinna reflex, pretreatment and daily during treatment with
antibiotics.
(AD) Suggested relationship between degree of kanamycin damage to cochlea
and daily dose rather than total dose.   (ENG)

340

Vestibular problems due to 150 mg daily of antituberculous agent, thiaceta-
zone (SM), in 15 of 75 humans with pulmonary tuberculosis.
Vestibular problems due to 0.75 to 1 g daily of antibiotic, streptomycin (SM)
(streptomycin sulfate), in 15 of 75 humans with pulmonary tuberculosis.
Vestibular problems due to 300 mg daily of antituberculous agent, isoniazid
(SM), in 15 of 75 humans with pulmonary tuberculosis.
(AD) Vestibulotoxic effects confirmed by vestibular function tests.
(AD) Statistical analysis showed higher occurrence of vestibular problems
in humans with thiacetazone in drug regimen than without thiacetazone.
(SL)

343

No hearing loss but decr in vestibular function, asymptomatic except for
dizziness in 1 case, due to 1 g daily of antibiotic, capreomycin (SM), for 4
months or more in 4 of 25 humans, adolescent, adult, and aged, range of 17 to
67 years age, male and female, 80 to 160 lb weight, with pulmonary tuberculosis and with kidney disorder in 2 cases.
Transient dizziness with no objective decr in vestibular function due to 1 g
daily of antibiotic, capreomycin (SM), for 4 months or more in 3 of 25 humans, adolescent, adult, and aged, range of 17 to 67 years age, male and
female, 80 to 160 lb weight, with pulmonary tuberculosis.
Simultaneous administration of 300 mg daily of antituberculous agent, isoniazid (SM), for 4 months or more in 25 humans, adolescent, adult, and aged,
range of 17 to 67 years age, male and female, 80 to 160 lb weight, with
pulmonary tuberculosis.
(CT) Pure tone audiometry, caloric tests, and cupulometry, pretreatment
and during treatment with capreomycin.
(AD) Study of clinical use and cochleo-vestibulotoxic effects of capreomycin.
Hearing loss, asymptomatic in 1 case and symptomatic in 1 case, due to 1 g
daily of antibiotic, viomycin, in 2 of 75 humans with pulmonary tuberculosis.
Objective decr in vestibular function due to 1 g daily of antibiotic, viomycin, in 21 of 75 humans with pulmonary tuberculosis.
Hearing loss, asymptomatic, due to 1 g daily of antibiotic, streptomycin, in
2 of 61 humans with pulmonary tuberculosis.
Objective decr in vestibular function due to 1 g daily of antibiotic, streptomycin, in 8 of 61 humans with pulmonary tuberculosis.
(CT) Audiometry and vestibular function tests, pretreatment and during
treatment with viomycin or streptomycin.
(AD) Results of study on capreomycin comp w results of previous study on
viomycin and streptomycin.   (ENG)

354

Vestibular problems due to 1 g daily, total doses of 1 to 115 g before onset
of ototoxicity, of antibiotic, streptomycin (SM), for several days to 9
months in 56 of 364 humans, adolescent and adult, 16 to 64 years age, female,
with tuberculosis of genitourinary system.
No specified ototoxic effects due to range of doses of antituberculous agent,
PAS (SM), for several days to 9 months in 13 of 369 humans, adolescent and
adult, 16 to 64 years age, female, with tuberculosis of genitourinary system.
Simultaneous administration of antituberculous agent, isoniazid (SM), in 274
humans, adolescent and adult, 16 to 64 years age, female, with tuberculosis
of genitourinary system. (ENG)

367

Auditory system problems due to oral administration of 150 mg daily of antituberculous agent, thiacetazone (CB), for 12 weeks in 47 of 581 humans,
adolescent and adult, 15 years or over age, male and female, with pulmonary
tuberculosis.
Auditory system problems due to oral administration of 150 mg daily of antituberculous agent, thiacetazone (CB) (IB), for 12 weeks in 39 of 584 humans,
adolescent and adult, 15 years or over age, male and female, with pulmonary
tuberculosis, with administration of vitamins and antihistamine.
Combined oral administration of 300 mg daily of antituberculous agent, i-
soniazid (CB), for 12 weeks in humans, adolescent and adult, 15 years or over
age, male and female, with pulmonary tuberculosis.
   (AD) Study of effect of inhibitors on toxicity of drugs in 1 group with
   drug regimen of thiacetazone and isoniazid in combination.
Auditory system problems due to parenteral administration of 1 g daily of
antibiotic, streptomycin (SM), for 12 weeks in 227 of 689 humans, adolescent
and adult, 15 years or over age, male and female, with pulmonary tuberculosis.
Auditory system problems due to parenteral administration of 1 g daily of
antibiotic, streptomycin (SM) (IB), for 12 weeks in 218 of 707 humans, adolescent and adult, 15 years or over age, male and female, with pulmonary tuberculosis, with administration of vitamins and antihistamine.
Auditory system problems due to simultaneous oral administration of 150 mg
daily of antituberculous agent, thiacetazone (SM), for 12 weeks in humans,
adolescent and adult, 15 years or over age, male and female, with pulmonary
tuberculosis.
Simultaneous oral administration of 300 mg daily of antituberculous agent,
isoniazid (SM), for 12 weeks in humans, adolescent and adult, 15 years or
over age, male and female, with pulmonary tuberculosis.
   (AD) Study of effect of inhibitors on toxicity of drugs in 1 group with
   drug regimen of streptomycin, thiacetazone, and isoniazid.
Auditory system problems due to parenteral administration of 1 g daily of
antibiotic, streptomycin (SM), for 12 weeks in 109 of 711 humans, adolescent
and adult, 15 years or over age, male and female, with pulmonary tuberculosis.
Auditory system problems due to parenteral administration of 1 g daily of
antibiotic, streptomycin (SM) (IB), for 12 weeks in 111 of 696 humans, adolescent and adult, 15 years or over age, male and female, with pulmonary tuberculosis, with administration of vitamins and antihistamine.
Simultaneous oral administration of 300 mg daily of antituberculous agent,
isoniazid (SM), for 12 weeks in humans, adolescent and adult, 15 years or
over age, male and female, with pulmonary tuberculosis.
   (AD) Study of effect of inhibitors on toxicity of drugs in 1 group with
   drug regimen of streptomycin and isoniazid.
   (AD) Study of effectiveness of inhibitors in prevention of toxic effects
   of thiacetazone and streptomycin.
   (AD) Study suggested that vitamins and antihistamine not effective in
   prevention of toxicity. (ENG)

377

Lesion of vestibular apparatus due to about 22 g of antibiotic, streptomycin
(SM), in human with pulmonary tuberculosis.
   (AD) Lesion of vestibular apparatus confirmed by vestibular function test.
Simultaneous administration of 185 g of antituberculous agent, PAS (SM), in
human with pulmonary tuberculosis.
Simultaneous administration of 16.5 g of antituberculous agent, isoniazid

(SM), in human with pulmonary tuberculosis.   (POL)

433

Dizziness due to 1 g daily of antibiotic, streptomycin (SM), for 6 months in
32 percent of 114 humans with pulmonary tuberculosis.
Dizziness due to 300 mg daily of antituberculous agent, isoniazid (SM), for 6
months with streptomycin and then 6 months alone in 32 percent of 114 humans
with pulmonary tuberculosis.
   (AD) Regimen of simultaneous administration of streptomycin and isoniazid
   for 6 months followed by administration of isoniazid only for 6 months.
Dizziness due to 1 g daily of antibiotic, streptomycin (SM), for 6 months in
54 percent of 94 humans with pulmonary tuberculosis.
Dizziness due to 150 mg daily of antituberculous agent, thiacetazone (SM),
for 6 months with streptomycin and isoniazid and then 6 months with isoniazid
in 54 percent of 94 humans with pulmonary tuberculosis.
Dizziness due to 300 mg daily of antituberculous agent, isoniazid (SM), for 6
months with streptomycin and thiacetazone and then 6 months with thiacetazone
in 54 percent of 94 humans with pulmonary tuberculosis.
   (AD) Regimen of simultaneous administration of streptomycin, thiacetazone,
   and isoniazid for 6 months followed by administration of thiacetazone and
   isoniazid for 6 months.
Dizziness due to 150 mg daily of antituberculous agent, thiacetazone (SM),
for 1 year in 13 percent of 78 humans with pulmonary tuberculosis.
Dizziness due to 300 mg daily of antituberculous agent, isoniazid (SM), for 1
year in 13 percent of 78 humans with pulmonary tuberculosis.
   (AD) Regimen of simultaneous administration of thiacetazone and isoniazid
   for 1 year.
   (AD) Study of role of drug regimens with thiacetazone in treatment of
   pulmonary tuberculosis.   (ENG)

447

Dizziness and tinnitus within first 14 weeks due to 150 mg daily in 2 divided
doses of antituberculous agent, thiacetazone (SM), for 26 weeks in 30 of 410
humans, adolescent and adult, 15 to over 55 years age, 30 to over 50 kg
weight, with tuberculosis.
No ototoxic effects due to 300 mg daily in 2 divided doses of antituberculous
agent, isoniazid (SM), for 26 weeks in 30 of 410 humans, adolescent and
adult, 15 to over 55 years age, 30 to over 50 kg weight, with tuberculosis.
   (AD) Study of toxicity of thiacetazone in treatment of tuberculosis.
   (ENG)

481

Damage to vestibular apparatus due to 1 g daily or twice daily of antibiotic,
streptomycin (SM), for maximum of 3 months in 9 of 108 humans, range of 2 to
86 years age, male and female, with pulmonary tuberculosis.
Simultaneous administration of 12 g daily of antituberculous agent, PAS (SM),
for 12 to 18 months in 108 humans, range of 2 to 86 years age, male and
female, with pulmonary tuberculosis.
Simultaneous administration of 300 mg daily of antituberculous agent, isoniazid (SM), for 12 to 18 months in 108 humans, range of 2 to 86 years age, male
and female, with pulmonary tuberculosis.   (ENG)

535

Dizziness due to parenteral administration of 0.75 g on 6 days a week for 3
months and then 1 g on 2 days a week with intervals of 2 to 3 days for 15
months of antibiotic, streptomycin (SM), for total of 18 months in 2 of 80
humans, adult, range of ages, female and male, 16 to 92 kg weight, with
pulmonary tuberculosis.
Dizziness due to 300 mg on 6 days a week for 3 months and then 600 mg on 2
days a week with intervals of 2 to 3 days for 15 months of antituberculous
agent, isoniazid (SM), for total of 18 months in 1 of 80 humans, adult, range
of ages, female and male, 16 to 92 kg weight, with pulmonary tuberculosis.
Simultaneous administration of 12 g on 6 days a week of antituberculous
agent, PAS (SM), for 3 months in 80 humans, adult, range of ages, female and
male, 16 to 92 kg weight, with pulmonary tuberculosis.   (ENG)

536

Damage to eighth cranial nerve and vertigo due to 1 g or 0.75 g daily of

antibiotic, streptomycin (SM), for about 3 months usually in less than 55 of
181 humans, adult and aged, primarily 50 years or over age, male and female,
with pulmonary tuberculosis.
Simultaneous administration of 300 mg daily of antituberculous agent, isoniazid (SM), for 18 months to 2 years usually in 181 humans, adult and aged,
primarily 50 years or over age, male and female, with pulmonary tuberculosis.
Simultaneous administration of 12 g daily of antituberculous agent, PAS (SM),
for 18 months to 2 years usually in 181 humans, adult and aged, primarily 50
years or over age, male and female, with pulmonary tuberculosis.   (ENG)

                                                                                537
Dizziness due to oral administration in tablet of 150 mg daily of antituberculous agent, thiacetazone (CB) (SM), in 1 of 147 humans, African, adolescent
and adult, 15 years or more age, with pulmonary tuberculosis and without
previous treatment.
Dizziness due to oral administration in tablet of 300 mg daily of antituberculous agent, isoniazid (CB) (SM), in 1 of 147 humans, African, adolescent
and adult, 15 years or more age, with pulmonary tuberculosis and without
previous treatment.
   (AD) Dizziness in 1 patient due to combined treatment with thiacetazone
   and isoniazid only.
Dizziness due to parenteral, intramuscular, administration of 1 g daily of
antibiotic, streptomycin (SM) (streptomycin sulfate), for first 2 weeks in 1
of 161 humans, African, adolescent and adult, 15 years or more age, with
pulmonary tuberculosis and without previous treatment.
   (AD) Dizziness in 1 patient due to simultaneous treatment with thiacetazone and isoniazid in 1 tablet and intramuscular streptomycin for 2 weeks.
Dizziness due to parenteral, intramuscular, administration of 1 g daily of
antibiotic, streptomycin (SM) (streptomycin sulfate), for first 8 weeks in 10
of 162 humans, African, adolescent and adult, 15 years or more age, with
pulmonary tuberculosis and without previous treatment.
   (AD) Dizziness in 10 patients due to simultaneous treatment with thiacetazone and isoniazid in 1 tablet and intramuscular streptomycin for 8 weeks.
   (AD) Study showed vestibulotoxic effects in total of 12 of 818 patients
   treated for pulmonary tuberculosis.   (ENG)

                                                                                538
Dizziness due to parenteral administration of 1 g daily for first 8 weeks and
then 1 g twice weekly for 12 weeks of antibiotic, streptomycin (SM), for
total of 20 weeks in 5 of 77 humans with pulmonary tuberculosis.
Simultaneous administration of 300 mg daily in single dose of antituberculous
agent, isoniazid (SM), in 77 humans with pulmonary tuberculosis.
Simultaneous administration of 15 mg per kg daily of antituberculous agent,
ethambutol (SM), in 77 humans with pulmonary tuberculosis.
No reported ototoxic effects due to 600 mg daily in single dose of antibiotic, rifampicin, in 157 humans with pulmonary tuberculosis.   (ENG)

                                                                                593
Vestibular problems due to 1 g in 24 hours of antibiotic, (SQ) streptomycin
(SM), in 1 human, adult, 32 years age, female, with tuberculosis.
Vestibular problems due to 450 mg of antituberculous agent, (SQ) isoniazid
(SM), in 1 human, adult, 32 years age, female, with tuberculosis.
Vestibular problems due to oral administration in tablets of 0.10 g of anti-
convulsant, (SQ) diphenylhydantoin, in 1 human, adult, 32 years age, female,
with tuberculosis.
Vestibular problems due to oral administration in tablets of 3 tablets of
0.10 g each daily of anticonvulsant, (SQ) diphenylhydantoin (SM), in 1 human,
adult, 49 years age, female, with tuberculosis.
Vestibular problems due to 300 mg of antituberculous agent, (SQ) isoniazid
(SM), in 1 human, adult, 49 years age, female, with tuberculosis.
Simultaneous administration of 500 cm of antituberculous agent, (SQ) PAS
(SM), in 1 human, adult, 49 years age, female, with tuberculosis.
   (AD) Report of vestibulotoxic effects in 2 patients due to diphenylhydan-
   toin with isoniazid or streptomycin.   (FR)

                                                                                615
Tinnitus, hearing loss, vertigo, and dizziness due to oral administration in
tablet of 150 mg daily of antituberculous agent, thiacetazone (CB) (SM), in

some of 1002 humans with tuberculosis.
Tinnitus, hearing loss, vertigo, and dizziness due to oral administration in
tablet of 300 mg daily of antituberculous agent, isoniazid (CB) (SM), in some
of 1002 humans with tuberculosis.
Tinnitus, hearing loss, vertigo, and dizziness due to parenteral administration of 1 g daily of antibiotic, streptomycin (SM), in some of 1002 humans
with tuberculosis.
    (AD) Reported 21.4 percent incidence of toxic effects in regimen of thia-
    cetazone, isoniazid, and streptomycin.
    (AD) Suggested that effects of streptomycin potentiated by thiacetazone.
Unspecified ototoxic effects due to oral administration of 300 mg daily of
antituberculous agent, isoniazid (SM), in 987 humans with tuberculosis.
Unspecified ototoxic effects due to parenteral administration of 1 g daily of
antibiotic, streptomycin (SM), in 987 humans with tuberculosis.
    (AD) Reported 7.8 percent incidence of toxic effects in regimen of isonia-
    zid and streptomycin without thiacetazone.   (ENG)

619

Tinnitus in 7 cases and vertigo in 2 cases due to 1 g twice weekly of antibiotic, streptomycin (SM), in total of 9 of 190 humans, Japanese, adult, 20
to 61 years age, male and female, with pulmonary tuberculosis and without
previous chemotherapy.
Tinnitus in 7 cases and vertigo in 2 cases due to about 7.5 mg per kg in
single dose daily of antituberculous agent, isoniazid (SM), in total of 9 of
190 humans, Japanese, adult, 20 to 61 years age, male and female, with pulmonary tuberculosis and without previous chemotherapy.
Simultaneous administration of 10 g daily in 3 divided doses of antituberculous agent, PAS (SM), in 190 humans, Japanese, adult, 20 to 61 years age,
male and female, with pulmonary tuberculosis and without previous chemotherapy.
Tinnitus in 3 cases and hearing loss in 2 cases due to 1 g twice weekly of
antibiotic, streptomycin (SM), in total of 5 of 160 humans, Japanese, adult,
20 to 61 years age, male and female, with pulmonary tuberculosis and without
previous chemotherapy.
Tinnitus in 3 cases and hearing loss in 2 cases due to 18 mg per kg in 3
divided doses of antituberculous agent, isoniazid (SM), in total of 5 of 160
humans, Japanese, adult, 20 to 61 years age, male and female, with pulmonary
tuberculosis and without previous chemotherapy.
Simultaneous administration of 10 g daily in 3 divided doses of antituberculous agent, PAS (SM), in 160 humans, Japanese, adult, 20 to 61 years age,
male and female, with pulmonary tuberculosis and without previous chemotherapy.
    (AD) Similar ototoxic effects in both drug regimens.   (ENG)

621

Primarily vestibular problems due to antibiotic, streptomycin, in humans.
Primarily hearing loss but also vestibular problems due to antibiotic, dihy-
drostreptomycin, in humans.
Primarily hearing loss but also vestibular problems due to antibiotic, kana-
mycin, in humans.
Primarily hearing loss but also vestibular problems due to antibiotic, neomy-
cin, in humans.
Primarily hearing loss but also vestibular problems due to antibiotic, genta-
micin, in humans.
Vertigo and ataxia due to antituberculous agent, isoniazid, in humans.
Hearing loss due to salicylate, aspirin, in humans.
Hearing loss and vertigo due to antimalarial, quinine, in humans.
Nystagmus due to barbiturates in humans.
Vestibular problems due to analgesic, morphine, in humans.
Nystagmus due to sedative, alcohol, in humans.
Nystagmus and hearing loss due to chemical agent, carbon monoxide, in humans.
Ototoxic effects due to antineoplastic, nitrogen mustard, in humans.
Ototoxic effects due to chemical agent, aniline, in humans.
Ototoxic effects due to chemical agent, tobacco, in humans.
Nystagmus due to chemical agent, nicotine, in humans.
Vestibular problems due to anticonvulsants in humans.
Vestibular problems due to anesthetics in humans.
Vestibular problems due to diuretics in humans.

(AD) Inclusion of comprehensive list of ototoxic agents.   (SP)

700

Dizziness or vertigo, during first 3 months in 7 cases and after 3 to 6
months in 5 cases, due to 1 g daily for first 3 months, and then 1 g 3 times
a week for second 3 months in patients 50 years age or less, or 1 g 3 times a
week for 6 months in patients over 50 years age, of antibiotic, streptomycin
(SM) (streptomycin sulfate), for 6 months in 12 (20 percent) of 59 humans,
adult and aged, 55 years or more age in most cases, male, with chronic pulmonary tuberculosis and pneumoconiosis.
    (AD) Reported 20 percent incidence of streptomycin ototoxicity in first
    year of therapy.
Incr hearing loss reported after 6 months due to 1 g daily for first 3
months, and then 1 g 3 times a week for second 3 months in patients 50 years
age or less, or 1 g 3 times a week for 6 months in patients over 50 years
age, of antibiotic, streptomycin (SM) (streptomycin sulfate), for 6 months in
1 of 59 humans, adult and aged, 55 years or more age in most cases, male,
with chronic pulmonary tuberculosis and pneumoconiosis and with previous
hearing loss.
    (AD) Reported 1 case of hearing loss due to streptomycin in first year of
    therapy.
Dizziness and tinnitus after 14 months due to 1 g daily for first 3 months,
and then 1 g 3 times a week for second 3 months in patients 50 years age or
less, or 1 g 3 times a week for 6 months in patients over 50 years age, of
antibiotic, streptomycin (SM) (streptomycin sulfate), for 6 months in 1 of 31
humans, male, with chronic pulmonary tuberculosis and pneumoconiosis.
    (AD) Reported 1 case with ototoxic effects within 18 months of therapy.
Simultaneous oral administration in cachets of 333 mg daily of antituberculous agent, isoniazid (SM) (CB), for 18 months or more in 59 humans, male,
with chronic pulmonary tuberculosis and pneumoconiosis.
Simultaneous oral administration in cachets of 15 g daily of antituberculous
agent, PAS (SM) (CB) (sodium PAS), for 18 months or more in 59 humans, male,
with chronic pulmonary tuberculosis and pneumoconiosis.   (ENG)

PAS

090

Tinnitus and vertigo due to unspecified method of administration of 0.75 g
daily of antibiotic, (SQ) streptomycin (SM), for 5 weeks in 1 human, adult,
38 years age, female, with pulmonary tuberculosis.
Simultaneous administration of antituberculous agent, (SQ) PAS (SM), in 1
human, adult, 38 years age, female, with pulmonary tuberculosis.
Simultaneous administration of antituberculous agent, (SQ) isoniazid (SM), in
1 human, adult, 38 years age, female, with pulmonary tuberculosis.
No reported ototoxic effects due to unspecified method of administration of
150 mg daily of antituberculous agent, (SQ) thiacetazone, for 11 months in 1
human, adult, 38 years age, female, with pulmonary tuberculosis.
    (AD) Hemolytic disease due to treatment with thiacetazone.   (ENG)

103

Cochleo-vestibulotoxic effects due to range of less than 50 g to 300 g of
antibiotic, streptomycin (SM) (streptomycin sulfate), for 6 to 8 months in
humans, adult, with tuberculous meningitis.
Simultaneous administration of antituberculous agent, PAS (SM), in humans,
adult, with tuberculous meningitis.
Simultaneous administration of antituberculous agent, isoniazid (SM), in
humans, adult, with tuberculous meningitis.
    (AD) Follow up study after average of 7 years.   (GER)

136

Vestibular problems due to oral administration of 150 mg daily of antituberculous agent, thiacetazone (CB), for 12 months in 4 of 150 humans with pulmonary tuberculosis and without previous treatment.
Combined oral administration of 30 mg daily of antituberculous agent, isoniazid (CB), for 12 months in 150 humans with pulmonary tuberculosis and without
previous treatment.
No vestibular problems due to 10 g daily in 2 doses of antituberculous agent,
PAS (CB) (sodium PAS), for 12 months in 100 humans with pulmonary tuberculo-

sis and without previous treatment.
Combined administration of 200 mg daily in 2 doses of antituberculous agent,
isoniazid (CB), for 12 months in 100 humans with pulmonary tuberculosis and
without previous treatment.
    (AD) Comparative study of effects of thiacetazone and PAS with isoniazid
    in treatment of tuberculosis.   (ENG)

                                                                          156
Sensorineural hearing loss due to unspecified method of administration of
high doses of antibiotic, streptomycin (SM), in 7 humans, infant and child,
with tuberculous meningitis.
Simultaneous administration of unspecified doses of antituberculous agent,
PAS (SM), in 7 humans, infant and child, with tuberculous meningitis.
Simultaneous administration of unspecified doses of antituberculous agent,
isoniazid (SM), in 7 humans, infant and child, with tuberculous meningitis.
Sensorineural hearing loss due to unspecified method of administration of
high doses of antibiotic, viomycin, in 7 humans, infant and child, with
tuberculous meningitis.
    (AD) Cochleotoxic effect due to antibiotic therapy or infection.   (ENG)

                                                                          198
Severe vertigo due to parenteral, intramuscular, administration of 1 g daily
in single dose of antibiotic, streptomycin (SM) (streptomycin sulfate), for 6
months in 2 of 41 humans, 108.2 lb average weight, with pulmonary tuberculosis and with previous streptomycin therapy in some.
Simultaneous oral administration of 15 g daily in single dose of antituberc-
lous agent, PAS (SM) (sodium PAS), for 6 months in 2 of 41 humans, 108.2 lb
average weight, with pulmonary tuberculosis and with previous streptomycin
therapy in some.
No vestibulotoxic effects due to parenteral, intramuscular, administration of
1 g daily in single dose of antibiotic, streptomycin (SM) (streptomycin
sulfate), for 6 months in 41 humans, 113.5 lb average weight, with pulmonary
tuberculosis and with previous streptomycin therapy in some.
Simultaneous oral administration of 15 g daily in 2 doses of antituberculous
agent, PAS (SM) (sodium PAS), for 6 months in 41 humans, 113.5 lb average
weight, with pulmonary tuberculosis and with previous streptomycin therapy in
some.
    (AD) Study of retreatment of pulmonary tuberculosis in humans with no
    response to previous chemotherapy.   (ENG)

                                                                          227
Bilateral tinnitus and sudden deafness possibly due to cardiovascular agent,
(SQ) hexadimethrine bromide, in 1 human, adult, 32 years age, female, with
chronic nephritis and treated with hemodialysis.
Previous administration of antituberculous agent, (SQ) PAS, in 1 human,
adult, 32 years age, female, with chronic nephritis and treated with hemodialysis.
Previous administration of antituberculous agent, (SQ) isoniazid, in 1 human,
adult, 32 years age, female, with chronic nephritis and treated with hemodialysis.
Damage to Reissner's membrane, degeneration of organ of Corti, stria vascularis, and spiral ganglion, and slight changes in vestibular apparatus possibly due to cardiovascular agent, (SQ) hexadimethrine bromide, in 1 human,
adult, 32 years age, female, with chronic nephritis and treated with hemodialysis.
Progressive severe sensorineural hearing loss possibly due to cardiovascular
agent, hexadimethrine bromide, in 4 humans, adolescent and adult, 17 to 40
years age, with kidney disorders and treated with hemodialysis.
    (AD) Association of hexadimethrine bromide with hearing loss only when
    used with hemodialysis in treatment of kidney disorder.
    (AD) No hearing loss in group treated with hemodialysis without hexadime-
    thrine bromide.   (ENG)

                                                                          290
Vestibular problems, sensorineural hearing loss, and tinnitus due to total
doses of 12 to 63 g of antibiotic, streptomycin, in 24 humans with tuberculosis.
    (AD) Subjects tested after streptomycin intoxication with audiology and

cupulometry.
(AD) Individual responses to streptomycin observed.
Changes in cupulometric curves for postrotatory nystagmus, showing changes in
vestibular apparatus, due to 0.5 g daily, total doses of 30 to 100 g, of
antibiotic, streptomycin (SM) (streptomycin sulfate), in 23 humans with
various infections.
Simultaneous administration of 0.5 g of antibiotic, dihydrostreptomycin (SM),
in 23 humans with various infections.
Simultaneous administration of antituberculous agent, PAS (SM), in 23 humans
with various infections.
(CT) Pretreatment vestibular function normal.
(CT) Subjects tested with audiology and cupulometry before and during
treatment with streptomycin.
(AD) Hearing loss in 1 subject in group with cupulometry during treatment
but in 5 subjects in other group with cupulometry only after treatment.
(AD) Suggested use of cupulometry for possible prevention of streptomycin
intoxication. (ENG)

                                                                   323
Progressive severe bilateral sensorineural hearing loss and vestibular problems due to parenteral administration of 1 g twice weekly of antibiotic, (SQ)
viomycin (viomycin pantothenate), for total of 10 weeks in 1 human, adult, 59
years age, female, with pulmonary tuberculosis and kidney disorder.
(AD) Cochleo-vestibulotoxic effects confirmed by audiometry at different
periods during and after treatment and by caloric test.
Previous administration of antibiotic, (SQ) chloramphenicol, in 1 human,
adult, 59 years age, female, for infection before diagnosis of tuberculosis.
Possible but not reported auditory system problems due to previous parenteral
administration of 0.5 g twice daily of antibiotic, (SQ) streptomycin, for 1
week in 1 human, adult, 59 years age, female, for infection before diagnosis
of tuberculosis.
(AD) Suggested that possible previous ototoxic effects of streptomycin
potentiated by viomycin (viomycin pantothenate).
Previous administration of antituberculous agent, (SQ) PAS, in 1 human,
adult, 59 years age, female, with pulmonary tuberculosis and kidney disorder.
(ENG)

                                                                   326
Hearing loss due to parenteral, intramuscular, administration of 1.0 g daily
of antibiotic, capreomycin (SM), for less than 6 months in 2 of 53 humans
with cavitary pulmonary tuberculosis and no previous chemotherapy.
No reported ototoxic effects due to oral administration of 12.0 g daily in 3
divided doses of antituberculous agent, PAS (SM), for up to 6 months in 53
humans with cavitary pulmonary tuberculosis and no previous chemotherapy.
(ENG)

                                                                   327
More severe hearing loss due to parenteral, intramuscular, administration of
1 g daily of antibiotic, (SQ) capreomycin (SM), for long period in 1 of 32
humans, male, with pulmonary tuberculosis and with previous antibiotic therapy.
Hearing loss before capreomycin treatment due to (SQ) antibiotics, aminoglycoside, in 1 of 32 humans, male, with pulmonary tuberculosis.
(AD) Hearing loss confirmed by audiogram.
Tinnitus due to parenteral, intramuscular, administration of 1 g daily of
antibiotic, (SQ) capreomycin (SM), for long period in 3 of 32 humans with
pulmonary tuberculosis.
Simultaneous administration of other (SQ) antituberculous agents (SM), in 32
humans, adult and aged, 20 to 69 years age, male and female, with pulmonary
tuberculosis.
Previous administration of antituberculous agent, (SQ) PAS, in 32 humans,
adult and aged, 20 to 69 years age, male and female, with pulmonary tubercu
losis. (ENG)

                                                                   332
No subjective hearing loss but objective hearing loss over 20 decibels and
tinnitus due to parenteral, intramuscular, administration of 1 g daily for
first 60 days and then 1 g twice a week of antibiotic, capreomycin (SM), for

6 months in 3 of 100 humans treated for pulmonary tuberculosis.
Hearing loss, tinnitus, or dizziness due to parenteral, intramuscular, administration of 1 g daily for first 60 days and then 1 g twice a week of
antibiotic, streptomycin (SM), for 6 months in 8 of 99 humans treated for
pulmonary tuberculosis.
Hearing loss over 20 decibels due to parenteral, intramuscular, administration of 1 g daily for first 60 days and then 1 g twice a week of antibiotic,
streptomycin (SM), for 6 months in 3 of 99 humans treated for pulmonary
tuberculosis.
Simultaneous oral administration of 0.3 g daily in 2 doses of antituberculous
agent, isoniazid (SM), for 6 months in humans treated for pulmonary tuberculosis.
Simultaneous administration of 10 g daily in 3 doses of antituberculous
agent, PAS (SM), for 6 months in humans treated for pulmonary tuberculosis.
    (AD) Report on ototoxic effects of antibiotics used in initial treatment
    of tuberculosis.
High frequency hearing loss, tinnitus, or dizziness due to parenteral, intramuscular, administration of 1 g daily for first 60 days and then 1 g twice a
week of antibiotic, capreomycin (SM), for 6 months in 6 of 66 humans retreated for pulmonary tuberculosis.
No subjective auditory system problems but objective hearing loss over 20
decibels due to parenteral, intramuscular, administration of 1 g 3 times a
week of antibiotic, kanamycin (SM), for 6 months in 4 of 40 humans retreated
for pulmonary tuberculosis.
No subjective auditory system problems but objective hearing loss over 20
decibels due to parenteral, intramuscular, administration of 1 g daily for
first 60 days and then 1 g twice a week of antibiotic, streptomycin (SM), for
6 months in 1 of 13 humans retreated for pulmonary tuberculosis.
Simultaneous oral administration of 0.3 g daily in 2 doses of antituberculous
agent, isoniazid (SM), for 6 months in humans retreated for pulmonary tuberculosis.
    (AD) Report on ototoxic effects of antibiotics used in retreatment of
    tuberculosis.
    (CT) Audiometry, pretreatment and during treatment, 2 times a month in
    first 2 months and then 1 time a month.
    (AD) Comparative study of clinical use and cochleo-vestibulotoxic effects
    of capreomycin and other antibiotics in treatment and retreatment of
    pulmonary tuberculosis. (ENG)

                                                                         354
Vestibular problems due to 1 g daily, total doses of 1 to 115 g before onset
of ototoxicity, of antibiotic, streptomycin (SM), for several days to 9
months in 56 of 364 humans, adolescent and adult, 16 to 64 years age, female,
with tuberculosis of genitourinary system.
No specified ototoxic effects due to range of doses of antituberculous agent,
PAS (SM), for several days to 9 months in 13 of 369 humans, adolescent and
adult, 16 to 64 years age, female, with tuberculosis of genitourinary system.
Simultaneous administration of antituberculous agent, isoniazid (SM), in 274
humans, adolescent and adult, 16 to 64 years age, female, with tuberculosis
of genitourinary system. (ENG)

                                                                         377
Lesion of vestibular apparatus due to about 22 g of antibiotic, streptomycin
(SM), in human with pulmonary tuberculosis.
    (AD) Lesion of vestibular apparatus confirmed by vestibular function test.
Simultaneous administration of 185 g of antituberculous agent, PAS (SM), in
human with pulmonary tuberculosis.
Simultaneous administration of 16.5 g of antituberculous agent, isoniazid
(SM), in human with pulmonary tuberculosis. (POL)

                                                                         446
Vestibular problems only in 5 and dizziness, tinnitus, and hearing loss in 1
due to parenteral, intramuscular, administration of 1 g daily in single
injection of antibiotic, streptomycin (SM) (streptomycin sulfate), for 6
months only in 6 (6 percent) of 65 humans, Negro, adolescent and adult, 15 to
over 55 years age, male and female, 80 to over 140 lb weight, for retreatment
of pulmonary tuberculosis.
Simultaneous oral administration of 15 g of antituberculous agent, PAS (SM)

(sodium PAS), for 1 year in 65 humans, Negro, adolescent and adult, 15 to
over 55 years age, male and female, 80 to over 140 lb weight, for retreatment
of pulmonary tuberculosis.
   (AD) Study of value of regimen of streptomycin, PAS, and pyrazinamide in
   retreatment of pulmonary tuberculosis. (ENG)

481

Damage to vestibular apparatus due to 1 g daily or twice daily of antibiotic,
streptomycin (SM), for maximum of 3 months in 9 of 108 humans, range of 2 to
86 years age, male and female, with pulmonary tuberculosis.
Simultaneous administration of 12 g daily of antituberculous agent, PAS (SM),
for 12 to 18 months in 108 humans, range of 2 to 86 years age, male and
female, with pulmonary tuberculosis.
Simultaneous administration of 300 mg daily of antituberculous agent, isoniazid (SM), for 12 to 18 months in 108 humans, range of 2 to 86 years age, male
and female, with pulmonary tuberculosis. (ENG)

535

Dizziness due to parenteral administration of 0.75 g on 6 days a week for 3
months and then 1 g on 2 days a week with intervals of 2 to 3 days for 15
months of antibiotic, streptomycin (SM), for total of 18 months in 2 of 80
humans, adult, range of ages, female and male, 16 to 92 kg weight, with
pulmonary tuberculosis.
Dizziness due to 300 mg on 6 days a week for 3 months and then 600 mg on 2
days a week with intervals of 2 to 3 days for 15 months of antituberculous
agent, isoniazid (SM), for total of 18 months in 1 of 80 humans, adult, range
of ages, female and male, 16 to 92 kg weight, with pulmonary tuberculosis.
Simultaneous administration of 12 g on 6 days a week of antituberculous
agent, PAS (SM), for 3 months in 80 humans, adult, range of ages, female and
male, 16 to 92 kg weight, with pulmonary tuberculosis. (ENG)

536

Damage to eighth cranial nerve and vertigo due to 1 g or 0.75 g daily of
antibiotic, streptomycin (SM), for about 3 months usually in less than 55 of
181 humans, adult and aged, primarily 50 years or over age, male and female,
with pulmonary tuberculosis.
Simultaneous administration of 300 mg daily of antituberculous agent, isoniazid (SM), for 18 months to 2 years usually in 181 humans, adult and aged,
primarily 50 years or over age, male and female, with pulmonary tuberculosis.
Simultaneous administration of 12 g daily of antituberculous agent, PAS (SM),
for 18 months to 2 years usually in 181 humans, adult and aged, primarily 50
years or over age, male and female, with pulmonary tuberculosis. (ENG)

593

Vestibular problems due to 1 g in 24 hours of antibiotic, (SQ) streptomycin
(SM), in 1 human, adult, 32 years age, female, with tuberculosis.
Vestibular problems due to 450 mg of antituberculous agent, (SQ) isoniazid
(SM), in 1 human, adult, 32 years age, female, with tuberculosis.
Vestibular problems due to oral administration in tablets of 0.10 g of anti-
convulsant, (SQ) diphenylhydantoin, in 1 human, adult, 32 years age, female,
with tuberculosis.
Vestibular problems due to oral administration in tablets of 3 tablets of
0.10 g each daily of anticonvulsant, (SQ) diphenylhydantoin (SM), in 1 human,
adult, 49 years age, female, with tuberculosis.
Vestibular problems due to 300 mg of antituberculous agent, (SQ) isoniazid
(SM), in 1 human, adult, 49 years age, female, with tuberculosis.
Simultaneous administration of 500 cm of antituberculous agent, (SQ) PAS
(SM), in 1 human, adult, 49 years age, female, with tuberculosis.
   (AD) Report of vestibulotoxic effects in 2 patients due to diphenylhydan-
   toin with isoniazid or streptomycin. (FR)

619

Tinnitus in 7 cases and vertigo in 2 cases due to 1 g twice weekly of antibiotic, streptomycin (SM), in total of 9 of 190 humans, Japanese, adult, 20
to 61 years age, male and female, with pulmonary tuberculosis and without
previous chemotherapy.
Tinnitus in 7 cases and vertigo in 2 cases due to about 7.5 mg per kg in
single dose daily of antituberculous agent, isoniazid (SM), in total of 9 of

190 humans, Japanese, adult, 20 to 61 years age, male and female, with pulmonary tuberculosis and without previous chemotherapy.
Simultaneous administration of 10 g daily in 3 divided doses of antituberculous agent, PAS (SM), in 190 humans, Japanese, adult, 20 to 61 years age,
male and female, with pulmonary tuberculosis and without previous chemotherapy.
Tinnitus in 3 cases and hearing loss in 2 cases due to 1 g twice weekly of
antibiotic, streptomycin (SM), in total of 5 of 160 humans, Japanese, adult,
20 to 61 years age, male and female, with pulmonary tuberculosis and without
previous chemotherapy.
Tinnitus in 3 cases and hearing loss in 2 cases due to 18 mg per kg in 3
divided doses of antituberculous agent, isoniazid (SM), in total of 5 of 160
humans, Japanese, adult, 20 to 61 years age, male and female, with pulmonary
tuberculosis and without previous chemotherapy.
Simultaneous administration of 10 g daily in 3 divided doses of antituberculous agent, PAS (SM), in 160 humans, Japanese, adult, 20 to 61 years age,
male and female, with pulmonary tuberculosis and without previous chemotherapy.
    (AD) Similar ototoxic effects in both drug regimens. (ENG)

                                                                         700
Dizziness or vertigo, during first 3 months in 7 cases and after 3 to 6
months in 5 cases, due to 1 g daily for first 3 months, and then 1 g 3 times
a week for second 3 months in patients 50 years age or less, or 1 g 3 times a
week for 6 months in patients over 50 years age, of antibiotic, streptomycin
(SM) (streptomycin sulfate), for 6 months in 12 (20 percent) of 59 humans,
adult and aged, 55 years or more age in most cases, male, with chronic pulmonary tuberculosis and pneumoconiosis.
    (AD) Reported 20 percent incidence of streptomycin ototoxicity in first
    year of therapy.
Incr hearing loss reported after 6 months due to 1 g daily for first 3
months, and then 1 g 3 times a week for second 3 months in patients 50 years
age or less, or 1 g 3 times a week for 6 months in patients over 50 years
age, of antibiotic, streptomycin (SM) (streptomycin sulfate), for 6 months in
1 of 59 humans, adult and aged, 55 years or more age in most cases, male,
with chronic pulmonary tuberculosis and pneumoconiosis and with previous
hearing loss.
    (AD) Reported 1 case of hearing loss due to streptomycin in first year of
    therapy.
Dizziness and tinnitus after 14 months due to 1 g daily for first 3 months,
and then 1 g 3 times a week for second 3 months in patients 50 years age or
less, or 1 g 3 times a week for 6 months in patients over 50 years age, of
antibiotic, streptomycin (SM) (streptomycin sulfate), for 6 months in 1 of 31
humans, male, with chronic pulmonary tuberculosis and pneumoconiosis.
    (AD) Reported 1 case with ototoxic effects within 18 months of therapy.
Simultaneous oral administration in cachets of 333 mg daily of antituberculous agent, isoniazid (SM) (CB), for 18 months or more in 59 humans, male,
with chronic pulmonary tuberculosis and pneumoconiosis.
Simultaneous oral administration in cachets of 15 g daily of antituberculous
agent, PAS (SM) (CB) (sodium PAS), for 18 months or more in 59 humans, male,
with chronic pulmonary tuberculosis and pneumoconiosis. (ENG)

                               Thiacetazone

                                                                         041
Cochleo-vestibulotoxic effects due to unspecified method of administration of
300 mg daily of antituberculous agent, isoniazid, for 6 to 18 months in 12.9
percent of 70 humans with tuberculosis.
Cochleo-vestibulotoxic effects due to unspecified method of administration of
300 mg of antituberculous agent, isoniazid (SM), for 6 to 18 months in 22
percent of 297 humans with tuberculosis.
Cochleo-vestibulotoxic effects due to unspecified method of administration of
150 mg of antituberculous agent, thiacetazone (SM), for 6 to 18 months in 22
percent of 297 humans with tuberculosis.
Cochleo-vestibulotoxic effects due to unspecified method of administration of
antituberculous agent, isoniazid (SM), for 6 to 18 months in 82.9 percent of
82 humans with tuberculosis.
Cochleo-vestibulotoxic effects due to unspecified method of administration of

antituberculous agent, thiacetazone (SM), for 6 to 8 months in 82.9 percent
of 82 humans with tuberculosis.
Cochleo-vestibulotoxic effects due to unspecified method of administration of
1 g of antibiotic, streptomycin (SM), for 6 to 18 months in 82.9 percent of
82 humans with tuberculosis.
Cochleo-vestibulotoxic effects due to unspecified method of administration of
300 mg of antituberculous agent, isoniazid (SM), for 6 to 18 months in 25
percent of 20 humans with tuberculosis.
Cochleo-vestibulotoxic effects due to unspecified method of administration of
1 g of antibiotic, streptomycin (SM), for 6 to 18 months in 25 percent of 20
humans with tuberculosis.
   (AD) Potentiation by thiacetazone of cochleo-vestibulotoxic effects of
   streptomycin suggested.
   (AD) Audiometry and vestibular function tests every 2 weeks for 6 to 18
   months in total of 469 humans with tuberculosis. (ENG)

                                                                        090
Tinnitus and vertigo due to unspecified method of administration of 0.75 g
daily of antibiotic, (SQ) streptomycin (SM), for 5 weeks in 1 human, adult,
38 years age, female, with pulmonary tuberculosis.
Simultaneous administration of antituberculous agent, (SQ) PAS (SM), in 1
human, adult, 38 years age, female, with pulmonary tuberculosis.
Simultaneous administration of antituberculous agent, (SQ) isoniazid (SM), in
1 human, adult, 38 years age, female, with pulmonary tuberculosis.
No reported ototoxic effects due to unspecified method of administration of
150 mg daily of antituberculous agent, (SQ) thiacetazone, for 11 months in 1
human, adult, 38 years age, female, with pulmonary tuberculosis.
   (AD) Hemolytic disease due to treatment with thiacetazone. (ENG)

                                                                        136
Vestibular problems due to oral administration of 150 mg daily of antituberculous agent, thiacetazone (CB), for 12 months in 4 of 150 humans with pulmonary tuberculosis and without previous treatment.
Combined oral administration of 30 mg daily of antituberculous agent, isoniazid (CB), for 12 months in 150 humans with pulmonary tuberculosis and without
previous treatment.
No vestibular problems due to 10 g daily in 2 doses of antituberculous agent,
PAS (CB) (sodium PAS), for 12 months in 100 humans with pulmonary tuberculosis and without previous treatment.
Combined administration of 200 mg daily in 2 doses of antituberculous agent,
isoniazid (CB), for 12 months in 100 humans with pulmonary tuberculosis and
without previous treatment.
   (AD) Comparative study of effects of thiacetazone and PAS with isoniazid
   in treatment of tuberculosis. (ENG)

                                                                        340
Vestibular problems due to 150 mg daily of antituberculous agent, thiaceta-
zone (SM), in 15 of 75 humans with pulmonary tuberculosis.
Vestibular problems due to 0.75 to 1 g daily of antibiotic, streptomycin (SM)
(streptomycin sulfate), in 15 of 75 humans with pulmonary tuberculosis.
Vestibular problems due to 300 mg daily of antituberculous agent, isoniazid
(SM), in 15 of 75 humans with pulmonary tuberculosis.
   (AD) Vestibulotoxic effects confirmed by vestibular function tests.
   (AD) Statistical analysis showed higher occurrence of vestibular problems
   in humans with thiacetazone in drug regimen than without thiacetazone.
   (SL)

                                                                        367
Auditory system problems due to oral administration of 150 mg daily of antituberculous agent, thiacetazone (CB), for 12 weeks in 47 of 581 humans,
adolescent and adult, 15 years or over age, male and female, with pulmonary
tuberculosis.
Auditory system problems due to oral administration of 150 mg daily of antituberculous agent, thiacetazone (CB) (IB), for 12 weeks in 39 of 584 humans,
adolescent and adult, 15 years or over age, male and female, with pulmonary
tuberculosis, with administration of vitamins and antihistamine.
Combined oral administration of 300 mg daily of antituberculous agent, i-
soniazid (CB), for 12 weeks in humans, adolescent and adult, 15 years or over

age, male and female, with pulmonary tuberculosis.

(AD) Study of effect of inhibitors on toxicity of drugs in 1 group with
drug regimen of thiacetazone and isoniazid in combination.

Auditory system problems due to parenteral administration of 1 g daily of
antibiotic, streptomycin (SM), for 12 weeks in 227 of 689 humans, adolescent
and adult, 15 years or over age, male and female, with pulmonary tuberculosis.

Auditory system problems due to parenteral administration of 1 g daily of
antibiotic, streptomycin (SM) (IB), for 12 weeks in 218 of 707 humans, adolescent and adult, 15 years or over age, male and female, with pulmonary tuberculosis, with administration of vitamins and antihistamine.

Auditory system problems due to simultaneous oral administration of 150 mg
daily of antituberculous agent, thiacetazone (SM), for 12 weeks in humans,
adolescent and adult, 15 years or over age, male and female, with pulmonary
tuberculosis.

Simultaneous oral administration of 300 mg daily of antituberculous agent,
isoniazid (SM), for 12 weeks in humans, adolescent and adult, 15 years or
over age, male and female, with pulmonary tuberculosis.

(AD) Study of effect of inhibitors on toxicity of drugs in 1 group with
drug regimen of streptomycin, thiacetazone, and isoniazid.

Auditory system problems due to parenteral administration of 1 g daily of
antibiotic, streptomycin (SM), for 12 weeks in 109 of 711 humans, adolescent
and adult, 15 years or over age, male and female, with pulmonary tuberculosis.

Auditory system problems due to parenteral administration of 1 g daily of
antibiotic, streptomycin (SM) (IB), for 12 weeks in 111 of 696 humans, adolescent and adult, 15 years or over age, male and female, with pulmonary tuberculosis, with administration of vitamins and antihistamine.

Simultaneous oral administration of 300 mg daily of antituberculous agent,
isoniazid (SM), for 12 weeks in humans, adolescent and adult, 15 years or
over age, male and female, with pulmonary tuberculosis.

(AD) Study of effect of inhibitors on toxicity of drugs in 1 group with
drug regimen of streptomycin and isoniazid.

(AD) Study of effectiveness of inhibitors in prevention of toxic effects
of thiacetazone and streptomycin.

(AD) Study suggested that vitamins and antihistamine not effective in
prevention of toxicity.   (ENG)

433

Dizziness due to 1 g daily of antibiotic, streptomycin (SM), for 6 months in
32 percent of 114 humans with pulmonary tuberculosis.

Dizziness due to 300 mg daily of antituberculous agent, isoniazid (SM), for 6
months with streptomycin and then 6 months alone in 32 percent of 114 humans
with pulmonary tuberculosis.

(AD) Regimen of simultaneous administration of streptomycin and isoniazid
for 6 months followed by administration of isoniazid only for 6 months.

Dizziness due to 1 g daily of antibiotic, streptomycin (SM), for 6 months in
54 percent of 94 humans with pulmonary tuberculosis.

Dizziness due to 150 mg daily of antituberculous agent, thiacetazone (SM),
for 6 months with streptomycin and isoniazid and then 6 months with isoniazid
in 54 percent of 94 humans with pulmonary tuberculosis.

Dizziness due to 300 mg daily of antituberculous agent, isoniazid (SM), for 6
months with streptomycin and thiacetazone and then 6 months with thiacetazone
in 54 percent of 94 humans with pulmonary tuberculosis.

(AD) Regimen of simultaneous administration of streptomycin, thiacetazone,
and isoniazid for 6 months followed by administration of thiacetazone and
isoniazid for 6 months.

Dizziness due to 150 mg daily of antituberculous agent, thiacetazone (SM),
for 1 year in 13 percent of 78 humans with pulmonary tuberculosis.

Dizziness due to 300 mg daily of antituberculous agent, isoniazid (SM), for 1
year in 13 percent of 78 humans with pulmonary tuberculosis.

(AD) Regimen of simultaneous administration of thiacetazone and isoniazid
for 1 year.

(AD) Study of role of drug regimens with thiacetazone in treatment of
pulmonary tuberculosis. (ENG)

447

Dizziness and tinnitus within first 14 weeks due to 150 mg daily in 2 divided

doses of antituberculous agent, thiacetazone (SM), for 26 weeks in 30 of 410
humans, adolescent and adult, 15 to over 55 years age, 30 to over 50 kg
weight, with tuberculosis.
No ototoxic effects due to 300 mg daily in 2 divided doses of antituberculous
agent, isoniazid (SM), for 26 weeks in 30 of 410 humans, adolescent and
adult, 15 to over 55 years age, 30 to over 50 kg weight, with tuberculosis.
  (AD) Study of toxicity of thiacetazone in treatment of tuberculosis.
  (ENG)

537

Dizziness due to oral administration in tablet of 150 mg daily of antituberculous agent, thiacetazone (CB) (SM), in 1 of 147 humans, African, adolescent
and adult, 15 years or more age, with pulmonary tuberculosis and without
previous treatment.
Dizziness due to oral administration in tablet of 300 mg daily of antituberculous agent, isoniazid (CB) (SM), in 1 of 147 humans, African, adolescent
and adult, 15 years or more age, with pulmonary tuberculosis and without
previous treatment.
  (AD) Dizziness in 1 patient due to combined treatment with thiacetazone
    and isoniazid only.
Dizziness due to parenteral, intramuscular, administration of 1 g daily of
antibiotic, streptomycin (SM) (streptomycin sulfate), for first 2 weeks in 1
of 161 humans, African, adolescent and adult, 15 years or more age, with
pulmonary tuberculosis and without previous treatment.
  (AD) Dizziness in 1 patient due to simultaneous treatment with thiaceta-
    zone and isoniazid in 1 tablet and intramuscular streptomycin for 2 weeks.
Dizziness due to parenteral, intramuscular, administration of 1 g daily of
antibiotic, streptomycin (SM) (streptomycin sulfate), for first 8 weeks in 10
of 162 humans, African, adolescent and adult, 15 years or more age, with
pulmonary tuberculosis and without previous treatment.
  (AD) Dizziness in 10 patients due to simultaneous treatment with thiaceta-
    zone and isoniazid in 1 tablet and intramuscular streptomycin for 8 weeks.
  (AD) Study showed vestibulotoxic effects in total of 12 of 818 patients
    treated for pulmonary tuberculosis.   (ENG)

615

Tinnitus, hearing loss, vertigo, and dizziness due to oral administration in
tablet of 150 mg daily of antituberculous agent, thiacetazone (CB) (SM), in
some of 1002 humans with tuberculosis.
Tinnitus, hearing loss, vertigo, and dizziness due to oral administration in
tablet of 300 mg daily of antituberculous agent, isoniazid (CB) (SM), in some
of 1002 humans with tuberculosis.
Tinnitus, hearing loss, vertigo, and dizziness due to parenteral administration of 1 g daily of antibiotic, streptomycin (SM), in some of 1002 humans
with tuberculosis.
  (AD) Reported 21.4 percent incidence of toxic effects in regimen of thia-
    cetazone, isoniazid, and streptomycin.
  (AD) Suggested that effects of streptomycin potentiated by thiacetazone.
Unspecified ototoxic effects due to oral administration of 300 mg daily of
antituberculous agent, isoniazid (SM), in 987 humans with tuberculosis.
Unspecified ototoxic effects due to parenteral administration of 1 g daily of
antibiotic, streptomycin (SM), in 987 humans with tuberculosis.
  (AD) Reported 7.8 percent incidence of toxic effects in regimen of isonia-
    zid and streptomycin without thiacetazone. (ENG)

634

Ototoxic effects due to antituberculous agent, thiacetazone, in humans with
tuberculosis.   (FR)

CARDIOVASCULAR AGENTS

Chromonar

530

Transient ototoxic effects due to cardiovascular agent, chromonar, in humans
treated for heart disorders.   (GER)

Digitalis

Sensorineural hearing loss, tinnitus, dizziness, and disorder of equilibrium due to cardiovascular agent, digitalis, in 1 human treated for heart disorder. (POL)

Hexadimethrine bromide

Bilateral tinnitus and sudden deafness possibly due to cardiovascular agent, (SQ) hexadimethrine bromide, in 1 human, adult, 32 years age, female, with chronic nephritis and treated with hemodialysis.
Previous administration of antituberculous agent, (SQ) PAS, in 1 human, adult, 32 years age, female, with chronic nephritis and treated with hemodialysis.
Previous administration of antituberculous agent, (SQ) isoniazid, in 1 human, adult, 32 years age, female, with chronic nephritis and treated with hemodialysis.
Damage to Reissner's membrane, degeneration of organ of Corti, stria vascularis, and spiral ganglion, and slight changes in vestibular apparatus possibly due to cardiovascular agent, (SQ) hexadimethrine bromide, in 1 human, adult, 32 years age, female, with chronic nephritis and treated with hemodialysis.
Progressive severe sensorineural hearing loss possibly due to cardiovascular agent, hexadimethrine bromide, in 4 humans, adolescent and adult, 17 to 40 years age, with kidney disorders and treated with hemodialysis.
  (AD) Association of hexadimethrine bromide with hearing loss only when used with hemodialysis in treatment of kidney disorder.
  (AD) No hearing loss in group treated with hemodialysis without hexadimethrine bromide. (ENG)

Usually transient hearing loss and no structural damage to organ of Corti, stria vascularis, and spiral ganglion due to oral or topical administration of salicylates in humans.
Hearing loss due to antimalarial, quinine, in humans.
Usually permanent hearing loss due to antimalarial, chloroquine, in humans.
Transient and permanent hearing loss and possible damage to hair cells of organ of Corti due to diuretic, ethacrynic acid, in humans.
Sensorineural hearing loss due to cardiovascular agent, hexadimethrine bromide, in humans with kidney disorder.
Sensorineural hearing loss and damage to organ of Corti due to topical administration of antineoplastic, nitrogen mustard, in humans.
Sensorineural hearing loss due to high doses of antibiotic, chloramphenicol, in humans.
Primary vestibular problems due to antibiotic, streptomycin, in humans.
Hearing loss due to high doses usually of antibiotic, streptomycin, in humans.
  (AD) Early detection of hearing loss by audiometry prevents permanent damage.
High frequency hearing loss and severe damage to outer hair cells and slight damage to inner hair cells of organ of Corti due to antibiotic, kanamycin, in humans.
Sensorineural hearing loss due to parenteral, oral, and topical administration of antibiotic, neomycin, in humans with or without kidney disorders.
Degeneration of hair cells of organ of Corti and of nerve process due to antibiotics, aminoglycoside, in animals.
  (AD) Literature review of physiological and structural cochleo-vestibulotoxic effects or ototoxic drugs.
  (AD) Discussion of suggested mechanism of ototoxicity and routes of drugs to inner ear.
Bilateral sensorineural hearing loss due to oral administration of antibiotic, neomycin, in 4 of 8 humans with liver disease.
Bilateral sensorineural hearing loss due to oral administration of range of doses of antibiotic, neomycin (SM), in 2 of 5 humans with liver disease.
Bilateral sensorineural hearing loss due to diuretics (SM), in 2 of 5 humans

with liver disease.
Transient progression of previous hearing loss due to parenteral, intravenous, administration of diuretic, ethacrynic acid (SM), in 1 injection in 1
of 5 humans with liver disease.
   (CT) Normal cochlear function in 6 humans, control group, with liver
   disease and not treated with neomycin or diuretics.
   (CT) Normal cochlear function in 13 humans, control group, with liver
   disease and treated with diuretics but not with neomycin.
   (AD) Hearing loss confirmed by audiometry.
   (AD) Reported that hearing loss due to neomycin or diuretics in humans
   with liver disease not related to dosage.
   (AD) Clinical study of effects of treatment with neomycin and diuretics in
   humans with liver disease.
Bilateral sensorineural hearing loss and vertigo due to antibiotic, ampicil-
lin, in 1 human, adolescent, 17 years age, female, with tonsillitis.
   (AD) Cited case report.
Severe sensorineural hearing loss and vertigo due to topical administration
in ear drops of antibiotic, framycetin, in 1 human, adult, 42 years age,
male, with previous slight high frequency hearing loss.
   (AD) Cited case report.
Atrophy of hair cells of organ of Corti and hearing loss due to antibiotic,
dihydrostreptomycin, in humans with tuberculous meningitis.
   (AD) Cited study.
Loss of inner hair cells and damage to outer hair cells due to 18 g of anti-
biotic, neomycin, for 18 days in 1 human.
   (AD) Cited case report. (ENG)

Propranolol

280

High frequency hearing loss 3 weeks after beginning of therapy due to oral
administration of 20 mg daily, then 60 mg daily for 1 week, with interval of
1 week, and then 30 mg daily for 12 days of cardiovascular agent, (SQ) propranolol, for total of 19 days in 1 human, aged, 68 years age, female, with
heart disorder, arteriosclerosis.
   (AD) Sensorineural hearing loss confirmed by audiometry.
   (AD) Some improvement in hearing sensitivity during 6 months after cessation of drug.
No reported ototoxic effects due to unspecified method of administration
about 2 years previously of unspecified dose of cardiovascular agent, (SQ)
quinidine, for unspecified period in 1 human, aged, 68 years age, female,
with heart disorder, arteriosclerosis.
   (AD) Effects on gastrointestinal system and skin rash due to quinidine.
   (AD) Patient had history of toxic effects of drugs.
   (AD) Suggested that possible previous hearing loss made more severe by
   propranolol. (ENG)

552

Tinnitus within several hours due to 10 mg twice daily of cardiovascular
agent, propranolol, for 4 days in 1 human, adult, 56 years age, female, with
mild hypertension.
   (AD) Case report of tinnitus for duration of dosage of 10 mg twice daily
   of propranolol.
   (AD) Cessation of tinnitus after decr in dosage to 10 mg daily of propranolol. (ENG)

Quinidine

280

High frequency hearing loss 3 weeks after beginning of therapy due to oral
administration of 20 mg daily, then 60 mg daily for 1 week, with interval of
1 week, and then 30 mg daily for 12 days of cardiovascular agent, (3Q) propranolol, for total of 19 days in 1 human, aged, 68 years age, female, with
heart disorder, arteriosclerosis.
   (AD) Sensorineural hearing loss confirmed by audiometry.
   (AD) Some improvement in hearing sensitivity during 6 months after cessation of drug.
No reported ototoxic effects due to unspecified method of administration

about 2 years previously of unspecified dose of cardiovascular agent, (SQ)
quinidine, for unspecified period in 1 human, aged, 68 years age, female,
with heart disorder, arteriosclerosis.
   (AD) Effects on gastrointestinal system and skin rash due to quinidine.
   (AD) Patient had history of toxic effects of drugs.
   (AD) Suggested that possible previous hearing loss made more severe by
   propranolol. (ENG)

                                                                    366
Possible auditory system problems due to cardiovascular agent, quinidine, in
humans.
No ototoxic effects due to 2.40 to 9.00 g of cardiovascular agent, quinidine,
in 150 humans, adolescent and adult, male and female, with auricular fibril-
lation.
   (AD) Other toxic effects in 46 of 150 humans but no ototoxic effects
   reported. (SP)

                                                                    597
Hearing loss due to salicylates in humans.
Hearing loss due to antimalarial, quinine, in humans.
Hearing loss due to antibiotic, streptomycin, in humans.
Tinnitus due to chemical agent, camphor, in humans.
Tinnitus due to chemical agent, tobacco, in humans.
Tinnitus due to cardiovascular agent, quinidine, in humans.
Tinnitus due to chemical agent, ergot, in humans.
Tinnitus due to chemical agent, alcohol, methyl, in humans.
   (AD) Discussion of toxic effects of drugs. (ENG)

                            CONTRACEPTIVES

                                                                    378
Total unilateral sensorineural hearing loss, tinnitus, and vertigo 7 days
after injection due to parenteral, (SQ) intramuscular, administration of 150
mg of (SQ) contraceptive, methoxy progesterone acetate, in 1 injection in 1
human, adult, 26 years age, female.
   (AD) Cochleo-vestibulotoxic effects confirmed by audiometry and vestibular
   function tests 1 month later.
   (AD) Suggested that ototoxic effects result of obstruction of cochlear
   artery due to contraceptive.
Dizziness due to previous (SQ) oral administration of other (SQ) contraceptives in 1 human, adult, 26 years age, female. (ENG)

                                                                    379
Sudden deafness, tinnitus, severe vertigo, and objective decr in vestibular
function due to oral administration of 2 mg daily of contraceptive, norethin-
drone (CB), for 3 months in 1 human, adult, 34 years age, female.
Sudden deafness, tinnitus, severe vertigo, and objective decr in vestibular
function due to oral administration of 2 mg daily of contraceptive, mestranol
(CB), for 3 months in 1 human, adult, 34 years age, female.
   (AD) Cochleo-vestibulotoxic effects confirmed by audiometry and vestibular
   function tests.
   (AD) Partial improvement in hearing 20 days later.
Severe bilateral sudden deafness, tinnitus, and dizziness due to oral admini-
stration of contraceptive, norethindrone (CB), for 2 years in 1 human, adult,
20 years age, female.
Severe bilateral sudden deafness, tinnitus, and dizziness due to oral administration of contraceptive, mestranol (CB), for 2 years in 1 human, adult, 20
years age, female.
   (AD) Audiometry and vestibular function tests 7 days after onset of ototoxic effects.
   (AD) Partial improvement in 1 ear and total recovery in other ear 30 days
   later.
   (AD) Suggested that ototoxic effects resulted from blood coagulation due
   to contraceptive. (ENG)

                                                                    402
Pressure in the ears due to contraceptives in 1 human, adult, 33 years age,
female.

(AD) Pressure possibly due to obstruction of Eustachian tube.
Possible vertigo, sudden deafness, and distortion of sound due to contraceptives in humans. (ENG)

DIURETICS

175

No change in potassium and sodium concentrations or in cation content of
endolymph due to parenteral, intravenous and intraperitoneal, administration
of range of doses of diuretics in 1 dose or multiple doses in animals, guinea
pigs, 250 to 400 g weight, with normal pinna reflex. (ENG)

621

Primarily vestibular problems due to antibiotic, streptomycin, in humans.
Primarily hearing loss but also vestibular problems due to antibiotic, dihy-
drostreptomycin, in humans.
Primarily hearing loss but also vestibular problems due to antibiotic, kana-
mycin, in humans.
Primarily hearing loss but also vestibular problems due to antibiotic, neomy-
cin, in humans.
Primarily hearing loss but also vestibular problems due to antibiotic, genta-
micin, in humans.
Vertigo and ataxia due to antituberculous agent, isoniazid, in humans.
Hearing loss due to salicylate, aspirin, in humans.
Hearing loss and vertigo due to antimalarial, quinine, in humans.
Nystagmus due to barbiturates in humans.
Vestibular problems due to analgesic, morphine, in humans.
Nystagmus due to sedative, alcohol, in humans.
Nystagmus and hearing loss due to chemical agent, carbon monoxide, in humans.
Ototoxic effects due to antineoplastic, nitrogen mustard, in humans.
Ototoxic effects due to chemical agent, aniline, in humans.
Ototoxic effects due to chemical agent, tobacco, in humans.
Nystagmus due to chemical agent, nicotine, in humans.
Vestibular problems due to anticonvulsants in humans.
Vestibular problems due to anesthetics in humans.
Vestibular problems due to diuretics in humans.
    (AD) Inclusion of comprehensive list of ototoxic agents.   (SP)

Acetazolamide

130

Decr in cochlear microphonic and neural potentials and incr in sodium and
glucose of endolymph due to parenteral, intravenous, administration of 30 to
60 mg per kg, in saline solution, of diuretic, ethacrynic acid, for 5 minute
period in animals, cats.
Changes in stria vascularis and damage to outer hair cells of organ of Corti
due to parenteral, intravenous, administration of 30 to 60 mg per kg, in
saline solution, of diuretic, ethacrynic acid, for 5 minute period in animals, cats.
No change in cochlear microphonic, no incr in endolymph glucose, and normal
endolymph chemical composition due to parenteral, intravenous, administration
of 50 mg per kg, in saline solution, of diuretic, acetazolamide, for 5 minute
period in animals, cats.
Slow decr in cochlear microphonic and neural potentials due to parenteral,
intravenous, administration of 200 mg per kg, in saline solution, of diuretic, acetazolamide, for 5 minute period in animals, cats.
    (CT) Same method using 7 cc per kg of saline solution in 14 cats, control
    group.
    (AD) Clinical significance of study of acetazolamide not determined due to
    lack of reports of hearing loss with use of drug.
Severe decr in cochlear microphonic and neural potentials but no changes in
electrolyte concentrations of endolymph or perilymph due to parenteral,
intravenous, administration of 30 mg per kg daily of diuretic, ethacrynic
acid, for 3 to 4 days in 3 animals, cats.
    (AD) Results of study suggest severe hearing loss.
Edema of stria vascularis and damage to outer hair cells of organ of Corti
but normal chemical composition of endolymph and perilymph due to parenteral,
intraperitoneal, administration of 30 mg per kg of diuretic, ethacrynic acid,

in 1 dose in 9 animals, cats.
  (AD) Study of effect of diuretics on chemical composition of fluids of
inner ear and relationship to cochlear microphonic and histopathology of
temporal bone. (ENG)

278

Histochemical changes in cochlea due to parenteral administration of 15 mg
per kg daily of diuretic, furosemide, for 8 to 14 days in animals, guinea
pigs, 300 g weight.
Histochemical changes in cochlea due to parenteral administration of 8 mg per
kg daily of diuretic, acetazolamide, for 8 to 14 days in animals, guinea
pigs, 300 g weight. (GER)

Ethacrynic acid

005

Transient primary decr in cochlear microphonic and action potential due to
parenteral, intravenous, administration of 10 mg per kg of diuretic, ethacrynic acid, in 1 injection in 20 animals, cats, adult.
Transient primary decr in cochlear microphonic and action potential due to
parenteral, intravenous, administration of 10 mg per kg of diuretic, furosemide, in 1 injection in 20 animals, cats, adult.
Delayed severe secondary decr in cochlear microphonic and action potential
due to parenteral, intravenous, administration of more than 10 mg per kg of
diuretic, ethacrynic acid, in animals, cats.
  (CT) Same method using 50 mg per kg and 100 mg per kg of diuretic, chlorothiazide, in cats, control group, showed no ototoxic effect.
Degeneration of outer hair cells of organ of Corti in basal and middle coils
of cochlea due to parenteral, intravenous, administration of 30 mg per kg of
diuretic, ethacrynic acid, in 1 injection in 2 animals, cats.
Degeneration of outer hair cells of organ of Corti due to parenteral, intramuscular, administration of 15 mg per kg of diuretic, ethacrynic acid, for 2
weeks in 1 animal, cat. (ENG)

010

Permanent sensorineural hearing loss due to parenteral, intramuscular, administration of low doses, less than 2 g, of antibiotic, (SQ) kanamycin
(kanamycin sulfate), for short period in 5 humans, adult, range of 33 to 47
years age, range of 90 to 177 lb weight, with kidney disorder.
Permanent sensorineural hearing loss due to parenteral, intramuscular, administration of low doses, less than 2 g, of antibiotic, (SQ) streptomycin,
for short period in 5 humans, adult, range of 33 to 47 years age, range of 90
to 177 lb weight, with kidney disorder.
Permanent sensorineural hearing loss due to parenteral, intramuscular, administration of low doses, less than 2 g, of antibiotic, (SQ) neomycin, for
short period in 5 humans, adult, range of 33 to 47 years age, range of 90 to
177 lb weight, with kidney disorder.
Permanent sensorineural hearing loss due to parenteral, intramuscular, administration of low doses, less than 2 g, of diuretic, (SQ) ethacrynic acid,
for short period in 5 humans, adult, range of 33 to 47 years age, range of 90
to 177 lb weight, with kidney disorder.
  (AD) Study of cochleotoxic effects of kanamycin with other antibiotics and
with ethacrynic acid. (ENG)

028

Bilateral sensorineural hearing loss and tinnitus due to parenteral, intravenous, administration of 100 mg of diuretic, ethacrynic acid (SM), in 2
doses in 1 human, adult, 24 years age, male, with kidney disorder.
Bilateral sensorineural hearing loss and tinnitus due to parenteral, intravenous, administration of 4 g of antibiotic, streptomycin (SM), for 5 days in
1 human, adult, 24 years age, male, with kidney disorder.
Bilateral sensorineural hearing loss due to parenteral, intravenous, administration of 500 mg of diuretic, ethacrynic acid (SM), for 4 days in 1 human,
adult, 35 years age, female, with kidney disorder.
Bilateral sensorineural hearing loss due to parenteral, intravenous, administration of 1.5 g of antibiotic, streptomycin (SM), for 4 days in 1 human,
adult, 35 years age, female, with kidney disorder.
Permanent hearing loss due to parenteral, intravenous, administration of 200

mg of diuretic, ethacrynic acid, in humans.   (ENG)

035

Transient and permanent hearing loss and vertigo due to oral and parenteral,
intravenous, administration of diuretic, ethacrynic acid, in 12 humans with
kidney disorders.
    (AD) Hearing loss not related to administration route or dosage.   (ENG)

038

Bilateral sensorineural hearing loss due to oral administration of 200 mg
twice a day of diuretic, (SQ) ethacrynic acid, for several weeks in 1 human,
adult, 40 years age, female, with kidney disorder.
Previous oral administration of 40 mg daily of diuretic, (SQ) furosemide
(SM), for unspecified period in 1 human, adult, 40 years age, female, with
kidney disorder.
Previous oral administration of 500 mg daily of diuretic, (SQ) chlorothiazide
(SM), for unspecified period in 1 human, adult, 40 years age, female, with
kidney disorder.
Sensorineural hearing loss and unsteady gait due to parenteral, intravenous,
administration of 200 mg of diuretic, (SQ) ethacrynic acid (SM), for unspeci-
fied period in 1 human, adult, 20 years age, female, with kidney disorder.
Simultaneous parenteral, intravenous, administration of 25 g of diuretic,
(SQ) mannitol (SM), for unspecified period in 1 human, adult, 20 years age,
female, with kidney disorder.
Previous administration of unspecified dose of chemical agent, (SQ) carbon
tetrachloride, for unspecified period in 1 human, adult, 20 years age, female, with kidney disorder.
Transient sensorineural hearing loss due to parenteral, intravenous, administration of 800 mg daily of diuretic, ethacrynic acid (SM), for unspecified
period in 1 human, adult, 25 years age, female, with chronic kidney disorder.
Simultaneous administration of unspecified doses of diuretic, chlorothiazide
(SM), for unspecified period in 1 human, adult, 25 years age, female, with
chronic kidney disorder.
Simultaneous administration of unspecified doses of diuretic, mannitol (SM),
for unspecified period in 1 human, adult, 25 years age, female, with chronic
kidney disorder.
Transient sensorineural hearing loss and dizziness due to parenteral, (SQ)
intravenous, administration of unspecified doses of diuretic, ethacrynic
acid, for unspecified period in 1 human, adult, 52 years age, female, with
kidney disorder.
Transient sensorineural hearing loss and dizziness due to (SQ) oral administration of 300 mg of diuretic, ethacrynic acid, for unspecified period in 1
human, adult, 52 years age, female, with kidney disorder.
Sensorineural hearing loss due to oral administration of 20 mg 3 times daily
of diuretic, ethacrynic acid, for 3 days in 1 human, adult, 28 years age,
male, with kidney disorder.
    (AD) Discussion of 5 case reports of ototoxic effects due to treatment
    with ethacrynic acid.   (ENG)

042

Transient bilateral sensorineural hearing loss due to parenteral, intravenous, administration of 50 mg of diuretic, (SQ) ethacrynic acid, in 1
injection in 1 human, adult, 45 years age, female, with lymphosarcoma and
with normal kidney function.
    (AD) Hearing loss reported 15 minutes after treatment with ethacrynic
    acid.
Previous parenteral, intramuscular, administration of 60 mg every 6 hours of
antibiotic, (SQ) gentamicin (gentamicin sulfate), for unspecified period in 1
human, adult, 45 years age, female, with lymphosarcoma and with normal kidney
function.
Bilateral sensorineural hearing loss due to parenteral, intravenous, administration of 100 mg of diuretic, (SQ) ethacrynic acid, in 2 injections of 50 mg
each 6 hours apart in 1 human, adult, 64 years age, female, with acute leukemia and with normal kidney function.
    (AD) Histological study after death showed no damage to inner ear.
Previous unspecified method of administration of unspecified dose of antibiotic, (SQ) polymyxin B (polymyxin B sulfate), in 1 human, adult, 64 years age,
female, with acute leukemia and with normal kidney function.

232   Ethacrynic acid

Previous parenteral, intramuscular, administration of 0.5 g every 12 hours of
antibiotic, (SQ) kanamycin (kanamycin sulfate), for unspecified period in 1
human, adult, 64 years age, female, with acute leukemia and with normal
kidney function.
   (AD) Suggested that hearing loss due to combined action of ethacrynic acid
   and antibiotics.   (ENG)

                                                                           055
Transient bilateral sensorineural hearing loss and tinnitus due to parenteral, intravenous, administration of 100 mg of diuretic, (SQ) ethacrynic
acid, in 1 injection in 1 human, adult, 64 years age, male, with kidney
disorder.
   (CT) Pretreatment audiology showed no auditory system problems.
   (AD) Hearing loss 5 minutes after administration of ethacrynic acid.
Previous parenteral, intravenous, administration of unspecified doses of
diuretic, (SQ) furosemide, for unspecified period in 1 human, adult, 64 years
age, male, with kidney disorder.   (ENG)

                                                                           060
Possible hearing loss due to high doses, as high as 200 mg, of diuretic,
ethacrynic acid, in humans with kidney disorders.
   (AD) Comment on risk of administration of high test doses of ethacrynic
   acid in humans with kidney disorder as suggested in recent study.   (ENG)

                                                                           061
Transient hearing loss due to high test dose, as high as 200 mg, of diuretic,
ethacrynic acid, in humans with kidney disorder
   (AD) Explanation of use of high test dose.
   (AD) Need for hydration before administration of test dose of ethacrynic
   acid.
   (AD) Procedure caused only 3 cases of transient hearing loss in 3 years.
   (ENG)

                                                                           089
Sudden deafness due to parenteral, intravenous, administration of 100 mg, in
100 ml saline solution, of diuretic, (SQ) ethacrynic acid, in 1 injection in
1 human, adult, 42 years age, female, quadriplegic, with kidney disorder.
Previous administration of unspecified dose of antibiotic, (SQ) chloramphenicol, for unspecified period in 1 human, adult, 42 years age, female, quadriplegic, with kidney disorder.
Previous administration of 1 g of antibiotic, (SQ) kanamycin, for unspecified
period in 1 human, adult, 42 years age, female, quadriplegic, with kidney
disorder and genitourinary system infection.   (ENG)

                                                                           097
Hearing loss due to diuretic, ethacrynic acid, in humans, female.
   (AD) Report on toxic effects of drugs.   (SW)

                                                                           098
Hearing loss due to parenteral, intravenous, administration of diuretic,
ethacrynic acid, in humans with kidney disorder.   (DAN)

                                                                           102
Progressive hearing loss and tinnitus due to diuretic, ethacrynic acid, in 1
human, adult, 48 years age, with kidney disorder.
   (AD) Hearing loss confirmed by audiometry.
   (AD) Need for audiometry with use of ethacrynic acid in humans with kidney
   disorder.   (FR)

                                                                           125
Sensorineural hearing loss due to parenteral, intravenous, administration of
range of 9.2 to 86 mg per kg of diuretic, ethacrynic acid (sodium ethacrynate), in 1 injection in 7 of 12 animals, guinea pigs, young, 240 to 489 g
weight.
   (AD) Hearing loss confirmed by loss of Preyer reflex 6 minutes after
   injection.
Primary damage to stria vascularis and some damage to outer hair cells of
organ of Corti due to parenteral, intravenous, administration of range of 9.2

to 86 mg per kg of diuretic, ethacrynic acid (sodium ethacrynate), in 1
injection in 12 animals, guinea pigs, young, 240 to 489 g weight.
    (AD) Electron microscopic study of cochlea.   (ENG)

                                                                           130
Decr in cochlear microphonic and neural potentials and incr in sodium and
glucose of endolymph due to parenteral, intravenous, administration of 30 to
60 mg per kg, in saline solution, of diuretic, ethacrynic acid, for 5 minute
period in animals, cats.
Changes in stria vascularis and damage to outer hair cells of organ of Corti
due to parenteral, intravenous, administration of 30 to 60 mg per kg, in
saline solution, of diuretic, ethacrynic acid, for 5 minute period in animals, cats.
No change in cochlear microphonic, no incr in endolymph glucose, and normal
endolymph chemical composition due to parenteral, intravenous, administration
of 50 mg per kg, in saline solution, of diuretic, acetazolamide, for 5 minute
period in animals, cats.
Slow decr in cochlear microphonic and neural potentials due to parenteral,
intravenous, administration of 200 mg per kg, in saline solution, of diuretic, acetazolamide, for 5 minute period in animals, cats.
    (CT) Same method using 7 cc per kg of saline solution in 14 cats, control
    group.
    (AD) Clinical significance of study of acetazolamide not determined due to
    lack of reports of hearing loss with use of drug.
Severe decr in cochlear microphonic and neural potentials but no changes in
electrolyte concentrations of endolymph or perilymph due to parenteral,
intravenous, administration of 30 mg per kg daily of diuretic, ethacrynic
acid, for 3 to 4 days in 3 animals, cats.
    (AD) Results of study suggest severe hearing loss.
Edema of stria vascularis and damage to outer hair cells of organ of Corti
but normal chemical composition of endolymph and perilymph due to parenteral,
intraperitoneal, administration of 30 mg per kg of diuretic, ethacrynic acid,
in 1 dose in 9 animals, cats.
    (AD) Study of effect of diuretics on chemical composition of fluids of
    inner ear and relationship to cochlear microphonic and histopathology of
    temporal bone.   (ENG)

                                                                           144
Moderate bilateral sensorineural hearing loss within 20 minutes and damage to
outer hair cells of organ of Corti due to unspecified method of administration of 50 mg of diuretic, ethacrynic acid, in 1 dose in humans with kidney
disorder.
    (AD) Hearing loss confirmed by audiogram.
Sensorineural hearing loss within 15 minutes due to unspecified method of
administration of 20 to 30 mg per kg daily of diuretic, ethacrynic acid, in
20 animals, cats.
    (AD) Ethacrynic acid not recommended for clinical use in humans with
    kidney disorders.   (ENG)

                                                                           148
Transient sensorineural hearing loss due to diuretic, ethacrynic acid, in 1
human, adult, male.   (FIN)

                                                                           171
Rapid significant decr in cochlear microphonic but no pathological changes in
cochlea after 1 hour due to parenteral, intravenous, administration of high
doses, 20, 30, or 40 mg per kg, in solution of physiological saline, of
diuretic, ethacrynic acid, in 1 injection for acute effects in 3 groups of 18
animals, guinea pigs, young, 250 g weight.
No detected decr in cochlear microphonic and no permanent physiological or
structural changes in cochlea after 3 weeks due to parenteral, intravenous,
administration of high doses, 30 mg per kg, of diuretic, ethacrynic acid, in
chronic intoxication in 6 animals, guinea pigs, young, 250 g weight. (ENG)

                                                                           178
Sensorineural hearing loss due to diuretic, ethacrynic acid, in humans,
adult, female and male, with kidney disorders.   (NOR)

206

Transient bilateral sensorineural hearing loss due to oral administration of
50 mg every 6 hours of diuretic, ethacrynic acid, for 4 days initially and
then again 2 weeks later for 2 days in 1 human, Negro, adult, 55 years age,
female, with diabetes mellitus and kidney disorder.
  (AD) Hearing loss confirmed by audiogram.
Transient sensorineural hearing loss and tinnitus due to (SQ) oral and parenteral, (SQ) intravenous, administration of 300,300,400, and 500 mg of diuretic, ethacrynic acid, in 4 doses in 1 human, Caucasian, adult, 40 years age,
female, with chronic kidney disorder.
No auditory system problems due to parenteral, intravenous, administration of
(SQ) unspecified doses of diuretic, (SQ) ethacrynic acid, in (SQ) 3 injections in 1 human, Caucasian, adult, 20 years age, female, with kidney disorder.
Transient severe bilateral tinnitus, sensorineural hearing loss, and bilateral nystagmus due to parenteral, intravenous, administration of (SQ) 50 and
100 mg of diuretic, (SQ) ethacrynic acid, in (SQ) 2 injections in 1 human,
Caucasian, adult, 20 years age, female, with kidney disorder.
Previous administration, 2 days before onset of ototoxic effects, of antibiotic, (SQ) colistin (sodium colistimethate), in 1 injection in 1 human, Caucasian, adult, 20 years age, female, with kidney disorder.
Transient sensorineural hearing loss within 12 hours of first dose due to
oral administration of 50 mg of diuretic, ethacrynic acid, in 4 doses in 1
human, Caucasian, aged, 76 years age, male, with kidney disorder and with
previous moderate hearing loss due to otosclerosis.
Severe tinnitus within 1 hour of first dose and sensorineural hearing loss
within 1 half hour of second dose due to parenteral, intravenous, administration of 50 and 100 mg of diuretic, (SQ) ethacrynic acid, in 2 injections in 1
human, Caucasian, adult, 57 years age, female, with leukemia and kidney
disorder.
Administration about 1 week previously of antibiotic, (SQ) streptomycin, in 1
human, Caucasian, adult, 57 years age, female, with leukemia and kidney
disorder, for pneumonitis.
Administration about 1 week previously of antibiotic, (SQ) colistin (sodium
colistimethate), in 1 human, Caucasian, adult, 57 years age, female, with
leukemia and kidney disorder, for pneumonitis.
  (AD) Discussion of 5 case reports of transient hearing loss due to treatment with ethacrynic acid. (ENG)

219

Cochleo-vestibulotoxic effects due to antibiotics in humans.
Transient and permanent sensorineural hearing loss due to diuretic, etha-
crynic acid, in humans.
Transient sensorineural hearing loss, tinnitus, and vertigo due to salicy-
late, aspirin, in humans.
Transient and permanent sensorineural hearing loss and dizziness due to
antimalarial, quinine, in humans.
Sensorineural hearing loss due to antimalarial, chloroquine, in humans.
Sensorineural hearing loss, tinnitus, and vertigo due to chemical agents in
humans.
  (AD) Literature review of ototoxic drugs with clinical and histopathologi-
  cal correlations.
  (AD) Comment on ototoxicity of some chemical agents.
  (AD) Review of theories of mechanism of action of ototoxic drugs. (ENG)

246

Some incr in perilymph potassium due to parenteral, intravenous, administration of 10 mg per kg of diuretic, ethacrynic acid, in 1 injection in 12 to 14
animals, guinea pigs, pigmented, young, 200 to 400 g weight.
Some incr in perilymph potassium due to parenteral, intravenous, administration with 10 mg per kg, total of 30 mg per kg, of diuretic. ethacrynic acid,
in 3 injections, over total of 24 hours, in 12 to 14 animals, guinea pigs,
pigmented, young, 200 to 400 g weight.
Significant incr in perilymph potassium due to parenteral, intravenous,
administration of 10 mg per kg, total of 50 mg per kg, of diuretic, ethacrynic acid, in 5 injections, over total of 48 hours, in 12 to 14 animals,
guinea pigs, pigmented, young, 200 to 400 g weight.
  (CT) Same method using normal saline equal in volume to ethacrynic acid

dosage in 12 to 14 guinea pigs, control group.
(AD) Suggested that cochleotoxic effects of ethacrynic acid result of
inhibition of cochlear duct membrane ATP. (ENG)

295
Hearing loss due to parenteral, intravenous, administration of 50 to 100 mg
of diuretic, ethacrynic acid, in humans with kidney disorder. (DAN)

303
Transient sensorineural hearing loss and tinnitus due to unspecified method
of administration of 300 mg of diuretic, (SQ) ethacrynic acid (SM), for first
24 hours in 1 human, adult, 22 years age, female, with preeclampsia during
pregnancy.
Transient sensorineural hearing loss and tinnitus due to unspecified method
of administration of 180 mg of diuretic, (SQ) furosemide (SM), for first 24
hours in 1 human, adult, 22 years age, female, with preeclampsia during
pregnancy.
Transient sensorineural hearing loss and tinnitus due to unspecified method
of administration of 100 mg of diuretic, (SQ) ethacrynic acid (SM), for 5
days in 1 human, adult, 22 years age, female, with preeclampsia during pregnancy.
Transient sensorineural hearing loss and tinnitus due to unspecified method
of administration of 80 mg of diuretic, (SQ) furosemide (SM), for 5 days in 1
human, adult, 22 years age, female, with preeclampsia during pregnancy.
(AD) Cochleotoxic effects confirmed by audiology. (ENG)

304
Possible hearing loss and vertigo due to diuretic, ethacrynic acid, in humans.
(AD) Discussion of chemistry, pharmacology, clinical use, and toxicity of
ethacrynic acid. (ENG)

320
Transient hearing loss after 3 days of treatment due to unspecified method of
administration of 50 mg twice daily of diuretic, ethacrynic acid, in 1 human,
adult, 56 years age, male, with rheumatic heart disorder and with normal
kidney function. (ENG)

339
Decr in potassium concentration and incr in sodium concentration of endolymph
within 10 minutes of treatment but no change in perilymph due to parenteral,
intravenous, administration of 1 to 5 mg per kg of diuretic, ethacrynic acid,
in 1 injection in 6 animals, dogs, young.
(CT) Study of potassium and sodium concentrations of endolymph and perilymph before injection of ethacrynic acid. (ENG)

373
Possible progressive sensorineural hearing loss due to antibiotics, aminogly-
coside, in humans.
Possible transient hearing loss due to high doses of salicylate, aspirin, in
humans.
Possible transient hearing loss due to high doses of antimalarial, quinine,
in humans.
Possible hearing loss due to diuretic, ethacrynic acid, in humans.
Bilateral sudden deafness due to antibiotic, kanamycin, in 4 humans, adult,
34 years average age, male and female.
(AD) Hearing loss due to ototoxic drugs usually progressive.
(AD) Sudden deafness due to ototoxic drugs possible in some cases, as in
humans with kidney disorder.
(AD) Literature review on etiology of sudden deafness. (ENG)

374
Decr in cochlear microphonic due to 4-300 mg per percent of solution of
diuretic, furosemide, in animals, guinea pigs.
Decr in cochlear microphonic due to 2-200 mg per percent of solution of
diuretic, ethacrynic acid, in animals, guinea pigs. (GER)

Usually transient hearing loss and no structural damage to organ of Corti,
stria vascularis, and spiral ganglion due to oral or topical administration
of salicylates in humans.
Hearing loss due to antimalarial, quinine, in humans.
Usually permanent hearing loss due to antimalarial, chloroquine, in humans.
Transient and permanent hearing loss and possible damage to hair cells of
organ of Corti due to diuretic, ethacrynic acid, in humans.
Sensorineural hearing loss due to cardiovascular agent, hexadimethrine
bromide, in humans with kidney disorder.
Sensorineural hearing loss and damage to organ of Corti due to topical ad-
ministration of antineoplastic, nitrogen mustard, in humans.
Sensorineural hearing loss due to high doses of antibiotic, chloramphenicol,
in humans.
Primary vestibular problems due to antibiotic, streptomycin, in humans.
Hearing loss due to high doses usually of antibiotic, streptomycin, in humans.
   (AD) Early detection of hearing loss by audiometry prevents permanent
   damage.
High frequency hearing loss and severe damage to outer hair cells and slight
damage to inner hair cells of organ of Corti due to antibiotic, kanamycin, in
humans.
Sensorineural hearing loss due to parenteral, oral, and topical administration of antibiotic, neomycin, in humans with or without kidney disorders.
Degeneration of hair cells of organ of Corti and of nerve process due to
antibiotics, aminoglycoside, in animals.
   (AD) Literature review of physiological and structural cochleo-vestibulotoxic effects of ototoxic drugs.
   (AD) Discussion of suggested mechanism of ototoxicity and routes of drugs
   to inner ear.
Bilateral sensorineural hearing loss due to oral administration of antibiotic, neomycin, in 4 of 8 humans with liver disease.
Bilateral sensorineural hearing loss due to oral administration of range of
doses of antibiotic, neomycin (SM), in 2 of 5 humans with liver disease.
Bilateral sensorineural hearing loss due to diuretics (SM), in 2 of 5 humans
with liver disease.
Transient progression of previous hearing loss due to parenteral, intravenous, administration of diuretic, ethacrynic acid (SM), in 1 injection in 1
of 5 humans with liver disease.
   (CT) Normal cochlear function in 6 humans, control group, with liver
   disease and not treated with neomycin or diuretics.
   (CT) Normal cochlear function in 13 humans, control group, with liver
   disease and treated with diuretics but not with neomycin.
   (AD) Hearing loss confirmed by audiometry.
   (AD) Reported that hearing loss due to neomycin or diuretics in humans
   with liver disease not related to dosage.
   (AD) Clinical study of effects of treatment with neomycin and diuretics in
   humans with liver disease.
Bilateral sensorineural hearing loss and vertigo due to antibiotic, ampicil-
lin, in 1 human, adolescent, 17 years age, female, with tonsillitis.
   (AD) Cited case report.
Severe sensorineural hearing loss and vertigo due to topical administration
in ear drops of antibiotic, framycetin, in 1 human, adult, 42 years age,
male, with previous slight high frequency hearing loss.
   (AD) Cited case report.
Atrophy of hair cells of organ of Corti and hearing loss due to antibiotic,
dihydrostreptomycin, in humans with tuberculous meningitis.
   (AD) Cited study.
Loss of inner hair cells and damage to outer hair cells due to 18 g of anti-
biotic, neomycin, for 18 days in 1 human.
   (AD) Cited case report.   (ENG)

                                                                    415
Transient and permanent hearing loss due to high doses of diuretic, etha-
crynic acid, in humans.
Transient hearing loss due to parenteral, intravenous, administration of high
doses, 600 to 1000 mg, of diuretic, furosemide, in humans with kidney disor-
ders.
   (AD) Literature review of clinical use and toxic effects of diuretics.
   (ENG)

457

Tinnitus and progressive sensorineural hearing loss due to parenteral, intramuscular, administration of antibiotic, (SQ) streptomycin, for 10 days in 1
human, adult, 38 years age, female, with infections and later development of
kidney disorder.
Tinnitus and progressive sensorineural hearing loss due to 13.2 g of antibiotic, (SQ) kanamycin, for 11 days in 1 human, adult, 38 years age, female,
with infections and kidney disorder.
Hearing loss due to antimalarial, (SQ) quinine, in 1 human, adult, 20 years
age, male, with various infections and later development of kidney disorder.
Hearing loss due to 400 mg 2 times daily, total dose of 6.5 g, of antibiotic,
(SQ) kanamycin (SM), for 8 days in 1 human, adult, 20 years age, male, with
various infections and later development of kidney disorder.
Hearing loss due to 150 mg 2 times daily, total dose of 2400 mg, of antibiotic, (SQ) colistin (SM), for 8 days in 1 human, adult, 20 years age, male,
with various infections and later development of kidney disorder.
Tinnitus, total bilateral hearing loss, and vestibular problems due to parenteral, intramuscular, administration of 4.0 g daily, total of 21 g, of antibiotic, (SQ) kanamycin (SM), for 5 days in 1 human, adult, 20 years age,
male, with infections and kidney disorder.
Tinnitus, total bilateral hearing loss, and vestibular problems due to 0.6 g
daily, total dose of 1.3 g, of antibiotic, (SQ) colistin (SM), for 2 days in
1 human, adult, 20 years age, male, with infections and kidney disorder.
Tinnitus, total bilateral hearing loss, and vestibular problems due to 2 g
and then 8 g per 24 hours in divided doses, total dose of 26.5 g, of antibiotic, (SQ) chloramphenicol, for 9 days in 1 human, adult, 20 years age, male,
with infections and kidney disorder.
Bilateral hearing loss due to 1 g daily of antibiotic, actinomycin (SM), for
5 days in 1 human, adult, 62 years age, male, with infections and kidney
disorder.
Bilateral hearing loss due to unknown dose of antibiotic, kanamycin (SM), for
5 days in 1 human, adult, 62 years age, male, with infections and kidney
disorder.
Bilateral hearing loss and vestibular problems due to parenteral administration of high doses of antibiotic, (SQ) neomycin, for total of 21 days in 1
human, adult, 25 years age, male, with infection from wound.
Previous administration of unspecified doses of antibiotic, (SQ) streptomycin, in 1 human, adult, 25 years age, male, with infection from wound.
Later administration of antibiotic, (SQ) chloramphenicol, in 1 human, adult,
25 years age, male, with infection from wound.
Tinnitus and rapidly progressive bilateral hearing loss due to parenteral,
intramuscular, administration of 0.5 g every 12 hours of antibiotic, (SQ)
streptomycin, for 5 days in 1 human, adult, 21 years age, male, with infection from wound.
Tinnitus and rapidly progressive bilateral hearing loss due to parenteral,
intramuscular, administration of 200 mg daily, total of 6.8 g, of antibiotic,
(SQ) colistin (SM), in 1 human, adult, 21 years age, male, with infection
from wound.
Tinnitus and rapidly progressive bilateral hearing loss due to parenteral
administration of unspecified doses of antibiotic, (SQ) neomycin (SM), for
about 35 days in 1 human, adult, 21 years age, male, with infection from
wound.
Tinnitus and progressive bilateral hearing loss due to parenteral administration of 2 l per 24 hours of 1 percent solution of antibiotic, (SQ) neomycin,
for 10 days in 1 human, adult, 26 years age, male, with infection from wound.
    (AD) Hearing loss confirmed by audiometry.
Previous administration of 500 mg four times a day of antibiotic, (SQ) ampicillin, in 1 human, adult, 26 years age, male, with infection from wound.
Bilateral sudden deafness due to administration in dialysis fluid of less
than 150 mg of antibiotic, neomycin (3M), in 1 human, adult, 44 years age,
female, with kidney disorder.
Bilateral sudden deafness due to 50 mg of diuretic, ethacrynic acid (SM), in
1 human, adult, 44 years age, female, with kidney disorder.
    (AD) Hearing loss confirmed by audiology.
Tinnitus and progressive bilateral hearing loss beginning after 8 days of
treatment due to parenteral administration of 1 l every 4 hours for 3 days

238   Ethacrynic acid

and then every 8 hours for 10 days of 1 percent solution of antibiotic,
neomycin, in 1 human, adult, 20 years age, male, with infection from wound.
     (AD) Hearing loss confirmed by audiology.
Tinnitus and bilateral sensorineural hearing loss due to parenteral, intramuscular, administration of 1 g and then 0.5 g every 12 hours of antibiotic,
streptomycin (SM), for 15 days in 1 human, adult, 23 years age, male, with
infection from wound.
Tinnitus and bilateral sensorineural hearing loss due to topical administration by irrigation of 1 percent solution every 12 hours of antibiotic, neomycin (SM), for 14 days in 1 human, adult, 23 years age, male, with infection
from wound.
     (AD) Hearing loss confirmed by audiometry.
     (AD) Discussion of 10 case reports.   (ENG)

                                                                       482
Decr in cochlear function and vestibular function due to parenteral, intramuscular, administration of 50 to 100 mg per kg of antibiotic, streptomycin
(streptomycin sulfate), for 35 days in animals, guinea pigs, pigmented, 400
to 500 g weight.
     (AD) More ototoxic effects with higher dosage.
Decr in cochlear function with both doses but decr in vestibular function
with only higher dose due to parenteral, intramuscular, administration of 50
to 100 mg per kg of antibiotic, dihydrostreptomycin (dihydrostreptomycin
sulfate), for 35 days in animals, guinea pigs, pigmented, 400 to 500 g
weight.
     (AD) More decr in cochlear function with higher dosage.
Decr in cochlear function in all animals but decr in vestibular function in 2
groups only due to parenteral, intramuscular, administration of 50 to 100 mg
per kg of antibiotic, kanamycin, for 35 days in animals, guinea pigs, pigmented, 400 to 500 g weight.
     (AD) More decr in cochlear function with higher dosage.
Decr in cochlear function due to parenteral, intramuscular, administration of
20 mg per kg of diuretic, ethacrynic acid, for 35 days in animals, guinea
pigs, pigmented, 400 to 500 g weight.
     (CT) Study of guinea pigs, control group, not treated with ototoxic drugs.
Decr in ototoxic effects due to parenteral, intramuscular, administration of
100 mg per kg of antibiotic, streptomycin (IB) (streptomycin sulfate), for 35
days in animals, guinea pigs, pigmented, 400 to 500 g weight, with administration of 1 mg per kg of various inhibitors.
Decr in ototoxic effects due to parenteral, intramuscular, administration of
100 mg per kg of antibiotic, dihydrostreptomycin (IB) (dihydrostreptomycin
sulfate), for 35 days in animals, guinea pigs, pigmented, 400 to 500 g
weight, with administration of 1 mg per kg of various inhibitors.
Decr in ototoxic effects due to parenteral, intramuscular, administration of
100 mg per kg of antibiotic, kanamycin (IB), for 35 days in animals, guinea
pigs, pigmented, 400 to 500 g weight, with administration of 1 mg per kg of
various inhibitors.
Decr in ototoxic effects due to parenteral, intramuscular, administration of
20 mg per kg of diuretic, ethacrynic acid (IB), for 35 days in animals,
guinea pigs, pigmented, 400 to 500 g weight, with administration of 1 mg per
kg of various inhibitors.
     (AD) Measurement of Preyer reflex and vestibular function tests.
Ototoxic effects, functional and structural, due to parenteral, intraperitoneal, administration of 100 mg per kg of antibiotic, streptomycin (streptomycin sulfate), for 50 days in animals, mice, male, 18 to 22 g weight.
No ototoxic effects due to parenteral, intraperitoneal, administration of 100
mg per kg of antibiotic, dihydrostreptomycin (dihydrostreptomycin sulfate),
for 50 days in animals, mice, male, 18 to 22 g weight.
Ototoxic effects, functional and structural, due to parenteral, intraperitoneal, administration of 100 mg per kg of antibiotic, kanamycin, for 50 days
in animals, mice, male, 18 to 22 g weight.
     (CT) Study of mice, control group, not treated with ototoxic drugs.
No ototoxic effects due to parenteral, intraperitoneal, administration of 100
mg per kg of antibiotic, streptomycin (IB) (streptomycin sulfate), for 50
days in animals, mice, male, 18 to 22 g weight, with administration of 1 mg
per kg of vitamin B.
No ototoxic effects due to parenteral, intraperitoneal, administration of 100
mg per kg of antibiotic, dihydrostreptomycin (IB) (dihydrostreptomycin sul-

fate), for 50 days in animals, mice, male, 18 to 22 g weight, with administration of 1 mg per kg of vitamin B.
No ototoxic effects due to parenteral, intraperitoneal, administration of 100
mg per kg of antibiotic, kanamycin (IB), for 50 days in animals, mice, male,
18 to 22 g weight, with administration of vitamin B.
   (AD) More ototoxic effects of aminoglycoside antibiotics in guinea pigs
   than in mice.
   (AD) Ototoxic effects of diuretic in guinea pigs. (IT)

                                                                         503
Transient hearing loss 30 minutes after injection and change in composition
of fluids of cochlea due to parenteral, intravenous, administration of 50 mg
of diuretic, ethacrynic acid, in 1 human, adult, 45 years age, female, with
kidney disorder. (FR)

                                                                         511
Transient severe sudden deafness due to 1 g of diuretic, (SQ) furosemide, in
1 human, Korean, adult, 26 years age, female, with lupus erythematosus.
Transient severe sudden deafness due to administration 2 months later of 100
mg of diuretic, (SQ) ethacrynic acid, in 1 human, Korean, adult, 26 years
age, female, with lupus erythematosus.
   (AD) Suggested that cochleotoxic effects related to potent diuretic action. (ENG)

                                                                         512
Transient bilateral sudden deafness due to parenteral, intravenous, administration of 50 mg of diuretic, (SQ) ethacrynic acid, in 1 human, adult, 42
years age, male, alcoholic, with liver disease.
Previous administration of 25 g of diuretic, (SQ) mannitol, in 1 human,
adult, 42 years age, male, alcoholic, with liver disease. (ENG)

                                                                         539
Transient unilateral or bilateral ototoxic effects, vestibular problems in
66.6 percent of cases, due to antibiotic, gentamicin, in 14 humans.
   (AD) Literature review showed small number of cases of gentamicin ototoxi-
   city reported in Germany.
   (AD) Primary factor in gentamicin ototoxicity is kidney disorder.
   (AD) Other factors in gentamicin ototoxicity include dosage and simul-
   taneous administration of other ototoxic drugs.
Hearing loss due to diuretic, ethacrynic acid, in humans with kidney disorder. (GER)

                                                                         547
Bilateral sensorineural hearing loss within 20 minutes but normal vestibular
function due to parenteral, intravenous, administration of 50 mg of diuretic,
ethacrynic acid (SM), in 1 injection in 1 human, adult, 53 years age, female,
with kidney disorder.
   (AD) Hearing loss confirmed by audiogram.
   (AD) Vestibular function tests showed normal vestibular function.
Simultaneous oral administration of 18 g of antibiotic, neomycin (SM), in 7
days in 1 human, adult, 53 years age, female, with kidney disorder.
Severe destruction of outer hair cells of organ of Corti in basal coil of
cochlea due to parenteral, intravenous, administration of 50 mg of diuretic,
ethacrynic acid (SM), in 1 injection in 1 human, adult, 53 years age, female,
with kidney disorder.
   (AD) Suggested that damage to hair cells possibly due to neomycin also.
   (AD) Suggested possible permanent hearing loss as result of ethacrynic
   acid treatment in patients with kidney disorders.
Transient and permanent total hearing loss within 15 minutes due to parenteral administration of diuretic, ethacrynic acid, in animals, cats. (ENG)

                                                                         559
Possible tinnitus and transient hearing loss due to diuretic, ethacrynic
acid, in humans.
   (AD) Literature review of use, action, and toxic effects of diuretics.
   (ENG)

628

Hearing loss due to parenteral, intravenous, administration of 1 mg per kg
initial dose and then 0.75 mg per kg every 6 hours, dissolved in 200 ml of 5
percent glucose solution, of antibiotic, (SQ) gentamicin (gentamicin sulfate), in 4 of 60 humans, child, adolescent, adult, and aged, 6 to 76 years
age, with carcinoma, lymphoma, or leukemia and with azotemia in 3 of 4 and
previous hearing loss in 1 of 4.
Hearing loss due to previous administration of diuretic, (SQ) ethacrynic
acid, in 1 of 4 humans with gentamicin hearing loss.
    (AD) Suggested that hearing loss in 1 patient due to both gentamicin and
    ethacrynic acid.   (ENG)

641

Possible damage to eighth cranial nerve due to antibiotic, capreomycin, in
humans.
Possible vestibular problems and hearing loss due to antibiotic, gentamicin,
in humans.
Possible delayed transient or permanent hearing loss due to antibiotic,
kanamycin (SM), in humans, in particular with kidney disorders or with simultaneous administration of ethacrynic acid.
Possible delayed transient or permanent hearing loss due to diuretic, ethacrynic acid (SM), in humans.
Possible delayed transient or permanent severe hearing loss due to oral,
parenteral, or topical administration of antibiotic, neomycin, in humans.
Possible damage to eighth cranial nerve, primarily hearing loss, due to
antibiotic, paromomycin, in humans.
Possible hearing loss due to antibiotic, rifampicin, in humans.
High risk of damage to eighth cranial nerve, primarily transient or permanent
vestibular problems but also hearing loss, due to antibiotic, streptomycin,
in humans.
Possible damage to eighth cranial nerve, primarily hearing loss, due to high
doses of antibiotic, vancomycin, for long period of more than 10 days in
humans, in particular with kidney disorders.
Risk of damage to eighth cranial nerve, vestibular problems and hearing loss,
due to high doses of antibiotic, viomycin, for long period of more than 10
days in humans, in particular with kidney disorders.
    (AD) Discussion of toxic effects of antibiotics.   (ENG)

660

Transient hearing loss, tinnitus, or vertigo due to diuretic, ethacrynic
acid, in humans.   (ENG)

706

Ototoxic effects due to chemical agents and heavy metals in humans.
    (AD) Literature review of ototoxic effects of nicotine, carbon monoxide,
    carbon tetrachloride, mercury, arsenic, and lead.
Cochleo-vestibulotoxic effects, functional and structural, due to antibiotics
in humans.
    (AD) Literature review of ototoxicity of streptomycin, dihydrostreptomy-
    cin, neomycin, kanamycin, gentamicin, capreomycin, rifampicin, viomycin,
    isoniazid, aminosidine, and framycetin.
Hearing loss due to salicylates in humans.
Hearing loss due to antimalarial, quinine, in humans.
Hearing loss due to diuretic, ethacrynic acid, in humans.
    (AD) Literature review of effects of various ototoxic agents.   (IT)

Furosemide

003

Transient sudden deafness, vertigo, and tinnitus due to parenteral, rapid
intravenous, administration of range of 800 to 3600 mg of diuretic, furosemide, for range of 9 hours to 6 days in 5 humans, adult, 37 to 64 years age,
male and female, with severe kidney disorder.   (ENG)

005

Transient primary decr in cochlear microphonic and action potential due to
parenteral, intravenous, administration of 10 mg per kg of diuretic, ethacrynic acid, in 1 injection in 20 animals, cats, adult.
Transient primary decr in cochlear microphonic and action potential due to

parenteral, intravenous, administration of 10 mg per kg of diuretic, furosemide, in 1 injection in 20 animals, cats, adult.
Delayed severe secondary decr in cochlear microphonic and action potential
due to parenteral, intravenous, administration of more than 10 mg per kg of
diuretic, ethacrynic acid, in animals, cats.
   (CT) Same method using 50 mg per kg and 100 mg per kg of diuretic, chlorothiazide, in cats, control group, showed no ototoxic effect.
Degeneration of outer hair cells of organ of Corti in basal and middle coils
of cochlea due to parenteral, intravenous, administration of 30 mg per kg of
diuretic, ethacrynic acid, in 1 injection in 2 animals, cats.
Degeneration of outer hair cells of organ of Corti due to parenteral, intramuscular, administration of 15 mg per kg of diuretic, ethacrynic acid, for 2
weeks in 1 animal, cat. (ENG)

038

Bilateral sensorineural hearing loss due to oral administration of 200 mg
twice a day of diuretic, (SQ) ethacrynic acid, for several weeks in 1 human,
adult, 40 years age, female, with kidney disorder.
Previous oral administration of 40 mg daily of diuretic, (SQ) furosemide
(SM), for unspecified period in 1 human, adult, 40 years age, female, with
kidney disorder.
Previous oral administration of 500 mg daily of diuretic, (SQ) chlorothiazide
(SM), for unspecified period in 1 human, adult, 40 years age, female, with
kidney disorder.
Sensorineural hearing loss and unsteady gait due to parenteral, intravenous,
administration of 200 mg of diuretic, (SQ) ethacrynic acid (SM), for unspeci-
fied period in 1 human, adult, 20 years age, female, with kidney disorder.
Simultaneous parenteral, intravenous, administration of 25 g of diuretic,
(SQ) mannitol (SM), for unspecified period in 1 human, adult, 20 years age,
female, with kidney disorder.
Previous administration of unspecified dose of chemical agent, (SQ) carbon
tetrachloride, for unspecified period in 1 human, adult, 20 years age, female, with kidney disorder.
Transient sensorineural hearing loss due to parenteral, intravenous, administration of 800 mg daily of diuretic, ethacrynic acid (SM), for unspecified
period in 1 human, adult, 25 years age, female, with chronic kidney disorder.
Simultaneous administration of unspecified doses of diuretic, chlorothiazide
(SM), for unspecified period in 1 human, adult, 25 years age, female, with
chronic kidney disorder.
Simultaneous administration of unspecified doses of diuretic, mannitol (SM),
for unspecified period in 1 human, adult, 25 years age, female, with chronic
kidney disorder.
Transient sensorineural hearing loss and dizziness due to parenteral, (SQ)
intravenous, administration of unspecified doses of diuretic, ethacrynic
acid, for unspecified period in 1 human, adult, 52 years age, female, with
kidney disorder.
Transient sensorineural hearing loss and dizziness due to (SQ) oral administration of 300 mg of diuretic, ethacrynic acid, for unspecified period in 1
human, adult, 52 years age, female, with kidney disorder.
Sensorineural hearing loss due to oral administration of 20 mg 3 times daily
of diuretic, ethacrynic acid, for 3 days in 1 human, adult, 28 years age,
male, with kidney disorder.
   (AD) Discussion of 5 case reports of ototoxic effects due to treatment
   with ethacrynic acid. (ENG)

054

Ototoxic effects due to diuretic, furosemide, in humans.
   (AD) Comment on need for audiology as documentation for reports of ototoxicity of furosemide. (ENG)

055

Transient bilateral sensorineural hearing loss and tinnitus due to parenteral, intravenous, administration of 100 mg of diuretic, (SQ) ethacrynic
acid, in 1 injection in 1 human, adult, 64 years age, male, with kidney
disorder.
   (CT) Pretreatment audiology showed no auditory system problems.
   (AD) Hearing loss 5 minutes after administration of ethacrynic acid.
Previous parenteral, intravenous, administration of unspecified doses of

diuretic, (SQ) furosemide, for unspecified period in 1 human, adult, 64 years
age, male, with kidney disorder.   (ENG)

                                                                          059

Bilateral sensorineural hearing loss due to oral administration of 0 to 12 g
daily, total of 2500 g, of antibiotic, neomycin, for 16 months in 1 human,
Caucasian, adult, 49 years age, female, chronic alcoholic, with hepatic
encephalopathy and normal kidney function.
Bilateral sensorineural hearing loss due to oral administration of 0 to 4 g
daily, total of 800 g, of antibiotic, (SQ) neomycin, for 21 months in 1
human, Caucasian, adult, 47 years age, female, chronic alcoholic, with hepatic encephalopathy and normal kidney function.
More severe sensorineural hearing loss due to oral administration of 6 g
daily, total of 111 g, of antibiotic, (SQ) paromomycin, for 9 months in 1
human, Caucasian, adult, 47 years age, female, chronic alcoholic, with hepatic encephalopathy and normal kidney function.
Sensorineural hearing loss due to oral administration of 0 to 12 g daily,
total of 1500 g, of antibiotic, neomycin, for 11 months in 1 human, Caucasian, adult, 39 years age, female, chronic alcoholic, with hepatic encephalopathy and some kidney disorder.
Sensorineural hearing loss in right ear due to oral administration of 3 to 4
g daily, total of 500 g, of antibiotic, (SQ) neomycin, for 8 months in 1
human, Caucasian, aged, 66 years age, female, with hepatic encephalopathy and
kidney disorder.
   (AD) Tinnitus and sudden deafness in left ear 27 years earlier.
Sensorineural hearing loss in right ear due to oral administration of total
of 240 g of antibiotic, (SQ) paromomycin, for long period in 1 human, Caucasian, aged, 66 years age, female, with hepatic encephalopathy and kidney
disorder.
Sequential administration of unspecified doses of diuretic, (SQ) furosemide,
for unspecified period in 1 human, Caucasian, aged, 66 years age, female,
with hepatic encephalopathy and kidney disorder.
Bilateral sensorineural hearing loss due to oral administration of 0 to 12 g
daily, total of 1000 to 1500 g, of antibiotic, (SQ) neomycin, for 28 months
in 1 human, Caucasian, adult, 60 years age, male, chronic alcoholic, with
hepatic encephalopathy and kidney disorder.
Bilateral sensorineural hearing loss due to oral administration of total of
300 g of antibiotic, (SQ) paromomycin, for long period in 1 human, Caucasian,
adult, 60 years age, male, chronic alcoholic, with hepatic encephalopathy and
kidney disorder.
Sequential administration of unspecified doses of (SQ) diuretics for unspecified period in 1 human, Caucasian, adult, 60 years age, male, chronic alcoholic, with hepatic encephalopathy and kidney disorder.
   (AD) Discussion of 5 case reports of hearing loss due to antibiotic therapy.
   (AD) Audiograms confirmed hearing loss in all cases.   (ENG)

                                                                          072

No reported ototoxic effects due to (SQ) oral administration of incr doses to
maximum of 3 g of diuretic, furosemide, for 10 days in 1 human, Puerto Rican,
adult, 32 years age, male, with kidney disorder.
Transient bilateral sensorineural hearing loss and dizziness due to parenteral, (SQ) intravenous, administration of 200 mg every 2 hours on first day
and 3 doses of 400 mg each on second day, total of 1.2 g, of diuretic, furosemide, for 2 days in 1 human, Puerto Rican, adult, 32 years age, male, with
kidney disorder.
   (AD) Hearing loss not confirmed by audiometry.   (ENG)

                                                                          124

Cochleo-vestibulotoxic effects due to diuretic, furosemide, in humans.
   (AD) Comment on use of audiology to confirm effects of ototoxic drugs.
   (AD) Explanation of previous study of furosemide without confirmation of
   ototoxic effects by audiology.   (ENG)

                                                                          151

Possible sensorineural hearing loss due to parenteral, intravenous, administration of high doses, 100 to 1000 mg, of diuretic, furosemide, for long
period in humans with kidney disorders.

(AD) Need for audiometry with clinical use of furosemide.
(AD) Recommended treatment with diuretics for long periods in humans with
kidney disorders only in severe cases with edema and cardiovascular system
problems.   (GER)

234

Transient sensorineural hearing loss due to parenteral, rapid intravenous,
administration of high dose, 1000 mg, of diuretic, furosemide, in 40 minutes
in humans with kidney disorder.
    (AD) Hearing loss confirmed by audiogram.   (GER)

278

Histochemical changes in cochlea due to parenteral administration of 15 mg
per kg daily of diuretic, furosemide, for 8 to 14 days in animals, guinea
pigs, 300 g weight.
Histochemical changes in cochlea due to parenteral administration of 8 mg per
kg daily of diuretic, acetazolamide, for 8 to 14 days in animals, guinea
pigs, 300 g weight.   (GER)

303

Transient sensorineural hearing loss and tinnitus due to unspecified method
of administration of 300 mg of diuretic, (SQ) ethacrynic acid (SM), for first
24 hours in 1 human, adult, 22 years age, female, with preeclampsia during
pregnancy.
Transient sensorineural hearing loss and tinnitus due to unspecified method
of administration of 180 mg of diuretic, (SQ) furosemide (SM), for first 24
hours in 1 human, adult, 22 years age, female, with preeclampsia during
pregnancy.
Transient sensorineural hearing loss and tinnitus due to unspecified method
of administration of 100 mg of diuretic, (SQ) ethacrynic acid (SM), for 5
days in 1 human, adult, 22 years age, female, with preeclampsia during pregnancy.
Transient sensorineural hearing loss and tinnitus due to unspecified method
of administration of 80 mg of diuretic, (SQ) furosemide (SM), for 5 days in 1
human, adult, 22 years age, female, with preeclampsia during pregnancy.
    (AD) Cochleotoxic effects confirmed by audiology.   (ENG)

313

Transient hearing loss and vestibular problems due to high doses, 1000 mg, of
diuretic, furosemide, for 40 minutes in humans with kidney disorder.   (ENG)

374

Decr in cochlear microphonic due to 4-300 mg per percent of solution of
diuretic, furosemide, in animals, guinea pigs.
Decr in cochlear microphonic due to 2-200 mg per percent of solution of
diuretic, ethacrynic acid, in animals, guinea pigs.   (GER)

414

Transient hearing loss in short time after injection due to parenteral,
intravenous, administration of (SQ) high doses, 500 mg each dose, of diuretic, (SQ) furosemide, in (SQ) total of 2 doses, each for duration of 3
minutes, on consecutive days in 1 human, adult, 49 years age, female, with
chronic kidney disorder.
    (AD) No observed hearing loss before treatment with furosemide.
    (AD) Normal hearing within 4 hours.
No hearing loss due to parenteral, intravenous, administration of (SQ) 240 mg
of diuretic, (SQ) furosemide, in (SQ) 1 dose for duration of 5 minutes in 1
human, adult, 49 years age, female, with chronic kidney disorder.
    (AD) Suggested that cochleotoxic effect of furosemide is dose related.
    (AD) Different individual responses to furosemide suggest other factors in
    ototoxic effects.
Previous administration of antibiotic, (SQ) nalidixic acid, in 1 human,
adult, 49 years age, female, with chronic kidney disorder.   (ENG)

415

Transient and permanent hearing loss due to high doses of diuretic, ethacrynic acid, in humans.
Transient hearing loss due to parenteral, intravenous, administration of high

doses, 600 to 1000 mg, of diuretic, furosemide, in humans with kidney disor-
ders.
   (AD) Literature review of clinical use and toxic effects of diuretics.
   (ENG)

                                                                      507

Bilateral sensorineural hearing loss and tinnitus due to parenteral, rapid
intravenous, administration of 240 mg of diuretic, furosemide, in 2 injections in 1 human, aged, 67 years age, male, after surgery.
   (AD) Hearing loss confirmed by audiogram. (ENG)

                                                                      511

Transient severe sudden deafness due to 1 g of diuretic, (SQ) furosemide, in
1 human, Korean, adult, 26 years age, female, with lupus erythematosus.
Transient severe sudden deafness due to administration 2 months later of 100
mg of diuretic, (SQ) ethacrynic acid, in 1 human, Korean, adult, 26 years
age, female, with lupus erythematosus.
   (AD) Suggested that cochleotoxic effects related to potent diuretic action. (ENG)

                                                                      513

Transient acute midfrequency hearing loss due to parenteral, rapid intra-
venous, administration of high doses, 1000 mg, of diuretic, furosemide, in 40
minutes in 8(50 percent) of 16 humans with kidney disorder.
   (CT) Audiometry, pretreatment and posttreatment.
   (AD) Maximum hearing loss in middle frequency suggests lesion in organ of
   Corti and not in CNS.
   (AD) Suggested that cochleotoxic effects related to rate of administration
   and dosage. (ENG)

                                                                      514

Transient tinnitus due to parenteral, intravenous, administration of high
doses, 100 to 3200 mg daily, progressive doses on successive days, of diuretic, (SQ) furosemide, in 30 minutes to 10 hours in some of 15 humans with
kidney disorder and on dialysis.
   (AD) Later study of 4 humans with tinnitus due to furosemide showed normal
   audiograms.
Previous parenteral, rapid intravenous, administration of total of 60 g of
diuretic, (SQ) mannitol, in 24 hours in 15 humans with kidney disorder and on
dialysis.
   (CT) Treatment of 13 humans, control group, with dialysis only.
   (AD) Prevention of depletion of sodium and potassium by monitoring fluid
   and electrolyte balance. (ENG)

                                                                      515

Bilateral hearing loss due to oral (SM) administration of 480 mg daily of
diuretic, furosemide (SM), for 10 days in 1 human with kidney disorder.
Bilateral hearing loss due to parenteral, intravenous (SM), administration of
600 mg daily of diuretic, furosemide (SM), for 10 days in 1 human with kidney
disorder.
Bilateral hearing loss due to 500 mg of antibiotic, kanamycin (SM) (kanamycin
sulfate), in 2 doses in 1 human with kidney disorder.
   (AD) No pretreatment audiogram.
   (AD) Posttreatment audiogram confirmed hearing loss.
   (AD) Suggested audiometry, pretreatment and during treatment, for humans,
   in particular with kidney disorder, treated with high doses of intravenous
   furosemide. (ENG)

                                                                      516

Possible ototoxic effects due to parenteral, intravenous, administration of
diuretic, furosemide, in less than every 4 hours in humans with kidney disorder. (ENG)

                                                                      517

Transient tinnitus and hearing loss due to parenteral administration of 2000
mg of diuretic, furosemide, in 30 minutes in humans with chronic kidney
disorder. (ENG)

625

No ototoxic effects due to oral administration of range of 40 mg daily to 8 mg twice a day, dosage increased at intervals until maximum diuretic response, of diuretic, furosemide, for range of 1 to over 45 weeks in 14 humans, adolescent, adult, and aged, 18 to 74 years age, male and female, with kidney disorder. (ENG)

HEAVY METALS

Arsenic

510

Changes in metabolism of inner ear due to heavy metal, arsenic, for chronic intoxication in animals, guinea pigs.   (GER)

Cobalt

299

Transient bilateral sensorineural hearing loss and dizziness due to 25 mg every other day, total of 18 g, of heavy metal, cobalt (cobalt chlorine), in 6 months in 1 human, adult, 35 years age, female, with kidney disorder and anemia.
   (AD) Cochleo-vestibulotoxic effects confirmed by audiometry and caloric
   tests.   (ENG)

Lead

034

Degeneration and demyelination of eighth cranial nerve due to parenteral, intraperitoneal, administration of 300 mg per kg of 1 percent solution of heavy metal, lead (lead acetate), for 1 time every 7 days for 7 weeks in 40 animals, guinea pigs, 300 to 350 g weight.
   (CT) Study of 10 guinea pigs, control group. (ENG)

078
122

Transient acute vertigo and nystagmus due to sufficient doses to produce 122 mcg per 100 ml blood level and 115 mcg per 24 hours urine level of heavy metal, lead, in 1 human, adult, 55 years age, male.
Transient acute vertigo and nystagmus due to oral ingestion of total of about 0.606 to 1.15 mg daily of heavy metal, lead, in 1 human, adult, 41 years age, male. (ENG)

467

Changes in succinic dehydrogenase of organ of Corti due to parenteral, subcutaneous, administration of 2 mg per kg of heavy metal, lead (lead acetate), for 28 days in 20 animals, guinea pigs.
   (CT) Study of 10 guinea pigs, control group.   (GER)

497

Primary damage to vestibular apparatus but also cochlear impairment due to chemical agent, carbon disulfide, in humans.
Primary damage to vestibular apparatus but also cochlear impairment due to chemical agent, carbon monoxide, in humans.
Primary damage to vestibular apparatus but also cochlear impairment due to heavy metal, lead, in humans.
Primary damage to vestibular apparatus but also cochlear impairment due to chemical agent, benzene, in humans.
Primary damage to vestibular apparatus but also cochlear impairment due to chemical agent, carbon tetrachloride, in humans.
   (AD) Report on cochleo-vestibulotoxic effects of chemical agents in industry.   (IT)

554

Possible damage to inner ear due to parenteral, intraperitoneal, administration of 500 mg per kg of heavy metal, lead (lead acetate), in acute intoxication in animals, guinea pigs.
Possible damage to inner ear due to parenteral, intraperitoneal, administration of 20 mg per kg 2 times per week of heavy metal, lead (lead acetate), in

chronic intoxication, over period of 4 to 6 weeks, in animals, guinea pigs.
(GER)

Lithium

691

Vertigo due to oral administration in tablets of 300 to 2400 mg daily of
heavy metal, lithium (lithium carbonate), for 1 to 30 months in some of 91
humans, adult and aged, 20 to 73 years age, male and female, with psychologi-
cal disorders. (ENG)

Mercury

167

Decr in concentrations of succinic dehydrogenase, esterases, and sulfhydryl
compounds due to parenteral, subcutaneous, administration of 1 mg per kg, in
1 ml distilled water, of heavy metal, mercury (mercuric chloride), for 28
days in animals, guinea pigs.
(CT) Study of guinea pigs, control group, not treated with mercury.
(AD) Report on relationship between changes in metabolism in inner ear due
to mercury and auditory system problems. (GER)

208

Hearing loss due to oral ingestion, in contaminated fish, of heavy metal,
mercury (organic methyl mercury), in humans.
(AD) Recommended international limit of 0.5 ppm of mercury (organic methyl
mercury) for humans.
(AD) Reported high levels of mercury (organic methyl mercury) in fetuses.
(ENG)

269

Vertigo due to heavy metal, mercury, in humans.
(AD) Report on vestibulotoxic effects of heavy metals in industry.
(AD) Vestibular problems confirmed by vestibular function tests. (JAP)

445

No specified ototoxic effects due to topical administration in (SQ) ointment
of sufficient dose, in 10 percent ammoniated ointment, to produce urine level
of 80 mcg per 100 mg of heavy metal, mercury, in 1 human, infant, 11 months
age, male, with skin rash.
Dizziness due to topical route, (SQ) inhalation, of about 0.17 mg per m, for
about 8 hours every night, of vapor concentration, sufficient to produce
urine level of 100 mcg per liter, of heavy metal, mercury, for long period in
1 human, child, 11 years age, male. (ENG)

465

Hearing loss, nystagmus, and vertigo due to heavy metal, mercury, organic, in
humans, adolescent, adult, and aged.
(AD) Auditory system problems confirmed by audiology and vestibular function tests. (JAP)

696

Dizziness due to heavy metal, mercury (inorganic mercury), in 1 month to 38
years exposure in 1 of 154 humans, adolescent and adult, 18 to 62 years age,
during work in industry.
(AD) Report on 10 years study of exposure to mercury (inorganic mercury).
(ENG)

Thorium dioxide

416

Delayed unilateral sensorineural hearing loss and vestibular problems detected 22 years after treatment due to heavy metal, thorium dioxide, in 1
human, adult, 36 years age when treated, female, during roentgenography.
Delayed tinnitus, unilateral sensorineural hearing loss, and damage to vestibular function detected 21 years after treatment due to heavy metal, thorium
dioxide, in 1 human, adult, 36 years age when treated, male, during roentgenography.

(AD) Cochleo-vestibulotoxic effects of thorium dioxide confirmed by audiology and vestibular function tests.
(AD) Case reports of delayed ototoxic effects of thorium dioxide. (ENG)

SEDATIVES AND TRANQUILIZERS

444

Changes in cochlear function and vestibular function due to analeptic, caffeine, in animals and humans.
Changes in cochlear function and vestibular function due to analeptic, amphetamine, in animals and humans.
Changes in cochlear function and vestibular function due to sedatives and
tranquilizers in animals and humans.
    (AD) Suggested mechanism of action of drugs.
    (AD) Literature review of ototoxic effects of drugs. (IT)

543

Transient decr in cochlear function due to tranquilizers in 44 humans.
    (AD) Auditory system problem detected by audiometry.
    (AD) Suggested transient cochleotoxic effect due to inhibition of reticu-
    lar formation by action of tranquilizers. (GER)

550

Decr in cochlear potentials due to parenteral, intraperitoneal, administration of 15 mg per kg of anesthetics (CB) in 2 groups of 15 animals, guinea
pigs, pigmented and albino, 300 g weight.
Decr in cochlear potentials due to parenteral, intraperitoneal, administration of 15 mg per kg of sedative, barbiturate (CB) in 2 groups of 15 animals,
guinea pigs, pigmented and albino, 300 g weight. (IT)

621

Primarily vestibular problems due to antibiotic, streptomycin, in humans.
Primarily hearing loss but also vestibular problems due to antibiotic, dihy-
drostreptomycin, in humans.
Primarily hearing loss but also vestibular problems due to antibiotic, kana-
mycin, in humans.
Primarily hearing loss but also vestibular problems due to antibiotic, neomy-
cin, in humans.
Primarily hearing loss but also vestibular problems due to antibiotic, genta-
micin, in humans.
Vertigo and ataxia due to antituberculous agent, isoniazid, in humans.
Hearing loss due to salicylate, aspirin, in humans.
Hearing loss and vertigo due to antimalarial, quinine, in humans.
Nystagmus due to barbiturates in humans.
Vestibular problems due to analgesic, morphine, in humans.
Nystagmus due to sedative, alcohol, in humans.
Nystagmus and hearing loss due to chemical agent, carbon monoxide, in humans.
Ototoxic effects due to antineoplastic, nitrogen mustard, in humans.
Ototoxic effects due to chemical agent, aniline, in humans.
Ototoxic effects due to chemical agent, tobacco, in humans.
Nystagmus due to chemical agent, nicotine, in humans.
Vestibular problems due to anticonvulsants in humans.
Vestibular problems due to anesthetics in humans.
Vestibular problems due to diuretics in humans.
    (AD) Inclusion of comprehensive list of ototoxic agents. (SP)

Alcohol

026

Hearing loss in speech range due to sedative, alcohol, ethyl, in 145 humans.
    (AD) Total of 200 tests conducted. (GER)

114

Vestibulotoxic effects due to oral ingestion of large amounts of sedative,
alcohol, ethyl, in humans.
    (AD) Effects of alcohol on vestibular apparatus determined by duration of
    nystagmus. (GER)

153

Less severe effects on vestibular apparatus due to oral ingestion of 80-proof
and 100-proof concentrations of sedative, alcohol, ethyl, in 4 humans, adult,
27 to 50 years age, male, with bilateral vestibular problems.
    (AD) Same test procedures used in previous study of normal subjects showed
    more severe effects of alcohol on vestibular apparatus.
    (AD) Subjects with vestibular problems less vulnerable to effects of
    alcohol than normal subjects.   (ENG)

172

Vertigo due to sedative, alcohol, ethyl, in humans.
Vertigo due to antibiotic, streptomycin, in humans.
    (AD) Report on etiology of vertigo.   (GER)

220

Significant effect on auditory time perception due to parenteral administration of 0.75 cc, in 500 cc normal saline, of 95 percent solution of sedative,
alcohol, ethyl, in humans, adolescent and adult, 18 to 38 years age, male and
female.
    (CT) Same method using 500 cc of normal saline in subjects, control group.
    (ENG)

248

Effect on vestibular threshold due to sedative, alcohol, ethyl, in humans.
    (CT)   Pretreatment and posttreatment vestibular function tests.   (ENG)

262

Possible damage to vestibular apparatus and organ of Corti due to oral ingestion of large amounts of chemical agent, alcohol, ethyl, for long period in 8
humans, adult and aged, 44 to 75 years age, male and female, chronic alcoholics.
    (AD) Report on results of temporal bone study.
    (AD) Previous observations of transient hearing loss and tinnitus during
    alcohol intoxication.
    (AD) Need for more study for interpretation of results.   (ENG)

463

Nystagmus due to oral ingestion of 50 to 340 cc (0.44 to 2.58 g per kg) of 40
or 45 proof concentration of sedative, alcohol, ethyl, in 20 or 25 minutes in
38 humans, adult, 19 to 42 years age, male and female, 55 to 70 kg weight.
    (AD) Vestibular problems confirmed by vestibular function tests.
    (AD) Discussion of individual differences in responses to ethyl alcohol.
    (FR)

508

High frequency and low amplitude nystagmus due to sedative, alcohol, ethyl,
in humans.
    (AD) Study of effects of alcohol on vertigo and nystagmus.   (ENG)

526

Decr in perilymph activity and slower permeation of NA-24 sodium isotope into
perilymph due to parenteral, intraperitoneal, administration of doses, corresponding to 1.4 g of 100 percent alcohol per 1 kg body weight, of 10 percent
concentration of sedative, alcohol, ethyl, in 1 injection in 40 animals,
guinea pigs, adult, with intraperitoneal administration of NA-24 sodium
isotope.
    (CT) Same method with administration of NA-24 sodium isotope only in 13
    guinea pigs, control group.   (ENG)

527

Decr in vestibular neurons due to parenteral, slow intravenous, administration of low doses, corresponding to 0.6 g per kg of 100 percent alcohol, of
diluted 30 percent concentration of sedative, alcohol, ethyl, in 1 injection
in animals, cats, adult, male and female, 3.0 kg weight.
    (AD) Suggested susceptibility of vestibular neurons to direct effects of
    alcohol.
    (AD) Suggested that clinical alcoholic intoxication, with nystagmus, due
    to direct action of alcohol on vestibular neurons.   (ENG)

572

Effect on vestibular function due to oral administration of 2.0 ml per kg, in
orange juice, of 100-proof of sedative, alcohol, ethyl, in 30 minutes in 10
humans.
   (CT) Same method using beverage without alcohol in subjects, control
  group.
   (AD) Study of effect of alcohol ingestion on human performance in static
  situations and during motion.
   (AD) Tests of visuomotor skill during angular acceleration, pretreatment
  and 1 to 10 hours posttreatment. (ENG)

604

Decr in middle ear muscle reflex due to oral administration of amount to
produce blood levels of 0.02 to 0.15 percent of sedative, alcohol, ethyl, in
9 humans, adult, 21 to 24 years age, with normal pure tone audiograms.
Decr in middle ear muscle reflex due to oral administration of 1.5 to 4.3 mg
per kg of sedative, pentobarbital (pentobarbital sodium), in 6 humans, adult,
21 to 24 years age, with normal pure tone audiograms.
   (AD) More risk of noise induced hearing loss due to decr in middle ear
  muscle reflex. (ENG)

621

Primarily vestibular problems due to antibiotic, streptomycin, in humans.
Primarily hearing loss but also vestibular problems due to antibiotic, dihy-
drostreptomycin, in humans.
Primarily hearing loss but also vestibular problems due to antibiotic, kana-
mycin, in humans.
Primarily hearing loss but also vestibular problems due to antibiotic, neomy-
cin, in humans.
Primarily hearing loss but also vestibular problems due to antibiotic, genta-
micin, in humans.
Vertigo and ataxia due to antituberculous agent, isoniazid, in humans.
Hearing loss due to salicylate, aspirin, in humans.
Hearing loss and vertigo due to antimalarial, quinine, in humans.
Nystagmus due to barbiturates in humans.
Vestibular problems due to analgesic, morphine, in humans.
Nystagmus due to sedative, alcohol, in humans.
Nystagmus and hearing loss due to chemical agent, carbon monoxide, in humans.
Ototoxic effects due to antineoplastic, nitrogen mustard, in humans.
Ototoxic effects due to chemical agent, aniline, in humans.
Ototoxic effects due to chemical agent, tobacco, in humans.
Nystagmus due to chemical agent, nicotine, in humans.
Vestibular problems due to anticonvulsants in humans.
Vestibular problems due to anesthetics in humans.
Vestibular problems due to diuretics in humans.
   (AD) Inclusion of comprehensive list of ototoxic agents. (SP)

627

Sensorineural hearing loss and vestibular problems due to parenteral, oral,
and topical administration of antibiotics in humans with and without kidney
disorder.
Degeneration of cochlea due to parenteral, intratympanic, administration of
antibiotic, neomycin, in animals, guinea pigs.
Transient sensorineural hearing loss due to high doses of salicylates in
humans.
Sensorineural hearing loss due to antimalarial, quinine, in humans.
Sensorineural hearing loss due to chemical agent, tobacco, in humans.
Sensorineural hearing loss due to sedative, alcohol, in humans.
   (AD) Discussion of ototoxicity of various drugs as 1 etiology of sen-
  sorineural hearing loss in adults. (ENG)

703

No nystagmus due to parenteral, intramuscular, administration of 0.150 mg of
analgesic, fentanyl, in 5 animals, rabbits, 2.5 to 3 kg weight.
Positional nystagmus within 15 to 30 minutes due to parenteral administration
of 4 ml per kg of 96 percent solution of sedative, alcohol, in 8 animals,
rabbits, 2.5 to 3 kg weight.
Positional nystagmus within 15 to 30 minutes due to parenteral administration

of 4 ml per kg of 96 percent solution of sedative, (SQ) alcohol, in 11 animals, rabbits, 2.5 to 3 kg weight.
Partial or total suppression of positional nystagmus due to parenteral,
intramuscular, administration of 0.150 mg of analgesic, (SQ) fentanyl, in 6
of 11 animals, rabbits, 2.5 to 3 kg weight.
Decr in positional nystagmus due to parenteral, intramuscular, administration
of 0.08 to 0.10 mg of analgesic, (SQ) fentanyl, in 5 of 11 animals, rabbits,
2.5 to 3 kg weight.   (IT)

                                                                          710
Effect on vestibular function due to sedative, alcohol, ethyl, in humans.
(ENG)

                                                                          716
Damage to cochlear function due to oral ingestion of amount to produce blood
levels of 0.8 to more than 1.0 percent of sedative, alcohol, ethyl, in acute
intoxication in humans.
    (AD) Study of the effects of alcohol on cochlear function.   (GER)

                                Droperidol

                                                                          265
Hearing loss due to analgesic, fentanyl (SM), in humans, treated before
ultrasound therapy for Meniere's disease.
Hearing loss due to tranquilizer, droperidol (SM), in humans, treated before
ultrasound therapy for Meniere's disease.
    (AD) More severe hearing loss with simultaneous use of droperidol and
    fentanyl than with use of local anesthetic only.   (ENG)

                                                                          310
Transient decr in vestibular function due to parenteral, intravenous, administration of 2 ml of tranquilizer, droperidol (CB), for 2 minutes in 18 of 21
humans, adolescent and adult, female and male.
Transient decr in vestibular function due to parenteral, intravenous, administration of 2 ml of analgesic, fentanyl (CB) (fentanyl citrate), for 2
minutes in 18 of 21 humans, adolescent and adult, female and male.
    (CT) Caloric tests, pretreatment and posttreatment.   (DAN)

                               Pentobarbital

                                                                          604
Decr in middle ear muscle reflex due to oral administration of amount to
produce blood levels of 0.02 to 0.15 percent of sedative, alcohol, ethyl, in
9 humans, adult, 21 to 24 years age, with normal pure tone audiograms.
Decr in middle ear muscle reflex due to oral administration of 1.5 to 4.3 mg
per kg of sedative, pentobarbital (pentobarbital sodium), in 6 humans, adult,
21 to 24 years age, with normal pure tone audiograms.
    (AD) More risk of noise induced hearing loss due to decr in middle ear
    muscle reflex.   (ENG)

                                Thalidomide

                                                                          661
Hearing loss in fetus due to sedative, thalidomide, in humans, female,
treated during pregnancy.   (GER)

                                                                          695
Hearing loss in fetus due to sedative, thalidomide, in humans, female,
treated during pregnancy.
    (AD) Congenital hearing loss in 5 of 34 humans, child, of mothers treated
    with thalidomide during pregnancy.   (ENG)

                        MISCELLANEOUS CHEMICAL AGENTS

                                                                          177
Sensorineural hearing loss due to topical route, inhalation, of chemical
agents, nitro and amino compounds, in humans from exposure in chemical industry.

(AD) Hearing loss confirmed by audiology. (POL)

219

Cochleo-vestibulotoxic effects due to antibiotics in humans.
Transient and permanent sensorineural hearing loss due to diuretic, etha-
crynic acid, in humans.
Transient sensorineural hearing loss, tinnitus, and vertigo due to salicy-
late, aspirin, in humans.
Transient and permanent sensorineural hearing loss and dizziness due to
antimalarial, quinine, in humans.
Sensorineural hearing loss due to antimalarial, chloroquine, in humans.
Sensorineural hearing loss, tinnitus, and vertigo due to chemical agents in
humans.
  (AD) Literature review of ototoxic drugs with clinical and histopathologi-
  cal correlations.
  (AD) Comment on ototoxicity of some chemical agents.
  (AD) Review of theories of mechanism of action of ototoxic drugs. (ENG)

532

Damage to vestibular apparatus due to chemical agent, nitro solvent, in 1
human.
  (AD) Vestibular problem confirmed by vestibular function test. (POL)

597

Hearing loss due to salicylates in humans.
Hearing loss due to antimalarial, quinine, in humans.
Hearing loss due to antibiotic, streptomycin, in humans.
Tinnitus due to chemical agent, camphor, in humans.
Tinnitus due to chemical agent, tobacco, in humans.
Tinnitus due to cardiovascular agent, quinidine, in humans.
Tinnitus due to chemical agent, ergot, in humans.
Tinnitus due to chemical agent, alcohol, methyl, in humans.
  (AD) Discussion of toxic effects of drugs. (ENG)

706

Ototoxic effects due to chemical agents and heavy metals in humans.
  (AD) Literature review of ototoxic effects of nicotine, carbon monoxide,
  carbon tetrachloride, mercury, arsenic, and lead.
Cochleo-vestibulotoxic effects, functional and structural, due to antibiotics
in humans.
  (AD) Literature review of ototoxicity of streptomycin, dihydrostreptomy-
  cin, neomycin, kanamycin, gentamicin, capreomycin, rifampicin, viomycin,
  isoniazid, aminosidine, and framycetin.
Hearing loss due to salicylates in humans.
Hearing loss due to antimalarial, quinine, in humans.
Hearing loss due to diuretic, ethacrynic acid, in humans.
  (AD) Literature review of effects of various ototoxic agents. (IT)

6-Aminonicotinic acid

719

Progressive severe degeneration primarily in organ of Corti beginning after
24 hours but also damage to spiral ganglion and effect on cochlear function
due to parenteral, intraperitoneal, administration of 10 or 20 mg per kg of
chemical agent, 6-aminonicotinic acid, in animals, mice, audiogenic seizure-
susceptible.
Decr in ototoxic effects due to parenteral, intraperitoneal, administration
of 10 mg per kg of chemical agent, 6-aminonicotinic acid, in animals, mice,
audiogenic seizure-susceptible, with administration 5 minutes previously of
10 mg per kg of nicotinamide. (ENG)

720

Damage to cochlear function and progressive severe degeneration in cochlear
duct, beginning after 24 hours in spiral ligament, with severe damage to
organ of Corti, and with later atrophy of spiral ganglion due to parenteral,
intraperitoneal, administration of 20 mg per kg, in concentration of 2 mg per
ml sterile water, of chemical agent, 6-aminonicotinic acid, in 1 injection in
9 animals, mice, male, audiogenic seizure-susceptible.

(CT) Same method using water in 3 mice, control group.
(CT) Same method using 2 mice, chronic control group, not treated.
Damage to cochlear function and degeneration in cochlea due to parenteral,
intraperitoneal, administration of 20 mg per kg of chemical agent, 6-aminoni-
cotinic acid, in 6 animals, mice, not audiogenic seizure-susceptible.
   (CT) Same method using water in 2 mice, control group, showed no histological changes. (ENG)

730

Damage to cochlear function due to parenteral, intraperitoneal, administration of 20, 10, or 5 mg per kg, in concentration of 2 mg per ml of sterile
distilled water, of chemical agent, 6-aminonicotinic acid, in 1 injection in
18 animals, mice, about 30 days age, male, audiogenic seizure-susceptible.
   (AD) More severe hearing loss in mice with higher doses of 6-aminonico-
tinic acid.
No damage to cochlear function due to parenteral, intraperitoneal, administration of 1 mg per kg, in concentration of 2 mg per ml of sterile distilled
water, of chemical agent, 6-aminonicotinic acid, in 1 injection in 4 animals,
mice, about 30 days age, male, audiogenic seizure-susceptible.
   (CT) Same method using intraperitoneal administration of same amount of
water in 8 mice, control group, showed no damage to cochlear function.
(ENG)

Aniline

621

Primarily vestibular problems due to antibiotic, streptomycin, in humans.
Primarily hearing loss but also vestibular problems due to antibiotic, dihy-
drostreptomycin, in humans.
Primarily hearing loss but also vestibular problems due to antibiotic, kana-
mycin, in humans.
Primarily hearing loss but also vestibular problems due to antibiotic, neomy-
cin, in humans.
Primarily hearing loss but also vestibular problems due to antibiotic, genta-
micin, in humans.
Vertigo and ataxia due to antituberculous agent, isoniazid, in humans.
Hearing loss due to salicylate, aspirin, in humans.
Hearing loss and vertigo due to antimalarial, quinine, in humans.
Nystagmus due to barbiturates in humans.
Vestibular problems due to analgesic, morphine, in humans.
Nystagmus due to sedative, alcohol, in humans.
Nystagmus and hearing loss due to chemical agent, carbon monoxide, in humans.
Ototoxic effects due to antineoplastic, nitrogen mustard, in humans.
Ototoxic effects due to chemical agent, aniline, in humans.
Ototoxic effects due to chemical agent, tobacco, in humans.
Nystagmus due to chemical agent, nicotine, in humans.
Vestibular problems due to anticonvulsants in humans.
Vestibular problems due to anesthetics in humans.
Vestibular problems due to diuretics in humans.
   (AD) Inclusion of comprehensive list of ototoxic agents. (SP)

Benzene

497

Primary damage to vestibular apparatus but also cochlear impairment due to
chemical agent, carbon disulfide, in humans.
Primary damage to vestibular apparatus but also cochlear impairment due to
chemical agent, carbon monoxide, in humans.
Primary damage to vestibular apparatus but also cochlear impairment due to
heavy metal, lead, in humans.
Primary damage to vestibular apparatus but also cochlear impairment due to
chemical agent, benzene, in humans.
Primary damage to vestibular apparatus but also cochlear impairment due to
chemical agent, carbon tetrachloride, in humans.
   (AD) Report on cochleo-vestibulotoxic effects of chemical agents in industry. (IT)

Carbon disulfide

228

Hearing loss due to topical route, inhalation, of chemical agent, carbon
disulfide, for long period in humans in industry. (SER)

497

Primary damage to vestibular apparatus but also cochlear impairment due to
chemical agent, carbon disulfide, in humans.
Primary damage to vestibular apparatus but also cochlear impairment due to
chemical agent, carbon monoxide, in humans.
Primary damage to vestibular apparatus but also cochlear impairment due to
heavy metal, lead, in humans.
Primary damage to vestibular apparatus but also cochlear impairment due to
chemical agent, benzene, in humans.
Primary damage to vestibular apparatus but also cochlear impairment due to
chemical agent, carbon tetrachloride, in humans.
    (AD) Report on cochleo-vestibulotoxic effects of chemical agents in indus-
    try. (IT)

718

Dizziness, nystagmus, and high frequency hearing loss due to chemical agent,
carbon disulfide, in chronic intoxication in humans working in industry.
    (AD) Audiograms showed decr in higher frequencies.
    (AD) Literature review of effects of carbon disulfide. (GER)

Carbon monoxide

030

Hearing loss due to chemical agent, carbon monoxide, in humans.
    (AD) Studies with audiometry on patients with u-shaped audiograms. (GER)

033

Damage to organ of Corti due to topical route, inhalation, of chemical agent,
carbon monoxide, in 40 exposures in 5 animals, rabbits. (GER)

162

Permanent unilateral sensorineural hearing loss due to topical route, inhalation, of chemical agent, carbon monoxide, in acute intoxication in 1 human.
    (AD) Hearing loss confirmed by audiogram. (POL)

163

Sensorineural hearing loss due to topical route, inhalation, of chemical
agent, carbon monoxide, in humans.
    (AD) Literature review on carbon monoxide poisoning. (POL)

180

Bilateral sensorineural hearing loss with partial improvement due to topical
route, inhalation, of large amounts, to produce carboxy-hemoglobin level of
25 percent of total hemoglobin, of chemical agent, carbon monoxide, in 1
human, adult, 22 years age, male, with previous high intensity noise exposure.
    (AD) Hearing loss confirmed by audiometry but vestibular function tests
    normal.
    (AD) Suggested that audiometric configuration not type due to acoustic
    trauma. (ENG)

186

Diplacusis due to antibiotics, aminoglycoside, in humans.
Diplacusis due to antimalarial, quinine, in humans.
Diplacusis due to salicylate, aspirin, in humans.
Diplacusis due to chemical agent, carbon monoxide, in humans.
    (AD) Report on etiology of diplacusis with comment on ototoxic drugs.
    (ENG)

209

Slight incr but no decr in auditory flutter fusion threshold due to topical

route, inhalation, of 250 ml in 500 l air, to produce concentration of 10
percent carboxyhemoglobin in blood, of chemical agent, carbon monoxide, for
65 minutes at intervals of 7 days in 8 humans, adult, 23 to 48 years age,
male, healthy, 7 without smoking habit.
   (CT) For period before test, 8 subjects had no caffeine, alcohol, drugs,
   or nicotine.
   (CT) Study with oral administration of 100 mg phenobarbitone and placebo
   to determine response of same subjects to drug with known effects.
   (AD) Subjects tested with interrupted white noise.   (ENG)

                                                                        224
Slight sensorineural hearing loss due to topical route, inhalation, of large
amount, to produce high carboxyhemoglobin level of 36 percent 1.5 days after
exposure, of chemical agent, carbon monoxide, in 1 human, adult, 21 years
age, male.
Moderate bilateral sensorineural hearing loss due to topical route, inhalation, of large amount, to produce high carboxyhemoglobin level of 48 percent
1.5 days after exposure, of chemical agent, carbon monoxide, in 1 human,
adolescent, 18 years age, male.   (ENG)

                                                                        233
Vestibular problems due to topical route, inhalation, of large amount, to
produce average carboxyhemoglobin level of 60 ml per l, of chemical agent,
carbon monoxide, in 20 humans, adult, 30 years average age.
   (AD) Vestibular problems determined by vestibular function tests.   (FR)

                                                                        423
More severe and more rapid progression of presbycusis due to antimalarial,
quinine, in humans, adult and aged.
More severe and more rapid progression of presbycusis due to antibiotics,
aminoglycoside, in humans, adult and aged.
More severe and more rapid progression of presbycusis due to salicylate,
aspirin, in humans, adult and aged.
More severe and more rapid progression of presbycusis due to chemical agent,
carbon monoxide, in humans, adult and aged.
   (AD) Discussion of factors resulting in more severe and more rapid progression of presbycusis.   (FR)

                                                                        436
Hearing loss and damage to organ of Corti due to topical route, inhalation,
of chemical agent, carbon monoxide, in animals.   (GER)

                                                                        472
Vertigo due to topical route, inhalation, of chemical agent, carbon monoxide,
in humans, adult.   (RUS)

                                                                        497
Primary damage to vestibular apparatus but also cochlear impairment due to
chemical agent, carbon disulfide, in humans.
Primary damage to vestibular apparatus but also cochlear impairment due to
chemical agent, carbon monoxide, in humans.
Primary damage to vestibular apparatus but also cochlear impairment due to
heavy metal, lead, in humans.
Primary damage to vestibular apparatus but also cochlear impairment due to
chemical agent, benzene, in humans.
Primary damage to vestibular apparatus but also cochlear impairment due to
chemical agent, carbon tetrachloride, in humans.
   (AD) Report on cochleo-vestibulotoxic effects of chemical agents in industry.   (IT)

                                                                        621
Primarily vestibular problems due to antibiotic, streptomycin, in humans.
Primarily hearing loss but also vestibular problems due to antibiotic, dihy-
drostreptomycin, in humans.
Primarily hearing loss but also vestibular problems due to antibiotic, kana-
mycin, in humans.
Primarily hearing loss but also vestibular problems due to antibiotic, neomy-
cin, in humans.

Primarily hearing loss but also vestibular problems due to antibiotic, genta-
micin, in humans.
Vertigo and ataxia due to antituberculous agent, isoniazid, in humans.
Hearing loss due to salicylate, aspirin, in humans.
Hearing loss and vertigo due to antimalarial, quinine, in humans.
Nystagmus due to barbiturates in humans.
Vestibular problems due to analgesic, morphine, in humans.
Nystagmus due to sedative, alcohol, in humans.
Nystagmus and hearing loss due to chemical agent, carbon monoxide, in humans.
Ototoxic effects due to antineoplastic, nitrogen mustard, in humans.
Ototoxic effects due to chemical agent, aniline, in humans.
Ototoxic effects due to chemical agent, tobacco, in humans.
Nystagmus due to chemical agent, nicotine, in humans.
Vestibular problems due to anticonvulsants in humans.
Vestibular problems due to anesthetics in humans.
Vestibular problems due to diuretics in humans.
   (AD) Inclusion of comprehensive list of ototoxic agents.   (SP)

                                                                   673

Dizziness and decr in cochlear function due to topical route, inhalation, of
large amounts to produce 20 to 30 percent carboxyhemoglobin of chemical
agent, carbon monoxide, in humans.   (ENG)

Carbon tetrachloride

                                                                   038

Bilateral sensorineural hearing loss due to oral administration of 200 mg
twice a day of diuretic, (SQ) ethacrynic acid, for several weeks in 1 human,
adult, 40 years age, female, with kidney disorder.
Previous oral administration of 40 mg daily of diuretic, (SQ) furosemide
(SM), for unspecified period in 1 human, adult, 40 years age, female, with
kidney disorder.
Previous oral administration of 500 mg daily of diuretic, (SQ) chlorothiazide
(SM), for unspecified period in 1 human, adult, 40 years age, female, with
kidney disorder.
Sensorineural hearing loss and unsteady gait due to parenteral, intravenous,
administration of 200 mg of diuretic, (SQ) ethacrynic acid (SM), for unspeci-
fied period in 1 human, adult, 20 years age, female, with kidney disorder.
Simultaneous parenteral, intravenous, administration of 25 g of diuretic,
(SQ) mannitol (SM), for unspecified period in 1 human, adult, 20 years age,
female, with kidney disorder.
Previous administration of unspecified dose of chemical agent, (SQ) carbon
tetrachloride, for unspecified period in 1 human, adult, 20 years age, female, with kidney disorder.
Transient sensorineural hearing loss due to parenteral, intravenous, administration of 800 mg daily of diuretic, ethacrynic acid (SM), for unspecified
period in 1 human, adult, 25 years age, female, with chronic kidney disorder.
Simultaneous administration of unspecified doses of diuretic, chlorothiazide
(SM), for unspecified period in 1 human, adult, 25 years age, female, with
chronic kidney disorder.
Simultaneous administration of unspecified doses of diuretic, mannitol (SM),
for unspecified period in 1 human, adult, 25 years age, female, with chronic
kidney disorder.
Transient sensorineural hearing loss and dizziness due to parenteral, (SQ)
intravenous, administration of unspecified doses of diuretic, ethacrynic
acid, for unspecified period in 1 human, adult, 52 years age, female, with
kidney disorder.
Transient sensorineural hearing loss and dizziness due to (SQ) oral administration of 300 mg of diuretic, ethacrynic acid, for unspecified period in 1
human, adult, 52 years age, female, with kidney disorder.
Sensorineural hearing loss due to oral administration of 20 mg 3 times daily
of diuretic, ethacrynic acid, for 3 days in 1 human, adult, 28 years age,
male, with kidney disorder.
   (AD) Discussion of 5 case reports of ototoxic effects due to treatment
   with ethacrynic acid.   (ENG)

                                                                   230

Vestibular problems due to chemical agent, carbon tetrachloride, in humans.

(AD) Vestibular function tests conducted to determine effects of carbon
tetrachloride.   (RUS)

                                                                      497
Primary damage to vestibular apparatus but also cochlear impairment due to
chemical agent, carbon disulfide, in humans.
Primary damage to vestibular apparatus but also cochlear impairment due to
chemical agent, carbon monoxide, in humans.
Primary damage to vestibular apparatus but also cochlear impairment due to
heavy metal, lead, in humans.
Primary damage to vestibular apparatus but also cochlear impairment due to
chemical agent, benzene, in humans.
Primary damage to vestibular apparatus but also cochlear impairment due to
chemical agent, carbon tetrachloride, in humans.
    (AD) Report on cochleo-vestibulotoxic effects of chemical agents in indus-
    try.   (IT)

                          Chlorophenothane

                                                                      567
Effect on sensory hair cells in lateral line organ due to concentrations of 1
to 4 ppm, in aquaria containing 15 l of water, of chemical agent, chlorophenothane, for 18 hours at temperature of 22 to 23 degrees C in animals,
clawed toads, Xenopus laevis.
    (AD) Sensory hair cells of lateral line organ of toad comparable to hair
    cells in inner ear of higher vertebrates.   (ENG)

                              Cyanide

                                                                      372
Transient and permanent decr in cochlear microphonic, eighth nerve action
potential, and endocochlear potential due to topical administration, perfusion of scala tympani and scala vestibuli, with 50 mM in Ringer's solution of
chemical agent, cyanide (sodium cyanide), in animals, guinea pigs.
    (CT) Same method using modified Ringer's solution in guinea pigs, control
    group, showed gradual decr in cochlear microphonic and eighth nerve action
    potential but no change in endocochlear potential.
    (CT) Measurement of cochlear potentials, before, during, and after perfu-
    sion with cyanide (sodium cyanide).
    (AD) Study of effect of cyanide (sodium cyanide) in perilymph on cochlear
    potentials of guinea pigs.   (ENG)

                                                                      438
Suppression of microphonic potentials of saccule due to topical, intraluminal, administration of antibiotic, streptomycin, in animals, goldfish.
Suppression of microphonic potentials of saccule due to topical, intraluminal, administration of antibiotic, kanamycin, in animals, goldfish.
Suppression of microphonic potentials of saccule due to topical, intraluminal
or extraluminal, administration of 0.5 mg of chemical agent, cyanide, in
animals, goldfish.
Suppression of microphonic potentials of saccule due to topical, intraluminal
or extraluminal, administration of 0.1 mg of antimalarial, quinine, in animals, goldfish.
Suppression of microphonic potentials of saccule due to topical, intraluminal
or extraluminal, administration of 2 mg of anesthetic, procaine, in animals,
goldfish.
No effect on microphonic potentials of saccule due to topical administration
of salicylates in animals, goldfish.   (ENG)

                                                                      562
Decr in microphonic potential of saccule due to topical, intraluminal, administration of antibiotic, streptomycin, in animals, goldfish.
Decr in microphonic potential of saccule due to topical, intraluminal, administration of antibiotic, kanamycin, in animals, goldfish.
Permanent decr in microphonic potential of saccule due to topical, intraluminal or extraluminal, administration of 0.5 mg per ml of chemical agent,
cyanide, in animals, goldfish.
Permanent decr in microphonic potential of saccule due to topical, intralu-

minal or extraluminal, administration of 0.1 mg per ml of antimalarial,
quinine, in animals, goldfish.
No effect on microphonic potential of saccule due to salicylate, aspirin, in
animals, goldfish.
Some decr in microphonic potential of saccule due to 2 mg per ml of anesthetic, procaine, in animals, goldfish.
   (AD) Study of effects of various agents on microphonic potential of saccule of goldfish. (JAP)

563

Effect on cochlear microphonic due to topical administration of chemical
agent, cyanide, in animals, birds.
   (AD) Study of cochlear potentials of various birds. (GER)

566

Gradual decr in cochlear microphonics and decr in endocochlear potentials,
but not significant, due to salicylate, acetylsalicylic acid, in animals,
guinea pigs, 250 to 400 g weight.
Severe decr in cochlear potentials due to 2.0 mM of chemical agent, cyanide
(potassium cyanide), in animals, guinea pigs, 250 to 400 g weight.
   (AD) Study of effects of various agents on cochlear potentials. (ENG)

Dimethyl sulfoxide

134

Decr in threshold shift of 20 db and damage to outer hair cells and inner
hair cells of organ of Corti due to topical administration to external auditory meatus of 50 percent solution of chemical agent, dimethyl sulfoxide, for
21 days in 7 animals, cats.
Damage to 40 percent of eighth cranial nerve action potential due to topical
administration to external auditory meatus of chemical agent, dimethyl sulfoxide, for 6 hours in 4 animals, cats.
Damage to 60 percent of eighth cranial nerve action potential due to topical
administration to middle ear of chemical agent, dimethyl sulfoxide, for 6
hours in 4 animals, cats.
   (CT) Control group of 4 cats used.
   (AD) Suggested that dimethyl sulfoxide new ototoxic drug. (GER)

192

Sensorineural hearing loss, dizziness, vertigo, and nystagmus due to topical,
cutaneous, administration in ointment of 0.3 percent concentration of antibiotic, (SQ) neomycin, for 5 months in 1 human, Caucasian, child, 9 years
age, with dermatomyositis.
Sensorineural hearing loss, dizziness, vertigo, and nystagmus due to topical,
cutaneous, administration in ointment of 1 percent concentration of antibiotic, (SQ) neomycin (CB), for 2 months in 1 human, Caucasian, child, 9 years
age, with dermatomyositis.
Sensorineural hearing loss, dizziness, vertigo, and nystagmus due to topical,
cutaneous, administration in ointment of 11 percent concentration of chemical
agent, (SQ) dimethyl sulfoxide (CB), for 2 months in 1 human, Caucasian,
child, 9 years age, with dermatomyositis.
   (AD) Potentiation of cochleo-vestibulotoxic effects of neomycin as result
   of incr cutaneous absorption due to dimethyl sulfoxide.
   (AD) Hearing loss confirmed by audiogram. (ENG)

351

No observed ototoxic effects due to topical administration of 1 drop of
chemical agent, dimethyl sulfoxide (CB), in humans as anesthetic for myringotomy.
No observed ototoxic effects due to topical administration of 1 drop of
anesthetic, tetracaine (CB) (tetracaine hydrochloride), in humans as anesthetic for myringotomy. (ENG)

Dinitrophenol

405

Decr in cochlear potentials due to parenteral, intravenous, administration of
total dose of 5 to 35 mg per kg of solution of chemical agent, dinitrophenol,

in several doses in animals, cats, young, 1.0 to 1.8 kg weight, normal.
   (AD) Use of various intensities of test tone of 2 kcps.
More decr in cochlear potentials due to topical administration to round
window of 1 drop at a time of 3 concentrations, in order of increasing concentration, of chemical agent, dinitrophenol, in animals, cats, young, 1.0 to
1.8 kg weight, normal.
   (AD) Use of various intensities of test tone of 2 kcps.
   (CT) Measurement of cochlear potentials before and after administration of
   chemical agent, dinitrophenol.
   (CT) Measurement of cochlear potentials for longer than usual before
   administration of chemical agent, dinitrophenol, in some animals, control
   group.
   (CT) Higher frequency test tone of 5 kcps used in some animals, control
   group.
   (CT) Same method with administration of intravenous 2 percent solution of
   sodium bicarbonate with chemical agent, dinitrophenol, in cats, control
   group, resulted in no decr in cochlear potentials. (ENG)

406

Incr in cochlear potentials due to parenteral, intravenous, administration of
1 dose of 10 mg per kg and then doses of 5 mg per kg of chemical agent,
dinitrophenol, in total of 5 doses in animals, cats, with acoustic trauma.
   (AD) Use of low intensity test tone of 2 kcps.
Decr in cochlear potentials due to topical administration to round window of
1 drop at a time of various concentrations of chemical agent, dinitrophenol,
in animals, cats, with acoustic trauma.
   (AD) Use of low intensity test tone of 2 kcps.
   (AD) No consistent difference in effect on cochlear potentials of topical
   administration of chemical agent, dinitrophenol, in cats with and without
   acoustic trauma.
Decr in cochlear potentials due to parenteral, intravenous, administration of
1 dose of 5 mg per kg, followed by 1 dose of 10 mg per kg, followed by other
doses of 5 mg per kg of chemical agent, dinitrophenol, in total of 4 doses in
animals, cats, with acoustic trauma.
   (AD) Use of high intensity test tone of 2 kcps.
   (CT) Measurement of cochlear potentials for longer than usual before
   administration of chemical agent, dinitrophenol, in some animals, control
   group.
   (CT) Same method with administration of intravenous 2 percent solution of
   sodium bicarbonate with chemical agent, dinitrophenol, in cats, control
   group. (ENG)

Lysergide

722

Effect on reaction time to acoustic stimuli due to parenteral, intraperitoneal, administration of 0.16 and 0.04 mg per kg of chemical agent, lysergide, in 3 animals, rats, albino, about 120 days age, male, 300 g weight.
   (CT) Same method using 0.05 cc saline in rats, control group. (ENG)

Nicotine

115

Permanent cochleo-vestibulotoxic effects due to antibiotics, aminoglycoside,
in humans.
Transient cochlear impairment due to salicylates in humans.
Ototoxic effects due to antimalarial, quinine, in humans.
Ototoxic effects due to chemical agent, nicotine, in humans.
   (AD) Report on ototoxic effects of various drugs.
   (AD) Need for audiometry and vestibular function tests with clinical use
   of ototoxic drugs. (FR)

504

Ototoxic effects due to chemical agent, nicotine, in humans. (POL)

621

Primarily vestibular problems due to antibiotic, streptomycin, in humans.
Primarily hearing loss but also vestibular problems due to antibiotic, dihy-

drostreptomycin, in humans.
Primarily hearing loss but also vestibular problems due to antibiotic, kana-
mycin, in humans.
Primarily hearing loss but also vestibular problems due to antibiotic, neomy-
cin, in humans.
Primarily hearing loss but also vestibular problems due to antibiotic, genta-
micin, in humans.
Vertigo and ataxia due to antituberculous agent, isoniazid, in humans.
Hearing loss due to salicylate, aspirin, in humans.
Hearing loss and vertigo due to antimalarial, quinine, in humans.
Nystagmus due to barbiturates in humans.
Vestibular problems due to analgesic, morphine, in humans.
Nystagmus due to sedative, alcohol, in humans.
Nystagmus and hearing loss due to chemical agent, carbon monoxide, in humans.
Ototoxic effects due to antineoplastic, nitrogen mustard, in humans.
Ototoxic effects due to chemical agent, aniline, in humans.
Ototoxic effects due to chemical agent, tobacco, in humans.
Nystagmus due to chemical agent, nicotine, in humans.
Vestibular problems due to anticonvulsants in humans.
Vestibular problems due to anesthetics in humans.
Vestibular problems due to diuretics in humans.
   (AD) Inclusion of comprehensive list of ototoxic agents.   (SP)

                              Tobacco

                                                                       597

Hearing loss due to salicylates in humans.
Hearing loss due to antimalarial, quinine, in humans.
Hearing loss due to antibiotic, streptomycin, in humans.
Tinnitus due to chemical agent, camphor, in humans.
Tinnitus due to chemical agent, tobacco, in humans.
Tinnitus due to cardiovascular agent, quinidine, in humans.
Tinnitus due to chemical agent, ergot, in humans.
Tinnitus due to chemical agent, alcohol, methyl, in humans.
   (AD) Discussion of toxic effects of drugs.   (ENG)

                                                                       621

Primarily vestibular problems due to antibiotic, streptomycin, in humans.
Primarily hearing loss but also vestibular problems due to antibiotic, dihy-
drostreptomycin, in humans.
Primarily hearing loss but also vestibular problems due to antibiotic, kana-
mycin, in humans.
Primarily hearing loss but also vestibular problems due to antibiotic, neomy-
cin, in humans.
Primarily hearing loss but also vestibular problems due to antibiotic, genta-
micin, in humans.
Vertigo and ataxia due to antituberculous agent, isoniazid, in humans.
Hearing loss due to salicylate, aspirin, in humans.
Hearing loss and vertigo due to antimalarial, quinine, in humans.
Nystagmus due to barbiturates in humans.
Vestibular problems due to analgesic, morphine, in humans.
Nystagmus due to sedative, alcohol, in humans.
Nystagmus and hearing loss due to chemical agent, carbon monoxide, in humans.
Ototoxic effects due to antineoplastic, nitrogen mustard, in humans.
Ototoxic effects due to chemical agent, aniline, in humans.
Ototoxic effects due to chemical agent, tobacco, in humans.
Nystagmus due to chemical agent, nicotine, in humans.
Vestibular problems due to anticonvulsants in humans.
Vestibular problems due to anesthetics in humans.
Vestibular problems due to diuretics in humans.
   (AD) Inclusion of comprehensive list of ototoxic agents.   (SP)

                                                                       627

Sensorineural hearing loss and vestibular problems due to parenteral, oral,
and topical administration of antibiotics in humans with and without kidney
disorder.
Degeneration of cochlea due to parenteral, intratympanic, administration of
antibiotic, neomycin, in animals, guinea pigs.

Transient sensorineural hearing loss due to high doses of salicylates in humans.
Sensorineural hearing loss due to antimalarial, quinine, in humans.
Sensorineural hearing loss due to chemical agent, tobacco, in humans.
Sensorineural hearing loss due to sedative, alcohol, in humans.
    (AD) Discussion of ototoxicity of various drugs as 1 etiology of sensorineural hearing loss in adults.   (ENG)

                                                                        728
Dizziness due to topical route, inhalation, of chemical agent, tobacco, in humans without smoking habit.
    (AD) Study of subjective symptoms of effects of tobacco on subjects without smoking habit.   (ENG)

Part II EFFECTS OF OTOTOXIC AGENTS

NON-SPECIFIC EFFECTS (Alcohol)

220

Significant effect on auditory time perception due to parenteral administration of 0.75 cc, in 500 cc normal saline, of 95 percent solution of sedative, alcohol, ethyl, in humans, adolescent and adult, 18 to 38 years age, male and female.
   (CT) Same method using 500 cc of normal saline in subjects, control group. (ENG)

526

Decr in perilymph activity and slower permeation of NA-24 sodium isotope into perilymph due to parenteral, intraperitoneal, administration of doses, corresponding to 1.4 g of 100 percent alcohol per 1 kg body weight, of 10 percent concentration of sedative, alcohol, ethyl, in 1 injection in 40 animals, guinea pigs, adult, with intraperitoneal administration of NA-24 sodium isotope.
   (CT) Same method with administration of NA-24 sodium isotope only in 13 guinea pigs, control group. (ENG)

127

Ototoxic effects due to antibiotics in humans with kidney tuberculosis.
   (AD) Literature review of ototoxic effects of streptomycin, viomycin, kanamycin, and capreomycin. (GER)

154

Ototoxic effects due to antibiotics in humans with tuberculosis.
   (AD) Literature review of some new antituberculous agents of 1968. (GER)

240

Ototoxic effects due to topical administration to inner ear of antibiotics, aminoglycoside, in 200 animals, guinea pigs, 250 g weight, with positive Preyer reflex.
   (CT) Study of guinea pigs, control group.
   (AD) Comparative study of ototoxicity of aminoglycoside antibiotics. (GER)

260

High antibiotic levels in perilymph due to topical administration to inner ear of antibiotics in animals, guinea pigs.
   (AD) Antibiotic levels in perilymph due to topical administration comp w levels due to intramuscular administration.
   (AD) Neomycin levels due to topical route higher than levels due to intramuscular route. (GER)

441

Ototoxic effects due to antibiotics in humans.
   (AD) Monogr on production of antibiotics, mechanism of action, clinical use, toxicity, and other aspects. (RUS)

545

Ototoxic effects due to antibiotics in humans with disorders.
   (AD) Literature review of clinical use and toxic effects of antibiotics. (IT)

592

Ototoxic effects due to antibiotics in humans.
   (AD) Discussion of effects of some drugs used in otolaryngology. (CZ)

609

Possible ototoxic effects due to antibiotics in humans with genitourinary system infections.
   (AD) Literature review of antibiotic therapy of genitourinary system

infections. (GER)

630

Ototoxic effects due to antibiotics in humans treated for infection. (ENG)

640

Ototoxic effects due to antibiotics in humans with tuberculosis.
   (AD) Literature review of chemotherapy of tuberculosis with comment on
   toxic effects of drugs. (GER)

712

Ototoxic effects due to antibiotics in humans in surgery. (HUN)

690

Ototoxic effects due to antituberculous agents in humans with tuberculosis.
(JAP)

510

Changes in metabolism of inner ear due to heavy metal, arsenic, for chronic
intoxication in animals, guinea pigs. (GER)

077

Moderate ototoxic effects due to unspecified method of administration of
range of 25 to 515 g of antibiotic, capreomycin, for long period in 3 of 82
humans with pulmonary tuberculosis.
   (AD) Preliminary study for primary study of kidney function in capreomycin
   treatment. (ENG)

331

Possible decr in ototoxicity due to decr dosage, from 1 g daily to 1 g 5 days
a week, of antibiotic, capreomycin, in humans with pulmonary tuberculosis.
(ENG)

501

Ototoxic effects due to antibiotic, capreomycin, in humans treated for tuberculosis.
   (AD) Capreomycin less ototoxic than streptomycin and viomycin. (ENG)

568

Mild ototoxic effects due to 1 g on 6 days a week or 0.75 g when body weight
below 50 kg, total of 30 to over 330 g, of antibiotic, capreomycin, for long
period in 3 of 82 humans, adult and aged, 21 to 80 years age, male and female, with chronic tuberculosis. (ENG)

590

Ototoxic effects due to antibiotic, capreomycin, in animals.
   (AD) In vivo and in vitro studies of capreomycin. (IT)

209

Slight incr but no decr in auditory flutter fusion threshold due to topical
route, inhalation, of 250 ml in 500 l air, to produce concentration of 10
percent carboxyhemoglobin in blood, of chemical agent, carbon monoxide, for
65 minutes at intervals of 7 days in 8 humans, adult, 23 to 48 years age,
male, healthy, 7 without smoking habit.
   (CT) For period before test, 8 subjects had no caffeine, alcohol, drugs,
   or nicotine.
   (CT) Study with oral administration of 100 mg phenobarbitone and placebo
   to determine response of same subjects to drug with known effects.
   (AD) Subjects tested with interrupted white noise. (ENG)

567

Effect on sensory hair cells in lateral line organ due to concentrations of 1
to 4 ppm, in aquaria containing 15 l of water, of chemical agent, chlorophenothane, for 18 hours at temperature of 22 to 23 degrees C in animals,
clawed toads, Xenopus laevis.
   (AD) Sensory hair cells of lateral line organ of toad comparable to hair
   cells in inner ear of higher vertebrates. (ENG)

530

Transient ototoxic effects due to cardiovascular agent, chromonar, in humans
treated for heart disorders.   (GER)

142

No toxic effects on eighth cranial nerve due to antibiotic, modified dihydrostreptomycin, in animals, guinea pigs and mice.
   (AD)   Decr in antibiotic action and toxicity due to modification of quanidine group of dihydrostreptomycin molecule.
   (AD) Study of effect of chemical modification of dihydrostreptomycin
   molecule on biological activity and toxic effects of antibiotic.   (RUS)

187

Unspecified ototoxic effects due to parenteral, intravenous, intramuscular,
and intraperitoneal, administration of 0.9 percent sodium chloride solution
of antibiotics, aminoglycoside, in animals, mice, albino, adult, male and
female, 15 to 30 g weight.
   (CT) Same method using 0.9 percent sodium chloride solution in mice,
   control group.
   (AD) Comment on relationship of study to ototoxicity of antibiotics.
Risk of ototoxic effects due to antibiotic, dihydrostreptomycin, in chronic
intoxication in humans. (ENG)

317

Possible decr in ototoxic effects due to antibiotic, dihydrostreptomycin
(IB), in humans, with administration of pantothenate salt.
   (AD) Discussion of clinical use of dihydrostreptomycin and possible decr
   in ototoxicity with use of pantothenate salt of antibiotic. (GER)

175

No change in potassium and sodium concentrations or in cation content of
endolymph due to parenteral, intravenous and intraperitoneal, administration
of range of doses of diuretics in 1 dose or multiple doses in animals, guinea
pigs, 250 to 400 g weight, with normal pinna reflex. (ENG)

054

Ototoxic effects due to diuretic, furosemide, in humans.
   (AD) Comment on need for audiology as documentation for reports of ototoxicity of furosemide. (ENG)

516

Possible ototoxic effects due to parenteral, intravenous, administration of
diuretic, furosemide, in less than every 4 hours in humans with kidney disorder. (ENG)

625

No ototoxic effects due to oral administration of range of 40 mg daily to 8
mg twice a day, dosage increased at intervals until maximum diuretic response, of diuretic, furosemide, for range of 1 to over 45 weeks in 14 humans,
adolescent, adult, and aged, 18 to 74 years age, male and female, with kidney
disorder. (ENG)

451

No eighth cranial nerve toxicity due to 80 mg every 6 or 8 hours, and lower
dosage in humans with kidney disorder, to produce serum levels of 5 to 8 mcg
per ml of antibiotic, gentamicin, in 104 humans, adult, aged, and child, 2 to
80 years age, with various infections.
   (AD) Suggested that prevention of ototoxicity due to daily assays of serum
   levels. (ENG)

528

No reported ototoxic effects due to parenteral, intravenous or intramuscular,
administration of 40 mg every 8 hours in 1 injection, to produce blood level
of 20 mcg per ml in 1 case, of antibiotic, (SQ) gentamicin (SM), for 3 to 10
days in 25 humans with pseudomonas infection.
Parenteral, intravenous, administration of 1 dose of 2 g and then 1 g every 2
hours for 12 hours, followed by 1 g every 3 hours for 3 to 7 days of antibiotic, (SQ) carbenicillin (SM), in 25 humans with pseudomonas infection.

(AD) Study of treatment of pseudomonas infection with gentamicin and carbenicillin.

(AD) Decr in blood level of gentamicin when used simultaneously with carbenicillin. (ENG)

578

No clinical evidence of ototoxic effects due to high doses, 3 to 6 mg per kg daily, of antibiotic, gentamicin, in 53 humans, child, adolescent, adult, and aged, 10 to 84 years age, male and female, with bacteremia due to gram-negative bacilli and with kidney disorder in 14 cases.

(AD) Monitored for clinical symptoms of ototoxic effects.

(AD) No audiology or vestibular function tests to determine ototoxic effects. (ENG)

579

No clinical evidence of ototoxic effects due to parenteral, intravenous, administration of 1.5 to 6 mg per kg daily, average of 3 mg per kg daily, of antibiotic, gentamicin, for as long as 36 days in 25 humans, child and adolescent, 2.5 to 15 years age, with acute leukemia and infections.

(AD) No audiology or vestibular function tests used to determine ototoxic effects. (ENG)

580

No observed ototoxic effects in follow up study of 10 months due to parenteral, intramuscular, administration of 4 or 5 mg per kg daily in 2 equal doses at 12 hour intervals, to produce blood levels of 4.9 mcg per ml or less, of antibiotic, gentamicin, for 1 to 31 days in 16 humans, newborn infant, 0 to 22 days age, less than 2500 g weight in 8 patients, with infections.

No observed ototoxic effects due to parenteral, intravenous and intraventricular, administration of 1.6 mg per kg of antibiotic, gentamicin, in 1 human, newborn infant, low birth weight, with infection.

(AD) Responses of newborn infants to sound monitored. (ENG)

582

No observed ototoxic effects due to 2 mg per kg daily of antibiotic, gentamicin, for 5 to 10 days in over 100 humans, child, with genitourinary system infections.

(AD) Patients observed for evidence of ototoxicity. (ENG)

583

No observed ototoxic effects but possible damage to inner ear due to parenteral, intramuscular, administration of 3.0 or 5.0 mg per kg daily, to produce serum levels as high as 7.8 mcg per ml, of antibiotic, gentamicin, for 6 to 7 days in 45 humans, newborn infant, 1.4 to 21 days average age, low birth weight, with infections.

(AD) Measurement of blood levels at 0.5, 1, 4, 8, and 12 hours after first injection and on third day.

(AD) Follow up studies with audiology planned to determine if ototoxic effects resulted from gentamicin therapy. (ENG)

584

No observed ototoxic effects due to parenteral, intramuscular, administration of 2.5 mg per kg every 12 hours or 1.7 mg per kg every 8 hours, daily total of 5 mg per kg, to produce blood levels of 6 mcg per ml or less, of antibiotic, gentamicin, for 10 days in 60 humans, infant, male and female, with genitourinary system infections.

(AD) Determination of blood levels at 1, 2, 4, and 8 hours after first injection and at 12 hours in group with administration of gentamicin every 12 hours.

(AD) Blood levels higher and for longer duration in group with administration every 12 hours.

(AD) Follow up studies with audiograms planned to determine if ototoxic effects resulted from gentamicin therapy. (ENG)

587

No ototoxic effects due to parenteral (SM) administration of 3 mg per kg every 24 hours of antibiotic, gentamicin (SM), for 5 to 132 days in 99 humans

with burns and with infection secondary to burns.
Simultaneous parenteral administration of other antibiotics (SM) in 99 humans
with burns and with infection secondary to burns.
No ototoxic effects due to topical, direct site (SM), administration in cream
or ointment of 0.1 percent of antibiotic, gentamicin, in 50 humans with burns
and with infection secondary to burns.
(AD) No topical gentamicin therapy in 2 patients.   (ENG)

588

No observed ototoxic effects due to parenteral, intramuscular, administration
of range of 1.36 to 7.00 mg per kg daily, in 6 dosage regimens, to produce
blood levels of 10.5 to 18.5 mcg per ml in 8 patients tested, of antibiotic,
gentamicin, for short period in 160 humans, Filipino, adolescent and adult,
15 to 62 years age, male, 78 to 168 lb weight, with venereal disease.
(AD) Clinical evaluation of vestibular function and cochlear function
after gentamicin therapy.   (ENG)

599

Unspecified ototoxic effects due to parenteral, intramuscular, administration
of 40 mg, to produce blood levels of 3.7 mcg per ml 1 hour after treatment to
less than 0.1 and 0.2 mcg per ml after 8 hours, of antibiotic, gentamicin
(gentamicin sulfate), in 1 dose in 10 humans, male and female, 59 to 87 kg
weight.
(AD) Risk of ototoxic effects with gentamicin.
(AD) Study in unpaid subjects of pharmacology and clinical use of gentamicin.   (GER)

600

No ototoxic effects due to parenteral, intramuscular or intravenous, administration of 40 or 80 mg daily of antibiotic, gentamicin, in humans with pseudomonas infection.
No ototoxic effects due to topical, direct site, administration in cream of
0.3 percent daily of antibiotic, gentamicin, in humans with pseudomonas
infection.   (GER)

624

Possible ototoxic effects due to antibiotic, gentamicin, in humans with
pseudomonas infections.   (ENG)

632

Ototoxic effects due to antibiotic, gentamicin, in humans with infections.
(AD) Suggested dosage of 1 to maximum of 1.5 mg per kg of gentamicin in
therapy.   (GER)

679

Damage to eighth cranial nerve due to antibiotic, gentamicin, in humans.
(AD) Factors in gentamicin ototoxicity include concurrent kidney disorders, total doses over 1 g, serum levels over 12 mcg per ml, 60 years or
more age, and previous administration of ototoxic drugs, antibiotics.
(ENG)

046

Concentration of kanamycin in perilymph for more than 24 hours due to parenteral administration of 400 mg per kg of antibiotic, kanamycin, in 1 injection in animals, guinea pigs.
(AD) Study of kanamycin levels in blood, cerebrospinal fluid, perilymph,
and endolymph.   (JAP)

058

Ototoxic effects due to parenteral, subcutaneous, administration of 250 mg
per kg daily of antibiotic, kanamycin (kanamycin sulfate), for 10 days in 60
animals, guinea pigs, 250 g average weight.
(AD) Tests made 30, 60, and 120 minutes after last injection.
Ototoxic effects due to parenteral, subcutaneous, administration of 250 mg
per kg daily of antibiotic, kanamycin (kanamycin sulfate), for 11 days in 20
animals, guinea pigs.
(AD) Tests made 5 or 12 hours after last injection.
(AD) High concentration of kanamycin in perilymph and, in particular,

endolymph.
(AD) High concentration and long period of action of kanamycin in inner
ear causes ototoxic effects. (GER)

129
Incr in sodium in perilymph but no significant change in potassium due to
parenteral, intraperitoneal, administration of 20 mg per kg and 200 mg per kg
of antibiotic, kanamycin (kanamycin sulfate), for about 5 days in animals,
guinea pigs, 400 to 600 g weight.
(CT) Control group of 5 guinea pigs used. (SP)

147
Protection from ototoxic effects on inner ear due to antibiotic, kanamycin
(IB), in animals, cats, with administration of vitamin B.
(AD) Preliminary study. (SP)

161
No reported ototoxic effects due to parenteral, intramuscular, administration
of 2 g of antibiotic, kanamycin, in 1 injection in 4 humans, adult, 27 to 36
years age, with rectal gonorrhea.
(AD) Audiogram after treatment with kanamycin within normal range. (ENG)

176
Possible ototoxic effects due to low doses of antibiotic, kanamycin, in
humans.
(AD) Literature review of infections with report on toxic effects of
antibiotic therapy. (ENG)

494
Accumulation in fluids of inner ear due to antibiotic, kanamycin, in animals,
guinea pigs.
(AD) Suggested that route of kanamycin to inner ear is through stria
vascularis, plexus cochlearis, and round window. (JAP)

496
Perilymph level of 2.5 mcg per ml and blood level of 36 mcg per ml due to
parenteral, subcutaneous, administration of 25 mg per kg of antibiotic,
kanamycin (kanamycin sulfate), in 1 injection in animals, guinea pigs.
Incr of 10 times of perilymph level and incr in blood level due to parenteral, subcutaneous, administration of 50 mg per kg of antibiotic, kanamycin
(kanamycin sulfate), in 1 injection in animals, guinea pigs.
No incr in perilymph level but incr in blood level due to parenteral, subcutaneous, administration of 250 mg per kg of antibiotic, kanamycin (kanamycin
sulfate), in 1 injection in animals, guinea pigs.
Some incr in inner ear level due to parenteral, subcutaneous, administration
of 250 mg per kg daily, total of 2500 mg per kg, of antibiotic, kanamycin
(kanamycin sulfate), for 10 days in animals, guinea pigs.
More incr in inner ear level due to parenteral, subcutaneous, administration
of total of 5000 mg per kg of antibiotic, kanamycin (kanamycin sulfate), for
20 days in animals, guinea pigs.
(AD) Continuous accumulation of kanamycin in inner ear due to treatment
with daily injections of long duration.
(AD) High concentration of kanamycin in fluids of inner ear and slow
elimination of more than 25 hours.
(AD) Results of study showed direct linear relationship between dosage of
kanamycin and concentration in blood.
(AD) Results of study showed initial rapid accumulation with 25 and 50 mg
per kg doses in single injections and later lack of accumulation of kanamycin in perilymph.
(AD) Rapid incr in kanamycin level of inner ear with small incr in dosage
significant for clinical use of drug.
(AD) Accumulation of kanamycin in inner ear due to membrane sealing effect
of antibiotic. (ENG)

601
Effect on eighth cranial nerve due to antibiotic, kanamycin, in humans with
infections and with or without kidney disorder.
(AD) Study of use of kanamycin for therapy of various infections. (ENG)

657

Possible ototoxic effects due to parenteral, intramuscular, administration of 2 g of antibiotic, kanamycin, in humans with gonorrhea, in particular with concurrent kidney disorders. (ENG)

034

Degeneration and demyelination of eighth cranial nerve due to parenteral, intraperitoneal, administration of 300 mg per kg of 1 percent solution of heavy metal, lead (lead acetate), for 1 time every 7 days for 7 weeks in 40 animals, guinea pigs, 300 to 350 g weight.
   (CT) Study of 10 guinea pigs, control group. (ENG)

554

Possible damage to inner ear due to parenteral, intraperitoneal, administration of 500 mg per kg of heavy metal, lead (lead acetate), in acute intoxication in animals, guinea pigs.
Possible damage to inner ear due to parenteral, intraperitoneal, administration of 20 mg per kg 2 times per week of heavy metal, lead (lead acetate), in chronic intoxication, over period of 4 to 6 weeks, in animals, guinea pigs. (GER)

722

Effect on reaction time to acoustic stimuli due to parenteral, intraperitoneal, administration of 0.16 and 0.04 mg per kg of chemical agent, lysergide, in 3 animals, rats, albino, about 120 days age, male, 300 g weight.
   (CT) Same method using 0.05 cc saline in rats, control group. (ENG)

052

Ototoxic effects due to parenteral, oral, and topical administration of antibiotic, neomycin, in humans.
   (AD) Discussion of neomycin ototoxicity due to all usual administration routes. (ENG)

053

Ototoxic effects due to topical administration of high doses of antibiotic, neomycin, in humans.
   (AD) Need for careful consideration of dosage of neomycin used in topical administration. (ENG)

376

High concentration of drug in fluids of ear for long period due to parenteral, intravenous, administration of 15000 units per kg of antibiotic, neomycin, in 22 animals, cats.
   (AD) Comparative study of neomycin level in fluids of ear and in other biological fluids. (RUS)

424

Effect on muscles of middle ear due to antibiotic, neomycin, in animals, guinea pigs. (CZ)

504

Ototoxic effects due to chemical agent, nicotine, in humans. (POL)

386

Possible damage to inner ear due to topical administration in ear drops of ototoxic drugs for long period in humans.
   (AD) Discussion of clinical use and possible toxic effects of ear drops. (GER)

442

Degeneration of inner ear due to ototoxic drugs in humans.
   (AD) Changes in inner ear due to virus infections comp w changes due to ototoxic drugs or circulation problems. (ENG)

479

Auditory system problems due to ototoxic drugs in humans.
   (AD) Discussion of drugs with possible toxic effects on ear. (FR)

366
Possible auditory system problems due to cardiovascular agent, quinidine, in
humans.
No ototoxic effects due to 2.40 to 9.00 g of cardiovascular agent, quinidine,
in 150 humans, adolescent and adult, male and female, with auricular fibril-
lation.
   (AD) Other toxic effects in 46 of 150 humans but no ototoxic effects
   reported. (SP)

484
No observed ototoxic effects in fetuses due to parenteral, intramuscular,
administration of 15, 30, or 50 mg per kg in 1 injection daily of antimalarial, quinine, for 30 days in 3 groups of 12 animals, dogs, during pregnancy.
   (CT) Study of 7 dogs, control group, not treated with quinine.
   (AD) Study of effects of quinine on fetuses of animals. (FR)

029
Concentration of streptomycin in blood and perilymph due to 250, 50, 25, and
15 mg per kg of antibiotic, streptomycin (streptomycin sulfate), in 4 injections in 325 animals, guinea pigs.
Concentration of streptomycin in blood and perilymph due to 250, 50, 25, and
15 mg per kg of antibiotic, streptomycin (IB) (streptomycin sulfate), in 4
injections in 325 animals, guinea pigs, with administration of ozothin.
   (AD) Protective action of ozothin not dependable. (GER)

296
Ototoxic effects due to antibiotic, streptomycin, in large number of humans.
(BUL)

319
Ototoxic effects due to antibiotic, streptomycin, in humans with infections
of ear.
   (AD) Literature review of clinical use and ototoxicity of streptomycin.
   (GER)

403
Risk of damage to function of eighth cranial nerve due to antibiotic, streptomycin, for long period in humans, adult and child, with tuberculous meningitis.
   (AD) Need for tests of function of eighth cranial nerve with clinical use
   of streptomycin.
   (AD) Literature review of treatment of infections of CNS. (ENG)

408
Ototoxic effects due to antibiotic, streptomycin, in humans.
   (AD) Discussion of streptomycin ototoxicity, 1 of topics at conference on
   various aspects of the ear and hearing. (FR)

620
Changes of various degrees of intensity in cerebellar vermis, including
Purkinje's cell, due to 30 mg per kg, total doses of 600 mg and 1200 mg, of
antibiotic, streptomycin, in 2 groups of 24 animals, pigeons. (POL)

631
Ototoxic effects due to antibiotic, streptomycin, in humans with pulmonary
tuberculosis. (BUL)

661
Hearing loss in fetus due to sedative, thalidomide, in humans, female,
treated during pregnancy. (GER)

634
Ototoxic effects due to antituberculous agent, thiacetazone, in humans with
tuberculosis. (FR)

013
No reported ototoxic effects due to antibiotic, neomycin (CB), in 26 humans

with inflammation of external auditory meatus.
No reported ototoxic effects due to antibiotic, polymyxin B (CB), in 26
humans with inflammation of external auditory meatus.
    (AD) Study of use of neomycin, polymyxin B, and fluocinolone acetonide in
    treatment of inflammation of external auditory meatus. (FR)

                                                                        076
Ototoxic effects due to parenteral, intramuscular, administration of 1 g
daily of antibiotic, capreomycin (SM), for 9 months in 4 of 65 humans, adult
and aged, range of 20 to 70 years age, male and female, with pulmonary tuberculosis.
Simultaneous administration of ethambutol (SM) in 65 humans, adult and aged,
range of 20 to 70 years age, male and female, with pulmonary tuberculosis.
Simultaneous administration of antibiotic, rifampicin (SM), in 65 humans,
adult and aged, range of 20 to 70 years age, male and female, with pulmonary
tuberculosis. (ENG)

                                                                        088
Ototoxic effects in fetus due to unspecified method of administration of
unspecified doses of antibiotic, streptomycin, for long period in humans,
female, treated for tuberculosis during pregnancy.
Ototoxic effects in fetus due to unspecified method of administration of
unspecified doses of antibiotic, dihydrostreptomycin, for long period in
humans, female, treated for tuberculosis during pregnancy. (ENG)

                                                                        091
Ototoxic effects due to antibiotic, streptomycin (streptomycin sulfate), in
humans with pulmonary tuberculosis.
Ototoxic effects due to antibiotic, dihydrostreptomycin, in humans with
pulmonary tuberculosis.
Ototoxic effects due to antibiotic, florimycin, in humans with pulmonary
tuberculosis.
Ototoxic effects due to antibiotic, kanamycin, in humans with pulmonary
tuberculosis.
    (AD) Comparative study of ototoxicity of different derivatives of antibio-
    tics. (RUS)

                                                                        164
Ototoxic effects not determined due to parenteral, intramuscular and intrathecal, administration of 1.5 mg per kg every 8 to 12 hours, to produce peak
serum levels of 2.5 to 5.0 mcg per ml, of antibiotic, (SQ) gentamicin, for 9
to 13 days in 5 humans, newborn infant, with infections.
Ototoxic effects not determined due to parenteral, intramuscular, administration of 7.5 mg per kg every 12 hours of antibiotic, (SQ) kanamycin, for 7 to
17 days in 3 of 5 humans, newborn infant, with infections.
    (AD) No follow up studies of gentamicin over long period to determine
    ototoxic effects.
    (AD) Need for audiometry and vestibular function tests after several
    months to determine ototoxic effects.
    (AD) Study of clinical pharmacology of gentamicin. (ENG)

                                                                        318
High risk of ototoxic effects due to antibiotic, dihydrostreptomycin, in
humans with bacterial infections.
Risk of ototoxic effects due to antibiotic, streptomycin, in humans with
bacterial infections, with administration of pantothenic acid.
    (AD) Literature review on clinical use and ototoxicity of streptomycin.
    (AD) Recommended use of streptomycin only for tuberculosis due to high
    risk of ototoxic effects. (GER)

                                                                        348
No ototoxic effects due to topical administration in ear drops of 3 to 4 ear
drops 3 times daily of fluocinolone acetonide (CB), for 5 to 10 days in 54
humans, child, adolescent, adult, and aged, male and female, with infections
of middle ear and external ear.
No ototoxic effects due to topical administration in ear drops of 3 to 4 ear
drops 3 times daily of antibiotic, polymyxin B (CB), for 5 to 10 days in 54
humans, child, adolescent, adult, and aged, male and female, with infections

of middle ear and external ear.
No ototoxic effects due to topical administration in ear drops of 3 to 4 ear
drops 3 times daily of antibiotic, neomycin (CB) (neomycin sulfate), for 5 to
10 days in 54 humans, child, adolescent, adult, and aged, male and female,
with infections of middle ear and external ear. (IT)

                                                                        351
No observed ototoxic effects due to topical administration of 1 drop of
chemical agent, dimethyl sulfoxide (CB), in humans as anesthetic for myringotomy.
No observed ototoxic effects due to topical administration of 1 drop of
anesthetic, tetracaine (CB) (tetracaine hydrochloride), in humans as anesthetic for myringotomy. (ENG)

                                                                        438
Suppression of microphonic potentials of saccule due to topical, intraluminal, administration of antibiotic, streptomycin, in animals, goldfish.
Suppression of microphonic potentials of saccule due to topical, intraluminal, administration of antibiotic, kanamycin, in animals, goldfish.
Suppression of microphonic potentials of saccule due to topical, intraluminal
or extraluminal, administration of 0.5 mg of chemical agent, cyanide, in
animals, goldfish.
Suppression of microphonic potentials of saccule due to topical, intraluminal
or extraluminal, administration of 0.1 mg of antimalarial, quinine, in animals, goldfish.
Suppression of microphonic potentials of saccule due to topical, intraluminal
or extraluminal, administration of 2 mg of anesthetic, procaine, in animals,
goldfish.
No effect on microphonic potentials of saccule due to topical administration
of salicylates in animals, goldfish. (ENG)

                                                                        485
High concentration in fluids of inner ear and ototoxic effects due to 250 mg
per kg of antibiotic, streptomycin, in animals, guinea pigs.
High concentration in fluids of inner ear and ototoxic effects due to 250 mg
per kg of antibiotic, kanamycin, in animals, guinea pigs.
Higher concentration in fluids of inner ear and more severe ototoxic effects
due to 250 mg per kg of antibiotic, dihydrostreptomycin, in animals, guinea
pigs.
Higher concentration in fluids of inner ear and more severe ototoxic effects
due to 100 mg per kg of antibiotic, neomycin, in animals, guinea pigs.
    (AD) High concentration of aminoglycoside antibiotics in fluids of inner
    ear due to low doses as well as high doses.
    (AD) Ototoxic effect of aminoglycoside antibiotics due to retention of
    high concentrations in inner ear for long period and slow elimination of
    drugs.
Significant decr in concentration in fluids of inner ear and in serum and
decr in ototoxicity due to 250 mg per kg or 100 mg per kg of antibiotics
(IB), aminoglycoside, in animals, guinea pigs, with administration of ozothin.
Decr in concentration in fluids of inner ear and decr in ototoxicity due to
250 mg per kg or 100 mg per kg of antibiotics (IB), aminoglycoside, in animals, guinea pigs, with administration of pantothenic acid. (GER)

                                                                        491
Changes in sensory epithelium of otocyst due to antibiotic, streptomycin, in
animals, chickens, embryo.
Changes in sensory epithelium of otocyst due to antibiotic, neomycin, in
animals, chickens, embryo.
Changes in sensory epithelium of otocyst due to antibiotic, kanamycin, in
animals, chickens, embryo.
    (CT) Study of otocysts of chickens, control group, not treated with amino-
    glycoside antibiotics.
    (AD) Neomycin and kanamycin more toxic to otocysts of chickens than strep-
    tomycin. (CZ)

                                                                        495
Ototoxic effects due to parenteral, intramuscular, administration of 100 mg

per kg of antibiotic, neomycin (neomycin sulfate), in 10 injections in 10
animals, guinea pigs.
Significant decr in ototoxic effects due to parenteral, intramuscular, administration of 100 mg per kg of antibiotic, neomycin (IB) (neomycin sulfate), in 10 injections in 10 animals, guinea pigs, with combined administration of 1.2 ml per kg of ozothin.
Ototoxic effects due to parenteral, intramuscular, administration of 250 mg
per kg of antibiotic, streptomycin (streptomycin sulfate), in 10 injections
in animals, guinea pigs.
Decr in ototoxic effects due to parenteral, intramuscular, administration of
250 mg per kg of antibiotic, streptomycin (IB) (streptomycin sulfate), in 10
injections in 15 animals, guinea pigs, with combined administration of 1.2 ml
per kg of ozothin.
No ototoxic effects due to parenteral, intramuscular, administration of 250
mg per kg of antibiotic, streptomycin (IB) (streptomycin sulfate), in 10
injections in 6 animals, guinea pigs, with previous intramuscular administration of 1.2 ml per kg of ozothin.
   (CT) Study of 12 guinea pigs, control group.
   (AD) Electrophysiological study of effects of ozothin on ototoxicity of
   aminoglycoside antibiotics. (GER)

                                                                    557
Ototoxic effects due to previous administration of antibiotic, (SQ) streptomycin, in 8 humans with pulmonary tuberculosis.
No ototoxic effects due to 1.0 g daily of antibiotic, (SQ) capreomycin (SM),
for long period in same 8 of 38 humans with pulmonary tuberculosis.
Simultaneous administration of antituberculous agent, (SQ) ethambutol (SM),
in 38 humans with pulmonary tuberculosis. (ENG)

                                                                    560
Ototoxic effects due to antibiotic, streptomycin, in humans with tuberculo-
sis.
Ototoxic effects due to antibiotic, kanamycin, in humans with tuberculosis.
   (AD) Reported 4 to 5 percent incidence in audiometry of ototoxicity from
   streptomycin and kanamycin.
   (AD) Decr in ototoxicity with administration of streptomycin or kanamycin
   in evening before sleeping. (JAP)

                                                                    562
Decr in microphonic potential of saccule due to topical, intraluminal, administration of antibiotic, streptomycin, in animals, goldfish.
Decr in microphonic potential of saccule due to topical, intraluminal, administration of antibiotic, kanamycin, in animals, goldfish.
Permanent decr in microphonic potential of saccule due to topical, intraluminal or extraluminal, administration of 0.5 mg per ml of chemical agent,
cyanide, in animals, goldfish.
Permanent decr in microphonic potential of saccule due to topical, intraluminal or extraluminal, administration of 0.1 mg per ml of antimalarial,
quinine, in animals, goldfish.
No effect on microphonic potential of saccule due to salicylate, aspirin, in
animals, goldfish.
Some decr in microphonic potential of saccule due to 2 mg per ml of anesthetic, procaine, in animals, goldfish.
   (AD) Study of effects of various agents on microphonic potential of saccule of goldfish. (JAP)

                                                                    577
No ototoxic effects due to parenteral, intramuscular, administration of 3 to
5 mg per kg daily in 3 or 4 divided doses, average total dose of 3.0 g, of
antibiotic, gentamicin, for 12.7 days average in 41 humans, adolescent,
adult, and aged, 14 to 87 years age, male and female, with genitourinary
system infections primarily and with kidney disorder in 13 cases.
No ototoxic effects due to parenteral, intramuscular, administration of 15 mg
per kg daily in 2 or 3 divided doses, average total dose of 6.6 g, of antibiotic, kanamycin (SM), for 8 days average in 34 humans, adult and aged, 40
to 81 years age, male and female, with genitourinary system infection and
with kidney disorder in 8 cases.
No ototoxic effects due to parenteral, intramuscular or intravenous adminis-

tration of 1.5 to 2.5 mg per kg daily in 2 to 4 divided doses, average total
dose of 1.0 g, of antibiotic, polymyxin B (SM), for 6 days average in 34
humans, adult and aged, 40 to 81 years age, male and female, with genitourinary system infection and with kidney disorder in 8 cases.
   (AD) Comparative study of effects of 3 antibiotics on infections due to
   gram-negative bacilli. (ENG)

          602
Effect on eighth cranial nerve due to antibiotic, streptomycin, in humans.
Effect on eighth cranial nerve due to antibiotic, dihydrostreptomycin, in
humans.
   (AD) Comparative study of effect of 2 antibiotics on eighth cranial nerve.
   (ENG)

          604
Decr in middle ear muscle reflex due to oral administration of amount to
produce blood levels of 0.02 to 0.15 percent of sedative, alcohol, ethyl, in
9 humans, adult, 21 to 24 years age, with normal pure tone audiograms.
Decr in middle ear muscle reflex due to oral administration of 1.5 to 4.3 mg
per kg of sedative, pentobarbital (pentobarbital sodium), in 6 humans, adult,
21 to 24 years age, with normal pure tone audiograms.
   (AD) More risk of noise induced hearing loss due to decr in middle ear
   muscle reflex. (ENG)

          637
Ototoxic effects due to antibiotic, streptomycin (CB), in humans.
Ototoxic effects due to antibiotic, penicillin (CB), in humans. (GER)

          653
Possible ototoxic effects due to antibiotic, kanamycin, in humans with acute
genitourinary system infections.
Possible ototoxic effects due to antibiotic, gentamicin, in humans with acute
genitourinary system infections.
   (AD) Need for careful consideration in use of kanamycin and gentamicin in
   therapy, in particular in patients with kidney disorders. (ENG)

          674
No ototoxic effects due to parenteral, intramuscular, administration of 1 g
twice daily for 1 to 2 days, followed by 1 g daily for 8 to 10 days, with
reduced doses in patients with kidney disorder, of antibiotic, kanamycin
(SM), for total of about 9 to 12 days in 28 humans, adult and aged, 26 to 80
years age, male and female, with severe infections due to gram-negative
bacilli, with bacteremia in 16 cases and kidney disorder in 8 cases.
Simultaneous administration of antibiotic, chloramphenicol (SM), in most of
16 humans with bacteremia.
   (AD) Use of kanamycin without ototoxic effects in patients with kidney
   disorders due to decr in dosage and tests of serum levels of antibiotic.
   (ENG)

PHYSIOLOGICAL EFFECTS

Cochlear function

          021
Transient bilateral sensorineural hearing loss due to unspecified method of
administration of as much as 5.2 g daily of salicylate, acetylsalicylic acid,
for unspecified period in 1 human, aged, 76 years age, female, with rheumatoid arthritis.
   (AD) Improvement in hearing after cessation of treatment with acetylsalicylic acid.
   (AD) Suggested that damage to stria vascularis due to presbycusis and not
   due to acetylsalicylic acid. (ENG)

          113
Transient sensorineural hearing loss but no vestibular problems due to 0.5 to
1.0 g 4 times daily of solution of salicylate, acetylsalicylic acid, in 8 (16
percent) of 50 humans after tonsillectomy.
   (AD) Audiology and vestibular function tests to determine ototoxic ef-

fects. (DAN)

315
Dysacusis due to oral administration of 9 tablets for 4 days, 6 tablets for 7
days, and 3 tablets for 2 days, each tablet containing 500 mg of salicylate,
aspirin (aspirin aluminum), for total of 13 days in 1 of 19 humans, adult, 21
years age, female, with rheumatoid arthritis.
Tinnitus and dysacusis due to oral administration of 6 tablets for 3 days, 12
tablets for 2 days, 8 tablets for 2 days, and 9 tablets for 15 days, each
tablet containing 500 mg of salicylate, aspirin (aspirin aluminum), for total
of 22 days in 1 human, adult, 37 years age, female, with rheumatoid arthritis.
    (AD) Loss of appetite also due to administration of aspirin (aspirin
    aluminum) for 22 days. (ENG)

026
Hearing loss in speech range due to sedative, alcohol, ethyl, in humans.
    (AD) Total of 200 tests conducted. (GER)

262
Possible damage to vestibular apparatus and organ of Corti due to oral ingestion of large amounts of chemical agent, alcohol, ethyl, for long period in 8
humans, adult and aged, 44 to 75 years age, male and female, chronic alcoholics.
    (AD) Report on results of temporal bone study.
    (AD) Previous observations of transient hearing loss and tinnitus during
    alcohol intoxication.
    (AD) Need for more study for interpretation of results. (ENG)

716
Damage to cochlear function due to oral ingestion of amount to produce blood
levels of 0.8 to more than 1.0 percent of sedative, alcohol, ethyl, in acute
intoxication in humans.
    (AD) Study of the effects of alcohol on cochlear function. (GER)

721
Decr in eighth cranial nerve action potential and change in Preyer reflex
threshold due to parenteral, subcutaneous, administration of 2 or 3 to 20 mg
per kg of anticonvulsant, amino-oxyacetic acid, in animals, guinea pigs.
    (CT) Same method using saline in guinea pigs, control group, showed no
    change in reflex threshold.
    (AD) Changes in Preyer reflex threshold in part due to effects on auditory
    pathway. (ENG)

417
No significant effects on threshold at any frequency due to 5 mg of analeptic, amphetamine (dextro-amphetamine sulfate), in humans, adult, range of 22
to 38 years age, male and female, with no history of auditory system problem.
    (CT) Audiometry before and 65 minutes after administration of drug.
    (CT) Same method using placebo in 12 subjects, control group.
    (CT) Same method using no drug in 12 subjects, control group.
    (AD) Study to determine effects, toxic or therapeutic, of amphetamine on
    auditory threshold of humans. (ENG)

032
Progressive permanent sensorineural hearing loss due to topical administration of unspecified doses of antibiotics for long period in 1 human, child, 6
years age, female, with severe burns on 80 percent of body. (ENG)

066
Hearing loss due to various methods of administration of antibiotics in
humans with acute otitis media. (RUS)

099
Hearing loss due to antibiotics in humans, adult and child, male and female,
with kidney disorder. (HUN)

132
Sensorineural hearing loss due to antibiotics in humans.
   (AD) Study of iatrogenic hearing loss.   (GER)

182
Sensorineural hearing loss, from frequency at 8000 cps to speech range, due
to antibiotics in humans.
   (AD) Specific audiometric configuration for hearing loss due to antibiotics.
   (AD) Use of level of 15 db at 8000 cps for detection of hearing loss due
   to antibiotics. (ENG)

193
Sensorineural hearing loss and structural damage to cochlea due to low doses
of antibiotics in humans.
   (AD) Report on clinical and pathological effects possible with use of
   antibiotics.
   (AD) Toxic levels in blood possible due to low doses in therapy.
   (AD) Need for audiometry, vestibular function tests, and determination of
   blood levels of antibiotics during treatment. (SER)

244
Hearing loss and damage to organ of Corti due to antibiotics, aminoglycoside,
in humans.
   (AD) Literature review of ototoxic effects of different aminoglycoside
   antibiotics. (GER)

272
Hearing loss and damage to organ of Corti due to antibiotics in humans.
   (AD) Literature review of ototoxic effects of antibiotics used in therapy.
   (FIN)

357
Hearing loss due to antibiotics in 60 (5.4 percent) of 1100 humans treated for
different disorders. (RUS)

422
Hearing loss due to antibiotics in humans, female, treated during pregnancy
or for disorders of genitourinary system. (RUS)

521
Hearing loss due to antibiotics in humans, child, with infections.
   (AD) Analysis of ototoxic effects due to antibiotics. (RUS)

608
Possible hearing loss due to antibiotics in humans with disorders.
   (AD) Evaluation of degree of hearing loss due to antibiotics possible with
   pretreatment and posttreatment audiometry. (HUN)

638
Hearing loss due to antibiotics in humans with disorders.   (RUS)

689
Hearing loss due to antibiotics in humans with tuberculosis.   (POL)

704
Functional damage to cochlea evident before changes in structure due to
antibiotics in animals.
   (AD) Need for correlation of various methods, morphological, electrophy-
   siological, and biochemical, in study of function of inner ear.
   (AD) Literature review of various methods of study of auditory system.
   (ENG)

713
Inhibition of oxygen consumption of cochlea due to antibiotics in animals,
guinea pigs.
   (AD) In vitro study using microrespirometer of effect of antibiotics on
   oxygen consumption in guinea pig cochlea. (JAP)

207
Cochleotoxic effects due to antibiotic, capreomycin, in humans with tubercu-
losis.
  (AD) Report on new antituberculous agents.
  (AD) Need for careful consideration before use of capreomycin in treatment
  of tuberculosis. (FR)

328
Moderate hearing loss, subjective, due to total dose of 100 g of antibiotic,
capreomycin (SM), for 31 days or more in 1 of 38 humans, Negro, adult, 63
years age, male, with tuberculosis.
  (CT) Audiometry, pretreatment and during treatment.
  (AD) Audiometry showed possible hearing loss due to capreomycin.
Simultaneous administration of antituberculous agent, ethionamide (SM), in 1
of 38 humans, Negro, adult, 63 years age, male, with tuberculosis. (ENG)

330
Hearing loss due to parenteral, intramuscular, administration of 31 mg per kg
or 62 mg per kg daily of antibiotic, capreomycin (capreomycin disulfate), for
more than 1000 days in 4 animals, dogs, male and female.
Hearing loss due to parenteral, subcutaneous, administration of 13 mg per kg
or 130 mg per kg daily of antibiotic, capreomycin (capreomycin tetrahydroch-
loride), for 91 days in 2 animals, cats, male.
  (AD) Hearing loss determined by response of animals to reproducible sound.
  (ENG)

400
Transient mild cochlear impairment due to parenteral, intramuscular, administration of 1 g daily, maximum dose of 100 g, of antibiotic, capreomycin, in 1
of 21 humans with chronic tuberculosis of genitourinary system.
  (AD) Report on clinical use and toxic effects of new drugs in treatment of
  tuberculosis of genitourinary system. (GER)

556
Moderate lesion of cochlea due to unspecified doses of antibiotic, capreomycin, for long period in 5 (12.5 percent) of 40 humans, in treatment or retreatment for pulmonary tuberculosis.
  (AD) Cochlear function monitored by audiometry. (ENG)

228
Hearing loss due to topical route, inhalation, of chemical agent, carbon
disulfide, for long period in humans in industry. (SER)

030
Hearing loss due to chemical agent, carbon monoxide, in humans.
  (AD) Studies with audiometry on patients with u-shaped audiograms. (GER)

162
Permanent unilateral sensorineural hearing loss due to topical route, inhala-
tion, of chemical agent, carbon monoxide, in acute intoxication in 1 human.
  (AD) Hearing loss confirmed by audiogram. (POL)

163
Sensorineural hearing loss due to topical route, inhalation, of chemical
agent, carbon monoxide, in humans.
  (AD) Literature review on carbon monoxide poisoning. (POL)

180
Bilateral sensorineural hearing loss with partial improvement due to topical
route, inhalation, of large amounts, to produce carboxy-hemoglobin level of
25 percent of total hemoglobin, of chemical agent, carbon monoxide, in 1
human, adult, 22 years age, male, with previous high intensity noise exposure.
  (AD) Hearing loss confirmed by audiometry but vestibular function tests
  normal.
  (AD) Suggested that audiometric configuration not type due to acoustic
  trauma. (ENG)

224

Slight sensorineural hearing loss due to topical route, inhalation, of large amount, to produce high carboxyhemoglobin level of 36 percent 1.5 days after exposure, of chemical agent, carbon monoxide, in 1 human, adult, 21 years age, male.
Moderate bilateral sensorineural hearing loss due to topical route, inhalation, of large amount, to produce high carboxyhemoglobin level of 48 percent 1.5 days after exposure, of chemical agent, carbon monoxide, in 1 human, adolescent, 18 years age, male. (ENG)

436

Hearing loss and damage to organ of Corti due to topical route, inhalation, of chemical agent, carbon monoxide, in animals. (GER)

177

Sensorineural hearing loss due to topical route, inhalation, of chemical agents, nitro and amino compounds, in humans from exposure in chemical industry.
(AD) Hearing loss confirmed by audiology. (POL)

069

Progressive decr in cochlear response due to topical administration by insufflation to round window in powder of 8 mg (only 0.5 mg actually fell on round window) of antibiotic, chloramphenicol, in 1 administration in 8 animals, guinea pigs, 459 to 996 g weight.
(CT) Same method using saline in 2 guinea pigs, control group.
(AD) Measurement of cochlear response at 15 minutes and 1, 5, and 20 hours after insufflation. (ENG)

289

Possible cochlear impairment due to antibiotic, chloramphenicol, in humans.
(AD) Report on toxic effects of chloramphenicol. (RUM)

732

Hearing loss and total degeneration of organ of Corti and moderate degeneration of spiral ganglion and nerve process in fetus due to oral ingestion of 250 mg daily of antimalarial, chloroquine (chloroquine phosphate), in humans, female, during pregnancy.
(AD) Histopathological study of inner ear after death. (ENG)

714

Decr in cochlear microphonics due to topical administration to bulla of concentrations of 1, 3, and 6 units, in 0.1 ml, of anti-inflammatory agent, chymotrypsin, in 40 animals, guinea pigs.
(CT) Same method using physiological sodium chloride solution in guinea pigs, control group.
(AD) Electrophysiological study showed more decr in cochlear potentials with incr in concentration of chymotrypsin.
(AD) Suggested careful consideration in clinical use of chymotrypsin in treatment of adhesive otitis media. (GER)

429

Necrosis of cells of organ of Corti and hearing loss, partial or total, due to parenteral, intramuscular, administration of high doses, 150,000 units per kg daily, of antibiotic, colistin (colistin sulfate), for 7 to 21 days in animals, guinea pigs. (RUS)

372

Transient and permanent decr in cochlear microphonic, eighth nerve action potential, and endocochlear potential due to topical administration, perfusion of scala tympani and scala vestibuli, with 50 mM in Ringer's solution of chemical agent, cyanide (sodium cyanide), in animals, guinea pigs.
(CT) Same method using modified Ringer's solution in guinea pigs, control group, showed gradual decr in cochlear microphonic and eighth nerve action potential but no change in endocochlear potential.
(CT) Measurement of cochlear potentials, before, during, and after perfusion with cyanide (sodium cyanide).
(AD) Study of effect of cyanide (sodium cyanide) in perilymph on cochlear

potentials of guinea pigs. (ENG)

563
Effect on cochlear microphonic due to topical administration of chemical
agent, cyanide, in animals, birds.
 (AD) Study of cochlear potentials of various birds. (GER)

044
Change in cochlear response and damage to hair cells of organ of Corti due to
100 mg per kg daily of antibiotic, dihydrostreptomycin, in animals, rabbits.
Change in cochlear response and damage to stria vascularis due to 250 mg per
kg daily and 500 mg per kg daily of antibiotic, dihydrostreptomycin, in 2
other groups of animals, rabbits. (JAP)

050
Higher concentrations of dihydrostreptomycin in perilymph than in endolymph
due to parenteral, intraperitoneal, administration of 20 to 30 mc per kg
concentration, tritium-labelled, of antibiotic, dihydrostreptomycin (dihydrostreptomycin sulfate), in 1 injection in 8 animals, guinea pigs, albino, 200
to 250 g weight.
 (CT) Control group of 3 guinea pigs used.
 (AD) Study showed that dihydrostreptomycin carried by blood stream to
 spiral ligament earlier than to stria vascularis. (ENG)

106
Severe sensorineural hearing loss due to antibiotic, dihydrostreptomycin, in
humans.
 (AD) Comment on risk of ototoxic effects with clinical use of dihydrostreptomycin. (NOR)

551
Sensorineural hearing loss due to parenteral administration of range of
doses, 3, 15, 25, and 40 g, of antibiotic, dihydrostreptomycin, in humans,
adult and child, range of ages, male and female, in 4 families.
 (AD) Study of familial incidence of dihydrostreptomycin hearing loss and
 hereditary susceptibility of cochlea.
 (AD) Suggested that administration of dihydrostreptomycin in humans with
 hereditary susceptibility of cochlea results in hearing loss. (ENG)

645
Permanent severe hearing loss due to antibiotic, dihydrostreptomycin, in
humans.
 (AD) Suggested that no preparations of dihydrostreptomycin be used in
 therapy. (ENG)

726
Effect on concentration of cytoplasmic RNS in organ of Corti due to parenteral, intramuscular, administration of 100 mg per kg of antibiotic, dihydrostreptomycin, for 20 days in 5 animals, guinea pigs.
 (AD) Study of effect of dihydrostreptomycin on concentration of cytoplasmic RNS in inner ear of guinea pigs. (GER)

134
Decr in threshold shift of 20 db and damage to outer hair cells and inner
hair cells of organ of Corti due to topical administration to external auditory meatus of 50 percent solution of chemical agent, dimethyl sulfoxide, for
21 days in 7 animals, cats.
Damage to 40 percent of eighth cranial nerve action potential due to topical
administration to external auditory meatus of chemical agent, dimethyl sulfoxide, for 6 hours in 4 animals, cats.
Damage to 60 percent of eighth cranial nerve action potential due to topical
administration to middle ear of chemical agent, dimethyl sulfoxide, for 6
hours in 4 animals, cats.
 (CT) Control group of 4 cats used.
 (AD) Suggested that dimethyl sulfoxide new ototoxic drug. (GER)

405
Decr in cochlear potentials due to parenteral, intravenous, administration of

total dose of 5 to 35 mg per kg of solution of chemical agent, dinitrophenol, in several doses in animals, cats, young, 1.0 to 1.8 kg weight, normal.
(AD) Use of various intensities of test tone of 2 kcps.
More decr in cochlear potentials due to topical administration to round window of 1 drop at a time of 3 concentrations, in order of increasing concentration, of chemical agent, dinitrophenol, in animals, cats, young, 1.0 to 1.8 kg weight, normal.
(AD) Use of various intensities of test tone of 2 kcps.
(CT) Measurement of cochlear potentials before and after administration of chemical agent, dinitrophenol.
(CT) Measurement of cochlear potentials for longer than usual before administration of chemical agent, dinitrophenol, in some animals, control group.
(CT) Higher frequency test tone of 5 kcps used in some animals, control group.
(CT) Same method with administration of intravenous 2 percent solution of sodium bicarbonate with chemical agent, dinitrophenol, in cats, control group, resulted in no decr in cochlear potentials. (ENG)

406

Incr in cochlear potentials due to parenteral, intravenous, administration of 1 dose of 10 mg per kg and then doses of 5 mg per kg of chemical agent, dinitrophenol, in total of 5 doses in animals, cats, with acoustic trauma.
(AD) Use of low intensity test tone of 2 kcps.
Decr in cochlear potentials due to topical administration to round window of 1 drop at a time of various concentrations of chemical agent, dinitrophenol, in animals, cats, with acoustic trauma.
(AD) Use of low intensity test tone of 2 kcps.
(AD) No consistent difference in effect on cochlear potentials of topical administration of chemical agent, dinitrophenol, in cats with and without acoustic trauma.
Decr in cochlear potentials due to parenteral, intravenous, administration of 1 dose of 5 mg per kg, followed by 1 dose of 10 mg per kg, followed by other doses of 5 mg per kg of chemical agent, dinitrophenol, in total of 4 doses in animals, cats, with acoustic trauma.
(AD) Use of high intensity test tone of 2 kcps.
(CT) Measurement of cochlear potentials for longer than usual before administration of chemical agent, dinitrophenol, in some animals, control group.
(CT) Same method with administration of intravenous 2 percent solution of sodium bicarbonate with chemical agent, dinitrophenol, in cats, control group. (ENG)

160

Tinnitus due to unspecified method of administration of 300 mg daily of anticonvulsant, diphenylhydantoin (diphenylhydantoin sodium), for 2 years in 1 human, aged, 77 years age, female, for dizziness.
(AD) No tinnitus after cessation of treatment with diphenylhydantoin (diphenylhydantoin sodium). (ENG)

060

Possible hearing loss due to high doses, as high as 200 mg, of diuretic, ethacrynic acid, in humans with kidney disorders.
(AD) Comment on risk of administration of high test doses of ethacrynic acid in humans with kidney disorder as suggested in recent study. (ENG)

061

Transient hearing loss due to high test dose, as high as 200 mg, of diuretic, ethacrynic acid, in humans with kidney disorder .
(AD) Explanation of use of high test dose.
(AD) Need for hydration before administration of test dose of ethacrynic acid.
(AD) Procedure caused only 3 cases of transient hearing loss in 3 years. (ENG)

097

Hearing loss due to diuretic, ethacrynic acid, in humans, female.
(AD) Report on toxic effects of drugs. (SW)

098
Hearing loss due to parenteral, intravenous, administration of diuretic, ethacrynic acid, in humans with kidney disorder. (DAN)

102
Progressive hearing loss and tinnitus due to diuretic, ethacrynic acid, in 1 human, adult, 48 years age, with kidney disorder.
(AD) Hearing loss confirmed by audiometry.
(AD) Need for audiometry with use of ethacrynic acid in humans with kidney disorder. (FR)

125
Sensorineural hearing loss due to parenteral, intravenous, administration of range of 9.2 to 86 mg per kg of diuretic, ethacrynic acid (sodium ethacrynate), in 1 injection in 7 of 12 animals, guinea pigs, young, 240 to 489 g weight.
(AD) Hearing loss confirmed by loss of Preyer reflex 6 minutes after injection.
Primary damage to stria vascularis and some damage to outer hair cells of organ of Corti due to parenteral, intravenous, administration of range of 9.2 to 86 mg per kg of diuretic, ethacrynic acid (sodium ethacrynate), in 1 injection in 12 animals, guinea pigs, young, 240 to 489 g weight.
(AD) Electron microscopic study of cochlea. (ENG)

144
Moderate bilateral sensorineural hearing loss within 20 minutes and damage to outer hair cells of organ of Corti due to unspecified method of administration of 50 mg of diuretic, ethacrynic acid, in 1 dose in humans with kidney disorder.
(AD) Hearing loss confirmed by audiogram.
Sensorineural hearing loss within 15 minutes due to unspecified method of administration of 20 to 30 mg per kg daily of diuretic, ethacrynic acid, in 20 animals, cats.
(AD) Ethacrynic acid not recommended for clinical use in humans with kidney disorders. (ENG)

148
Transient sensorineural hearing loss due to diuretic, ethacrynic acid, in 1 human, adult, male. (FIN)

171
Rapid significant decr in cochlear microphonic but no pathological changes in cochlea after 1 hour due to parenteral, intravenous, administration of high doses, 20, 30, or 40 mg per kg, in solution of physiological saline, of diuretic, ethacrynic acid, in 1 injection for acute effects in 3 groups of 18 animals, guinea pigs, young, 250 g weight.
No detected decr in cochlear microphonic and no permanent physiological or structural changes in cochlea after 3 weeks due to parenteral, intravenous, administration of high doses, 30 mg per kg, of diuretic, ethacrynic acid, in chronic intoxication in 6 animals, guinea pigs, young, 250 g weight. (ENG)

178
Sensorineural hearing loss due to diuretic, ethacrynic acid, in humans, adult, female and male, with kidney disorders. (NOR)

246
Some incr in perilymph potassium due to parenteral, intravenous, administration of 10 mg per kg of diuretic, ethacrynic acid, in 1 injection in 12 to 14 animals, guinea pigs, pigmented, young, 200 to 400 g weight.
Some incr in perilymph potassium due to parenteral, intravenous, administration with 10 mg per kg, total of 30 mg per kg, of diuretic, ethacrynic acid, in 3 injections, over total of 24 hours, in 12 to 14 animals, guinea pigs, pigmented, young, 200 to 400 g weight.
Significant incr in perilymph potassium due to parenteral, intravenous, administration of 10 mg per kg, total of 50 mg per kg, of diuretic, ethacrynic acid, in 5 injections, over total of 48 hours, in 12 to 14 animals, guinea pigs, pigmented, young, 200 to 400 g weight.
(CT) Same method using normal saline equal in volume to ethacrynic acid

dosage in 12 to 14 guinea pigs, control group.
(AD) Suggested that cochleotoxic effects of ethacrynic acid result of
inhibition of cochlear duct membrane ATP. (ENG)

295
Hearing loss due to parenteral, intravenous, administration of 50 to 100 mg
of diuretic, ethacrynic acid, in humans with kidney disorder. (DAN)

320
Transient hearing loss after 3 days of treatment due to unspecified method of
administration of 50 mg twice daily of diuretic, ethacrynic acid, in 1 human,
adult, 56 years age, male, with rheumatic heart disorder and with normal
kidney function. (ENG)

339
Decr in potassium concentration and incr in sodium concentration of endolymph
within 10 minutes of treatment but no change in perilymph due to parenteral,
intravenous, administration of 1 to 5 mg per kg of diuretic, ethacrynic acid,
in 1 injection in 6 animals, dogs, young.
(CT) Study of potassium and sodium concentrations of endolymph and perilymph before injection of ethacrynic acid. (ENG)

503
Transient hearing loss 30 minutes after injection and change in composition
of fluids of cochlea due to parenteral, intravenous, administration of 50 mg
of diuretic, ethacrynic acid, in 1 human, adult, 45 years age, female, with
kidney disorder. (FR)

512
Transient bilateral sudden deafness due to parenteral, intravenous, administration of 50 mg of diuretic, (SQ) ethacrynic acid, in 1 human, adult, 42
years age, male, alcoholic, with liver disease.
Previous administration of 25 g of diuretic, (SQ) mannitol, in 1 human,
adult, 42 years age, male, alcoholic, with liver disease. (ENG)

559
Possible tinnitus and transient hearing loss due to diuretic, ethacrynic
acid, in humans.
(AD) Literature review of use, action, and toxic effects of diuretics.
(ENG)

603
Tinnitus due to oral administration of 25 mg twice a day, total of 50 mg per
kg, of anti-inflammatory agent, fluorometholone (NSC-33001), for 8 weeks in 1
of 112 humans, adult, 25 years average age, with tumors. (ENG)

151
Possible sensorineural hearing loss due to parenteral, intravenous, administration of high doses, 100 to 1000 mg, of diuretic, furosemide, for long
period in humans with kidney disorders.
(AD) Need for audiometry with clinical use of furosemide.
(AD) Recommended treatment with diuretics for long periods in humans with
kidney disorders only in severe cases with edema and cardiovascular system
problems. (GER)

234
Transient sensorineural hearing loss due to parenteral, rapid intravenous,
administration of high dose, 1000 mg, of diuretic, furosemide, in 40 minutes
in humans with kidney disorder.
(AD) Hearing loss confirmed by audiogram. (GER)

507
Bilateral sensorineural hearing loss and tinnitus due to parenteral, rapid
intravenous, administration of 240 mg of diuretic, furosemide, in 2 injections in 1 human, aged, 67 years age, male, after surgery.
(AD) Hearing loss confirmed by audiogram. (ENG)

513
Transient acute midfrequency hearing loss due to parenteral, rapid intra-
venous, administration of high doses, 1000 mg, of diuretic, furosemide, in 40
minutes in 8(50 percent) of 16 humans with kidney disorder.
  (CT) Audiometry, pretreatment and posttreatment.
  (AD) Maximum hearing loss in middle frequency suggests lesion in organ of
  Corti and not in CNS.
  (AD) Suggested that cochleotoxic effects related to rate of administration
  and dosage. (ENG)

514
Transient tinnitus due to parenteral, intravenous, administration of high
doses, 100 to 3200 mg daily, progressive doses on successive days, of diuretic, (SQ) furosemide, in 30 minutes to 10 hours in some of 15 humans with
kidney disorder and on dialysis.
  (AD) Later study of 4 humans with tinnitus due to furosemide showed normal
  audiograms.
Previous parenteral, rapid intravenous, administration of total of 60 g of
diuretic, (SQ) mannitol, in 24 hours in 15 humans with kidney disorder and on
dialysis.
  (CT) Treatment of 13 humans, control group, with dialysis only.
  (AD) Prevention of depletion of sodium and potassium by monitoring fluid
  and electrolyte balance. (ENG)

517
Transient tinnitus and hearing loss due to parenteral administration of 2000
mg of diuretic, furosemide, in 30 minutes in humans with chronic kidney
disorder. (ENG)

190
Sudden deafness and tinnitus due to topical administration of anesthetic,
garrot, in 1 human, adult, 36 years age, female, with previous hearing loss.
  (AD) Need for careful consideration in use of topical garrot in humans
  with history of auditory system problems or vestibular problems. (FR)

079
Hearing loss and range of degree of damage to hair cells of organ of Corti
due to parenteral, intramuscular, administration of 50, 80, 110, and 140 mg
per kg daily of antibiotic, gentamicin (gentamicin sulfate), for 7 to 28 days
in 4 groups of 12 animals, guinea pigs, adult, 250 to 500 g weight.
  (AD) Comparative study showed that degree of damage determined by dosage.
  (AD) Hearing loss determined by Preyer reflex. (ENG)

119
Damage to hair cells of organ of Corti and change in action potential due to
parenteral, intramuscular, administration of 20 mg per kg and 150 mg per kg
of antibiotic, gentamicin (gentamicin sulfate), in 2 groups of 59 animals,
guinea pigs.
  (CT) Control group of 26 guinea pigs used.
  (AD) More severe damage due to 150 mg per kg of gentamicin than due to 20
  mg per kg. (GER)

581
No hearing loss detected due to parenteral, intrathecal (SM), administration
of 1 mg daily of antibiotic, gentamicin, in 13 humans, infant.
No hearing loss detected due to parenteral, intramuscular (SM), administration of 2 mg per kg daily of antibiotic, gentamicin, in 13 humans, infant.
  (AD) Evaluation of cochlear function difficult in infants but no hearing
  loss detected after gentamicin therapy. (ENG)

585
High frequency hearing loss due to parenteral, intramuscular, administration
of 3.0 mg per kg daily or less of antibiotic, (SQ) gentamicin (gentamicin
sulfate), for several days in 1 of 215 humans, child, with genitourinary
system infection.
High frequency hearing loss due to previous administration of (SQ) other
antibiotics in 1 of 215 humans, child, with genitourinary system infection.
  (AD) Clinical evaluation of effect of gentamicin on eighth cranial nerve
  in patients and audiometry and vestibular function tests when indicated.
  (ENG)

586

Mild sensorineural hearing loss due to parenteral administration of 4 mg per kg every 24 hours in 4 divided doses, total doses of 1000 and 7788 mg, of antibiotic, gentamicin (gentamicin sulfate), for 25 to 138 days in 1 of 10 humans with infection secondary to burns.
  (AD) Audiology in 10 patients with therapy of long duration confirmed hearing loss in 1 patient.
No reported ototoxic effects due to parenteral (SM) administration of 4 mg per kg every 24 hours in 4 divided doses of antibiotic, gentamicin (gentamicin sulfate), for several days to over 30 days in other 85 humans, newborn infant, infant, child, and adolescent, 0 to 16 years age, with infection secondary to burns.
Simultaneous topical, direct site (SM), administration in cream of 0.1 percent of antibiotic, gentamicin (gentamicin sulfate), in some of 95 humans, newborn infant, infant, child, and adolescent, 0 to 16 years age, with infection secondary to burns. (ENG)

595

Bilateral hearing loss due to parenteral, intramuscular, administration of 80 mg daily of antibiotic, gentamicin, in 1 human, adult, 38 years age, male, with pulmonary infection.
  (AD) Hearing loss confirmed by audiogram. (FR)

702

Permanent total bilateral sensorineural hearing loss 5 days after cessation of treatment but no vestibular problems due to parenteral, intramuscular, administration of total dose of 0.32 g of antibiotic, gentamicin, in 16 single injections in 1 human, adult, 27 years age, male, with severe bilateral kidney disorder.
  (AD) Hearing loss confirmed by audiology. (GER)

725

Damage to eighth cranial nerve due to 20, 40, or 150 mg per kg of antibiotic, gentamicin (gentamicin sulfate), in 10 injections in animals, guinea pigs.
  (CT) Study of normal guinea pigs, control group. (GER)

397

Sensorineural hearing loss possibly due to antidiabetic, insulin, in humans treated for diabetes.
  (AD) Reported that hearing loss in many humans treated with insulin for diabetes.
  (AD) Hearing loss confirmed by audiometry. (ENG)

094

Inhibition of RNA metabolism in cells of Reissner's membrane due to unspecified method of administration of 400 mg per kg daily of antibiotic, kanamycin (kanamycin sulfate), for 14 days in 15 animals, guinea pigs, albino, 300 g weight. (ENG)

121

Tinnitus and high frequency hearing loss and damage to organ of Corti due to antibiotic, kanamycin, in humans.
  (AD) Literature review of kanamycin, use in therapy and toxic effects.
  (AD) Suggested clinical procedures for use of kanamycin with minimum risk of ototoxicity. (ENG)

126

Decr in acid mucopolysaccharides in stria vascularis and spiral ligament due to parenteral, subcutaneous, administration of 400 mg per kg daily for 5 days a week of antibiotic, kanamycin (kanamycin sulfate), for 10 days in 60 animals, guinea pigs, pigmented, 250 to 350 g weight, with normal pinna reflex.
  (CT) Control group of 8 guinea pigs used.
  (AD) Study of role of mucopolysaccharides in hearing. (ENG)

131

Severe sensorineural hearing loss due to antibiotic, kanamycin, in humans,

adult and child, female and male.
    (AD) Hearing loss confirmed by audiometry. (JAP)

146
Cochleotoxic effects due to antibiotic, kanamycin, in chronic intoxication in
animals, rabbits.
    (AD) Electrophysiological study of ototoxicity of kanamycin. (JAP)

159
Hearing loss due to antibiotic, kanamycin, in humans with infections. (JAP)

173
Decr in oxygen consumption of cochlea due to parenteral, intraperitoneal,
administration of 400 mg per kg daily of antibiotic, kanamycin (kanamycin
sulfate), for 5,10, and 20 days in 3 groups of 22 animals, guinea pigs,
white, 300 to 400 g weight.
    (CT) Study of oxygen consumption in 35 guinea pigs, control group, not
    treated with kanamycin.
    (AD) Measurement of oxygen consumption with differential type of microres-
    pirometer. (ENG)

199
Progressive high frequency hearing loss due to parenteral, intramuscular,
administration of 500 mg twice a day of antibiotic, kanamycin, in 1 human,
aged, male, with diabetes mellitus, vascular disorder, and osteomyelitis.
    (AD) Hearing loss confirmed by audiogram.
    (AD) Report on clinical use and toxicity of antibiotics. (ENG)

203
Permanent high frequency hearing loss due to range of less than 30 g to more
than 180 g of antibiotic, kanamycin, for long period in 55.6 percent of 72
humans with tuberculosis.
    (AD) Need for audiometry during treatment with kanamycin for prevention of
    more severe hearing loss. (GER)

204
Incr then decr in activity of 3 lysosomal enzymes in gradual permanent degeneration of hair cells of organ of Corti due to parenteral, intraperitoneal, administration of 250 mg per kg daily, total doses of 1750 to 10500
mg per kg, of antibiotic, kanamycin (kanamycin sulfate), for 1 to 6 weeks in
36 animals, guinea pigs, 250 to 300 g weight, with normal pinna reflex and no
middle ear infection.
Transient incr then decr in activity of 3 lysosomal enzymes in spiral ganglion due to parenteral, intraperitoneal, administration of 250 mg per kg
daily, total doses of 1750 to 10500 mg per kg, of antibiotic, kanamycin
(kanamycin sulfate), for 1 to 6 weeks in 36 animals, guinea pigs, 250 to 300
g weight, with normal pinna reflex and no middle ear infection.
    (CT) Study of 9 guinea pigs, control group, not treated with kanamycin.
    (AD) Suggested that histochemical changes in spiral ganglion independent
    of damage to organ of Corti. (ENG)

223
Sensorineural hearing loss due to antibiotic, kanamycin, in 1 human, adult,
female.
    (AD) Claim of negligence in treatment with kanamycin. (JAP)

229
Auditory system problems due to parenteral, intramuscular, administration of
high doses of antibiotic, kanamycin, for long period in humans, infant, for
infections.
    (AD) Recommended kanamycin dosage for infants of 7.5 mg per kg daily in
    divided doses every 12 hours by intramuscular administration for 12 days
    at most. (ENG)

241
Risk of damage to organ of Corti and hearing loss due to antibiotic, kanamycin, in humans, infant.
    (AD) Study of dose response relationships.

(AD)   Recommended dose of 15 mg per kg daily every 12 hours for infants.
(ENG)

242

Variations in decr in cochlear microphonic due to parenteral, intraperitoneal, administration of 100 mg per kg of antibiotic, kanamycin, for period
until measurement of cochlear microphonic not possible in 12 animals, rabbits, adult, normal.
Changes in outer hair cells and supporting cells, in particular in basal coil
of cochlea, and slight damage to inner hair cells of organ of Corti due to
parenteral, intraperitoneal, administration of 100 mg per kg of antibiotic,
kanamycin, for period until measurement of cochlear microphonic not possible
in 12 animals, rabbits, adult, normal.
    (AD) Serial observations on beginning and progression of cochleotoxic
    effects of kanamycin by daily measurement of cochlear microphonic and
    study of correlations between electrophysiological and histopathological
    changes.
    (AD) Variations in response of cochlea to kanamycin but correlation bet-
    ween electrophysiological and histopathological changes.   (ENG)

267

Degeneration of outer hair cells of organ of Corti and damage to spiral
ganglion due to 400 mg per kg daily of antibiotic, kanamycin, for 14 days in
animals, guinea pigs.
Permanent histological changes in cochlea due to 100 mg per kg of antibiotic,
kanamycin, in animals, guinea pigs.
Damage to organ of Corti of fetuses due to 200 mg per kg of antibiotic,
kanamycin, in animals, guinea pigs, treated during pregnancy.
    (AD) Report on previous results of experimentation.
Cochleotoxic effects due to antibiotic, kanamycin, in average of 30 percent
of more than 1000 humans, adult.
    (AD) Discussion of relationship between kanamycin ototoxicity and dosage,
    duration of treatment, age, previous auditory system problems, administra-
    tion of other ototoxic drugs, kidney function, and individual responses to
    drug.   (ENG)

268

Hearing loss due to antibiotic, kanamycin, in humans, adult.
    (AD) Discussion on incidence of hearing loss due to kanamycin, correlation
    between blood levels and ototoxicity, and relationship between kidney
    function and cochleotoxic effects.   (ENG)

286

Decr in cochlear microphonic due to antibiotic, kanamycin (kanamycin sulfate), in animals, guinea pigs.
Minimum effect on cochlear microphonic due to antibiotic, kanamycin (IB)
(kanamycin sulfate), in animals, guinea pigs, with administration of pantothenic acid.   (GER)

287

Cochlear impairment in fetus due to antibiotic, kanamycin, in humans, female,
treated during pregnancy.
    (AD) Discussion of cochleotoxic effects of kanamycin in newborn infants
    and infants.   (JAP)

307

No sensorineural hearing loss due to unspecified method of administration of
5 to 21 mg per kg daily, total doses of 30 to 450 mg, of antibiotic, kanamycin, for 3 to 11 days in 20 humans, infant and child, 1 to 4 years age,
treated when newborn infant for various infections.
    (CT) Study of 7 children, control group, treated with other antibiotics
    during neonatal period for similar infections.
    (AD) Use of pure tone audiometry or clinical evaluation only to determine
    hearing loss.
    (AD) Study to determine cochleotoxic effects of kanamycin when used in
    treatment of newborn infants.   (ENG)

Shifts in cochlear microphonic and action potential thresholds and loss of
Preyer reflex due to parenteral, subcutaneous, administration of 400 mg per
kg daily of antibiotic, kanamycin, for 10, 14, or 20 days in 3 groups of
animals, guinea pigs, adult, male.
    (CT) Study of guinea pigs, control group.
    (AD) Correlation between duration of dosage and decr in function.
    (AD) Study of guinea pigs showed individual responses to kanamycin.
Shifts in cochlear microphonic and action potential thresholds and loss of
Preyer reflex due to parenteral, subcutaneous, administration of 400 mg per
kg daily of antibiotic, kanamycin, for 10, 14, or 20 days in 3 groups of
animals, rats, adult, male.
    (CT) Study of rats, control group.
    (AD) Results of study of rats showed high degree of individual response to
kanamycin or technical difficulty in recording from round window of rat.
Shifts in cochlear microphonic and action potential thresholds and loss of
Preyer reflex due to parenteral, subcutaneous, administration of 400 mg per
kg daily of antibiotic, kanamycin, for 10, 14, or 20 days in 3 groups of
animals, rabbits, adult, male.
    (CT) Study of rabbits, control group.
    (AD) Similarity between cochlear impairment of rabbit and hearing loss in
humans due to kanamycin.
Destruction of hair cells of organ of Corti in all coils of cochlea and
damage to stria vascularis and spiral ganglion due to unspecified method of
administration of 200 mg per kg of antibiotic, kanamycin, for 20 days in
animals, guinea pigs.
    (AD) Difference in pattern and degree of cochlear impairment in different
species of animals.
    (AD) Suggested that physiological changes precede histological changes and
so show more clearly the ototoxic effects of the drug. (ENG)

349
Effect on hearing loss due to antibiotic, kanamycin (IB), in animals, rabbits, with administration of vitamin B derivatives.
    (AD) Study of effects of vitamin B derivatives on cochleotoxic effects of
kanamycin. (JAP)

391
Hearing loss in 15 fetuses due to parenteral, intramuscular, administration
of 200 mg per kg daily of antibiotic, kanamycin, for 15 days in animals,
rats, Wistar strain, female, about 150 g weight, during pregnancy.
    (AD) Test of Preyer reflex of rats, newborn infant, 30 days after birth.
No hearing loss due to 20 mg per kg daily of antibiotic, kanamycin, for 1 to
5 days in 15 humans, newborn infant.
    (CT) EEG in newborn infants, before and about 1 month after kanamycin
administration.
No hearing loss in fetuses due to antibiotic, kanamycin, in humans, female,
treated for pulmonary tuberculosis during pregnancy.
    (AD) Follow up study for 3 years after birth showed no hearing loss in
children.
    (AD) Discussion of clinical and experimental studies on effects of kanamy-
cin.
Hearing loss due to range of 30 to 100 mg per kg daily of antibiotic, kanamycin, for range of 3 to 46 days in 9 of 391 humans, newborn infant.
No hearing loss due to less than 60 mg per kg daily of antibiotic, kanamycin,
for less than 11 days in 382 humans, newborn infant.
    (AD) Discussion of reports from 100 hospitals in Japan on effects of
kanamycin in newborn infants.
    (AD) Relationship between cochleotoxic effects of kanamycin and daily
dosage and duration of treatment. (ENG)

393
Severe hearing loss due to parenteral administration of 1 to 2 g daily, total
doses of 30, 40, 21, and 4 g, of antibiotic, kanamycin, in 4 humans, adult,
53, 20, 32, and 37 years age, female and male, with kidney disorders.
    (AD) Case reports of cochleotoxic effects of kanamycin in humans with
kidney disorders. (ENG)

435

Decr in cochlear microphonic, summating potential, and eighth nerve action
potential due to parenteral, subcutaneous, administration of 800 mg per kg
daily of antibiotic, kanamycin, for 5 to 7 days in 8 animals, guinea pigs.
Slow decr of endocochlear potential in cochlear duct and low maximum negative
value of endocochlear potential due to parenteral, subcutaneous, administration of 800 mg per kg daily of antibiotic, kanamycin, for 5 to 7 days in 8
animals, guinea pigs, with anoxia.
    (AD) Longer survival time of endocochlear potential with severe decr in
    cochlear microphonic.
    (AD) Study of negative potential in cochlear duct of guinea pig during
    anoxia. (ENG)

439

Decr in cochlear potentials due to parenteral, intramuscular, administration
of 400 mg per kg of antibiotic, kanamycin, for 10 days in 8 animals, guinea
pigs. (FR)

440

Possible damage to organ of Corti in fetuses due to antibiotic, kanamycin, in
animals, guinea pigs, adult, during pregnancy.
    (AD) Study of transmission of drugs from mother to fetus.
    (AD) Serum levels of kanamycin in fetus about 7 percent of serum levels in
    mother and not related to variations in dosage.
    (AD) Slow elimination of kanamycin from fetus. (ENG)

489

Loss of Preyer reflex and progressive damage to hair cells of organ of Corti
beginning with basal coil of cochlea due to 400 mg per kg of antibiotic,
kanamycin (kanamycin sulfate), in 3 to 18 injections in 25 animals, guinea
pigs, adult, 250 to 350 g weight, with normal Preyer reflex.
    (CT) Daily administration of Ringer's solution in 4 guinea pigs, control
    group.
    (AD) Discussion of difference between ototoxic effects of kanamycin and
    streptomycin on organ of Corti. (ENG)

493

Decr in cochlear microphonics due to parenteral, intramuscular, administration of 400 or 200 mg per kg daily of antibiotic, kanamycin, in animals,
guinea pigs.
Decr in cochlear microphonics due to parenteral, intravenous, administration
of 100 mg per kg daily of antibiotic, kanamycin, for 3 to 10 days in animals,
guinea pigs.
No ototoxic effect in fetuses due to antibiotic, kanamycin, in animals,
guinea pigs, female, treated during pregnancy.
    (AD) More rapid and severe ototoxic effect with intravenous administration
    than with intramuscular administration. (ENG)

617

Hearing loss observed after several years possibly due to high doses, 125 mg
per kg daily, total of 10.75 g, of antibiotic, kanamycin, for total of 43
days in 1 human, child, treated after surgery for congenital intestinal
atresia when newborn infant.
    (AD) Hearing loss possibly congenital and not due to kanamycin therapy.
Bilateral hearing loss detected after 8 to 10 years but no subjective symptoms due to 100 mg per kg daily of antibiotic, kanamycin, for 8 to 14 days in
1 of 51 humans, child, treated for disorder when infant.
    (AD) Study with audiometry of effects of kanamycin used in treatment of 51
    newborn infants and infants.
    (CT) Study of 43 children, control group, without kanamycin therapy.
    (AD) Suggested that high doses of kanamycin not be used.
    (AD) Suggested that less ototoxic effects due to kanamycin in infants and
    children than in adults. (ENG)

618

Hearing loss due to parenteral, intramuscular, administration of 2 g in 2
doses, twice weekly, of antibiotic, kanamycin, in 7(1.1 percent) of 608
humans with pulmonary tuberculosis.
    (AD) Relationship between hearing loss and total dosage of kanamycin.

No hearing loss due to parenteral, intravenous, administration of 1 g twice weekly, dissolved in 300 ml of saline solution, of antibiotic, kanamycin, for long period in 1 human, adult, 40 years age, male, with pulmonary tuberculosis.
(AD) Cochlear function monitored by audiometry during therapy.
(AD) Higher blood levels of kanamycin with intravenous route than with intramuscular route. (ENG)

633
Cochlear impairment due to antibiotic, kanamycin, in humans, female, treated for gynecologic infections. (FR)

635
Effect on cochlear impairment due to antibiotic, kanamycin (IB), in animals, rabbits, with administration of derivative of thiamine. (JAP)

662
Hearing loss due to 250 mg of antibiotic, kanamycin (kanamycin sulfate), for 8 days in animals, guinea pigs, 200 to 300 g weight with exposure to noise.
(CT) Same method using 0.9 percent sodium chloride in guinea pigs, control group.
(AD) Study of ototoxic effects of kanamycin when administered to guinea pigs with exposure to noise. (GER)

675
Possible total hearing loss due to parenteral administration of antibiotic, kanamycin (kanamycin sulfate), in humans with genitourinary system infections and with concurrent kidney disorder. (ENG)

688
Hearing loss due to antibiotic, kanamycin, in 2 (8 percent) of 26 humans after 3 months and in 1 (5 percent) of 21 humans after 6 months of retreatment for pulmonary tuberculosis.
(CT) Audiograms, pretreatment and posttreatment.
Hearing loss due to antibiotic, kanamycin, for 6 months in 14.9 percent of humans during retreatment for pulmonary tuberculosis.
(AD) Hearing loss confirmed by audiograms. (ENG)

692
Bilateral sensorineural hearing loss possibly due to topical, direct site, administration in vertebral canal of 500 mg, in 2 cc water, of antibiotic, kanamycin (kanamycin sulfate), in 1 dose in 1 human, aged, 67 years age, male, with previous hearing loss, during surgery for lumbar disc.
(AD) Case report of hearing loss possibly due to kanamycin.
(AD) Hearing loss confirmed by audiometry.
(AD) Neurotoxic effects resulted from kanamycin administration. (ENG)

699
Permanent hearing loss due to parenteral, intramuscular, administration of 0.5 g at 6-hour intervals for 48 hours and then at 12-hour intervals for 5 days, total dose of more than 12 g, to produce peak serum levels of 10 to 30 mcg per ml after 12 hours, of antibiotic, kanamycin, for about 7 days in 2 of about 300 humans with various infections.
(AD) Higher risk of kanamycin ototoxicity in patients with dehydration or kidney disorder or with total doses of about 20 g.
(AD) Prevention or decr in ototoxic effects with regulation of daily dose and duration of therapy and with tests of kidney function. (ENG)

701
Hearing loss due to antibiotic, kanamycin, in humans.
(AD) Study of clinical use of vitamin K-1 in hearing loss due to kanamycin. (JAP)

724
Hearing loss due to antibiotic, kanamycin, in humans in dental treatment. (ENG)

727

Decr in cochleotoxic effects due to parenteral, subcutaneous, administration
of antibiotic, kanamycin (IB), in animals, cats, with administration of
pantothenic acid.
   (AD) Electrophysiological study of effect of pantothenic acid on kanamycin
   ototoxicity in cats.   (GER)

467

Changes in succinic dehydrogenase of organ of Corti due to parenteral, subcutaneous, administration of 2 mg per kg of heavy metal, lead (lead acetate),
for 28 days in 20 animals, guinea pigs.
   (CT) Study of 10 guinea pigs, control group.   (GER)

553

Tinnitus and distortion of sound due to parenteral, rapid intravenous, administration to arm of 2.5 mg per kg of 0.5 percent concentration of anesthetic, lidocaine, in 1 injection, with release of tourniquet 5 minutes after
injection, in 9 of 10 humans, unpaid subjects.   (ENG)

531

Hearing loss due to antibiotic, lincomycin, in 1 human treated with hemodialysis after bilateral nephrectomy for kidney disorder.
   (AD) Hearing loss confirmed by audiogram.   (CZ)

525

No loss of Preyer reflex and no structural changes in organ of Corti and
stria vascularis due to parenteral, intraperitoneal, administration of 3 to 5
mg per kg, in aqueous solution, of antineoplastic, mechlorethamine, for 5
days to 5 weeks in animals, 8 guinea pigs, adult, 300 to 400 g weight, and 6
mice, adult, 25 to 35 g weight, with normal Preyer reflex.
Loss of Preyer reflex and severe destruction of outer hair cells of organ of
Corti in basal and middle coils of cochlea but little or no change in stria
vascularis, spiral ganglion, and cochlear nerve due to parenteral, intraperitoneal, administration of 10 to 30 mg per kg, in aqueous solution, of antineoplastic, mechlorethamine, for 1 day to 5 weeks in animals, 7 guinea
pigs, adult, 300 to 400 g weight, and 19 mice, adult, 25 to 35 g weight, with
normal Preyer reflex.
   (CT) Same method using same volume of Ringer's solution in 5 animals,
   control group.
   (AD) Electron microscopic study of degeneration of cochlea in mechlorethamine intoxicated animals and in animals with congenital hearing loss to
   determine the mechanism of degeneration.
   (AD) Suggested possible effect on protein synthesis in hair cells of organ
   of Corti in early stages of mechlorethamine ototoxicity.   (ENG)

167

Decr in concentrations of succinic dehydrogenase, esterases, and sulfhydryl
compounds due to parenteral, subcutaneous, administration of 1 mg per kg, in
1 ml distilled water, of heavy metal, mercury (mercuric chloride), for 28
days in animals, guinea pigs.
   (CT) Study of guinea pigs, control group, not treated with mercury.
   (AD) Report on relationship between changes in metabolism in inner ear due
   to mercury and auditory system problems.   (GER)

208

Hearing loss due to oral ingestion, in contaminated fish, of heavy metal,
mercury (organic methyl mercury), in humans.
   (AD) Recommended international limit of 0.5 ppm of mercury (organic methyl
   mercury) for humans.
   (AD) Reported high levels of mercury (organic methyl mercury) in fetuses.
   (ENG)

001

Permanent bilateral high frequency hearing loss due to topical administration
by irrigation of joint cavity of left knee with 50 cc of 10 percent solution
of antibiotic, neomycin, for every 3 hours for 3 days and every 6 hours for 5
days in 1 human, child, 6 years age, male, 56 lb weight.
   (CT) Pretreatment audiogram showed normal bilateral hearing sensitivity.
   (ENG)

004
Bilateral sensorineural hearing loss due to oral administration of total of
600 g of antibiotic, neomycin, in 300 days in 1 human, child, 11 years age,
male, with chronic colitis.
   (AD) Literature review showed 4 other case reports of hearing loss due to
   oral administration of neomycin. (ENG)

025
Effect on electrical response of cochlea due to 300 mg per kg and 50 mg per
kg of antibiotic, neomycin, for 6 days and 10 days respectively in 2 groups
of animals, guinea pigs.
Decr in cochleotoxic effect due to antibiotic, neomycin (IB), in animals,
guinea pigs, with administration of ATP. (GER)

064
Risk of hearing loss due to topical administration of more than 1 g of antibiotic, neomycin, in more than 7 days in humans.
   (AD) Comment on risk of hearing loss with topical administration of neomycin. (ENG)

104
Hearing loss due to 1.5 g daily, total of 12 g, of antibiotic, neomycin, in 1
human, aged, 90 years age.
   (AD) Cochleotoxic effect due to negligence of physician. (SW)

150
Total sensorineural hearing loss due to topical administration by irrigation
of mediastinum with 2400 ml per 24 hours, total of 72 g, of 0.3 percent
solution of antibiotic, neomycin, for 11 days in 1 human, adult, 60 years
age, male, with purulent mediastinitis.
   (AD) High serum neomycin concentrations decr by hemodialysis. (ENG)

231
No hearing loss due to 8 g and then 12 g daily of antibiotic, neomycin
(neomycin sulfate), for total of 19 months in 1 human, adult, 48 years age,
male, chronic alcoholic, treated for infections. (ENG)

238
Sensorineural hearing loss due to oral administration of 50 to 100 mg per kg
of antibiotic, neomycin, in 9 of 17 humans, child, 2.5 to 7 years age, with
dyspepsia.
   (AD) Hearing loss determined by audiometry. (FR)

254
Hearing loss due to antibiotic, neomycin, in humans, infant.
   (AD) Routine use of neomycin for gastroenteritis in infants not recom-
   mended. (ENG)

381
Degeneration of organ of Corti and hearing loss due to various methods of
administration of antibiotic, neomycin, in humans.
   (AD) Literature review of toxic effects of new antibiotics. (GER)

385
Possible hearing loss due to oral administration of antibiotic, neomycin, in
humans, infant, with enteritis.
   (AD) Literature review of possible toxic effects of antibiotics in treatment of enteritis. (GER)

387
Risk of hearing loss due to parenteral and oral administration of antibiotic,
neomycin, in humans.
Possible hearing loss due to topical, rectal, administration of antibiotic,
neomycin, in humans.
   (AD) Study of rectal administration as possible route for neomycin therapy. (ENG)

469
Hearing loss due to parenteral administration of antibiotic, neomycin, in
humans. (FR)

498
Severe hearing loss 8 days after first dose due to oral administration of 7 g
on first day followed by 4 g on second day, total dose of 11 g, of antibiotic, neomycin, for total of 2 days in 1 human, adult, 45 years age, female,
treated before surgery.
    (AD) Case report of severe hearing loss due to neomycin therapy.
    (AD) Hearing clinically normal before neomycin treatment.
    (AD) Audiometry 1.5 years later confirmed auditory system problem. (ENG)

518
Hearing loss and damage to hair cells of organ of Corti but no histological
changes in vascular strip of spiral fissure due to antibiotic, neomycin, in
animals, guinea pigs.
    (CT) Study of guinea pigs, control group, not treated with neomycin.
    (RUS)

048
Severe sensorineural hearing loss and loss of hair cells of organ of Corti in
basal and middle coils of cochlea due to parenteral, intravenous, administration of high doses, 1.0 mg per kg, of antineoplastic, nitrogen mustard, in 1
injection in animals, cats, conditioned. (ENG)

138
Sensorineural hearing loss due to antiparasitic, oil of chenopodium, in 1
human, adult, 56 years age, male.
    (AD) Hearing loss confirmed by audiograms. (POL)

352
Severe hearing loss due to ototoxic drugs in humans, newborn infant.
    (AD) Comment on previous report on ototoxicity in premature infants.
    (AD) Discussion of decr in congenital hearing loss and prelingual hearing
    loss due to ototoxic drugs and other etiologic factors. (ENG)

398
Effect on auditory threshold due to parenteral, subcutaneous, administration
of ototoxic drugs in 4 animals, dogs, 1 to 2 years age, 7 to 10 kg weight,
conditioned.
    (CT) Determined standard deviation of auditory threshold in dogs by mea-
    surement of changes without administration of drugs.
    (CT) Measurement of auditory threshold before and after administration of
    drugs. (ENG)

407
Hearing loss due to ototoxic drugs in humans.
    (AD) Discussion of cochleotoxic effects of ototoxic drugs. (FR)

499
Sensorineural hearing loss due to ototoxic drugs in humans.
    (AD) Management of hearing loss includes prevention of ototoxicity due to
    drugs. (ENG)

505
Congenital hearing loss due to ototoxic drugs in humans, newborn infant.
    (AD) Discussion of etiology of congenital hearing loss. (ENG)

717
Hearing loss in fetus due to ototoxic drugs in humans treated during pregnancy.
    (AD) Discussion of etiology of hearing loss in risk children. (GER)

292
Cochlear impairment due to parenteral, intramuscular, administration of 1.2,
10, or 1 ml of antibiotic, penicillin (procaine penicillin G), in humans,
adult, with various infections.
    (AD) Discussion of 3 case reports. (SL)

418

Hearing loss within 2 to 3 minutes after injection and tinnitus due to parenteral, intravenous, administration of anesthetic, procaine (procaine hydrochloride), in 30 humans with normal hearing and treated for disorders.
  (AD) Study of effect on hearing loss and tinnitus of manual compression of
  neurovascular bundle.
  (AD) No effect on tinnitus or hearing loss of manual compression of neurovascular bundle before and during injection of procaine.
  (AD) Disappearance of tinnitus due to unilateral manual compression of
  neurovascular bundle after injection of procaine in 23 subjects.
  (AD) Suppression of tinnitus only during manual compression of neurovascular bundle in other subjects.
  (AD) Less effect on hearing loss of manual compression of neurovascular
  bundle after injection of procaine. (FR)

552

Tinnitus within several hours due to 10 mg twice daily of cardiovascular
agent, propranolol, for 4 days in 1 human, adult, 56 years age, female, with
mild hypertension.
  (AD) Case report of tinnitus for duration of dosage of 10 mg twice daily
  of propranolol.
  (AD) Cessation of tinnitus after decr in dosage to 10 mg daily of propranolol. (ENG)

239

Transient sensorineural hearing loss due to oral ingestion in tablets of 3 to
5 g (10 to 15 tablets) of antimalarial, quinine, in 1 human, adult, 26 years
age, male, with alcohol intoxication.
  (AD) Case of attempted suicide.
  (AD) Hearing loss confirmed by audiogram. (GER)

258

Cessation of blood flow in some capillaries of basilar membrane due to parenteral, intraperitoneal, administration of 125 mg of antimalarial, quinine
(quinine dihydrochloride), in 1 dose in animals, guinea pigs, 500 g weight.
Transient cessation of blood flow in some capillaries of basilar membrane due
to parenteral, intraperitoneal, administration of 62.5 mg per dose, total of
125 mg, of antimalarial, quinine (quinine dihydrochloride), in gradual doses
in animals, guinea pigs, 500 g weight.
  (CT) Study of guinea pigs, control group.
  (AD) Transient hearing loss due to quinine (quinine dihydrochloride) known
  from previous studies.
  (AD) Drugs known to produce hearing loss also produce cessation of blood
  flow in capillaries of basilar membrane. (ENG)

291

Cochlear impairment due to 5.0 g of antimalarial, quinine (quinine hydroch-
loride), in humans.
Cochlear impairment due to antimalarial, quinine (quinine hydrochloride), in
animals, cats and rabbits.
  (AD) Comparative animal studies and clinical case reports.
  (AD) Study of ocular toxicity with comment on ototoxicity. (GER)

388

Hearing loss in 2 fetuses, twin, male, due to oral ingestion of high doses of
antimalarial, quinine, for unspecified period in 1 human, female, at end of
first trimester of pregnancy to induce abortion.
  (AD) No visual perception defect in twins due to ingestion of quinine by
  mother during pregnancy.
  (AD) Suggested vascular or neural mechanism of ototoxic effects of
  quinine. (ENG)

607

Transient tinnitus and hearing loss after 2 hours due to oral ingestion of 6
g of antimalarial, quinine (quinine sulfate), in 1 dose in 1 human, adult, 26
years age, female, in suicide attempt.
Transient tinnitus and sensorineural hearing loss within 5 hours due to oral
ingestion of 12 g, to produce serum level of 9.2 mg per l, of antimalarial,

quinine (quinine sulfate), in 1 human, adult, 24 years age, female, during
pregnancy in attempt to induce abortion. (ENG)

174

Transient high frequency hearing loss and tinnitus after 4 hours due to oral
administration of 1 g daily of antidiabetic, (SQ) R 94, for 28 days at most
in 26 humans, adolescent and adult, 15 to 55 years age, male, with moderate
to severe diabetes.
Incr in high frequency hearing loss due to oral administration of 1 g of
antidiabetic, (SQ) R 94, for 7 days after onset of hearing loss in 9 of 26
humans, adolescent and adult, 15 to 55 years age, male, with moderate to
severe diabetes.
Decr and complete reversal of hearing loss due to oral administration of 1 g
of antidiabetic, (SQ) R 94 (IB), in 15 of 26 humans, adolescent and adult, 15
to 55 years age, male, with moderate to severe diabetes, with administration
of 100 and 200 mg of nicotinic acid.
    (AD) Reversal of hearing loss after cessation of treatment with R 94 or
    with administration of nicotinic acid.
    (CT) Use of subjects with no recent treatment with ototoxic drugs.
    (CT) Audiometry, pretreatment and 4 hours after every daily dose.
    (AD) Vestibular function tests normal. (ENG)

622

Possible transient hearing loss due to antibiotic, rifampicin, in humans.
(ENG)

626

Transient hearing loss during therapy due to 300 mg 3 times a day of antibiotic, rifampicin, for 14 days in 2 of 27 humans, adult and aged, 20 to 79
years age, female and male, with genitourinary system infections. (ENG)

401

Possible TTS(auditory) of 24 hours duration due to high doses of salicylates
in humans.
Obstruction of capillaries of spiral vessels of basilar membrane due to high
doses of salicylates in humans.
    (AD) Same obstruction of capillaries due to sound stimulation.
    (AD) TTS(auditory) possibly due to obstruction of capillaries by salicy-
    lates or sound.
Susceptibility to PTS(auditory) due to salicylates in humans exposed to
noise.
    (AD) Conclusions based on animal experimentation. (ENG)

448

Significant decr in ATP levels of Reissner's membrane but no change in P-
creatine due to parenteral, intraperitoneal, administration of high doses,
400 mg per kg, of salicylate in animals, guinea pigs, young, about 200 g
weight.
Incr in ATP of cochlear nerve and incr in P-creatine of stria vascularis due
to parenteral, intraperitoneal, administration of high doses, 400 mg per kg,
of salicylate in animals, guinea pigs, young, 200 g weight.
    (CT) Same method using 0.9 percent saline in 3 guinea pigs, control group.
    (AD) Suggested that ototoxicity of salicylate possibly due to impairment
    of energy metabolism of Reissner's membrane. (ENG)

596

Tinnitus due to high doses of salicylates in humans.
    (AD) Tinnitus early symptom of salicylate intoxication in some cases.
    (AD) Discussion of etiology, symptoms, diagnosis and evaluation, treat-
    ment, and prevention of salicylate intoxication. (ENG)

686

Decr in ATP and p-creatine of organ of Corti, spiral ganglion, cochlear
nerve, stria vascularis, and Reissner's membrane only after 3 days of exposure due to range of doses of salicylate in animals, guinea pigs.
    (AD) Results of study suggest that ototoxicity of salicylates not due to
    impairment of energy metabolism of cochlea. (ENG)

168

Appearance of salicylate in blood vessels of stria vascularis and spiral ligament after 15 minutes due to parenteral, intravenous and intraperitoneal, administration of 6.6 to 49.5 mc per kg, tritium-labelled solution, of salicylate, salicylic acid, in 5 animals, guinea pigs, albino, adult, 300 to 320 g weight.
Concentration of salicylate in stria vascularis and spiral ligament and diffusion into organ of Corti and Rosenthal's canal after 1 hour due to parenteral, intravenous and intraperitoneal, administration of 6.6 to 49.5 mc per kg, tritium-labelled solution, of salicylate, salicylic acid, in 5 animals, guinea pigs, albino, adult, 300 to 320 g weight.
Small amount of salicylate after 6 hours and no salicylate after 13 hours in cochlea due to parenteral, intravenous and intraperitoneal, administration of 6.6 to 49.5 mc per kg, tritium-labelled solution, of salicylate, salicylic acid, in 5 animals, guinea pigs, albino, adult, 300 to 320 g weight.
  (AD) Autoradiographical study to determine mechanism of salicylate ototoxicity by localization of tritiated salicylate in cochlea of guinea pigs.
  (AD) Salicylate levels in cochlea due to vascular route and diffusion into cochlear duct and not due to accumulation in specific areas. (ENG)

312

Transient bilateral sensorineural hearing loss of 60 and 50 decibels due to topical, direct site, administration of ointment with 5 percent of salicylate, salicylic acid, for 3 times daily in 2 humans, female, with psoriasis. (ENG)

082

Transient threshold shift due to parenteral, intraperitoneal, administration of 300 mg per kg (equivalent to 65 aspirin tablets for 70 kg man),in saline solution, of salicylate, sodium salicylate, in 1 injection in animals, guinea pigs.
  (CT) Electrophysiological measurement of hearing sensitivity before and after salicylate injection.
Transient threshold shift due to parenteral, intraperitoneal, administration of 100 to 250 mg per kg of salicylate, sodium salicylate, in animals, guinea pigs, conditioned. (ENG)

166

Decr in succinic dehydrogenase concentration, in particular in stria vascularis and outer hair cells of organ of Corti, and decr in esterases and sulfhydryl compounds due to parenteral, subcutaneous, administration of 100 mg per kg daily, in 2 ml distilled water, of salicylate, sodium salicylate, for 28 days in animals, guinea pigs.
  (CT) Study of guinea pigs, control group, not treated with sodium salicylate.
  (AD) Report on relationship between changes in metabolism in inner ear due to sodium salicylate and auditory system problems. (GER)

189

Threshold shift due to parenteral, intraperitoneal, administration of 300 mg per kg of salicylate, sodium salicylate, in 1 dose in 4 animals, cats.
Small threshold shift of about 3 decibels due to parenteral, intraperitoneal, administration of 125 mg per kg daily of salicylate, sodium salicylate, for total of 28 injections in 4 animals, cats.
Threshold shift due to parenteral, intraperitoneal, administration of (SQ) 300 mg per kg of salicylate, sodium salicylate, in (SQ) 1 dose in 6 animals, guinea pigs.
Small threshold shift of about 4 decibels due to parenteral, intraperitoneal, administration of (SQ) 150,225, or 300 mg per kg daily of salicylate, sodium salicylate, for (SQ) total of 10 injections in 6 animals, guinea pigs. (ENG)

205

Changes in biochemical composition of endolymph and perilymph due to parenteral, intraperitoneal, administration of 350 mg per kg of salicylate, sodium salicylate, in 1 injection in 6 animals, cats.
  (CT) Same method using 10 ml saline solution in 3 cats, control group.
Decr in cochlear microphonic and neural potential due to parenteral, intraperitoneal, administration of 350 mg per kg of salicylate, sodium salicylate,

in 1 injection in 7 animals, cats.
  (CT) Baseline cochlear microphonic and neural potential obtained.
  (AD) Suggested that hearing loss in salicylate intoxication due to bioche-
mical changes in cochlea. (ENG)

023

No degeneration in inner hair cells and outer hair cells of organ of Corti
due to parenteral, intramuscular, administration of 200 mg per kg daily of
antibiotic, streptomycin (streptomycin sulfate), for 10 days in 15 animals,
guinea pigs, 150 to 200 g weight.
  (CT) Study of 5 guinea pigs, control group.
Changes in succinic dehydrogenase activity in hair cells of organ of Corti
due to parenteral, intramuscular, administration of 200 mg per kg daily of
antibiotic, streptomycin (streptomycin sulfate), for 10 days in 15 animals,
guinea pigs, 150 to 200 g weight.
  (CT) Study of 10 guinea pigs, control group.
  (AD) Difference between inner hair cells and outer hair cells discussed.
(ENG)

031

Damage to cochlea due to antibiotic, streptomycin, in animals, guinea pigs.
  (AD) Study of RNA and protein in cochlea for evaluation of streptomycin
  ototoxicity. (GER)

037

Progressive hearing loss due to 0.75 to 1 g daily of antibiotic, streptomycin, for long period in 7.2 percent of 125 humans. (GER)

040

Sensorineural hearing loss due to parenteral, intramuscular, administration
of 1 g twice a week of antibiotic, streptomycin (streptomycin sulfate), for
335 days in 1 human, adult, 63 years age, male, with bone tuberculosis.
  (AD) Pretreatment hearing loss reported.
Sensorineural hearing loss due to parenteral, intramuscular, administration
of 0.5 g twice a week of antibiotic, streptomycin (streptomycin sulfate), for
333 days in 1 human, child, 3 years age, with bone tuberculosis. (ENG)

067

High frequency hearing loss in 11.4 percent of fetuses due to 10 g to more
than 100 g of antibiotic, streptomycin, in 44 humans, female, treated for
tuberculosis during pregnancy.
  (AD) Hearing loss confirmed by audiogram.
  (AD) Damage most often due to streptomycin treatment during first trimester. (GER)

100

Hearing loss due to antibiotic, streptomycin, in human, male.
  (AD) Court case on ototoxic effects due to streptomycin. (GER)

112

Permanent inhibition of cochlear microphonic due to parenteral administration
of high doses of antibiotic, streptomycin, in animals, guinea pigs and rabbits.
Rapid decr in cochlear potentials due to lower doses of antibiotic, streptomycin, in animals, guinea pigs and rabbits, sensitized with horse serum.
  (AD) Study to show pathogenesis of cochlear neuritis in association with
  streptomycin treatment. (RUS)

133

Sensorineural hearing loss due to antibiotic, streptomycin, in 6 of 420
humans, child, with suppurative meningitis. (RUS)

200

Moderate to profound sensorineural hearing loss, possibly due to 25 mg per kg
every 12 hours of antibiotic, streptomycin (streptomycin sulfate), in 8 doses
in 16 of 17 humans, child, about 4 years age, treated in neonatal period for
hemolytic disease or hyperbilirubinemia.
  (AD) Hearing loss determined by pure tone audiometry using play audiometry

methods.
(AD) Reported that not possible to determine role of streptomycin independent of high bilirubin level in hearing loss of 16 children. (ENG)

217
Sensorineural hearing loss due to antibiotic, streptomycin, in humans.
(AD) Comment on ototoxic effects of drugs. (FIN)

259
Damage to hair cells of organ of Corti and decr in action potentials due to
parenteral, intramuscular, administration of 250 mg per kg, in distilled
water, of antibiotic, streptomycin (streptomycin sulfate), in 10 doses in 1
group of total of over 100 animals, guinea pigs, 200 g average weight.
Normal hair cells of organ of Corti and no decr in action potentials due to
parenteral, intramuscular, administration of 250 mg per kg of antibiotic,
streptomycin (IB) (streptomycin sulfate), in 10 doses in 1 group of total of
over 100 animals, guinea pigs, 200 g average weight, with administration of
1.2 ml of ozothin.
(CT) Study of guinea pigs, control group.
(AD) Significant decr in ototoxicity of streptomycin due to administration
of ozothin. (ENG)

271
Sensorineural hearing loss due to antibiotic, streptomycin, in humans, child.
(AD) Statistical analysis of etiology and occurrence of sensorineural
hearing loss in children. (JAP)

347
Delayed hearing loss at 2 different times due to 15 g each time of antibiotic, streptomycin, in 1 human, child, male, treated at 8 years age for rheu-
matism and at 13 years age for pneumonia.
(AD) Similar audiograms after 2 periods of treatment.
Delayed hearing loss due to 6 and 8 g of antibiotic, streptomycin, in 2
humans, adult and child, female, mother and daughter.
Delayed hearing loss due to 6 and 5 g of antibiotic, streptomycin, in 2
humans, adult, 34 and 36 years age, female, sisters.
Delayed hearing loss due to 10 and 8 g of antibiotic, streptomycin, in 2
humans, adult, 23 and 24 years age, female, sisters.
Sensorineural hearing loss due to 10 and 4 g of antibiotic, streptomycin, in
3 humans, female, sisters.
Delayed hearing loss due to low doses of antibiotic, streptomycin, in 3
humans, adult and child, 50, 26, and 8 years age, female, mother, daughter,
and granddaughter.
(AD) Suggested familial and constitutional predisposition in streptomycin
ototoxicity. (FR)

363
Decr in hearing loss due to antibiotic, streptomycin (IB), in 9 of 40 humans
with administration of ATP, vitamin A, vitamin E, ascorbic acid, or nicotinic
acid.
Decr in hearing loss due to other antibiotics (IB) in 9 of 40 humans with
administration of ATP, vitamin A, vitamin E, ascorbic acid, or nicotinic
acid.
(CT) Audiology before and 5 to 6 days after administration of inhibitors.
(AD) Study of effectiveness of treatment of auditory system problems due
to ototoxic drugs. (RUS)

364
Damage to organ of Corti, spiral ganglion, and cochlear nuclei of medulla
oblongata 15 days after beginning of treatment due to 100 mg per kg of antibiotic, streptomycin, in 38 animals, guinea pigs.
Decr in damage to spiral ganglion and cochlear nuclei of medulla oblongata
due to 100 mg per kg of antibiotic, streptomycin (IB), in 8 of 18 animals,
guinea pigs, with simultaneous administration of 2 ml of 5 percent unitiol
for 30 to 60 days.
Decr in hearing loss due to ototoxic drugs (IB) in 3 of 25 humans with administration of unitiol.
No hearing loss due to antibiotic, streptomycin (IB), in 25 humans with

pulmonary tuberculosis with administration of unitiol.
   (AD) Study of effect of inhibitor, unitiol, on streptomycin ototoxicity.
   (RUS)

                                                                          375
Possible hearing loss due to antibiotic, streptomycin, in humans.
   (AD) Discussion of value of experimentation with animals to determine use
   and effects of drugs in humans.
   (AD) Possible to determine total hearing loss due to drugs in dogs and
   monkeys but more difficult to determine partial hearing loss in animals.
   (AD) Possible that high doses of drugs used in experimentation help to
   determine effects in therapeutic doses. (ENG)

                                                                          390
Sensorineural hearing loss due to antibiotic, streptomycin, in 2.2 percent of
3250 humans with pulmonary tuberculosis.
   (AD) Symptoms of cochlear impairment more delayed than symptoms of disorder of vestibular function. (RUS)

                                                                          452
Hearing loss due to 0.5 g daily, total of 30 to 50 g, of antibiotic, strep-
tomycin, in some of 187 humans, child, adolescent, and adult, 12 to 20 years
age, with tuberculosis.
   (AD) Audiogram confirmed hearing loss.
   (AD) Inclusion of 3 case reports. (HUN)

                                                                          490
No hearing loss due to average dose of 36.8 mg per kg daily, average total
dose of 118.9 mg per kg, of antibiotic, streptomycin (streptomycin sulfate),
for short period, average of 3.2 days, in 98 humans, child, 7 and 8 years
age, female and male, treated when newborn infants.
   (AD) Follow up study with audiometry of children treated in neonatal
   period with streptomycin.
   (CT) Study of 102 children, control group, not treated in neonatal period
   with ototoxic drugs.
   (AD) Sensorineural hearing loss detected in 3 of 98 children treated with
   streptomycin not attributed to antibiotic. (ENG)

                                                                          500
Sensorineural hearing loss due to antibiotic, streptomycin, in humans, new-
born infant.
   (AD) Discussion of etiology of hearing loss in children. (ENG)

                                                                          509
Hearing loss due to high doses of antibiotic, streptomycin, for long period
in humans. (POL)

                                                                          524
Damage to eighth cranial nerve due to antibiotics in 8 of 103 humans with
kidney disorder.
Hearing loss due to antibiotic, streptomycin, in 6 of 103 humans with kidney
disorder.
   (AD) Study of effects of ototoxic drugs in humans with kidney disorder.
   (ENG)

                                                                          542
Deaf-mutism in fetus due to antibiotic, streptomycin, in human, female,
treated during pregnancy.
   (AD) Case report of congenital hearing loss due to streptomycin therapy in
   mother during pregnancy. (ENG)

                                                                          561
Sensorineural hearing loss due to antibiotic, streptomycin, in humans.
   (AD) Study of incidence of various types of hearing loss.
   (AD) Reported that some cases of sensorineural hearing loss of unknown
   etiology possibly due to streptomycin therapy. (JAP)

612
Hearing loss due to parenteral administration of antibiotic, streptomycin, in
humans.
  (AD) Literature review of ototoxic effects of streptomycin.
  (AD) Ototoxic effects of neomycin and kanamycin comp w effects of strep-
  tomycin and dihydrostreptomycin. (SP)

695
Hearing loss in fetus due to sedative, thalidomide, in humans, female,
treated during pregnancy.
  (AD) Congenital hearing loss in 5 of 34 humans, child, of mothers treated
  with thalidomide during pregnancy. (ENG)

049
Hearing loss and damage to hair cells of organ of Corti due to parenteral,
(SQ) intraperitoneal, administration of 200 mg per kg daily of antibiotic,
tobramycin (nebramycin (factor 6)), for 6 days in 13 animals, guinea pigs,
220 to 260 g weight.
Hearing loss and damage to hair cells of organ of Corti due to parenteral,
(SQ) subcutaneous, administration of 150 mg per kg daily of antibiotic,
tobramycin (nebramycin (factor 6)), for 6 weeks in 13 animals, guinea pigs,
220 to 260 g weight.
  (CT) Control group of 5 guinea pigs used.
  (AD) Loss of Preyer reflex showed hearing loss. (ENG)

543
Transient decr in cochlear function due to tranquilizers in 44 humans.
  (AD) Auditory system problem detected by audiometry.
  (AD) Suggested transient cochleotoxic effect due to inhibition of reticu-
  lar formation by action of tranquilizers. (GER)

214
Hearing loss due to high blood levels of 90 mcg per ml or more of antibiotic,
vancomycin, in humans.
  (AD) Report on chemical composition, mechanism of action, clinical use,
  and toxicity of vancomycin. (ENG)

120
Sensorineural hearing loss and damage to eighth cranial nerve due to paren-
teral, intramuscular, administration of 1 g daily of antibiotic, viomycin
(IB), for 1 month or more in 5 percent of 60 humans with pulmonary tuberculo-
sis and treated with vitamin B.
  (AD) Need for audiometry with clinical use of viomycin. (POL)

719
Progressive severe degeneration primarily in organ of Corti beginning after
24 hours but also damage to spiral ganglion and effect on cochlear function
due to parenteral, intraperitoneal, administration of 10 or 20 mg per kg of
chemical agent, 6-aminonicotinic acid, in animals, mice, audiogenic seizure-
susceptible.
Decr in ototoxic effects due to parenteral, intraperitoneal, administration
of 10 mg per kg of chemical agent, 6-aminonicotinic acid, in animals, mice,
audiogenic seizure-susceptible, with administration 5 minutes previously of
10 mg per kg of nicotinamide. (ENG)

720
Damage to cochlear function and progressive severe degeneration in cochlear
duct, beginning after 24 hours in spiral ligament, with severe damage to
organ of Corti, and with later atrophy of spiral ganglion due to parenteral,
intraperitoneal, administration of 20 mg per kg, in concentration of 2 mg per
ml sterile water, of chemical agent, 6-aminonicotinic acid, in 1 injection in
9 animals, mice, male, audiogenic seizure-susceptible.
  (CT) Same method using water in 3 mice, control group.
  (CT) Same method using 2 mice, chronic control group, not treated.
Damage to cochlear function and degeneration in cochlea due to parenteral,
intraperitoneal, administration of 20 mg per kg of chemical agent, 6-aminoni-
cotinic acid, in 6 animals, mice, not audiogenic seizure-susceptible.
  (CT) Same method using water in 2 mice, control group, showed no histological changes. (ENG)

730

Damage to cochlear function due to parenteral, intraperitoneal, administration of 20, 10, or 5 mg per kg, in concentration of 2 mg per ml of sterile
distilled water, of chemical agent, 6-aminonicotinic acid, in 1 injection in
18 animals, mice, about 30 days age, male, audiogenic seizure-susceptible.
   (AD) More severe hearing loss in mice with higher doses of 6-aminonico-
tinic acid.
No damage to cochlear function due to parenteral, intraperitoneal, administration of 1 mg per kg, in concentration of 2 mg per ml of sterile distilled
water, of chemical agent, 6-aminonicotinic acid, in 1 injection in 4 animals,
mice, about 30 days age, male, audiogenic seizure-susceptible.
   (CT) Same method using intraperitoneal administration of same amount of
   water in 8 mice, control group, showed no damage to cochlear function.
   (ENG)

005

Transient primary decr in cochlear microphonic and action potential due to
parenteral, intravenous, administration of 10 mg per kg of diuretic, ethacrynic acid, in 1 injection in 20 animals, cats, adult.
Transient primary decr in cochlear microphonic and action potential due to
parenteral, intravenous, administration of 10 mg per kg of diuretic, furosemide, in 1 injection in 20 animals, cats, adult.
Delayed severe secondary decr in cochlear microphonic and action potential
due to parenteral, intravenous, administration of more than 10 mg per kg of
diuretic, ethacrynic acid, in animals, cats.
   (CT) Same method using 50 mg per kg and 100 mg per kg of diuretic, chlorothiazide, in cats, control group, showed no ototoxic effect.
Degeneration of outer hair cells of organ of Corti in basal and middle coils
of cochlea due to parenteral, intravenous, administration of 30 mg per kg of
diuretic, ethacrynic acid, in 1 injection in 2 animals, cats.
Degeneration of outer hair cells of organ of Corti due to parenteral, intramuscular, administration of 15 mg per kg of diuretic, ethacrynic acid, for 2
weeks in 1 animal, cat. (ENG)

010

Permanent sensorineural hearing loss due to parenteral, intramuscular, administration of low doses, less than 2 g, of antibiotic, (SQ) kanamycin
(kanamycin sulfate), for short period in 5 humans, adult, range of 33 to 47
years age, range of 90 to 177 lb weight, with kidney disorder.
Permanent sensorineural hearing loss due to parenteral, intramuscular, administration of low doses, less than 2 g, of antibiotic, (SQ) streptomycin,
for short period in 5 humans, adult, range of 33 to 47 years age, range of 90
to 177 lb weight, with kidney disorder.
Permanent sensorineural hearing loss due to parenteral, intramuscular, administration of low doses, less than 2 g, of antibiotic, (SQ) neomycin, for
short period in 5 humans, adult, range of 33 to 47 years age, range of 90 to
177 lb weight, with kidney disorder.
Permanent sensorineural hearing loss due to parenteral, intramuscular, administration of low doses, less than 2 g, of diuretic, (SQ) ethacrynic acid,
for short period in 5 humans, adult, range of 33 to 47 years age, range of 90
to 177 lb weight, with kidney disorder.
   (AD) Study of cochleotoxic effects of kanamycin with other antibiotics and
   with ethacrynic acid. (ENG)

012

Permanent sensorineural hearing loss due to parenteral, intramuscular, administration of high doses, about 100 mg per kg daily, total of more than 6 g
of antibiotic, (SQ) neomycin (neomycin sulfate), for 7 days in 1 human,
Caucasian, infant, 13 months age.
Unspecified effects due to parenteral, intramuscular, administration of about
12 mg per kg daily recommended dosage, total of 20 mg, of antibiotic, (SQ)
kanamycin (kanamycin sulfate), for less than 24 hours in 1 human, Caucasian,
infant, 13 months age.
   (CT) Normal response to acoustic stimulus before administration of antibiotics.
   (AD) Suggested that ototoxicity of neomycin not potentiated by administration of kanamycin in this case. (ENG)

018

Hearing loss due to parenteral administration of low doses, 1 g daily, of antibiotic, (SQ) streptomycin, in 3 injections in 1 human, adult, 22 years age, male, with pulmonary tuberculosis.
Unspecified effects due to previous administration of 3 unspecified doses of antimalarial, (SO) quinine, in 1 human, adult, 22 years age, male, with pulmonary tuberculosis. (ENG)

019

Progressive severe sensorineural hearing loss and tinnitus due to unspecified method of administration of 0.5 g twice daily, total of 16 g, of antibiotic, kanamycin, for 16 days in 1 human, Caucasian, adult, 25 years age, male, with kidney disorder and treated with peritoneal dialysis.
   (AD) Audiograms showed hearing loss and recruitment test showed reversed
   recruitment.
Severe sensorineural hearing loss due to unspecified method of administration of 0.5 g daily for 40 days and then 0.5 g 3 times a week for 3 weeks of antibiotic, streptomycin, for total period of about 9 weeks in 1 human, Negro, child, 9 years age, male, with pulmonary tuberculosis and kidney disorder.
   (AD) No record of hearing loss before treatment with streptomycin.
Delayed severe bilateral high frequency hearing loss due to unspecified method of administration of 0.5 g daily for 8 months and then 0.5 g every 3 days for 4 months, followed by a break of 3.5 months, and then 0.5 g every 3 days for 1.5 months, total of 153 g of antibiotic, dihydrostreptomycin, for total period of about 13.5 months in 1 human, Negro, infant, 16 months age, female, with tuberculosis.
   (AD) Hearing loss detected at 13 years age.
Hearing loss and tinnitus due to unspecified method of administration of 1 g daily of antibiotic, streptomycin, for 10 weeks and possibly for a longer period after discharge in 1 human, Negro, adult, 23 years age, male, treated for infection in tuberculosis hospital.
   (AD) Hearing loss detected 1 month after treatment with streptomycin.
Progressive severe sensorineural hearing loss due to unspecified method of administration of 0.5 g 3 times a week, total of 61 g of antibiotic, streptomycin, for about 10 months in 1 human, Negro, child, 9 years age, female, with pulmonary tuberculosis.
   (AD) Discussion of 5 case reports. (ENG)

027

Progressive bilateral high frequency hearing loss and tinnitus due to topical administration by irrigation of wound with 80 ml every 4 hours for 2 weeks and then 40 ml every 4 hours of 0.5 percent solution of antibiotic, (SQ) neomycin (SM), in 1 human, adult, 24 years age, male, paraplegic, with infection of ulcer of left hip.
Progressive bilateral high frequency hearing loss and tinnitus due to topical administration by irrigation of wound with 80 ml every 4 hours for 2 weeks and then 40 ml every 4 hours of 0.1 percent solution of antibiotic, (SQ) polymyxin B (SM), in 1 human, adult, 24 years age, male, paraplegic, with infection of ulcer of left hip.
No reported ototoxic effects due to unspecified method of administration of 1 g daily of antibiotic, (SQ) streptomycin, for 5 days in 1 human, adult, 24 years age, male, paraplegic, with infection of ulcer of left hip. (ENG)

028

Bilateral sensorineural hearing loss and tinnitus due to parenteral, intravenous, administration of 100 mg of diuretic, ethacrynic acid (SM), in 2 doses in 1 human, adult, 24 years age, male, with kidney disorder.
Bilateral sensorineural hearing loss and tinnitus due to parenteral, intravenous, administration of 4 g of antibiotic, streptomycin (SM), for 5 days in 1 human, adult, 24 years age, male, with kidney disorder.
Bilateral sensorineural hearing loss due to parenteral, intravenous, administration of 500 mg of diuretic, ethacrynic acid (SM), for 4 days in 1 human, adult, 35 years age, female, with kidney disorder.
Bilateral sensorineural hearing loss due to parenteral, intravenous, administration of 1.5 g of antibiotic, streptomycin (SM), for 4 days in 1 human, adult, 35 years age, female, with kidney disorder.
Permanent hearing loss due to parenteral, intravenous, administration of 200

mg of diuretic, ethacrynic acid, in humans.   (ENG)

042

Transient bilateral sensorineural hearing loss due to parenteral, intravenous, administration of 50 mg of diuretic, (SQ) ethacrynic acid, in 1
injection in 1 human, adult, 45 years age, female, with lymphosarcoma and
with normal kidney function.
   (AD) Hearing loss reported 15 minutes after treatment with ethacrynic
   acid.
Previous parenteral, intramuscular, administration of 60 mg every 6 hours of
antibiotic, (SQ) gentamicin (gentamicin sulfate), for unspecified period in 1
human, adult, 45 years age, female, with lymphosarcoma and with normal kidney
function.
Bilateral sensorineural hearing loss due to parenteral, intravenous, administration of 100 mg of diuretic, (SQ) ethacrynic acid, in 2 injections of 50 mg
each 6 hours apart in 1 human, adult, 64 years age, female, with acute leukemia and with normal kidney function.
   (AD) Histological study after death showed no damage to inner ear.
Previous unspecified method of administration of unspecified dose of antibiotic, (SQ) polymyxin B (polymyxin B sulfate), in 1 human, adult, 64 years age,
female, with acute leukemia and with normal kidney function.
Previous parenteral, intramuscular, administration of 0.5 g every 12 hours of
antibiotic, (SQ) kanamycin (kanamycin sulfate), for unspecified period in 1
human, adult, 64 years age, female, with acute leukemia and with normal
kidney function.
   (AD) Suggested that hearing loss due to combined action of ethacrynic acid
   and antibiotics. (ENG)

051

Progressive permanent sensorineural hearing loss and tinnitus due to topical
administration to joint of left knee and parenteral, intramuscular, administration of high doses, total of 42.5 g, of antibiotic, (SQ) neomycin, for
long period, 19 days, in 1 human, adult, with infection of left knee.
Previous administration of high doses of antibiotic, (SQ) chloramphenicol,
for unspecified period in 1 human, adult, with infection of left knee.
   (AD) Report of case in court with claim of negligence for administration
   of high doses of neomycin that resulted in hearing loss. (ENG)

055

Transient bilateral sensorineural hearing loss and tinnitus due to parenteral, intravenous, administration of 100 mg of diuretic, (SQ) ethacrynic
acid, in 1 injection in 1 human, adult, 64 years age, male, with kidney
disorder.
   (CT) Pretreatment audiology showed no auditory system problems.
   (AD) Hearing loss 5 minutes after administration of ethacrynic acid.
Previous parenteral, intravenous, administration of unspecified doses of
diuretic, (SQ) furosemide, for unspecified period in 1 human, adult, 64 years
age, male, with kidney disorder. (ENG)

056

Range of degree of hearing loss due to range of 40 to 300 g of antibiotic,
(SQ) streptomycin, in 59 of 338 humans, male and female, with no previous
treatment with streptomycin.
   (AD) No auditory system problems before treatment.
   (AD) Hearing loss often detected in alcoholics in group.
Range of degree of hearing loss due to range of 40 to 100 g of antibiotic,
(SQ) streptomycin, in 8 of 32 humans with previous treatment with streptomy-
cin.
   (AD) No reported auditory system problems before treatment.
   (AD) More severe hearing loss with administration of 100 g or more of
   streptomycin in both groups.
   (AD) More severe hearing loss in group with previous streptomycin treat-
   ment.
No reported ototoxic effects due to high doses of antibiotic, (SQ) dihydros-
treptomycin, in some of total of 370 humans treated with streptomycin. (SER)

059

Bilateral sensorineural hearing loss due to oral administration of 0 to 12 g

daily, total of 2500 g, of antibiotic, neomycin, for 16 months in 1 human, Caucasian, adult, 49 years age, female, chronic alcoholic, with hepatic encephalopathy and normal kidney function.
Bilateral sensorineural hearing loss due to oral administration of 0 to 4 g daily, total of 800 g, of antibiotic, (SQ) neomycin, for 21 months in 1 human, Caucasian, adult, 47 years age, female, chronic alcoholic, with hepatic encephalopathy and normal kidney function.
More severe sensorineural hearing loss due to oral administration of 6 g daily, total of 111 g, of antibiotic, (SQ) paromomycin, for 9 months in 1 human, Caucasian, adult, 47 years age, female, chronic alcoholic, with hepatic encephalopathy and normal kidney function.
Sensorineural hearing loss due to oral administration of 0 to 12 g daily, total of 1500 g, of antibiotic, neomycin, for 11 months in 1 human, Caucasian, adult, 39 years age, female, chronic alcoholic, with hepatic encephalopathy and some kidney disorder.
Sensorineural hearing loss in right ear due to oral administration of 3 to 4 g daily, total of 500 g, of antibiotic, (SQ) neomycin, for 8 months in 1 human, Caucasian, aged, 66 years age, female, with hepatic encephalopathy and kidney disorder.
    (AD) Tinnitus and sudden deafness in left ear 27 years earlier.
Sensorineural hearing loss in right ear due to oral administration of total of 240 g of antibiotic, (SQ) paromomycin, for long period in 1 human, Caucasian, aged, 66 years age, female, with hepatic encephalopathy and kidney disorder.
Sequential administration of unspecified doses of diuretic, (SQ) furosemide, for unspecified period in 1 human, Caucasian, aged, 66 years age, female, with hepatic encephalopathy and kidney disorder.
Bilateral sensorineural hearing loss due to oral administration of 0 to 12 g daily, total of 1000 to 1500 g, of antibiotic, (SQ) neomycin, for 28 months in 1 human, Caucasian, adult, 60 years age, male, chronic alcoholic, with hepatic encephalopathy and kidney disorder.
Bilateral sensorineural hearing loss due to oral administration of total of 300 g of antibiotic, (SQ) paromomycin, for long period in 1 human, Caucasian, adult, 60 years age, male, chronic alcoholic, with hepatic encephalopathy and kidney disorder.
Sequential administration of unspecified doses of (SQ) diuretics for unspecified period in 1 human, Caucasian, adult, 60 years age, male, chronic alcoholic, with hepatic encephalopathy and kidney disorder.
    (AD) Discussion of 5 case reports of hearing loss due to antibiotic therapy.
    (AD) Audiograms confirmed hearing loss in all cases.   (ENG)

                                                                    062
High frequency hearing loss and tinnitus due to parenteral, intramuscular, administration of 1 g daily for first 60 days and then 1 g daily for 2 days each week of antibiotic, capreomycin (SM), for 1 year in 7 of 89 humans, range of ages, male and female, with pulmonary tuberculosis.
    (CT) No auditory system problems before treatment.
    (CT) Audiometry 1 time each month for duration of treatment.
    (AD) Previous resistance to primary antituberculous agents reported.
Simultaneous oral administration of 25 mg per kg daily for first 60 days and then 15 mg per kg daily of antituberculous agent, ethambutol (SM), for 1 year in 89 humans, range of ages, male and female, with pulmonary tuberculosis.
No reported ototoxic effects due to oral administration of 300 mg daily of antituberculous agent, isoniazid (SM), for 1 year in 89 humans, range of ages, male and female, with pulmonary tuberculosis.
    (AD) Previous resistance to isoniazid reported.   (ENG)

                                                                    063
Progressive permanent bilateral sensorineural hearing loss due to topical administration by irrigation of wound with 1000 ml of 1 percent solution (6.5 g) of antibiotic, neomycin (CB) (neomycin sulfate), in 1 administration in 1 human, Caucasian, adolescent, 18 years age, male, with gunshot wound of abdomen.
    (AD) Hearing loss reported 21 days after treatment.
Progressive permanent bilateral sensorineural hearing loss due to topical administration by irrigation of wound with 1000 ml of 0.1 percent solution (650 mg) of antibiotic, polymyxin B (CB) (polymyxin B sulfate), in 1 adminis-

tration in 1 human, Caucasian, adolescent, 18 years age, male, with gunshot
wound of abdomen.
   (AD) Study reported that ototoxic effects only due to neomycin.
   (AD) Hemodialysis 24 hours after treatment for prevention of hearing loss
   not satisfactory.
Progressive permanent bilateral sensorineural hearing loss due to topical
administration by irrigation of wound with high doses of 1 percent solution
of antibiotic, (SQ) neomycin, for 22 days in 1 human, Caucasian, adult, 20
years age, male, with gunshot wounds.
   (AD) Hearing loss reported after 19 days of treatment.
Previous administration of unspecified dose of antibiotic, (SQ) streptomycin,
for 6 days in 1 human, Caucasian, adult, 20 years age, male, with gunshot
wounds.
Progressive permanent bilateral sensorineural hearing loss due to topical
administration by irrigation of wound with total of 4000 ml of 1 percent
solution of antibiotic, neomycin (CB) (neomycin sulfate), in 4 days in 1
human, Caucasian, adult, 39 years age, male, with wounds.
   (AD) Hearing loss reported within 5 days.
Progressive permanent bilateral sensorineural hearing loss due to topical
administration by irrigation of wound with total of 4000 ml of 0.1 percent
solution of antibiotic, polymyxin B (CB) (polymyxin B sulfate), in 4 days in
1 human, Caucasian, adult, 39 years age, male, with wounds.
   (AD) Discussion of 3 case reports of hearing loss due to topical administration of antibiotics. (ENG)

068

Hearing loss and tinnitus or hyperacusis due to oral administration of 1 g
daily of antibiotic, (SQ) capreomycin, for 2 years in 3 of first group of 34
humans with tuberculosis.
No reported ototoxic effects due to previous unspecified method of administration of unspecified doses of antibiotic, (SQ) streptomycin, in first group
of 34 humans with tuberculosis.
Hearing loss due to previous unspecified method of administration of unspecified doses of antibiotic, (SQ) streptomycin, in 9 of second group of 31
humans with tuberculosis.
More severe hearing loss due to oral administration of 1 g daily of antibiotic, (SQ) capreomycin, for 2 years in 1 of second group of 31 humans with
tuberculosis. (ENG)

073

Permanent hearing loss due to 10 to 35 mg per kg daily or twice daily of
antibiotic, dihydrostreptomycin, in 23(26.4 percent) of 87 humans, child,
with pulmonary and meningeal tuberculosis.
Permanent hearing loss due to 15 to 35 mg per kg daily or twice daily of
antibiotic, streptomycin, in 1(5.2 percent)of 19 humans, child, with pulmonary and meningeal tuberculosis.
   (AD) More ototoxic effects with 1 dose per day than with 2 doses per day.
Permanent hearing loss due to 15 to 20 mg per kg daily or twice daily of
antibiotic, dihydrostreptomycin (CB), in 4(18.6 percent) of 46 humans, child,
with pulmonary and meningeal tuberculosis.
Permanent hearing loss due to 15 to 20 mg per kg daily or twice daily of
antibiotic, streptomycin (CB), in 4(18.6 percent) of 46 humans, child, with
pulmonary and meningeal tuberculosis.
   (CT) No hearing loss in 14 children, control group, treated with PAS and
   isoniazid.
   (AD) Need to confirm hearing loss with audiometry discussed. (SER)

074

Decr in cochlear microphonic due to topical administration to round window of
range of 210 to 680 g of antibiotic, streptomycin, in animals, guinea pigs.
Decr in cochlear microphonic due to topical administration to round window of
range of 210 to 680 g of antibiotic, kanamycin, in animals, guinea pigs.
No decr in cochlear microphonic due to topical administration to round window
of range of 210 to 680 g of antibiotic, neomycin, in animals, guinea pigs.
   (POL)

075

Hearing loss due to previous administration of antibiotic, (SQ) streptomycin,

in 18 of total of 67 humans with tuberculosis.
More severe hearing loss, tinnitus, or hyperacusis due to unspecified method
of administration of unspecified doses of antibiotic, (SQ) capreomycin, for
long period in 4 of 45 humans with tuberculosis.
No ototoxic effects due to unspecified method of administration of unspecified doses of antibiotic, (SQ) capreomycin, for short period in other 22
humans with tuberculosis. (ENG)

085

Hearing loss due to antibiotic, viomycin, in 17.7 percent of 152 humans with
tuberculosis.
(CT) Systematic controls with audiology.
Hearing loss due to antibiotic, viomycin (IB), in only 5.3 percent of 36
humans with previous hearing loss with administration of nialamid.
Hearing loss due to antibiotic, kanamycin, in 20 percent of 55 humans with
tuberculosis.
Hearing loss due to antibiotic, kanamycin (IB), in 0 of 25 humans with previous hearing loss with administration of nialamid.
Lesion of inner ear due to antibiotic, neomycin (IB), in only 1 human with
previous hearing loss with administration of nialamid. (GER)

089

Sudden deafness due to parenteral, intravenous, administration of 100 mg, in
100 ml saline solution, of diuretic, (SQ) ethacrynic acid, in 1 injection in
1 human, adult, 42 years age, female, quadriplegic, with kidney disorder.
Previous administration of unspecified dose of antibiotic, (SQ) chloramphenicol, for unspecified period in 1 human, adult, 42 years age, female, quadriplegic, with kidney disorder.
Previous administration of 1 g of antibiotic, (SQ) kanamycin, for unspecified
period in 1 human, adult, 42 years age, female, quadriplegic, with kidney
disorder and genitourinary system infection. (ENG)

130

Decr in cochlear microphonic and neural potentials and incr in sodium and
glucose of endolymph due to parenteral, intravenous, administration of 30 to
60 mg per kg, in saline solution, of diuretic, ethacrynic acid, for 5 minute
period in animals, cats.
Changes in stria vascularis and damage to outer hair cells of organ of Corti
due to parenteral, intravenous, administration of 30 to 60 mg per kg, in
saline solution, of diuretic, ethacrynic acid, for 5 minute period in animals, cats.
No change in cochlear microphonic, no incr in endolymph glucose, and normal
endolymph chemical composition due to parenteral, intravenous, administration
of 50 mg per kg, in saline solution, of diuretic, acetazolamide, for 5 minute
period in animals, cats.
Slow decr in cochlear microphonic and neural potentials due to parenteral,
intravenous, administration of 200 mg per kg, in saline solution, of diuretic, acetazolamide, for 5 minute period in animals, cats.
   (CT) Same method using 7 cc per kg of saline solution in 14 cats, control
   group.
   (AD) Clinical significance of study of acetazolamide not determined due to
   lack of reports of hearing loss with use of drug.
Severe decr in cochlear microphonic and neural potentials but no changes in
electrolyte concentrations of endolymph or perilymph due to parenteral,
intravenous, administration of 30 mg per kg daily of diuretic, ethacrynic
acid, for 3 to 4 days in 3 animals, cats.
   (AD) Results of study suggest severe hearing loss.
Edema of stria vascularis and damage to outer hair cells of organ of Corti
but normal chemical composition of endolymph and perilymph due to parenteral,
intraperitoneal, administration of 30 mg per kg of diuretic, ethacrynic acid,
in 1 dose in 9 animals, cats.
   (AD) Study of effect of diuretics on chemical composition of fluids of
   inner ear and relationship to cochlear microphonic and histopathology of
   temporal bone. (ENG)

139

Cochleotoxic effects due to antibiotic, kanamycin, in humans and animals,
guinea pigs.

Cochleotoxic effects due to antibiotic, streptomycin, in humans and animals, guinea pigs.

   (AD) Literature review of mechanism of action of ototoxic antibiotics. (POL)

140

Total bilateral sensorineural hearing loss due to 40 mg daily, total of 1.80 g, of antibiotic, gentamicin, for 45 days in 1 human, aged, 69 years age, female, with kidney disorder.

   (AD) Hearing loss confirmed by audiogram.

Sensorineural hearing loss due to parenteral administration of 40 mg in 2 injections daily, total of 480 mg, of antibiotic, gentamicin (SM), in 1 human, aged, 65 years age, male.

Simultaneous administration of antibiotic, transcycline (SM), in 1 human, aged, 65 years age, male.

Simultaneous administration of antibiotic, colistin (SM) (colistimethate), in 1 human, aged, 65 years age, male.

Sensorineural hearing loss due to 40 mg daily, total of 0.84 g, of antibiotic, gentamicin, for 21 days in 1 human, adult, 50 years age, male, with normal kidney function.

   (AD) Hearing loss confirmed by audiogram.

   (AD) Discussion of 3 case reports of gentamicin ototoxicity. (FR)

156

Sensorineural hearing loss due to unspecified method of administration of high doses of antibiotic, streptomycin (SM), in 7 humans, infant and child, with tuberculous meningitis.

Simultaneous administration of unspecified doses of antituberculous agent, PAS (SM), in 7 humans, infant and child, with tuberculous meningitis.

Simultaneous administration of unspecified doses of antituberculous agent, isoniazid (SM), in 7 humans, infant and child, with tuberculous meningitis.

Sensorineural hearing loss due to unspecified method of administration of high doses of antibiotic, viomycin, in 7 humans, infant and child, with tuberculous meningitis.

   (AD) Cochleotoxic effect due to antibiotic therapy or infection. (ENG)

158

No reported ototoxic effects due to 5 g of antibiotic, (SQ) streptomycin, in 1 human, adult, 63 years age, male, with bronchopleural fistula and staphylococcal empyema.

Progressive total bilateral sensorineural hearing loss due to topical administration by irrigation of empyema cavity with (SQ) 1200 ml of 1 percent solution of antibiotic, (SQ) neomycin, for 10 days, total of 33 irrigations, in 1 human, adult, 63 years age, male, with bronchopleural fistula and staphylococcal empyema.

Progressive total bilateral sensorineural hearing loss due to topical administration by irrigation of empyema cavity with (SQ) 700 ml of 1 percent solution, total of 403 g in all, of antibiotic, (SQ) neomycin, in 1 administration in 1 human, adult, 63 years age, male, at time of surgery to close cavity.

Sequential parenteral, intramuscular, administration of total of 4 g of antibiotic, (SQ) streptomycin (streptomycin sulfate), for 4 to 5 days in 1 human, adult, 63 years age, male, after closure of empyema cavity.

   (AD) No hearing loss before closure of cavity.

   (AD) Hearing loss confirmed by audiogram but no vestibular problems detected by vestibular function tests.

   (AD) Suggested that hearing loss due to neomycin only and not to streptomycin. (ENG)

169

Progressive sensorineural hearing loss, complete range of degrees of damage to organ of Corti, and degeneration in cochlear nuclei due to parenteral, intramuscular, administration of 15 to 100 mg per kg daily of antibiotic, kanamycin (kanamycin sulfate), for 28 to 180 days in 3 animals, monkeys, young, 2 to 6 years age, male and female, 3 to 9 kg weight, conditioned.

High frequency hearing loss and damage to organ of Corti due to parenteral, intramuscular, administration of 100 mg per kg daily of antibiotic, neomycin (neomycin sulfate), for 5 days in 1 animal, monkey, young, conditioned.

Delayed severe sensorineural hearing loss after 2 months and severe damage to
organ of Corti due to parenteral, intramuscular, administration of 50 mg per
kg of antibiotic, neomycin (neomycin sulfate), for 15 days in 1 animal,
monkey, young, conditioned.
   (CT) Pretreatment hearing baseline determined.
   (AD) Study showed correlation of measurement of hearing loss and histopathology of cochlea in same subject.
   (AD) Cochleograms made to show patterns of cell loss.
   (AD) Reported that neomycin more ototoxic than kanamycin. (ENG)

                                                                           170
Sensorineural hearing loss due to topical administration in ear drops of
antibiotic, neomycin, in humans with no other explanation for hearing loss.
Sensorineural hearing loss due to topical administration in ear drops of
antibiotic, chloramphenicol, in humans with no other explanation for hearing
loss.
Sensorineural hearing loss due to topical administration in ear drops of
antibiotic, framycetin, in humans with no other explanation for hearing loss.
   (AD) Comment on topical use of antibiotics and possible risk of cochleotoxic effects. (ENG)

                                                                           179
Progressive high frequency hearing loss and tinnitus due to 1 g daily of
antibiotic, kanamycin, in 3 humans, adolescent and adult, male, with tuberculosis and with previous treatment with ototoxic drugs but with no report of
toxic effects.
Less severe sensorineural hearing loss and no tinnitus due to 1 g 5 times a
week of antibiotic, kanamycin, in 1 human, male, with tuberculosis and with
previous treatment with ototoxic drugs.
Sensorineural hearing loss and tinnitus due to 6 g of antibiotic, kanamycin
(SM), in 1 human, male, with tuberculosis and with previous treatment with
ototoxic drugs.
Sensorineural hearing loss and tinnitus due to parenteral administration of
1000 mg per day of antibiotic, streptomycin (SM), in 1 human, male, with
tuberculosis and with previous treatment with ototoxic drugs.
No high frequency hearing loss due to parenteral administration of 1 g daily
of antibiotic, streptomycin, in 1 human, female, with tuberculosis and with
previous treatment with ototoxic drugs.
High frequency hearing loss but no tinnitus due to 750 mg daily of antibiotic, streptomycin, in 1 human, female, with tuberculosis and with previous
treatment with ototoxic drugs.
Simultaneous administration of range of doses of other antituberculous agents
(SM) in total of 7 humans, adolescent and adult, 13 to 49 years age, male and
female, with tuberculosis and with previous treatment with ototoxic drugs.
   (AD) Study using high frequency audiometry and conventional audiometry.
   (CT) Pretreatment audiograms obtained. (ENG)

                                                                           181
Decr in succinic dehydrogenase in outer hair cells of organ of Corti due to
parenteral, intratympanic, administration of 200 mg per ml solution of antibiotic, kanamycin (kanamycin sulfate), in animals, guinea pigs, adult.
Decr in succinic dehydrogenase in outer hair cells of organ of Corti due to
parenteral, intratympanic, administration of 200 mg per ml solution of antibiotic, dihydrostreptomycin (dihydrostreptomycin sulfate), in animals, guinea
pigs, adult.
Decr in succinic dehydrogenase in outer hair cells of organ of Corti due to
parenteral, intratympanic, administration of 200 mg per ml solution of antibiotic, chloramphenicol (chloramphenicol succinate), in animals, guinea pigs,
adult.
   (AD) Same type of damage to organ of Corti due to all 3 antibiotics.
Severe decr in succinic dehydrogenase in organ of Corti, in particular in
outer hair cells, and atrophy of outer hair cells due to saturated solution
of antimalarial, quinine (quinine hydrochloride), in animals, guinea pigs.
Complete degeneration of organ of Corti due to saturated solution of antimalarial, quinine (quinine hydrochloride), in animals, guinea pigs.
   (AD) Damage to organ of Corti more severe due to quinine than to antibiotics.
   (AD) Activity of succinic dehydrogenase often higher in outer hair cells.

(AD) Possible that damage to outer hair cells due to higher rate of metabolism. (ENG)

183

Inhibition of oxygen consumption of cochlea due to 0.04 mg of antibiotic,
chloramphenicol (chloramphenicol sodium succinate), in animals, guinea pigs,
adult, 300 g weight, with normal Preyer reflex.
More inhibition of oxygen consumption of cochlea due to 0.04 mg of antibiotic, kanamycin (kanamycin sulfate), in animals, guinea pigs, adult, 300 g
weight, with normal Preyer reflex.
    (CT) Study of oxygen consumption in normal cochlea.
    (AD) Measurement of oxygen consumption with differential type of microres-
    pirometer.
    (AD) In vitro study.
No detected change in Preyer reflex due to parenteral, intracutaneous, administration of 400 mg per kg of antibiotic, chloramphenicol, for 20 days in
animals, guinea pigs.
    (AD) In vivo study.
    (AD) Results with chloramphenicol in vivo not same as results in vitro.
    (ENG)

186

Diplacusis due to antibiotics, aminoglycoside, in humans.
Diplacusis due to antimalarial, quinine, in humans.
Diplacusis due to salicylate, aspirin, in humans.
Diplacusis due to chemical agent, carbon monoxide, in humans.
    (AD) Report on etiology of diplacusis with comment on ototoxic drugs.
    (ENG)

188

Possible hearing loss due to antibiotics in humans, child, treated when
newborn infant.
    (AD) Reported that 23 percent of 46 children with idiopathic hearing loss
    treated with antibiotics in neonatal period.
    (CT) Reported that 2 percent of 54 children with normal hearing treated
    with antibiotics in neonatal period.
Possible hearing loss in fetus due to salicylate, aspirin, in humans, female,
during pregnancy.
    (AD) Ingestion of salicylate, aspirin, during pregnancy by mothers of 2
    percent of total of 118 children with hearing loss.
    (CT) Ingestion of salicylate, aspirin, during pregnancy by mothers of 0 of
    54 children with normal hearing.
    (AD) Study of etiology of hearing loss in children. (ENG)

196

Sensorineural hearing loss due to unspecified doses of antibiotic, streptomycin, in 8.9 percent of 2917 humans, child, adolescent, and adult, 10 to 34
years age, with pulmonary tuberculosis.
Sensorineural hearing loss due to unspecified doses of antibiotic, streptomycin (SM), in high percent of 608 humans, child, adolescent, and adult, 10 to
34 years age, with pulmonary tuberculosis.
Sensorineural hearing loss due to unspecified doses of antibiotic, kanamycin
(SM), in high percent of 608 humans, child, adolescent, and adult, 10 to 34
years age, with pulmonary tuberculosis.
    (CT) Study of 314 humans, control group, without pulmonary tuberculosis.
    (CT) No subjective hearing loss before treatment with antibiotics.
    (CT) Hearing loss after antibiotic treatment confirmed by audiometry.
    (AD) Statistical analysis of 3525 cases with antibiotic therapy.
    (AD) Highest incidence of hearing loss in 30 to 34 years age group.
    (AD) Higher incidence of severe hearing loss in group treated with two
    antibiotics than in group treated with streptomycin only. (ENG)

227

Bilateral tinnitus and sudden deafness possibly due to cardiovascular agent,
(SQ) hexadimethrine bromide, in 1 human, adult, 32 years age, female, with
chronic nephritis and treated with hemodialysis.
Previous administration of antituberculous agent, (SQ) PAS, in 1 human,
adult, 32 years age, female, with chronic nephritis and treated with hemodia-

lysis.
Previous administration of antituberculous agent, (SQ) isoniazid, in 1 human, adult, 32 years age, female, with chronic nephritis and treated with hemodialysis.
Damage to Reissner's membrane, degeneration of organ of Corti, stria vascularis, and spiral ganglion, and slight changes in vestibular apparatus possibly due to cardiovascular agent, (SQ) hexadimethrine bromide, in 1 human, adult, 32 years age, female, with chronic nephritis and treated with hemodialysis.
Progressive severe sensorineural hearing loss possibly due to cardiovascular agent, hexadimethrine bromide, in 4 humans, adolescent and adult, 17 to 40 years age, with kidney disorders and treated with hemodialysis.
  (AD) Association of hexadimethrine bromide with hearing loss only when used with hemodialysis in treatment of kidney disorder.
  (AD) No hearing loss in group treated with hemodialysis without hexadimethrine bromide. (ENG)

236

Bilateral high frequency hearing loss due to parenteral, intramuscular, administration of high dose, 90 mg per kg daily, total of 99.2 g, of antibiotic, kanamycin, for 62 days in 1 human, child, with miliary tuberculosis.
High frequency hearing loss due to parenteral, intramuscular, administration of high dose, 25 mg per kg daily, total of 22.2 g, of antibiotic, kanamycin, for 148 days in 1 human, child, with miliary tuberculosis.
Permanent severe sensorineural hearing loss due to parenteral, intramuscular, administration of high doses of antibiotic, kanamycin, in 1 human, child, with multiple infections.
Progressive sensorineural hearing loss due to oral administration of antibiotic, neomycin, for 11 months in 1 human, child, 11.5 years age, male, with severe ulcerative ileocolitis.
  (AD) Hearing loss confirmed by audiogram.
  (AD) Discussion of 4 case reports of ototoxic effects due to kanamycin or neomycin.
  (AD) Suggested that risk of kanamycin ototoxicity less in children than in adults.
Sensorineural hearing loss due to 10 to 100 mg per kg daily of antibiotic, kanamycin, for 5 to 95 days in 5 of 30 humans, child and infant, with infections.
  (CT) Study of 30 children and infants, control group, not treated with kanamycin.
  (AD) Suggested that cochleotoxic effects related to total dose of kanamycin.
  (AD) Report on studies made during 8 years of clinical use of kanamycin. (ENG)

237

Hearing loss due to parenteral, intramuscular, administration of 15 mg per kg daily of antibiotic, kanamycin, for 6 to 10 days in 5.1 percent of 143 humans, child, treated when newborn infant for infection.
Hearing loss due to parenteral, intramuscular, administration of 40 mg per kg daily of antibiotic, streptomycin, for 6 to 12 days in 5.6 percent of 93 humans, child, treated when newborn infant for infection.
  (CT) Hearing loss in 4.4 percent of 170 children, control group, without antibiotic therapy.
  (AD) Hearing loss confirmed by audiogram.
  (AD) Suggested low kanamycin ototoxicity in newborn infants with use of recommended dosage. (ENG)

265

Hearing loss due to analgesic, fentanyl (SM), in humans, treated before ultrasound therapy for Meniere's disease.
Hearing loss due to tranquilizer, droperidol (SM), in humans, treated before ultrasound therapy for Meniere's disease.
  (AD) More severe hearing loss with simultaneous use of droperidol and fentanyl than with use of local anesthetic only. (ENG)

278

Histochemical changes in cochlea due to parenteral administration of 15 mg

per kg daily of diuretic, furosemide, for 8 to 14 days in animals, guinea pigs, 300 g weight.
Histochemical changes in cochlea due to parenteral administration of 8 mg per kg daily of diuretic, acetazolamide, for 8 to 14 days in animals, guinea pigs, 300 g weight. (GER)

280
High frequency hearing loss 3 weeks after beginning of therapy due to oral administration of 20 mg daily, then 60 mg daily for 1 week, with interval of 1 week, and then 30 mg daily for 12 days of cardiovascular agent, (SQ) propranolol, for total of 19 days in 1 human, aged, 68 years age, female, with heart disorder, arteriosclerosis.
(AD) Sensorineural hearing loss confirmed by audiometry.
(AD) Some improvement in hearing sensitivity during 6 months after cessation of drug.
No reported ototoxic effects due to unspecified method of administration about 2 years previously of unspecified dose of cardiovascular agent, (SQ) quinidine, for unspecified period in 1 human, aged, 68 years age, female, with heart disorder, arteriosclerosis.
(AD) Effects on gastrointestinal system and skin rash due to quinidine.
(AD) Patient had history of toxic effects of drugs.
(AD) Suggested that possible previous hearing loss made more severe by propranolol. (ENG)

282
Limited effects on blood vessels of stria vascularis and spiral prominence due to 300 mg per kg daily of antibiotic, kanamycin, for 4 to 9 days in animals, guinea pigs.
Limited effects on blood vessels of stria vascularis and spiral prominence due to 30 mg per kg daily of antibiotic, dihydrostreptomycin, for 4 to 9 days in animals, guinea pigs.
Limited effects on blood vessels of stria vascularis and spiral prominence due to 30 mg per kg daily of antibiotic, chloramphenicol, for 4 to 9 days in animals, guinea pigs.
(CT) Study of guinea pigs, control group. (JAP)

284
Hearing loss due to antibiotics, aminoglycoside, in humans.
Hearing loss due to salicylate, sodium salicylate, in humans.
Hearing loss due to antimalarial, quinine, in humans.
(AD) Discussion of clinical use and cochleotoxic effects of ototoxic drugs in humans. (FR)

288
Changes in cochlear microphonic due to parenteral, intramuscular, administration of 300 mg per kg daily of antibiotic, kanamycin, in animals, cats.
Changes in cochlear microphonic due to parenteral, intramuscular, administration of 200 and 100 mg per kg daily of antibiotic, streptomycin, in animals, cats.
Hearing loss due to 300 mg per kg daily of antibiotic, kanamycin, in humans.
Hearing loss due to range of 50 to 200 mg per kg daily of antibiotic, streptomycin, in humans.
(CT) Study of subjects, control group, not treated with aminoglycoside antibiotics.
(AD) Hearing loss confirmed by audiogram. (JAP)

303
Transient sensorineural hearing loss and tinnitus due to unspecified method of administration of 300 mg of diuretic, (SQ) ethacrynic acid (SM), for first 24 hours in 1 human, adult, 22 years age, female, with preeclampsia during pregnancy.
Transient sensorineural hearing loss and tinnitus due to unspecified method of administration of 180 mg of diuretic, (SQ) furosemide (SM), for first 24 hours in 1 human, adult, 22 years age, female, with preeclampsia during pregnancy.
Transient sensorineural hearing loss and tinnitus due to unspecified method of administration of 100 mg of diuretic, (SQ) ethacrynic acid (SM), for 5 days in 1 human, adult, 22 years age, female, with preeclampsia during preg-

nancy.
Transient sensorineural hearing loss and tinnitus due to unspecified method
of administration of 80 mg of diuretic, (SQ) furosemide (SM), for 5 days in 1
human, adult, 22 years age, female, with preeclampsia during pregnancy.
    (AD) Cochleotoxic effects confirmed by audiology.   (ENG)

314

Loss of enzymes, succinic dehydrogenase and DPN diaphorase, in outer hair
cells of organ of Corti but usually no enzyme loss in inner hair cells due to
topical administration to bulla of 200 mg per ml of antibiotic, kanamycin
(kanamycin sulfate), in 1 injection in animals, guinea pigs.
Loss of enzymes, succinic dehydrogenase and DPN diaphorase, in outer hair
cells of organ of Corti but usually no enzyme loss in inner hair cells due to
topical administration to bulla of 200 mg per ml of antibiotic, dihydrostreptomycin (dihydrostreptomycin sulfate), in 1 injection in animals, guinea
pigs.
Loss of enzymes, succinic dehydrogenase and DPN diaphorase, in outer hair
cells of organ of Corti but usually no enzyme loss in inner hair cells due to
topical administration to bulla of 200 mg per ml of antibiotic, chloramphenicol (chloramphenicol succinate), in 1 injection in animals, guinea pigs.
More severe effects on enzymes, succinic hydrogenase and DPN diaphorase, in
outer hair cells of organ of Corti due to topical administration to bulla of
saturated solution of antimalarial, quinine (quinine hydrochloride), in 1
injection in animals, guinea pigs.
    (CT) Activity of succinic dehydrogenase often higher in outer hair cells
    than in inner hair cells of organ of Corti in guinea pigs, control group.
    (AD) Suggested correlation between cochleotoxic effects of drugs and
    metabolic activity of hair cells.   (ENG)

326

Hearing loss due to parenteral, intramuscular, administration of 1.0 g daily
of antibiotic, capreomycin (SM), for less than 6 months in 2 of 53 humans
with cavitary pulmonary tuberculosis and no previous chemotherapy.
No reported ototoxic effects due to oral administration of 12.0 g daily in 3
divided doses of antituberculous agent, PAS (SM), for up to 6 months in 53
humans with cavitary pulmonary tuberculosis and no previous chemotherapy.
(ENG)

327

More severe hearing loss due to parenteral, intramuscular, administration of
1 g daily of antibiotic, (SQ) capreomycin (SM), for long period in 1 of 32
humans, male, with pulmonary tuberculosis and with previous antibiotic therapy.
Hearing loss before capreomycin treatment due to (SQ) antibiotics, aminoglycoside, in 1 of 32 humans, male, with pulmonary tuberculosis.
    (AD) Hearing loss confirmed by audiogram.
Tinnitus due to parenteral, intramuscular, administration of 1 g daily of
antibiotic, (SQ) capreomycin (SM), for long period in 3 of 32 humans with
pulmonary tuberculosis.
Simultaneous administration of other (SQ) antituberculous agents (SM), in 32
humans, adult and aged, 20 to 69 years age, male and female, with pulmonary
tuberculosis.
Previous administration of antituberculous agent, (SQ) PAS, in 32 humans,
adult and aged, 20 to 69 years age, male and female, with pulmonary tuberculosis.   (ENG)

334

Effect on organ of Corti of fetuses due to parenteral, intraperitoneal,
administration of daily doses of antibiotic, streptomycin, in animals, rats,
female, during pregnancy.
Effect on organ of Corti of fetuses due to parenteral, intraperitoneal,
administration of daily doses of antibiotic, dihydrostreptomycin, in animals,
rats, female, during pregnancy.
    (AD) Determined concentration of antibiotic in blood of fetus.   (GER)

338

No loss of pinna reflex and no significant histological changes due to parenteral, subcutaneous, administration of 400 mg per kg daily in 1 injection of

antibiotic, dihydrostreptomycin, for 8 to 37 injections in 8 animals, guinea pigs, young, 200 to 290 g weight.
Hearing loss after 64 injections and moderate damage to hair cells of cochlea due to parenteral, subcutaneous, administration of 600 mg per kg daily, total dose of 38.4 g, of antibiotic, dihydrostreptomycin, for 9 to 64 injections in 1 of 5 animals, guinea pigs, young, 200 to 290 g weight.
No loss of pinna reflex and no significant histological changes due to 50 mg per kg daily of antibiotic, kanamycin, for 64 injections in 10 animals, guinea pigs.
   (CT) Test of pinna reflex, pretreatment and daily during treatment with antibiotics.
   (AD) Suggested relationship between degree of kanamycin damage to cochlea and daily dose rather than total dose. (ENG)

342
More severe sensorineural hearing loss of 20 decibels or more due to paren- (SQ) teral administration of total doses of 173 and 172 g of antibiotic, (SQ) capreomycin, for long period, range of 2 to 18 months, in 2 of 294 humans, male and female, with pulmonary tuberculosis and with previous hearing loss.
   (CT) Audiometry, pretreatment and during treatment.
   (AD) Suggested that occurrence of auditory system problems due to ca-
      preomycin not high.
Sensorineural hearing loss due to previous administration of antibiotic, (SQ) streptomycin, in 1 of 294 humans with pulmonary tuberculosis. (ENG)

350
Cochleotoxic effects due to 0.75 or 1 g daily, total doses of 30.0 to 116.75 g, of antibiotic, streptomycin, in 9(7.2 percent)of 125 humans with disor-ders.
Cochleotoxic effects due to 1 g daily, total of less than 30 to over 180 g, of antibiotic, kanamycin, in 40 (55.6 percent) of 72 humans with disorders.
   (AD) Comparative study of ototoxic effects of 2 aminoglycoside antibio-
      tics. (GER)

355
Tinnitus and hearing loss due to previous oral administration of (SQ) 4.5 g daily of salicylate, (SQ) aspirin, in 4 of 6 humans with rheumatoid arthri-tis.
Tinnitus and hearing loss due to oral administration of (SQ) 3.6 g daily of salicylate, (SQ) aspirin, for short period, 2 weeks, in 1 of 6 humans with rheumatoid arthritis.
No ototoxic effects due to oral administration of 0.3, 0.6, and 0.9 g daily of anti-inflammatory agent, (SQ) ibuprofen, for short period, 2 weeks, in 6 humans with rheumatoid arthritis.
No ototoxic effects due to range of 200 to 1200 mg daily, average of 600 mg daily, of anti-inflammatory agent, ibuprofen, for long period, 3 months to over 12 months, in 27 humans, adult, 60.6 years average age, male and female, with rheumatoid arthritis.
   (AD) Comparative study of effectiveness of aspirin and ibuprofen in treat-
      ment of rheumatoid arthritis. (ENG)

356
Hearing loss due to antibiotic, streptomycin, in 120 of 150 humans, child, 2 to 4 years age, most treated when newborn infant or infant for different disorders.
Hearing loss due to antibiotic, streptomycin (SM), in 30 of 150 humans, child, 2 to 4 years age, most treated when newborn infant or infant for different disorders.
Hearing loss due to antibiotic, neomycin (SM), in 30 of 150 humans, child, 2 to 4 years age, most treated when newborn infant or infant for different disorders.
Hearing loss due to other antibiotics (SM) in 30 of 150 humans, child, 2 to 4 years age, most treated when newborn infant or infant for different disor-ders.
   (AD) Hearing loss determined by play audiometry.
   (AD) No relationship between hearing loss and dosage or duration of treat-
      ment with antibiotics.
   (AD) No improvement in hearing after 1 to 2 years. (RUS)

359

Hearing loss due to oral administration of 400, 600, or 800 mg of anti-inflammatory agent, ibuprofen, for 2 weeks in 2 of 30 humans, adult and aged, 30
to 79 years age, female and male, with rheumatoid arthritis.
Unspecified ototoxic effects due to oral administration of 2.4, 3.6, or 4.8 g
daily of salicylate, aspirin, for 2 weeks in 18 of 30 humans, adult and aged,
30 to 79 years age, female and male, with rheumatoid arthritis.
   (AD) Comparative study of ibuprofen, aspirin, and placebo in treatment of
   rheumatoid arthritis. (ENG)

362

Hearing loss due to high and low doses of antibiotic, streptomycin, in humans, child and adult, with different disorders and with previous hearing
loss in 2 humans.
Hearing loss due to high doses of antibiotic, neomycin, in humans, child and
adult, with different disorders.
   (AD) Need for daily audiometry and vestibular function tests with administration of aminoglycoside antibiotics.
   (AD) If ototoxic effect observed, need to withdraw ototoxic drug or ad-
   minister vitamins, glucose, dimedrol, calcium chloride, or electrophoresis
   with potassium iodide. (RUS)

373

Possible progressive sensorineural hearing loss due to antibiotics, aminogly-
coside, in humans.
Possible transient hearing loss due to high doses of salicylate, aspirin, in
humans.
Possible transient hearing loss due to high doses of antimalarial, quinine,
in humans.
Possible hearing loss due to diuretic, ethacrynic acid, in humans.
Bilateral sudden deafness due to antibiotic, kanamycin, in 4 humans, adult,
34 years average age, male and female.
   (AD) Hearing loss due to ototoxic drugs usually progressive.
   (AD) Sudden deafness due to ototoxic drugs possible in some cases, as in
   humans with kidney disorder.
   (AD) Literature review on etiology of sudden deafness. (ENG)

374

Decr in cochlear microphonic due to 4-300 mg per percent of solution of
diuretic, furosemide, in animals, guinea pigs.
Decr in cochlear microphonic due to 2-200 mg per percent of solution of
diuretic, ethacrynic acid, in animals, guinea pigs. (GER)

394

Tinnitus and hearing loss due to total of 50 to 100 g, in some cases, of
antibiotic, (SQ) kanamycin, in 176(9 percent) of 2054 humans with surgery for
pulmonary tuberculosis.
   (AD) Improvement in hearing in only 30 percent of humans.
Possible hearing loss due to previous administration of antibiotic, (SQ)
streptomycin, for long period in 176 of 2054 humans before surgery for pulmonary tuberculosis. (ENG)

413

Decr in threshold of detection of acoustic stimuli of shorter duration than
16 msec due to 0.4 g of analeptic, caffeine, in humans, adult, and animals.
Decr in threshold of detection of acoustic stimuli of longer duration than 16
msec due to 0.015 to 0.02 g of analeptic, amphetamine, in humans, adult, and
animals. (RUS)

414

Transient hearing loss in short time after injection due to parenteral,
intravenous, administration of (SQ) high doses, 500 mg each dose, of diuretic, (SQ) furosemide, in (SQ) total of 2 doses, each for duration of 3
minutes, on consecutive days in 1 human, adult, 49 years age, female, with
chronic kidney disorder.
   (AD) No observed hearing loss before treatment with furosemide.
   (AD) Normal hearing within 4 hours.
No hearing loss due to parenteral, intravenous, administration of (SQ) 240 mg

of diuretic, (SQ) furosemide, in (SQ) 1 dose for duration of 5 minutes in 1
human, adult, 49 years age, female, with chronic kidney disorder.
   (AD) Suggested that cochleotoxic effect of furosemide is dose related.
   (AD) Different individual responses to furosemide suggest other factors in
ototoxic effects.
Previous administration of antibiotic, (SQ) nalidixic acid, in 1 human,
adult, 49 years age, female, with chronic kidney disorder. (ENG)

415
Transient and permanent hearing loss due to high doses of diuretic, etha-
crynic acid, in humans.
Transient hearing loss due to parenteral, intravenous, administration of high
doses, 600 to 1000 mg, of diuretic, furosemide, in humans with kidney disor-
ders.
   (AD) Literature review of clinical use and toxic effects of diuretics.
   (ENG)

423
More severe and more rapid progression of presbycusis due to antimalarial,
quinine, in humans, adult and aged.
More severe and more rapid progression of presbycusis due to antibiotics,
aminoglycoside, in humans, adult and aged.
More severe and more rapid progression of presbycusis due to salicylate,
aspirin, in humans, adult and aged.
More severe and more rapid progression of presbycusis due to chemical agent,
carbon monoxide, in humans, adult and aged.
   (AD) Discussion of factors resulting in more severe and more rapid progression of presbycusis. (FR)

430
Permanent hearing loss, partial or total, due to parenteral, intramuscular,
administration of 200,000 units per kg daily of antibiotic, streptomycin, for
30 days in animals, guinea pigs.
Permanent hearing loss, partial or total, due to parenteral, intramuscular,
administration of 150,000 units per kg daily of antibiotic, colistin (colistin sulfate), for 7 to 21 days in animals, guinea pigs. (RUS)

437
Hearing loss and damage to cochlea due to antibiotic, neomycin, in animals,
guinea pigs and monkeys, and humans.
Hearing loss and damage to cochlea due to antibiotic, streptomycin, in animals, guinea pigs and monkeys, and humans.
   (AD) Discussion of findings on decr of ototoxicity of aminoglycoside
   antibiotics. (GER)

443
Decr in summating potential and threshold shift due to topical administration
to round window of 2 percent solution of anesthetic, tetracaine, in animals,
guinea pigs.
Decr in summating potential and threshold shift due to topical administration
to round window of 4 percent solution of anesthetic, lidocaine, in animals,
guinea pigs.
   (AD) More changes in summating potential and threshold due to tetracaine
   than to lidocaine.
   (AD) Partial recovery of summating potential after 60 minutes in guinea
   pigs treated with lidocaine. (GER)

468
Complete inhibition of acetylcholine induced decr in cochlear potential due
to parenteral, intravenous, administration of 1.0 mg of antibiotic, streptomycin (streptomycin sulfate), in 1 injection in 5 animals, cats, male and
female, 1.5 to 2.8 kg weight, with injection of acetylcholine.
Minimum inhibition of acetylcholine induced decr in cochlear potential due to
parenteral, intravenous, administration of 1.0 mg of antibiotic, dihydrostreptomycin (dihydrostreptomycin sulfate), in 1 injection in 5 animals, cats,
male and female, 1.5 to 2.8 kg weight, with injection of acetylcholine.
Complete inhibition of acetylcholine induced decr in cochlear potential due
to parenteral, intravenous, administration of 1.0 mg of antibiotic, kanamycin

(kanamycin sulfate), in 1 injection in 5 animals, cats, male and female, 1.5
to 2.8 kg weight, with injection of acetylcholine.
Complete inhibition of acetylcholine induced decr in cochlear potential due
to parenteral, intravenous, administration of 1.0 mg of antibiotic, neomycin
(neomycin sulfate), in 1 injection in 5 animals, cats, male and female, 1.5
to 2.8 kg weight, with injection of acetylcholine.
Acute inhibition of acetylcholine induced decr in cochlear potential due to
parenteral, intravenous, administration of 1.0 mg of antimalarial, quinine
(quinine hydrochloride), in 1 injection in 5 animals, cats, male and female,
1.5 to 2.8 kg weight, with injection of acetylcholine.
    (CT) Injections of 0.1 ml isotonic saline in cats, control group.
Inhibition of acetylcholine induced decr in cochlear potential due to parenteral, subcutaneous, administration of 300 mg per kg daily of antibiotic,
streptomycin, for 7 to 9 days in 10 animals, cats.
Inhibition of acetylcholine induced decr in cochlear potential due to parenteral, subcutaneous, administration of 100 mg per kg daily of antibiotic,
neomycin, for 7 to 9 days in 10 animals, cats.
    (CT) Study of 7 cats, control group, not treated with antibiotics.
    (AD) Study of effect of acetylcholine on cochlear potential after acute
    and chronic administration of ototoxic drugs.
    (AD) Suggested relationship between change in acetylcholine activity and
    ototoxic drugs.
    (AD) Suggested that ototoxicity partially due to disruption of efferent
    effect on cochlea. (ENG)

                                                                          477
Significant decr in oxygen consumption of cochlea due to high doses of antibiotic, kanamycin, in animals, guinea pigs.
Significant decr in oxygen consumption of cochlea due to high doses of antibiotic, streptomycin, in animals, guinea pigs.
Incr followed by significant decr in oxygen consumption of cochlea due to
high doses of antibiotic, dihydrostreptomycin, in animals, guinea pigs.
    (CT) Determination of oxygen consumption of guinea pigs, control group,
    not treated with ototoxic drugs.
    (AD) Suggested that ototoxicity of aminoglycoside antibiotics due to
    inhibition of respiratory enzymes of cells of inner ear. (ENG)

                                                                          511
Transient severe sudden deafness due to 1 g of diuretic, (SQ) furosemide, in
1 human, Korean, adult, 26 years age, female, with lupus erythematosus.
Transient severe sudden deafness due to administration 2 months later of 100
mg of diuretic, (SQ) ethacrynic acid, in 1 human, Korean, adult, 26 years
age, female, with lupus erythematosus.
    (AD) Suggested that cochleotoxic effects related to potent diuretic ac-
    tion. (ENG)

                                                                          515
Bilateral hearing loss due to oral (SM) administration of 480 mg daily of
diuretic, furosemide (SM), for 10 days in 1 human with kidney disorder.
Bilateral hearing loss due to parenteral, intravenous (SM), administration of
600 mg daily of diuretic, furosemide (SM), for 10 days in 1 human with kidney
disorder.
Bilateral hearing loss due to 500 mg of antibiotic, kanamycin (SM) (kanamycin
sulfate), in 2 doses in 1 human with kidney disorder.
    (AD) No pretreatment audiogram.
    (AD) Posttreatment audiogram confirmed hearing loss.
    (AD) Suggested audiometry, pretreatment and during treatment, for humans,
    in particular with kidney disorder, treated with high doses of intravenous
    furosemide. (ENG)

                                                                          520
Decr in time of latency with incr in intensity of acoustic stimuli due to
parenteral, intraperitoneal, administration of 80 mg per kg daily, total of
480 mg, of antibiotic, cephalothin (cephalothin sodium), for 15 days in 10
animals, guinea pigs, albino.
Decr in time of latency with incr in intensity of acoustic stimuli due to
parenteral, intraperitoneal, administration of 20 mg per kg daily, total of
120 mg, of antibiotic, lincomycin (lincomycin chloride), for 15 days in 10

animals, guinea pigs, albino.
Decr in time of latency with incr in intensity of acoustic stimuli due to
parenteral, intraperitoneal, administration of 50 mg per kg daily, total of
300 mg, of antibiotic, cephaloridine, for 15 days in 10 animals, guinea pigs,
albino.
  (CT) Study of guinea pigs, control group, not treated with antibiotics.
  (AD) Study of response of guinea pigs to acoustic stimuli after treatment
  with antibiotics. (IT)

                                                                          522
Hearing loss due to antibiotic, kanamycin, for 2 to 10 months in 30.4 percent
of 56 humans with chronic pulmonary tuberculosis and treated previously with
other drugs.
No significant ototoxic effects due to antibiotic, florimycin, for 2 to 10
months in 50 humans with chronic pulmonary tuberculosis and treated previously with other drugs.
  (AD) Study of effects of kanamycin and florimycin in treatment of pulmonary tuberculosis. (RUS)

                                                                          547
Bilateral sensorineural hearing loss within 20 minutes but normal vestibular
function due to parenteral, intravenous, administration of 50 mg of diuretic,
ethacrynic acid (SM), in 1 injection in 1 human, adult, 53 years age, female,
with kidney disorder.
  (AD) Hearing loss confirmed by audiogram.
  (AD) Vestibular function tests showed normal vestibular function.
Simultaneous oral administration of 18 g of antibiotic, neomycin (SM), in 7
days in 1 human, adult, 53 years age, female, with kidney disorder.
Severe destruction of outer hair cells of organ of Corti in basal coil of
cochlea due to parenteral, intravenous, administration of 50 mg of diuretic,
ethacrynic acid (SM), in 1 injection in 1 human, adult, 53 years age, female,
with kidney disorder.
  (AD) Suggested that damage to hair cells possibly due to neomycin also.
  (AD) Suggested possible permanent hearing loss as result of ethacrynic
  acid treatment in patients with kidney disorders.
Transient and permanent total hearing loss within 15 minutes due to parenteral administration of diuretic, ethacrynic acid, in animals, cats. (ENG)

                                                                          550
Decr in cochlear potentials due to parenteral, intraperitoneal, administration of 15 mg per kg of anesthetics (CB) in 2 groups of 15 animals, guinea
pigs, pigmented and albino, 300 g weight.
Decr in cochlear potentials due to parenteral, intraperitoneal, administration of 15 mg per kg of sedative, barbiturate (CB) in 2 groups of 15 animals,
guinea pigs, pigmented and albino, 300 g weight. (IT)

                                                                          558
Severe hearing loss due to antibiotic, kanamycin (SM), in 1 human, adult, 44
years age, female, with basilar meningitis.
Simultaneous administration of 1 g daily of antituberculous agent, ethambutol
(SM), in 1 human, adult, 44 years age, female, with basilar meningitis.
(ENG)

                                                                          564
Hearing loss due to antibiotic, kanamycin (SM), for long period in 3 of 4
humans, adult, range of ages, male and female, during retreatment for pulmonary tuberculosis.
Simultaneous administration of 25 mg per kg for 2 months and then 15 mg per
kg of antituberculous agent, ethambutol (SM), in 4 humans, adult, range of
ages, male and female, during retreatment for pulmonary tuberculosis.
  (CT) Treatment with ethambutol and 2 other antituberculous agents in
  humans, control group. (ENG)

                                                                          565
Inhibition of oxygen consumption of cochlea due to 0.04 M of antibiotic,
kanamycin (kanamycin sulfate), in animals, guinea pigs, adult, 300 g weight,
with normal Preyer reflex.
Inhibition of oxygen consumption of cochlea due to 0.04 M of antibiotic,

chloramphenicol (chloramphenicol sodium succinate), in animals, guinea pigs, adult, 300 g weight, with normal Preyer reflex.

(AD) Less inhibition of oxygen consumption by chloramphenicol than by kanamycin.

Incr inhibition of oxygen consumption of cochlea due to 0.04 M of antibiotic, kanamycin (SM) (kanamycin sulfate), in animals, guinea pigs, adult, 300 g weight, with normal Preyer reflex.

Incr inhibition of oxygen consumption of cochlea due to 0.04 M of antibiotic, chloramphenicol (SM) (chloramphenicol sodium succinate), in animals, guinea pigs, adult, 300 g weight, with normal Preyer reflex.

(CT) Measurement of oxygen consumption of normal cochlea without administration of ototoxic drugs.

(AD) In vitro study using microrespirometer of effect of interaction of kanamycin and chloramphenicol on oxygen consumption in guinea pig cochlea.

(AD) Potentiation of inhibition of oxygen consumption of cochlea with simultaneous administration of kanamycin and chloramphenicol.

(AD) Suggested risk of ototoxicity in clinical use of kanamycin and chloramphenicol. (ENG)

566

Gradual decr in cochlear microphonics and decr in endocochlear potentials, but not significant, due to salicylate, acetylsalicylic acid, in animals, guinea pigs, 250 to 400 g weight.

Severe decr in cochlear potentials due to 2.0 mM of chemical agent, cyanide (potassium cyanide), in animals, guinea pigs, 250 to 400 g weight.

(AD) Study of effects of various agents on cochlear potentials. (ENG)

569

Slight hearing loss due to 1 g daily in single dose of antibiotic, capreomycin (SM), in 2 of 31 humans with chronic pulmonary tuberculosis.

(AD) Audiometry and vestibular function tests every 4 weeks and then every 6 weeks.

(AD) Cessation of treatment with capreomycin in 4 cases to prevent hearing loss.

Simultaneous administration of 25 mg per kg daily in single dose for 12 weeks and then 15 mg per kg of antituberculous agent, ethambutol (SM), in 31 humans with chronic pulmonary tuberculosis.

Simultaneous oral administration of 1 other antituberculous agent (SM), in 31 humans with chronic pulmonary tuberculosis. (ENG)

570

Transient slight hearing loss due to parenteral, intramuscular, administration of 1 g daily, maximum dose of 90 g, of antibiotic, capreomycin (SM), in 1 of 16 humans with chronic tuberculosis of genitourinary system.

Simultaneous administration of 2 other antituberculous agents (SM), in 16 humans with chronic tuberculosis of genitourinary system.

Hearing loss due to 1 g daily average dose of antibiotic, capreomycin (SM), for long period in 1 of 20 humans, adult, male and female, with chronic tuberculosis, and 5 also alcoholics.

Simultaneous administration of other antituberculous agents (SM), in 20 humans, adult, male and female, with chronic tuberculosis, and 5 also alcoholics.

(AD) Discussion of various reports of auditory system problems due to capreomycin therapy. (ENG)

597

Hearing loss due to salicylates in humans.
Hearing loss due to antimalarial, quinine, in humans.
Hearing loss due to antibiotic, streptomycin, in humans.
Tinnitus due to chemical agent, camphor, in humans.
Tinnitus due to chemical agent, tobacco, in humans.
Tinnitus due to cardiovascular agent, quinidine, in humans.
Tinnitus due to chemical agent, ergot, in humans.
Tinnitus due to chemical agent, alcohol, methyl, in humans.

(AD) Discussion of toxic effects of drugs. (ENG)

611

Hearing loss due to range of 0.8 to 15 g of antibiotic, neomycin (SM), in 9

humans, child, adult, and aged, 4 or less to 65 years age, with various
infections.
Simultaneous administration of antibiotic, streptomycin (SM), in 6 humans,
child, adult, and aged, 4 or less to 65 years age, with various infections.
Simultaneous administration of antibiotic, polymyxin (SM), in 1 human, child,
less than 4 years age, with various infections.
  (AD) Hearing loss confirmed by audiograms.
  (AD) Discussion of 9 case reports. (HUN)

613

Significant decr in cochlear microphonic due to topical administration to
round window of 10 percent concentration of anesthetic, cocaine, in 15
minutes in animals, guinea pigs, 400 to 600 g weight.
Less, but permanent, decr in cochlear microphonic due to topical administration to round window of 2 percent concentration of anesthetic, tetracaine, in
15 minutes in animals, guinea pigs, 400 to 600 g weight.
  (AD) Need for careful consideration in use of topical anesthetic within
  middle ear.
  (AD) Suggested that cocaine not be used within middle ear. (GER)

628

Hearing loss due to parenteral, intravenous, administration of 1 mg per kg
initial dose and then 0.75 mg per kg every 6 hours, dissolved in 200 ml of 5
percent glucose solution, of antibiotic, (SQ) gentamicin (gentamicin sulfate), in 4 of 60 humans, child, adolescent, adult, and aged, 6 to 76 years
age, with carcinoma, lymphoma, or leukemia and with azotemia in 3 of 4 and
previous hearing loss in 1 of 4.
Hearing loss due to previous administration of diuretic, (SQ) ethacrynic
acid, in 1 of 4 humans with gentamicin hearing loss.
  (AD) Suggested that hearing loss in 1 patient due to both gentamicin and
  ethacrynic acid. (ENG)

698

Hearing loss, after 3 months in most cases, due to parenteral administration
of 0.5 g twice daily for 7 days a week of antibiotic, kanamycin, in 29 (39
percent) of 75 humans with pulmonary tuberculosis.
Damage to eighth cranial nerve due to parenteral administration of 1 g twice
daily for 2 days a week of antibiotic, kanamycin, for more than 12 months in
5 (7 percent) of 64 humans with pulmonary tuberculosis.
  (AD) Low incidence of ototoxic effects reported in study possibly due to
  administration of kanamycin only 2 days a week.
Damage to eighth cranial nerve due to parenteral administration of 15 mg per
kg daily of antibiotic, kanamycin, in 4 (6 percent) of 65 humans with pulmonary tuberculosis and with previous hearing loss.
Hearing loss due to parenteral administration of 15 to 20 mg per kg for 5
days a week of antibiotic, (SQ) kanamycin, in 19 (22 percent) of 82 humans
with pulmonary tuberculosis and with previous hearing loss in 10 cases.
  (AD) Hearing loss confirmed by audiometry.
  (AD) Ototoxic effects in patients 50 years or over age in 15 of 19 cases.
Previous administration of antibiotic, (SQ) streptomycin, for long period in
82 humans with pulmonary tuberculosis.
Previous administration of antibiotic, (SQ) viomycin, in 10 of 82 humans with
pulmonary tuberculosis.
  (AD) Discussion of ototoxic effects of kanamycin reported in 4 studies.
  (AD) Significant factors in kanamycin ototoxicity reported to be age over
  50 years, high daily dose of more than 20 mg per kg, high serum level of
  more than 25 mcg per ml, concurrent kidney disorders, and previous hearing
  loss. (ENG)

715

Loss of outer hair cells of organ of Corti in lower part of first coil of
cochlea due to parenteral, intramuscular, administration of 400 mg per kg of
antibiotic, capreomycin, for 28 days in 40 percent of 10 animals, guinea
pigs, albino, 300 g weight.
Severe loss of outer hair cells of organ of Corti from lower part of basal
coil to upper coil of cochlea due to parenteral, intramuscular, administration of 400 mg per kg of antibiotic, kanamycin, for 28 days in 100 percent of
11 animals, guinea pigs, albino, 300 g weight.

(CT) Test of Preyer reflex before, during, and after administration of antibiotics.
(AD) Study suggested that capreomycin less ototoxic than kanamycin in guinea pigs.
(AD) No observed damage to vestibular apparatus. (JAP)

Vestibular function

143

Transient unsteady gait and dizziness due to oral administration of high doses, 12 to 30 tablets per day, of salicylate, aspirin, in 1 human, adult, 44 years age, male, self treatment for pain after accident.
(AD) EEG abnormal for 5 weeks. (ENG)

114

Vestibulotoxic effects due to oral ingestion of large amounts of sedative, alcohol, ethyl, in humans.
(AD) Effects of alcohol on vestibular apparatus determined by duration of nystagmus. (GER)

153

Less severe effects on vestibular apparatus due to oral ingestion of 80-proof and 100-proof concentrations of sedative, alcohol, ethyl, in 4 humans, adult, 27 to 50 years age, male, with bilateral vestibular problems.
(AD) Same test procedures used in previous study of normal subjects showed more severe effects of alcohol on vestibular apparatus.
(AD) Subjects with vestibular problems less vulnerable to effects of alcohol than normal subjects. (ENG)

248

Effect on vestibular threshold due to sedative, alcohol, ethyl, in humans.
(CT) Pretreatment and posttreatment vestibular function tests. (ENG)

463

Nystagmus due to oral ingestion of 50 to 340 cc (0.44 to 2.58 g per kg) of 40 or 45 proof concentration of sedative, alcohol, ethyl, in 20 or 25 minutes in 38 humans, adult, 19 to 42 years age, male and female, 55 to 70 kg weight.
(AD) Vestibular problems confirmed by vestibular function tests.
(AD) Discussion of individual differences in responses to ethyl alcohol.
(FR)

508

High frequency and low amplitude nystagmus due to sedative, alcohol, ethyl, in humans.
(AD) Study of effects of alcohol on vertigo and nystagmus. (ENG)

527

Decr in vestibular neurons due to parenteral, slow intravenous, administration of low doses, corresponding to 0.6 g per kg of 100 percent alcohol, of diluted 30 percent concentration of sedative, alcohol, ethyl, in 1 injection in animals, cats, adult, male and female, 3.0 kg weight.
(AD) Suggested susceptibility of vestibular neurons to direct effects of alcohol.
(AD) Suggested that clinical alcoholic intoxication, with nystagmus, due to direct action of alcohol on vestibular neurons. (ENG)

572

Effect on vestibular function due to oral administration of 2.0 ml per kg, in orange juice, of 100-proof of sedative, alcohol, ethyl, in 30 minutes in 10 humans.
(CT) Same method using beverage without alcohol in subjects, control group.
(AD) Study of effect of alcohol ingestion on human performance in static situations and during motion.
(AD) Tests of visuomotor skill during angular acceleration, pretreatment and 1 to 10 hours posttreatment. (ENG)

710
Effect on vestibular function due to sedative, alcohol, ethyl, in humans.
(ENG)

279
Transient inhibition of endorgan of ampulla of semicircular canal due to
range of doses of antibiotics, aminoglycoside, in animals, frogs.
   (CT) Study of frogs, control group.
   (AD) In vitro study of effect of antibiotics on function of ampullar
   endorgan of semicircular canal of frog. (IT)

711
Vestibular problems due to antibiotic, capreomycin, for more than 3 months in
1 of 35 humans with pulmonary tuberculosis. (POL)

665
Transient slight dizziness and equilibrium disorder due to oral administration in tablets of range of less than 600 mg to 1200 mg daily, of anticonvulsant, carbamazepine, for long period in large group of humans, adult and
aged, 30 to over 80 years age, male and female, with facial pain.
Severe dizziness due to oral administration in tablets of range of less than
600 mg to 1200 mg daily, of anticonvulsant, carbamazepine, for long period in
2 of 71 humans, adult and aged, 30 to over 80 years age, male and female,
with facial pain and with concurrent multiple sclerosis in 1 and cerebral
arteriosclerosis in other. (ENG)

669
Possible transient dizziness due to anticonvulsant, carbamazepine, in humans
with trigeminal neuralgia. (ENG)

233
Vestibular problems due to topical route, inhalation, of large amount, to
produce average carboxyhemoglobin level of 60 ml per 1, of chemical agent,
carbon monoxide, in 20 humans, adult, 30 years average age.
   (AD) Vestibular problems determined by vestibular function tests. (FR)

472
Vertigo due to topical route, inhalation, of chemical agent, carbon monoxide,
in humans, adult. (RUS)

230
Vestibular problems due to chemical agent, carbon tetrachloride, in humans.
   (AD) Vestibular function tests conducted to determine effects of carbon
   tetrachloride. (RUS)

532
Damage to vestibular apparatus due to chemical agent, nitro solvent, in 1
human.
   (AD) Vestibular problem confirmed by vestibular function test. (POL)

478
Nystagmus due to parenteral, intramuscular, administration of 0.5 g daily,
total dose of 50 g, of antibiotic, dihydrostreptomycin, in 6 humans with
pulmonary tuberculosis.
Nystagmus due to parenteral, intramuscular, administration of total doses of
105 to 300 g of antibiotic, dihydrostreptomycin, in 10 humans with pulmonary
tuberculosis.
   (AD) Case report included.
   (AD) Study using cupulometry of vestibular problems due to dihydrostreptomycin therapy. (GER)

344
No significant change in perrotatory neuronal response of medial vestibular
nucleus due to parenteral, intravenous, administration of 2, 8, or 20 mg per
kg of antihistamine, dimenhydrinate, in animals, cats, adult, 2.5 kg average
weight.
Significant decr in perrotatory neuronal response of medial vestibular nucleus due to parenteral, intravenous, administration of 0.4 mg per kg of
diazepan in animals, cat s, adult, 2.5 kg average weight.

(CT) Same method using 1 ml Ringer's solution in cats, control group, showed no significant changes.
(AD) Possible peripheral or central location, or both, of action of dimenhydrinate.
(AD) Study to determine if changes in perrotatory response of medial vestibular nucleus is result of action on vestibular apparatus.
(AD) Suggest that endorgan not location of action of dimenhydrinate. (ENG)

654
Possible ataxia due to high doses to produce blood level of 3 mg per 100 ml or more of anticonvulsant, diphenylhydantoin, in humans, child and adult, with epilepsy.
Possible nystagmus due to doses to produce blood level of more than 2 mg per 100 ml of anticonvulsant, diphenylhydantoin, in humans, child and adult, with epilepsy. (ENG)

655
Possible ataxia and nystagmus due to anticonvulsant, diphenylhydantoin, in humans with convulsive disorders. (ENG)

658
Vertigo due to parenteral, intravenous, administration of 250 mg of anticonvulsant, diphenylhydantoin, in some of 123 humans, adult and aged, male and female, with heart disorders. (GER)

664
Nystagmus due to parenteral, intramuscular or intravenous, administration of 1000 to 1500 mg on first day, and then 400 to 1500 mg on second day, followed by 400 to 600 mg, to produce blood levels of 8.6 to 35.0 mcg per ml, of anticonvulsant, diphenylhydantoin, in 8 of 10 humans, adult and aged, 40 to 65 years age, male and female, 50-94 kg weight, with heart disorders. (ENG)

671
Nystagmus due to anticonvulsant, diphenylhydantoin, in humans, child and adult, male and female, with epilepsy. (FIN)

544
Vertigo due to antituberculous agent, ethambutol, in 2 of 187 humans treated for pulmonary tuberculosis.
(AD) Literature review showed report of 2 cases of vertigo due to ethambutol. (FR)

036
Damage to vestibular apparatus due to parenteral or topical administration of antibiotic, gentamicin (gentamicin sulfate), in humans. (ENG)

218
Transient vertigo due to parenteral, intramuscular, administration of 2 x 40 mg of antibiotic, gentamicin, for 15 days in 1 human, adult, 39 years age, 72 kg weight, with diabetes mellitus and chronic pyelonephritis. (GER)

300
Possible vestibular problems due to more than recommended 240 mg daily of antibiotic, gentamicin, in humans, in particular with kidney disorder or 40 years or over age.
(AD) More risk of ototoxicity with gentamicin than with other aminoglycoside antibiotics.
(AD) Need for study of relationship between vestibular problems and dosage and duration of therapy. (ENG)

301
Severe vertigo 2 days after cessation of treatment due to topical (SM) administration of 0.1 percent solution of antibiotic, gentamicin, for 4 weeks in 1 human, aged, 65 years age, male, with mild kidney disorder.
Severe vertigo 2 days after cessation of treatment due to parenteral (SM) administration of 40 mg every 6 hours of antibiotic, gentamicin (gentamicin sulfate), for 4 weeks in 1 human, aged, 65 years age, male, with mild kidney

disorder.
(CT) Study of gentamicin serum levels in normal subjects and humans
treated for pseudomonas infections with recommended dose of gentamicin.
(AD) Case report of vestibulotoxic effect of gentamicin. (ENG)

302
Transient dizziness due to parenteral, intramuscular, administration of 120
mg 2 or 3 times daily of antibiotic, gentamicin, for several weeks in 4 of 23
humans, adult and aged, range of 50 to over 70 years age, male, with bronchial infections and with normal kidney function.
(AD) Vestibulotoxic effect confirmed by caloric tests. (ENG)

426
Damage to vestibular function due to sufficient doses to produce blood level
of over 10 mcg per ml of antibiotic, gentamicin, in humans with or without
kidney disorders.
(AD) High blood levels due to kidney disorders or due to high doses or
long period of treatment in humans with normal kidney function.
(AD) Comment on study that reported vestibulotoxic effects of gentamicin
with blood levels lower than 10 mcg per ml. (ENG)

427
Damage to vestibular function due to high doses of antibiotic, gentamicin, in
humans with normal kidney function.
Damage to vestibular function due to antibiotic, gentamicin, in humans with
kidney disorder.
(AD) Risk of gentamicin ototoxicity with blood levels of over 10 mcg per
ml.
(AD) Suggested that gentamicin ototoxicity is dose related.
(AD) Comment on study that reported vestibulotoxic effects of gentamicin
with blood levels lower than 10 mcg per ml. (ENG)

428
Possible damage to eighth cranial nerve due to high blood level of over 10
mcg per ml of antibiotic, gentamicin, in humans.
(AD) Need for serum assays and other tests in clinical use of gentamicin.
(AD) Comment on study that reported vestibulotoxic effects of gentamicin
with blood levels lower than 10 mcg per ml. (ENG)

471
Damage to vestibular apparatus due to antibiotic, gentamicin, in humans with
genitourinary system infections.
(AD) Comment on risk of vestibulotoxic effects in clinical use of gentamicin. (GER)

474
Transient dizziness due to parenteral, intramuscular, administration of 80
mg, to produce serum level of 12 mcg per ml, of antibiotic, gentamicin, in 1
injection in 1 human, adult, 62 years age, female, 46.5 kg weight. (ENG)

475
Possible damage to eighth cranial nerve with vestibular problems due to
parenteral administration of low doses to produce recommended serum levels of
antibiotic, gentamicin, in humans with genitourinary system infections.
(ENG)

548
Transient vestibular problems due to parenteral administration of antibiotic,
gentamicin, in humans. (GER)

573
Bilateral vestibular problems, ataxia, and damage to hair cells of organ of
Corti in basal coil of cochlea and of cristae and maculae due to parenteral,
intramuscular, administration of 80 or 50 mg per kg on 5 days a week of
antibiotic, gentamicin, in 5 animals, squirrel monkeys, Saimiri sciureus,
about 2 years age, male and female.
Loss of equilibrium, ataxia, damage to hair cells of cristae and maculae, and
some degeneration of nerve process near hair cells due to parenteral, subcu-

taneous, administration of 60, 30, or 20 mg per kg on 7 days a week of antibiotic, gentamicin, in 7 animals, squirrel monkeys, Saimiri sciureus, about 2
years age, male and female.

(AD) Type 1 hair cells of cristae and maculae more vulnerable to gentamicin than type 2 hair cells.

(CT) Squirrel monkey rail method and test of nystagmus, pretreatment and
posttreatment.

(AD) Earlier onset of equilibrium disorders with high daily doses than
with low daily doses.

(AD) Total doses before onset of ataxia slightly more in group with high
daily doses.

(AD) Less ototoxic effects and slower onset with administration of gentamicin 5 days a week than 7 days a week.

(AD) Lower doses in group with injections 7 days a week resulted in more
severe and earlier onset of loss of equilibrium.

(AD) Damage to vestibular apparatus slightly more severe in animals with
higher daily doses.

(AD) Correlation between equilibrium test and electron microscopic findings. (ENG)

574

Ataxia due to parenteral, subcutaneous, administration of 20, 40, or 60 mg
per kg daily, dissolved in distilled water in volume of 0.5 ml per kg, of
antibiotic, gentamicin (gentamicin sulfate), for 10 to 70 days in animals,
cats, male, 2.5 to 5.0 kg weight.

(AD) Tests to determine ataxia conducted.

(AD) Relationship between onset of ataxia and dosage.

Permanent ataxia due to parenteral, subcutaneous, administration of 40 mg per
kg daily of antibiotic, gentamicin (gentamicin sulfate), for 16, 18, or 19
days, followed by a rest for 29 to 32 days, and then 19 to 20 days more in 3
animals, cats.

(AD) Ataxia persisted during period without gentamicin treatment.

Ataxia due to parenteral, subcutaneous, administration of 20, 40, or 60 mg
per kg daily, total doses of 600 to about 900 mg per kg, of antibiotic,
gentamicin (gentamicin sulfate), in animals, cats.

(AD) Occurrence of ataxia after smaller average total dose at lower dosage
levels than at higher levels.

(AD) Inverse relationship between onset of ataxia and total dosage suggests that duration of treatment possibly significant factor at dosage
levels studied.

Ataxia after 25 days due to parenteral, subcutaneous, administration of 40 mg
per kg daily of antibiotic, gentamicin (gentamicin sulfate), for 5 days in 5
animals, cats.

Ataxia after 18 days due to parenteral, subcutaneous, administration of 40 mg
per kg daily of antibiotic, gentamicin (gentamicin sulfate), for 7 days in 5
animals, cats.

(AD) Results of experiment suggest significance of total dosage and duration of treatment.

Ataxia after 17 days due to parenteral, subcutaneous, administration of 40 mg
per kg 1 time daily, average total of 680 mg per kg, of antibiotic, gentamicin (gentamicin sulfate), in 6 animals, cats.

Ataxia after 19.4 days due to parenteral, subcutaneous, administration of 20
mg per kg twice daily, average total of 776 mg per kg of antibiotic, gentamicin (gentamicin sulfate), in 5 animals, cats.

(AD) Average total dose to produce ataxia higher with 2 doses daily than
with single daily dose.

Ataxia after 16 days due to parenteral, (SQ) subcutaneous, administration of
40 mg per kg daily, to produce blood levels of 100 mcg per ml 30 minutes
after treatment, of antibiotic, gentamicin (gentamicin sulfate), in 1 dose in
2 animals, cats.

(AD) Rapid decr in blood levels 24 hours after treatment.

Ataxia after 16 days due to parenteral, (SQ) intraarterial, administration of
40 mg per kg daily of antibiotic, gentamicin (gentamicin sulfate), in 2
animals, cats.

(AD) Blood levels monitored daily.

(AD) Peak blood levels with intraarterial administration 2 to 6 times as
high as with subcutaneous route and decr rapidly to less than 1 mcg per ml
24 hours after treatment.

(AD) Decr in kidney function at time of occurrence of ataxia.
(AD) Report on various experiments in study of factors in effect of gentamicin on vestibular function in cats.
(AD) Suggested that total dosage and duration of treatment possibly more
significant factors than peak blood levels with reference to time of onset
of ataxia at dosage levels studied. (ENG)

605

Decr in ototoxic effects due to parenteral, subcutaneous, administration of
high doses of antibiotic, gentamicin (IB) (gentamicin sulfate), in acute
intoxication in 20 animals, mice, male, 20 g weight, with simultaneous subcutaneous administration of calcium chloride.
    (CT) Same method using 8 mg of calcium chloride in mice, control group,
    showed no ototoxic effects.
    (CT) Same method using 12.5 mg of gentamicin (gentamicin sulfate) in mice,
    control group, showed ototoxic effects.
Decr in ototoxic effects due to parenteral, subcutaneous or intravenous,
administration of 25 mg per ml solution of antibiotic, gentamicin (IB) (gentamicin sulfate), in acute intoxication in animals, mice, male, 20 g weight,
with combined administration of 1, 2, 4, 8, 16, or 32 mg per ml concentrations of calcium chloride.
Decr in ototoxic effects due to parenteral, subcutaneous, administration of
antibiotic, gentamicin (IB) (gentamicin hydrochloride), in acute intoxication
in animals, mice, male, 20 g weight, with combined administration of complex
of calcium chloride.
    (AD) Decr in ototoxic effects in mice to less than 0.2 of effects of
    gentamicin (gentamicin hydrochloride) and to less than 0.5 of effects of
    gentamicin (gentamicin sulfate) due to calcium chloride.
Ataxia and equilibrium disorder due to parenteral, subcutaneous, administration of 60 and 120 mg per kg 1 time daily of antibiotic, gentamicin (gentamicin sulfate), in chronic intoxication in 20 animals, cats, male and female.
    (CT) Same method using saline in cats, control group.
Ataxia and equilibrium disorder due to parenteral, subcutaneous, administration of 60 and 120 mg per kg 1 time daily of antibiotic, gentamicin (IB)
(gentamicin hydrochloride), in chronic intoxication in 20 animals, cats, male
and female, with administration of complex of calcium chloride.
    (AD) No decr in ototoxicity due to calcium chloride in cats. (ENG)

642

Possible transient or permanent damage to eighth cranial nerve, primarily
vestibular problems, due to parenteral, intramuscular, administration of high
doses of antibiotic, gentamicin (gentamicin sulfate), for long period in
humans, in particular with kidney disorders.
    (AD) Need to monitor vestibular function and cochlear function with doses
    over 3 mg per kg daily or with administration of gentamicin for more than
    10 days.
    (AD) Recommended that serum concentrations of gentamicin not be higher
    than 10 mcg per ml.
    (AD) Dizziness possibly early symptom of ototoxicity. (ENG)

651

No vestibular problems due to 4 to 6 mg per kg daily of antibiotic, gentamicin, in 100 humans, infant, 3 to 12 months age, with various severe infections.
    (AD) Vestibular function tests used to determine vestibulotoxic effects.
    (ENG)

678

Primarily transient but also permanent severe vestibular problems due to
doses to produce serum levels over 12 mcg per ml of antibiotic, gentamicin,
in humans.
    (AD) Study of in vitro activity of gentamicin only or gentamicin combined
    with other antibiotics. (ENG)

360

Transient dizziness due to 0.9 or 0.6 g daily of anti-inflammatory agent,
ibuprofen, for 7 or 14 days in 1 of 39 humans, adult, range of ages, male and
female, with arthritis.

(AD) Comparative study of ibuprofen and placebo in treatment of arthritis.
(ENG)

396

No hearing loss but decr in vestibular function due to parenteral, intramuscular, administration of 25 mg of antidepressant, imipramine hydrochloride,
in 20 humans.   (IT)

659

Possible dizziness due to anti-inflammatory agent, indomethacin, in humans.
(ENG)

668

Possible vertigo due to anti-inflammatory agent, indomethacin, in humans,
adult.
    (AD) High incidence of vertigo due to indomethacin reported in studies.
    (AD) Incidence and degree of effect usually dose related. (ENG)

707

Dizziness due to 75 mg daily of anti-inflammatory agent, indomethacin, in 1
of 24 humans with bone and joint disorder. (CZ)

078

Transient acute vertigo and nystagmus due to sufficient doses to produce 122
mcg per 100 ml blood level and 115 mcg per 24 hours urine level of heavy
metal, lead, in 1 human, adult, 55 years age, male.
Transient acute vertigo and nystagmus due to oral ingestion of total of about
0.606 to 1.15 mg daily of heavy metal, lead, in 1 human, adult, 41 years age,
male. (ENG)

691

Vertigo due to oral administration in tablets of 300 to 2400 mg daily of
heavy metal, lithium (lithium carbonate), for 1 to 30 months in some of 91
humans, adult and aged, 20 to 73 years age, male and female, with psychologi-
cal disorders. (ENG)

269

Vertigo due to heavy metal, mercury, in humans.
    (AD) Report on vestibulotoxic effects of heavy metals in industry.
    (AD) Vestibular problems confirmed by vestibular function tests. (JAP)

445

No specified ototoxic effects due to topical administration in (SQ) ointment
of sufficient dose, in 10 percent ammoniated ointment, to produce urine level
of 80 mcg per 100 mg of heavy metal, mercury, in 1 human, infant, 11 months
age, male, with skin rash.
Dizziness due to topical route, (SQ) inhalation, of about 0.17 mg per m, for
about 8 hours every night, of vapor concentration, sufficient to produce
urine level of 100 mcg per liter, of heavy metal, mercury, for long period in
1 human, child, 11 years age, male. (ENG)

696

Dizziness due to heavy metal, mercury (inorganic mercury), in 1 month to 38
years exposure in 1 of 154 humans, adolescent and adult, 18 to 62 years age,
during work in industry.
    (AD) Report on 10 years study of exposure to mercury (inorganic mercury).
    (ENG)

623

Vertigo due to oral administration of antibiotic, nalidixic acid, in humans.
(ENG)

281

Vestibular neuritis due to ototoxic agents in humans. (SER)

682

Possible dizziness and ataxia due to high blood levels of over 5 mcg per ml
of antibiotic, polymyxin B, in humans, adult.

(AD) Discussion of clinical pharmacology, dosage, toxic effects, and use
in therapy of polymyxins. (ENG)

636

Inhibition of potentials of endorgan of ampulla of posterior semicircular
canal due to 2.5, 10, or 20 mcg per ml, in Tyrode solution, of antimalarial,
quinine (quinine hydrochloride), in animals, frogs.
    (CT) Study of effect on potentials of Tyrode solution without quinine.
    (AD) Electrophysiological study of effect of quinine on potentials of
    endorgan of ampulla of posterior semicircular canal.
    (AD) Some recovery of potentials after cessation of quinine administra-
    tion.
    (AD) Suggested that toxic effects on endorgan of semicircular canal result
    from administration of quinine. (ENG)

571

No significant effect on vestibular apparatus due to oral administration of
50 or 150 mg per kg daily, total of 1.55 and 4.65 g per kg, of antibiotic,
rifampicin, for 5 weeks in 2 groups of 7 animals, rabbits, male.
    (CT) Same method using 1 percent carboxymethyl-cellulose in rabbits,
    control group.
    (AD) Measurement of horizontal nystagmus 2, 3, 4, and 5 weeks after begin-
    ning of treatment.
No accumulation in perilymph due to oral administration of 100 mg per kg of
antibiotic, rifampicin, for 1 dose in animals, guinea pigs.
    (AD) Determination of rifampicin concentration in perilymph and blood
    after 2, 6, and 24 hours.
    (AD) Study of vestibulotoxic effects and retention in inner ear of rifam-
    picin. (ENG)

647

No damage to eighth cranial nerve observed but possible dizziness due to
parenteral administration of antibiotic, spectinomycin, in humans with gonorrhea.
    (AD) New antibiotic for treatment of gonorrhea.
    (AD) Spectinomycin chemically related to ototoxic drugs as streptomycin
    and kanamycin. (ENG)

024

Suppression of semicircular canal function due to parenteral administration
of range of 22.5 to 54 g, total doses, of antibiotic, streptomycin (streptomycin sulfate), for range of 7.5 to 26 days in 4 humans, adult, male and
female, treated for Meniere's disease.
    (AD) Use of ototoxic effect of streptomycin in treatment of Meniere's
    disease. (ENG)

092

Decr of enzyme activity in vestibular apparatus due to topical administration
to bulla of 0.2 cc of 50 percent solution of antibiotic, streptomycin, in 10
animals, guinea pigs. (GER)

110

Nystagmus and other vestibular problems due to topical administration to
bulla of 0.5 g of antibiotic, streptomycin, in 1 injection in cats.
    (AD) Suggested route of streptomycin in cat from bulla by way of large
    membrane of round window to inner ear.
Changes in chromatin in hair cells, type 1, of maculae due to topical administration to bulla of 0.5 g of antibiotic, streptomycin, in 1 injection in
cats.
    (AD) Suggested that destruction of hair cells due to changes in protein
    metabolism as result of action of streptomycin. (ENG)

211

Severe and slight vertigo due to total of 29 to 57 g of antibiotic, streptomycin, for long period in 14 of 180 humans, adult, 50 years or less age,
male, with pneumoconiosis. (ENG)

216
Damage to hair cells and decr in excitation of vestibular apparatus due to
parenteral, intramuscular, administration of 250 mg per kg of antibiotic,
streptomycin (streptomycin sulfate), for 10 and 30 days in animals, guinea
pigs.
Damage to hair cells and decr in excitation of vestibular apparatus due to
parenteral, intramuscular, administration of 250 mg per kg of antibiotic,
streptomycin (IB) (streptomycin sulfate), for 10 and 30 days in animals,
guinea pigs, with intramuscular administration of 1.25 ml per kg of ozothin.
   (CT) Study of 14 guinea pigs, control group, with 1.25 ml per kg or 2.5 ml
   per kg daily of ozothin.
   (AD) No decr in streptomycin damage to hair cells of vestibular apparatus
   with administration of ozothin.
   (AD) Evaluation of damage with cytovestibulogram and caloric test.
   (AD) Vestibulotoxic effects depend on total dosage of streptomycin used.
   (GER)

253
Severe vestibular problems, as nystagmus, after 3 to 6 hours due to topical
administration to middle ear and parenteral administration of high doses of
antibiotic, streptomycin, for range of 1 to 7 days in 28 animals, cats.
Decr in ribosomes of cytoplasm of type 1 hair cells of vestibular apparatus
due to topical administration to middle ear and parenteral administration of
high doses of antibiotic, streptomycin, for range of 1 to 7 days in 28 animals, cats.
   (CT) Study of cats, control group.
   (AD) Suggested that primary location of action of streptomycin is protein
   synthesis of cells.   (GER)

321
Vestibular problems due to antibiotic, streptomycin, in humans.
   (AD) Use of ENG to determine extent of vestibular problems due to strep-
   tomycin. (RUM)

336
Damage to type 1 hair cells of vestibular apparatus and vestibular problems
due to topical administration to middle ear of antibiotic, streptomycin, in 1
injection in animals.
   (AD) Destruction of hair cells and ototoxicity result of effect of streptomycin on protein synthesis of cells.   (FR)

341
Transient vestibular problems due to 1.0 g daily of antibiotic, streptomycin
(streptomycin sulfate), for short period, 1 or 2 months, in 32 of 84 humans
with tuberculosis.
   (AD) Vestibulotoxic effects determined by ENG.
   (AD) Slight vestibular problem in only 2 humans 1 year after cessation of
   treatment. (POL)

399
Risk of vestibular problems due to antibiotic, streptomycin, in humans,
adult, with tuberculous meningitis.
   (AD) Report on treatment of meningitis and possible toxic effects of drugs
   used. (GER)

449
Vertigo due to antibiotic, streptomycin, in 1 human, adult, female. (JAP)

453
Damage to vestibular function due to antibiotic, streptomycin, in 2 humans,
adult, 20 and 60 years age, male, with tuberculosis.
   (AD) Vestibular problem confirmed by vestibular function tests.
   (AD) Discussion of restoration of vestibular function after damage due to
   streptomycin therapy. (GER)

470
Damage to vestibular apparatus due to antibiotic, streptomycin, in humans.
   (AD) Study of effect of drugs on kidney function and vestibular function.
   (FR)

476
Vestibulotoxic effects due to 100 mg per kg of antibiotic, streptomycin, in animals, pigeons.
Some decr in vestibulotoxic effects due to 100 mg per kg of antibiotic, streptomycin (IB), for 30 days in animals, pigeons, with administration of 25000 units of vitamin A.
    (AD) Structural damage similar in both groups of pigeons.   (POL)

480
Changes in acid phosphatase activity of vestibular apparatus due to antibiotic, streptomycin (streptomycin sulfate), in animals.
    (AD) Study using electron microscopy of acid phosphatase activity of vestibular apparatus.   (JAP)

534
Dizziness within 6 weeks due to parenteral, intramuscular, administration of 0.75 g daily of antibiotic, streptomycin, in 8 (31 percent) of 27 humans, child, adult, and aged, 12 to 76 years age, female and male, 34 to 89 kg weight, with tuberculosis.
    (AD) Use of vestibular function tests in patients reporting dizziness.
    (AD) Study showed significant relationship between higher 24 hour serum levels and dizziness.
    (AD) Suggested decr in dosage when serum streptomycin more than 3 mcg per ml at 24 hours.
    (AD) More risk of vestibulotoxic effects due to streptomycin in patients over 45 years age.   (ENG)

648
Vertigo due to antibiotic, streptomycin, in 3 humans with tuberculosis.
    (AD) Report on testing with ENG of 191 patients with vertigo of various etiologies.   (ENG)

667
Possible vertigo due to antiparasitic, thiabendazole, in humans with parasitic disorder.   (ENG)

728
Dizziness due to topical route, inhalation, of chemical agent, tobacco, in humans without smoking habit.
    (AD) Study of subjective symptoms of effects of tobacco on subjects without smoking habit.   (ENG)

095
Ototoxic effects due to unspecified method of administration of (SQ) 0.75 g daily of antibiotic, streptomycin (SM), for (SQ) 3 months initial treatment in 6 of 140 humans with tuberculosis.
Simultaneous unspecified method of administration of (SQ) 300 mg of antituberculous agent, isoniazid (SM), in 140 humans with tuberculosis.
Ototoxic effects due to unspecified method of administration of (SQ) 1 g 3 days a week of antibiotic, streptomycin (SM), for (SQ) 18 months following initial treatment in 24 of 140 humans with tuberculosis.
Dizziness due to simultaneous unspecified method of administration of (SQ) 600 mg of antituberculous agent, isoniazid (SM), in unspecified number of humans with tuberculosis and with other toxic effects due to isoniazid.
(ENG)

107
Vertigo and nystagmus due to antibiotic, kanamycin, in humans, male and female.
Vertigo and nystagmus due to antibiotic, streptomycin, in humans, male and female.
    (AD) Preclinical detection of vestibular problems by ENG.   (FR)

118
Nystagmus and unsteady gait due to unspecified doses of antibiotics (SM) in 1 human, adult, 47 years age, male, with epilepsy.
Simultaneous administration of anticonvulsant, primidone (SM), in 1 human, adult, 47 years age, male, with epilepsy.

Simultaneous administration of antihistamine, dimenhydrinate (SM), in 1 human, adult, 47 years age, male, with epilepsy. (ENG)

136

Vestibular problems due to oral administration of 150 mg daily of antituberculous agent, thiacetazone (CB), for 12 months in 4 of 150 humans with pulmonary tuberculosis and without previous treatment.
Combined oral administration of 30 mg daily of antituberculous agent, isoniazid (CB), for 12 months in 150 humans with pulmonary tuberculosis and without previous treatment.
No vestibular problems due to 10 g daily in 2 doses of antituberculous agent, PAS (CB) (sodium PAS), for 12 months in 100 humans with pulmonary tuberculosis and without previous treatment.
Combined administration of 200 mg daily in 2 doses of antituberculous agent, isoniazid (CB), for 12 months in 100 humans with pulmonary tuberculosis and without previous treatment.
   (AD) Comparative study of effects of thiacetazone and PAS with isoniazid
   in treatment of tuberculosis. (ENG)

137

Vestibular problems due to 1 g daily of antibiotic, capreomycin (SM), for long period in 2 of 20 humans with tuberculosis.
Simultaneous administration of 25 mg per kg for first 60 days and then 15 mg per kg of antituberculous agent, ethambutol (SM), in 20 humans with tuberculosis.
Simultaneous administration of 300 mg twice daily for several months and then 450 mg in 1 dose of antibiotic, rifampicin (SM), in 20 humans with tuberculosis. (ENG)

172

Vertigo due to sedative, alcohol, ethyl, in humans.
Vertigo due to antibiotic, streptomycin, in humans.
   (AD) Report on etiology of vertigo. (GER)

198

Severe vertigo due to parenteral, intramuscular, administration of 1 g daily in single dose of antibiotic, streptomycin (SM) (streptomycin sulfate), for 6 months in 2 of 41 humans, 108.2 lb average weight, with pulmonary tuberculosis and with previous streptomycin therapy in some.
Simultaneous oral administration of 15 g daily in single dose of antituberculous agent, PAS (SM) (sodium PAS), for 6 months in 2 of 41 humans, 108.2 lb average weight, with pulmonary tuberculosis and with previous streptomycin therapy in some.
No vestibulotoxic effects due to parenteral, intramuscular, administration of 1 g daily in single dose of antibiotic, streptomycin (SM) (streptomycin sulfate), for 6 months in 41 humans, 113.5 lb average weight, with pulmonary tuberculosis and with previous streptomycin therapy in some.
Simultaneous oral administration of 15 g daily in 2 doses of antituberculous agent, PAS (SM) (sodium PAS), for 6 months in 41 humans, 113.5 lb average weight, with pulmonary tuberculosis and with previous streptomycin therapy in some.
   (AD) Study of retreatment of pulmonary tuberculosis in humans with no
   response to previous chemotherapy. (ENG)

276

Decr in vestibular responses due to parenteral, intramuscular, administration of 250 mg per kg of antibiotic, streptomycin (streptomycin sulfate), in 10 or 25 injections in 13 animals, guinea pigs, 250 to 300 g weight.
Decr in vestibular responses for several hours due to parenteral, intraperitoneal, administration of 1.5, 3.0, or 4.5 mg of analeptic, dimorpholamine, in 17 animals, guinea pigs, 250 to 300 g weight. (GER)

285

Transient inhibition of endorgan of ampulla due to range of doses of antibiotic, streptomycin (streptomycin sulfate), in animals, frogs.
Transient inhibition of endorgan of ampulla due to range of doses of antibiotic, dihydrostreptomycin (dihydrostreptomycin sulfate), in animals, frogs.
Transient inhibition of endorgan of ampulla due to range of doses of antibio-

tic, neomycin (neomycin sulfate), in animals, frogs.
Transient inhibition of endorgan of ampulla due to range of doses of antibio-
tic, kanamycin (kanamycin sulfate), in animals, frogs.
   (CT) Study of frogs, control group.
   (AD) More inhibition of endorgan of ampulla with streptomycin than with
   other aminoglycoside antibiotics.
   (AD) Agreement between in vivo and in vitro observations of intensity of
   action on endorgans of vestibular apparatus. (ENG)

                                                                        310
Transient decr in vestibular function due to parenteral, intravenous, administration of 2 ml of tranquilizer, droperidol (CB), for 2 minutes in 18 of 21
humans, adolescent and adult, female and male.
Transient decr in vestibular function due to parenteral, intravenous, administration of 2 ml of analgesic, fentanyl (CB) (fentanyl citrate), for 2
minutes in 18 of 21 humans, adolescent and adult, female and male.
   (CT) Caloric tests, pretreatment and posttreatment. (DAN)

                                                                        340
Vestibular problems due to 150 mg daily of antituberculous agent, thiaceta-
zone (SM), in 15 of 75 humans with pulmonary tuberculosis.
Vestibular problems due to 0.75 to 1 g daily of antibiotic, streptomycin (SM)
(streptomycin sulfate), in 15 of 75 humans with pulmonary tuberculosis.
Vestibular problems due to 300 mg daily of antituberculous agent, isoniazid
(SM), in 15 of 75 humans with pulmonary tuberculosis.
   (AD) Vestibulotoxic effects confirmed by vestibular function tests.
   (AD) Statistical analysis showed higher occurrence of vestibular problems
   in humans with thiacetazone in drug regimen than without thiacetazone.
   (SL)

                                                                        346
Temporary inhibition of oxygen consumption at level of mitochondria of cen-
tral vestibular nuclei due to antibiotic, streptomycin, in animals.
Temporary inhibition of oxygen consumption at level of mitochondria of cen-
tral vestibular nuclei due to antibiotic, rifampicin, in animals.
   (AD) Discussion of chronic and acute vestibular toxicity. (ENG)

                                                                        354
Vestibular problems due to 1 g daily, total doses of 1 to 115 g before onset
of ototoxicity, of antibiotic, streptomycin (SM), for several days to 9
months in 56 of 364 humans, adolescent and adult, 16 to 64 years age, female,
with tuberculosis of genitourinary system.
No specified ototoxic effects due to range of doses of antituberculous agent,
PAS (SM), for several days to 9 months in 13 of 369 humans, adolescent and
adult, 16 to 64 years age, female, with tuberculosis of genitourinary system.
Simultaneous administration of antituberculous agent, isoniazid (SM), in 274
humans, adolescent and adult, 16 to 64 years age, female, with tuberculosis
of genitourinary system. (ENG)

                                                                        377
Lesion of vestibular apparatus due to about 22 g of antibiotic, streptomycin
(SM), in human with pulmonary tuberculosis.
   (AD) Lesion of vestibular apparatus confirmed by vestibular function test.
Simultaneous administration of 185 g of antituberculous agent, PAS (SM), in
human with pulmonary tuberculosis.
Simultaneous administration of 16.5 g of antituberculous agent, isoniazid
(SM), in human with pulmonary tuberculosis. (POL)

                                                                        433
Dizziness due to 1 g daily of antibiotic, streptomycin (SM), for 6 months in
32 percent of 114 humans with pulmonary tuberculosis.
Dizziness due to 300 mg daily of antituberculous agent, isoniazid (SM), for 6
months with streptomycin and then 6 months alone in 32 percent of 114 humans
with pulmonary tuberculosis.
   (AD) Regimen of simultaneous administration of streptomycin and isoniazid
   for 6 months followed by administration of isoniazid only for 6 months.
Dizziness due to 1 g daily of antibiotic, streptomycin (SM), for 6 months in
54 percent of 94 humans with pulmonary tuberculosis.

Dizziness due to 150 mg daily of antituberculous agent, thiacetazone (SM), for 6 months with streptomycin and isoniazid and then 6 months with isoniazid in 54 percent of 94 humans with pulmonary tuberculosis.
Dizziness due to 300 mg daily of antituberculous agent, isoniazid (SM), for 6 months with streptomycin and thiacetazone and then 6 months with thiacetazone in 54 percent of 94 humans with pulmonary tuberculosis.
   (AD) Regimen of simultaneous administration of streptomycin, thiacetazone, and isoniazid for 6 months followed by administration of thiacetazone and isoniazid for 6 months.
Dizziness due to 150 mg daily of antituberculous agent, thiacetazone (SM), for 1 year in 13 percent of 78 humans with pulmonary tuberculosis.
Dizziness due to 300 mg daily of antituberculous agent, isoniazid (SM), for 1 year in 13 percent of 78 humans with pulmonary tuberculosis.
   (AD) Regimen of simultaneous administration of thiacetazone and isoniazid for 1 year.
   (AD) Study of role of drug regimens with thiacetazone in treatment of pulmonary tuberculosis. (ENG)

473
Possible vestibular problems due to antibiotic, viomycin, in humans with infections.
Possible vestibular problems due to antibiotic, capreomycin, in humans with infections.
   (AD) Experiments to find new derivatives of viomycin and capreomycin with biological activity but with less toxic effects. (ENG)

481
Damage to vestibular apparatus due to 1 g daily or twice daily of antibiotic, streptomycin (SM), for maximum of 3 months in 9 of 108 humans, range of 2 to 86 years age, male and female, with pulmonary tuberculosis.
Simultaneous administration of 12 g daily of antituberculous agent, PAS (SM), for 12 to 18 months in 108 humans, range of 2 to 86 years age, male and female, with pulmonary tuberculosis.
Simultaneous administration of 300 mg daily of antituberculous agent, isoniazid (SM), for 12 to 18 months in 108 humans, range of 2 to 86 years age, male and female, with pulmonary tuberculosis. (ENG)

519
Dizziness but no other ototoxic effects due to parenteral, intramuscular, administration of 1 g daily in single dose of antibiotic, capreomycin (SM), for long period in 1 of 33 humans, adult and aged, 21 to over 70 years age, with pulmonary tuberculosis of long duration and with previous treatment with other drugs.
Simultaneous oral administration of 25 mg per kg during first 60 days and then 15 mg per kg of antituberculous agent, ethambutol (SM), in 1 of 33 humans, adult and aged, 21 to over 70 years age, with pulmonary tuberculosis of long duration and with previous treatment with other drugs.
Simultaneous administration of 600 mg of antibiotic, rifampicin (SM), in 1 of 33 humans, adult and aged, 21 to over 70 years age, with pulmonary tuberculosis of long duration and with previous treatment with other drugs.
   (AD) Otoneurology tests every 4 to 8 weeks. (ENG)

535
Dizziness due to parenteral administration of 0.75 g on 6 days a week for 3 months and then 1 g on 2 days a week with intervals of 2 to 3 days for 15 months of antibiotic, streptomycin (SM), for total of 18 months in 2 of 80 humans, adult, range of ages, female and male, 16 to 92 kg weight, with pulmonary tuberculosis.
Dizziness due to 300 mg on 6 days a week for 3 months and then 600 mg on 2 days a week with intervals of 2 to 3 days for 15 months of antituberculous agent, isoniazid (SM), for total of 18 months in 1 of 80 humans, adult, range of ages, female and male, 16 to 92 kg weight, with pulmonary tuberculosis.
Simultaneous administration of 12 g on 6 days a week of antituberculous agent, PAS (SM), for 3 months in 80 humans, adult, range of ages, female and male, 16 to 92 kg weight, with pulmonary tuberculosis. (ENG)

536
Damage to eighth cranial nerve and vertigo due to 1 g or 0.75 g daily of

antibiotic, streptomycin (SM), for about 3 months usually in less than 55 of
181 humans, adult and aged, primarily 50 years or over age, male and female,
with pulmonary tuberculosis.
Simultaneous administration of 300 mg daily of antituberculous agent, isoniazid (SM), for 18 months to 2 years usually in 181 humans, adult and aged,
primarily 50 years or over age, male and female, with pulmonary tuberculosis.
Simultaneous administration of 12 g daily of antituberculous agent, PAS (SM),
for 18 months to 2 years usually in 181 humans, adult and aged, primarily 50
years or over age, male and female, with pulmonary tuberculosis. (ENG)

537

Dizziness due to oral administration in tablet of 150 mg daily of antituberculous agent, thiacetazone (CB) (SM), in 1 of 147 humans, African, adolescent
and adult, 15 years or more age, with pulmonary tuberculosis and without
previous treatment.
Dizziness due to oral administration in tablet of 300 mg daily of antituberculous agent, isoniazid (CB) (SM), in 1 of 147 humans, African, adolescent
and adult, 15 years or more age, with pulmonary tuberculosis and without
previous treatment.
   (AD) Dizziness in 1 patient due to combined treatment with thiacetazone
   and isoniazid only.
Dizziness due to parenteral, intramuscular, administration of 1 g daily of
antibiotic, streptomycin (SM) (streptomycin sulfate), for first 2 weeks in 1
of 161 humans, African, adolescent and adult, 15 years or more age, with
pulmonary tuberculosis and without previous treatment.
   (AD) Dizziness in 1 patient due to simultaneous treatment with thiacetazone and isoniazid in 1 tablet and intramuscular streptomycin for 2 weeks.
Dizziness due to parenteral, intramuscular, administration of 1 g daily of
antibiotic, streptomycin (SM) (streptomycin sulfate), for first 8 weeks in 10
of 162 humans, African, adolescent and adult, 15 years or more age, with
pulmonary tuberculosis and without previous treatment.
   (AD) Dizziness in 10 patients due to simultaneous treatment with thiacetazone and isoniazid in 1 tablet and intramuscular streptomycin for 8 weeks.
   (AD) Study showed vestibulotoxic effects in total of 12 of 818 patients
   treated for pulmonary tuberculosis. (ENG)

538

Dizziness due to parenteral administration of 1 g daily for first 8 weeks and
then 1 g twice weekly for 12 weeks of antibiotic, streptomycin (SM), for
total of 20 weeks in 5 of 77 humans with pulmonary tuberculosis.
Simultaneous administration of 300 mg daily in single dose of antituberculous
agent, isoniazid (SM), in 77 humans with pulmonary tuberculosis.
Simultaneous administration of 15 mg per kg daily of antituberculous agent,
ethambutol (SM), in 77 humans with pulmonary tuberculosis.
No reported ototoxic effects due to 600 mg daily in single dose of antibiotic, rifampicin, in 157 humans with pulmonary tuberculosis. (ENG)

593

Vestibular problems due to 1 g in 24 hours of antibiotic, (SQ) streptomycin
(SM), in 1 human, adult, 32 years age, female, with tuberculosis.
Vestibular problems due to 450 mg of antituberculous agent, (SQ) isoniazid
(SM), in 1 human, adult, 32 years age, female, with tuberculosis.
Vestibular problems due to oral administration in tablets of 0.10 g of anti-
convulsant, (SQ) diphenylhydantoin, in 1 human, adult, 32 years age, female,
with tuberculosis.
Vestibular problems due to oral administration in tablets of 3 tablets of
0.10 g each daily of anticonvulsant, (SQ) diphenylhydantoin (SM), in 1 human,
adult, 49 years age, female, with tuberculosis.
Vestibular problems due to 300 mg of antituberculous agent, (SQ) isoniazid
(SM), in 1 human, adult, 49 years age, female, with tuberculosis.
Simultaneous administration of 500 cm of antituberculous agent, (SQ) PAS
(SM), in 1 human, adult, 49 years age, female, with tuberculosis.
   (AD) Report of vestibulotoxic effects in 2 patients due to diphenylhydan-
   toin with isoniazid or streptomycin. (FR)

614

Vertigo due to parenteral administration of 0.5 g twice daily of antibiotic,
streptomycin (SM), for 7 days in 3 of 59 humans, aged, 70 years or over age,

with chronic bronchitis.
Simultaneous administration of 3,000,000 units twice daily of antibiotic, penicillin (SM), for 14 days in 3 of 59 humans, aged, 70 years or over age, with chronic bronchitis.   (ENG)

681

Degrees of inhibition of potential of endorgan of ampulla of posterior semi-circular canal due to 50, 200, 300, and 500 mcg per cc, in Tyrode solution, of antibiotic, streptomycin (streptomycin sulfate), in animals, frogs.
Degrees of inhibition of potential of endorgan of ampulla of posterior semi-circular canal due to 100, 200, and 500 mcg per cc, in Tyrode solution, of antibiotic, dihydrostreptomycin, in animals, frogs.
   (AD) Recovery of potential after cessation of administration of antibio-
   tics. (IT)

685

Total loss of vestibular function but no hearing loss due to total of 840 mg of antibiotic, gentamicin (SM), in 47 day period in 1 of 181 humans, aged, 70 years age, female, with kidney disorder.
Total loss of vestibular function but no hearing loss due to 2 g of antibio-tic, streptomycin (SM), in 47 day period in 1 of 181 humans, aged, 70 years age, female, with kidney disorder.
Permanent vestibular problems due to 2.56 g of antibiotic, (SQ) gentamicin, for 18 days in 1 of 181 humans, adult, 39 years age, female, with kidney disorder.
Vestibular problems due to previous administration of antibiotic, (SQ) strep-tomycin, in 1 of 181 humans, adult, 39 years age, female, with kidney disor-der.
Permanent vestibular problems, with dizziness, due to antibiotic, gentamicin, in 1 of 181 humans, adult, 38 years age, female, with kidney disorder.
Transient dizziness after 3 days due to antibiotic, gentamicin, in 1 of 181 humans, adolescent, 16 years age, female, with kidney disorder.
   (AD) Serial vestibular function tests and audiometry not conducted in 181
   patients.
Vestibular problems due to parenteral, intramuscular, administration of 1 g daily of antibiotic, (SQ) streptomycin (SM), in 1 human, adult, 19 years age, male, with pseudomonas infection.
   (AD) Vestibular problems due to previous streptomycin therapy.
Simultaneous administration of 300 mg daily of antibiotic, (SQ) colistin (SM) (colistimethate), for 15 days in 1 human, adult, 19 years age, male, with pseudomonas infection.
Sequential parenteral, intramuscular, administration of 40 mg 3 times a day of antibiotic, (SQ) gentamicin, for 36 days in 1 human, adult, 19 years age, male, with pseudomonas infection.
Dizziness after 4 days due to parenteral, intramuscular, administration of 40 mg 4 times a day, total of 2.56 g, of antibiotic, gentamicin, for 16 days in 1 human, adult, 30 years age, female, with kidney disorder.
   (AD) Discussion of 6 case reports of vestibulotoxic effects of gentamicin.
   (ENG)

703

No nystagmus due to parenteral, intramuscular, administration of 0.150 mg of analgesic, fentanyl, in 5 animals, rabbits, 2.5 to 3 kg weight.
Positional nystagmus within 15 to 30 minutes due to parenteral administration of 4 ml per kg of 96 percent solution of sedative, alcohol, in 8 animals, rabbits, 2.5 to 3 kg weight.
Positional nystagmus within 15 to 30 minutes due to parenteral administration of 4 ml per kg of 96 percent solution of sedative, (SQ) alcohol, in 11 ani-mals, rabbits, 2.5 to 3 kg weight.
Partial or total suppression of positional nystagmus due to parenteral, intramuscular, administration of 0.150 mg of analgesic, (SQ) fentanyl, in 6 of 11 animals, rabbits, 2.5 to 3 kg weight.
Decr in positional nystagmus due to parenteral, intramuscular, administration of 0.08 to 0.10 mg of analgesic, (SQ) fentanyl, in 5 of 11 animals, rabbits, 2.5 to 3 kg weight. (IT)

708

Vertigo due to oral administration in capsules of 75 mg in 2 capsules 3 times

daily of anti-inflammatory agent, indomethacin, in 2 of 18 humans during treatment for arthritis.
Vertigo due to oral administration in capsules of 75 mg in 2 capsules 3 times daily of anti-inflammatory agent, indomethacin, for 4 weeks in 1 of 7 humans after treatment for arthritis.
Vertigo due to oral administration in capsules of 1500 mg daily in 2 capsules 3 times daily of anti-inflammatory agent, mefenamic acid, for 4 weeks in 1 of 39 humans after treatment for arthritis. (ENG)

Cochleo-vestibular function

594
Transient severe vertigo due to oral administration in tablets of 50 mg per kg of 500 mg tablets of antiparasitic, A-16612, for 2 days in 1 human, adult, with schistosomiasis.
Auditory hallucination due to 100 mg per kg daily of antiparasitic, A-16612, for 3 days in 1 human, adult, with schistosomiasis.
  (AD) Study of chemotherapy of schistosomiasis with new antiparasitic agent, A-16612. (ENG)

007
Permanent unilateral sensorineural hearing loss and transient vertigo and tinnitus due to oral administration of range of 0.6 to 0.9 g of salicylate, aspirin, for every 2 hours for 3 days in 1 human, adult, 19 years age, female, with pain after tooth extraction.
  (AD) Literature review showed 2 other case reports of hearing loss due to aspirin. (ENG)

105
Transient bilateral incr in pure tone threshold but without tone decay and without difference limen and decr in duration of nystagmus and in slow phase velocity of nystagmus due to oral administration of incr doses to about 6 to 8 g per day, until subjective hearing loss observed, of salicylate, aspirin (CB), in 12 humans, adult and aged, range of 23 to 68 years age, with rheumatoid arthritis.
Combined administration of magnesium aluminum hydroxide (CB) in 12 humans, adult and aged, range of 23 to 68 years age, with rheumatoid arthritis.
  (CT) Withdrawal of salicylates before treatment for standardization of salicylate level.
  (CT) Audiometry and vestibular function tests before, during, and after treatment with salicylate.
  (AD) Serum salicylate level determined when subjective hearing loss reported.
Transient sensorineural hearing loss but no damage to hair cells of organ of Corti or to membranous labyrinth due to oral administration of high doses, as high as 7 to 10 g per day, of salicylates for long period in 1 human, Caucasian, adult, 62 years age, female, with previous progressive hearing loss.
Transient sensorineural hearing loss but no damage to organ of Corti, spiral ganglion, or membranous labyrinth due to oral administration of high doses, as high as 5 g per day, of salicylate, aspirin, for 15 years in 1 human, adult, 61 years age, female, with rheumatoid arthritis. (ENG)

128
Transient tinnitus due to oral administration of 2 tablets every 4 hours or more frequently, to produce serum salicylate level of 92 mg per 100 ml, of salicylate, aspirin, for about 6 days in 1 human, Caucasian, adolescent, 14 years age, female, self treatment for upper respiratory system infection.
Tinnitus and dizziness due to oral administration of about 5 bottles of 100 tablets each, to produce serum salicylate levels of 72 mg per 100 ml after 3 to 4 hours, 59 mg per 100 ml after 6 to 7 hours, 150 mg per 100 ml after 14 to 15 hours, of salicylate, aspirin, in 1 dose in 1 human, Caucasian, adult, 19 years age, female, suicide.
Loss of equilibrium due to oral administration of 62.5 mg per teaspoon of colic medicine of salicylate in 1 human, Caucasian, infant, 3 months age, male, with colic.
  (AD) Low serum salicylate level in infant.
  (AD) Discussion of 3 case reports of salicylate ototoxicity. (ENG)

411

Total bilateral hearing loss and within 48 hours, unilateral hearing loss, due to oral ingestion of 46 tablets of salicylate, aspirin, in 1 dose in 1 human, in suicide attempt.
Vestibular problems due to oral ingestion of 46 tablets of salicylate, aspirin, in 1 dose in 1 human, in suicide attempt.
   (AD) Case report of cochleo-vestibulotoxic effects of high dose of aspirin in suicide attempt.   (FR)

649

Transient tinnitus, hearing loss, or dizziness due to oral administration in tablets of 1.4 g, in 4 tablets, in 3 initial doses at 7 hour intervals and then daily, to produce high serum levels of 20.5 to 28.0 mg per 100 ml, of salicylate, aspirin, for 2 to 3 weeks in 9 of 20 humans, adolescent, adult, and aged, 15 to 70 years age, female and male, with bone and joint disorders.
   (AD) Report on use of new sustained release aspirin in treatment of bone and joint disorders.   (ENG)

247

No ototoxic effects due to parenteral, subcutaneous, administration of low doses used in therapy, 20 mg per kg daily in 2 doses every 12 hours, of antibiotic, aminosidine (aminosidine sulfate), for 60 days in 20 animals, guinea pigs, adult, 300 g average weight.
   (CT) Study of 5 guinea pigs, control group.
   (CT) Test for Preyer reflex and vestibular function tests, pretreatment and during treatment.
   (AD) Previous studies showed ototoxic effects of high doses of aminosidine in animals.
   (AD) Suggested clinical use of aminosidine in low doses for short periods.
   (IT)

251

Damage to organ of Corti and crista ampullaris due to parenteral, subcutaneous, administration of 200 or 400 mg per kg daily in 3 doses every 8 hours of antibiotic, aminosidine (aminosidine sulfate), for 30 days in 2 groups of 16 animals, guinea pigs, 300 g weight.
Less damage to organ of Corti and crista ampullaris due to parenteral, subcutaneous, administration of 50 or 100 mg per kg daily in 3 doses every 8 hours of antibiotic, aminosidine (aminosidine sulfate), for 30 days in 2 groups of 16 animals, guinea pigs, 300 g weight.
   (CT) Study of 8 guinea pigs, control group.
   (CT) Observation of function of cochlea and vestibular apparatus, pretreatment and during treatment.   (IT)

252

No cochlear impairment or vestibular problems due to parenteral, intramuscular, administration of average daily dose of 16 mg per kg in 2 doses every 12 hours of antibiotic, aminosidine (aminosidine sulfate), for range of 10 to 30 days in 118 humans, adult, male and female, with disorders.
   (CT) Audiometry and vestibular function tests, pretreatment and posttreatment, immediately after cessation of treatment and 1 month later.   (IT)

083

Cochleo-vestibulotoxic effects due to parenteral, oral, and topical administration of antibiotics in humans, with normal kidney function and with kidney disorder.
   (AD) Literature review of ototoxic effects of antibiotics.
   (AD) Recommended dosage and duration of dosage of antibiotics discussed.
   (ENG)

123

Sensorineural hearing loss and vestibular problems due to range of doses of antibiotics in humans.
   (AD) Report on cochleo-vestibulotoxic effects of antibiotics used clinically.   (ENG)

135

Vertigo and sensorineural hearing loss due to antibiotics, aminoglycoside, in

humans.
   (AD) Possible permanent damage due to low doses of streptomycin, dihydros-
   treptomycin, or kanamycin.
   (AD) Report on etiology of vertigo. (ENG)

                                                                      201
Vertigo and sensorineural hearing loss due to antibiotics, aminoglycoside, in
humans.
   (AD) Report on risks in clinical use of different antibiotics.
   (AD) Need for audiometry and vestibular function tests in antibiotic
   therapy over long period.
   (AD) Cochleo-vestibulotoxic effects due to daily and total dosage of
   antibiotics. (FR)

                                                                      202
Risk of cochleo-vestibulotoxic effects due to antibiotics, aminoglycoside, in
humans, child, treated for tuberculosis and in particular with kidney disor-
ders.
   (AD) Good prognosis for vestibular problems in children.
   (AD) Need for early detection of hearing loss in children.
   (AD) Comment on maximum doses of antibiotics. (FR)

                                                                      210
Risk of cochleo-vestibulotoxic effects due to oral or parenteral administration of antibiotics, aminoglycoside, in humans with normal kidney function
and with kidney disorder.
Risk of cochleo-vestibulotoxic effects due to topical administration of low
doses of antibiotics, aminoglycoside, in humans.
   (AD) Literature review of auditory system problems due to aminoglycoside
   antibiotics.
   (AD) Need to determine dosage of antibiotics on basis of body weight,
   kidney function, and age.
   (AD) Need for audiometry, vestibular function tests, determination of
   blood levels, and tests of kidney function during treatment with antibiotics. (SW)

                                                                      221
Cochleo-vestibulotoxic effects due to antibiotics, aminoglycoside, in humans
with tuberculosis of genitourinary system.
   (AD) Need for multiple antibiotic therapy in tuberculosis but risk of
   ototoxic effects. (IT)

                                                                      222
Cochleo-vestibulotoxic effects due to antibiotics in humans treated for
tuberculosis.
   (AD) Report on ototoxic effects of antibiotics used in tuberculosis chemotherapy and control of ototoxic effects. (GER)

                                                                      264
Cochleo-vestibulotoxic effects due to antibiotics in humans.
   (AD) Comment on complications due to antibiotics after head and neck
   surgery. (ENG)

                                                                      294
Hearing loss and vestibular problems due to antibiotics in humans, adult,
male and female, with chronic kidney disorder. (RUS)

                                                                      458
Damage to cochlear function and vestibular function and structural damage to
cochlea and vestibular apparatus due to antibiotics in animals, guinea pigs.
   (AD) Use of Preyer reflex, vestibular function tests, and measurement of
   cochlear microphonics to determine ototoxic effects of antibiotics on
   function of inner ear.
   (AD) Histological study to determine structural damage to inner ear.
   (ENG)

                                                                      462
Damage to hair cells of organ of Corti, stria vascularis, nerve process,

spiral ganglion, limbus, and cochlear wall due to antibiotics in animals, guinea pigs.
   (AD) Ototoxic effects result of retention of antibiotics in inner ear longer than in blood due to slower elimination.
   (AD) More active cells of cochlea more sensitive to ototoxic antibiotics.
   (AD) Neomycin most ototoxic, followed by kanamycin, viomycin, streptomycin, and capreomycin.
   (AD) Study of effect of inhibitors, nialamide, pantothenic acid, methylated compounds, and vitamin B on ototoxicity of antibiotics.
   (AD) Electrophysiological and histological study of cochleo-vestibulotoxic effects of antibiotics in guinea pig. (ENG)

523
Cochleo-vestibulotoxic effects due to topical, parenteral, or oral administration of antibiotics, aminoglycoside, in humans. (NOR)

549
Cochleo-vestibulotoxic effects due to antibiotics in humans with disorders. (RUS)

297
Possible vestibular problems and hearing loss due to recommended 1 g daily of antibiotic, capreomycin, in humans with tuberculosis.
   (AD) Ototoxicity due to capreomycin similar to ototoxicity due to streptomycin. (ENG)

329
Hearing loss or dizziness due to parenteral, intramuscular, administration of 1 g daily, total doses of 20 to 445 g, of antibiotic, (SQ) capreomycin (SM), for range of 20 days to over 18 months in 5 of 43 humans, adult and aged, 24 to 83 years age, male and female, with pulmonary tuberculosis and with previous treatment with antituberculous agents.
   (CT) Audiometry, pretreatment and during treatment.
Simultaneous administration of 500 to 1000 mg daily in single or divided doses of antituberculous agent, (SQ) ethionamide (SM), for range of 20 days to over 18 months in 43 humans, adult and aged, 24 to 83 years age, male and female, with pulmonary tuberculosis and with previous treatment with antituberculous agents.
Previous administration of other (SQ) antituberculous agents in 43 humans, adult and aged, 24 to 83 years age, male and female, with pulmonary tuberculosis. (ENG)

555
Cochlear impairment due to parenteral, intramuscular, administration of 100 mg per kg 3 times per week or 25 or 50 mg per kg daily of antibiotic, capreomycin, for 2 years in several animals, dogs.
Vestibular problems due to parenteral, subcutaneous, administration of 125 mg per kg daily of antibiotic, capreomycin, for 84 days in several animals, cats.
   (AD) Discussion of chemistry of capreomycin, results of in vitro and in vivo studies, and toxicity of capreomycin in animals. (ENG)

541
Vertigo due to anticonvulsant, carbamazepine, in 58(11.4 percent) of humans treated for paroxysmal trigeminal neuralgia.
Tinnitus due to anticonvulsant, carbamazepine, in 1(0.2 percent)of humans treated for paroxysmal trigeminal neuralgia.
   (AD) Need to monitor use of carbamazepine in therapy. (ENG)

718
Dizziness, nystagmus, and high frequency hearing loss due to chemical agent, carbon disulfide, in chronic intoxication in humans working in industry.
   (AD) Audiograms showed decr in higher frequencies.
   (AD) Literature review of effects of carbon disulfide. (GER)

673
Dizziness and decr in cochlear function due to topical route, inhalation, of large amounts to produce 20 to 30 percent carboxyhemoglobin of chemical

agent, carbon monoxide, in humans. (ENG)

365
Possible vertigo and tinnitus due to high doses, 300 mg daily, of antimalarial, chloroquine (chloroquine sulfate), in humans with tuberculoid lepro-
sy. (FR)

299
Transient bilateral sensorineural hearing loss and dizziness due to 25 mg
every other day, total of 18 g, of heavy metal, cobalt (cobalt chlorine), in
6 months in 1 human, adult, 35 years age, female, with kidney disorder and
anemia.
    (AD) Cochleo-vestibulotoxic effects confirmed by audiometry and caloric
    tests. (ENG)

378
Total unilateral sensorineural hearing loss, tinnitus, and vertigo 7 days
after injection due to parenteral, (SQ) intramuscular, administration of 150
mg of (SQ) contraceptive, methoxy progesterone acetate, in 1 injection in 1
human, adult, 26 years age, female.
    (AD) Cochleo-vestibulotoxic effects confirmed by audiometry and vestibular
    function tests 1 month later.
    (AD) Suggested that ototoxic effects result of obstruction of cochlear
    artery due to contraceptive.
Dizziness due to previous (SQ) oral administration of other (SQ) contraceptives in 1 human, adult, 26 years age, female. (ENG)

379
Sudden deafness, tinnitus, severe vertigo, and objective decr in vestibular
function due to oral administration of 2 mg daily of contraceptive, norethin-
drone (CB), for 3 months in 1 human, adult, 34 years age, female.
Sudden deafness, tinnitus, severe vertigo, and objective decr in vestibular
function due to oral administration of 2 mg daily of contraceptive, mestranol
(CB), for 3 months in 1 human, adult, 34 years age, female.
    (AD) Cochleo-vestibulotoxic effects confirmed by audiometry and vestibular
    function tests.
    (AD) Partial improvement in hearing 20 days later.
Severe bilateral sudden deafness, tinnitus, and dizziness due to oral administration of contraceptive, norethindrone (CB), for 2 years in 1 human, adult,
20 years age, female.
Severe bilateral sudden deafness, tinnitus, and dizziness due to oral administration of contraceptive, mestranol (CB), for 2 years in 1 human, adult, 20
years age, female.
    (AD) Audiometry and vestibular function tests 7 days after onset of ototo-
    xic effects.
    (AD) Partial improvement in 1 ear and total recovery in other ear 30 days
    later.
    (AD) Suggested that ototoxic effects resulted from blood coagulation due
    to contraceptive. (ENG)

402
Pressure in the ears due to contraceptives in 1 human, adult, 33 years age,
female.
    (AD) Pressure possibly due to obstruction of Eustachian tube.
Possible vertigo, sudden deafness, and distortion of sound due to contraceptives in humans. (ENG)

533
Sensorineural hearing loss, tinnitus, dizziness, and disorder of equilibrium
due to cardiovascular agent, digitalis, in 1 human treated for heart disorder. (POL)

383
Nystagmus and cochlear impairment due to high doses of anticonvulsant, diphenylhydantoin, in humans, infant and child.
    (AD) Literature review of toxic risks of antibiotics and other drugs.
    (GER)

035
Transient and permanent hearing loss and vertigo due to oral and parenteral, intravenous, administration of diuretic, ethacrynic acid, in 12 humans with kidney disorders.
(AD) Hearing loss not related to administration route or dosage. (ENG)

304
Possible hearing loss and vertigo due to diuretic, ethacrynic acid, in humans.
(AD) Discussion of chemistry, pharmacology, clinical use, and toxicity of ethacrynic acid. (ENG)

660
Transient hearing loss, tinnitus, or vertigo due to diuretic, ethacrynic acid, in humans. (ENG)

003
Transient sudden deafness, vertigo, and tinnitus due to parenteral, rapid intravenous, administration of range of 800 to 3600 mg of diuretic, furosemide, for range of 9 hours to 6 days in 5 humans, adult, 37 to 64 years age, male and female, with severe kidney disorder. (ENG)

072
No reported ototoxic effects due to (SQ) oral administration of incr doses to maximum of 3 g of diuretic, furosemide, for 10 days in 1 human, Puerto Rican, adult, 32 years age, male, with kidney disorder.
Transient bilateral sensorineural hearing loss and dizziness due to parenteral, (SQ) intravenous, administration of 200 mg every 2 hours on first day and 3 doses of 400 mg each on second day, total of 1.2 g, of diuretic, furosemide, for 2 days in 1 human, Puerto Rican, adult, 32 years age, male, with kidney disorder.
(AD) Hearing loss not confirmed by audiometry. (ENG)

124
Cochleo-vestibulotoxic effects due to diuretic, furosemide, in humans.
(AD) Comment on use of audiology to confirm effects of ototoxic drugs.
(AD) Explanation of previous study of furosemide without confirmation of ototoxic effects by audiology. (ENG)

313
Transient hearing loss and vestibular problems due to high doses, 1000 mg, of diuretic, furosemide, for 40 minutes in humans with kidney disorder. (ENG)

008
Severe vestibular problems and bilateral sensorineural hearing loss due to unspecified method of administration of more than 1 mg per kg recommended daily dosage of antibiotic, gentamicin (gentamicin sulfate), for unspecified period in 5 humans with kidney disorder.
(AD) No pretreatment tests conducted.
Severe vestibular problems and unilateral sensorineural hearing loss due to unspecified method of administration of more than 1 mg per kg recommended daily dosage of antibiotic, gentamicin (gentamicin sulfate), for unspecified period in 3 humans with kidney disorder.
(CT) Pretreatment vestibular function tests and audiometry showed normal vestibular function and normal hearing.
Transient vestibular problems only due to unspecified method of administration of more than 1 mg per kg recommended daily dosage of antibiotic, gentamicin (gentamicin sulfate), for unspecified period in 2 humans with normal kidney function.
(CT) Pretreatment vestibular function tests showed normal vestibular function. (ENG)

081
Dizziness, tinnitus, and high frequency hearing loss due to parenteral, intramuscular, administration of 40 mg daily, total of 1470 mg intermittently, of antibiotic, gentamicin, in 74 days in 1 human, adolescent, 15 years age, male, with kidney disorder.
(AD) Hearing loss confirmed by audiogram.

(AD) Loss of hair and visual perception defect due to gentamicin treatment. (ENG)

093
Cochleo-vestibulotoxic effects due to parenteral administration of 50 to 100
mg per kg daily of antibiotic, gentamicin (gentamicin sulfate), for 20 days
in humans and animals, cats and guinea pigs.
(AD) Literature review showed ototoxic effects of gentamicin in 2.8 percent of cases reported. (ENG)

101
Primary damage to vestibular apparatus but also cochlear impairment due to
parenteral, intramuscular, administration of 40 mg every 8 hours and 80 mg
every 8 hours of antibiotic, gentamicin, in 7 of 16(2 groups of 8) humans,
adult, male and female, with normal kidney function.
Primary damage to vestibular apparatus but also cochlear impairment due to
parenteral, intramuscular, administration of 40 mg daily of antibiotic,
gentamicin, in 7 of 8 humans, adult, male and female, with kidney disorder.
Primary damage to vestibular apparatus but also cochlear impairment due to
parenteral, intravenous, administration of 80 mg of antibiotic, gentamicin,
in 6 of 7 humans, adult, male and female, with chronic kidney disorder and
treated with hemodialysis.
(AD) Comparative study of humans with normal kidney function and with
kidney disorder.
(AD) Higher incidence of ototoxic effects due to gentamicin in humans with
kidney disorder.
(AD) Cochleo-vestibulotoxic effects confirmed by audiometry and vestibular
function tests. (FR)

117
Transient sensorineural hearing loss due to parenteral, intramuscular, administration of 80 mg daily, total of 320 mg, of antibiotic, gentamicin, for
1 to 4 days in 1 of 339 humans, adult, female, with chronic pyelonephritis.
Transient sensorineural hearing loss due to parenteral, intramuscular, administration of 80 mg daily, total of 1200 mg, of antibiotic, gentamicin, for
1 to 15 days in 1 of 339 humans, adult, female.
Transient vestibular problem due to 80 mg daily, total of 560 mg, of antibiotic, gentamicin, for 7 days in 1 of 339 humans, adult, female, with kidney
disorder.
(AD) Need for vestibular function tests with use of gentamicin in humans
with kidney disorder.
(AD) Report of results of 33 investigations. (ENG)

195
Damage to vestibular nerve and cochlear nerve due to antibiotic, gentamicin,
in humans.
(AD) Comment on use in therapy and cochleo-vestibulotoxic effects of
gentamicin. (ENG)

225
Vestibular problems, in particular dizziness, due to antibiotic, gentamicin,
in 19 of 1327 humans, range of ages, with normal kidney function and with
kidney disorder.
Vestibular problems and high frequency hearing loss due to antibiotic, gentamicin, in 8 of 1327 humans, range of ages, with normal kidney function and
with kidney disorder.
High frequency hearing loss due to antibiotic, gentamicin, in 4 of 1327
humans, range of ages, with normal kidney function and with kidney disorder.
(AD) Kidney disorders in 33.3 percent of patients, previous or simultaneous treatment with other ototoxic drugs in 50 percent, and 50 years or
more age in about 50 percent.
(AD) Comparison of incidence of ototoxicity due to gentamicin and other
aminoglycoside antibiotics. (ENG)

277
Sensorineural hearing loss due to parenteral administration of total doses of
160 mg to more than 4000 mg of antibiotic, gentamicin, in 52 humans.
Vestibular problems due to parenteral administration of total doses of 160 mg

to more than 4000 mg of antibiotic, gentamicin, in 34 humans.
  (CT) Audiometry and vestibular function tests before and after treatment
  with gentamicin. (GER)

298

Possible vestibular problems and high frequency hearing loss due to more than
225 mg daily of antibiotic, gentamicin, in humans.
  (AD) Report on chemistry, pharmacology, clinical use, and cochleo-vestibulotoxic effects of gentamicin.
  (AD) More risk of ototoxicity with gentamicin, dose for dose, than with
  other aminoglycoside antibiotics.
Range of degrees of vestibular problems 1 to 14 days after cessation of
treatment due to total doses of 0.74 to 3.15 g of antibiotic, gentamicin, in
5 of 57 humans with kidney disorder.
  (AD) Report of cases in previous study. (ENG)

306

Vestibular problems due to unspecified dose of antibiotic, gentamicin, for 10
days in 1 human.
Significant vestibular problems and hearing loss due to antibiotic, gentamicin, in 14 of 27 humans, some with kidney disorders, with previous treatment
with ototoxic drugs, or over 40 years age.
  (AD) Vestibular problems confirmed by vestibular function tests.
  (AD) Report on clinical pharmacology, clinical use, and cochleo-vestibulotoxic effects of gentamicin.
  (AD) Reported 2.5 percent incidence in USA of vestibular problems due to
  gentamicin.
  (AD) Suggested that ototoxicity of gentamicin is dose related. (ENG)

369

Rapid loss of Preyer reflex and more gradual changes in vestibular function
due to parenteral, intramuscular, administration of 100 mg per kg daily in 2
doses of antibiotic, gentamicin, for 6 to 49 days in 8 animals, guinea pigs.
Loss of Preyer reflex and changes in vestibular function due to parenteral,
intramuscular, administration of 75 mg per kg daily in 2 doses of antibiotic,
gentamicin, for 15 to 52 days in 8 animals, guinea pigs.
Less effect on Preyer reflex and vestibular function due to parenteral,
intramuscular, administration of 50 mg per kg daily in 2 doses of antibiotic,
gentamicin, for 35 to 53 days in 8 animals, guinea pigs.
  (CT) Use of 6 guinea pigs, control group.
  (CT) Determination of Preyer reflex and vestibular function, pretreatment
  and during treatment with audiometry and vestibular function tests.
  (AD) Relationship but not precise correlation between cochleo-vestibuloto-
  xic effects of gentamicin and daily dosage and duration of treatment.
  (IT)

431

No vestibular problems or hearing loss due to parenteral, intravenous, administration for 30 to 45 minutes of high doses, 4 to 5 mg per kg daily,
diluted in 30 to 50 cc of sterile water, to produce blood levels of 6.25 mcg
per ml or less, of antibiotic, gentamicin (gentamicin sulfate), for total of
20 days in 1 human, adolescent, 13 years age, with cystic fibrosis.
No vestibular problems or hearing loss due to parenteral, intravenous, administration for 30 to 45 minutes of high doses, 4 to 5 mg per kg daily,
diluted in 30 to 50 cc of sterile water, to produce blood levels of 6.25 mcg
per ml or less of antibiotic, gentamicin (SM) (gentamicin sulfate), for range
of 2 to 13 days in 4 humans, adolescent and child, 2 to 13 years age, with
cystic fibrosis.
Simultaneous parenteral, intravenous, administration of high doses, 100 to
600 mg per kg every 4 hours, of antibiotic, carbenicillin (SM) (disodium
carbenicillin), for range of 2 to 19 days in 4 humans, adolescent and child,
2 to 13 years age, with cystic fibrosis.
  (CT) Audiograms and vestibular function tests before and after treatment
  with gentamicin.
  (AD) Comment on high doses of gentamicin without toxicity. (ENG)

575

Transient and permanent vestibular problems only in 29 cases, hearing loss

only in 7 cases, and vestibular problems and hearing loss in 8 cases, beginning less than 10 to 14 days after treatment, due to antibiotic, gentamicin,
in 44 humans, with kidney disorder in 64 percent of cases.
    (AD) Survey of clinical experience in USA with gentamicin ototoxicity.
    (AD) Statistical analysis of administration of gentamicin with and without
ototoxic effects to determine significant factors in ototoxicity.
    (AD) Reported 2 percent incidence of ototoxicity due to gentamicin.
    (AD) Kidney disorders in patients and size of daily dose, mg per kg,
reported most significant factors in gentamicin ototoxicity.
    (AD) Relationship between daily dose and ototoxicity suggests that blood
level of gentamicin possibly significant factor in ototoxicity.
    (AD) Previous therapy with gentamicin or other ototoxic drugs, total dose,
mg and mg per kg, and duration of therapy reported significant factors in
gentamicin ototoxicity in patients with kidney disorder.
    (AD) Occurrence of gentamicin ototoxicity in patients with kidney disor-
ders at younger age than in patients with normal kidney function.
    (AD) Suggested highest risk of gentamicin ototoxicity in younger patients
with kidney disorder. (ENG)

                                                                          606
Transient vertigo after 7 days due to doses to produce blood level of 20 mcg
per ml of antibiotic, gentamicin, in 1 human, adult, 53 years age, male, with
kidney disorder and with previous hearing loss due to other aminoglycoside
antibiotics.
Transient vertigo after 5 days due to doses to produce blood level of 10 mcg
per ml of antibiotic, gentamicin, in 1 human, adult, 32 years age, female,
with chronic pyelonephritis.
Transient vertigo and hearing loss after 6 days due to high doses to produce
blood level of 40 mcg per ml of antibiotic, gentamicin, in 1 human, adult, 20
years age, male, with kidney disorder and severe pseudomonas infection.
    (CT) Audiometry and vestibular function tests, pretreatment and posttreat-
ment.
    (AD) Ototoxic effects in 3 of 58 patients in study.
Unilateral vestibular problem with dizziness due to high daily doses and high
total doses to produce blood levels of 4 to 32 mcg per ml of antibiotic,
gentamicin, in 10 of 40 humans, 7 with kidney disorders.
    (CT) Audiometry and vestibular function tests, pretreatment and posttreat-
ment in 5 patients.
    (AD) Ototoxic effects in 10 of 40 patients in study.
    (AD) Bilateral high frequency hearing loss in 2 patients without pretreat-
ment audiograms possibly not due to gentamicin.
Unilateral tinnitus possibly due to topical, (SQ) direct site, administration
of 40 mg of antibiotic, gentamicin, in 1 human with previous noise induced
hearing loss.
Unilateral tinnitus possibly due to parenteral, (SQ) intramuscular, administration of total of 160 mg of antibiotic, gentamicin, in 1 human with previous noise induced hearing loss.
    (AD) Tinnitus, as well as hearing loss, possibly present before adminis-
tration of gentamicin.
Incr vertigo due to 120 mg daily of antibiotic, gentamicin, in 1 human,
adult, 36 years age, male, with previous vertigo.
    (CT) Audiometry and vestibular function tests, pretreatment and posttreat-
ment.
    (AD) Ototoxic effects in possibly 2 of 148 patients in study treated with
topical or parenteral gentamicin.
    (AD) Discussion of 3 studies of ototoxic effects of gentamicin. (ENG)

                                                                          629
Hearing loss and vestibular problems due to antibiotic, (SQ) gentamicin
(gentamicin sulfate), in 16(2.8 percent) of 565 humans, with kidney disorder
in 10 cases and with previous treatment with ototoxic drugs in 7 cases.
Possible ototoxic effects due to previous administration of other (SQ) ototoxic drugs in 7 of 16 humans.
Hearing loss and vestibular problems due to antibiotic, gentamicin, in 23(2
percent) of 1152 humans.
    (AD) Discussion of incidence of ototoxicity due to gentamicin reported in
2 studies. (ENG)

639

Hearing loss in 6 cases and vestibular problems in 17 cases due to parenteral administration of antibiotic, gentamicin, in 23 (2 percent) of 1152 humans. (ENG)

650

Transient bilateral hearing loss and moderate dizziness after 6 days due to 0.8 mg per kg daily of antibiotic, gentamicin, in 1 of 44 humans with various infections and with normal kidney function.
(CT) Vestibular function tests and audiometry, before, during, and after gentamicin treatment. (ENG)

652

No vestibular problems or hearing loss observed due to parenteral, intravenous, administration of 1 mg per kg initial dose, and then 0.75 mg per kg every 6 hours, in 200 ml dextrose solution over 2 hour period, of antibiotic, gentamicin (SM), for 2 weeks minimum or for 5 days after cessation of fever, whichever longer, in 23 humans, adolescent, adult, and aged, 13 to 68 years age, with acute leukemia or metastatic cancer and with previous treatment with other antibiotics in some.
(AD) No vestibular function tests or audiometry used to determine if ototoxic effects.
Simultaneous parenteral, intravenous, administration of 4 g every 4 hours of antibiotic, carbenicillin (SM), for 2 weeks minimum or for 5 days after cessation of fever, whichever longer, in 23 humans, adolescent, adult, and aged, 13 to 68 years age, with acute leukemia or metastatic cancer and with previous treatment with other antibiotics in some. (ENG)

677

Transient or permanent, bilateral or unilateral, vestibular problems primarily but also possible high frequency hearing loss due to parenteral administration of high doses to produce serum levels over 10 mcg per ml of antibiotic, gentamicin, in humans, in particular with kidney disorders.
(AD) Gentamicin ototoxicity also in patients with previous treatment with ototoxic drugs or with previous auditory system problems.
(AD) Reported 2 to 2.5 percent incidence of vestibular problems due to parenteral gentamicin.
(AD) Literature review of mechanism of action, pharmacology, dosage, clinical use, and toxic effects of gentamicin. (ENG)

683

Primarily transient or permanent, unilateral or bilateral, vestibular problems but also high frequency hearing loss due to parenteral administration of high doses to produce blood levels over 10 mcg per ml of antibiotic, gentamicin, in humans, in particular with kidney disorders or with previous treatment with ototoxic drugs, or with previous auditory system problems.
(AD) Discussion of chemical structure, antibiotic activity, clinical pharmacology, use in therapy, and toxic effects.
(AD) Reported 2 to 2.5 percent incidence of vestibular problems due to parenteral gentamicin.
(AD) Unilateral vestibular problems in 50 percent of patients tested. (ENG)

684

Possible permanent severe vestibular problems and some hearing loss due to antibiotic, gentamicin, in humans.
(AD) Possible to use potential ototoxic drugs with minimum risk of permanent ototoxic effects by regulation of dosage and cessation of therapy at first symptom of ototoxicity. (ENG)

729

No hearing loss or vestibular problems due to parenteral, intramuscular, administration of total dose of 160 to more than 4000 mg of antibiotic, gentamicin, for 2 to 40 days in 72 humans with various infections.
No hearing loss or vestibular problems due to topical administration in solution or ointment of antibiotic, gentamicin, for 2 to 40 days in 55 humans with various infections or in surgery. (GER)

263
Possible dizziness, tinnitus, and hearing loss due to anti-inflammatory
agent, ibuprofen, in humans. (ENG)

693
Tinnitus due to oral administration in capsules of 75 mg daily of anti-inflammatory agent, indomethacin, for 4 weeks in 1 of 14 humans, male and female, with rheumatoid arthritis.
Dizziness due to oral administration in capsules of 75 mg daily of anti-
inflammatory agent, indomethacin, for 4 weeks in 1 of 14 humans, male and
female, with rheumatoid arthritis. (ENG)

697
Dizziness in 12 cases and hearing loss in 1 case due to oral (SM) administration in capsules of 25 mg twice a day for 2 days and then 4 times a day for 2
days, followed by 50 mg 3 times a day for 2 days and then 4 times a day, of
anti-inflammatory agent, indomethacin, for 12 weeks in 12 (40 percent) of 30
humans with bone and joint disorder.
Dizziness in 12 cases and hearing loss in 1 case due to topical, rectal (SM),
administration in suppositories of 100 mg daily of anti-inflammatory agent,
indomethacin, for first 6 days in 12 (40 percent) of 30 humans with bone and
joint disorder. (ENG)

165
Hearing loss, tinnitus, or vertigo due to parenteral administration of 36.0
mg per kg daily, total of 46.7 g, of antibiotic, kanamycin, for 20.3 average
days in 22 of 106 humans, adult, 50.8 years average age.
   (AD) Report on case study from previous study.
   (AD) Literature review of clinical and experimental studies. (ENG)

309
Bilateral sensorineural hearing loss and tinnitus, tinnitus only, or vertigo
due to parenteral, intramuscular, administration of 1 g daily in 2 doses or
15 mg per kg, total doses of 6 to 9 g, of antibiotic, kanamycin, for 6 to 9
days in 5 of 17 humans, adult and aged, female and male, with genitourinary
system infections and normal kidney function.
Bilateral sensorineural hearing loss, tinnitus, and vertigo due to parenteral, intramuscular, administration of less than normal dosage of antibiotic, kanamycin, for 6 to 9 days in 2 of 17 humans, adult, male and female,
with genitourinary system infections and kidney disorder.
   (CT) Pure tone audiometry, pretreatment, during treatment, and posttreatment.
   (AD) Discussion of case reports.
   (AD) Prospective study to determine clinical effectiveness of kanamycin in
   genitourinary system infections. (ENG)

459
No significant decr in cochlear microphonic due to parenteral, subcutaneous,
administration of 100 mg per kg daily for 5 days a week, total dose of 3 g
per kg, of antibiotic, kanamycin (kanamycin sulfate), for 30 days in animals,
guinea pigs.
Decr in cochlear microphonics in 14 of 15 ears, damage to hair cells of organ
of Corti and to stria vascularis, slight to severe damage to spiral ganglion,
damage to macula utriculi, and slight damage to crista ampullaris and macula
sacculi due to parenteral, subcutaneous, administration of 250 mg per kg
daily for 5 days a week, total dose of 5 g per kg, of antibiotic, kanamycin
(kanamycin sulfate), for 20 days in animals, guinea pigs.
Significant decr in cochlear microphonics in all ears, damage to outer hair
cells of organ of Corti and to stria vascularis, and slight damage to spiral
ganglion due to parenteral, subcutaneous, administration of 200 mg per kg
daily for 5 days a week, total dose of 6 g per kg, of antibiotic, kanamycin
(kanamycin sulfate), for 30 days in animals, guinea pigs.
Significant decr in cochlear microphonics due to parenteral, subcutaneous,
administration of 200 mg per kg daily for 5 days a week, total dose of 6 g
per kg, of antibiotic, kanamycin (IB) (kanamycin sulfate), for 30 days in
animals, guinea pigs, with subcutaneous administration of 1.5 mg per kg of
nialamide.
Significant decr in cochlear microphonics, damage to hair cells of organ of

Corti and to stria vascularis, and slight damage to spiral ganglion due to parenteral, subcutaneous, administration of 200 mg per kg daily for 5 days a week, total dose of 6 g per kg, of antibiotic, kanamycin (IB) (kanamycin sulfate), for 30 days in animals, guinea pigs, with subcutaneous administration of 8 mg per kg of nialamide.
Significant decr in cochlear microphonics, damage to hair cells of organ of Corti and to stria vascularis, slight to severe damage to spiral ganglion, slight damage to limbus, and slight damage to macula utriculi and cristae due to parenteral, subcutaneous, administration of 200 mg per kg daily for 5 days a week, total dose of 6 g per kg, of antibiotic, kanamycin (IB) (kanamycin sulfate), for 30 days in animals, guinea pigs, with subcutaneous administration of 15 mg per kg of nialamide.
   (AD) No prevention of kanamycin effects on cochlear microphonics with administration of nialamide.
Less decr in cochlear microphonics in 6, 10, and 11 of 3 groups of 15 ears, damage to hair cells of organ of Corti and to stria vascularis, slight damage to spiral ganglion and to limbus, damage to macula utriculi, and slight damage to crista ampullaris due to parenteral, subcutaneous, administration of 250 mg per kg daily for 5 days a week, total dose of 5 g per kg, of antibiotic, kanamycin (IB), for 20 days in 3 groups of animals, guinea pigs, with pantothenic acid.
   (CT) Same method using daily subcutaneous administration of 0.25 cc of isotonic saline in guinea pigs, control group.
   (AD) Decr in kanamycin effects on cochlear microphonics with pantothenic acid.
   (AD) Study of functional and structural cochleo-vestibulotoxic effects of kanamycin with and without inhibitors.
   (AD) Statistical analysis of results.   (ENG)

                                                                    152
Transient moderate dizziness due to parenteral, intravenous, administration of 1.0 mg per kg of 1 percent concentration of anesthetic, lidocaine, for 30 seconds in 23 humans.
Transient severe dizziness and tinnitus due to parenteral, intravenous, administration of 1.5 mg per kg of 1 percent concentration of anesthetic, lidocaine, for 30 seconds in 6 humans.
   (CT) Same study without lidocaine injection in 9 humans, control group.
   (AD) Auditory system problems due to lidocaine reported in previous studies.   (ENG)

                                                                    646
Possible vertigo and tinnitus due to parenteral, intravenous, administration of 2 percent solution of anesthetic, lidocaine, in humans with heart disorder.   (ENG)

                                                                    465
Hearing loss, nystagmus, and vertigo due to heavy metal, mercury, organic, in humans, adolescent, adult, and aged.
   (AD) Auditory system problems confirmed by audiology and vestibular function tests.   (JAP)

                                                                    273
Vertigo and hearing loss due to topical administration in ear drops of 500,000 ED in distilled water, in 6 to 8 ear drops daily, of antibiotic, neomycin, for 8 days in 1 human with suppuration from right ear.
   (AD) Hearing loss confirmed by audiometry.   (RUS)

                                                                    461
Destruction of cochlear microphonics, destruction of hair cells of organ of Corti in basal coil of cochlea, severe damage to stria vascularis, damage to nuclei of limbus, and slight damage to macula utriculi due to parenteral, subcutaneous, administration of 100 mg per kg daily for 5 days a week, total dose of 3 g per kg, of antibiotic, neomycin (neomycin sulfate), for 30 days in animals, guinea pigs.
No damage to cochlear microphonics and no structural damage to cochlea or vestibular apparatus due to parenteral, subcutaneous, administration of 100 mg per kg daily for 5 days a week, total dose of 3 g per kg, of antibiotic, neomycin (methylneomycin), for 30 days in animals, guinea pigs.

Decr in cochlear microphonics due to parenteral, subcutaneous, administration
of 100 mg per kg daily for 5 days a week, total dose of 1.5 g per kg, of
antibiotic, neomycin (neomycin sulfate), for 15 days in animals, guinea pigs.
Decr in cochlear microphonics due to parenteral, subcutaneous, administration
of 200 mg per kg daily for 5 days a week, total dose of 2 g per kg, of antibiotic, neomycin (neomycin sulfate), for 10 days in animals, guinea pigs.
Decr in cochlear microphonics due to parenteral, subcutaneous, administration
of 200 mg per kg daily for 5 days a week, total dose of 2 g per kg, of antibiotic, neomycin (IB) (neomycin sulfate), for 10 days in animals, guinea
pigs, with administration of vitamin B.
   (CT) Same method with daily subcutaneous administration of 0.25 cc isotonic saline in guinea pigs, control group.
   (AD) No decr in ototoxic effects of neomycin on cochlear microphonics with
   administration of vitamin B.
   (AD) Study of functional and structural cochleo-vestibulotoxic effects of
   neomycin.
   (AD) Statistical analysis of results. (ENG)

                                                                      194
Vestibular problems, primary effect, and bilateral sensorineural hearing loss
due to antineoplastic, nitrogen mustard, for long periods in 24 humans with
malignant tumors and lupus erythematosus.
   (AD) Auditory system problems confirmed by audiometry and vestibular
   function tests.
   (AD) Cochleo-vestibulotoxic effects after treatment with nitrogen mustard
   due to dosage, duration of treatment, and route of administration. (SP)

                                                                      709
Possible hearing loss and vertigo after 10 to 48 hours due to antiparasitic,
oil of chenopodium, in humans. (FR)

                                                                      450
Hearing loss and vertigo due to high doses of antimalarial, quinine, in
humans, adult, female and male, in suicide attempt.
   (AD) Study with EEG of acute quinine ototoxicity. (IT)

                                                                      502
Possible transient hearing loss or dizziness due to antibiotic, rifampicin,
in humans treated for tuberculosis or other infections.
   (AD) Literature review of clinical use, pharmacology, toxicity, and other
   aspects of rifampicin. (ENG)

                                                                      014
No permanent sensorineural hearing loss or damage to cochlea or vestibular
apparatus due to 20 to 30 mg per kg daily, total of 2 to 39 g, of antibiotic,
streptomycin, for 6 months to 5 years in 205 humans, child and adolescent,
range of 6 to 14 years age, with various disorders. (POL)

                                                                      017
Ototoxic effects, vestibular problems and cochlear impairment in 78 percent,
vestibular problems only in 14 percent, and cochlear impairment only in 8
percent due to unspecified method of administration of unspecified doses of
antibiotic, streptomycin (streptomycin sulfate), for unspecified period in
100 humans with tuberculosis and other infections.
   (CT) No symptoms of damage to cochlea or vestibular apparatus before
   treatment with streptomycin.
   (AD) Recommendation of audiometry and vestibular function test, pretreatment and during treatment, for early detection of ototoxic effects. (ENG)

                                                                      070
Cochleo-vestibulotoxic effects due to range of less than 50 g to more than
200 g of antibiotic, streptomycin, in 127 humans with pulmonary tuberculosis
and 1 human with croupous pneumonia.
   (AD) Statistical analysis showed correlation between ototoxic effects and
   dosage.
   (AD) Vestibular problems detected earlier than hearing loss.
   (AD) Suggested use of audiometry before streptomycin treatment and every
   10 to 15 days during treatment. (RUS)

071
Cochleo-vestibulotoxic effects due to antibiotic, streptomycin (SM) (streptomycin sulfate), in 65.5 percent of 553 humans, child and adolescent, 3 to
15 years age, with pulmonary tuberculosis.
Simultaneous administration of other unspecified antituberculous agents (SM)
in 553 humans, child and adolescent, 3 to 15 years age, with pulmonary tuberculosis.
    (CT) No cochleo-vestibulotoxic effects in 113 humans, child and adoles-
    cent, control group, not treated with streptomycin.
    (AD) Analysis by audiometry of ototoxic effects of streptomycin in chil-
    dren and adolescents. (SER)

155
Suppression of function of semicircular canal due to parenteral, intramuscular, administration of range of 1100 to 4600 mg total doses of antibiotic,
streptomycin (streptomycin sulfate), for 16 to 23 doses in 8 animals, squirrel monkeys, with normal semicircular canal function.
    (CT) Vestibular function tests used to confirm pretreatment normal func-
    tion of semicircular canal.
Moderate to severe damage to hair cells of cristae and organ of Corti and
some changes in spiral ganglion and maculae due to parenteral, intramuscular,
administration of range of 1100 to 4600 mg total doses of antibiotic, streptomycin (streptomycin sulfate), for 16 to 23 doses in 8 animals, squirrel
monkeys, with normal semicircular canal function.
    (AD) Report on 8 case studies to show clinical and pathological correla-
    tions. (ENG)

191
Vestibular problems due to unspecified method of administration of unspecified doses of antibiotic, streptomycin, for long period in 9 of 155 humans
with tuberculosis.
Cochlear impairment due to unspecified method of administration of unspecified doses of antibiotic, streptomycin, for long period in 4 of 155 humans
with tuberculosis.
Vestibular problems and cochlear impairment due to unspecified method of
administration of unspecified doses of antibiotic, streptomycin, for long
period in 1 of 155 humans with tuberculosis. (ENG)

215
Primary damage to vestibular function but also cochlear impairment due to
blood levels over 25 mcg per ml of antibiotic, streptomycin, in humans.
    (AD) Report on dosage, clinical use, and toxicity of streptomycin.
    (AD) Relationship between cochleo-vestibulotoxic effects and daily dosage
    and duration of treatment.
    (AD) Need for audiometry and vestibular function tests during treatment
    and for 6 months after treatment with streptomycin. (ENG)

243
Hearing loss and vestibular problems due to 1.5 g of antibiotic, streptomycin
(streptomycin pantothenate), in 1 human, child, male.
    (AD) Literature review of pharmacology and toxicology of aminoglycoside
    antibiotics, streptomycin, dihydrostreptomycin, kanamycin, and neomycin.
    (GER)

380
Unilateral loss of vestibular function and no ataxia due to parenteral administration, infusion into carotid artery, of 150 cc in Ringer's Lactate
every 24 hours, total dose of 0.84 to 1.5 g per kg, of antibiotic, streptomycin (streptomycin sulfate), for 3 to 10 days in 5 animals, cat s, adult, 1.9
to 3.1 kg weight.
Bilateral loss of vestibular function with ataxia and destruction of hair
cells of crista ampullaris and semicircular canal due to parenteral administration, infusion into carotid artery, of 150 cc in Ringer's Lactate every 24
hours, total dose of 1.2 to 2.5 g per kg, of antibiotic, streptomycin (streptomycin sulfate), for 6 to 12 days in 5 animals, cats, adult, 2.3 to 5.1 kg
weight.
No hearing loss and no damage to hair cells of organ of Corti due to parenteral administration, infusion into carotid artery, of 150 cc in Ringer's

Lactate every 24 hours, total dose of 0.84 to 2.5 g per kg, of antibiotic,
streptomycin (streptomycin sulfate), for 3 to 12 days in 10 animals, cats,
adult, 1.9 to 5.1 kg weight.
Decr in cochlear microphonic but no damage to hair cells of organ of Corti
due to parenteral administration, infusion into carotid artery, of 150 cc in
Ringer's Lactate every 24 hours, total dose of 1.0 g per kg, of antibiotic,
streptomycin (streptomycin sulfate), for 4 days in 1 animal, cat, adult, 3.0
kg weight.
  (CT) Measurement of cochlear function and vestibular function before and
  after infusion of streptomycin.
  (AD) Type of loss of vestibular function due to total dosage of streptomycin and duration of administration.
  (AD) Unilateral destruction of vestibular function without cochlear impairment is goal in treatment of Meniere's disease. (ENG)

                                                                        395
Damage first to outer hair cells of organ of Corti in basal coil of cochlea
due to high doses of antibiotics, aminoglycoside, in animals, guinea pigs.
  (AD) Same damage due to x-ray radiation.
Primary damage to central areas of crista ampullaris, crista neglecta, and
macula due to antibiotics, aminoglycoside, in animals, guinea pigs.
  (AD) Damage to peripheral areas of crista ampullaris, crista neglecta, and
  macula due to x-ray radiation.
Disturbance of protein synthesis due to topical administration to bulla of
antibiotic, streptomycin, in animals, guinea pigs.
  (AD) Similar electron microscopy findings for streptomycin administration
  to bulla and for x-ray radiation.
  (AD) Cochleo-vestibulotoxic effects due to x-ray radiation comp w effects
  due to antibiotics. (ENG)

                                                                        421
Damage to cochlear function and vestibular function due to antibiotic, streptomycin, in humans, adult, with tuberculosis. (RUS)

                                                                        425
Decr in ototoxic effect on organ of Corti and crista ampullaris due to topical administration to bulla of 0.2 ccm of 50 percent solution of antibiotic,
streptomycin (IB) (streptomycin sulfate), in 10 animals, guinea pigs with
intramuscular administration of 1 ml per 100 g ozothin.
  (AD) Histochemical study of effect of ozothin on ototoxicity of streptomycin in guinea pigs. (GER)

                                                                        487
Severe vestibular problems due to parenteral, intramuscular, administration
of antibiotic, streptomycin (streptomycin sulfate), for long period in 8
percent of 600 humans with tuberculosis and with previous hearing loss in
some cases.
Transient hearing loss in most cases due to parenteral, intramuscular, administration of antibiotic, streptomycin (streptomycin sulfate), for long
period in some of 600 humans with tuberculosis and with previous hearing loss
in some cases.
  (CT) Audiometry and vestibular function tests before, during, and after
  streptomycin treatment.
  (AD) Improvement in vestibular function after cessation of streptomycin
  treatment.
  (AD) Transient hearing loss in most cases due to early detection with
  audiology. (GER)

                                                                        488
Permanent cochleo-vestibulotoxic effects due to range of doses of antibiotic,
streptomycin (streptomycin sulfate), in some of 1198 humans treated for
tuberculosis and other disorders.
  (AD) Auditory system problems detected by audiology.
  (AD) Comment on differences in individual responses to streptomycin.
  (SER)

                                                                        643
Possible transient or permanent damage to eighth cranial nerve, vestibular

problems and hearing loss, due to antibiotic, streptomycin, in humans with tuberculosis and in particular with concurrent kidney disorders.
 (AD) Need for careful consideration in use of streptomycin in therapy. (ENG)

663

Vertigo due to antibiotic, streptomycin, in 2 humans.
Tinnitus and sensorineural hearing loss but no vertigo due to antibiotic, streptomycin, in 3 humans.
 (AD) Treatment with dogmatil of vestibular problems and hearing loss due to streptomycin. (FR)

687

Vestibular problems and hearing loss due to high doses of antibiotic, streptomycin, in humans.
 (AD) Discussion of toxic effects of drugs. (GER)

723

Possible sensorineural hearing loss and vestibular problems due to antibiotic, streptomycin, in humans treated for tuberculosis during pregnancy. (GER)

266

Effect on enzymes of cochlea and vestibular apparatus due to topical administration to bulla of 0.2 ml of 2 percent solution of anesthetic, tetracaine (tetracaine hydrochloride), in animals, guinea pigs.
 (CT) Study of guinea pigs, control group, not treated with tetracaine. (GER)

416

Delayed unilateral sensorineural hearing loss and vestibular problems detected 22 years after treatment due to heavy metal, thorium dioxide, in 1 human, adult, 36 years age when treated, female, during roentgenography.
Delayed tinnitus, unilateral sensorineural hearing loss, and damage to vestibular function detected 21 years after treatment due to heavy metal, thorium dioxide, in 1 human, adult, 36 years age when treated, male, during roentgenography.
 (AD) Cochleo-vestibulotoxic effects of thorium dioxide confirmed by audiology and vestibular function tests.
 (AD) Case reports of delayed ototoxic effects of thorium dioxide. (ENG)

404

No cochleo-vestibulotoxic effects due to parenteral, intravenous, administration of 1 g, dissolved in 250 ml isotonic saline, of antibiotic, vancomycin, for every 14 days for long period, more than 60 days, in 25 humans with chronic kidney disorder and treated with intermittent hemodialysis.
 (AD) Audiometry every 12 weeks.
 (AD) Previous reports of severe ototoxicity due to vancomycin.
 (AD) Previous report suggested occurrence of ototoxicity with vancomycin serum levels over 80 mcg per ml.
 (AD) Suggested that vancomycin ototoxicity not related to total dosage or duration of treatment. (ENG)

122

Damage to eighth cranial nerve and sensorineural hearing loss and vestibular problems due to unspecified doses of antibiotic, viomycin, for long period in humans.
 (AD) Literature review of viomycin, use in therapy and toxic effects.
 (AD) Recommended intramuscular administration of 1 to 2 g daily dose of viomycin for 2 to 3 weeks for minimum risk of ototoxicity. (ENG)

598

Vertigo or tinnitus due to oral administration in tablets of 1 to 3 tablets of 200 mg each, total of 200 to 600 mg, of antimalarial, 16-126 RP, in 1 dose in 3 of 20 humans, African, child, 4 or less to over 9 years age, with malaria.
Vertigo due to oral administration in tablets of 2 to 6 tablets of 200 mg each, total of 400 to 1200 mg, of antimalarial, 16-126 RP, for 2 days in 1 of

15 humans, African, child, 4 or less to over 9 years age, with malaria.   (FR)

009

Delayed permanent sensorineural hearing loss and damage to outer hair cells of basal and middle coils of cochlea due to unspecified doses of antibiotic, dihydrostreptomycin, in humans.

Vertigo and dizziness due to unspecified method of administration of 2 to 3 g daily of antibiotic, streptomycin (streptomycin sulfate), for 30 to 50 days in humans with tuberculosis.

Hearing loss due to unspecified method of administration of high doses of antibiotic, streptomycin (streptomycin sulfate), for long period in humans.

Gradual high frequency hearing loss and tinnitus and degeneration of hair cells of organ of Corti in basal coil of cochlea due to unspecified doses of antibiotic, kanamycin, in humans.

Delayed severe high frequency hearing loss due to parenteral, oral, or topical administration by inhalation of unspecified doses of antibiotic, neomycin, for unspecified period in humans with kidney disorder.

Complete degeneration of inner hair cells due to unspecified method of administration of 18 g of antibiotic, neomycin, for unspecified period in humans with bacterial endocarditis.

Lesions in organ of Corti due to parenteral administration of unspecified doses of antibiotic, polymyxin B, for unspecified period in animals, guinea pigs.

Sensorineural hearing loss due to parenteral, intravenous, administration of 80 to 95 mg per ml of antibiotic, vancomycin, for unspecified period in humans with kidney disorder.

   (AD) Sensorineural hearing loss and vestibular problems due to 6 antibiotics in humans and animals, guinea pigs.

   (AD) Literature review of ototoxic effects of antibiotics. (ENG)

011

Transient cochleo-vestibulotoxic effects due to topical administration by inhalation and parenteral, intramuscular, administration of 0.5 g twice a day for 6 days, followed by a 1-day break, of antibiotic, (SQ) kanamycin (kanamycin sulfate), for 1 to 3 months in 2 of 17 humans treated for tuberculosis.

   (CT) Pretreatment audiometry and vestibular function tests conducted.

Ototoxic effects due to previous administration of antibiotic, (SQ) streptomycin, in 2 of 17 humans with tuberculosis. (RUS)

016

Progressive bilateral sensorineural hearing loss and vertigo due to unspecified method of administration of total of 3 g of antibiotic, (SQ) streptomycin (SM), for unspecified period in 1 human, Caucasian, adult, 32 years age, male, with kidney disorder and on intermittent hemodialysis.

Progressive bilateral sensorineural hearing loss and vertigo due to unspecified method of administration of antibiotic, (SQ) colistin (SM), for unspecified period in 1 human, Caucasian, adult, 32 years age, male, with kidney disorder and on intermittent hemodialysis.

Permanent sensorineural hearing loss due to parenteral, intravenous, administration of 1.6 mg per kg 2 times daily, total of 500 mg of antibiotic, (SQ) gentamicin, for unspecified period in 1 human, Caucasian, adult, 32 years age, male, with kidney disorder and on intermittent hemodialysis.

No definite ototoxic effects reported due to unspecified method of administration of 1 g every 2 weeks, total of 12 g, of antibiotic, (SQ) vancomycin, for about 6 months in 1 human, Caucasian, adult, 32 years age, male, with kidney disorder and on intermittent hemodialysis.

   (AD) Hearing loss due to streptomycin and colistin potentiated by gentamicin.   (ENG)

020

Effect on function of inner ear due to parenteral, subcutaneous, administration of high doses, range of 30 to 75 mg per kg of antibiotic, gentamicin, for about 8 to 20 days in 11 animals, cats.

   (AD) Preliminary study of dosage levels.

Damage to semicircular canal, membranous labyrinth, and outer hair cells and inner hair cells of the cochlea due to parenteral, subcutaneous, administration of high doses, range of 30 to 75 mg per kg of antibiotic, gentamicin, for about 8 to 20 days in 11 animals, cats, with kidney damage resulting from

gentamicin.
   (AD) Preliminary study of dosage levels.
Partial hearing loss due to parenteral, subcutaneous, administration of 20 mg
per kg of antibiotic, gentamicin, for 14 days in 1 out of 15 animals, cats.
Complete degeneration of outer hair cells of organ of Corti due to parenteral, subcutaneous, administration of 20 mg per kg of antibiotic, gentamicin, for 14 days in 1 out of 15 animals, cats.
Range of degree of damage, transient and permanent, to vestibular apparatus
due to parenteral, subcutaneous, administration of 20 mg per kg of antibiotic, gentamicin, for 14 days in 15 animals, cats.
Complete damage to vestibular apparatus due to parenteral, subcutaneous,
administration of 200 mg per kg of antibiotic, streptomycin, for 9 days in
animals, cats.
Higher incidence and earlier symptoms of ototoxic effects due to parenteral,
subcutaneous, administration of 20 mg per kg of antibiotic, gentamicin, for
14 days in 66.6 percent of 15 animals, cats, with kidney damage than in cats
with normal kidney function.
   (AD) Study of correlation of functional and histological effects of gentamicin.
   (AD) Comparative study of effect on vestibular apparatus of gentamicin and
   streptomycin. (ENG)

                                                                        038
Bilateral sensorineural hearing loss due to oral administration of 200 mg
twice a day of diuretic, (SQ) ethacrynic acid, for several weeks in 1 human,
adult, 40 years age, female, with kidney disorder.
Previous oral administration of 40 mg daily of diuretic, (SQ) furosemide
(SM), for unspecified period in 1 human, adult, 40 years age, female, with
kidney disorder.
Previous oral administration of 500 mg daily of diuretic, (SQ) chlorothiazide
(SM), for unspecified period in 1 human, adult, 40 years age, female, with
kidney disorder.
Sensorineural hearing loss and unsteady gait due to parenteral, intravenous,
administration of 200 mg of diuretic, (SQ) ethacrynic acid (SM), for unspeci-
fied period in 1 human, adult, 20 years age, female, with kidney disorder.
Simultaneous parenteral, intravenous, administration of 25 g of diuretic,
(SQ) mannitol (SM), for unspecified period in 1 human, adult, 20 years age,
female, with kidney disorder.
Previous administration of unspecified dose of chemical agent, (SQ) carbon
tetrachloride, for unspecified period in 1 human, adult, 20 years age, female, with kidney disorder.
Transient sensorineural hearing loss due to parenteral, intravenous, administration of 800 mg daily of diuretic, ethacrynic acid (SM), for unspecified
period in 1 human, adult, 25 years age, female, with chronic kidney disorder.
Simultaneous administration of unspecified doses of diuretic, chlorothiazide
(SM), for unspecified period in 1 human, adult, 25 years age, female, with
chronic kidney disorder.
Simultaneous administration of unspecified doses of diuretic, mannitol (SM),
for unspecified period in 1 human, adult, 25 years age, female, with chronic
kidney disorder.
Transient sensorineural hearing loss and dizziness due to parenteral, (SQ)
intravenous, administration of unspecified doses of diuretic, ethacrynic
acid, for unspecified period in 1 human, adult, 52 years age, female, with
kidney disorder.
Transient sensorineural hearing loss and dizziness due to (SQ) oral administration of 300 mg of diuretic, ethacrynic acid, for unspecified period in 1
human, adult, 52 years age, female, with kidney disorder.
Sensorineural hearing loss due to oral administration of 20 mg 3 times daily
of diuretic, ethacrynic acid, for 3 days in 1 human, adult, 28 years age,
male, with kidney disorder.
   (AD) Discussion of 5 case reports of ototoxic effects due to treatment
   with ethacrynic acid. (ENG)

                                                                        041
Cochleo-vestibulotoxic effects due to unspecified method of administration of
300 mg daily of antituberculous agent, isoniazid, for 6 to 18 months in 12.9
percent of 70 humans with tuberculosis.
Cochleo-vestibulotoxic effects due to unspecified method of administration of

300 mg of antituberculous agent, isoniazid (SM), for 6 to 18 months in 22 percent of 297 humans with tuberculosis.
Cochleo-vestibulotoxic effects due to unspecified method of administration of 150 mg of antituberculous agent, thiacetazone (SM), for 6 to 18 months in 22 percent of 297 humans with tuberculosis.
Cochleo-vestibulotoxic effects due to unspecified method of administration of antituberculous agent, isoniazid (SM), for 6 to 18 months in 82.9 percent of 82 humans with tuberculosis.
Cochleo-vestibulotoxic effects due to unspecified method of administration of antituberculous agent, thiacetazone (SM), for 6 to 8 months in 82.9 percent of 82 humans with tuberculosis.
Cochleo-vestibulotoxic effects due to unspecified method of administration of 1 g of antibiotic, streptomycin (SM), for 6 to 18 months in 82.9 percent of 82 humans with tuberculosis.
Cochleo-vestibulotoxic effects due to unspecified method of administration of 300 mg of antituberculous agent, isoniazid (SM), for 6 to 18 months in 25 percent of 20 humans with tuberculosis.
Cochleo-vestibulotoxic effects due to unspecified method of administration of 1 g of antibiotic, streptomycin (SM), for 6 to 18 months in 25 percent of 20 humans with tuberculosis.
  (AD) Potentiation by thiacetazone of cochleo-vestibulotoxic effects of streptomycin suggested.
  (AD) Audiometry and vestibular function tests every 2 weeks for 6 to 18 months in total of 469 humans with tuberculosis. (ENG)

                                                                              057
No ototoxic effects within 2 months due to antibiotic, dihydrostreptomycin (dihydrostreptomycin ascorbinate), in humans with pulmonary tuberculosis.
  (AD) Audiometry used to determine ototoxic effects.
Tinnitus and vertigo due to antibiotic, streptomycin (streptomycin sulfate), in humans with pulmonary tuberculosis.
  (AD) Comparative study of effects of 2 antibiotics used in treatment of pulmonary tuberculosis. (RUS)

                                                                              080
Hearing loss and vertigo due to parenteral administration of antibiotic, streptomycin, in humans, child and adult, with normal kidney function and with kidney disorder.
  (AD) Suggested use for severe infections only.
Delayed permanent hearing loss due to antibiotic, dihydrostreptomycin, in humans.
  (AD) High risk of ototoxic effects with clinical use.
Hearing loss due to oral administration of antibiotic, paromomycin, in humans.
Progressive permanent hearing loss and tinnitus due to parenteral administration of antibiotic, kanamycin, in humans.
Progressive permanent hearing loss and tinnitus due to parenteral and topical administration of antibiotic, neomycin, in humans.
  (AD) Need for careful consideration in use of paromomycin, kanamycin, and neomycin due to potential ototoxicity.
  (AD) Discussion of ototoxic effects of 5 antibiotics. (ENG)

                                                                              087
High frequency hearing loss and tinnitus due to antibiotics in humans, particularly infant and aged, and humans with kidney disorder.
Degeneration in hair cells of organ of Corti due to antibiotics in humans.
Vertigo and unsteady gait due to antibiotic, streptomycin, in humans.
Bilateral damage to vestibular apparatus due to antibiotic, streptomycin, in humans.
  (AD) Literature review of physiological and structural cochleo-vestibulotoxic effects of antibiotics.
  (AD) Degree of damage determined by dosage and duration of dosage of antibiotics. (ENG)

                                                                              090
Tinnitus and vertigo due to unspecified method of administration of 0.75 g daily of antibiotic, (SQ) streptomycin (SM), for 5 weeks in 1 human, adult, 38 years age, female, with pulmonary tuberculosis.

Simultaneous administration of antituberculous agent, (SQ) PAS (SM), in 1 human, adult, 38 years age, female, with pulmonary tuberculosis.
Simultaneous administration of antituberculous agent, (SQ) isoniazid (SM), in 1 human, adult, 38 years age, female, with pulmonary tuberculosis.
No reported ototoxic effects due to unspecified method of administration of 150 mg daily of antituberculous agent, (SQ) thiacetazone, for 11 months in 1 human, adult, 38 years age, female, with pulmonary tuberculosis.
  (AD) Hemolytic disease due to treatment with thiacetazone. (ENG)

103

Cochleo-vestibulotoxic effects due to range of less than 50 g to 300 g of antibiotic, streptomycin (SM) (streptomycin sulfate), for 6 to 8 months in humans, adult, with tuberculous meningitis.
Simultaneous administration of antituberculous agent, PAS (SM), in humans, adult, with tuberculous meningitis.
Simultaneous administration of antituberculous agent, isoniazid (SM), in humans, adult, with tuberculous meningitis.
  (AD) Follow up study after average of 7 years. (GER)

115

Permanent cochleo-vestibulotoxic effects due to antibiotics, aminoglycoside, in humans.
Transient cochlear impairment due to salicylates in humans.
Ototoxic effects due to antimalarial, quinine, in humans.
Ototoxic effects due to chemical agent, nicotine, in humans.
  (AD) Report on ototoxic effects of various drugs.
  (AD) Need for audiometry and vestibular function tests with clinical use of ototoxic drugs. (FR)

116

Moderate unilateral sensorineural hearing loss in 1 of 36 fetuses due to total of 13 g of antibiotic, dihydrostreptomycin, in 33 humans, female, treated during pregnancy for tuberculosis.
  (AD) Child not treated with dihydrostreptomycin or streptomycin.
Sensorineural hearing loss due to 1 g daily for the first 30 days and then 1 g twice a week of antibiotic, dihydrostreptomycin (CB), in 8 (24 percent) of 33 humans, female, treated during pregnancy for tuberculosis.
Sensorineural hearing loss due to 1 g daily for the first 30 days and then 1 g twice a week of antibiotic, streptomycin (CB), in 8 (24 percent) of 33 humans, female, treated during pregnancy for tuberculosis.
Vestibular problems due to antibiotic, (SQ) dihydrostreptomycin, in 1 of 33 humans, female, treated during pregnancy for tuberculosis and chronic pyelonephritis.
Vestibular problems due to antibiotic, (SQ) streptomycin, in 1 of 33 humans, female, treated during pregnancy for tuberculosis and chronic pyelonephritis.
  (AD) Case histories, audiometry, and vestibular function tests for children and adults. (ENG)

141

Total bilateral sensorineural hearing loss, tinnitus, and vestibular problems due to 120 mg daily, total of 1.2 g, of antibiotic, gentamicin (SM), for 10 days in 1 human, adult, 22 years age, female, 46 kg weight, with purulent pleurisy after surgery.
Total bilateral sensorineural hearing loss, tinnitus, and vestibular problems due to 1 g every 2 days, total of 9 g, of antibiotic, kanamycin (SM), for 18 days in 1 human, adult, 22 years age, female, 46 kg weight, with purulent pleurisy after surgery.
Total bilateral sensorineural hearing loss and vestibular problems due to high doses, 160 mg daily, of antibiotic, gentamicin, for long period, 47 days, in 1 human, adult, 35 years age, with pleurisy.
Total bilateral sensorineural hearing loss and vestibular problems due to 1 g every 2 days of antibiotic, kanamycin, for 26 days in 1 human, adult, 35 years age, with pleurisy.
Total bilateral sensorineural hearing loss and vestibular problems due to 160 mg daily of antibiotic, gentamicin (SM), for 12 days in 1 human, adult, 35 years age, with pleurisy.
Total bilateral sensorineural hearing loss and vestibular problems due to 1 g every 2 days of antibiotic, kanamycin (SM), for 12 days in 1 human, adult, 35

years age, with pleurisy.
   (AD) Hearing loss confirmed by audiogram.
   (AD) Discussion of 2 case reports of gentamicin ototoxicity.   (FR)

184
Incr in ATP hydrolyzing system in stria vascularis and spiral ligament and
incr in ATP activity in membranous labyrinth due to parenteral, intraperitoneal, administration of 400 mg per kg 5 days a week of antibiotic, kanamycin (kanamycin sulfate), for 20 days in animals, guinea pigs, adult, with
normal pinna reflex.
Incr in ATP hydrolyzing system in stria vascularis and spiral ligament due to
parenteral, intraperitoneal, administration of 400 mg per kg 5 days a week of
antibiotic, streptomycin (streptomycin sulfate), for 20 days in animals,
guinea pigs, adult, with normal pinna reflex.
Decr in ATP hydrolyzing system in stria vascularis and spiral ligament and
decr in ATP activity in membranous labyrinth due to parenteral, intraperitoneal, administration of 400 mg per kg 5 days a week of antibiotic, dihydrostreptomycin (dihydrostreptomycin sulfate), for 20 days in animals, guinea
pigs, adult, with normal pinna reflex.
   (CT) Study of normal activity of ATP hydrolyzing system.   (ENG)

185
Ataxia, damage to hair cells of macula, and damage to hair cells of organ of
Corti due to parenteral, subcutaneous, administration of 10 to 80 mg per kg
daily of antibiotic, gentamicin (gentamicin sulfate), for 19 to 120 days in
animals, cats.
Ataxia due to 100 and 200 mg per kg daily of antibiotic, streptomycin (streptomycin sulfate), for 8 to 40 days in animals, cats.
Loss of Preyer reflex, decr in cochlear potential and eighth cranial nerve
action potential, and loss of outer hair cells of organ of Corti due to 80 to
200 mg per kg daily of antibiotic, gentamicin (gentamicin sulfate), in animals, guinea pigs.
Damage to cochlea due to 100 and 200 mg per kg of antibiotic, kanamycin
(kanamycin sulfate), in animals, guinea pigs.
   (AD) Comparative study of ototoxicity of gentamicin and other aminoglycoside antibiotics.
   (AD) Study suggested low risk of ototoxicity when gentamicin used in
   recommended clinical dose of 1 to 3 mg per kg.   (ENG)

192
Sensorineural hearing loss, dizziness, vertigo, and nystagmus due to topical,
cutaneous, administration in ointment of 0.3 percent concentration of antibiotic, (SQ) neomycin, for 5 months in 1 human, Caucasian, child, 9 years
age, with dermatomyositis.
Sensorineural hearing loss, dizziness, vertigo, and nystagmus due to topical,
cutaneous, administration in ointment of 1 percent concentration of antibiotic, (SQ) neomycin (CB), for 2 months in 1 human, Caucasian, child, 9 years
age, with dermatomyositis.
Sensorineural hearing loss, dizziness, vertigo, and nystagmus due to topical,
cutaneous, administration in ointment of 11 percent concentration of chemical
agent, (SQ) dimethyl sulfoxide (CB), for 2 months in 1 human, Caucasian,
child, 9 years age, with dermatomyositis.
   (AD) Potentiation of cochleo-vestibulotoxic effects of neomycin as result
   of incr cutaneous absorption due to dimethyl sulfoxide.
   (AD) Hearing loss confirmed by audiogram.   (ENG)

206
Transient bilateral sensorineural hearing loss due to oral administration of
50 mg every 6 hours of diuretic, ethacrynic acid, for 4 days initially and
then again 2 weeks later for 2 days in 1 human, Negro, adult, 55 years age,
female, with diabetes mellitus and kidney disorder.
   (AD) Hearing loss confirmed by audiogram.
Transient sensorineural hearing loss and tinnitus due to (SQ) oral and parenteral, (SQ) intravenous, administration of 300,300,400, and 500 mg of diuretic, ethacrynic acid, in 4 doses in 1 human, Caucasian, adult, 40 years age,
female, with chronic kidney disorder.
No auditory system problems due to parenteral, intravenous, administration of
(SQ) unspecified doses of diuretic, (SQ) ethacrynic acid, in (SQ) 3 injec-

tions in 1 human, Caucasian, adult, 20 years age, female, with kidney disorder.
Transient severe bilateral tinnitus, sensorineural hearing loss, and bilateral nystagmus due to parenteral, intravenous, administration of (SQ) 50 and 100 mg of diuretic, (SQ) ethacrynic acid, in (SQ) 2 injections in 1 human, Caucasian, adult, 20 years age, female, with kidney disorder.
Previous administration, 2 days before onset of ototoxic effects, of antibiotic, (SQ) colistin (sodium colistimethate), in 1 injection in 1 human, Caucasian, adult, 20 years age, female, with kidney disorder.
Transient sensorineural hearing loss within 12 hours of first dose due to oral administration of 50 mg of diuretic, ethacrynic acid, in 4 doses in 1 human, Caucasian, aged, 76 years age, male, with kidney disorder and with previous moderate hearing loss due to otosclerosis.
Severe tinnitus within 1 hour of first dose and sensorineural hearing loss within 1 half hour of second dose due to parenteral, intravenous, administration of 50 and 100 mg of diuretic, (SQ) ethacrynic acid, in 2 injections in 1 human, Caucasian, adult, 57 years age, female, with leukemia and kidney disorder.
Administration about 1 week previously of antibiotic, (SQ) streptomycin, in 1 human, Caucasian, adult, 57 years age, female, with leukemia and kidney disorder, for pneumonitis.
Administration about 1 week previously of antibiotic, (SQ) colistin (sodium colistimethate), in 1 human, Caucasian, adult, 57 years age, female, with leukemia and kidney disorder, for pneumonitis.
   (AD)   Discussion of 5 case reports of transient hearing loss due to treatment with ethacrynic acid.   (ENG)

213
Dizziness due to antibiotic, polymyxin B (polymyxin B sulfate), in humans.
Dizziness due to antibiotic, colistin (sodium colistimethate), in humans.
Ototoxic effects due to antibiotic, ristocetin, in humans.
Hearing loss due to antibiotic, vancomycin, in humans.
   (AD)   Report on pharmacology, clinical use, and toxicity of antibiotics. (ENG)

219
Cochleo-vestibulotoxic effects due to antibiotics in humans.
Transient and permanent sensorineural hearing loss due to diuretic, ethacrynic acid, in humans.
Transient sensorineural hearing loss, tinnitus, and vertigo due to salicylate, aspirin, in humans.
Transient and permanent sensorineural hearing loss and dizziness due to antimalarial, quinine, in humans.
Sensorineural hearing loss due to antimalarial, chloroquine, in humans.
Sensorineural hearing loss, tinnitus, and vertigo due to chemical agents in humans.
   (AD) Literature review of ototoxic drugs with clinical and histopathological correlations.
   (AD) Comment on ototoxicity of some chemical agents.
   (AD) Review of theories of mechanism of action of ototoxic drugs.   (ENG)

249
Cochleo-vestibulotoxic effects due to antibiotics, aminoglycoside, in humans.
Cochlear impairment due to antimalarial, quinine, in humans.
Transient cochlear impairment and vestibular problems due to salicylates in humans.
   (AD)   Occurrence of ototoxic effects with different dosages due to individual responses to drugs.
   (AD)   Need for observation and tests with clinical use of ototoxic drugs. (FR)

250
Damage to vestibular apparatus due to more than 1 g daily of antibiotic, streptomycin, for 60 to 120 days in 25 percent of humans.
Dizziness 5 days after cessation of treatment due to parenteral, intramuscular, administration of 1 g every 12 hours of antibiotic, streptomycin (SM), for 9 days in 1 human, adult, 44 years age, female, with peritonitis.
Simultaneous parenteral, intravenous, administration of 600 mg every 18 hours

of antibiotic, lincomycin (SM), for 9 days in 1 human, adult, 44 years age, female, with peritonitis.

(AD) Case report of vestibular problem due to streptomycin.
Damage to cochlea due to antibiotic, dihydrostreptomycin, for more than 1 week in 4 to 15 percent of humans.
Sensorineural hearing loss and damage to organ of Corti due to antibiotic, kanamycin, in humans.
Sensorineural hearing loss and damage to organ of Corti due to antibiotic, vancomycin, in humans.

(AD) Discussion of cochleo-vestibulotoxic effects due to antibiotic therapy in surgery. (ENG)

255

Slight hearing loss and vertigo due to parenteral, intramuscular, administration of 1 g every 24 hours of antibiotic, capreomycin (SM), for range of 5 to 12 months in 4 of 21 humans, adult, with pulmonary tuberculosis and without pretreatment audiometric changes.
Slight and severe hearing loss and vertigo due to parenteral, intramuscular, administration of 1 g every 24 hours of antibiotic, capreomycin (SM), for range of 5 to 12 months in 12 of 40 humans, adult, with pulmonary tuberculosis and with pretreatment audiometric changes.
Simultaneous administration of antituberculous agent, ethambutol (SM), in all of 61 humans, adult, with pulmonary tuberculosis.

(AD) Treatment with capreomycin discontinued in 4 humans with severe ototoxic effects.
(AD) Audiometry every 4 weeks during treatment. (ENG)

261

Nystagmus, ataxia, and loss of pinna reflex after 4 to 5 hours due to parenteral, intratympanic, administration of 5 to 20 mg, in 0.1 ml Ringer's solution, of antibiotic, streptomycin (streptomycin sulfate), in 1 ear of 15 animals, guinea pigs, pigmented, 250 to 350 g weight, with normal pinna reflex.

(CT) Use of other ear of 15 guinea pigs, control group.
No detected vestibular problems due to parenteral administration of 300 mg per kg daily of antibiotic, kanamycin (kanamycin sulfate), for 8 to 15 days in 5 animals, guinea pigs, pigmented, 250 to 350 g weight, with normal pinna reflex.
Degeneration of hair cells of vestibular apparatus and organ of Corti due to parenteral, intratympanic, administration of 5 to 20 mg, in 0.1 ml Ringer's solution, of antibiotic, streptomycin (streptomycin sulfate), in all 15 animals, guinea pigs, pigmented, 250 to 350 g weight, with normal pinna reflex.

(AD) Suggested relationship between histological changes and streptomycin dosage.
Degeneration of hair cells of vestibular apparatus and organ of Corti due to parenteral administration of 300 mg per kg daily of antibiotic, kanamycin (kanamycin sulfate), for 8 to 15 days in 4 out of 5 animals, guinea pigs, pigmented, 250 to 350 g weight, with normal pinna reflex.

(AD) Same pattern of degeneration in vestibular apparatus due to streptomycin and kanamycin.
(AD) Hair cells of vestibular apparatus more sensitive to streptomycin and hair cells of organ of Corti more sensitive to kanamycin. (ENG)

283

Effect on action potentials and cochlear microphonic and on vestibular apparatus due to range of doses of antibiotic, streptomycin, for range of periods in animals, cats.
Effect on action potentials and cochlear microphonic and on vestibular apparatus due to range of doses of antibiotic, kanamycin, for range of periods in animals, cats. (IT)

290

Vestibular problems, sensorineural hearing loss, and tinnitus due to total doses of 12 to 63 g of antibiotic, streptomycin, in 24 humans with tuberculosis.

(AD) Subjects tested after streptomycin intoxication with audiology and cupulometry.

(AD) Individual responses to streptomycin observed.
Changes in cupulometric curves for postrotatory nystagmus, showing changes in vestibular apparatus, due to 0.5 g daily, total doses of 30 to 100 g, of antibiotic, streptomycin (SM) (streptomycin sulfate), in 23 humans with various infections.
Simultaneous administration of 0.5 g of antibiotic, dihydrostreptomycin (SM), in 23 humans with various infections.
Simultaneous administration of antituberculous agent, PAS (SM), in 23 humans with various infections.
  (CT) Pretreatment vestibular function normal.
  (CT) Subjects tested with audiology and cupulometry before and during treatment with streptomycin.
  (AD) Hearing loss in 1 subject in group with cupulometry during treatment but in 5 subjects in other group with cupulometry only after treatment.
  (AD) Suggested use of cupulometry for possible prevention of streptomycin intoxication. (ENG)

293
Cochleo-vestibulotoxic effects due to antibiotic, streptomycin (SM), in humans, range of ages, with pulmonary tuberculosis.
Simultaneous administration of other antituberculous agents (SM) in humans, range of ages, with pulmonary tuberculosis.
  (AD) Report on toxic effects due to simultaneous treatment with various antituberculous agents. (BUL)

305
Dizziness, vertigo, tinnitus, and hearing loss due to oral administration of 50, 100, 150, and then 200 mg, incr daily doses each week, of anti-inflammatory agent, indomethacin, for 4 weeks in 7 of 24 humans, adult and aged, range of 23 to 69 years age, male and female, with rheumatoid arthritis.
Dizziness, vertigo, tinnitus, and hearing loss due to oral administration of 1.6, 3.2, 4.8, and then 6.4 g, incr daily doses each week, of salicylate, acetylsalicylic acid, for 4 weeks in 18 of 24 humans, adult and aged, range of 23 to 69 years age, male and female, with rheumatoid arthritis.
  (AD) Comparative study of effectiveness of indomethacin and acetylsalicylic acid in treatment of rheumatoid arthritis. (ENG)

308
Possible hearing loss due to antibiotic, kanamycin, in humans with tuberculosis.
Possible vestibular problems and cochlear impairment due to antibiotic, capreomycin, in humans with tuberculosis.
  (AD) Comment on possible cochleo-vestibulotoxic effects of antibiotics used in treatment of tuberculosis. (ENG)

311
Vertigo or hearing loss of 10 to 20 decibels due to antibiotic, streptomycin, in 14 of 67 humans with pulmonary tuberculosis.
Vertigo or hearing loss of 30 to 40 decibels due to antibiotic, streptomycin (CB), in 12 of 59 humans with pulmonary tuberculosis.
Vertigo or hearing loss of 30 to 40 decibels due to antibiotic, dihydrostreptomycin (CB), in 12 of 59 humans with pulmonary tuberculosis.
  (AD) Hearing loss confirmed by audiometry. (DUT)

316
Possible vestibular problems and cochlear impairment due to more than recommended dose of 15 to 30 mg per kg daily of antibiotic, streptomycin, for long period in humans.
Hearing loss due to parenteral, intramuscular, administration of total doses of 5 to 6 g of antibiotic, kanamycin, in humans, adult, with kidney disorder.
Possible hearing loss due to parenteral, topical, or oral administration of high doses of antibiotic, neomycin, for long period in humans.
Possible hearing loss due to high doses of antibiotic, framycetin, for long period in humans.
Possible hearing loss due to antibiotic, vancomycin, in humans.
Possible hearing loss and vestibular problems due to antibiotic, viomycin, in humans.
  (AD) High risk of ototoxicity with simultaneous administration of viomycin

and streptomycin.
Possible vestibular problems due to antibiotic, gentamicin, in humans.
   (AD) Administration of gentamicin not recommended for newborn infants, for
   humans during pregnancy, and for humans treated with other ototoxic drugs.
Ataxia and hearing loss due to antibiotic, colistin, in humans.
   (AD) Literature review on ototoxic antibiotics.
   (AD) Results of studies on use of pantothenate salt of some antibiotics
   for decr in ototoxicity not clear.
   (AD) Suggested effect of ototoxic antibiotics on breakdown of glucose on
   which hair cells of inner ear depend for energy.   (ENG)

                                                                          322
Cochleo-vestibulotoxic effects due to parenteral, intramuscular, administra-
tion of 1 g daily and then 1 g every other day of antibiotic, (SQ) capreomycin (SM), for 6 months in 3 of 36 humans, adult and aged, range of 20 to 80
years age, male and female, with pulmonary tuberculosis.
   (AD) Ototoxic effects confirmed by audiogram.
Simultaneous administration of 600 mg daily of antibiotic, (SQ) rifampicin
(SM), for 6 months in 36 humans, adult and aged, range of 20 to 80 years age,
male and female, with pulmonary tuberculosis.
Simultaneous administration of 25 mg per kg daily and then 15 mg per kg daily
of antituberculous agent, (SQ) ethambutol (SM), for 6 months in 36 humans,
adult and aged, range of 20 to 80 years age, male and female, with pulmonary
tuberculosis.
Cochleo-vestibulotoxic effects due to previous administration of (SQ) antibiotics, aminoglycoside, in 36 humans, adult and aged, range of 20 to 80
years age, male and female, with pulmonary tuberculosis.
   (AD) Therapy with antibiotics not satisfactory.   (FR)

                                                                          323
Progressive severe bilateral sensorineural hearing loss and vestibular problems due to parenteral administration of 1 g twice weekly of antibiotic, (SQ)
viomycin (viomycin pantothenate), for total of 10 weeks in 1 human, adult, 59
years age, female, with pulmonary tuberculosis and kidney disorder.
   (AD) Cochleo-vestibulotoxic effects confirmed by audiometry at different
   periods during and after treatment and by caloric test.
Previous administration of antibiotic, (SQ) chloramphenicol, in 1 human,
adult, 59 years age, female, for infection before diagnosis of tuberculosis.
Possible but not reported auditory system problems due to previous parenteral
administration of 0.5 g twice daily of antibiotic, (SQ) streptomycin, for 1
week in 1 human, adult, 59 years age, female, for infection before diagnosis
of tuberculosis.
   (AD) Suggested that possible previous ototoxic effects of streptomycin
   potentiated by viomycin (viomycin pantothenate).
Previous administration of antituberculous agent, (SQ) PAS, in 1 human,
adult, 59 years age, female, with pulmonary tuberculosis and kidney disorder.
(ENG)

                                                                          324
Ataxia, vestibular problems with improvement in some, and damage to hair
cells of vestibular apparatus due to parenteral, subcutaneous, administration
of 20 mg per kg of antibiotic, gentamicin (gentamicin sulfate), for 19 days
maximum for acute intoxication and 14 days for chronic intoxication in 15
animals, cats.
Hearing loss and damage to hair cells of cochlea due to parenteral, subcutaneous, administration of 20 mg per kg of antibiotic, gentamicin (gentamicin
sulfate), for 19 days maximum for acute intoxication and 14 days for chronic
intoxication in 1 of 15 animals, cats.
   (AD) Preliminary study to determine minimum toxic level of gentamicin by
   parenteral route made previously.
   (AD) Cochleo-vestibulotoxic effects determined by audiometry and vestibular function tests.
Permanent severe vestibular problems and damage to hair cells of vestibular
apparatus due to parenteral, subcutaneous, administration of 200 mg per kg of
antibiotic, streptomycin (streptomycin sulfate), in 3 animals, cats.
Hearing loss and damage to hair cells of cochlea due to parenteral, subcutaneous, administration of 200 mg per kg of antibiotic, streptomycin (streptomycin sulfate), in 2 of 3 animals, cats.

Ataxia, vestibular problems, and damage to hair cells of vestibular apparatus
due to topical administration to bulla in solution of 6 percent concentration
in water of antibiotic, gentamicin (gentamicin sulfate), for 19 days in 1
animal, cat.
Ataxia, vestibular problems, and more severe damage to hair cells of vestibular apparatus due to topical administration to bulla in solution of 6 percent
concentration in Monex of antibiotic, gentamicin (gentamicin sulfate), for 5
days in 3 animals, cats.
   (CT) Same method using water or Monex without gentamicin in 11 cats,
   control group, showed no ototoxic effects.
   (AD) Preliminary study to determine concentration of gentamicin for topical route made previously.
Vestibular problems due to topical administration to bulla in solution of 6
percent concentration in water of antibiotic, neomycin, for 31 days in 2
animals, cats.
   (AD) Comparative study of effects of gentamicin and other aminoglycoside
   antibiotics.
   (AD) Ototoxicity of gentamicin dose related. (ENG)

325

High frequency hearing loss due to parenteral, intramuscular, administration
of total of 15 mg per kg in 2 doses 5 times a week of antibiotic, (SQ) capreomycin (SM), for 37 and 45 days in 2 of 70 humans, adult, 35 and 64 years
age, with pulmonary tuberculosis and with previous treatment with other
ototoxic drugs.
Transient vertigo due to parenteral, intramuscular, administration of total
of 15 mg per kg in 2 doses 5 times a week of antibiotic, (SQ) capreomycin
(SM), for 5, 25, and 94 days in 3 of 70 humans, adult, 39, 61, and 62 years
age, with pulmonary tuberculosis and with previous treatment with streptomycin.
Simultaneous administration of other (SQ) antituberculous agents (SM), in 70
humans, adult, male and female, with pulmonary tuberculosis.
Possible ototoxic effects due to previous administration of antibiotic, (SQ)
streptomycin, in 3 of 70 humans, adult, 39, 61, and 62 years age, with pulmonary tuberculosis. (ENG)

332

No subjective hearing loss but objective hearing loss over 20 decibels and
tinnitus due to parenteral, intramuscular, administration of 1 g daily for
first 60 days and then 1 g twice a week of antibiotic, capreomycin (SM), for
6 months in 3 of 100 humans treated for pulmonary tuberculosis.
Hearing loss, tinnitus, or dizziness due to parenteral, intramuscular, administration of 1 g daily for first 60 days and then 1 g twice a week of
antibiotic, streptomycin (SM), for 6 months in 8 of 99 humans treated for
pulmonary tuberculosis.
Hearing loss over 20 decibels due to parenteral, intramuscular, administration of 1 g daily for first 60 days and then 1 g twice a week of antibiotic,
streptomycin (SM), for 6 months in 3 of 99 humans treated for pulmonary
tuberculosis.
Simultaneous oral administration of 0.3 g daily in 2 doses of antituberculous
agent, isoniazid (SM), for 6 months in humans treated for pulmonary tuberculosis.
Simultaneous administration of 10 g daily in 3 doses of antituberculous
agent, PAS (SM), for 6 months in humans treated for pulmonary tuberculosis.
   (AD) Report on ototoxic effects of antibiotics used in initial treatment
   of tuberculosis.
High frequency hearing loss, tinnitus, or dizziness due to parenteral, intramuscular, administration of 1 g daily for first 60 days and then 1 g twice a
week of antibiotic, capreomycin (SM), for 6 months in 6 of 66 humans retreated for pulmonary tuberculosis.
No subjective auditory system problems but objective hearing loss over 20
decibels due to parenteral, intramuscular, administration of 1 g 3 times a
week of antibiotic, kanamycin (SM), for 6 months in 4 of 40 humans retreated
for pulmonary tuberculosis.
No subjective auditory system problems but objective hearing loss over 20
decibels due to parenteral, intramuscular, administration of 1 g daily for
first 60 days and then 1 g twice a week of antibiotic, streptomycin (SM), for
6 months in 1 of 13 humans retreated for pulmonary tuberculosis.

Simultaneous oral administration of 0.3 g daily in 2 doses of antituberculous agent, isoniazid (SM), for 6 months in humans retreated for pulmonary tuberculosis.
   (AD) Report on ototoxic effects of antibiotics used in retreatment of tuberculosis.
   (CT) Audiometry, pretreatment and during treatment, 2 times a month in first 2 months and then 1 time a month.
   (AD) Comparative study of clinical use and cochleo-vestibulotoxic effects of capreomycin and other antibiotics in treatment and retreatment of pulmonary tuberculosis. (ENG)

                                                                        333
Vestibular problems due to antibiotic, streptomycin, in humans.
Severe cochlear impairment due to antibiotic, dihydrostreptomycin, in humans.
Loss of hair cells in organ of Corti and hearing loss due to antibiotics, aminoglycoside, in humans.
Hearing loss in fetus due to antimalarial, quinine, in humans, female, treated during pregnancy.
Transient hearing loss due to high doses of salicylate, aspirin, for long period in humans.
   (AD) Discussion of possible cochleo-vestibulotoxic effects of ototoxic drugs.
   (AD) Ototoxic effects related to concurrent disorders, dosage, duration of treatment, and age of individuals. (ENG)

                                                                        335
Vestibular problems due to antibiotic, streptomycin, in humans.
Severe cochlear impairment due to antibiotic, dihydrostreptomycin, in humans.
Cochlear impairment due to parenteral, oral, and topical administration of antibiotic, neomycin, in humans.
Tinnitus and hearing loss due to antibiotic, kanamycin, in humans.
Vestibular problems and hearing loss due to antibiotic, gentamicin, in humans.
   (AD) Discussion of clinical use and possible cochleo-vestibulotoxic effects of aminoglycoside antibiotics. (SP)

                                                                        343
No hearing loss but decr in vestibular function, asymptomatic except for dizziness in 1 case, due to 1 g daily of antibiotic, capreomycin (SM), for 4 months or more in 4 of 25 humans, adolescent, adult, and aged, range of 17 to 67 years age, male and female, 80 to 160 lb weight, with pulmonary tuberculosis and with kidney disorder in 2 cases.
Transient dizziness with no objective decr in vestibular function due to 1 g daily of antibiotic, capreomycin (SM), for 4 months or more in 3 of 25 humans, adolescent, adult, and aged, range of 17 to 67 years age, male and female, 80 to 160 lb weight, with pulmonary tuberculosis.
Simultaneous administration of 300 mg daily of antituberculous agent, isoniazid (SM), for 4 months or more in 25 humans, adolescent, adult, and aged, range of 17 to 67 years age, male and female, 80 to 160 lb weight, with pulmonary tuberculosis.
   (CT) Pure tone audiometry, caloric tests, and cupulometry, pretreatment and during treatment with capreomycin.
   (AD) Study of clinical use and cochleo-vestibulotoxic effects of capreomycin.
Hearing loss, asymptomatic in 1 case and symptomatic in 1 case, due to 1 g daily of antibiotic, viomycin, in 2 of 75 humans with pulmonary tuberculosis.
Objective decr in vestibular function due to 1 g daily of antibiotic, viomycin, in 21 of 75 humans with pulmonary tuberculosis.
Hearing loss, asymptomatic, due to 1 g daily of antibiotic, streptomycin, in 2 of 61 humans with pulmonary tuberculosis.
Objective decr in vestibular function due to 1 g daily of antibiotic, streptomycin, in 8 of 61 humans with pulmonary tuberculosis.
   (CT) Audiometry and vestibular function tests, pretreatment and during treatment with viomycin or streptomycin.
   (AD) Results of study on capreomycin comp w results of previous study on viomycin and streptomycin. (ENG)

Transient hearing loss and vestibular problem due to salicylate, aspirin, in humans.
Decr in cochlear microphonic and action potential and decr in malic dehydrogenase in endolymph and perilymph due to salicylate, aspirin, in humans.
  (AD) Suggested that cochleo-vestibulotoxic effects of salicylates due to electrophysiological and biochemical changes and not structural changes.
Primary distribution in stria vascularis and spiral ligament due to salicylate, aspirin, in humans.
  (AD) Possible but not definite location of toxic activity of aspirin.
High concentration in inner ear after 5 to 7 hours due to parenteral, intraperitoneal, administration of salicylate, sodium salicylate, in animals, cats.
  (AD) Report on clinical use and ototoxic effects of aspirin. (ENG)

353
Dizziness due to oral administration of 600 mg of analgesic, clonixin, in 1 dose in 2 of 24 humans, adult and aged, 21 to 68 years age, male and female, 126 to 210 lb weight, treated after surgery.
Hearing loss due to parenteral, intramuscular, administration of 6 mg of analgesic, morphine (morphine sulfate), in 1 dose in 1 of 24 humans, adult and aged, 21 to 68 years age, male and female, 126 to 210 lb weight, treated after surgery.
  (AD) Comparative study of effectiveness of oral clonixin and parenteral morphine in treatment after surgery. (ENG)

358
Severe to total hearing loss due to antibiotic, paromomycin, in most of humans treated.
Severe to total hearing loss due to antibiotic, streptomycin, in most of humans treated.
Severe to total hearing loss due to antibiotic, neomycin, in most of humans treated.
Objective but no subjective vestibular problems due to antibiotic, streptomycin, in 2 humans. (RUS)

361
Transient dizziness and tinnitus due to oral administration of 750 mg daily of anti-inflammatory agent, ibuprofen, for 5 days in 1 of 9 humans, adult and aged, 37 to 67 years age, male and female, with rheumatoid arthritis.
  (AD) Ibuprofen therapy discontinued after 5 days.
Hearing loss and tinnitus due to oral administration of 5 g daily of salicylate, aspirin, for 1 week in 3 of 9 humans, adult and aged, 37 to 67 years age, male and female, with rheumatoid arthritis.
  (AD) Comparative study of ibuprofen, aspirin, and prednisolone in treatment of rheumatoid arthritis. (ENG)

367
Auditory system problems due to oral administration of 150 mg daily of antituberculous agent, thiacetazone (CB), for 12 weeks in 47 of 581 humans, adolescent and adult, 15 years or over age, male and female, with pulmonary tuberculosis.
Auditory system problems due to oral administration of 150 mg daily of antituberculous agent, thiacetazone (CB) (IB), for 12 weeks in 39 of 584 humans, adolescent and adult, 15 years or over age, male and female, with pulmonary tuberculosis, with administration of vitamins and antihistamine.
Combined oral administration of 300 mg daily of antituberculous agent, isoniazid (CB), for 12 weeks in humans, adolescent and adult, 15 years or over age, male and female, with pulmonary tuberculosis.
  (AD) Study of effect of inhibitors on toxicity of drugs in 1 group with drug regimen of thiacetazone and isoniazid in combination.
Auditory system problems due to parenteral administration of 1 g daily of antibiotic, streptomycin (SM), for 12 weeks in 227 of 689 humans, adolescent and adult, 15 years or over age, male and female, with pulmonary tuberculosis.
Auditory system problems due to parenteral administration of 1 g daily of antibiotic, streptomycin (SM) (IB), for 12 weeks in 218 of 707 humans, adolescent and adult, 15 years or over age, male and female, with pulmonary tuberculosis, with administration of vitamins and antihistamine.

Auditory system problems due to simultaneous oral administration of 150 mg daily of antituberculous agent, thiacetazone (SM), for 12 weeks in humans, adolescent and adult, 15 years or over age, male and female, with pulmonary tuberculosis.

Simultaneous oral administration of 300 mg daily of antituberculous agent, isoniazid (SM), for 12 weeks in humans, adolescent and adult, 15 years or over age, male and female, with pulmonary tuberculosis.

   (AD) Study of effect of inhibitors on toxicity of drugs in 1 group with
   drug regimen of streptomycin, thiacetazone, and isoniazid.

Auditory system problems due to parenteral administration of 1 g daily of antibiotic, streptomycin (SM), for 12 weeks in 109 of 711 humans, adolescent and adult, 15 years or over age, male and female, with pulmonary tuberculosis.

Auditory system problems due to parenteral administration of 1 g daily of antibiotic, streptomycin (SM) (IB), for 12 weeks in 111 of 696 humans, adolescent and adult, 15 years or over age, male and female, with pulmonary tuberculosis, with administration of vitamins and antihistamine.

Simultaneous oral administration of 300 mg daily of antituberculous agent, isoniazid (SM), for 12 weeks in humans, adolescent and adult, 15 years or over age, male and female, with pulmonary tuberculosis.

   (AD) Study of effect of inhibitors on toxicity of drugs in 1 group with
   drug regimen of streptomycin and isoniazid.

   (AD) Study of effectiveness of inhibitors in prevention of toxic effects
   of thiacetazone and streptomycin.

   (AD) Study suggested that vitamins and antihistamine not effective in
   prevention of toxicity. (ENG)

                                                                          368
Possible vestibular problems and hearing loss due to antibiotic, streptomycin, in humans with tuberculosis.

Permanent hearing loss due to antibiotic, dihydrostreptomycin, in humans with tuberculosis.

Possible permanent hearing loss due to antibiotic, kanamycin, in humans with tuberculosis.

Possible vestibular problems and hearing loss due to antibiotic, viomycin, in humans with tuberculosis.

Possible damage to eighth cranial nerve due to antibiotic, capreomycin, in humans with tuberculosis.

   (AD) Discussion of primary and secondary drugs used in tuberculosis chemotherapy. (FR)

                                                                          384
Usually transient hearing loss and no structural damage to organ of Corti, stria vascularis, and spiral ganglion due to oral or topical administration of salicylates in humans.

Hearing loss due to antimalarial, quinine, in humans.

Usually permanent hearing loss due to antimalarial, chloroquine, in humans.

Transient and permanent hearing loss and possible damage to hair cells of organ of Corti due to diuretic, ethacrynic acid, in humans.

Sensorineural hearing loss due to cardiovascular agent, hexadimethrine bromide, in humans with kidney disorder.

Sensorineural hearing loss and damage to organ of Corti due to topical administration of antineoplastic, nitrogen mustard, in humans.

Sensorineural hearing loss due to high doses of antibiotic, chloramphenicol, in humans.

Primary vestibular problems due to antibiotic, streptomycin, in humans.

Hearing loss due to high doses usually of antibiotic, streptomycin, in humans.

   (AD) Early detection of hearing loss by audiometry prevents permanent
   damage.

High frequency hearing loss and severe damage to outer hair cells and slight damage to inner hair cells of organ of Corti due to antibiotic, kanamycin, in humans.

Sensorineural hearing loss due to parenteral, oral, and topical administration of antibiotic, neomycin, in humans with or without kidney disorders.

Degeneration of hair cells of organ of Corti and of nerve process due to antibiotics, aminoglycoside, in animals.

   (AD) Literature review of physiological and structural cochleo-vestibulotoxic effects of ototoxic drugs.

(AD)   Discussion of suggested mechanism of ototoxicity and routes of drugs to inner ear.

Bilateral sensorineural hearing loss due to oral administration of antibiotic, neomycin, in 4 of 8 humans with liver disease.

Bilateral sensorineural hearing loss due to oral administration of range of doses of antibiotic, neomycin (SM), in 2 of 5 humans with liver disease.

Bilateral sensorineural hearing loss due to diuretics (SM), in 2 of 5 humans with liver disease.

Transient progression of previous hearing loss due to parenteral, intravenous, administration of diuretic, ethacrynic acid (SM), in 1 injection in 1 of 5 humans with liver disease.

(CT)   Normal cochlear function in 6 humans, control group, with liver disease and not treated with neomycin or diuretics.

(CT)   Normal cochlear function in 13 humans, control group, with liver disease and treated with diuretics but not with neomycin.

(AD)   Hearing loss confirmed by audiometry.

(AD)   Reported that hearing loss due to neomycin or diuretics in humans with liver disease not related to dosage.

(AD)   Clinical study of effects of treatment with neomycin and diuretics in humans with liver disease.

Bilateral sensorineural hearing loss and vertigo due to antibiotic, ampicillin, in 1 human, adolescent, 17 years age, female, with tonsillitis.

(AD)   Cited case report.

Severe sensorineural hearing loss and vertigo due to topical administration in ear drops of antibiotic, framycetin, in 1 human, adult, 42 years age, male, with previous slight high frequency hearing loss.

(AD)   Cited case report.

Atrophy of hair cells of organ of Corti and hearing loss due to antibiotic, dihydrostreptomycin, in humans with tuberculous meningitis.

(AD)   Cited study.

Loss of inner hair cells and damage to outer hair cells due to 18 g of antibiotic, neomycin, for 18 days in 1 human.

(AD)   Cited case report.   (ENG)

392

No hearing loss but tinnitus due to parenteral, intramuscular, administration of range of 0.05 to 1.0 g daily according to age of antibiotic, kanamycin, for short period in 4 of 125 humans, infant, child, and adult, with acute otorhinolaryngological infections.

(AD)   Audiograms showed no hearing loss.

Hearing loss, subjective in 1 case and latent in others, but no vestibular problems due to 1.0 g daily 2 times a week of antibiotic, (SQ) kanamycin, for long period in 15 of 66 humans, adolescent and adult, 15 to 55 years age, with pulmonary tuberculosis and with previous streptomycin treatment.

(CT)   Audiogram before and during treatment with kanamycin.

Hearing loss due to previous administration of antibiotic, (SQ) streptomycin, in 31 of 272 humans.

Sensorineural hearing loss due to previous administration of total of 600 g of antibiotic, (SQ) streptomycin, in 1 human, adult, 27 years age.

More severe sensorineural hearing loss, subjective, due to total of 136 g of antibiotic, (SQ) kanamycin, in 1 human, adult, 27 years age.

(AD)   Case report of hearing loss due to streptomycin potentiated by treatment with kanamycin.

Hearing loss, latent, and tinnitus, but no vestibular problems due to total of over 20 g to over 300 g of antibiotic, kanamycin, for long period in 10 of 70 humans with pulmonary tuberculosis and no previous chemotherapy.

(CT)   Audiogram before and during treatment with kanamycin.

(AD)   Clinical studies of effects of treatment with kanamycin for short and long periods.

Vestibular problems after 10 to 12 days due to parenteral administration of 100 mg per kg daily of antibiotic, streptomycin, in 3 animals, cats, 2 kg weight.

Slight vestibular problems after 30 days due to 300 mg per kg daily of antibiotic, kanamycin, in 3 animals, cats, 2 kg weight.

Decr in cochlear microphonic due to 200 mg per kg daily of antibiotic, streptomycin, in 11 injections in animals, cats.

Slight decr in cochlear microphonic due to 300 mg per kg daily of antibiotic,

kanamycin, in 11 to 60 injections in animals, cats.
(AD) Comparative experimental studies of cochleo-vestibulotoxic effects of
kanamycin and streptomycin in cats.
(AD) Different effects of 2 aminoglycoside antibiotics on vestibular
function but similar effects on cochlear function. (ENG)

409

Primary damage to hair cells of organ of Corti, hearing loss, and possible
vestibular problems due to antibiotic, viomycin, in humans.
Damage to hair cells of organ of Corti and hearing loss due to antibiotic,
neomycin, in humans.
Damage to hair cells of organ of Corti and hearing loss due to antibiotic,
kanamycin, in humans.
Primary damage to vestibular apparatus, vestibular problems, and possible
hearing loss due to antibiotic, streptomycin, in humans.
Primary damage to vestibular apparatus, vestibular problems, and possible
hearing loss due to antibiotic, gentamicin, in humans.
(AD) Need for audiometry and vestibular function tests, pretreatment and
during treatment, with clinical use of aminoglycoside antibiotics.
(AD) Incr in blood levels and ototoxicity of antibiotics in humans with
kidney disorders. (ENG)

419

Hearing loss and vestibular problems due to antibiotic, streptomycin, in
humans with various disorders.
Hearing loss and vestibular problems due to other ototoxic drugs in humans
with various disorders.
(AD) Discussion of cochleo-vestibulotoxic effects of ototoxic drugs used
in therapy for various disorders. (GER)

420

Acute hearing loss due to 10 mg on first day and then 60 mg daily for 3 days,
total of 220 mg, of antibiotic, (SQ) gentamicin, in total of 4 days in 1
human, adolescent, 16 years age, with kidney disorder.
(AD) Hearing loss confirmed by audiogram.
Previous administration of antibiotic, (SQ) colistin, in 1 human, adolescent,
16 years age, with kidney disorder.
Vestibular problems due to 40 mg daily, total of 400 mg, of antibiotic,
gentamicin, in total of 10 days in 1 human, aged, 68 years age, with kidney
disorder. (GER)

434

Slight ototoxic effects due to range of doses of antibiotic, streptomycin, in
8 of 40 humans, female, treated for tuberculosis during pregnancy.
Slight ototoxic effects due to range of doses of antibiotic, dihydrostreptomycin, in 2 of 40 humans, female, treated for tuberculosis during pregnancy.
Vestibular problems and sensorineural hearing loss in mother and vestibular
problems in fetus due to total of 27 g of antibiotic, streptomycin (CB), for
2.5 months in 1 human, adult, 28 years age, female, treated for pulmonary
tuberculosis at end of pregnancy.
Vestibular problems and sensorineural hearing loss in mother and vestibular
problems in fetus due to total of 27 g of antibiotic, dihydrostreptomycin
(CB), for 2.5 months in 1 human, adult, 28 years age, female, treated for
pulmonary tuberculosis at end of pregnancy.
(AD) Pure tone audiometry and vestibular function tests in child, female,
at 10 years age.
Mixed hearing loss in mother and severe sensorineural hearing loss and vestibular problems in fetus due to total of 28 g of antibiotic, (SQ) dihydrostreptomycin, for 2.5 months in 1 human, adult, 22 years age, female, treated for
tuberculosis at beginning of pregnancy.
Mixed hearing loss in mother and severe sensorineural hearing loss and vestibular problems in fetus due to total of 28 g of antibiotic, (SQ) streptomycin, for 2.5 months in 1 human, adult, 22 years age, female, treated for
tuberculosis at beginning of pregnancy.
(AD) Pure tone audiometry and vestibular function tests in child, female,
at 10 years age. (ENG)

444

Changes in cochlear function and vestibular function due to analeptic, caffeine, in animals and humans.
Changes in cochlear function and vestibular function due to analeptic, amphetamine, in animals and humans.
Changes in cochlear function and vestibular function due to sedatives and tranquilizers in animals and humans.
  (AD) Suggested mechanism of action of drugs.
  (AD) Literature review of ototoxic effects of drugs.   (IT)

446

Vestibular problems only in 5 and dizziness, tinnitus, and hearing loss in 1 due to parenteral, intramuscular, administration of 1 g daily in single injection of antibiotic, streptomycin (SM) (streptomycin sulfate), for 6 months only in 6 (6 percent) of 65 humans, Negro, adolescent and adult, 15 to over 55 years age, male and female, 80 to over 140 lb weight, for retreatment of pulmonary tuberculosis.
Simultaneous oral administration of 15 g of antituberculous agent, PAS (SM) (sodium PAS), for 1 year in 65 humans, Negro, adolescent and adult, 15 to over 55 years age, male and female, 80 to over 140 lb weight, for retreatment of pulmonary tuberculosis.
  (AD) Study of value of regimen of streptomycin, PAS, and pyrazinamide in retreatment of pulmonary tuberculosis.   (ENG)

447

Dizziness and tinnitus within first 14 weeks due to 150 mg daily in 2 divided doses of antituberculous agent, thiacetazone (SM), for 26 weeks in 30 of 410 humans, adolescent and adult, 15 to over 55 years age, 30 to over 50 kg weight, with tuberculosis.
No ototoxic effects due to 300 mg daily in 2 divided doses of antituberculous agent, isoniazid (SM), for 26 weeks in 30 of 410 humans, adolescent and adult, 15 to over 55 years age, 30 to over 50 kg weight, with tuberculosis.
  (AD) Study of toxicity of thiacetazone in treatment of tuberculosis.   (ENG)

457

Tinnitus and progressive sensorineural hearing loss due to parenteral, intramuscular, administration of antibiotic, (SQ) streptomycin, for 10 days in 1 human, adult, 38 years age, female, with infections and later development of kidney disorder.
Tinnitus and progressive sensorineural hearing loss due to 13.2 g of antibiotic, (SQ) kanamycin, for 11 days in 1 human, adult, 38 years age, female, with infections and kidney disorder.
Hearing loss due to antimalarial, (SQ) quinine, in 1 human, adult, 20 years age, male, with various infections and later development of kidney disorder.
Hearing loss due to 400 mg 2 times daily, total dose of 6.5 g, of antibiotic, (SQ) kanamycin (SM), for 8 days in 1 human, adult, 20 years age, male, with various infections and later development of kidney disorder.
Hearing loss due to 150 mg 2 times daily, total dose of 2400 mg, of antibiotic, (SQ) colistin (SM), for 8 days in 1 human, adult, 20 years age, male, with various infections and later development of kidney disorder.
Tinnitus, total bilateral hearing loss, and vestibular problems due to parenteral, intramuscular, administration of 4.0 g daily, total of 21 g, of antibiotic, (SQ) kanamycin (SM), for 5 days in 1 human, adult, 20 years age, male, with infections and kidney disorder.
Tinnitus, total bilateral hearing loss, and vestibular problems due to 0.6 g daily, total dose of 1.3 g, of antibiotic, (SQ) colistin (SM), for 2 days in 1 human, adult, 20 years age, male, with infections and kidney disorder.
Tinnitus, total bilateral hearing loss, and vestibular problems due to 2 g and then 8 g per 24 hours in divided doses, total dose of 26.5 g, of antibiotic, (SQ) chloramphenicol, for 9 days in 1 human, adult, 20 years age, male, with infections and kidney disorder.
Bilateral hearing loss due to 1 g daily of antibiotic, actinomycin (SM), for 5 days in 1 human, adult, 62 years age, male, with infections and kidney disorder.
Bilateral hearing loss due to unknown dose of antibiotic, kanamycin (SM), for 5 days in 1 human, adult, 62 years age, male, with infections and kidney disorder.

Bilateral hearing loss and vestibular problems due to parenteral administration of high doses of antibiotic, (SQ) neomycin, for total of 21 days in 1 human, adult, 25 years age, male, with infection from wound.
Previous administration of unspecified doses of antibiotic, (SQ) streptomycin, in 1 human, adult, 25 years age, male, with infection from wound.
Later administration of antibiotic, (SQ) chloramphenicol, in 1 human, adult, 25 years age, male, with infection from wound.
Tinnitus and rapidly progressive bilateral hearing loss due to parenteral, intramuscular, administration of 0.5 g every 12 hours of antibiotic, (SQ) streptomycin, for 5 days in 1 human, adult, 21 years age, male, with infection from wound.
Tinnitus and rapidly progressive bilateral hearing loss due to parenteral, intramuscular, administration of 200 mg daily, total of 6.8 g, of antibiotic, (SQ) colistin (SM), in 1 human, adult, 21 years age, male, with infection from wound.
Tinnitus and rapidly progressive bilateral hearing loss due to parenteral administration of unspecified doses of antibiotic, (SQ) neomycin (SM), for about 35 days in 1 human, adult, 21 years age, male, with infection from wound.
Tinnitus and progressive bilateral hearing loss due to parenteral administration of 2 l per 24 hours of 1 percent solution of antibiotic, (SQ) neomycin, for 10 days in 1 human, adult, 26 years age, male, with infection from wound.
    (AD) Hearing loss confirmed by audiometry.
Previous administration of 500 mg four times a day of antibiotic, (SQ) ampicillin, in 1 human, adult, 26 years age, male, with infection from wound.
Bilateral sudden deafness due to administration in dialysis fluid of less than 150 mg of antibiotic, neomycin (SM), in 1 human, adult, 44 years age, female, with kidney disorder.
Bilateral sudden deafness due to 50 mg of diuretic, ethacrynic acid (SM), in 1 human, adult, 44 years age, female, with kidney disorder.
    (AD) Hearing loss confirmed by audiology.
Tinnitus and progressive bilateral hearing loss beginning after 8 days of treatment due to parenteral administration of 1 l every 4 hours for 3 days and then every 8 hours for 10 days of 1 percent solution of antibiotic, neomycin, in 1 human, adult, 20 years age, male, with infection from wound.
    (AD) Hearing loss confirmed by audiology.
Tinnitus and bilateral sensorineural hearing loss due to parenteral, intramuscular, administration of 1 g and then 0.5 g every 12 hours of antibiotic, streptomycin (SM), for 15 days in 1 human, adult, 23 years age, male, with infection from wound.
Tinnitus and bilateral sensorineural hearing loss due to topical administration by irrigation of 1 percent solution every 12 hours of antibiotic, neomycin (SM), for 14 days in 1 human, adult, 23 years age, male, with infection from wound.
    (AD) Hearing loss confirmed by audiometry.
    (AD) Discussion of 10 case reports. (ENG)

                                                                    460
No significant decr in cochlear microphonics due to parenteral, subcutaneous, administration of 100 mg per kg daily for 5 days a week, total dose of 7.5 g per kg, of antibiotic, streptomycin (streptomycin sulfate), for 75 days in animals, guinea pigs.
Statistically significant decr in cochlear microphonics at 1 of 18 points examined, damage to hair cells of organ of Corti, slight damage to stria vascularis and spiral ganglion, damage to macula utriculi and cristae, slight damage to macula sacculi, and vestibular problems due to parenteral, subcutaneous, administration of 200 mg per kg daily, then 400 mg per kg, followed by return to 200 mg per kg, total dose of 15 g per kg, of antibiotic, streptomycin (streptomycin sulfate), for 58 days in animals, guinea pigs.
    (AD) Vestibular problems confirmed by vestibular function tests.
No significant decr in cochlear microphonics due to parenteral, subcutaneous, administration of 100 mg per kg daily for 5 days a week, total dose of 7.5 g per kg, of antibiotic, viomycin (viomycin sulfate), for 75 days in animals, guinea pigs.
Significant decr in cochlear microphonics, damage to hair cells of organ of Corti and to stria vascularis, slight damage to spiral ganglion, and slight damage to macula utriculi and crista ampullaris due to parenteral, subcutaneous, administration of 200 mg per kg daily for 5 days a week, then 400 mg

per kg, total dose of 15 g per kg, of antibiotic, viomycin (viomycin sulfate), for total of 67 days in animals, guinea pigs.
   (AD) Most toxicity for cochlear microphonics in guinea pig due to viomycin.
No significant decr in cochlear microphonics due to parenteral, subcutaneous,
administration of 100 mg per kg daily for 5 days each week, total dose of 7.5
g per kg, of antibiotic, capreomycin (capreomycin sulfate), for 75 days in
animals, guinea pigs.
No significant decr in cochlear microphonics, slight damage to outer hair
cells of organ of Corti and to stria vascularis, and no damage to vestibular
apparatus due to parenteral, subcutaneous, administration of 200 mg per kg
daily for 5 days a week, then 400 mg per kg, total dose of 15 g per kg, of
antibiotic, capreomycin (capreomycin sulfate), for total of 67 days in animals, guinea pigs.
   (CT) Same method using subcutaneous administration of 0.25 cc daily of
   isotonic saline in guinea pigs, control group.
   (AD) Least toxicity for inner ear of guinea pig due to capreomycin.
   (AD) Study of functional and structural cochleo-vestibulotoxic effects of
   streptomycin, viomycin, and capreomycin.
   (AD) Statistical analysis of results.   (ENG)

                                                                          482
Decr in cochlear function and vestibular function due to parenteral, intramuscular, administration of 50 to 100 mg per kg of antibiotic, streptomycin
(streptomycin sulfate), for 35 days in animals, guinea pigs, pigmented, 400
to 500 g weight.
   (AD) More ototoxic effects with higher dosage.
Decr in cochlear function with both doses but decr in vestibular function
with only higher dose due to parenteral, intramuscular, administration of 50
to 100 mg per kg of antibiotic, dihydrostreptomycin (dihydrostreptomycin
sulfate), for 35 days in animals, guinea pigs, pigmented, 400 to 500 g
weight.
   (AD) More decr in cochlear function with higher dosage.
Decr in cochlear function in all animals but decr in vestibular function in 2
groups only due to parenteral, intramuscular, administration of 50 to 100 mg
per kg of antibiotic, kanamycin, for 35 days in animals, guinea pigs, pigmented, 400 to 500 g weight.
   (AD) More decr in cochlear function with higher dosage.
Decr in cochlear function due to parenteral, intramuscular, administration of
20 mg per kg of diuretic, ethacrynic acid, for 35 days in animals, guinea
pigs, pigmented, 400 to 500 g weight.
   (CT) Study of guinea pigs, control group, not treated with ototoxic drugs.
Decr in ototoxic effects due to parenteral, intramuscular, administration of
100 mg per kg of antibiotic, streptomycin (IB) (streptomycin sulfate), for 35
days in animals, guinea pigs, pigmented, 400 to 500 g weight, with administration of 1 mg per kg of various inhibitors.
Decr in ototoxic effects due to parenteral, intramuscular, administration of
100 mg per kg of antibiotic, dihydrostreptomycin (IB) (dihydrostreptomycin
sulfate), for 35 days in animals, guinea pigs, pigmented, 400 to 500 g
weight, with administration of 1 mg per kg of various inhibitors.
Decr in ototoxic effects due to parenteral, intramuscular, administration of
100 mg per kg of antibiotic, kanamycin (IB), for 35 days in animals, guinea
pigs, pigmented, 400 to 500 g weight, with administration of 1 mg per kg of
various inhibitors.
Decr in ototoxic effects due to parenteral, intramuscular, administration of
20 mg per kg of diuretic, ethacrynic acid (IB), for 35 days in animals,
guinea pigs, pigmented, 400 to 500 g weight, with administration of 1 mg per
kg of various inhibitors.
   (AD) Measurement of Preyer reflex and vestibular function tests.
Ototoxic effects, functional and structural, due to parenteral, intraperitoneal, administration of 100 mg per kg of antibiotic, streptomycin (streptomycin sulfate), for 50 days in animals, mice, male, 18 to 22 g weight.
No ototoxic effects due to parenteral, intraperitoneal, administration of 100
mg per kg of antibiotic, dihydrostreptomycin (dihydrostreptomycin sulfate),
for 50 days in animals, mice, male, 18 to 22 g weight.
Ototoxic effects, functional and structural, due to parenteral, intraperitoneal, administration of 100 mg per kg of antibiotic, kanamycin, for 50 days
in animals, mice, male, 18 to 22 g weight.

(CT) Study of mice, control group, not treated with ototoxic drugs.
No ototoxic effects due to parenteral, intraperitoneal, administration of 100
mg per kg of antibiotic, streptomycin (IB) (streptomycin sulfate), for 50
days in animals, mice, male, 18 to 22 g weight, with administration of 1 mg
per kg of vitamin B.
No ototoxic effects due to parenteral, intraperitoneal, administration of 100
mg per kg of antibiotic, dihydrostreptomycin (IB) (dihydrostreptomycin sulfate), for 50 days in animals, mice, male, 18 to 22 g weight, with administration of 1 mg per kg of vitamin B.
No ototoxic effects due to parenteral, intraperitoneal, administration of 100
mg per kg of antibiotic, kanamycin (IB), for 50 days in animals, mice, male,
18 to 22 g weight, with administration of vitamin B.
    (AD) More ototoxic effects of aminoglycoside antibiotics in guinea pigs
than in mice.
    (AD) Ototoxic effects of diuretic in guinea pigs.   (IT)

                                                                    483
Possible damage to vestibular nerve and cochlear nerve due to antibiotic,
streptomycin, in humans with or without kidney disorder.
Possible damage to vestibular nerve and cochlear nerve due to antibiotic,
gentamicin, in humans with or without kidney disorder.
Possible damage to vestibular nerve and cochlear nerve due to antibiotic,
kanamycin, in humans with or without kidney disorder.
Possible damage to vestibular nerve and cochlear nerve due to antibiotic,
neomycin, in humans with or without kidney disorder.
    (AD) Incidence of effects on vestibular function highest in streptomycin,
    followed by gentamicin, kanamycin, and neomycin.
    (AD) Incidence of effects on cochlear function highest in neomycin, fol-
    lowed by kanamycin, gentamicin, and streptomycin.
    (AD) Need for careful consideration in clinical use of aminoglycoside
    antibiotics.
Possible cochlear impairment and vestibular problems due to antibiotic,
paromomycin, in humans.
Possible dizziness and ataxia due to antibiotic, polymyxin B, in humans.
Possible but rare dizziness and vertigo due to antibiotic, nalidixic acid, in
humans.   (ENG)

                                                                    486
Incr in ATP activity of stria vascularis and spiral ligament but no pattern
of enzyme changes observed in membranous labyrinth due to 400 mg per kg daily
of antibiotic, kanamycin, for 3 weeks in animals, guinea pigs.
Incr in ATP activity of stria vascularis and spiral ligament but no pattern
of enzyme changes observed in membranous labyrinth due to 400 mg per kg daily
of antibiotic, streptomycin, for 3 weeks in animals, guinea pigs.
Decr in ATP activity of stria vascularis and spiral ligament but no pattern
of enzyme changes observed in membranous labyrinth due to 400 mg per kg daily
of antibiotic, dihydrostreptomycin, for 3 weeks in animals, guinea pigs.
    (CT) Study of guinea pigs, control group, not treated with aminoglycoside
    antibiotics.
    (AD) Study of effects of ototoxic drugs on ATP activity of inner ear of
    guinea pigs.   (JAP)

                                                                    497
Primary damage to vestibular apparatus but also cochlear impairment due to
chemical agent, carbon disulfide, in humans.
Primary damage to vestibular apparatus but also cochlear impairment due to
chemical agent, carbon monoxide, in humans.
Primary damage to vestibular apparatus but also cochlear impairment due to
heavy metal, lead, in humans.
Primary damage to vestibular apparatus but also cochlear impairment due to
chemical agent, benzene, in humans.
Primary damage to vestibular apparatus but also cochlear impairment due to
chemical agent, carbon tetrachloride, in humans.
    (AD) Report on cochleo-vestibulotoxic effects of chemical agents in indus-
    try.   (IT)

                                                                    529
Total loss of Preyer reflex within several days but no vestibular problems

due to parenteral, subcutaneous, administration of range of high doses to more than 1000 mg per kg daily of antibiotic, kanamycin (kanamycin sulfate), in animals, rats, Wistar, albino, female, 50 g weight.

(AD) Linear relationship between hearing loss and kanamycin dosage.

Loss of Preyer reflex but no vestibular problems due to parenteral, subcutaneous, administration of range of high doses to more than 600 mg per kg daily of antibiotic, neomycin, in animals, rats, Wistar, albino, female, 50 g weight.

(AD) Linear relationship between hearing loss and neomycin dosage.

(AD) Hearing loss observed with lower doses of neomycin than kanamycin.

Moderate to severe vestibular problems but cochlear impairment in only 1 case due to parenteral, subcutaneous, administration of high doses, 471, 583, 720, 887, and 1089 mg per kg daily, of antibiotic, streptomycin (streptomycin sulfate), in animals, rats, Wistar, albino, female, 50 g weight.

(AD) Linear realtionship between vestibular problems and streptomycin dosage.

Transient moderate to severe vestibular problems but cochlear impairment in only 1 case due to parenteral, subcutaneous, administration of high doses, 765, 940, 1151, and 1377 mg per kg daily, of antibiotic, dihydrostreptomycin (dihydrostreptomycin sulfate), in 40 animals, rats, Wistar, albino, female, 50 g weight.

(CT) Same method using saline in 30 rats, control group, showed no cochleo-vestibulotoxic effects.

Hearing loss due to parenteral, subcutaneous, administration of 500 mg per kg daily of antibiotic, kanamycin (SM), in animals, rats, Wistar, albino, female, 50 g weight.

Hearing loss due to parenteral, subcutaneous, administration of range of doses of antibiotic, neomycin (SM), in animals, rats, Wistar, albino, female, 50 g weight.

(AD) Incr in ototoxicity of neomycin due to kanamycin.

Hearing loss but no vestibular problems due to parenteral, subcutaneous, administration of 500 mg per kg of antibiotic, kanamycin (SM), in animals, rats, Wistar, albino, female, 50 g weight.

Hearing loss but no vestibular problems due to parenteral, subcutaneous, administration of 200, 270, 364.5, and 492 mg per kg daily of antibiotic, streptomycin (SM), in animals, rats, Wistar, albino, female, 50 g weight.

Hearing loss but no vestibular problems due to parenteral, subcutaneous, administration of 500 mg per kg daily of antibiotic, kanamycin (SM), in animals, rats, Wistar, albino, female, 50 g weight.

Hearing loss but no vestibular problems due to parenteral, subcutaneous, administration of 350, 472.5, 637.9, and 861.1 mg per kg daily of antibiotic, dihydrostreptomycin (SM), in animals, rats, Wistar, albino, female, 50 g weight.

(AD) Tests of cochlear function and vestibular function, pretreatment and daily during treatment.

(AD) Comparative study of ototoxic effects of aminoglycoside antibiotics in Wistar rats.

(AD) Report of hearing loss in 321 (43.4 percent) of total of 740 rats in study.

(AD) Suggested that ototoxic effects of kanamycin and neomycin due to different mechanisms of action than ototoxic effects of streptomycin and dihydrostreptomycin. (ENG)

539

Transient unilateral or bilateral ototoxic effects, vestibular problems in 66.6 percent of cases, due to antibiotic, gentamicin, in 14 humans.

(AD) Literature review showed small number of cases of gentamicin ototoxicity reported in Germany.

(AD) Primary factor in gentamicin ototoxicity is kidney disorder.

(AD) Other factors in gentamicin ototoxicity include dosage and simultaneous administration of other ototoxic drugs.

Hearing loss due to diuretic, ethacrynic acid, in humans with kidney disorder. (GER)

576

Progressive ataxia beginning after 4 days of treatment due to topical administration to bulla of 0.4 ml daily of aqueous solution of 10 percent concentration, to produce blood level of 7 mcg per ml, of antibiotic, gentamicin,

for 19 days maximum in 1 of 2 animals, cats.
Minimal transient ataxia beginning after 10 to 18 days of treatment and
moderate damage to cristae and maculae but normal cochlea due to topical
administration to bulla of 0.4 ml daily of aqueous solution of 3 percent
concentration, to produce blood levels of less than 0.5 mcg per ml, of antibiotic, gentamicin, for 19 days maximum in 1 of 3 animals, cats.
 (AD) Preliminary studies of topical gentamicin in cats.
 (AD) Not possible to obtain audiograms due to administration of gentamicin
 in middle ear so evaluation of cochlear function depended on histological
 study of cochlea.
 (AD) Evaluation of vestibular function with vestibular function tests.
Ataxia beginning after 12 days of treatment, decr in duration of rotatory
nystagmus, change in ENG, and loss of hair cells of cristae and of organ of
Corti in basal coil of cochlea due to topical administration to bulla of 0.4
ml daily of aqueous solution of 6 percent concentration of antibiotic, gentamicin, for 19 days maximum in 4 animals, cats.
No clinical vestibular problems and no significant change in duration of
rotatory nystagmus and in ENG but degeneration of cochlea and spiral ganglion
and changes in saccule due to topical administration to bulla of 0.4 ml daily
of aqueous solution of 3 percent concentration of antibiotic, gentamicin, for
30 days maximum in 5 animals, cats.
 (AD) Direct relationship between onset of ataxia and concentration of
 gentamicin solution.
 (AD) Correlation between duration of rotatory nystagmus and ataxia.
 (AD) Topical gentamicin most toxic to cochlea and saccule.
 (AD) Need to monitor clinical use of gentamicin with audiology.
No clinical vestibular problems, transient decr in duration of rotatory
nystagmus, transient bilateral decr in ENG, and loss of hair cells of organ
of Corti in basal coil of cochlea but normal vestibular apparatus due to
topical administration to bulla of 0.4 ml daily of solution of 6 percent
concentration of antibiotic, neomycin, for 30 days maximum in 2 animals,
cats.
 (AD) Comparative study of effects of topical gentamicin and neomycin.
 (CT) Same methods using 0.4 ml distilled water for 30 days in 7 cats,
 control group, showed no clinical vestibular problems and no histological
 changes. (ENG)

589
Dizziness during or after 5 or 6 injections but no evidence of hearing loss
due to parenteral, intramuscular and then intravenous (SM), administration of
7 mg per kg total daily, not exceeding 180 mg total dose every 24 hours, of
antibiotic, (SQ) gentamicin, for as long as 30 days in 5 of 80 humans, infant, child, and adult, 8 months to 36 years age, with cystic fibrosis and
severe pulmonary infection.
 (AD) Audiology in 40 of 80 patients showed no evidence of hearing loss.
 (AD) Dizziness possibly due to rapid administration of gentamicin.
High frequency hearing loss before gentamicin therapy possibly due to previous administration of (SQ) ototoxic drugs in some of 80 humans, infant,
child, and adult, 8 months to 36 years age, with cystic fibrosis and severe
pulmonary infection.
Dizziness due to topical administration by inhalation (SM) of 16 to 20 mg up
to 4 times a day, in 2 ml of 0.125 percent phenylephrine hydrochloride and
propylene glycol, of antibiotic, (SQ) gentamicin (CB), in some of 80 humans,
infant, child, and adult, 8 months to 36 years age, with cystic fibrosis and
severe pulmonary infection.
Dizziness due to topical administration by inhalation (SM) of 16 to 20 mg up
to 4 times a day, in 2 ml of 0.125 percent phenylephrine hydrochloride and
propylene glycol, of antibiotic, (SQ) neomycin (CB), in some of 80 humans,
infant, child, and adult, 8 months to 36 years age, with cystic fibrosis and
severe pulmonary infection. (ENG)

591
Hearing loss due to antibiotic, capreomycin, for long period in 2 of 28
humans with tuberculosis.
 (AD) Results of 1 study of effects of capreomycin.
No ototoxic effects due to antibiotic, (SQ) capreomycin, for 1 to 24 months
in 16 humans with tuberculosis.
 (AD) Results of other study of effects of capreomycin.

Vestibular problems due to previous administration of antibiotic, (SQ) streptomycin, in 8 of 16 humans with tuberculosis.
   (AD) Suggested that less ototoxicity due to capreomycin than to streptomycin. (ENG)

610
Possible ototoxic effects due to antibiotic, capreomycin, in humans with
tuberculosis of genitourinary system.
Possible hearing loss due to antibiotic, kanamycin, in humans with tuberculo-
sis of genitourinary system.
Possible hearing loss and vestibular problems due to antibiotic, viomycin, in
humans with tuberculosis of genitourinary system.
   (AD) Discussion of treatment of tuberculosis of genitourinary system.
   (GER)

615
Tinnitus, hearing loss, vertigo, and dizziness due to oral administration in
tablet of 150 mg daily of antituberculous agent, thiacetazone (CB) (SM), in
some of 1002 humans with tuberculosis.
Tinnitus, hearing loss, vertigo, and dizziness due to oral administration in
tablet of 300 mg daily of antituberculous agent, isoniazid (CB) (SM), in some
of 1002 humans with tuberculosis.
Tinnitus, hearing loss, vertigo, and dizziness due to parenteral administration of 1 g daily of antibiotic, streptomycin (SM), in some of 1002 humans
with tuberculosis.
   (AD) Reported 21.4 percent incidence of toxic effects in regimen of thiacetazone, isoniazid, and streptomycin.
   (AD) Suggested that effects of streptomycin potentiated by thiacetazone.
Unspecified ototoxic effects due to oral administration of 300 mg daily of
antituberculous agent, isoniazid (SM), in 987 humans with tuberculosis.
Unspecified ototoxic effects due to parenteral administration of 1 g daily of
antibiotic, streptomycin (SM), in 987 humans with tuberculosis.
   (AD) Reported 7.8 percent incidence of toxic effects in regimen of isoniazid and streptomycin without thiacetazone. (ENG)

619
Tinnitus in 7 cases and vertigo in 2 cases due to 1 g twice weekly of antibiotic, streptomycin (SM), in total of 9 of 190 humans, Japanese, adult, 20
to 61 years age, male and female, with pulmonary tuberculosis and without
previous chemotherapy.
Tinnitus in 7 cases and vertigo in 2 cases due to about 7.5 mg per kg in
single dose daily of antituberculous agent, isoniazid (SM), in total of 9 of
190 humans, Japanese, adult, 20 to 61 years age, male and female, with pulmonary tuberculosis and without previous chemotherapy.
Simultaneous administration of 10 g daily in 3 divided doses of antituberculous agent, PAS (SM), in 190 humans, Japanese, adult, 20 to 61 years age,
male and female, with pulmonary tuberculosis and without previous chemotherapy.
Tinnitus in 3 cases and hearing loss in 2 cases due to 1 g twice weekly of
antibiotic, streptomycin (SM), in total of 5 of 160 humans, Japanese, adult,
20 to 61 years age, male and female, with pulmonary tuberculosis and without
previous chemotherapy.
Tinnitus in 3 cases and hearing loss in 2 cases due to 18 mg per kg in 3
divided doses of antituberculous agent, isoniazid (SM), in total of 5 of 160
humans, Japanese, adult, 20 to 61 years age, male and female, with pulmonary
tuberculosis and without previous chemotherapy.
Simultaneous administration of 10 g daily in 3 divided doses of antituberculous agent, PAS (SM), in 160 humans, Japanese, adult, 20 to 61 years age,
male and female, with pulmonary tuberculosis and without previous chemotherapy.
   (AD) Similar ototoxic effects in both drug regimens. (ENG)

621
Primarily vestibular problems due to antibiotic, streptomycin, in humans.
Primarily hearing loss but also vestibular problems due to antibiotic, dihy-
drostreptomycin, in humans.
Primarily hearing loss but also vestibular problems due to antibiotic, kana-
mycin, in humans.

Primarily hearing loss but also vestibular problems due to antibiotic, neomycin, in humans.
Primarily hearing loss but also vestibular problems due to antibiotic, gentamicin, in humans.
Vertigo and ataxia due to antituberculous agent, isoniazid, in humans.
Hearing loss due to salicylate, aspirin, in humans.
Hearing loss and vertigo due to antimalarial, quinine, in humans.
Nystagmus due to barbiturates in humans.
Vestibular problems due to analgesic, morphine, in humans.
Nystagmus due to sedative, alcohol, in humans.
Nystagmus and hearing loss due to chemical agent, carbon monoxide, in humans.
Ototoxic effects due to antineoplastic, nitrogen mustard, in humans.
Ototoxic effects due to chemical agent, aniline, in humans.
Ototoxic effects due to chemical agent, tobacco, in humans.
Nystagmus due to chemical agent, nicotine, in humans.
Vestibular problems due to anticonvulsants in humans.
Vestibular problems due to anesthetics in humans.
Vestibular problems due to diuretics in humans.
    (AD) Inclusion of comprehensive list of ototoxic agents. (SP)

627
Sensorineural hearing loss and vestibular problems due to parenteral, oral, and topical administration of antibiotics in humans with and without kidney disorder.
Degeneration of cochlea due to parenteral, intratympanic, administration of antibiotic, neomycin, in animals, guinea pigs.
Transient sensorineural hearing loss due to high doses of salicylates in humans.
Sensorineural hearing loss due to antimalarial, quinine, in humans.
Sensorineural hearing loss due to chemical agent, tobacco, in humans.
Sensorineural hearing loss due to sedative, alcohol, in humans.
    (AD) Discussion of ototoxicity of various drugs as 1 etiology of sensorineural hearing loss in adults. (ENG)

641
Possible damage to eighth cranial nerve due to antibiotic, capreomycin, in humans.
Possible vestibular problems and hearing loss due to antibiotic, gentamicin, in humans.
Possible delayed transient or permanent hearing loss due to antibiotic, kanamycin (SM), in humans, in particular with kidney disorders or with simultaneous administration of ethacrynic acid.
Possible delayed transient or permanent hearing loss due to diuretic, ethacrynic acid (SM), in humans.
Possible delayed transient or permanent severe hearing loss due to oral, parenteral, or topical administration of antibiotic, neomycin, in humans.
Possible damage to eighth cranial nerve, primarily hearing loss, due to antibiotic, paromomycin, in humans.
Possible hearing loss due to antibiotic, rifampicin, in humans.
High risk of damage to eighth cranial nerve, primarily transient or permanent vestibular problems but also hearing loss, due to antibiotic, streptomycin, in humans.
Possible damage to eighth cranial nerve, primarily hearing loss, due to high doses of antibiotic, vancomycin, for long period of more than 10 days in humans, in particular with kidney disorders.
Risk of damage to eighth cranial nerve, vestibular problems and hearing loss, due to high doses of antibiotic, viomycin, for long period of more than 10 days in humans, in particular with kidney disorders.
    (AD) Discussion of toxic effects of antibiotics. (ENG)

644
Possible vertigo due to antimalarial, amodiaquine (amodiaquine dihydrochloride), in humans with parasitic infections.
Possible sensorineural hearing loss due to antimalarial, chloroquine (chloroquine hydrochloride) (chloroquine phosphate), in humans with parasitic infections.
Possible vertigo and ataxia due to antiparasitic, metronidazole, in humans with parasitic infections.

Dizziness due to antiparasitic, quinacrine (quinacrine hydrochloride), in humans with parasitic infections.
Tinnitus due to antimalarial, quinine (quinine dihydrochloride) (quinine sulfate), in humans with parasitic infections.
Possible vertigo and tinnitus due to antiparasitic, thiabendazole, in humans with parasitic infections.
Possible tinnitus due to antiparasitic, tryparsamide, in humans with parasitic infections.
   (AD) Discussion of clinical use and toxic effects of drugs used for parasitic infections. (ENG)

656

Possible permanent severe damage to eighth cranial nerve, primarily vestibular problems but also hearing loss, due to parenteral administration of antibiotic, streptomycin, in humans with tuberculosis, in particular with concurrent kidney disorder.
Possible permanent severe damage to eighth cranial nerve due to parenteral administration of antibiotic, viomycin, in humans with tuberculosis.
Possible permanent severe damage to eighth cranial nerve due to parenteral administration of antibiotic, kanamycin, in humans with tuberculosis.
Possible permanent severe damage to eighth cranial nerve due to parenteral administration of antibiotic, capreomycin, in humans with tuberculosis.
   (AD) Discussion of primary and secondary drugs used in treatment of tuberculosis. (ENG)

666

Permanent severe and possibly delayed and progressive hearing loss and vestibular problems due to parenteral administration of antibiotic, kanamycin, in humans, in particular with severe kidney disorders.
Permanent severe and possibly delayed and progressive hearing loss and vestibular problems due to parenteral administration of antibiotic, neomycin, in humans, in particular with severe kidney disorders.
   (AD) Cochleo-vestibulotoxic effects of kanamycin and neomycin usually dose related but occur also after low doses.
   (AD) Higher risk of ototoxic effects due to kanamycin and neomycin in older patients.
   (AD) Need for audiometry 2 times a week with administration of antibiotics for more than 7 days.
   (AD) Recommended adult dose of 1.5 g daily for not more than 1 week and lower doses in patients with kidney disorder and dehydration.
   (AD) Suggested use of kanamycin and neomycin for only severe infections.
   (AD) Kanamycin reported less toxic than neomycin.
Hearing loss due to oral administration of antibiotic, neomycin, in humans. (ENG)

670

Possible vestibular problems due to parenteral administration of antibiotic, gentamicin, in humans.
Damage to eighth cranial nerve, primarily hearing loss, usually permanent, due to parenteral administration of high doses of antibiotic, kanamycin, for more than 10 days in humans, in particular with kidney disorders.
Damage to eighth cranial nerve, primarily hearing loss, usually permanent, due to parenteral administration of high doses of antibiotic, neomycin, for more than 10 days in humans, in particular with kidney disorders.
Possible damage to eighth cranial nerve, primarily hearing loss, due to parenteral administration of antibiotic, paromomycin, in humans.
Transient or permanent vestibular problems due to parenteral administration of antibiotic, streptomycin, in humans.
Permanent severe hearing loss due to parenteral administration of antibiotic, dihydrostreptomycin, in humans.
Damage to eighth cranial nerve, primarily hearing loss, due to parenteral administration of high doses of antibiotic, vancomycin, for more than 10 days in humans, in particular with kidney disorders.
Damage to eighth cranial nerve, vestibular problems and hearing loss, due to parenteral administration of high doses of antibiotic, viomycin, for more than 10 days in humans, in particular with kidney disorders.
   (AD) Discussion of toxic effects of antibiotics. (ENG)

672

Possible sensorineural hearing loss due to parenteral administration of antibiotic, kanamycin, in humans with kidney disorders.
  (AD) Need for decr in dosage and 3 to 4 days interval between doses in patients with kidney disorders.
Possible vestibular problems and hearing loss due to parenteral administration of antibiotic, streptomycin, in humans with kidney disorders.
  (AD) Need for decr in dosage and 3 to 4 days interval between doses in patients with kidney disorders.
Possible vestibular problems due to parenteral administration of antibiotic, gentamicin, in humans with kidney disorders.
  (AD) Need for decr in dosage and unknown period between doses in patients with kidney disorders.
Possible hearing loss due to parenteral administration of antibiotic, vancomycin, in humans with kidney disorders.
  (AD) Need for decr in dosage and 9 days interval between doses in patients with kidney disorders.
  (AD) Report on use of antibiotics in patients with kidney disorders.
  (AD) Need for total initial dose followed by 50 percent of initial dose at recommended intervals.
  (AD) Change in dosage based on serum half-life of antibiotic.
  (AD) Literature review of effect of antibiotics in patients with kidney disorders. (ENG)

676

Vestibular problems due to antibiotic, streptomycin, in humans.
  (AD) Ototoxic effects of streptomycin particularly with high doses, long period of treatment, concurrent kidney disorders, and in older patients.
Hearing loss due to antibiotic, dihydrostreptomycin, in humans.
Hearing loss due to antibiotic, viomycin, in humans.
  (AD) Discussion of toxic effects of various antibiotics.
  (AD) Comment that effect of some inhibitors on ototoxicity not known definitely. (FR)

694

Vertigo and tinnitus due to oral administration in 3 tablets of 750 mg daily of anti-inflammatory agent, (SQ) monophenylbutazone, for 5 days in 1 of 10 humans, male, with rheumatoid arthritis.
Previous oral administration in 3 tablets of 840 mg daily of salicylate, (SQ) acetylsalicylic acid, for 2 weeks in 1 of 10 humans, male, with rheumatoid arthritis. (ENG)

700

Dizziness or vertigo, during first 3 months in 7 cases and after 3 to 6 months in 5 cases, due to 1 g daily for first 3 months, and then 1 g 3 times a week for second 3 months in patients 50 years age or less, or 1 g 3 times a week for 6 months in patients over 50 years age, of antibiotic, streptomycin (SM) (streptomycin sulfate), for 6 months in 12 (20 percent) of 59 humans, adult and aged, 55 years or more age in most cases, male, with chronic pulmonary tuberculosis and pneumoconiosis.
  (AD) Reported 20 percent incidence of streptomycin ototoxicity in first year of therapy.
Incr hearing loss reported after 6 months due to 1 g daily for first 3 months, and then 1 g 3 times a week for second 3 months in patients 50 years age or less, or 1 g 3 times a week for 6 months in patients over 50 years age, of antibiotic, streptomycin (SM) (streptomycin sulfate), for 6 months in 1 of 59 humans, adult and aged, 55 years or more age in most cases, male, with chronic pulmonary tuberculosis and pneumoconiosis and with previous hearing loss.
  (AD) Reported 1 case of hearing loss due to streptomycin in first year of therapy.
Dizziness and tinnitus after 14 months due to 1 g daily for first 3 months, and then 1 g 3 times a week for second 3 months in patients 50 years age or less, or 1 g 3 times a week for 6 months in patients over 50 years age, of antibiotic, streptomycin (SM) (streptomycin sulfate), for 6 months in 1 of 31 humans, male, with chronic pulmonary tuberculosis and pneumoconiosis.
  (AD) Reported 1 case with ototoxic effects within 18 months of therapy.
Simultaneous oral administration in cachets of 333 mg daily of antitubercu-

lous   agent,   isoniazid   (SM) (CB), for 18 months or more in 59 humans, male,
with chronic pulmonary tuberculosis and pneumoconiosis.
Simultaneous oral administration in cachets of 15 g daily of antituberculous
agent, PAS (SM) (CB) (sodium PAS), for 18 months or more in 59 humans, male,
with chronic pulmonary tuberculosis and pneumoconiosis.   (ENG)

706

Ototoxic effects due to chemical agents and heavy metals in humans.
   (AD)   Literature review of ototoxic effects of nicotine, carbon monoxide,
   carbon tetrachloride, mercury, arsenic, and lead.
Cochleo-vestibulotoxic effects, functional and structural, due to antibiotics
in humans.
   (AD)   Literature review of ototoxicity of streptomycin, dihydrostreptomy-
   cin, neomycin, kanamycin, gentamicin, capreomycin, rifampicin, viomycin,
   isoniazid, aminosidine, and framycetin.
Hearing loss due to salicylates in humans.
Hearing loss due to antimalarial, quinine, in humans.
Hearing loss due to diuretic, ethacrynic acid, in humans.
   (AD) Literature review of effects of various ototoxic agents.   (IT)

731

Possible damage to eighth cranial nerve, vestibular problems, due to antibiotic, streptomycin, in humans with gram-negative bacilli.
Possible damage to eighth cranial nerve, hearing loss, due to antibiotic,
kanamycin, in humans with gram-negative bacilli.
Possible damage to eighth cranial nerve, hearing loss, due to antibiotic,
neomycin, in humans with gram-negative bacilli.
Possible damage to eighth cranial nerve, vestibular problems, due to antibio-
tic, gentamicin, in humans with gram-negative bacilli.
Possible ototoxic effects due to antibiotic, vancomycin, in humans with gram-
positive cocci.
   (AD) Need to decr dosage of antibiotics in patients with kidney disorders.
   (AD) Discussion of possible toxic effects of antibiotics used in surgery.
   (ENG)

STRUCTURAL EFFECTS

Cochlear findings

021

Transient bilateral sensorineural hearing loss due to unspecified method of
administration of as much as 5.2 g daily of salicylate, acetylsalicylic acid,
for unspecified period in 1 human, aged, 76 years age, female, with rheumatoid arthritis.
   (AD) Improvement in hearing after cessation of treatment with acetylsalicylic acid.
   (AD) Suggested that damage to stria vascularis due to presbycusis and not
   due to acetylsalicylic acid.   (ENG)

065

Prevention of destruction of organ of Corti due to low doses of antibiotics
(IB) in animals, guinea pigs, with administration of vitamin B and amino
acids.
   (AD) Need for histological studies to determine method for prevention of
   ototoxicity.   (FR)

149

Damage to organ of Corti due to antibiotics in humans.
   (AD) Discussion of ototoxicity in humans based on animal experimentation.
   (FR)

193

Sensorineural hearing loss and structural damage to cochlea due to low doses
of antibiotics in humans.
   (AD) Report on clinical and pathological effects possible with use of
   antibiotics.
   (AD) Toxic levels in blood possible due to low doses in therapy.
   (AD) Need for audiometry, vestibular function tests, and determination of

blood levels of antibiotics during treatment.   (SER)

244
Hearing loss and damage to organ of Corti due to antibiotics, aminoglycoside,
in humans.
   (AD)   Literature   review   of   ototoxic effects of different aminoglycoside
   antibiotics.   (GER)

272
Hearing loss and damage to organ of Corti due to antibiotics in humans.
   (AD) Literature review of ototoxic effects of antibiotics used in therapy.
   (FIN)

410
Damage   to   organ   of   Corti   of   fetus due to antibiotics in humans, female,
during pregnancy.
   (AD) Discussion of etiology of damage to organ of Corti in fetus.   (FR)

704
Functional   damage   to   cochlea   evident   before   changes in structure due to
antibiotics in animals.
   (AD)   Need   for correlation of various methods, morphological, electrophy-
   siological, and biochemical, in study of function of inner ear.
   (AD)   Literature   review   of   various methods of study of auditory system.
   (ENG)

033
Damage to organ of Corti due to topical route, inhalation, of chemical agent,
carbon monoxide, in 40 exposures in 5 animals, rabbits.   (GER)

436
Hearing   loss   and damage to organ of Corti due to topical route, inhalation,
of chemical agent, carbon monoxide, in animals.   (GER)

002
Damage   to   organ of Corti and stria vascularis due to topical administration
to   round   window   of   16   mg of 1.44M solution and 8 mg of 0.72M solution of
antibiotic, chloramphenicol (chloramphenicol succinate), for 30 minutes in 11
animals, guinea pigs, adult, for each solution.
   (CT)   Same   method   using 1.44M solution of sodium (sodium succinate) in 8
   guinea pigs, control group, showed no histological damage.   (ENG)

732
Hearing   loss and total degeneration of organ of Corti and moderate degeneration   of   spiral ganglion and nerve process in fetus due to oral ingestion of
250 mg daily of antimalarial, chloroquine (chloroquine phosphate), in humans,
female, during pregnancy.
   (AD) Histopathological study of inner ear after death.   (ENG)

412
Damage to organ of Corti and eighth cranial nerve due to parenteral, intramu-
scular, administration of antibiotic, colistin, in animals, guinea pigs.
   (AD) Study showed individual differences in response to colistin.
   (AD)   Administration of colistin to guinea pigs in study of toxic neuritis
   of eighth cranial nerve.   (RUS)

429
Necrosis   of   cells of organ of Corti and hearing loss, partial or total, due
to parenteral, intramuscular, administration of high doses, 150,000 units per
kg daily,   of   antibiotic,   colistin (colistin sulfate), for 7 to 21 days in
animals, guinea pigs.   (RUS)

044
Change in cochlear response and damage to hair cells of organ of Corti due to
100 mg per kg daily of antibiotic, dihydrostreptomycin, in animals, rabbits.
Change   in cochlear response and damage to stria vascularis due to 250 mg per
kg   daily   and   500   mg per kg daily of antibiotic, dihydrostreptomycin, in 2
other groups of animals, rabbits.   (JAP)

382

Damage to hair cells of organ of Corti and nervous tissue of osseous spiral lamina due to topical administration to inner ear of 9.8 percent tritium-labelled solution, in same amount of Ringer's solution, of antibiotic, dihydrostreptomycin, in animals, guinea pigs, 250 to 450 g weight.
(AD) Autoradiographical study of distribution of dihydrostreptomycin in cochlear duct.
(AD) Suggested that ototoxicity of dihydrostreptomycin due to retention of drug for long period in perilymph and specific accumulation of drug in hair cells and nervous tissue of organ of Corti. (ENG)

464

Possible decr in damage to organ of Corti and eighth cranial nerve due to antibiotic, dihydrostreptomycin (IB), in animals, guinea pigs, with administration of citrobioflavonoid complex. (IT)

134

Decr in threshold shift of 20 db and damage to outer hair cells and inner hair cells of organ of Corti due to topical administration to external auditory meatus of 50 percent solution of chemical agent, dimethyl sulfoxide, for 21 days in 7 animals, cats.
Damage to 40 percent of eighth cranial nerve action potential due to topical administration to external auditory meatus of chemical agent, dimethyl sulfoxide, for 6 hours in 4 animals, cats.
Damage to 60 percent of eighth cranial nerve action potential due to topical administration to middle ear of chemical agent, dimethyl sulfoxide, for 6 hours in 4 animals, cats.
(CT) Control group of 4 cats used.
(AD) Suggested that dimethyl sulfoxide new ototoxic drug. (GER)

125

Sensorineural hearing loss due to parenteral, intravenous, administration of range of 9.2 to 86 mg per kg of diuretic, ethacrynic acid (sodium ethacrynate), in 1 injection in 7 of 12 animals, guinea pigs, young, 240 to 489 g weight.
(AD) Hearing loss confirmed by loss of Preyer reflex 6 minutes after injection.
Primary damage to stria vascularis and some damage to outer hair cells of organ of Corti due to parenteral, intravenous, administration of range of 9.2 to 86 mg per kg of diuretic, ethacrynic acid (sodium ethacrynate), in 1 injection in 12 animals, guinea pigs, young, 240 to 489 g weight.
(AD) Electron microscopic study of cochlea. (ENG)

144

Moderate bilateral sensorineural hearing loss within 20 minutes and damage to outer hair cells of organ of Corti due to unspecified method of administration of 50 mg of diuretic, ethacrynic acid, in 1 dose in humans with kidney disorder.
(AD) Hearing loss confirmed by audiogram.
Sensorineural hearing loss within 15 minutes due to unspecified method of administration of 20 to 30 mg per kg daily of diuretic, ethacrynic acid, in 20 animals, cats.
(AD) Ethacrynic acid not recommended for clinical use in humans with kidney disorders. (ENG)

171

Rapid significant decr in cochlear microphonic but no pathological changes in cochlea after 1 hour due to parenteral, intravenous, administration of high doses, 20, 30, or 40 mg per kg, in solution of physiological saline, of diuretic, ethacrynic acid, in 1 injection for acute effects in 3 groups of 18 animals, guinea pigs, young, 250 g weight.
No detected decr in cochlear microphonic and no permanent physiological or structural changes in cochlea after 3 weeks due to parenteral, intravenous, administration of high doses, 30 mg per kg, of diuretic, ethacrynic acid, in chronic intoxication in 6 animals, guinea pigs, young, 250 g weight. (ENG)

079

Hearing loss and range of degree of damage to hair cells of organ of Corti

due to parenteral, intramuscular, administration of 50, 80, 110, and 140 mg
per kg daily of antibiotic, gentamicin (gentamicin sulfate), for 7 to 28 days
in 4 groups of 12 animals, guinea pigs, adult, 250 to 500 g weight.
  (AD) Comparative study showed that degree of damage determined by dosage.
  (AD) Hearing loss determined by Preyer reflex. (ENG)

                                                                    119
Damage to hair cells of organ of Corti and change in action potential due to
parenteral, intramuscular, administration of 20 mg per kg and 150 mg per kg
of antibiotic, gentamicin (gentamicin sulfate), in 2 groups of 59 animals,
guinea pigs.
  (CT) Control group of 26 guinea pigs used.
  (AD) More severe damage due to 150 mg per kg of gentamicin than due to 20
  mg per kg. (GER)

                                                                    256
Loss of outer hair cells of organ of Corti in basal coil of cochlea due to
parenteral, intramuscular, administration of 110 mg per kg daily of antibiotic, gentamicin, for 28 days in animals, guinea pigs.
Less damage to hair cells of organ of Corti in second and third coils of
cochlea due to parenteral, intramuscular, administration of 110 mg per kg
daily of antibiotic, gentamicin, for 19 days in animals, guinea pigs.
  (AD) Suggested relationship between duration of administration of gentamicin and degree of damage to inner ear. (ENG)

                                                                    616
Range of degrees of damage to hair cells of organ of Corti due to parenteral,
intramuscular, administration of 50 to 140 mg per kg daily of antibiotic,
gentamicin, for 7 to 20 days in 4 groups of animals, guinea pigs.
  (AD) Relationship between hair cell damage and dosage of gentamicin.
  (ENG)

                                                                    043
Histochemical and electron microscopic changes in Reissner's membrane due to
parenteral, intramuscular, administration of 400 mg per kg daily of antibiotic, kanamycin, for 15 days in 10 animals, guinea pigs, 300 to 400 g weight.
  (ENG)

                                                                    086
Damage to organ of Corti due to parenteral, subcutaneous, administration of
150 mg per kg and 250 mg per kg of antibiotic, kanamycin, in 10 days in
animals, cats.
  (AD) Comparative study of ototoxicity of 4 compounds of kanamycin. (GER)

                                                                    096
Loss of outer hair cells and inner hair cells and damage to reticular membrane of organ of Corti due to parenteral, intraperitoneal (SM), administration of 400 mg per kg (SM) of antibiotic, kanamycin (kanamycin sulfate), in 5
days in animals, 15 cats, adult, 2.5 kg weight, and 30 guinea pigs, young,
300 g weight.
Simultaneous topical (SM) administration to middle ear cavity of 0.6 ml of 20
percent solution (SM) of antibiotic, kanamycin (kanamycin sulfate), for 1 day
in animals, 15 cats, adult, 2.5 kg weight, and 30 guinea pigs, young, 300 g
weight.
  (AD) Study of repair pattern in reticular membrane after loss of hair
  cells. (ENG)

                                                                    108
Degeneration of outer hair cells of organ of Corti due to parenteral, intramuscular, administration of 400 mg per kg daily of antibiotic, kanamycin, for
14 days in animals, guinea pigs.
Degeneration of outer hair cells of organ of Corti due to parenteral, intramuscular, administration of 400 mg per kg daily of antibiotic, kanamycin, in
animals, guinea pigs, after acoustic trauma.
More severe damage to outer hair cells and inner hair cells of organ of Corti
due to parenteral, intramuscular, administration of 400 mg per kg daily of
antibiotic, kanamycin, in animals, guinea pigs, before acoustic trauma.
  (AD) More severe cochleotoxic effects due to treatment with kanamycin

before acoustic trauma.   (FR)

121
Tinnitus and high frequency hearing loss and damage to organ of Corti due to
antibiotic, kanamycin, in humans.
    (AD) Literature review of kanamycin, use in therapy and toxic effects.
    (AD) Suggested clinical procedures for use of kanamycin with minimum risk
    of ototoxicity. (ENG)

145
Decr of only 33.3 percent in cells of spiral ganglion due to 12 g of antibiotic, kanamycin, for 8 days in 1 human with kidney disorder.
    (AD) Temporal bone study of number of cells of spiral ganglion after
    treatment with kanamycin.
    (AD) Near normal number of spiral ganglion cells after treatment with
    ototoxic drug. (ENG)

241
Risk of damage to organ of Corti and hearing loss due to antibiotic, kanamycin, in humans, infant.
    (AD) Study of dose response relationships.
    (AD) Recommended dose of 15 mg per kg daily every 12 hours for infants.
    (ENG)

242
Variations in decr in cochlear microphonic due to parenteral, intraperitoneal, administration of 100 mg per kg of antibiotic, kanamycin, for period
until measurement of cochlear microphonic not possible in 12 animals, rabbits, adult, normal.
Changes in outer hair cells and supporting cells, in particular in basal coil
of cochlea, and slight damage to inner hair cells of organ of Corti due to
parenteral, intraperitoneal, administration of 100 mg per kg of antibiotic,
kanamycin, for period until measurement of cochlear microphonic not possible
in 12 animals, rabbits, adult, normal.
    (AD) Serial observations on beginning and progression of cochleotoxic
    effects of kanamycin by daily measurement of cochlear microphonic and
    study of correlations between electrophysiological and histopathological
    changes.
    (AD) Variations in response of cochlea to kanamycin but correlation bet-
    ween electrophysiological and histopathological changes.   (ENG)

267
Degeneration of outer hair cells of organ of Corti and damage to spiral
ganglion due to 400 mg per kg daily of antibiotic, kanamycin, for 14 days in
animals, guinea pigs.
Permanent histological changes in cochlea due to 100 mg per kg of antibiotic,
kanamycin, in animals, guinea pigs.
Damage to organ of Corti of fetuses due to 200 mg per kg of antibiotic,
kanamycin, in animals, guinea pigs, treated during pregnancy.
    (AD) Report on previous results of experimentation.
Cochleotoxic effects due to antibiotic, kanamycin, in average of 30 percent
of more than 1000 humans, adult.
    (AD) Discussion of relationship between kanamycin ototoxicity and dosage,
    duration of treatment, age, previous auditory system problems, administra-
    tion of other ototoxic drugs, kidney function, and individual responses to
    drug. (ENG)

270
Damage to organ of Corti due to antibiotic, kanamycin, in animals, guinea
pigs.   (JAP)

274
Degrees of damage, from loss of hair cells to complete destruction of organ
of Corti, but with partial replacement of organ of Corti by other structures
due to parenteral, intraperitoneal, administration of 200 mg per kg 5 days a
week of antibiotic, kanamycin (kanamycin sulfate), for 10, 15, and 20 days in
3 groups of 30 animals, guinea pigs, pigmented, young, 300 g weight.
    (AD) Report on degeneration and regeneration processes of organ of Corti.

(AD) Study of patterns of replacement structure of reticular membrane.
(ENG)

337

Shifts in cochlear microphonic and action potential thresholds and loss of
Preyer reflex due to parenteral, subcutaneous, administration of 400 mg per
kg daily of antibiotic, kanamycin, for 10, 14, or 20 days in 3 groups of
animals, guinea pigs, adult, male.
   (CT) Study of guinea pigs, control group.
   (AD) Correlation between duration of dosage and decr in function.
   (AD) Study of guinea pigs showed individual responses to kanamycin.
Shifts in cochlear microphonic and action potential thresholds and loss of
Preyer reflex due to parenteral, subcutaneous, administration of 400 mg per
kg daily of antibiotic, kanamycin, for 10, 14, or 20 days in 3 groups of
animals, rats, adult, male.
   (CT) Study of rats, control group.
   (AD) Results of study of rats showed high degree of individual response to
   kanamycin or technical difficulty in recording from round window of rat.
Shifts in cochlear microphonic and action potential thresholds and loss of
Preyer reflex due to parenteral, subcutaneous, administration of 400 mg per
kg daily of antibiotic, kanamycin, for 10, 14, or 20 days in 3 groups of
animals, rabbits, adult, male.
   (CT) Study of rabbits, control group.
   (AD) Similarity between cochlear impairment of rabbit and hearing loss in
   humans due to kanamycin.
Destruction of hair cells of organ of Corti in all coils of cochlea and
damage to stria vascularis and spiral ganglion due to unspecified method of
administration of 200 mg per kg of antibiotic, kanamycin, for 20 days in
animals, guinea pigs.
   (AD) Difference in pattern and degree of cochlear impairment in different
   species of animals.
   (AD) Suggested that physiological changes precede histological changes and
   so show more clearly the ototoxic effects of the drug. (ENG)

371

Damage to hair cells of organ of Corti due to parenteral administration of
150 mg per kg of antibiotic, kanamycin (kanamycin sulfate), for 20 and 30
injections in animals, guinea pigs.
Decr in damage to hair cells of organ of Corti due to parenteral administration of 150 mg per kg of antibiotic, kanamycin (IB), for 20 and 30 injections
in animals, guinea pigs, with administration of pantothenic acid.
Slight decr in damage to hair cells of organ of Corti due to parenteral
administration of 150 mg per kg of antibiotic, kanamycin (IB) (kanamycin
sulfate), for 20 injections in animals, guinea pigs, with administration of
ozothin.
Slight decr in damage to hair cells of organ of Corti due to parenteral
administration of 150 mg per kg of antibiotic, kanamycin (IB), for 20 injections in animals, guinea pigs, with administration of pantothenic acid and
ozothin.
   (AD) Study of cochleotoxic effects of kanamycin without and with pantothenic acid and ozothin. (GER)

440

Possible damage to organ of Corti in fetuses due to antibiotic, kanamycin, in
animals, guinea pigs, adult, during pregnancy.
   (AD) Study of transmission of drugs from mother to fetus.
   (AD) Serum levels of kanamycin in fetus about 7 percent of serum levels in
   mother and not related to variations in dosage.
   (AD) Slow elimination of kanamycin from fetus. (ENG)

466

Possible decr in damage to organ of Corti due to antibiotic, kanamycin (IB),
in animals, guinea pigs, with administration of vitamin B, nialamide, dexamethasone, or glutathione. (FR)

489

Loss of Preyer reflex and progressive damage to hair cells of organ of Corti
beginning with basal coil of cochlea due to 400 mg per kg of antibiotic,

kanamycin (kanamycin sulfate), in 3 to 18 injections in 25 animals, guinea pigs, adult, 250 to 350 g weight, with normal Preyer reflex.
   (CT) Daily administration of Ringer's solution in 4 guinea pigs, control group.
   (AD) Discussion of difference between ototoxic effects of kanamycin and streptomycin on organ of Corti. (ENG)

492

Damage to hair cells of organ of Corti due to 400, 200, or 100 mg per kg daily of antibiotic, kanamycin, for 14 days in animals, guinea pigs.
   (CT) Study of normal guinea pigs, control group, not treated with aminoglycoside antibiotic.
Possible protection of organ of Corti from damage due to antibiotic, kanamycin (IB), in animals, guinea pigs with administration of inhibitor.
   (AD) Electrophysiological and histological study of effect of ototoxic drug on cochlea of guinea pigs. (FR)

493

Decr in cochlear microphonics due to parenteral, intramuscular, administration of 400 or 200 mg per kg daily of antibiotic, kanamycin, in animals, guinea pigs.
Decr in cochlear microphonics due to parenteral, intravenous, administration of 100 mg per kg daily of antibiotic, kanamycin, for 3 to 10 days in animals, guinea pigs.
No ototoxic effect in fetuses due to antibiotic, kanamycin, in animals, guinea pigs, female, treated during pregnancy.
   (AD) More rapid and severe ototoxic effect with intravenous administration than with intramuscular administration. (ENG)

705

No significant loss of hair cells of organ of Corti due to 15, 50, or 100 mg per kg daily of antibiotic, kanamycin, for 3 or 5 weeks in animals, guinea pigs.
No significant loss of hair cells of organ of Corti due to 15 or 50 mg per kg daily of antibiotic, kanamycin, for 3 weeks in animals, guinea pigs, with exposure to low level noise, 68 to 72 decibels at 125 Hz.
Damage to outer hair cells primarily in apical coil of cochlea due to 15 or 50 mg per kg daily of antibiotic, kanamycin, for 5 weeks in animals, guinea pigs, with exposure to low level noise, 68 to 72 decibels at 125 Hz.
Damage to outer hair cells primarily in apical coil of cochlea due to 100 mg per kg daily of antibiotic, kanamycin, for 3 weeks in animals, guinea pigs, with exposure to low level noise, 68 to 72 decibels at 125 Hz.
   (AD) Earlier occurrence of hair cell damage with incr in dosage of kanamycin in guinea pigs with exposure to low level noise.
   (AD) Study of sensitization by low level noise of hair cells of cochlea to damage by low doses of kanamycin. (ENG)

525

No loss of Preyer reflex and no structural changes in organ of Corti and stria vascularis due to parenteral, intraperitoneal, administration of 3 to 5 mg per kg, in aqueous solution, of antineoplastic, mechlorethamine, for 5 days to 5 weeks in animals, 8 guinea pigs, adult, 300 to 400 g weight, and 6 mice, adult, 25 to 35 g weight, with normal Preyer reflex.
Loss of Preyer reflex and severe destruction of outer hair cells of organ of Corti in basal and middle coils of cochlea but little or no change in stria vascularis, spiral ganglion, and cochlear nerve due to parenteral, intraperitoneal, administration of 10 to 30 mg per kg, in aqueous solution, of antineoplastic, mechlorethamine, for 1 day to 5 weeks in animals, 7 guinea pigs, adult, 300 to 400 g weight, and 19 mice, adult, 25 to 35 g weight, with normal Preyer reflex.
   (CT) Same method using same volume of Ringer's solution in 5 animals, control group.
   (AD) Electron microscopic study of degeneration of cochlea in mechlorethamine intoxicated animals and in animals with congenital hearing loss to determine the mechanism of degeneration.
   (AD) Suggested possible effect on protein synthesis in hair cells of organ of Corti in early stages of mechlorethamine ototoxicity. (ENG)

257
Degeneration of hair cells of organ of Corti due to parenteral, intramuscular, administration of 200 mg per kg of antibiotic, neomycin (neomycin sulfate), for 6 days in 15 animals, guinea pigs, albino.
  (CT) Study of 7 guinea pigs, control group.
  (AD) Use of surface specimen technique in study of cochleotoxic effects of neomycin. (ENG)

381
Degeneration of organ of Corti and hearing loss due to various methods of administration of antibiotic, neomycin, in humans.
  (AD) Literature review of toxic effects of new antibiotics. (GER)

518
Hearing loss and damage to hair cells of organ of Corti but no histological changes in vascular strip of spiral fissure due to antibiotic, neomycin, in animals, guinea pigs.
  (CT) Study of guinea pigs, control group, not treated with neomycin. (RUS)

048
Severe sensorineural hearing loss and loss of hair cells of organ of Corti in basal and middle coils of cochlea due to parenteral, intravenous, administration of high doses, 1.0 mg per kg, of antineoplastic, nitrogen mustard, in 1 injection in animals, cats, conditioned. (ENG)

540
Effect on cells of cochlea due to antineoplastic, nitrogen mustard, in animals. (JAP)

023
No degeneration in inner hair cells and outer hair cells of organ of Corti due to parenteral, intramuscular, administration of 200 mg per kg daily of antibiotic, streptomycin (streptomycin sulfate), for 10 days in 15 animals, guinea pigs, 150 to 200 g weight.
  (CT) Study of 5 guinea pigs, control group.
Changes in succinic dehydrogenase activity in hair cells of organ of Corti due to parenteral, intramuscular, administration of 200 mg per kg daily of antibiotic, streptomycin (streptomycin sulfate), for 10 days in 15 animals, guinea pigs, 150 to 200 g weight.
  (CT) Study of 10 guinea pigs, control group.
  (AD) Difference between inner hair cells and outer hair cells discussed. (ENG)

259
Damage to hair cells of organ of Corti and decr in action potentials due to parenteral, intramuscular, administration of 250 mg per kg, in distilled water, of antibiotic, streptomycin (streptomycin sulfate), in 10 doses in 1 group of total of over 100 animals, guinea pigs, 200 g average weight.
Normal hair cells of organ of Corti and no decr in action potentials due to parenteral, intramuscular, administration of 250 mg per kg of antibiotic, streptomycin (IB) (streptomycin sulfate), in 10 doses in 1 group of total of over 100 animals, guinea pigs, 200 g average weight, with administration of 1.2 ml of ozothin.
  (CT) Study of guinea pigs, control group.
  (AD) Significant decr in ototoxicity of streptomycin due to administration of ozothin. (ENG)

364
Damage to organ of Corti, spiral ganglion, and cochlear nuclei of medulla oblongata 15 days after beginning of treatment due to 100 mg per kg of antibiotic, streptomycin, in 38 animals, guinea pigs.
Decr in damage to spiral ganglion and cochlear nuclei of medulla oblongata due to 100 mg per kg of antibiotic, streptomycin (IB), in 8 of 18 animals, guinea pigs, with simultaneous administration of 2 ml of 5 percent unitiol for 30 to 60 days.
Decr in hearing loss due to ototoxic drugs (IB) in 3 of 25 humans with administration of unitiol.

No hearing loss due to antibiotic, streptomycin (IB), in 25 humans with pulmonary tuberculosis with administration of unitiol.
   (AD) Study of effect of inhibitor, unitiol, on streptomycin ototoxicity. (RUS)

389

Damage to epithelial cells of round window due to 1 percent solution of anesthetic, tetracaine, in animals, guinea pigs, 250 to 500 g weight. (GER)

049

Hearing loss and damage to hair cells of organ of Corti due to parenteral, (SQ) intraperitoneal, administration of 200 mg per kg daily of antibiotic, tobramycin (nebramycin (factor 6)), for 6 days in 13 animals, guinea pigs, 220 to 260 g weight.
Hearing loss and damage to hair cells of organ of Corti due to parenteral, (SQ) subcutaneous, administration of 150 mg per kg daily of antibiotic, tobramycin (nebramycin (factor 6)), for 6 weeks in 13 animals, guinea pigs, 220 to 260 g weight.
   (CT) Control group of 5 guinea pigs used.
   (AD) Loss of Preyer reflex showed hearing loss. (ENG)

719

Progressive severe degeneration primarily in organ of Corti beginning after 24 hours but also damage to spiral ganglion and effect on cochlear function due to parenteral, intraperitoneal, administration of 10 or 20 mg per kg of chemical agent, 6-aminonicotinic acid, in animals, mice, audiogenic seizure-susceptible.
Decr in ototoxic effects due to parenteral, intraperitoneal, administration of 10 mg per kg of chemical agent, 6-aminonicotinic acid, in animals, mice, audiogenic seizure-susceptible, with administration 5 minutes previously of 10 mg per kg of nicotinamide. (ENG)

720

Damage to cochlear function and progressive severe degeneration in cochlear duct, beginning after 24 hours in spiral ligament, with severe damage to organ of Corti, and with later atrophy of spiral ganglion due to parenteral, intraperitoneal, administration of 20 mg per kg, in concentration of 2 mg per ml sterile water, of chemical agent, 6-aminonicotinic acid, in 1 injection in 9 animals, mice, male, audiogenic seizure-susceptible.
   (CT) Same method using water in 3 mice, control group.
   (CT) Same method using 2 mice, chronic control group, not treated.
Damage to cochlear function and degeneration in cochlea due to parenteral, intraperitoneal, administration of 20 mg per kg of chemical agent, 6-aminonicotinic acid, in 6 animals, mice, not audiogenic seizure-susceptible.
   (CT) Same method using water in 2 mice, control group, showed no histological changes. (ENG)

005

Transient primary decr in cochlear microphonic and action potential due to parenteral, intravenous, administration of 10 mg per kg of diuretic, ethacrynic acid, in 1 injection in 20 animals, cats, adult.
Transient primary decr in cochlear microphonic and action potential due to parenteral, intravenous, administration of 10 mg per kg of diuretic, furosemide, in 1 injection in 20 animals, cats, adult.
Delayed severe secondary decr in cochlear microphonic and action potential due to parenteral, intravenous, administration of more than 10 mg per kg of diuretic, ethacrynic acid, in animals, cats.
   (CT) Same method using 50 mg per kg and 100 mg per kg of diuretic, chlorothiazide, in cats, control group, showed no ototoxic effect.
Degeneration of outer hair cells of organ of Corti in basal and middle coils of cochlea due to parenteral, intravenous, administration of 30 mg per kg of diuretic, ethacrynic acid, in 1 injection in 2 animals, cats.
Degeneration of outer hair cells of organ of Corti due to parenteral, intramuscular, administration of 15 mg per kg of diuretic, ethacrynic acid, for 2 weeks in 1 animal, cat. (ENG)

006

Range of degrees of degeneration of endorgan of organ of Corti due to paren-

teral, intratympanic, administration of range of 1 to 100 mg per ml concentration of antibiotic, neomycin, in 1 injection in animals, guinea pigs,
young, 250 g average weight.
Range of degrees of degeneration of endorgan of organ of Corti due to parenteral, intratympanic, administration of range of 1 to 100 mg per ml concentration of antibiotic, polymyxin B, in 1 injection in animals, guinea pigs,
young, 250 g average weight.
Range of degrees of degeneration of endorgan of organ of Corti due to parenteral, intratympanic, administration of range of 1 to 100 mg per ml concentration of antibiotic, colistin, in 1 injection in animals, guinea pigs,
young, 250 g average weight.
   (CT) Same method using comparable concentration of saline solution or
   solution of glucose or sodium G penicillin in guinea pigs, control group,
   showed no histological damage.
Degeneration of endorgan of organ of Corti due to topical administration to
ear canal of range of 5 to 100 mg per ml 1 time daily of antibiotic, neomycin, for 8 to 25 days in 14 animals, guinea pigs. (ENG)

                                                                        009
Delayed permanent sensorineural hearing loss and damage to outer hair cells
of basal and middle coils of cochlea due to unspecified doses of antibiotic,
dihydrostreptomycin, in humans.
Vertigo and dizziness due to unspecified method of administration of 2 to 3 g
daily of antibiotic, streptomycin (streptomycin sulfate), for 30 to 50 days
in humans with tuberculosis.
Hearing loss due to unspecified method of administration of high doses of
antibiotic, streptomycin (streptomycin sulfate), for long period in humans.
Gradual high frequency hearing loss and tinnitus and degeneration of hair
cells of organ of Corti in basal coil of cochlea due to unspecified doses of
antibiotic, kanamycin, in humans.
Delayed severe high frequency hearing loss due to parenteral, oral, or topical administration by inhalation of unspecified doses of antibiotic, neomycin, for unspecified period in humans with kidney disorder.
Complete degeneration of inner hair cells due to unspecified method of administration of 18 g of antibiotic, neomycin, for unspecified period in
humans with bacterial endocarditis.
Lesions in organ of Corti due to parenteral administration of unspecified
doses of antibiotic, polymyxin B, for unspecified period in animals, guinea
pigs.
Sensorineural hearing loss due to parenteral, intravenous, administration of
80 to 95 mg per ml of antibiotic, vancomycin, for unspecified period in
humans with kidney disorder.
   (AD) Sensorineural hearing loss and vestibular problems due to 6 antibiotics in humans and animals, guinea pigs.
   (AD) Literature review of ototoxic effects of antibiotics. (ENG)

                                                                        042
Transient bilateral sensorineural hearing loss due to parenteral, intravenous, administration of 50 mg of diuretic, (SQ) ethacrynic acid, in 1
injection in 1 human, adult, 45 years age, female, with lymphosarcoma and
with normal kidney function.
   (AD) Hearing loss reported 15 minutes after treatment with ethacrynic
   acid.
Previous parenteral, intramuscular, administration of 60 mg every 6 hours of
antibiotic, (SQ) gentamicin (gentamicin sulfate), for unspecified period in 1
human, adult, 45 years age, female, with lymphosarcoma and with normal kidney
function.
Bilateral sensorineural hearing loss due to parenteral, intravenous, administration of 100 mg of diuretic, (SQ) ethacrynic acid, in 2 injections of 50 mg
each 6 hours apart in 1 human, adult, 64 years age, female, with acute leukemia and with normal kidney function.
   (AD) Histological study after death showed no damage to inner ear.
Previous unspecified method of administration of unspecified dose of antibiotic, (SQ) polymyxin B (polymyxin B sulfate), in 1 human, adult, 64 years age,
female, with acute leukemia and with normal kidney function.
Previous parenteral, intramuscular, administration of 0.5 g every 12 hours of
antibiotic, (SQ) kanamycin (kanamycin sulfate), for unspecified period in 1
human, adult, 64 years age, female, with acute leukemia and with normal

kidney function.
   (AD) Suggested that hearing loss due to combined action of ethacrynic acid
   and antibiotics.   (ENG)

                                                                      045
Progressive degeneration of endorgan of cochlea due to low doses of antibiotic, dihydrostreptomycin, in animals, guinea pigs.
Progressive degeneration of endorgan of cochlea due to low doses of antibiotic, neomycin, in animals, guinea pigs.   (JAP)

                                                                      084
Decr in damage to organ of Corti due to topical administration of antibiotic,
kanamycin (IB), in animals, guinea pigs, 300 to 500 g weight, with intravenous administration of cytochrome C.
Decr in damage to organ of Corti due to topical administration of antibiotic,
streptomycin (IB) (streptomycin sulfate), in animals, guinea pigs, 300 to 500
g weight, with intravenous administration of cytochrome C.   (POL)

                                                                      130
Decr in cochlear microphonic and neural potentials and incr in sodium and
glucose of endolymph due to parenteral, intravenous, administration of 30 to
60 mg per kg, in saline solution, of diuretic, ethacrynic acid, for 5 minute
period in animals, cats.
Changes in stria vascularis and damage to outer hair cells of organ of Corti
due to parenteral, intravenous, administration of 30 to 60 mg per kg, in
saline solution, of diuretic, ethacrynic acid, for 5 minute period in animals, cats.
No change in cochlear microphonic, no incr in endolymph glucose, and normal
endolymph chemical composition due to parenteral, intravenous, administration
of 50 mg per kg, in saline solution, of diuretic, acetazolamide, for 5 minute
period in animals, cats.
Slow decr in cochlear microphonic and neural potentials due to parenteral,
intravenous, administration of 200 mg per kg, in saline solution, of diuretic, acetazolamide, for 5 minute period in animals, cats.
   (CT) Same method using 7 cc per kg of saline solution in 14 cats, control
   group.
   (AD) Clinical significance of study of acetazolamide not determined due to
   lack of reports of hearing loss with use of drug.
Severe decr in cochlear microphonic and neural potentials but no changes in
electrolyte concentrations of endolymph or perilymph due to parenteral,
intravenous, administration of 30 mg per kg daily of diuretic, ethacrynic
acid, for 3 to 4 days in 3 animals, cats.
   (AD) Results of study suggest severe hearing loss.
Edema of stria vascularis and damage to outer hair cells of organ of Corti
but normal chemical composition of endolymph and perilymph due to parenteral,
intraperitoneal, administration of 30 mg per kg of diuretic, ethacrynic acid,
in 1 dose in 9 animals, cats.
   (AD) Study of effect of diuretics on chemical composition of fluids of
   inner ear and relationship to cochlear microphonic and histopathology of
   temporal bone.   (ENG)

                                                                      169
Progressive sensorineural hearing loss, complete range of degrees of damage
to organ of Corti, and degeneration in cochlear nuclei due to parenteral,
intramuscular, administration of 15 to 100 mg per kg daily of antibiotic,
kanamycin (kanamycin sulfate), for 28 to 180 days in 3 animals, monkeys,
young, 2 to 6 years age, male and female, 3 to 9 kg weight, conditioned.
High frequency hearing loss and damage to organ of Corti due to parenteral,
intramuscular, administration of 100 mg per kg daily of antibiotic, neomycin
(neomycin sulfate), for 5 days in 1 animal, monkey, young, conditioned.
Delayed severe sensorineural hearing loss after 2 months and severe damage to
organ of Corti due to parenteral, intramuscular, administration of 50 mg per
kg of antibiotic, neomycin (neomycin sulfate), for 15 days in 1 animal,
monkey, young, conditioned.
   (CT) Pretreatment hearing baseline determined.
   (AD) Study showed correlation of measurement of hearing loss and histopathology of cochlea in same subject.
   (AD) Cochleograms made to show patterns of cell loss.

(AD) Reported that neomycin more ototoxic than kanamycin. (ENG)

181
Decr in succinic dehydrogenase in outer hair cells of organ of Corti due to parenteral, intratympanic, administration of 200 mg per ml solution of antibiotic, kanamycin (kanamycin sulfate), in animals, guinea pigs, adult.
Decr in succinic dehydrogenase in outer hair cells of organ of Corti due to parenteral, intratympanic, administration of 200 mg per ml solution of antibiotic, dihydrostreptomycin (dihydrostreptomycin sulfate), in animals, guinea pigs, adult.
Decr in succinic dehydrogenase in outer hair cells of organ of Corti due to parenteral, intratympanic, administration of 200 mg per ml solution of antibiotic, chloramphenicol (chloramphenicol succinate), in animals, guinea pigs, adult.
   (AD) Same type of damage to organ of Corti due to all 3 antibiotics.
Severe decr in succinic dehydrogenase in organ of Corti, in particular in outer hair cells, and atrophy of outer hair cells due to saturated solution of antimalarial, quinine (quinine hydrochloride), in animals, guinea pigs.
Complete degeneration of organ of Corti due to saturated solution of antimalarial, quinine (quinine hydrochloride), in animals, guinea pigs.
   (AD) Damage to organ of Corti more severe due to quinine than to antibiotics.
   (AD) Activity of succinic dehydrogenase often higher in outer hair cells.
   (AD) Possible that damage to outer hair cells due to higher rate of metabolism. (ENG)

197
Progressive degeneration of organ of Corti beginning at base of cochlea due to antibiotic, neomycin, in animals, guinea pigs.
Progressive degeneration of organ of Corti beginning at base of cochlea due to antibiotic, kanamycin, in animals, guinea pigs.
Progressive degeneration of organ of Corti beginning at base of cochlea due to antibiotic, framycetin, in animals, guinea pigs.
No damage to hair cells of organ of Corti due to parenteral administration of high doses of antibiotic, dihydrostreptomycin, for long periods in animals, guinea pigs.
   (AD) Surface specimen technique used in study of organ of Corti.
   (AD) Damage to organ of Corti due to ototoxic drugs different from that due to noise. (ENG)

226
Changes in hair cells of inner ear but no damage to stria vascularis due to parenteral, intramuscular, administration of 300 mg per kg of antibiotic, streptomycin (streptomycin sulfate), in animals, guinea pigs.
Damage to hair cells, then complete degeneration of organ of Corti, and degeneration of spiral ganglion due to parenteral, intramuscular, administration of 200 or 300 mg per kg daily of antibiotic, kanamycin (kanamycin sulfate), for range of 7 to 29 injections in 28 animals, guinea pigs.
   (AD) Studies using electron microscopy and light microscopy.
   (AD) Study of transport in cochlea.
   (AD) Suggested that debris from degeneration in cochlea removed by Claudius cells and Reissner's membrane. (ENG)

245
Degeneration of outer hair cells of organ of Corti and changes in supporting cells due to 400 mg per kg daily of antibiotic, kanamycin, for 14 days in animals, guinea pigs.
Degeneration of organ of Corti due to 400 mg per kg daily of antibiotic, dihydrostreptomycin, for 14 days in animals, guinea pigs.
   (AD) Comparative study of cochleotoxic effects of kanamycin and dihydrostreptomycin. (FR)

333
Vestibular problems due to antibiotic, streptomycin, in humans.
Severe cochlear impairment due to antibiotic, dihydrostreptomycin, in humans.
Loss of hair cells in organ of Corti and hearing loss due to antibiotics, aminoglycoside, in humans.
Hearing loss in fetus due to antimalarial, quinine, in humans, female,

treated during pregnancy.
Transient hearing loss due to high doses of salicylate, aspirin, for long
period in humans.
(AD) Discussion of possible cochleo-vestibulotoxic effects of ototoxic
drugs.
(AD) Ototoxic effects related to concurrent disorders, dosage, duration of
treatment, and age of individuals. (ENG)

338
No loss of pinna reflex and no significant histological changes due to parenteral, subcutaneous, administration of 400 mg per kg daily in 1 injection of
antibiotic, dihydrostreptomycin, for 8 to 37 injections in 8 animals, guinea
pigs, young, 200 to 290 g weight.
Hearing loss after 64 injections and moderate damage to hair cells of cochlea
due to parenteral, subcutaneous, administration of 600 mg per kg daily, total
dose of 38.4 g, of antibiotic, dihydrostreptomycin, for 9 to 64 injections in
1 of 5 animals, guinea pigs, young, 200 to 290 g weight.
No loss of pinna reflex and no significant histological changes due to 50 mg
per kg daily of antibiotic, kanamycin, for 64 injections in 10 animals,
guinea pigs.
(CT) Test of pinna reflex, pretreatment and daily during treatment with
antibiotics.
(AD) Suggested relationship between degree of kanamycin damage to cochlea
and daily dose rather than total dose. (ENG)

437
Hearing loss and damage to cochlea due to antibiotic, neomycin, in animals,
guinea pigs and monkeys, and humans.
Hearing loss and damage to cochlea due to antibiotic, streptomycin, in animals, guinea pigs and monkeys, and humans.
(AD) Discussion of findings on decr of ototoxicity of aminoglycoside
antibiotics. (GER)

547
Bilateral sensorineural hearing loss within 20 minutes but normal vestibular
function due to parenteral, intravenous, administration of 50 mg of diuretic,
ethacrynic acid (SM), in 1 injection in 1 human, adult, 53 years age, female,
with kidney disorder.
(AD) Hearing loss confirmed by audiogram.
(AD) Vestibular function tests showed normal vestibular function.
Simultaneous oral administration of 18 g of antibiotic, neomycin (SM), in 7
days in 1 human, adult, 53 years age, female, with kidney disorder.
Severe destruction of outer hair cells of organ of Corti in basal coil of
cochlea due to parenteral, intravenous, administration of 50 mg of diuretic,
ethacrynic acid (SM), in 1 injection in 1 human, adult, 53 years age, female,
with kidney disorder.
(AD) Suggested that damage to hair cells possibly due to neomycin also.
(AD) Suggested possible permanent hearing loss as result of ethacrynic
acid treatment in patients with kidney disorders.
Transient and permanent total hearing loss within 15 minutes due to parenteral administration of diuretic, ethacrynic acid, in animals, cats. (ENG)

627
Sensorineural hearing loss and vestibular problems due to parenteral, oral,
and topical administration of antibiotics in humans with and without kidney
disorder.
Degeneration of cochlea due to parenteral, intratympanic, administration of
antibiotic, neomycin, in animals, guinea pigs.
Transient sensorineural hearing loss due to high doses of salicylates in
humans.
Sensorineural hearing loss due to antimalarial, quinine, in humans.
Sensorineural hearing loss due to chemical agent, tobacco, in humans.
Sensorineural hearing loss due to sedative, alcohol, in humans.
(AD) Discussion of ototoxicity of various drugs as 1 etiology of sen-
sorineural hearing loss in adults. (ENG)

715
Loss of outer hair cells of organ of Corti in lower part of first coil of

cochlea due to parenteral, intramuscular, administration of 400 mg per kg of antibiotic, capreomycin, for 28 days in 40 percent of 10 animals, guinea pigs, albino, 300 g weight.
Severe loss of outer hair cells of organ of Corti from lower part of basal coil to upper coil of cochlea due to parenteral, intramuscular, administration of 400 mg per kg of antibiotic, kanamycin, for 28 days in 100 percent of 11 animals, guinea pigs, albino, 300 g weight.
(CT) Test of Preyer reflex before, during, and after administration of antibiotics.
(AD) Study suggested that capreomycin less ototoxic than kanamycin in guinea pigs.
(AD) No observed damage to vestibular apparatus. (JAP)

Vestibular findings

454
Damage to vestibular apparatus due to high doses of antibiotic, gentamicin, in animals, guinea pigs.
Damage to vestibular apparatus due to low doses of antibiotic, gentamicin, in humans with disorders. (GER)

546
Degeneration and fusion of hair cells of crista ampullaris, first in central part and later in peripheral parts, due to topical administration to bulla of 0.2 ml in 1 injection daily of 0.3 percent solution of antibiotic, gentamicin (gentamicin sulfate), for total of 7 injections in animals, guinea pigs.
(AD) Electron microscopic study of effects of gentamicin on vestibular apparatus.
(AD) Study showed more damage to type 1 hair cells than to type 2 hair cells. (ENG)

110
Nystagmus and other vestibular problems due to topical administration to bulla of 0.5 g of antibiotic, streptomycin, in 1 injection in cats.
(AD) Suggested route of streptomycin in cat from bulla by way of large membrane of round window to inner ear.
Changes in chromatin in hair cells, type 1, of maculae due to topical administration to bulla of 0.5 g of antibiotic, streptomycin, in 1 injection in cats.
(AD) Suggested that destruction of hair cells due to changes in protein metabolism as result of action of streptomycin. (ENG)

216
Damage to hair cells and decr in excitation of vestibular apparatus due to parenteral, intramuscular, administration of 250 mg per kg of antibiotic, streptomycin (streptomycin sulfate), for 10 and 30 days in animals, guinea pigs.
Damage to hair cells and decr in excitation of vestibular apparatus due to parenteral, intramuscular, administration of 250 mg per kg of antibiotic, streptomycin (IB) (streptomycin sulfate), for 10 and 30 days in animals, guinea pigs, with intramuscular administration of 1.25 ml per kg of ozothin.
(CT) Study of 14 guinea pigs, control group, with 1.25 ml per kg or 2.5 ml per kg daily of ozothin.
(AD) No decr in streptomycin damage to hair cells of vestibular apparatus with administration of ozothin.
(AD) Evaluation of damage with cytovestibulogram and caloric test.
(AD) Vestibulotoxic effects depend on total dosage of streptomycin used. (GER)

253
Severe vestibular problems, as nystagmus, after 3 to 6 hours due to topical administration to middle ear and parenteral administration of high doses of antibiotic, streptomycin, for range of 1 to 7 days in 28 animals, cats.
Decr in ribosomes of cytoplasm of type 1 hair cells of vestibular apparatus due to topical administration to middle ear and parenteral administration of high doses of antibiotic, streptomycin, for range of 1 to 7 days in 28 animals, cats.
(CT) Study of cats, control group.

(AD) Suggested that primary location of action of streptomycin is protein synthesis of cells. (GER)

336

Damage to type 1 hair cells of vestibular apparatus and vestibular problems due to topical administration to middle ear of antibiotic, streptomycin, in 1 injection in animals.
(AD) Destruction of hair cells and ototoxicity result of effect of streptomycin on protein synthesis of cells. (FR)

380

Unilateral loss of vestibular function and no ataxia due to parenteral administration, infusion into carotid artery, of 150 cc in Ringer's Lactate every 24 hours, total dose of 0.84 to 1.5 g per kg, of antibiotic, streptomycin (streptomycin sulfate), for 3 to 10 days in 5 animals, cat s, adult, 1.9 to 3.1 kg weight.
Bilateral loss of vestibular function with ataxia and destruction of hair cells of crista ampullaris and semicircular canal due to parenteral administration, infusion into carotid artery, of 150 cc in Ringer's Lactate every 24 hours, total dose of 1.2 to 2.5 g per kg, of antibiotic, streptomycin (streptomycin sulfate), for 6 to 12 days in 5 animals, cats, adult, 2.3 to 5.1 kg weight.
No hearing loss and no damage to hair cells of organ of Corti due to parenteral administration, infusion into carotid artery, of 150 cc in Ringer's Lactate every 24 hours, total dose of 0.84 to 2.5 g per kg, of antibiotic, streptomycin (streptomycin sulfate), for 3 to 12 days in 10 animals, cats, adult, 1.9 to 5.1 kg weight.
Decr in cochlear microphonic but no damage to hair cells of organ of Corti due to parenteral administration, infusion into carotid artery, of 150 cc in Ringer's Lactate every 24 hours, total dose of 1.0 g per kg, of antibiotic, streptomycin (streptomycin sulfate), for 4 days in 1 animal, cat, adult, 3.0 kg weight.
(CT) Measurement of cochlear function and vestibular function before and after infusion of streptomycin.
(AD) Type of loss of vestibular function due to total dosage of streptomycin and duration of administration.
(AD) Unilateral destruction of vestibular function without cochlear impairment is goal in treatment of Meniere's disease. (ENG)

456

Damage to type 1 hair cells of cristae and macula utriculi, no significant changes in macula sacculi, and no changes in type 2 hair cells of vestibular apparatus due to parenteral, intramuscular, administration of 200 mg per kg daily, total doses of 1600 to 3800 mg per kg, of antibiotic, streptomycin (streptomycin sulfate), for range of 10 to 26 days, until decline in caloric threshold values of 2 to 10 degrees C, in 4 animals, squirrel monkeys, 500 to 600 g weight.
Severe damage to type 1 and 2 hair cells of cristae, loss of type 1 hair cells of macula utriculi, and slight changes in macula sacculi due to parenteral, intramuscular, administration of 200 mg per kg daily, total doses of 2000 and 2600 mg per kg, of antibiotic, streptomycin (streptomycin sulfate), for 14 and 18 days, until complete suppression of vestibular function, in 2 animals, squirrel monkeys, 500 to 600 g weight.
(AD) Damage to vestibular function determined by vestibular function tests.
(AD) Relative mild damage in early period of intoxication result of low concentration of streptomycin in endolymph due to intramuscular route.
(AD) Suggested mechanism of streptomycin action is damage to enzyme system, damage to cytoplasmic membrane, and inhibition of protein synthesis and ribosome function. (ENG)

476

Vestibulotoxic effects due to 100 mg per kg of antibiotic, streptomycin, in animals, pigeons.
Some decr in vestibulotoxic effects due to 100 mg per kg of antibiotic, streptomycin (IB), for 30 days in animals, pigeons, with administration of 25000 units of vitamin A.
(AD) Structural damage similar in both groups of pigeons. (POL)

015

Damage to cells of ampulla due to range of doses of antibiotic, viomycin, in
animals.
  (AD) Electron microscopic study of effects of viomycin on vestibular
  apparatus. (JAP)

047

Range of degree of damage to crista ampullaris and macula due to parenteral,
intramuscular, administration of 150 mg per kg daily of antibiotic, viomycin
(viomycin sulfate), for about 2 to 3 weeks in 3 animals, squirrel monkeys.
Range of degree of damage to crista ampullaris and macula due to parenteral,
intramuscular, administration of 200 to 300 mg per kg daily of antibiotic,
viomycin (viomycin sulfate), for about 2 to 3 weeks in 3 animals, cats.
More severe damage to crista ampullaris and macula due to topical administration in solution of range of 113 mg per ml to 500 mg per ml solution of
antibiotic, viomycin (viomycin sulfate), in 1 or 2 doses in 9 animals, cats.
  (CT) Control group of 2 monkeys and 2 cats used. (ENG)

232

Degeneration of hair cells of vestibular apparatus due to parenteral administration of antibiotic, kanamycin, in animals, guinea pigs.
Degeneration of hair cells of vestibular apparatus due to administration to
middle ear of antibiotic, streptomycin, in animals, guinea pigs.
  (AD) Study using surface specimen technique. (ENG)

275

Loss of some hair cells of crista ampullaris with replacement by supporting
cells due to parenteral, intraperitoneal, administration of 250 mg per kg
every other day of antibiotic, streptomycin (streptomycin sulfate), for 8
weeks in 1 group of 48 animals, guinea pigs, pigmented, young, 300 g average
weight.
Loss of some hair cells of crista ampullaris with replacement by supporting
cells due to parenteral, intraperitoneal, administration of 250 mg per kg
every other day of antibiotic, kanamycin (kanamycin sulfate), for 8 weeks in
1 group of 48 animals, guinea pigs, pigmented, young, 300 g average weight.
Loss of some hair cells of crista ampullaris with replacement by supporting
cells due to topical administration to middle ear of 0.6 ml of 250 mg per kg
of antibiotic, streptomycin (streptomycin sulfate), for 3 times with interval
of 1 week in 1 group of 48 animals, guinea pigs, pigmented, young, 300 g
average weight.
Loss of some hair cells of crista ampullaris with replacement by supporting
cells due to topical administration to middle ear of 0.6 ml of 250 mg per kg
of antibiotic, kanamycin (kanamycin sulfate), for 3 times with interval of 1
week in 1 group of 48 animals, guinea pigs, pigmented, young, 300 g average
weight.
  (AD) Degeneration of hair cells of crista ampullaris most severe in group
  with topical administration of streptomycin to middle ear.
  (AD) Degeneration of hair cells of crista ampullaris least severe in group
  with intraperitoneal administration of kanamycin. (ENG)

432

Damage to sensory epithelia of macula utriculi and macula sacculi due to
parenteral, intraperitoneal, administration of 250 mg per kg every other day
of antibiotic, streptomycin (streptomycin sulfate), for 8 weeks in 12 animals, guinea pigs, pigmented, young, about 300 g weight.
Least severe damage to sensory epithelia of macula utriculi and macula sacculi due to parenteral, intraperitoneal, administration of 250 mg per kg every
day of antibiotic, kanamycin (kanamycin sulfate), for 8 weeks in 12 animals,
guinea pigs, pigmented, young, about 300 g weight.
Most severe damage to sensory epithelia of macula utriculi and macula sacculi
due to topical administration to middle ear cavity through tympanic membrane
of about 0.6 ml of concentration of 250 mg per kg of antibiotic, streptomycin
(streptomycin sulfate), in 8 injections, with interval of 1 week between
injections, in 12 animals, guinea pigs, pigmented, young, about 300 g weight.
Damage to sensory epithelia of macula utriculi and macula sacculi due to
topical administration to middle ear cavity through tympanic membrane of
about 0.6 ml of concentration of 250 mg per kg of antibiotic, kanamycin
(kanamycin sulfate), in 8 injections, with interval of 1 week between injec-

tions, in 12 animals, guinea pigs, pigmented, young, about 300 g weight.
(AD)   More damage to vestibular apparatus due to topical administration
than due to parenteral administration of antibiotics.
(AD) More loss of hair cells in sensory epithelium of macula utriculi than
in that of macula sacculi.
(AD) Type 1 hair cells more vulnerable to aminoglycoside antibiotics than
type 2 hair cells.
(AD) Comment on morphological and phylogenetical vulnerability of hair
cells.
(AD) Replacement of hair cells of vestibular apparatus by supporting
cells. (ENG)

455

Damage to sensory epithelia of vestibular apparatus due to 250 mg per kg of
antibiotic, streptomycin, in animals.
Damage to sensory epithelia of vestibular apparatus due to 250 mg per kg of
antibiotic, kanamycin, in animals. (JAP)

Cochleo-vestibular findings

105

Transient bilateral incr in pure tone threshold but without tone decay and
without difference limen and decr in duration of nystagmus and in slow phase
velocity of nystagmus due to oral administration of incr doses to about 6 to
8 g per day, until subjective hearing loss observed, of salicylate, aspirin
(CB), in 12 humans, adult and aged, range of 23 to 68 years age, with rheumatoid arthritis.
Combined administration of magnesium aluminum hydroxide (CB) in 12 humans,
adult and aged, range of 23 to 68 years age, with rheumatoid arthritis.
(CT) Withdrawal of salicylates before treatment for standardization of
salicylate level.
(CT) Audiometry and vestibular function tests before, during, and after
treatment with salicylate.
(AD) Serum salicylate level determined when subjective hearing loss reported.
Transient sensorineural hearing loss but no damage to hair cells of organ of
Corti or to membranous labyrinth due to oral administration of high doses, as
high as 7 to 10 g per day, of salicylates for long period in 1 human, Caucasian, adult, 62 years age, female, with previous progressive hearing loss.
Transient sensorineural hearing loss but no damage to organ of Corti, spiral
ganglion, or membranous labyrinth due to oral administration of high doses,
as high as 5 g per day, of salicylate, aspirin, for 15 years in 1 human,
adult, 61 years age, female, with rheumatoid arthritis. (ENG)

262

Possible damage to vestibular apparatus and organ of Corti due to oral ingestion of large amounts of chemical agent, alcohol, ethyl, for long period in 8
humans, adult and aged, 44 to 75 years age, male and female, chronic alcoholics.
(AD) Report on results of temporal bone study.
(AD) Previous observations of transient hearing loss and tinnitus during
alcohol intoxication.
(AD) Need for more study for interpretation of results. (ENG)

251

Damage to organ of Corti and crista ampullaris due to parenteral, subcutaneous, administration of 200 or 400 mg per kg daily in 3 doses every 8
hours of antibiotic, aminosidine (aminosidine sulfate), for 30 days in 2
groups of 16 animals, guinea pigs, 300 g weight.
Less damage to organ of Corti and crista ampullaris due to parenteral, subcutaneous, administration of 50 or 100 mg per kg daily in 3 doses every 8 hours
of antibiotic, aminosidine (aminosidine sulfate), for 30 days in 2 groups of
16 animals, guinea pigs, 300 g weight.
(CT) Study of 8 guinea pigs, control group.
(CT) Observation of function of cochlea and vestibular apparatus, pretreatment and during treatment. (IT)

039

Damage to endorgan of cochlea and vestibular apparatus due to parenteral or oral administration of high doses of antibiotics for long periods in humans. No reported ototoxic effects due to topical administration of unspecified doses of antibiotics for unspecified period in humans. (ENG)

458

Damage to cochlear function and vestibular function and structural damage to cochlea and vestibular apparatus due to antibiotics in animals, guinea pigs.
   (AD) Use of Preyer reflex, vestibular function tests, and measurement of cochlear microphonics to determine ototoxic effects of antibiotics on function of inner ear.
   (AD) Histological study to determine structural damage to inner ear. (ENG)

462

Damage to hair cells of organ of Corti, stria vascularis, nerve process, spiral ganglion, limbus, and cochlear wall due to antibiotics in animals, guinea pigs.
   (AD) Ototoxic effects result of retention of antibiotics in inner ear longer than in blood due to slower elimination.
   (AD) More active cells of cochlea more sensitive to ototoxic antibiotics.
   (AD) Neomycin most ototoxic, followed by kanamycin, viomycin, streptomycin, and capreomycin.
   (AD) Study of effect of inhibitors, nialamide, pantothenic acid, methylated compounds, and vitamin B on ototoxicity of antibiotics.
   (AD) Electrophysiological and histological study of cochleo-vestibulotoxic effects of antibiotics in guinea pig. (ENG)

506

Damage to hair cells of vestibular apparatus and cochlea due to antibiotics in humans and animals.
   (AD) Discussion of relationship between elimination of drugs and damage to ear.
   (AD) Need for careful consideration in use of aminoglycoside antibiotics. (ENG)

022

Progressive degeneration of hair cells of organ of Corti and membranous labyrinth due to topical administration to middle ear of 0.2 ml 1 time daily of 50 percent saline solution of antibiotic, gentamicin, for 1 to 4 days in animals, guinea pigs.
Severe damage to sensory epithelia of vestibular apparatus and degeneration of hair cells of cochlea due to topical administration to middle ear of 0.2 ml of 0.3 percent solution of antibiotic, gentamicin, for 13 days in animals, guinea pigs.
   (AD) Degeneration due to topical administration of low concentration of gentamicin for long period similar to degeneration due to intramuscular injections of high doses of gentamicin for long period in other studies.
   (AD) Study includes literature review of clinical and experimental ototoxicity. (ENG)

370

Severe damage to hair cells of organ of Corti, supporting cells, stria vascularis, Reissner's membrane, spiral ganglion, crista ampullaris, and semicircular canal due to parenteral, intramuscular, administration of 100 mg per kg daily of antibiotic, gentamicin, for 28, 35, or 49 days in 4 animals, guinea pigs.
Damage to hair cells of organ of Corti in basal coil of cochlea, supporting cells, and spiral ganglion, and severe damage to crista ampullaris and semicircular canal due to parenteral, intramuscular, administration of 75 mg per kg daily of antibiotic, gentamicin, for 35, 42, or 49 days in 3 animals, guinea pigs.
Moderate damage to hair cells of organ of Corti in basal coil of cochlea, supporting cells, spiral ganglion, crista ampullaris, and semicircular canal due to parenteral, intramuscular, administration of 50 mg per kg daily of antibiotic, gentamicin, for 38 or 46 days in 2 animals, guinea pigs.
   (CT) Normal function of cochlea and vestibular apparatus in 3 guinea pigs, control group, not treated with gentamicin.

(AD) Relationship but not precise correlation between cochleo-vestibuloto-xic effects of gentamicin and dosage and duration of treatment.
(AD) Individual differences in response to same doses of gentamicin for same period.
(AD) Not precise correlation between results of histological study and results of previous functional study. (IT)

573

Bilateral vestibular problems, ataxia, and damage to hair cells of organ of Corti in basal coil of cochlea and of cristae and maculae due to parenteral, intramuscular, administration of 80 or 50 mg per kg on 5 days a week of antibiotic, gentamicin, in 5 animals, squirrel monkeys, Saimiri sciureus, about 2 years age, male and female.
Loss of equilibrium, ataxia, damage to hair cells of cristae and maculae, and some degeneration of nerve process near hair cells due to parenteral, subcutaneous, administration of 60, 30, or 20 mg per kg on 7 days a week of antibiotic, gentamicin, in 7 animals, squirrel monkeys, Saimiri sciureus, about 2 years age, male and female.
    (AD) Type 1 hair cells of cristae and maculae more vulnerable to gentamicin than type 2 hair cells.
    (CT) Squirrel monkey rail method and test of nystagmus, pretreatment and posttreatment.
    (AD) Earlier onset of equilibrium disorders with high daily doses than with low daily doses.
    (AD) Total doses before onset of ataxia slightly more in group with high daily doses.
    (AD) Less ototoxic effects and slower onset with administration of gentamicin 5 days a week than 7 days a week.
    (AD) Lower doses in group with injections 7 days a week resulted in more severe and earlier onset of loss of equilibrium.
    (AD) Damage to vestibular apparatus slightly more severe in animals with higher daily doses.
    (AD) Correlation between equilibrium test and electron microscopic findings. (ENG)

680

Damage to vestibular apparatus and cochlea due to high doses of antibiotic, gentamicin, for several weeks in animals, guinea pigs.
    (AD) Electron microscopical study of effects of gentamicin on inner ear of guinea pig. (ENG)

459

No significant decr in cochlear microphonic due to parenteral, subcutaneous, administration of 100 mg per kg daily for 5 days a week, total dose of 3 g per kg, of antibiotic, kanamycin (kanamycin sulfate), for 30 days in animals, guinea pigs.
Decr in cochlear microphonics in 14 of 15 ears, damage to hair cells of organ of Corti and to stria vascularis, slight to severe damage to spiral ganglion, damage to macula utriculi, and slight damage to crista ampullaris and macula sacculi due to parenteral, subcutaneous, administration of 250 mg per kg daily for 5 days a week, total dose of 5 g per kg, of antibiotic, kanamycin (kanamycin sulfate), for 20 days in animals, guinea pigs.
Significant decr in cochlear microphonics in all ears, damage to outer hair cells of organ of Corti and to stria vascularis, and slight damage to spiral ganglion due to parenteral, subcutaneous, administration of 200 mg per kg daily for 5 days a week, total dose of 6 g per kg, of antibiotic, kanamycin (kanamycin sulfate), for 30 days in animals, guinea pigs.
Significant decr in cochlear microphonics due to parenteral, subcutaneous, administration of 200 mg per kg daily for 5 days a week, total dose of 6 g per kg, of antibiotic, kanamycin (IB) (kanamycin sulfate), for 30 days in animals, guinea pigs, with subcutaneous administration of 1.5 mg per kg of nialamide.
Significant decr in cochlear microphonics, damage to hair cells of organ of Corti and to stria vascularis, and slight damage to spiral ganglion due to parenteral, subcutaneous, administration of 200 mg per kg daily for 5 days a week, total dose of 6 g per kg, of antibiotic, kanamycin (IB) (kanamycin sulfate), for 30 days in animals, guinea pigs, with subcutaneous administration of 8 mg per kg of nialamide.

Significant decr in cochlear microphonics, damage to hair cells of organ of Corti and to stria vascularis, slight to severe damage to spiral ganglion, slight damage to limbus, and slight damage to macula utriculi and cristae due to parenteral, subcutaneous, administration of 200 mg per kg daily for 5 days a week, total dose of 6 g per kg, of antibiotic, kanamycin (IB) (kanamycin sulfate), for 30 days in animals, guinea pigs, with subcutaneous administration of 15 mg per kg of nialamide.

(AD) No prevention of kanamycin effects on cochlear microphonics with administration of nialamide.

Less decr in cochlear microphonics in 6, 10, and 11 of 3 groups of 15 ears, damage to hair cells of organ of Corti and to stria vascularis, slight damage to spiral ganglion and to limbus, damage to macula utriculi, and slight damage to crista ampullaris due to parenteral, subcutaneous, administration of 250 mg per kg daily for 5 days a week, total dose of 5 g per kg, of antibiotic, kanamycin (IB), for 20 days in 3 groups of animals, guinea pigs, with pantothenic acid.

(CT) Same method using daily subcutaneous administration of 0.25 cc of isotonic saline in guinea pigs, control group.

(AD) Decr in kanamycin effects on cochlear microphonics with pantothenic acid.

(AD) Study of functional and structural cochleo-vestibulotoxic effects of kanamycin with and without inhibitors.

(AD) Statistical analysis of results.   (ENG)

157

Damage to hair cells of organ of Corti and membranous labyrinth and to neurons of spiral ganglion due to parenteral, subcutaneous, administration of 100 mg per kg, in physiological saline, of antibiotic, neomycin (neomycin sulfate), in 5 and 7 doses in 21 animals, guinea pigs, albino, 250 to 700 g weight.

Moderate damage to organ of Corti, less degeneration of hair cells of membranous labyrinth, and decr in number of neurons of spiral ganglion due to parenteral, subcutaneous, administration of 100 mg per kg of antibiotic, neomycin (neomycin sulfate), in 10,12,14,15, and 20 doses in 33 animals, guinea pigs, albino, 250 to 700 g weight.

Range of degrees of degeneration up to complete destruction of organ of Corti and disappearance of most of neurons of spiral ganglion due to parenteral, subcutaneous, administration of 100 mg per kg of antibiotic, neomycin (neomycin sulfate), in 30 doses in 6 animals, guinea pigs, albino, 250 to 700 g weight.

Range of degrees of degeneration up to complete destruction of organ of Corti and disappearance of most of neurons of spiral ganglion due to parenteral, subcutaneous, administration of 150 mg per kg of antibiotic, neomycin (neomycin sulfate), in 10 and 20 doses in 4 animals, guinea pigs, albino, 250 to 700 g weight.

(CT) Study of 19 guinea pigs, control group.

(AD) Damage due to high doses for shorter period similar to damage due to low doses for longer period.   (ENG)

461

Destruction of cochlear microphonics, destruction of hair cells of organ of Corti in basal coil of cochlea, severe damage to stria vascularis, damage to nuclei of limbus, and slight damage to macula utriculi due to parenteral, subcutaneous, administration of 100 mg per kg daily for 5 days a week, total dose of 3 g per kg, of antibiotic, neomycin (neomycin sulfate), for 30 days in animals, guinea pigs.

No damage to cochlear microphonics and no structural damage to cochlea or vestibular apparatus due to parenteral, subcutaneous, administration of 100 mg per kg daily for 5 days a week, total dose of 3 g per kg, of antibiotic, neomycin (methylneomycin), for 30 days in animals, guinea pigs.

Decr in cochlear microphonics due to parenteral, subcutaneous, administration of 100 mg per kg daily for 5 days a week, total dose of 1.5 g per kg, of antibiotic, neomycin (neomycin sulfate), for 15 days in animals, guinea pigs.

Decr in cochlear microphonics due to parenteral, subcutaneous, administration of 200 mg per kg daily for 5 days a week, total dose of 2 g per kg, of antibiotic, neomycin (neomycin sulfate), for 10 days in animals, guinea pigs.

Decr in cochlear microphonics due to parenteral, subcutaneous, administration of 200 mg per kg daily for 5 days a week, total dose of 2 g per kg, of anti-

biotic, neomycin (IB) (neomycin sulfate), for 10 days in animals, guinea pigs, with administration of vitamin B.
   (CT) Same method with daily subcutaneous administration of 0.25 cc iso-tonic saline in guinea pigs, control group.
   (AD) No decr in ototoxic effects of neomycin on cochlear microphonics with administration of vitamin B.
   (AD) Study of functional and structural cochleo-vestibulotoxic effects of neomycin.
   (AD) Statistical analysis of results.   (ENG)

235

Effect on hair cells of vestibular apparatus and organ of Corti due to ototo-xic drugs in humans and animals.
   (AD) Suggested role of hair cells of vestibular apparatus and organ of Corti as sensory meters with relative resistance to drugs.
   (AD) Literature review of effects of drugs on sensory endings.   (ENG)

111

Damage to organ of Corti and vestibular apparatus due to antibiotic, strep-tomycin, in humans and animals, guinea pigs.
   (AD) Comparative study of ototoxic effects of streptomycin in humans and animals. (GER)

155

Suppression of function of semicircular canal due to parenteral, intramuscu-lar, administration of range of 1100 to 4600 mg total doses of antibiotic, streptomycin (streptomycin sulfate), for 16 to 23 doses in 8 animals, squir-rel monkeys, with normal semicircular canal function.
   (CT) Vestibular function tests used to confirm pretreatment normal func-tion of semicircular canal.
Moderate to severe damage to hair cells of cristae and organ of Corti and some changes in spiral ganglion and maculae due to parenteral, intramuscular, administration of range of 1100 to 4600 mg total doses of antibiotic, strep-tomycin (streptomycin sulfate), for 16 to 23 doses in 8 animals, squirrel monkeys, with normal semicircular canal function.
   (AD) Report on 8 case studies to show clinical and pathological correla-tions. (ENG)

212

Changes in hair cells of vestibular apparatus due to 250 mg per kg daily of antibiotic, streptomycin (streptomycin sulfate), for 10 or 20 days in 9 animals, guinea pigs, 140 to 300 g weight.
Decr in damage to cochlea due to 250 mg per kg daily of antibiotic, strep-tomycin (IB) (streptomycin sulfate), for 10 or 15 days in 10 animals, guinea pigs, 140 to 300 g weight, with intramuscular administration of 1.25 ml per kg daily of ozothin.
   (CT) Study of 10 guinea pigs, control group, 5 normal and 5 with paren-teral administration of 2.5 ml per kg daily of ozothin for 10 days.
   (AD) Study not show decr in streptomycin damage to vestibular apparatus with administration of ozothin.   (GER)

395

Damage first to outer hair cells of organ of Corti in basal coil of cochlea due to high doses of antibiotics, aminoglycoside, in animals, guinea pigs.
   (AD) Same damage due to x-ray radiation.
Primary damage to central areas of crista ampullaris, crista neglecta, and macula due to antibiotics, aminoglycoside, in animals, guinea pigs.
   (AD) Damage to peripheral areas of crista ampullaris, crista neglecta, and macula due to x-ray radiation.
Disturbance of protein synthesis due to topical administration to bulla of antibiotic, streptomycin, in animals, guinea pigs.
   (AD) Similar electron microscopy findings for streptomycin administration to bulla and for x-ray radiation.
   (AD) Cochleo-vestibulotoxic effects due to x-ray radiation comp w effects due to antibiotics.   (ENG)

020

Effect on function of inner ear due to parenteral, subcutaneous, administra-

tion of high doses, range of 30 to 75 mg per kg of antibiotic, gentamicin, for about 8 to 20 days in 11 animals, cats.
   (AD) Preliminary study of dosage levels.
Damage to semicircular canal, membranous labyrinth, and outer hair cells and inner hair cells of the cochlea due to parenteral, subcutaneous, administration of high doses, range of 30 to 75 mg per kg of antibiotic, gentamicin, for about 8 to 20 days in 11 animals, cats, with kidney damage resulting from gentamicin.
   (AD) Preliminary study of dosage levels.
Partial hearing loss due to parenteral, subcutaneous, administration of 20 mg per kg of antibiotic, gentamicin, for 14 days in 1 out of 15 animals, cats.
Complete degeneration of outer hair cells of organ of Corti due to parenteral, subcutaneous, administration of 20 mg per kg of antibiotic, gentamicin, for 14 days in 1 out of 15 animals, cats.
Range of degree of damage, transient and permanent, to vestibular apparatus due to parenteral, subcutaneous, administration of 20 mg per kg of antibiotic, gentamicin, for 14 days in 15 animals, cats.
Complete damage to vestibular apparatus due to parenteral, subcutaneous, administration of 200 mg per kg of antibiotic, streptomycin, for 9 days in animals, cats.
Higher incidence and earlier symptoms of ototoxic effects due to parenteral, subcutaneous, administration of 20 mg per kg of antibiotic, gentamicin, for 14 days in 66.6 percent of 15 animals, cats, with kidney damage than in cats with normal kidney function.
   (AD) Study of correlation of functional and histological effects of gentamicin.
   (AD) Comparative study of effect on vestibular apparatus of gentamicin and streptomycin. (ENG)

                                                                              087
High frequency hearing loss and tinnitus due to antibiotics in humans, particularly infant and aged, and humans with kidney disorder.
Degeneration in hair cells of organ of Corti due to antibiotics in humans.
Vertigo and unsteady gait due to antibiotic, streptomycin, in humans.
Bilateral damage to vestibular apparatus due to antibiotic, streptomycin, in humans.
   (AD) Literature review of physiological and structural cochleo-vestibulotoxic effects of antibiotics.
   (AD) Degree of damage determined by dosage and duration of dosage of antibiotics. (ENG)

                                                                              109
Damage to hair cells in organ of Corti due to topical administration of 300 mg per kg of antibiotic, kanamycin, in 14 injections in animals, guinea pigs.
Severe degeneration of hair cells of organ of Corti and membranous labyrinth due to topical administration to middle ear of low doses of antibiotics in animals, guinea pigs.
   (AD) Report on studies of several years on cochleo-vestibulotoxic effects due to antibiotics. (ENG)

                                                                              185
Ataxia, damage to hair cells of macula, and damage to hair cells of organ of Corti due to parenteral, subcutaneous, administration of 10 to 80 mg per kg daily of antibiotic, gentamicin (gentamicin sulfate), for 19 to 120 days in animals, cats.
Ataxia due to 100 and 200 mg per kg daily of antibiotic, streptomycin (streptomycin sulfate), for 8 to 40 days in animals, cats.
Loss of Preyer reflex, decr in cochlear potential and eighth cranial nerve action potential, and loss of outer hair cells of organ of Corti due to 80 to 200 mg per kg daily of antibiotic, gentamicin (gentamicin sulfate), in animals, guinea pigs.
Damage to cochlea due to 100 and 200 mg per kg of antibiotic, kanamycin (kanamycin sulfate), in animals, guinea pigs.
   (AD) Comparative study of ototoxicity of gentamicin and other aminoglycoside antibiotics.
   (AD) Study suggested low risk of ototoxicity when gentamicin used in recommended clinical dose of 1 to 3 mg per kg. (ENG)

219

Cochleo-vestibulotoxic effects due to antibiotics in humans.
Transient and permanent sensorineural hearing loss due to diuretic, etha-
crynic acid, in humans.
Transient sensorineural hearing loss, tinnitus, and vertigo due to salicy-
late, aspirin, in humans.
Transient and permanent sensorineural hearing loss and dizziness due to
antimalarial, quinine, in humans.
Sensorineural hearing loss due to antimalarial, chloroquine, in humans.
Sensorineural hearing loss, tinnitus, and vertigo due to chemical agents in
humans.
   (AD) Literature review of ototoxic drugs with clinical and histopathologi-
   cal correlations.
   (AD) Comment on ototoxicity of some chemical agents.
   (AD) Review of theories of mechanism of action of ototoxic drugs. (ENG)

227

Bilateral tinnitus and sudden deafness possibly due to cardiovascular agent,
(SQ) hexadimethrine bromide, in 1 human, adult, 32 years age, female, with
chronic nephritis and treated with hemodialysis.
Previous administration of antituberculous agent, (SQ) PAS, in 1 human,
adult, 32 years age, female, with chronic nephritis and treated with hemodialysis.
Previous administration of antituberculous agent, (SQ) isoniazid, in 1 human,
adult, 32 years age, female, with chronic nephritis and treated with hemodialysis.
Damage to Reissner's membrane, degeneration of organ of Corti, stria vascularis, and spiral ganglion, and slight changes in vestibular apparatus possibly due to cardiovascular agent, (SQ) hexadimethrine bromide, in 1 human,
adult, 32 years age, female, with chronic nephritis and treated with hemodialysis.
Progressive severe sensorineural hearing loss possibly due to cardiovascular
agent, hexadimethrine bromide, in 4 humans, adolescent and adult, 17 to 40
years age, with kidney disorders and treated with hemodialysis.
   (AD) Association of hexadimethrine bromide with hearing loss only when
   used with hemodialysis in treatment of kidney disorder.
   (AD) No hearing loss in group treated with hemodialysis without hexadimethrine bromide. (ENG)

250

Damage to vestibular apparatus due to more than 1 g daily of antibiotic,
streptomycin, for 60 to 120 days in 25 percent of humans.
Dizziness 5 days after cessation of treatment due to parenteral, intramuscular, administration of 1 g every 12 hours of antibiotic, streptomycin (SM),
for 9 days in 1 human, adult, 44 years age, female, with peritonitis.
Simultaneous parenteral, intravenous, administration of 600 mg every 18 hours
of antibiotic, lincomycin (SM), for 9 days in 1 human, adult, 44 years age,
female, with peritonitis.
   (AD) Case report of vestibular problem due to streptomycin.
Damage to cochlea due to antibiotic, dihydrostreptomycin, for more than 1
week in 4 to 15 percent of humans.
Sensorineural hearing loss and damage to organ of Corti due to antibiotic,
kanamycin, in humans.
Sensorineural hearing loss and damage to organ of Corti due to antibiotic,
vancomycin, in humans.
   (AD) Discussion of cochleo-vestibulotoxic effects due to antibiotic therapy in surgery. (ENG)

261

Nystagmus, ataxia, and loss of pinna reflex after 4 to 5 hours due to parenteral, intratympanic, administration of 5 to 20 mg, in 0.1 ml Ringer's solution, of antibiotic, streptomycin (streptomycin sulfate), in 1 ear of 15
animals, guinea pigs, pigmented, 250 to 350 g weight, with normal pinna
reflex.
   (CT) Use of other ear of 15 guinea pigs, control group.
No detected vestibular problems due to parenteral administration of 300 mg
per kg daily of antibiotic, kanamycin (kanamycin sulfate), for 8 to 15 days
in 5 animals, guinea pigs, pigmented, 250 to 350 g weight, with normal pinna

reflex.
Degeneration of hair cells of vestibular apparatus and organ of Corti due to
parenteral, intratympanic, administration of 5 to 20 mg, in 0.1 ml Ringer's
solution, of antibiotic, streptomycin (streptomycin sulfate), in all 15
animals, guinea pigs, pigmented, 250 to 350 g weight, with normal pinna
reflex.
   (AD) Suggested relationship between histological changes and streptomycin
   dosage.
Degeneration of hair cells of vestibular apparatus and organ of Corti due to
parenteral administration of 300 mg per kg daily of antibiotic, kanamycin
(kanamycin sulfate), for 8 to 15 days in 4 out of 5 animals, guinea pigs,
pigmented, 250 to 350 g weight, with normal pinna reflex.
   (AD) Same pattern of degeneration in vestibular apparatus due to streptomycin and kanamycin.
   (AD) Hair cells of vestibular apparatus more sensitive to streptomycin and
   hair cells of organ of Corti more sensitive to kanamycin. (ENG)

                                                                        324
Ataxia, vestibular problems with improvement in some, and damage to hair
cells of vestibular apparatus due to parenteral, subcutaneous, administration
of 20 mg per kg of antibiotic, gentamicin (gentamicin sulfate), for 19 days
maximum for acute intoxication and 14 days for chronic intoxication in 15
animals, cats.
Hearing loss and damage to hair cells of cochlea due to parenteral, subcutaneous, administration of 20 mg per kg of antibiotic, gentamicin (gentamicin
sulfate), for 19 days maximum for acute intoxication and 14 days for chronic
intoxication in 1 of 15 animals, cats.
   (AD) Preliminary study to determine minimum toxic level of gentamicin by
   parenteral route made previously.
   (AD) Cochleo-vestibulotoxic effects determined by audiometry and vestibular function tests.
Permanent severe vestibular problems and damage to hair cells of vestibular
apparatus due to parenteral, subcutaneous, administration of 200 mg per kg of
antibiotic, streptomycin (streptomycin sulfate), in 3 animals, cats.
Hearing loss and damage to hair cells of cochlea due to parenteral, subcutaneous, administration of 200 mg per kg of antibiotic, streptomycin (streptomycin sulfate), in 2 of 3 animals, cats.
Ataxia, vestibular problems, and damage to hair cells of vestibular apparatus
due to topical administration to bulla in solution of 6 percent concentration
in water of antibiotic, gentamicin (gentamicin sulfate), for 19 days in 1
animal, cat.
Ataxia, vestibular problems, and more severe damage to hair cells of vestibular apparatus due to topical administration to bulla in solution of 6 percent
concentration in Monex of antibiotic, gentamicin (gentamicin sulfate), for 5
days in 3 animals, cats.
   (CT) Same method using water or Monex without gentamicin in 11 cats,
   control group, showed no ototoxic effects.
   (AD) Preliminary study to determine concentration of gentamicin for topical route made previously.
Vestibular problems due to topical administration to bulla in solution of 6
percent concentration in water of antibiotic, neomycin, for 31 days in 2
animals, cats.
   (AD) Comparative study of effects of gentamicin and other aminoglycoside
   antibiotics.
   (AD) Ototoxicity of gentamicin dose related. (ENG)

                                                                        384
Usually transient hearing loss and no structural damage to organ of Corti,
stria vascularis, and spiral ganglion due to oral or topical administration
of salicylates in humans.
Hearing loss due to antimalarial, quinine, in humans.
Usually permanent hearing loss due to antimalarial, chloroquine, in humans.
Transient and permanent hearing loss and possible damage to hair cells of
organ of Corti due to diuretic, ethacrynic acid, in humans.
Sensorineural hearing loss due to cardiovascular agent, hexadimethrine
bromide, in humans with kidney disorder.
Sensorineural hearing loss and damage to organ of Corti due to topical ad-
ministration of antineoplastic, nitrogen mustard, in humans.

Sensorineural hearing loss due to high doses of antibiotic, chloramphenicol, in humans.
Primary vestibular problems due to antibiotic, streptomycin, in humans.
Hearing loss due to high doses usually of antibiotic, streptomycin, in humans.
   (AD) Early detection of hearing loss by audiometry prevents permanent damage.
High frequency hearing loss and severe damage to outer hair cells and slight damage to inner hair cells of organ of Corti due to antibiotic, kanamycin, in humans.
Sensorineural hearing loss due to parenteral, oral, and topical administration of antibiotic, neomycin, in humans with or without kidney disorders.
Degeneration of hair cells of organ of Corti and of nerve process due to antibiotics, aminoglycoside, in animals.
   (AD) Literature review of physiological and structural cochleo-vestibulo-toxic effects of ototoxic drugs.
   (AD) Discussion of suggested mechanism of ototoxicity and routes of drugs to inner ear.
Bilateral sensorineural hearing loss due to oral administration of antibiotic, neomycin, in 4 of 8 humans with liver disease.
Bilateral sensorineural hearing loss due to oral administration of range of doses of antibiotic, neomycin (SM), in 2 of 5 humans with liver disease.
Bilateral sensorineural hearing loss due to diuretics (SM), in 2 of 5 humans with liver disease.
Transient progression of previous hearing loss due to parenteral, intravenous, administration of diuretic, ethacrynic acid (SM), in 1 injection in 1 of 5 humans with liver disease.
   (CT) Normal cochlear function in 6 humans, control group, with liver disease and not treated with neomycin or diuretics.
   (CT) Normal cochlear function in 13 humans, control group, with liver disease and treated with diuretics but not with neomycin.
   (AD) Hearing loss confirmed by audiometry.
   (AD) Reported that hearing loss due to neomycin or diuretics in humans with liver disease not related to dosage.
   (AD) Clinical study of effects of treatment with neomycin and diuretics in humans with liver disease.
Bilateral sensorineural hearing loss and vertigo due to antibiotic, ampicillin, in 1 human, adolescent, 17 years age, female, with tonsillitis.
   (AD) Cited case report.
Severe sensorineural hearing loss and vertigo due to topical administration in ear drops of antibiotic, framycetin, in 1 human, adult, 42 years age, male, with previous slight high frequency hearing loss.
   (AD) Cited case report.
Atrophy of hair cells of organ of Corti and hearing loss due to antibiotic, dihydrostreptomycin, in humans with tuberculous meningitis.
   (AD) Cited study.
Loss of inner hair cells and damage to outer hair cells due to 18 g of antibiotic, neomycin, for 18 days in 1 human.
   (AD) Cited case report. (ENG)

                                                               409
Primary damage to hair cells of organ of Corti, hearing loss, and possible vestibular problems due to antibiotic, viomycin, in humans.
Damage to hair cells of organ of Corti and hearing loss due to antibiotic, neomycin, in humans.
Damage to hair cells of organ of Corti and hearing loss due to antibiotic, kanamycin, in humans.
Primary damage to vestibular apparatus, vestibular problems, and possible hearing loss due to antibiotic, streptomycin, in humans.
Primary damage to vestibular apparatus, vestibular problems, and possible hearing loss due to antibiotic, gentamicin, in humans.
   (AD) Need for audiometry and vestibular function tests, pretreatment and during treatment, with clinical use of aminoglycoside antibiotics.
   (AD) Incr in blood levels and ototoxicity of antibiotics in humans with kidney disorders. (ENG)

                                                               460
No significant decr in cochlear microphonics due to parenteral, subcutaneous,

administration of 100 mg per kg daily for 5 days a week, total dose of 7.5 g
per kg, of antibiotic, streptomycin (streptomycin sulfate), for 75 days in
animals, guinea pigs.
Statistically significant decr in cochlear microphonics at 1 of 18 points
examined, damage to hair cells of organ of Corti, slight damage to stria
vascularis and spiral ganglion, damage to macula utriculi and cristae, slight
damage to macula sacculi, and vestibular problems due to parenteral, subcutaneous, administration of 200 mg per kg daily, then 400 mg per kg, followed
by return to 200 mg per kg, total dose of 15 g per kg, of antibiotic, streptomycin (streptomycin sulfate), for 58 days in animals, guinea pigs.
  (AD) Vestibular problems confirmed by vestibular function tests.
No significant decr in cochlear microphonics due to parenteral, subcutaneous,
administration of 100 mg per kg daily for 5 days a week, total dose of 7.5 g
per kg, of antibiotic, viomycin (viomycin sulfate), for 75 days in animals,
guinea pigs.
Significant decr in cochlear microphonics, damage to hair cells of organ of
Corti and to stria vascularis, slight damage to spiral ganglion, and slight
damage to macula utriculi and crista ampullaris due to parenteral, subcutaneous, administration of 200 mg per kg daily for 5 days a week, then 400 mg
per kg, total dose of 15 g per kg, of antibiotic, viomycin (viomycin sulfate), for total of 67 days in animals, guinea pigs.
  (AD) Most toxicity for cochlear microphonics in guinea pig due to viomycin.
No significant decr in cochlear microphonics due to parenteral, subcutaneous,
administration of 100 mg per kg daily for 5 days each week, total dose of 7.5
g per kg, of antibiotic, capreomycin (capreomycin sulfate), for 75 days in
animals, guinea pigs.
No significant decr in cochlear microphonics, slight damage to outer hair
cells of organ of Corti and to stria vascularis, and no damage to vestibular
apparatus due to parenteral, subcutaneous, administration of 200 mg per kg
daily for 5 days a week, then 400 mg per kg, total dose of 15 g per kg, of
antibiotic, capreomycin (capreomycin sulfate), for total of 67 days in animals, guinea pigs.
  (CT) Same method using subcutaneous administration of 0.25 cc daily of
  isotonic saline in guinea pigs, control group.
  (AD) Least toxicity for inner ear of guinea pig due to capreomycin.
  (AD) Study of functional and structural cochleo-vestibulotoxic effects of
  streptomycin, viomycin, and capreomycin.
  (AD) Statistical analysis of results.   (ENG)

482

Decr in cochlear function and vestibular function due to parenteral, intramuscular, administration of 50 to 100 mg per kg of antibiotic, streptomycin
(streptomycin sulfate), for 35 days in animals, guinea pigs, pigmented, 400
to 500 g weight.
  (AD) More ototoxic effects with higher dosage.
Decr in cochlear function with both doses but decr in vestibular function
with only higher dose due to parenteral, intramuscular, administration of 50
to 100 mg per kg of antibiotic, dihydrostreptomycin (dihydrostreptomycin
sulfate), for 35 days in animals, guinea pigs, pigmented, 400 to 500 g
weight.
  (AD) More decr in cochlear function with higher dosage.
Decr in cochlear function in all animals but decr in vestibular function in 2
groups only due to parenteral, intramuscular, administration of 50 to 100 mg
per kg of antibiotic, kanamycin, for 35 days in animals, guinea pigs, pigmented, 400 to 500 g weight.
  (AD) More decr in cochlear function with higher dosage.
Decr in cochlear function due to parenteral, intramuscular, administration of
20 mg per kg of diuretic, ethacrynic acid, for 35 days in animals, guinea
pigs, pigmented, 400 to 500 g weight.
  (CT) Study of guinea pigs, control group, not treated with ototoxic drugs.
Decr in ototoxic effects due to parenteral, intramuscular, administration of
100 mg per kg of antibiotic, streptomycin (IB) (streptomycin sulfate), for 35
days in animals, guinea pigs, pigmented, 400 to 500 g weight, with administration of 1 mg per kg of various inhibitors.
Decr in ototoxic effects due to parenteral, intramuscular, administration of
100 mg per kg of antibiotic, dihydrostreptomycin (IB) (dihydrostreptomycin
sulfate), for 35 days in animals, guinea pigs, pigmented, 400 to 500 g

weight, with administration of 1 mg per kg of various inhibitors.
Decr in ototoxic effects due to parenteral, intramuscular, administration of
100 mg per kg of antibiotic, kanamycin (IB), for 35 days in animals, guinea
pigs, pigmented, 400 to 500 g weight, with administration of 1 mg per kg of
various inhibitors.
Decr in ototoxic effects due to parenteral, intramuscular, administration of
20 mg per kg of diuretic, ethacrynic acid (IB), for 35 days in animals,
guinea pigs, pigmented, 400 to 500 g weight, with administration of 1 mg per
kg of various inhibitors.
    (AD) Measurement of Preyer reflex and vestibular function tests.
Ototoxic effects, functional and structural, due to parenteral, intraperitoneal, administration of 100 mg per kg of antibiotic, streptomycin (streptomycin sulfate), for 50 days in animals, mice, male, 18 to 22 g weight.
No ototoxic effects due to parenteral, intraperitoneal, administration of 100
mg per kg of antibiotic, dihydrostreptomycin (dihydrostreptomycin sulfate),
for 50 days in animals, mice, male, 18 to 22 g weight.
Ototoxic effects, functional and structural, due to parenteral, intraperitoneal, administration of 100 mg per kg of antibiotic, kanamycin, for 50 days
in animals, mice, male, 18 to 22 g weight.
    (CT) Study of mice, control group, not treated with ototoxic drugs.
No ototoxic effects due to parenteral, intraperitoneal, administration of 100
mg per kg of antibiotic, streptomycin (IB) (streptomycin sulfate), for 50
days in animals, mice, male, 18 to 22 g weight, with administration of 1 mg
per kg of vitamin B.
No ototoxic effects due to parenteral, intraperitoneal, administration of 100
mg per kg of antibiotic, dihydrostreptomycin (IB) (dihydrostreptomycin sulfate), for 50 days in animals, mice, male, 18 to 22 g weight, with administration of 1 mg per kg of vitamin B.
No ototoxic effects due to parenteral, intraperitoneal, administration of 100
mg per kg of antibiotic, kanamycin (IB), for 50 days in animals, mice, male,
18 to 22 g weight, with administration of vitamin B.
    (AD) More ototoxic effects of aminoglycoside antibiotics in guinea pigs
    than in mice.
    (AD) Ototoxic effects of diuretic in guinea pigs. (IT)

576

Progressive ataxia beginning after 4 days of treatment due to topical administration to bulla of 0.4 ml daily of aqueous solution of 10 percent concentration, to produce blood level of 7 mcg per ml, of antibiotic, gentamicin,
for 19 days maximum in 1 of 2 animals, cats.
Minimal transient ataxia beginning after 10 to 18 days of treatment and
moderate damage to cristae and maculae but normal cochlea due to topical
administration to bulla of 0.4 ml daily of aqueous solution of 3 percent
concentration, to produce blood levels of less than 0.5 mcg per ml, of antibiotic, gentamicin, for 19 days maximum in 1 of 3 animals, cats.
    (AD) Preliminary studies of topical gentamicin in cats.
    (AD) Not possible to obtain audiograms due to administration of gentamicin
    in middle ear so evaluation of cochlear function depended on histological
    study of cochlea.
    (AD) Evaluation of vestibular function with vestibular function tests.
Ataxia beginning after 12 days of treatment, decr in duration of rotatory
nystagmus, change in ENG, and loss of hair cells of cristae and of organ of
Corti in basal coil of cochlea due to topical administration to bulla of 0.4
ml daily of aqueous solution of 6 percent concentration of antibiotic, gentamicin, for 19 days maximum in 4 animals, cats.
No clinical vestibular problems and no significant change in duration of
rotatory nystagmus and in ENG but degeneration of cochlea and spiral ganglion
and changes in saccule due to topical administration to bulla of 0.4 ml daily
of aqueous solution of 3 percent concentration of antibiotic, gentamicin, for
30 days maximum in 5 animals, cats.
    (AD) Direct relationship between onset of ataxia and concentration of
    gentamicin solution.
    (AD) Correlation between duration of rotatory nystagmus and ataxia.
    (AD) Topical gentamicin most toxic to cochlea and saccule.
    (AD) Need to monitor clinical use of gentamicin with audiology.
No clinical vestibular problems, transient decr in duration of rotatory
nystagmus, transient bilateral decr in ENG, and loss of hair cells of organ
of Corti in basal coil of cochlea but normal vestibular apparatus due to

topical administration to bulla of 0.4 ml daily of solution of 6 percent concentration of antibiotic, neomycin, for 30 days maximum in 2 animals, cats.

(AD) Comparative study of effects of topical gentamicin and neomycin.

(CT) Same methods using 0.4 ml distilled water for 30 days in 7 cats, control group, showed no clinical vestibular problems and no histological changes. (ENG)

706

Ototoxic effects due to chemical agents and heavy metals in humans.

(AD) Literature review of ototoxic effects of nicotine, carbon monoxide, carbon tetrachloride, mercury, arsenic, and lead.

Cochleo-vestibulotoxic effects, functional and structural, due to antibiotics in humans.

(AD) Literature review of ototoxicity of streptomycin, dihydrostreptomycin, neomycin, kanamycin, gentamicin, capreomycin, rifampicin, viomycin, isoniazid, aminosidine, and framycetin.

Hearing loss due to salicylates in humans.

Hearing loss due to antimalarial, quinine, in humans.

Hearing loss due to diuretic, ethacrynic acid, in humans.

(AD) Literature review of effects of various ototoxic agents. (IT)

Part III SPECIES AFFECTED BY OTOTOXIC AGENTS

HUMANS

113

Transient sensorineural hearing loss but no vestibular problems due to 0.5 to 1.0 g 4 times daily of solution of salicylate, acetylsalicylic acid, in 8 (16 percent) of 50 humans after tonsillectomy.
   (AD) Audiology and vestibular function tests to determine ototoxic effects.   (DAN)

411

Total bilateral hearing loss and within 48 hours, unilateral hearing loss, due to oral ingestion of 46 tablets of salicylate, aspirin, in 1 dose in 1 human, in suicide attempt.
Vestibular problems due to oral ingestion of 46 tablets of salicylate, aspirin, in 1 dose in 1 human, in suicide attempt.
   (AD) Case report of cochleo-vestibulotoxic effects of high dose of aspirin in suicide attempt.   (FR)

026

Hearing loss in speech range due to sedative, alcohol, ethyl, in 145 humans.
   (AD) Total of 200 tests conducted.   (GER)

114

Vestibulotoxic effects due to oral ingestion of large amounts of sedative, alcohol, ethyl, in humans.
   (AD) Effects of alcohol on vestibular apparatus determined by duration of nystagmus.   (GER)

248

Effect on vestibular threshold due to sedative, alcohol, ethyl, in humans.
   (CT) Pretreatment and posttreatment vestibular function tests.   (ENG)

508

High frequency and low amplitude nystagmus due to sedative, alcohol, ethyl, in humans.
   (AD) Study of effects of alcohol on vertigo and nystagmus.   (ENG)

572

Effect on vestibular function due to oral administration of 2.0 ml per kg, in orange juice, of 100-proof of sedative, alcohol, ethyl, in 30 minutes in 10 humans.
   (CT) Same method using beverage without alcohol in subjects, control group.
   (AD) Study of effect of alcohol ingestion on human performance in static situations and during motion.
   (AD) Tests of visuomotor skill during angular acceleration, pretreatment and 1 to 10 hours posttreatment.   (ENG)

710

Effect on vestibular function due to sedative, alcohol, ethyl, in humans. (ENG)

716

Damage to cochlear function due to oral ingestion of amount to produce blood levels of 0.8 to more than 1.0 percent of sedative, alcohol, ethyl, in acute intoxication in humans.
   (AD) Study of the effects of alcohol on cochlear function.   (GER)

039

Damage to endorgan of cochlea and vestibular apparatus due to parenteral or

oral administration of high doses of antibiotics for long periods in humans.
No reported ototoxic effects due to topical administration of unspecified
doses of antibiotics for unspecified period in humans. (ENG)

066
Hearing loss due to various methods of administration of antibiotics in
humans with acute otitis media. (RUS)

083
Cochleo-vestibulotoxic effects due to parenteral, oral, and topical administration of antibiotics in humans, with normal kidney function and with kidney
disorder.
    (AD) Literature review of ototoxic effects of antibiotics.
    (AD) Recommended dosage and duration of dosage of antibiotics discussed.
    (ENG)

123
Sensorineural hearing loss and vestibular problems due to range of doses of
antibiotics in humans.
    (AD) Report on cochleo-vestibulotoxic effects of antibiotics used clini-
    cally. (ENG)

127
Ototoxic effects due to antibiotics in humans with kidney tuberculosis.
    (AD) Literature review of ototoxic effects of streptomycin, viomycin,
    kanamycin, and capreomycin. (GER)

132
Sensorineural hearing loss due to antibiotics in humans.
    (AD) Study of iatrogenic hearing loss. (GER)

135
Vertigo and sensorineural hearing loss due to antibiotics, aminoglycoside, in
humans.
    (AD) Possible permanent damage due to low doses of streptomycin, dihydros-
    treptomycin, or kanamycin.
    (AD) Report on etiology of vertigo. (ENG)

149
Damage to organ of Corti due to antibiotics in humans.
    (AD) Discussion of ototoxicity in humans based on animal experimentation.
    (FR)

154
Ototoxic effects due to antibiotics in humans with tuberculosis.
    (AD) Literature review of some new antituberculous agents of 1968. (GER)

182
Sensorineural hearing loss, from frequency at 8000 cps to speech range, due
to antibiotics in humans.
    (AD) Specific audiometric configuration for hearing loss due to antibio-
    tics.
    (AD) Use of level of 15 db at 8000 cps for detection of hearing loss due
    to antibiotics. (ENG)

193
Sensorineural hearing loss and structural damage to cochlea due to low doses
of antibiotics in humans.
    (AD) Report on clinical and pathological effects possible with use of
    antibiotics.
    (AD) Toxic levels in blood possible due to low doses in therapy.
    (AD) Need for audiometry, vestibular function tests, and determination of
    blood levels of antibiotics during treatment. (SER)

201
Vertigo and sensorineural hearing loss due to antibiotics, aminoglycoside, in
humans.
    (AD) Report on risks in clinical use of different antibiotics.

(AD) Need for audiometry and vestibular function tests in antibiotic therapy over long period.
(AD) Cochleo-vestibulotoxic effects due to daily and total dosage of antibiotics. (FR)

210
Risk of cochleo-vestibulotoxic effects due to oral or parenteral administration of antibiotics, aminoglycoside, in humans with normal kidney function and with kidney disorder.
Risk of cochleo-vestibulotoxic effects due to topical administration of low doses of antibiotics, aminoglycoside, in humans.
(AD) Literature review of auditory system problems due to aminoglycoside antibiotics.
(AD) Need to determine dosage of antibiotics on basis of body weight, kidney function, and age.
(AD) Need for audiometry, vestibular function tests, determination of blood levels, and tests of kidney function during treatment with antibiotics. (SW)

221
Cochleo-vestibulotoxic effects due to antibiotics, aminoglycoside, in humans with tuberculosis of genitourinary system.
(AD) Need for multiple antibiotic therapy in tuberculosis but risk of ototoxic effects. (IT)

222
Cochleo-vestibulotoxic effects due to antibiotics in humans treated for tuberculosis.
(AD) Report on ototoxic effects of antibiotics used in tuberculosis chemotherapy and control of ototoxic effects. (GER)

244
Hearing loss and damage to organ of Corti due to antibiotics, aminoglycoside, in humans.
(AD) Literature review of ototoxic effects of different aminoglycoside antibiotics. (GER)

264
Cochleo-vestibulotoxic effects due to antibiotics in humans.
(AD) Comment on complications due to antibiotics after head and neck surgery. (ENG)

272
Hearing loss and damage to organ of Corti due to antibiotics in humans.
(AD) Literature review of ototoxic effects of antibiotics used in therapy. (FIN)

357
Hearing loss due to antibiotics in 60(5.4 percent) of 1100 humans treated for different disorders. (RUS)

410
Damage to organ of Corti of fetus due to antibiotics in humans, female, during pregnancy.
(AD) Discussion of etiology of damage to organ of Corti in fetus. (FR)

422
Hearing loss due to antibiotics in humans, female, treated during pregnancy or for disorders of genitourinary system. (RUS)

441
Ototoxic effects due to antibiotics in humans.
(AD) Monogr on production of antibiotics, mechanism of action, clinical use, toxicity, and other aspects. (RUS)

506
Damage to hair cells of vestibular apparatus and cochlea due to antibiotics in humans and animals.

(AD) Discussion of relationship between elimination of drugs and damage to
ear.
(AD) Need for careful consideration in use of aminoglycoside antibiotics.
(ENG)

523
Cochleo-vestibulotoxic effects due to topical, parenteral, or oral administration of antibiotics, aminoglycoside, in humans.   (NOR)

545
Ototoxic effects due to antibiotics in humans with disorders.
   (AD) Literature review of clinical use and toxic effects of antibiotics.
   (IT)

549
Cochleo-vestibulotoxic effects due to antibiotics in humans with disorders.
(RUS)

592
Ototoxic effects due to antibiotics in humans.
   (AD) Discussion of effects of some drugs used in otolaryngology.   (CZ)

608
Possible hearing loss due to antibiotics in humans with disorders.
   (AD) Evaluation of degree of hearing loss due to antibiotics possible with
   pretreatment and posttreatment audiometry.   (HUN)

609
Possible ototoxic effects due to antibiotics in humans with genitourinary
system infections.
   (AD) Literature review of antibiotic therapy of genitourinary system
   infections.   (GER)

630
Ototoxic effects due to antibiotics in humans treated for infection.   (ENG)

638
Hearing loss due to antibiotics in humans with disorders.   (RUS)

640
Ototoxic effects due to antibiotics in humans with tuberculosis.
   (AD) Literature review of chemotherapy of tuberculosis with comment on
   toxic effects of drugs.   (GER)

689
Hearing loss due to antibiotics in humans with tuberculosis.   (POL)

712
Ototoxic effects due to antibiotics in humans in surgery.   (HUN)

690
Ototoxic effects due to antituberculous agents in humans with tuberculosis.
(JAP)

077
Moderate ototoxic effects due to unspecified method of administration of
range of 25 to 515 g of antibiotic, capreomycin, for long period in 3 of 82
humans with pulmonary tuberculosis.
   (AD) Preliminary study for primary study of kidney function in capreomycin
   treatment.   (ENG)

207
Cochleotoxic effects due to antibiotic, capreomycin, in humans with tubercu-
losis.
   (AD) Report on new antituberculous agents.
   (AD) Need for careful consideration before use of capreomycin in treatment
   of tuberculosis.   (FR)

297
Possible vestibular problems and hearing loss due to recommended 1 g daily of antibiotic, capreomycin, in humans with tuberculosis.
(AD) Ototoxicity due to capreomycin similar to ototoxicity due to streptomycin. (ENG)

331
Possible decr in ototoxicity due to decr dosage, from 1 g daily to 1 g 5 days a week, of antibiotic, capreomycin, in humans with pulmonary tuberculosis. (ENG)

400
Transient mild cochlear impairment due to parenteral, intramuscular, administration of 1 g daily, maximum dose of 100 g, of antibiotic, capreomycin, in 1 of 21 humans with chronic tuberculosis of genitourinary system.
(AD) Report on clinical use and toxic effects of new drugs in treatment of tuberculosis of genitourinary system. (GER)

501
Ototoxic effects due to antibiotic, capreomycin, in humans treated for tuberculosis.
(AD) Capreomycin less ototoxic than streptomycin and viomycin. (ENG)

556
Moderate lesion of cochlea due to unspecified doses of antibiotic, capreomycin, for long period in 5(12.5 percent) of 40 humans, in treatment or retreatment for pulmonary tuberculosis.
(AD) Cochlear function monitored by audiometry. (ENG)

711
Vestibular problems due to antibiotic, capreomycin, for more than 3 months in 1 of 35 humans with pulmonary tuberculosis. (POL)

541
Vertigo due to anticonvulsant, carbamazepine, in 58(11.4 percent) of humans treated for paroxysmal trigeminal neuralgia.
Tinnitus due to anticonvulsant, carbamazepine, in 1(0.2 percent)of humans treated for paroxysmal trigeminal neuralgia.
(AD) Need to monitor use of carbamazepine in therapy. (ENG)

669
Possible transient dizziness due to anticonvulsant, carbamazepine, in humans with trigeminal neuralgia. (ENG)

228
Hearing loss due to topical route, inhalation, of chemical agent, carbon disulfide, for long period in humans in industry. (SER)

718
Dizziness, nystagmus, and high frequency hearing loss due to chemical agent, carbon disulfide, in chronic intoxication in humans working in industry.
(AD) Audiograms showed decr in higher frequencies.
(AD) Literature review of effects of carbon disulfide. (GER)

030
Hearing loss due to chemical agent, carbon monoxide, in humans.
(AD) Studies with audiometry on patients with u-shaped audiograms. (GER)

162
Permanent unilateral sensorineural hearing loss due to topical route, inhalation, of chemical agent, carbon monoxide, in acute intoxication in 1 human.
(AD) Hearing loss confirmed by audiogram. (POL)

163
Sensorineural hearing loss due to topical route, inhalation, of chemical agent, carbon monoxide, in humans.
(AD) Literature review on carbon monoxide poisoning. (POL)

673
Dizziness and decr in cochlear function due to topical route, inhalation, of
large amounts to produce 20 to 30 percent carboxyhemoglobin of chemical
agent, carbon monoxide, in humans. (ENG)

230
Vestibular problems due to chemical agent, carbon tetrachloride, in humans.
  (AD) Vestibular function tests conducted to determine effects of carbon
  tetrachloride. (RUS)

177
Sensorineural hearing loss due to topical route, inhalation, of chemical
agents, nitro and amino compounds, in humans from exposure in chemical industry.
  (AD) Hearing loss confirmed by audiology. (POL)

532
Damage to vestibular apparatus due to chemical agent, nitro solvent, in 1
human.
  (AD) Vestibular problem confirmed by vestibular function test. (POL)

289
Possible cochlear impairment due to antibiotic, chloramphenicol, in humans.
  (AD) Report on toxic effects of chloramphenicol. (RUM)

365
Possible vertigo and tinnitus due to high doses, 300 mg daily, of antimalarial, chloroquine (chloroquine sulfate), in humans with tuberculoid lepro-
sy. (FR)

732
Hearing loss and total degeneration of organ of Corti and moderate degeneration of spiral ganglion and nerve process in fetus due to oral ingestion of
250 mg daily of antimalarial, chloroquine (chloroquine phosphate), in humans,
female, during pregnancy.
  (AD) Histopathological study of inner ear after death. (ENG)

530
Transient ototoxic effects due to cardiovascular agent, chromonar, in humans
treated for heart disorders. (GER)

533
Sensorineural hearing loss, tinnitus, dizziness, and disorder of equilibrium
due to cardiovascular agent, digitalis, in 1 human treated for heart disorder. (POL)

106
Severe sensorineural hearing loss due to antibiotic, dihydrostreptomycin, in
humans.
  (AD) Comment on risk of ototoxic effects with clinical use of dihydrostreptomycin. (NOR)

187
Unspecified ototoxic effects due to parenteral, intravenous, intramuscular,
and intraperitoneal, administration of 0.9 percent sodium chloride solution
of antibiotics, aminoglycoside, in animals, mice, albino, adult, male and
female, 15 to 30 g weight.
  (CT) Same method using 0.9 percent sodium chloride solution in mice,
  control group.
  (AD) Comment on relationship of study to ototoxicity of antibiotics.
Risk of ototoxic effects due to antibiotic, dihydrostreptomycin, in chronic
intoxication in humans. (ENG)

317
Possible decr in ototoxic effects due to antibiotic, dihydrostreptomycin
(IB), in humans, with administration of pantothenate salt.
  (AD) Discussion of clinical use of dihydrostreptomycin and possible decr
  in ototoxicity with use of pantothenate salt of antibiotic. (GER)

478

Nystagmus due to parenteral, intramuscular, administration of 0.5 g daily, total dose of 50 g, of antibiotic, dihydrostreptomycin, in 6 humans with pulmonary tuberculosis.
Nystagmus due to parenteral, intramuscular, administration of total doses of 105 to 300 g of antibiotic, dihydrostreptomycin, in 10 humans with pulmonary tuberculosis.
  (AD) Case report included.
  (AD) Study using cupulometry of vestibular problems due to dihydrostreptomycin therapy. (GER)

645

Permanent severe hearing loss due to antibiotic, dihydrostreptomycin, in humans.
  (AD) Suggested that no preparations of dihydrostreptomycin be used in therapy. (ENG)

655

Possible ataxia and nystagmus due to anticonvulsant, diphenylhydantoin, in humans with convulsive disorders. (ENG)

035

Transient and permanent hearing loss and vertigo due to oral and parenteral, intravenous, administration of diuretic, ethacrynic acid, in 12 humans with kidney disorders.
  (AD) Hearing loss not related to administration route or dosage. (ENG)

060

Possible hearing loss due to high doses, as high as 200 mg, of diuretic, ethacrynic acid, in humans with kidney disorders.
  (AD) Comment on risk of administration of high test doses of ethacrynic acid in humans with kidney disorder as suggested in recent study. (ENG)

061

Transient hearing loss due to high test dose, as high as 200 mg, of diuretic, ethacrynic acid, in humans with kidney disorder .
  (AD) Explanation of use of high test dose.
  (AD) Need for hydration before administration of test dose of ethacrynic acid.
  (AD) Procedure caused only 3 cases of transient hearing loss in 3 years. (ENG)

097

Hearing loss due to diuretic, ethacrynic acid, in humans, female.
  (AD) Report on toxic effects of drugs. (SW)

098

Hearing loss due to parenteral, intravenous, administration of diuretic, ethacrynic acid, in humans with kidney disorder. (DAN)

144

Moderate bilateral sensorineural hearing loss within 20 minutes and damage to outer hair cells of organ of Corti due to unspecified method of administration of 50 mg of diuretic, ethacrynic acid, in 1 dose in humans with kidney disorder.
  (AD) Hearing loss confirmed by audiogram.
Sensorineural hearing loss within 15 minutes due to unspecified method of administration of 20 to 30 mg per kg daily of diuretic, ethacrynic acid, in 20 animals, cats.
  (AD) Ethacrynic acid not recommended for clinical use in humans with kidney disorders. (ENG)

295

Hearing loss due to parenteral, intravenous, administration of 50 to 100 mg of diuretic, ethacrynic acid, in humans with kidney disorder. (DAN)

304

Possible hearing loss and vertigo due to diuretic, ethacrynic acid, in hu-

mans.
    (AD)   Discussion of chemistry, pharmacology, clinical use, and toxicity of
ethacrynic acid.   (ENG)

                                                                            559
Possible tinnitus and transient hearing loss due to diuretic, ethacrynic
acid, in humans.
    (AD)   Literature review of use, action, and toxic effects of diuretics.
(ENG)

                                                                            660
Transient hearing loss, tinnitus, or vertigo due to diuretic, ethacrynic
acid, in humans.   (ENG)

                                                                            544
Vertigo due to antituberculous agent, ethambutol, in 2 of 187 humans treated
for pulmonary tuberculosis.
    (AD) Literature review showed report of 2 cases of vertigo due to ethambu-
tol.   (FR)

                                                                            054
Ototoxic effects due to diuretic, furosemide, in humans.
    (AD)   Comment on need for audiology as documentation for reports of ototo-
xicity of furosemide.   (ENG)

                                                                            124
Cochleo-vestibulotoxic effects due to diuretic, furosemide, in humans.
    (AD) Comment on use of audiology to confirm effects of ototoxic drugs.
    (AD) Explanation of previous study of furosemide without confirmation of
ototoxic effects by audiology.   (ENG)

                                                                            151
Possible sensorineural hearing loss due to parenteral, intravenous, administration of high doses, 100 to 1000 mg, of diuretic, furosemide, for long
period in humans with kidney disorders.
    (AD) Need for audiometry with clinical use of furosemide.
    (AD) Recommended treatment with diuretics for long periods in humans with
kidney disorders only in severe cases with edema and cardiovascular system
problems.   (GER)

                                                                            234
Transient sensorineural hearing loss due to parenteral, rapid intravenous,
administration of high dose, 1000 mg, of diuretic, furosemide, in 40 minutes
in humans with kidney disorder.
    (AD) Hearing loss confirmed by audiogram.   (GER)

                                                                            313
Transient hearing loss and vestibular problems due to high doses, 1000 mg, of
diuretic, furosemide, for 40 minutes in humans with kidney disorder.   (ENG)

                                                                            513
Transient acute midfrequency hearing loss due to parenteral, rapid intravenous, administration of high doses, 1000 mg, of diuretic, furosemide, in 40
minutes in 8(50 percent) of 16 humans with kidney disorder.
    (CT) Audiometry, pretreatment and posttreatment.
    (AD) Maximum hearing loss in middle frequency suggests lesion in organ of
Corti and not in CNS.
    (AD) Suggested that cochleotoxic effects related to rate of administration
and dosage.   (ENG)

                                                                            514
Transient tinnitus due to parenteral, intravenous, administration of high
doses, 100 to 3200 mg daily, progressive doses on successive days, of diuretic, (SQ) furosemide, in 30 minutes to 10 hours in some of 15 humans with
kidney disorder and on dialysis.
    (AD) Later study of 4 humans with tinnitus due to furosemide showed normal
    audiograms.
Previous parenteral, rapid intravenous, administration of total of 60 g of

diuretic, (SQ) mannitol, in 24 hours in 15 humans with kidney disorder and on dialysis.
  (CT) Treatment of 13 humans, control group, with dialysis only.
  (AD) Prevention of depletion of sodium and potassium by monitoring fluid and electrolyte balance. (ENG)

516
Possible ototoxic effects due to parenteral, intravenous, administration of diuretic, furosemide, in less than every 4 hours in humans with kidney disorder. (ENG)

517
Transient tinnitus and hearing loss due to parenteral administration of 2000 mg of diuretic, furosemide, in 30 minutes in humans with chronic kidney disorder. (ENG)

008
Severe vestibular problems and bilateral sensorineural hearing loss due to unspecified method of administration of more than 1 mg per kg recommended daily dosage of antibiotic, gentamicin (gentamicin sulfate), for unspecified period in 5 humans with kidney disorder.
  (AD) No pretreatment tests conducted.
Severe vestibular problems and unilateral sensorineural hearing loss due to unspecified method of administration of more than 1 mg per kg recommended daily dosage of antibiotic, gentamicin (gentamicin sulfate), for unspecified period in 3 humans with kidney disorder.
  (CT) Pretreatment vestibular function tests and audiometry showed normal vestibular function and normal hearing.
Transient vestibular problems only due to unspecified method of administration of more than 1 mg per kg recommended daily dosage of antibiotic, gentamicin (gentamicin sulfate), for unspecified period in 2 humans with normal kidney function.
  (CT) Pretreatment vestibular function tests showed normal vestibular function. (ENG)

036
Damage to vestibular apparatus due to parenteral or topical administration of antibiotic, gentamicin (gentamicin sulfate), in humans. (ENG)

093
Cochleo-vestibulotoxic effects due to parenteral administration of 50 to 100 mg per kg daily of antibiotic, gentamicin (gentamicin sulfate), for 20 days in humans and animals, cats and guinea pigs.
  (AD) Literature review showed ototoxic effects of gentamicin in 2.8 percent of cases reported. (ENG)

195
Damage to vestibular nerve and cochlear nerve due to antibiotic, gentamicin, in humans.
  (AD) Comment on use in therapy and cochleo-vestibulotoxic effects of gentamicin. (ENG)

225
Vestibular problems, in particular dizziness, due to antibiotic, gentamicin, in 19 of 1327 humans, range of ages, with normal kidney function and with kidney disorder.
Vestibular problems and high frequency hearing loss due to antibiotic, gentamicin, in 8 of 1327 humans, range of ages, with normal kidney function and with kidney disorder.
High frequency hearing loss due to antibiotic, gentamicin, in 4 of 1327 humans, range of ages, with normal kidney function and with kidney disorder.
  (AD) Kidney disorders in 33.3 percent of patients, previous or simultaneous treatment with other ototoxic drugs in 50 percent, and 50 years or more age in about 50 percent.
  (AD) Comparison of incidence of ototoxicity due to gentamicin and other aminoglycoside antibiotics. (ENG)

277

Sensorineural hearing loss due to parenteral administration of total doses of
160 mg to more than 4000 mg of antibiotic, gentamicin, in 52 humans.
Vestibular problems due to parenteral administration of total doses of 160 mg
to more than 4000 mg of antibiotic, gentamicin, in 34 humans.
   (CT) Audiometry and vestibular function tests before and after treatment
   with gentamicin. (GER)

298

Possible vestibular problems and high frequency hearing loss due to more than
225 mg daily of antibiotic, gentamicin, in humans.
   (AD) Report on chemistry, pharmacology, clinical use, and cochleo-vestibulotoxic effects of gentamicin.
   (AD) More risk of ototoxicity with gentamicin, dose for dose, than with
   other aminoglycoside antibiotics.
Range of degrees of vestibular problems 1 to 14 days after cessation of
treatment due to total doses of 0.74 to 3.15 g of antibiotic, gentamicin, in
5 of 57 humans with kidney disorder.
   (AD) Report of cases in previous study. (ENG)

300

Possible vestibular problems due to more than recommended 240 mg daily of
antibiotic, gentamicin, in humans, in particular with kidney disorder or 40
years or over age.
   (AD) More risk of ototoxicity with gentamicin than with other aminoglycoside antibiotics.
   (AD) Need for study of relationship between vestibular problems and dosage
   and duration of therapy. (ENG)

306

Vestibular problems due to unspecified dose of antibiotic, gentamicin, for 10
days in 1 human.
Significant vestibular problems and hearing loss due to antibiotic, gentamicin, in 14 of 27 humans, some with kidney disorders, with previous treatment
with ototoxic drugs, or over 40 years age.
   (AD) Vestibular problems confirmed by vestibular function tests.
   (AD) Report on clinical pharmacology, clinical use, and cochleo-vestibulotoxic effects of gentamicin.
   (AD) Reported 2.5 percent incidence in USA of vestibular problems due to
   gentamicin.
   (AD) Suggested that ototoxicity of gentamicin is dose related. (ENG)

426

Damage to vestibular function due to sufficient doses to produce blood level
of over 10 mcg per ml of antibiotic, gentamicin, in humans with or without
kidney disorders.
   (AD) High blood levels due to kidney disorders or due to high doses or
   long period of treatment in humans with normal kidney function.
   (AD) Comment on study that reported vestibulotoxic effects of gentamicin
   with blood levels lower than 10 mcg per ml. (ENG)

427

Damage to vestibular function due to high doses of antibiotic, gentamicin, in
humans with normal kidney function.
Damage to vestibular function due to antibiotic, gentamicin, in humans with
kidney disorder.
   (AD) Risk of gentamicin ototoxicity with blood levels of over 10 mcg per
   ml.
   (AD) Suggested that gentamicin ototoxicity is dose related.
   (AD) Comment on study that reported vestibulotoxic effects of gentamicin
   with blood levels lower than 10 mcg per ml. (ENG)

428

Possible damage to eighth cranial nerve due to high blood level of over 10
mcg per ml of antibiotic, gentamicin, in humans.
   (AD) Need for serum assays and other tests in clinical use of gentamicin.
   (AD) Comment on study that reported vestibulotoxic effects of gentamicin
   with blood levels lower than 10 mcg per ml. (ENG)

454
Damage to vestibular apparatus due to high doses of antibiotic, gentamicin,
in animals, guinea pigs.
Damage to vestibular apparatus due to low doses of antibiotic, gentamicin, in
humans with disorders. (GER)

471
Damage to vestibular apparatus due to antibiotic, gentamicin, in humans with
genitourinary system infections.
   (AD) Comment on risk of vestibulotoxic effects in clinical use of gentamicin. (GER)

475
Possible damage to eighth cranial nerve with vestibular problems due to
parenteral administration of low doses to produce recommended serum levels of
antibiotic, gentamicin, in humans with genitourinary system infections.
(ENG)

528
No reported ototoxic effects due to parenteral, intravenous or intramuscular,
administration of 40 mg every 8 hours in 1 injection, to produce blood level
of 20 mcg per ml in 1 case, of antibiotic, (SQ) gentamicin (SM), for 3 to 10
days in 25 humans with pseudomonas infection.
Parenteral, intravenous, administration of 1 dose of 2 g and then 1 g every 2
hours for 12 hours, followed by 1 g every 3 hours for 3 to 7 days of antibiotic, (SQ) carbenicillin (SM), in 25 humans with pseudomonas infection.
   (AD) Study of treatment of pseudomonas infection with gentamicin and
   carbenicillin.
   (AD) Decr in blood level of gentamicin when used simultaneously with
   carbenicillin. (ENG)

548
Transient vestibular problems due to parenteral administration of antibiotic,
gentamicin, in humans. (GER)

575
Transient and permanent vestibular problems only in 29 cases, hearing loss
only in 7 cases, and vestibular problems and hearing loss in 8 cases, begin-
ning less than 10 to 14 days after treatment, due to antibiotic, gentamicin,
in 44 humans, with kidney disorder in 64 percent of cases.
   (AD) Survey of clinical experience in USA with gentamicin ototoxicity.
   (AD) Statistical analysis of administration of gentamicin with and without
   ototoxic effects to determine significant factors in ototoxicity.
   (AD) Reported 2 percent incidence of ototoxicity due to gentamicin.
   (AD) Kidney disorders in patients and size of daily dose, mg per kg,
   reported most significant factors in gentamicin ototoxicity.
   (AD) Relationship between daily dose and ototoxicity suggests that blood
   level of gentamicin possibly significant factor in ototoxicity.
   (AD) Previous therapy with gentamicin or other ototoxic drugs, total dose,
   mg and mg per kg, and duration of therapy reported significant factors in
   gentamicin ototoxicity in patients with kidney disorder.
   (AD) Occurrence of gentamicin ototoxicity in patients with kidney disorders at younger age than in patients with normal kidney function.
   (AD) Suggested highest risk of gentamicin ototoxicity in younger patients
   with kidney disorder. (ENG)

587
No ototoxic effects due to parenteral (SM) administration of 3 mg per kg
every 24 hours of antibiotic, gentamicin (SM), for 5 to 132 days in 99 humans
with burns and with infection secondary to burns.
Simultaneous parenteral administration of other antibiotics (SM) in 99 humans
with burns and with infection secondary to burns.
No ototoxic effects due to topical, direct site (SM), administration in cream
or ointment of 0.1 percent of antibiotic, gentamicin, in 50 humans with burns
and with infection secondary to burns.
   (AD) No topical gentamicin therapy in 2 patients. (ENG)

599

Unspecified ototoxic effects due to parenteral, intramuscular, administration
of 40 mg, to produce blood levels of 3.7 mcg per ml 1 hour after treatment to
less than 0.1 and 0.2 mcg per ml after 8 hours, of antibiotic, gentamicin
(gentamicin sulfate), in 1 dose in 10 humans, male and female, 59 to 87 kg
weight.
  (AD) Risk of ototoxic effects with gentamicin.
  (AD) Study in unpaid subjects of pharmacology and clinical use of gentamicin. (GER)

600

No ototoxic effects due to parenteral, intramuscular or intravenous, administration of 40 or 80 mg daily of antibiotic, gentamicin, in humans with pseudomonas infection.
No ototoxic effects due to topical, direct site, administration in cream of
0.3 percent daily of antibiotic, gentamicin, in humans with pseudomonas
infection. (GER)

624

Possible ototoxic effects due to antibiotic, gentamicin, in humans with
pseudomonas infections. (ENG)

629

Hearing loss and vestibular problems due to antibiotic, (SQ) gentamicin
(gentamicin sulfate), in 16 (2.8 percent) of 565 humans, with kidney disorder
in 10 cases and with previous treatment with ototoxic drugs in 7 cases.
Possible ototoxic effects due to previous administration of other (SQ) ototoxic drugs in 7 of 16 humans.
Hearing loss and vestibular problems due to antibiotic, gentamicin, in 23 (2
percent) of 1152 humans.
  (AD) Discussion of incidence of ototoxicity due to gentamicin reported in
  2 studies. (ENG)

632

Ototoxic effects due to antibiotic, gentamicin, in humans with infections.
  (AD) Suggested dosage of 1 to maximum of 1.5 mg per kg of gentamicin in
  therapy. (GER)

639

Hearing loss in 6 cases and vestibular problems in 17 cases due to parenteral
administration of antibiotic, gentamicin, in 23 (2 percent) of 1152 humans.
(ENG)

642

Possible transient or permanent damage to eighth cranial nerve, primarily
vestibular problems, due to parenteral, intramuscular, administration of high
doses of antibiotic, gentamicin (gentamicin sulfate), for long period in
humans, in particular with kidney disorders.
  (AD) Need to monitor vestibular function and cochlear function with doses
  over 3 mg per kg daily or with administration of gentamicin for more than
  10 days.
  (AD) Recommended that serum concentrations of gentamicin not be higher
  than 10 mcg per ml.
  (AD) Dizziness possibly early symptom of ototoxicity. (ENG)

650

Transient bilateral hearing loss and moderate dizziness after 6 days due to
0.8 mg per kg daily of antibiotic, gentamicin, in 1 of 44 humans with various
infections and with normal kidney function.
  (CT) Vestibular function tests and audiometry, before, during, and after
  gentamicin treatment. (ENG)

677

Transient or permanent, bilateral or unilateral, vestibular problems primarily but also possible high frequency hearing loss due to parenteral administration of high doses to produce serum levels over 10 mcg per ml of antibiotic, gentamicin, in humans, in particular with kidney disorders.
  (AD) Gentamicin ototoxicity also in patients with previous treatment with
  ototoxic drugs or with previous auditory system problems.

(AD) Reported 2 to 2.5 percent incidence of vestibular problems due to parenteral gentamicin.
(AD) Literature review of mechanism of action, pharmacology, dosage, clinical use, and toxic effects of gentamicin. (ENG)

678

Primarily transient but also permanent severe vestibular problems due to doses to produce serum levels over 12 mcg per ml of antibiotic, gentamicin, in humans.
(AD) Study of in vitro activity of gentamicin only or gentamicin combined with other antibiotics. (ENG)

679

Damage to eighth cranial nerve due to antibiotic, gentamicin, in humans.
(AD) Factors in gentamicin ototoxicity include concurrent kidney disorders, total doses over 1 g, serum levels over 12 mcg per ml, 60 years or more age, and previous administration of ototoxic drugs, antibiotics. (ENG)

683

Primarily transient or permanent, unilateral or bilateral, vestibular problems but also high frequency hearing loss due to parenteral administration of high doses to produce blood levels over 10 mcg per ml of antibiotic, gentamicin, in humans, in particular with kidney disorders or with previous treatment with ototoxic drugs, or with previous auditory system problems.
(AD) Discussion of chemical structure, antibiotic activity, clinical pharmacology, use in therapy, and toxic effects.
(AD) Reported 2 to 2.5 percent incidence of vestibular problems due to parenteral gentamicin.
(AD) Unilateral vestibular problems in 50 percent of patients tested. (ENG)

684

Possible permanent severe vestibular problems and some hearing loss due to antibiotic, gentamicin, in humans.
(AD) Possible to use potential ototoxic drugs with minimum risk of permanent ototoxic effects by regulation of dosage and cessation of therapy at first symptom of ototoxicity. (ENG)

729

No hearing loss or vestibular problems due to parenteral, intramuscular, administration of total dose of 160 to more than 4000 mg of antibiotic, gentamicin, for 2 to 40 days in 72 humans with various infections.
No hearing loss or vestibular problems due to topical administration in solution or ointment of antibiotic, gentamicin, for 2 to 40 days in 55 humans with various infections or in surgery. (GER)

263

Possible dizziness, tinnitus, and hearing loss due to anti-inflammatory agent, ibuprofen, in humans. (ENG)

396

No hearing loss but decr in vestibular function due to parenteral, intramuscular, administration of 25 mg of antidepressant, imipramine hydrochloride, in 20 humans. (IT)

659

Possible dizziness due to anti-inflammatory agent, indomethacin, in humans. (ENG)

693

Tinnitus due to oral administration in capsules of 75 mg daily of anti-inflammatory agent, indomethacin, for 4 weeks in 1 of 14 humans, male and female, with rheumatoid arthritis.
Dizziness due to oral administration in capsules of 75 mg daily of anti-inflammatory agent, indomethacin, for 4 weeks in 1 of 14 humans, male and female, with rheumatoid arthritis. (ENG)

697
Dizziness in 12 cases and hearing loss in 1 case due to oral (SM) administration in capsules of 25 mg twice a day for 2 days and then 4 times a day for 2
days, followed by 50 mg 3 times a day for 2 days and then 4 times a day, of
anti-inflammatory agent, indomethacin, for 12 weeks in 12 (40 percent) of 30
humans with bone and joint disorder.
Dizziness in 12 cases and hearing loss in 1 case due to topical, rectal (SM),
administration in suppositories of 100 mg daily of anti-inflammatory agent,
indomethacin, for first 6 days in 12(40 percent) of 30 humans with bone and
joint disorder. (ENG)

707
Dizziness due to 75 mg daily of anti-inflammatory agent, indomethacin, in 1
of 24 humans with bone and joint disorder. (CZ)

397
Sensorineural hearing loss possibly due to antidiabetic, insulin, in humans
treated for diabetes.
   (AD) Reported that hearing loss in many humans treated with insulin for
   diabetes.
   (AD) Hearing loss confirmed by audiometry. (ENG)

121
Tinnitus and high frequency hearing loss and damage to organ of Corti due to
antibiotic, kanamycin, in humans.
   (AD) Literature review of kanamycin, use in therapy and toxic effects.
   (AD) Suggested clinical procedures for use of kanamycin with minimum risk
   of ototoxicity. (ENG)

145
Decr of only 33.3 percent in cells of spiral ganglion due to 12 g of antibiotic, kanamycin, for 8 days in 1 human with kidney disorder.
   (AD) Temporal bone study of number of cells of spiral ganglion after
   treatment with kanamycin.
   (AD) Near normal number of spiral ganglion cells after treatment with
   ototoxic drug. (ENG)

159
Hearing loss due to antibiotic, kanamycin, in humans with infections. (JAP)

176
Possible ototoxic effects due to low doses of antibiotic, kanamycin, in
humans.
   (AD) Literature review of infections with report on toxic effects of
   antibiotic therapy. (ENG)

203
Permanent high frequency hearing loss due to range of less than 30 g to more
than 180 g of antibiotic, kanamycin, for long period in 55.6 percent of 72
humans with tuberculosis.
   (AD) Need for audiometry during treatment with kanamycin for prevention of
   more severe hearing loss. (GER)

287
Cochlear impairment in fetus due to antibiotic, kanamycin, in humans, female,
treated during pregnancy.
   (AD) Discussion of cochleotoxic effects of kanamycin in newborn infants
   and infants. (JAP)

601
Effect on eighth cranial nerve due to antibiotic, kanamycin, in humans with
infections and with or without kidney disorder.
   (AD) Study of use of kanamycin for therapy of various infections. (ENG)

633
Cochlear impairment due to antibiotic, kanamycin, in humans, female, treated
for gynecologic infections. (FR)

657

Possible ototoxic effects due to parenteral, intramuscular, administration of 2 g of antibiotic, kanamycin, in humans with gonorrhea, in particular with concurrent kidney disorders. (ENG)

675

Possible total hearing loss due to parenteral administration of antibiotic, kanamycin (kanamycin sulfate), in humans with genitourinary system infections and with concurrent kidney disorder. (ENG)

688

Hearing loss due to antibiotic, kanamycin, in 2 (8 percent) of 26 humans after 3 months and in 1 (5 percent) of 21 humans after 6 months of retreatment for pulmonary tuberculosis.
    (CT) Audiograms, pretreatment and posttreatment.
Hearing loss due to antibiotic, kanamycin, for 6 months in 14.9 percent of humans during retreatment for pulmonary tuberculosis.
    (AD) Hearing loss confirmed by audiograms. (ENG)

699

Permanent hearing loss due to parenteral, intramuscular, administration of 0.5 g at 6-hour intervals for 48 hours and then at 12-hour intervals for 5 days, total dose of more than 12 g, to produce peak serum levels of 10 to 30 mcg per ml after 12 hours, of antibiotic, kanamycin, for about 7 days in 2 of about 300 humans with various infections.
    (AD) Higher risk of kanamycin ototoxicity in patients with dehydration or kidney disorder or with total doses of about 20 g.
    (AD) Prevention or decr in ototoxic effects with regulation of daily dose and duration of therapy and with tests of kidney function. (ENG)

701

Hearing loss due to antibiotic, kanamycin, in humans.
    (AD) Study of clinical use of vitamin K-1 in hearing loss due to kanamycin. (JAP)

724

Hearing loss due to antibiotic, kanamycin, in humans in dental treatment. (ENG)

152

Transient moderate dizziness due to parenteral, intravenous, administration of 1.0 mg per kg of 1 percent concentration of anesthetic, lidocaine, for 30 seconds in 23 humans.
Transient severe dizziness and tinnitus due to parenteral, intravenous, administration of 1.5 mg per kg of 1 percent concentration of anesthetic, lidocaine, for 30 seconds in 6 humans.
    (CT) Same study without lidocaine injection in 9 humans, control group.
    (AD) Auditory system problems due to lidocaine reported in previous studies. (ENG)

553

Tinnitus and distortion of sound due to parenteral, rapid intravenous, administration to arm of 2.5 mg per kg of 0.5 percent concentration of anesthetic, lidocaine, in 1 injection, with release of tourniquet 5 minutes after injection, in 9 of 10 humans, unpaid subjects. (ENG)

646

Possible vertigo and tinnitus due to parenteral, intravenous, administration of 2 percent solution of anesthetic, lidocaine, in humans with heart disorder. (ENG)

531

Hearing loss due to antibiotic, lincomycin, in 1 human treated with hemodialysis after bilateral nephrectomy for kidney disorder.
    (AD) Hearing loss confirmed by audiogram. (CZ)

208

Hearing loss due to oral ingestion, in contaminated fish, of heavy metal,

mercury (organic methyl mercury), in humans.
   (AD) Recommended international limit of 0.5 ppm of mercury (organic methyl
   mercury) for humans.
   (AD) Reported high levels of mercury (organic methyl mercury) in fetuses.
   (ENG)

                                                                          269
Vertigo due to heavy metal, mercury, in humans.
   (AD) Report on vestibulotoxic effects of heavy metals in industry.
   (AD) Vestibular problems confirmed by vestibular function tests. (JAP)

                                                                          623
Vertigo due to oral administration of antibiotic, nalidixic acid, in humans.
   (ENG)

                                                                          052
Ototoxic effects due to parenteral, oral, and topical administration of
antibiotic, neomycin, in humans.
   (AD) Discussion of neomycin ototoxicity due to all usual administration
   routes. (ENG)

                                                                          053
Ototoxic effects due to topical administration of high doses of antibiotic,
neomycin, in humans.
   (AD) Need for careful consideration of dosage of neomycin used in topical
   administration. (ENG)

                                                                          064
Risk of hearing loss due to topical administration of more than 1 g of antibiotic, neomycin, in more than 7 days in humans.
   (AD) Comment on risk of hearing loss with topical administration of neomycin. (ENG)

                                                                          273
Vertigo and hearing loss due to topical administration in ear drops of
500,000 ED in distilled water, in 6 to 8 ear drops daily, of antibiotic,
neomycin, for 8 days in 1 human with suppuration from right ear.
   (AD) Hearing loss confirmed by audiometry. (RUS)

                                                                          381
Degeneration of organ of Corti and hearing loss due to various methods of
administration of antibiotic, neomycin, in humans.
   (AD) Literature review of toxic effects of new antibiotics. (GER)

                                                                          387
Risk of hearing loss due to parenteral and oral administration of antibiotic,
neomycin, in humans.
Possible hearing loss due to topical, rectal, administration of antibiotic,
neomycin, in humans.
   (AD) Study of rectal administration as possible route for neomycin therapy. (ENG)

                                                                          469
Hearing loss due to parenteral administration of antibiotic, neomycin, in
humans. (FR)

                                                                          504
Ototoxic effects due to chemical agent, nicotine, in humans. (POL)

                                                                          194
Vestibular problems, primary effect, and bilateral sensorineural hearing loss
due to antineoplastic, nitrogen mustard, for long periods in 24 humans with
malignant tumors and lupus erythematosus.
   (AD) Auditory system problems confirmed by audiometry and vestibular
   function tests.
   (AD) Cochleo-vestibulotoxic effects after treatment with nitrogen mustard
   due to dosage, duration of treatment, and route of administration. (SP)

709

Possible hearing loss and vertigo after 10 to 48 hours due to antiparasitic, oil of chenopodium, in humans. (FR)

235

Effect on hair cells of vestibular apparatus and organ of Corti due to ototoxic drugs in humans and animals.
(AD) Suggested role of hair cells of vestibular apparatus and organ of Corti as sensory meters with relative resistance to drugs.
(AD) Literature review of effects of drugs on sensory endings. (ENG)

281

Vestibular neuritis due to ototoxic agents in humans. (SER)

386

Possible damage to inner ear due to topical administration in ear drops of ototoxic drugs for long period in humans.
(AD) Discussion of clinical use and possible toxic effects of ear drops. (GER)

407

Hearing loss due to ototoxic drugs in humans.
(AD) Discussion of cochleotoxic effects of ototoxic drugs. (FR)

442

Degeneration of inner ear due to ototoxic drugs in humans.
(AD) Changes in inner ear due to virus infections comp w changes due to ototoxic drugs or circulation problems. (ENG)

479

Auditory system problems due to ototoxic drugs in humans.
(AD) Discussion of drugs with possible toxic effects on ear. (FR)

499

Sensorineural hearing loss due to ototoxic drugs in humans.
(AD) Management of hearing loss includes prevention of ototoxicity due to drugs. (ENG)

717

Hearing loss in fetus due to ototoxic drugs in humans treated during pregnancy.
(AD) Discussion of etiology of hearing loss in risk children. (GER)

418

Hearing loss within 2 to 3 minutes after injection and tinnitus due to parenteral, intravenous, administration of anesthetic, procaine (procaine hydrochloride), in 30 humans with normal hearing and treated for disorders.
(AD) Study of effect on hearing loss and tinnitus of manual compression of neurovascular bundle.
(AD) No effect on tinnitus or hearing loss of manual compression of neurovascular bundle before and during injection of procaine.
(AD) Disappearance of tinnitus due to unilateral manual compression of neurovascular bundle after injection of procaine in 23 subjects.
(AD) Suppression of tinnitus only during manual compression of neurovascular bundle in other subjects.
(AD) Less effect on hearing loss of manual compression of neurovascular bundle after injection of procaine. (FR)

291

Cochlear impairment due to 5.0 g of antimalarial, quinine (quinine hydrochloride), in humans.
Cochlear impairment due to antimalarial, quinine (quinine hydrochloride), in animals, cats and rabbits.
(AD) Comparative animal studies and clinical case reports.
(AD) Study of ocular toxicity with comment on ototoxicity. (GER)

388

Hearing loss in 2 fetuses, twin, male, due to oral ingestion of high doses of

antimalarial, quinine, for unspecified period in 1 human, female, at end of
first trimester of pregnancy to induce abortion.
  (AD) No visual perception defect in twins due to ingestion of quinine by
  mother during pregnancy.
  (AD) Suggested vascular or neural mechanism of ototoxic effects of
  quinine. (ENG)

                                                                         502
Possible transient hearing loss or dizziness due to antibiotic, rifampicin,
in humans treated for tuberculosis or other infections.
  (AD) Literature review of clinical use, pharmacology, toxicity, and other
  aspects of rifampicin. (ENG)

                                                                         622
Possible transient hearing loss due to antibiotic, rifampicin, in humans.
(ENG)

                                                                         401
Possible TTS(auditory) of 24 hours duration due to high doses of salicylates
in humans.
Obstruction of capillaries of spiral vessels of basilar membrane due to high
doses of salicylates in humans.
  (AD) Same obstruction of capillaries due to sound stimulation.
  (AD) TTS(auditory) possibly due to obstruction of capillaries by salicy-
  lates or sound.
Susceptibility to PTS(auditory) due to salicylates in humans exposed to
noise.
  (AD) Conclusions based on animal experimentation. (ENG)

                                                                         596
Tinnitus due to high doses of salicylates in humans.
  (AD) Tinnitus early symptom of salicylate intoxication in some cases.
  (AD) Discussion of etiology, symptoms, diagnosis and evaluation, treat-
  ment, and prevention of salicylate intoxication. (ENG)

                                                                         312
Transient bilateral sensorineural hearing loss of 60 and 50 decibels due to
topical, direct site, administration of ointment with 5 percent of salicylate, salicylic acid, for 3 times daily in 2 humans, female, with psoriasis.
(ENG)

                                                                         647
No damage to eighth cranial nerve observed but possible dizziness due to
parenteral administration of antibiotic, spectinomycin, in humans with gonorrhea.
  (AD) New antibiotic for treatment of gonorrhea.
  (AD) Spectinomycin chemically related to ototoxic drugs as streptomycin
  and kanamycin. (ENG)

                                                                         017
Ototoxic effects, vestibular problems and cochlear impairment in 78 percent,
vestibular problems only in 14 percent, and cochlear impairment only in 8
percent due to unspecified method of administration of unspecified doses of
antibiotic, streptomycin (streptomycin sulfate), for unspecified period in
100 humans with tuberculosis and other infections.
  (CT) No symptoms of damage to cochlea or vestibular apparatus before
  treatment with streptomycin.
  (AD) Recommendation of audiometry and vestibular function test, pretreatment and during treatment, for early detection of ototoxic effects. (ENG)

                                                                         037
Progressive hearing loss due to 0.75 to 1 g daily of antibiotic, streptomycin, for long period in 7.2 percent of 125 humans. (GER)

                                                                         067
High frequency hearing loss in 11.4 percent of fetuses due to 10 g to more
than 100 g of antibiotic, streptomycin, in 44 humans, female, treated for
tuberculosis during pregnancy.

(AD) Hearing loss confirmed by audiogram.
(AD) Damage most often due to streptomycin treatment during first trimester. (GER)

070
Cochleo-vestibulotoxic effects due to range of less than 50 g to more than
200 g of antibiotic, streptomycin, in 127 humans with pulmonary tuberculosis
and 1 human with croupous pneumonia.
(AD) Statistical analysis showed correlation between ototoxic effects and
dosage.
(AD) Vestibular problems detected earlier than hearing loss.
(AD) Suggested use of audiometry before streptomycin treatment and every
10 to 15 days during treatment. (RUS)

100
Hearing loss due to antibiotic, streptomycin, in human, male.
(AD) Court case on ototoxic effects due to streptomycin. (GER)

111
Damage to organ of Corti and vestibular apparatus due to antibiotic, streptomycin, in humans and animals, guinea pigs.
(AD) Comparative study of ototoxic effects of streptomycin in humans and
animals. (GER)

191
Vestibular problems due to unspecified method of administration of unspecified doses of antibiotic, streptomycin, for long period in 9 of 155 humans
with tuberculosis.
Cochlear impairment due to unspecified method of administration of unspecified doses of antibiotic, streptomycin, for long period in 4 of 155 humans
with tuberculosis.
Vestibular problems and cochlear impairment due to unspecified method of
administration of unspecified doses of antibiotic, streptomycin, for long
period in 1 of 155 humans with tuberculosis. (ENG)

215
Primary damage to vestibular function but also cochlear impairment due to
blood levels over 25 mcg per ml of antibiotic, streptomycin, in humans.
(AD) Report on dosage, clinical use, and toxicity of streptomycin.
(AD) Relationship between cochleo-vestibulotoxic effects and daily dosage
and duration of treatment.
(AD) Need for audiometry and vestibular function tests during treatment
and for 6 months after treatment with streptomycin. (ENG)

217
Sensorineural hearing loss due to antibiotic, streptomycin, in humans.
(AD) Comment on ototoxic effects of drugs. (FIN)

296
Ototoxic effects due to antibiotic, streptomycin, in large number of humans.
(BUL)

319
Ototoxic effects due to antibiotic, streptomycin, in humans with infections
of ear.
(AD) Literature review of clinical use and ototoxicity of streptomycin.
(GER)

321
Vestibular problems due to antibiotic, streptomycin, in humans.
(AD) Use of ENG to determine extent of vestibular problems due to strep-
tomycin. (RUM)

341
Transient vestibular problems due to 1.0 g daily of antibiotic, streptomycin
(streptomycin sulfate), for short period, 1 or 2 months, in 32 of 84 humans
with tuberculosis.
(AD) Vestibulotoxic effects determined by ENG.

(AD) Slight vestibular problem in only 2 humans 1 year after cessation of treatment. (POL)

363

Decr in hearing loss due to antibiotic, streptomycin (IB), in 9 of 40 humans with administration of ATP, vitamin A, vitamin E, ascorbic acid, or nicotinic acid.
Decr in hearing loss due to other antibiotics (IB) in 9 of 40 humans with administration of ATP, vitamin A, vitamin E, ascorbic acid, or nicotinic acid.
   (CT) Audiology before and 5 to 6 days after administration of inhibitors.
   (AD) Study of effectiveness of treatment of auditory system problems due to ototoxic drugs. (RUS)

364

Damage to organ of Corti, spiral ganglion, and cochlear nuclei of medulla oblongata 15 days after beginning of treatment due to 100 mg per kg of antibiotic, streptomycin, in 38 animals, guinea pigs.
Decr in damage to spiral ganglion and cochlear nuclei of medulla oblongata due to 100 mg per kg of antibiotic, streptomycin (IB), in 8 of 18 animals, guinea pigs, with simultaneous administration of 2 ml of 5 percent unitiol for 30 to 60 days.
Decr in hearing loss due to ototoxic drugs (IB) in 3 of 25 humans with administration of unitiol.
No hearing loss due to antibiotic, streptomycin (IB), in 25 humans with pulmonary tuberculosis with administration of unitiol.
   (AD) Study of effect of inhibitor, unitiol, on streptomycin ototoxicity. (RUS)

375

Possible hearing loss due to antibiotic, streptomycin, in humans.
   (AD) Discussion of value of experimentation with animals to determine use and effects of drugs in humans.
   (AD) Possible to determine total hearing loss due to drugs in dogs and monkeys but more difficult to determine partial hearing loss in animals.
   (AD) Possible that high doses of drugs used in experimentation help to determine effects in therapeutic doses. (ENG)

390

Sensorineural hearing loss due to antibiotic, streptomycin, in 2.2 percent of 3250 humans with pulmonary tuberculosis.
   (AD) Symptoms of cochlear impairment more delayed than symptoms of disorder of vestibular function. (RUS)

408

Ototoxic effects due to antibiotic, streptomycin, in humans.
   (AD) Discussion of streptomycin ototoxicity, 1 of topics at conference on various aspects of the ear and hearing. (FR)

470

Damage to vestibular apparatus due to antibiotic, streptomycin, in humans.
   (AD) Study of effect of drugs on kidney function and vestibular function. (FR)

487

Severe vestibular problems due to parenteral, intramuscular, administration of antibiotic, streptomycin (streptomycin sulfate), for long period in 8 percent of 600 humans with tuberculosis and with previous hearing loss in some cases.
Transient hearing loss in most cases due to parenteral, intramuscular, administration of antibiotic, streptomycin (streptomycin sulfate), for long period in some of 600 humans with tuberculosis and with previous hearing loss in some cases.
   (CT) Audiometry and vestibular function tests before, during, and after streptomycin treatment.
   (AD) Improvement in vestibular function after cessation of streptomycin treatment.
   (AD) Transient hearing loss in most cases due to early detection with

audiology.   (GER)

488

Permanent cochleo-vestibulotoxic effects due to range of doses of antibiotic, streptomycin (streptomycin sulfate), in some of 1198 humans treated for tuberculosis and other disorders.
   (AD) Auditory system problems detected by audiology.
   (AD) Comment on differences in individual responses to streptomycin.
   (SER)

509

Hearing loss due to high doses of antibiotic, streptomycin, for long period in humans.   (POL)

524

Damage to eighth cranial nerve due to antibiotics in 8 of 103 humans with kidney disorder.
Hearing loss due to antibiotic, streptomycin, in 6 of 103 humans with kidney disorder.
   (AD) Study of effects of ototoxic drugs in humans with kidney disorder.
   (ENG)

542

Deaf-mutism in fetus due to antibiotic, streptomycin, in human, female, treated during pregnancy.
   (AD) Case report of congenital hearing loss due to streptomycin therapy in mother during pregnancy.   (ENG)

561

Sensorineural hearing loss due to antibiotic, streptomycin, in humans.
   (AD) Study of incidence of various types of hearing loss.
   (AD) Reported that some cases of sensorineural hearing loss of unknown etiology possibly due to streptomycin therapy.   (JAP)

612

Hearing loss due to parenteral administration of antibiotic, streptomycin, in humans.
   (AD) Literature review of ototoxic effects of streptomycin.
   (AD) Ototoxic effects of neomycin and kanamycin comp w effects of streptomycin and dihydrostreptomycin.   (SP)

631

Ototoxic effects due to antibiotic, streptomycin, in humans with pulmonary tuberculosis.   (BUL)

643

Possible transient or permanent damage to eighth cranial nerve, vestibular problems and hearing loss, due to antibiotic, streptomycin, in humans with tuberculosis and in particular with concurrent kidney disorders.
   (AD) Need for careful consideration in use of streptomycin in therapy.
   (ENG)

648

Vertigo due to antibiotic, streptomycin, in 3 humans with tuberculosis.
   (AD) Report on testing with ENG of 191 patients with vertigo of various etiologies.   (ENG)

663

Vertigo due to antibiotic, streptomycin, in 2 humans.
Tinnitus and sensorineural hearing loss but no vertigo due to antibiotic, streptomycin, in 3 humans.
   (AD) Treatment with dogmatil of vestibular problems and hearing loss due to streptomycin.   (FR)

687

Vestibular problems and hearing loss due to high doses of antibiotic, streptomycin, in humans.
   (AD) Discussion of toxic effects of drugs.   (GER)

723

Possible sensorineural hearing loss and vestibular problems due to antibiotic, streptomycin, in humans treated for tuberculosis during pregnancy.
(GER)

661

Hearing loss in fetus due to sedative, thalidomide, in humans, female,
treated during pregnancy. (GER)

695

Hearing loss in fetus due to sedative, thalidomide, in humans, female,
treated during pregnancy.
   (AD) Congenital hearing loss in 5 of 34 humans, child, of mothers treated
with thalidomide during pregnancy. (ENG)

667

Possible vertigo due to antiparasitic, thiabendazole, in humans with parasitic disorder. (ENG)

634

Ototoxic effects due to antituberculous agent, thiacetazone, in humans with
tuberculosis. (FR)

728

Dizziness due to topical route, inhalation, of chemical agent, tobacco, in
humans without smoking habit.
   (AD) Study of subjective symptoms of effects of tobacco on subjects without smoking habit. (ENG)

543

Transient decr in cochlear function due to tranquilizers in 44 humans.
   (AD) Auditory system problem detected by audiometry.
   (AD) Suggested transient cochleotoxic effect due to inhibition of reticu-
lar formation by action of tranquilizers. (GER)

214

Hearing loss due to high blood levels of 90 mcg per ml or more of antibiotic,
vancomycin, in humans.
   (AD) Report on chemical composition, mechanism of action, clinical use,
and toxicity of vancomycin. (ENG)

404

No cochleo-vestibulotoxic effects due to parenteral, intravenous, administration of 1 g, dissolved in 250 ml isotonic saline, of antibiotic, vancomycin,
for every 14 days for long period, more than 60 days, in 25 humans with
chronic kidney disorder and treated with intermittent hemodialysis.
   (AD) Audiometry every 12 weeks.
   (AD) Previous reports of severe ototoxicity due to vancomycin.
   (AD) Previous report suggested occurrence of ototoxicity with vancomycin
serum levels over 80 mcg per ml.
   (AD) Suggested that vancomycin ototoxicity not related to total dosage or
duration of treatment. (ENG)

120

Sensorineural hearing loss and damage to eighth cranial nerve due to parenteral, intramuscular, administration of 1 g daily of antibiotic, viomycin
(IB), for 1 month or more in 5 percent of 60 humans with pulmonary tuberculosis and treated with vitamin B.
   (AD) Need for audiometry with clinical use of viomycin. (POL)

122

Damage to eighth cranial nerve and sensorineural hearing loss and vestibular
problems due to unspecified doses of antibiotic, viomycin, for long period in
humans.
   (AD) Literature review of viomycin, use in therapy and toxic effects.
   (AD) Recommended intramuscular administration of 1 to 2 g daily dose of
viomycin for 2 to 3 weeks for minimum risk of ototoxicity. (ENG)

009

Delayed permanent sensorineural hearing loss and damage to outer hair cells of basal and middle coils of cochlea due to unspecified doses of antibiotic, dihydrostreptomycin, in humans.
Vertigo and dizziness due to unspecified method of administration of 2 to 3 g daily of antibiotic, streptomycin (streptomycin sulfate), for 30 to 50 days in humans with tuberculosis.
Hearing loss due to unspecified method of administration of high doses of antibiotic, streptomycin (streptomycin sulfate), for long period in humans.
Gradual high frequency hearing loss and tinnitus and degeneration of hair cells of organ of Corti in basal coil of cochlea due to unspecified doses of antibiotic, kanamycin, in humans.
Delayed severe high frequency hearing loss due to parenteral, oral, or topical administration by inhalation of unspecified doses of antibiotic, neomycin, for unspecified period in humans with kidney disorder.
Complete degeneration of inner hair cells due to unspecified method of administration of 18 g of antibiotic, neomycin, for unspecified period in humans with bacterial endocarditis.
Lesions in organ of Corti due to parenteral administration of unspecified doses of antibiotic, polymyxin B, for unspecified period in animals, guinea pigs.
Sensorineural hearing loss due to parenteral, intravenous, administration of 80 to 95 mg per ml of antibiotic, vancomycin, for unspecified period in humans with kidney disorder.
   (AD) Sensorineural hearing loss and vestibular problems due to 6 antibiotics in humans and animals, guinea pigs.
   (AD) Literature review of ototoxic effects of antibiotics. (ENG)

011

Transient cochleo-vestibulotoxic effects due to topical administration by inhalation and parenteral, intramuscular, administration of 0.5 g twice a day for 6 days, followed by a 1-day break, of antibiotic, (SQ) kanamycin (kanamycin sulfate), for 1 to 3 months in 2 of 17 humans treated for tuberculosis.
   (CT) Pretreatment audiometry and vestibular function tests conducted.
Ototoxic effects due to previous administration of antibiotic, (SQ) streptomycin, in 2 of 17 humans with tuberculosis. (RUS)

013

No reported ototoxic effects due to antibiotic, neomycin (CB), in 26 humans with inflammation of external auditory meatus.
No reported ototoxic effects due to antibiotic, polymyxin B (CB), in 26 humans with inflammation of external auditory meatus.
   (AD) Study of use of neomycin, polymyxin B, and fluocinolone acetonide in treatment of inflammation of external auditory meatus. (FR)

041

Cochleo-vestibulotoxic effects due to unspecified method of administration of 300 mg daily of antituberculous agent, isoniazid, for 6 to 18 months in 12.9 percent of 70 humans with tuberculosis.
Cochleo-vestibulotoxic effects due to unspecified method of administration of 300 mg of antituberculous agent, isoniazid (SM), for 6 to 18 months in 22 percent of 297 humans with tuberculosis.
Cochleo-vestibulotoxic effects due to unspecified method of administration of 150 mg of antituberculous agent, thiacetazone (SM), for 6 to 18 months in 22 percent of 297 humans with tuberculosis.
Cochleo-vestibulotoxic effects due to unspecified method of administration of antituberculous agent, isoniazid (SM), for 6 to 18 months in 82.9 percent of 82 humans with tuberculosis.
Cochleo-vestibulotoxic effects due to unspecified method of administration of antituberculous agent, thiacetazone (SM), for 6 to 8 months in 82.9 percent of 82 humans with tuberculosis.
Cochleo-vestibulotoxic effects due to unspecified method of administration of 1 g of antibiotic, streptomycin (SM), for 6 to 18 months in 82.9 percent of 82 humans with tuberculosis.
Cochleo-vestibulotoxic effects due to unspecified method of administration of 300 mg of antituberculous agent, isoniazid (SM), for 6 to 18 months in 25 percent of 20 humans with tuberculosis.
Cochleo-vestibulotoxic effects due to unspecified method of administration of

1 g of antibiotic, streptomycin (SM), for 6 to 18 months in 25 percent of 20
humans with tuberculosis.
  (AD) Potentiation by thiacetazone of cochleo-vestibulotoxic effects of
  streptomycin suggested.
  (AD) Audiometry and vestibular function tests every 2 weeks for 6 to 18
  months in total of 469 humans with tuberculosis. (ENG)

                                                                          056
Range of degree of hearing loss due to range of 40 to 300 g of antibiotic,
(SQ) streptomycin, in 59 of 338 humans, male and female, with no previous
treatment with streptomycin.
  (AD) No auditory system problems before treatment.
  (AD) Hearing loss often detected in alcoholics in group.
Range of degree of hearing loss due to range of 40 to 100 g of antibiotic,
(SQ) streptomycin, in 8 of 32 humans with previous treatment with streptomy-
cin.
  (AD) No reported auditory system problems before treatment.
  (AD) More severe hearing loss with administration of 100 g or more of
  streptomycin in both groups.
  (AD) More severe hearing loss in group with previous streptomycin treat-
  ment.
No reported ototoxic effects due to high doses of antibiotic, (SQ) dihydros-
treptomycin, in some of total of 370 humans treated with streptomycin. (SER)

                                                                          057
No ototoxic effects within 2 months due to antibiotic, dihydrostreptomycin
(dihydrostreptomycin ascorbinate), in humans with pulmonary tuberculosis.
  (AD) Audiometry used to determine ototoxic effects.
Tinnitus and vertigo due to antibiotic, streptomycin (streptomycin sulfate),
in humans with pulmonary tuberculosis.
  (AD) Comparative study of effects of 2 antibiotics used in treatment of
  pulmonary tuberculosis. (RUS)

                                                                          062
High frequency hearing loss and tinnitus due to parenteral, intramuscular,
administration of 1 g daily for first 60 days and then 1 g daily for 2 days
each week of antibiotic, capreomycin (SM), for 1 year in 7 of 89 humans,
range of ages, male and female, with pulmonary tuberculosis.
  (CT) No auditory system problems before treatment.
  (CT) Audiometry 1 time each month for duration of treatment.
  (AD) Previous resistance to primary antituberculous agents reported.
Simultaneous oral administration of 25 mg per kg daily for first 60 days and
then 15 mg per kg daily of antituberculous agent, ethambutol (SM), for 1 year
in 89 humans, range of ages, male and female, with pulmonary tuberculosis.
No reported ototoxic effects due to oral administration of 300 mg daily of
antituberculous agent, isoniazid (SM), for 1 year in 89 humans, range of
ages, male and female, with pulmonary tuberculosis.
  (AD) Previous resistance to isoniazid reported. (ENG)

                                                                          068
Hearing loss and tinnitus or hyperacusis due to oral administration of 1 g
daily of antibiotic, (SQ) capreomycin, for 2 years in 3 of first group of 34
humans with tuberculosis.
No reported ototoxic effects due to previous unspecified method of administration of unspecified doses of antibiotic, (SQ) streptomycin, in first group
of 34 humans with tuberculosis.
Hearing loss due to previous unspecified method of administration of unspecified doses of antibiotic, (SQ) streptomycin, in 9 of second group of 31
humans with tuberculosis.
More severe hearing loss due to oral administration of 1 g daily of antibiotic, (SQ) capreomycin, for 2 years in 1 of second group of 31 humans with
tuberculosis. (ENG)

                                                                          075
Hearing loss due to previous administration of antibiotic, (SQ) streptomycin,
in 18 of total of 67 humans with tuberculosis.
More severe hearing loss, tinnitus, or hyperacusis due to unspecified method
of administration of unspecified doses of antibiotic, (SQ) capreomycin, for

long period in 4 of 45 humans with tuberculosis.
No ototoxic effects due to unspecified method of administration of unspecified doses of antibiotic, (SQ) capreomycin, for short period in other 22
humans with tuberculosis. (ENG)

085
Hearing loss due to antibiotic, viomycin, in 17.7 percent of 152 humans with
tuberculosis.
   (CT) Systematic controls with audiology.
Hearing loss due to antibiotic, viomycin (IB), in only 5.3 percent of 36
humans with previous hearing loss with administration of nialamid.
Hearing loss due to antibiotic, kanamycin, in 20 percent of 55 humans with
tuberculosis.
Hearing loss due to antibiotic, kanamycin (IB), in 0 of 25 humans with pre-
vious hearing loss with administration of nialamid.
Lesion of inner ear due to antibiotic, neomycin (IB), in only 1 human with
previous hearing loss with administration of nialamid. (GER)

088
Ototoxic effects in fetus due to unspecified method of administration of
unspecified doses of antibiotic, streptomycin, for long period in humans,
female, treated for tuberculosis during pregnancy.
Ototoxic effects in fetus due to unspecified method of administration of
unspecified doses of antibiotic, dihydrostreptomycin, for long period in
humans, female, treated for tuberculosis during pregnancy. (ENG)

091
Ototoxic effects due to antibiotic, streptomycin (streptomycin sulfate), in
humans with pulmonary tuberculosis.
Ototoxic effects due to antibiotic, dihydrostreptomycin, in humans with
pulmonary tuberculosis.
Ototoxic effects due to antibiotic, florimycin, in humans with pulmonary
tuberculosis.
Ototoxic effects due to antibiotic, kanamycin, in humans with pulmonary
tuberculosis.
   (AD) Comparative study of ototoxicity of different derivatives of antibiotics. (RUS)

095
Ototoxic effects due to unspecified method of administration of (SQ) 0.75 g
daily of antibiotic, streptomycin (SM), for (SQ) 3 months initial treatment
in 6 of 140 humans with tuberculosis.
Simultaneous unspecified method of administration of (SQ) 300 mg of antituberculous agent, isoniazid (SM), in 140 humans with tuberculosis.
Ototoxic effects due to unspecified method of administration of (SQ) 1 g 3
days a week of antibiotic, streptomycin (SM), for (SQ) 18 months following
initial treatment in 24 of 140 humans with tuberculosis.
Dizziness due to simultaneous unspecified method of administration of (SQ)
600 mg of antituberculous agent, isoniazid (SM), in unspecified number of
humans with tuberculosis and with other toxic effects due to isoniazid.
(ENG)

107
Vertigo and nystagmus due to antibiotic, kanamycin, in humans, male and
female.
Vertigo and nystagmus due to antibiotic, streptomycin, in humans, male and
female.
   (AD) Preclinical detection of vestibular problems by ENG. (FR)

115
Permanent cochleo-vestibulotoxic effects due to antibiotics, aminoglycoside,
in humans.
Transient cochlear impairment due to salicylates in humans.
Ototoxic effects due to antimalarial, quinine, in humans.
Ototoxic effects due to chemical agent, nicotine, in humans.
   (AD) Report on ototoxic effects of various drugs.
   (AD) Need for audiometry and vestibular function tests with clinical use
   of ototoxic drugs. (FR)

116

Moderate unilateral sensorineural hearing loss in 1 of 36 fetuses due to total of 13 g of antibiotic, dihydrostreptomycin, in 33 humans, female, treated during pregnancy for tuberculosis.
(AD) Child not treated with dihydrostreptomycin or streptomycin.
Sensorineural hearing loss due to 1 g daily for the first 30 days and then 1 g twice a week of antibiotic, dihydrostreptomycin (CB), in 8(24 percent)of 33 humans, female, treated during pregnancy for tuberculosis.
Sensorineural hearing loss due to 1 g daily for the first 30 days and then 1 g twice a week of antibiotic, streptomycin (CB), in 8(24 percent)of 33 humans, female, treated during pregnancy for tuberculosis.
Vestibular problems due to antibiotic, (SQ) dihydrostreptomycin, in 1 of 33 humans, female, treated during pregnancy for tuberculosis and chronic pyelonephritis.
Vestibular problems due to antibiotic, (SQ) streptomycin, in 1 of 33 humans, female, treated during pregnancy for tuberculosis and chronic pyelonephritis.
   (AD) Case histories, audiometry, and vestibular function tests for chil-
   dren and adults. (ENG)

136

Vestibular problems due to oral administration of 150 mg daily of antituber-culous agent, thiacetazone (CB), for 12 months in 4 of 150 humans with pul-monary tuberculosis and without previous treatment.
Combined oral administration of 30 mg daily of antituberculous agent, isonia-zid (CB), for 12 months in 150 humans with pulmonary tuberculosis and without previous treatment.
No vestibular problems due to 10 g daily in 2 doses of antituberculous agent, PAS (CB) (sodium PAS), for 12 months in 100 humans with pulmonary tuberculo-sis and without previous treatment.
Combined administration of 200 mg daily in 2 doses of antituberculous agent, isoniazid (CB), for 12 months in 100 humans with pulmonary tuberculosis and without previous treatment.
   (AD) Comparative study of effects of thiacetazone and PAS with isoniazid
   in treatment of tuberculosis. (ENG)

137

Vestibular problems due to 1 g daily of antibiotic, capreomycin (SM), for long period in 2 of 20 humans with tuberculosis.
Simultaneous administration of 25 mg per kg for first 60 days and then 15 mg per kg of antituberculous agent, ethambutol (SM), in 20 humans with tubercu-losis.
Simultaneous administration of 300 mg twice daily for several months and then 450 mg in 1 dose of antibiotic, rifampicin (SM), in 20 humans with tuberculo-sis. (ENG)

139

Cochleotoxic effects due to antibiotic, kanamycin, in humans and animals, guinea pigs.
Cochleotoxic effects due to antibiotic, streptomycin, in humans and animals, guinea pigs.
   (AD) Literature review of mechanism of action of ototoxic antibiotics.
   (POL)

170

Sensorineural hearing loss due to topical administration in ear drops of antibiotic, neomycin, in humans with no other explanation for hearing loss.
Sensorineural hearing loss due to topical administration in ear drops of antibiotic, chloramphenicol, in humans with no other explanation for hearing loss.
Sensorineural hearing loss due to topical administration in ear drops of antibiotic, framycetin, in humans with no other explanation for hearing loss.
   (AD) Comment on topical use of antibiotics and possible risk of cochleoto-
   xic effects. (ENG)

172

Vertigo due to sedative, alcohol, ethyl, in humans.
Vertigo due to antibiotic, streptomycin, in humans.
   (AD) Report on etiology of vertigo. (GER)

186

Diplacusis due to antibiotics, aminoglycoside, in humans.
Diplacusis due to antimalarial, quinine, in humans.
Diplacusis due to salicylate, aspirin, in humans.
Diplacusis due to chemical agent, carbon monoxide, in humans.
(AD) Report on etiology of diplacusis with comment on ototoxic drugs.
(ENG)

198

Severe vertigo due to parenteral, intramuscular, administration of 1 g daily
in single dose of antibiotic, streptomycin (SM) (streptomycin sulfate), for 6
months in 2 of 41 humans, 108.2 lb average weight, with pulmonary tuberculosis and with previous streptomycin therapy in some.
Simultaneous oral administration of 15 g daily in single dose of antituberculo-
lous agent, PAS (SM) (sodium PAS), for 6 months in 2 of 41 humans, 108.2 lb
average weight, with pulmonary tuberculosis and with previous streptomycin
therapy in some.
No vestibulotoxic effects due to parenteral, intramuscular, administration of
1 g daily in single dose of antibiotic, streptomycin (SM) (streptomycin
sulfate), for 6 months in 41 humans, 113.5 lb average weight, with pulmonary
tuberculosis and with previous streptomycin therapy in some.
Simultaneous oral administration of 15 g daily in 2 doses of antituberculous
agent, PAS (SM) (sodium PAS), for 6 months in 41 humans, 113.5 lb average
weight, with pulmonary tuberculosis and with previous streptomycin therapy in
some.
(AD) Study of retreatment of pulmonary tuberculosis in humans with no
response to previous chemotherapy. (ENG)

213

Dizziness due to antibiotic, polymyxin B (polymyxin B sulfate), in humans.
Dizziness due to antibiotic, colistin (sodium colistimethate), in humans.
Ototoxic effects due to antibiotic, ristocetin, in humans.
Hearing loss due to antibiotic, vancomycin, in humans.
(AD) Report on pharmacology, clinical use, and toxicity of antibiotics.
(ENG)

219

Cochleo-vestibulotoxic effects due to antibiotics in humans.
Transient and permanent sensorineural hearing loss due to diuretic, etha-
crynic acid, in humans.
Transient sensorineural hearing loss, tinnitus, and vertigo due to salicy-
late, aspirin, in humans.
Transient and permanent sensorineural hearing loss and dizziness due to
antimalarial, quinine, in humans.
Sensorineural hearing loss due to antimalarial, chloroquine, in humans.
Sensorineural hearing loss, tinnitus, and vertigo due to chemical agents in
humans.
(AD) Literature review of ototoxic drugs with clinical and histopathologi-
cal correlations.
(AD) Comment on ototoxicity of some chemical agents.
(AD) Review of theories of mechanism of action of ototoxic drugs. (ENG)

249

Cochleo-vestibulotoxic effects due to antibiotics, aminoglycoside, in humans.
Cochlear impairment due to antimalarial, quinine, in humans.
Transient cochlear impairment and vestibular problems due to salicylates in
humans.
(AD) Occurrence of ototoxic effects with different dosages due to indivi-
dual responses to drugs.
(AD) Need for observation and tests with clinical use of ototoxic drugs.
(FR)

265

Hearing loss due to analgesic, fentanyl (SM), in humans, treated before
ultrasound therapy for Meniere's disease.
Hearing loss due to tranquilizer, droperidol (SM), in humans, treated before
ultrasound therapy for Meniere's disease.
(AD) More severe hearing loss with simultaneous use of droperidol and

fentanyl than with use of local anesthetic only.   (ENG)

284

Hearing loss due to antibiotics, aminoglycoside, in humans.
Hearing loss due to salicylate, sodium salicylate, in humans.
Hearing loss due to antimalarial, quinine, in humans.
    (AD) Discussion of clinical use and cochleotoxic effects of ototoxic drugs
    in humans. (FR)

288

Changes in cochlear microphonic due to parenteral, intramuscular, administration of 300 mg per kg daily of antibiotic, kanamycin, in animals, cats.
Changes in cochlear microphonic due to parenteral, intramuscular, administration of 200 and 100 mg per kg daily of antibiotic, streptomycin, in animals,
cats.
Hearing loss due to 300 mg per kg daily of antibiotic, kanamycin, in humans.
Hearing loss due to range of 50 to 200 mg per kg daily of antibiotic, streptomycin, in humans.
    (CT) Study of subjects, control group, not treated with aminoglycoside
    antibiotics.
    (AD) Hearing loss confirmed by audiogram. (JAP)

290

Vestibular problems, sensorineural hearing loss, and tinnitus due to total
doses of 12 to 63 g of antibiotic, streptomycin, in 24 humans with tuberculosis.
    (AD) Subjects tested after streptomycin intoxication with audiology and
    cupulometry.
    (AD) Individual responses to streptomycin observed.
Changes in cupulometric curves for postrotatory nystagmus, showing changes in
vestibular apparatus, due to 0.5 g daily, total doses of 30 to 100 g, of
antibiotic, streptomycin (SM) (streptomycin sulfate), in 23 humans with
various infections.
Simultaneous administration of 0.5 g of antibiotic, dihydrostreptomycin (SM),
in 23 humans with various infections.
Simultaneous administration of antituberculous agent, PAS (SM), in 23 humans
with various infections.
    (CT) Pretreatment vestibular function normal.
    (CT) Subjects tested with audiology and cupulometry before and during
    treatment with streptomycin.
    (AD) Hearing loss in 1 subject in group with cupulometry during treatment
    but in 5 subjects in other group with cupulometry only after treatment.
    (AD) Suggested use of cupulometry for possible prevention of streptomycin
    intoxication. (ENG)

293

Cochleo-vestibulotoxic effects due to antibiotic, streptomycin (SM), in
humans, range of ages, with pulmonary tuberculosis.
Simultaneous administration of other antituberculous agents (SM) in humans,
range of ages, with pulmonary tuberculosis.
    (AD) Report on toxic effects due to simultaneous treatment with various
    antituberculous agents. (BUL)

308

Possible hearing loss due to antibiotic, kanamycin, in humans with tuberculosis.
Possible vestibular problems and cochlear impairment due to antibiotic,
capreomycin, in humans with tuberculosis.
    (AD) Comment on possible cochleo-vestibulotoxic effects of antibiotics
    used in treatment of tuberculosis. (ENG)

311

Vertigo or hearing loss of 10 to 20 decibels due to antibiotic, streptomycin,
in 14 of 67 humans with pulmonary tuberculosis.
Vertigo or hearing loss of 30 to 40 decibels due to antibiotic, streptomycin
(CB), in 12 of 59 humans with pulmonary tuberculosis.
Vertigo or hearing loss of 30 to 40 decibels due to antibiotic, dihydrostrep-
tomycin (CB), in 12 of 59 humans with pulmonary tuberculosis.

(AD) Hearing loss confirmed by audiometry.   (DUT)

                                                                    318
High risk of ototoxic effects due to antibiotic, dihydrostreptomycin, in
humans with bacterial infections.
Risk of ototoxic effects due to antibiotic, streptomycin, in humans with
bacterial infections, with administration of pantothenic acid.
   (AD) Literature review on clinical use and ototoxicity of streptomycin.
   (AD) Recommended use of streptomycin only for tuberculosis due to high
   risk of ototoxic effects. (GER)

                                                                    326
Hearing loss due to parenteral, intramuscular, administration of 1.0 g daily
of antibiotic, capreomycin (SM), for less than 6 months in 2 of 53 humans
with cavitary pulmonary tuberculosis and no previous chemotherapy.
No reported ototoxic effects due to oral administration of 12.0 g daily in 3
divided doses of antituberculous agent, PAS (SM), for up to 6 months in 53
humans with cavitary pulmonary tuberculosis and no previous chemotherapy.
(ENG)

                                                                    332
No subjective hearing loss but objective hearing loss over 20 decibels and
tinnitus due to parenteral, intramuscular, administration of 1 g daily for
first 60 days and then 1 g twice a week of antibiotic, capreomycin (SM), for
6 months in 3 of 100 humans treated for pulmonary tuberculosis.
Hearing loss, tinnitus, or dizziness due to parenteral, intramuscular, administration of 1 g daily for first 60 days and then 1 g twice a week of
antibiotic, streptomycin (SM), for 6 months in 8 of 99 humans treated for
pulmonary tuberculosis.
Hearing loss over 20 decibels due to parenteral, intramuscular, administration of 1 g daily for first 60 days and then 1 g twice a week of antibiotic,
streptomycin (SM), for 6 months in 3 of 99 humans treated for pulmonary
tuberculosis.
Simultaneous oral administration of 0.3 g daily in 2 doses of antituberculous
agent, isoniazid (SM), for 6 months in humans treated for pulmonary tuberculosis.
Simultaneous administration of 10 g daily in 3 doses of antituberculous
agent, PAS (SM), for 6 months in humans treated for pulmonary tuberculosis.
   (AD) Report on ototoxic effects of antibiotics used in initial treatment
   of tuberculosis.
High frequency hearing loss, tinnitus, or dizziness due to parenteral, intramuscular, administration of 1 g daily for first 60 days and then 1 g twice a
week of antibiotic, capreomycin (SM), for 6 months in 6 of 66 humans retreated for pulmonary tuberculosis.
No subjective auditory system problems but objective hearing loss over 20
decibels due to parenteral, intramuscular, administration of 1 g 3 times a
week of antibiotic, kanamycin (SM), for 6 months in 4 of 40 humans retreated
for pulmonary tuberculosis.
No subjective auditory system problems but objective hearing loss over 20
decibels due to parenteral, intramuscular, administration of 1 g daily for
first 60 days and then 1 g twice a week of antibiotic, streptomycin (SM), for
6 months in 1 of 13 humans retreated for pulmonary tuberculosis.
Simultaneous oral administration of 0.3 g daily in 2 doses of antituberculous
agent, isoniazid (SM), for 6 months in humans retreated for pulmonary tuberculosis.
   (AD) Report on ototoxic effects of antibiotics used in retreatment of
   tuberculosis.
   (CT) Audiometry, pretreatment and during treatment, 2 times a month in
   first 2 months and then 1 time a month.
   (AD) Comparative study of clinical use and cochleo-vestibulotoxic effects
   of capreomycin and other antibiotics in treatment and retreatment of
   pulmonary tuberculosis. (ENG)

                                                                    333
Vestibular problems due to antibiotic, streptomycin, in humans.
Severe cochlear impairment due to antibiotic, dihydrostreptomycin, in humans.
Loss of hair cells in organ of Corti and hearing loss due to antibiotics,
aminoglycoside, in humans.

Hearing loss in fetus due to antimalarial, quinine, in humans, female,
treated during pregnancy.
Transient hearing loss due to high doses of salicylate, aspirin, for long
period in humans.
   (AD) Discussion of possible cochleo-vestibulotoxic effects of ototoxic
   drugs.
   (AD) Ototoxic effects related to concurrent disorders, dosage, duration of
   treatment, and age of individuals. (ENG)

335

Vestibular problems due to antibiotic, streptomycin, in humans.
Severe cochlear impairment due to antibiotic, dihydrostreptomycin, in humans.
Cochlear impairment due to parenteral, oral, and topical administration of
antibiotic, neomycin, in humans.
Tinnitus and hearing loss due to antibiotic, kanamycin, in humans.
Vestibular problems and hearing loss due to antibiotic, gentamicin, in hu-
mans.
   (AD) Discussion of clinical use and possible cochleo-vestibulotoxic ef-
   fects of aminoglycoside antibiotics. (SP)

340

Vestibular problems due to 150 mg daily of antituberculous agent, thiaceta-
zone (SM), in 15 of 75 humans with pulmonary tuberculosis.
Vestibular problems due to 0.75 to 1 g daily of antibiotic, streptomycin (SM)
(streptomycin sulfate), in 15 of 75 humans with pulmonary tuberculosis.
Vestibular problems due to 300 mg daily of antituberculous agent, isoniazid
(SM), in 15 of 75 humans with pulmonary tuberculosis.
   (AD) Vestibulotoxic effects confirmed by vestibular function tests.
   (AD) Statistical analysis showed higher occurrence of vestibular problems
   in humans with thiacetazone in drug regimen than without thiacetazone.
   (SL)

342

More severe sensorineural hearing loss of 20 decibels or more due to parenteral administration of total doses of 173 and 172 g of antibiotic, (SQ)
capreomycin, for long period, range of 2 to 18 months, in 2 of 294 humans,
male and female, with pulmonary tuberculosis and with previous hearing loss.
   (CT) Audiometry, pretreatment and during treatment.
   (AD) Suggested that occurrence of auditory system problems due to capreomycin not high.
Sensorineural hearing loss due to previous administration of antibiotic, (SQ)
streptomycin, in 1 of 294 humans with pulmonary tuberculosis. (ENG)

345

Transient hearing loss and vestibular problem due to salicylate, aspirin, in
humans.
Decr in cochlear microphonic and action potential and decr in malic dehydrogenase in endolymph and perilymph due to salicylate, aspirin, in humans.
   (AD) Suggested that cochleo-vestibulotoxic effects of salicylates due to
   electrophysiological and biochemical changes and not structural changes.
Primary distribution in stria vascularis and spiral ligament due to salicylate, aspirin, in humans.
   (AD) Possible but not definite location of toxic activity of aspirin.
High concentration in inner ear after 5 to 7 hours due to parenteral, intraperitoneal, administration of salicylate, sodium salicylate, in animals,
cats.
   (AD) Report on clinical use and ototoxic effects of aspirin. (ENG)

350

Cochleotoxic effects due to 0.75 or 1 g daily, total doses of 30.0 to 116.75
g, of antibiotic, streptomycin, in 9(7.2 percent)of 125 humans with disorders.
Cochleotoxic effects due to 1 g daily, total of less than 30 to over 180 g,
of antibiotic, kanamycin, in 40 (55.6 percent) of 72 humans with disorders.
   (AD) Comparative study of ototoxic effects of 2 aminoglycoside antibiotics. (GER)

351
No observed ototoxic effects due to topical administration of 1 drop of
chemical agent, dimethyl sulfoxide (CB), in humans as anesthetic for myringotomy.
No observed ototoxic effects due to topical administration of 1 drop of
anesthetic, tetracaine (CB) (tetracaine hydrochloride), in humans as anesthetic for myringotomy. (ENG)

358
Severe to total hearing loss due to antibiotic, paromomycin, in most of
humans treated.
Severe to total hearing loss due to antibiotic, streptomycin, in most of
humans treated.
Severe to total hearing loss due to antibiotic, neomycin, in most of humans
treated.
Objective but no subjective vestibular problems due to antibiotic, streptomycin, in 2 humans. (RUS)

368
Possible vestibular problems and hearing loss due to antibiotic, streptomy-
cin, in humans with tuberculosis.
Permanent hearing loss due to antibiotic, dihydrostreptomycin, in humans with
tuberculosis.
Possible permanent hearing loss due to antibiotic, kanamycin, in humans with
tuberculosis.
Possible vestibular problems and hearing loss due to antibiotic, viomycin, in
humans with tuberculosis.
Possible damage to eighth cranial nerve due to antibiotic, capreomycin, in
humans with tuberculosis.
   (AD) Discussion of primary and secondary drugs used in tuberculosis chemotherapy. (FR)

377
Lesion of vestibular apparatus due to about 22 g of antibiotic, streptomycin
(SM), in human with pulmonary tuberculosis.
   (AD) Lesion of vestibular apparatus confirmed by vestibular function test.
Simultaneous administration of 185 g of antituberculous agent, PAS (SM), in
human with pulmonary tuberculosis.
Simultaneous administration of 16.5 g of antituberculous agent, isoniazid
(SM), in human with pulmonary tuberculosis. (POL)

394
Tinnitus and hearing loss due to total of 50 to 100 g, in some cases, of
antibiotic, (SQ) kanamycin, in 176(9 percent) of 2054 humans with surgery for
pulmonary tuberculosis.
   (AD) Improvement in hearing in only 30 percent of humans.
Possible hearing loss due to previous administration of antibiotic, (SQ)
streptomycin, for long period in 176 of 2054 humans before surgery for pulmonary tuberculosis. (ENG)

409
Primary damage to hair cells of organ of Corti, hearing loss, and possible
vestibular problems due to antibiotic, viomycin, in humans.
Damage to hair cells of organ of Corti and hearing loss due to antibiotic,
neomycin, in humans.
Damage to hair cells of organ of Corti and hearing loss due to antibiotic,
kanamycin, in humans.
Primary damage to vestibular apparatus, vestibular problems, and possible
hearing loss due to antibiotic, streptomycin, in humans.
Primary damage to vestibular apparatus, vestibular problems, and possible
hearing loss due to antibiotic, gentamicin, in humans.
   (AD) Need for audiometry and vestibular function tests, pretreatment and
   during treatment, with clinical use of aminoglycoside antibiotics.
   (AD) Incr in blood levels and ototoxicity of antibiotics in humans with
   kidney disorders. (ENG)

415
Transient and permanent hearing loss due to high doses of diuretic, ethacrynic acid, in humans.

Transient hearing loss due to parenteral, intravenous, administration of high
doses, 600 to 1000 mg, of diuretic, furosemide, in humans with kidney disorders.
   (AD) Literature review of clinical use and toxic effects of diuretics.
   (ENG)

                                                                           419
Hearing loss and vestibular problems due to antibiotic, streptomycin, in
humans with various disorders.
Hearing loss and vestibular problems due to other ototoxic drugs in humans
with various disorders.
   (AD) Discussion of cochleo-vestibulotoxic effects of ototoxic drugs used
   in therapy for various disorders. (GER)

                                                                           433
Dizziness due to 1 g daily of antibiotic, streptomycin (SM), for 6 months in
32 percent of 114 humans with pulmonary tuberculosis.
Dizziness due to 300 mg daily of antituberculous agent, isoniazid (SM), for 6
months with streptomycin and then 6 months alone in 32 percent of 114 humans
with pulmonary tuberculosis.
   (AD) Regimen of simultaneous administration of streptomycin and isoniazid
   for 6 months followed by administration of isoniazid only for 6 months.
Dizziness due to 1 g daily of antibiotic, streptomycin (SM), for 6 months in
54 percent of 94 humans with pulmonary tuberculosis.
Dizziness due to 150 mg daily of antituberculous agent, thiacetazone (SM),
for 6 months with streptomycin and isoniazid and then 6 months with isoniazid
in 54 percent of 94 humans with pulmonary tuberculosis.
Dizziness due to 300 mg daily of antituberculous agent, isoniazid (SM), for 6
months with streptomycin and thiacetazone and then 6 months with thiacetazone
in 54 percent of 94 humans with pulmonary tuberculosis.
   (AD) Regimen of simultaneous administration of streptomycin, thiacetazone,
   and isoniazid for 6 months followed by administration of thiacetazone and
   isoniazid for 6 months.
Dizziness due to 150 mg daily of antituberculous agent, thiacetazone (SM),
for 1 year in 13 percent of 78 humans with pulmonary tuberculosis.
Dizziness due to 300 mg daily of antituberculous agent, isoniazid (SM), for 1
year in 13 percent of 78 humans with pulmonary tuberculosis.
   (AD) Regimen of simultaneous administration of thiacetazone and isoniazid
   for 1 year.
   (AD) Study of role of drug regimens with thiacetazone in treatment of
   pulmonary tuberculosis. (ENG)

                                                                           437
Hearing loss and damage to cochlea due to antibiotic, neomycin, in animals,
guinea pigs and monkeys, and humans.
Hearing loss and damage to cochlea due to antibiotic, streptomycin, in animals, guinea pigs and monkeys, and humans.
   (AD) Discussion of findings on decr of ototoxicity of aminoglycoside
   antibiotics. (GER)

                                                                           444
Changes in cochlear function and vestibular function due to analeptic, caf-
feine, in animals and humans.
Changes in cochlear function and vestibular function due to analeptic, amphe-
tamine, in animals and humans.
Changes in cochlear function and vestibular function due to sedatives and
tranquilizers in animals and humans.
   (AD) Suggested mechanism of action of drugs.
   (AD) Literature review of ototoxic effects of drugs. (IT)

                                                                           473
Possible vestibular problems due to antibiotic, viomycin, in humans with
infections.
Possible vestibular problems due to antibiotic, capreomycin, in humans with
infections.
   (AD) Experiments to find new derivatives of viomycin and capreomycin with
   biological activity but with less toxic effects. (ENG)

481

Damage to vestibular apparatus due to 1 g daily or twice daily of antibiotic, streptomycin (SM), for maximum of 3 months in 9 of 108 humans, range of 2 to 86 years age, male and female, with pulmonary tuberculosis.
Simultaneous administration of 12 g daily of antituberculous agent, PAS (SM), for 12 to 18 months in 108 humans, range of 2 to 86 years age, male and female, with pulmonary tuberculosis.
Simultaneous administration of 300 mg daily of antituberculous agent, isoniazid (SM), for 12 to 18 months in 108 humans, range of 2 to 86 years age, male and female, with pulmonary tuberculosis. (ENG)

483

Possible damage to vestibular nerve and cochlear nerve due to antibiotic, streptomycin, in humans with or without kidney disorder.
Possible damage to vestibular nerve and cochlear nerve due to antibiotic, gentamicin, in humans with or without kidney disorder.
Possible damage to vestibular nerve and cochlear nerve due to antibiotic, kanamycin, in humans with or without kidney disorder.
Possible damage to vestibular nerve and cochlear nerve due to antibiotic, neomycin, in humans with or without kidney disorder.
   (AD) Incidence of effects on vestibular function highest in streptomycin, followed by gentamicin, kanamycin, and neomycin.
   (AD) Incidence of effects on cochlear function highest in neomycin, followed by kanamycin, gentamicin, and streptomycin.
   (AD) Need for careful consideration in clinical use of aminoglycoside antibiotics.
Possible cochlear impairment and vestibular problems due to antibiotic, paromomycin, in humans.
Possible dizziness and ataxia due to antibiotic, polymyxin B, in humans.
Possible but rare dizziness and vertigo due to antibiotic, nalidixic acid, in humans. (ENG)

497

Primary damage to vestibular apparatus but also cochlear impairment due to chemical agent, carbon disulfide, in humans.
Primary damage to vestibular apparatus but also cochlear impairment due to chemical agent, carbon monoxide, in humans.
Primary damage to vestibular apparatus but also cochlear impairment due to heavy metal, lead, in humans.
Primary damage to vestibular apparatus but also cochlear impairment due to chemical agent, benzene, in humans.
Primary damage to vestibular apparatus but also cochlear impairment due to chemical agent, carbon tetrachloride, in humans.
   (AD) Report on cochleo-vestibulotoxic effects of chemical agents in industry. (IT)

515

Bilateral hearing loss due to oral (SM) administration of 480 mg daily of diuretic, furosemide (SM), for 10 days in 1 human with kidney disorder.
Bilateral hearing loss due to parenteral, intravenous (SM), administration of 600 mg daily of diuretic, furosemide (SM), for 10 days in 1 human with kidney disorder.
Bilateral hearing loss due to 500 mg of antibiotic, kanamycin (SM) (kanamycin sulfate), in 2 doses in 1 human with kidney disorder.
   (AD) No pretreatment audiogram.
   (AD) Posttreatment audiogram confirmed hearing loss.
   (AD) Suggested audiometry, pretreatment and during treatment, for humans, in particular with kidney disorder, treated with high doses of intravenous furosemide. (ENG)

522

Hearing loss due to antibiotic, kanamycin, for 2 to 10 months in 30.4 percent of 56 humans with chronic pulmonary tuberculosis and treated previously with other drugs.
No significant ototoxic effects due to antibiotic, florimycin, for 2 to 10 months in 50 humans with chronic pulmonary tuberculosis and treated previously with other drugs.
   (AD) Study of effects of kanamycin and florimycin in treatment of pul-

monary tuberculosis.   (RUS)

538
Dizziness due to parenteral administration of 1 g daily for first 8 weeks and
then 1 g twice weekly for 12 weeks of antibiotic, streptomycin (SM), for
total of 20 weeks in 5 of 77 humans with pulmonary tuberculosis.
Simultaneous administration of 300 mg daily in single dose of antituberculous
agent, isoniazid (SM), in 77 humans with pulmonary tuberculosis.
Simultaneous administration of 15 mg per kg daily of antituberculous agent,
ethambutol (SM), in 77 humans with pulmonary tuberculosis.
No reported ototoxic effects due to 600 mg daily in single dose of antibiotic, rifampicin, in 157 humans with pulmonary tuberculosis. (ENG)

539
Transient unilateral or bilateral ototoxic effects, vestibular problems in
66.6 percent of cases, due to antibiotic, gentamicin, in 14 humans.
    (AD) Literature review showed small number of cases of gentamicin ototoxi-
    city reported in Germany.
    (AD) Primary factor in gentamicin ototoxicity is kidney disorder.
    (AD) Other factors in gentamicin ototoxicity include dosage and simul-
    taneous administration of other ototoxic drugs.
Hearing loss due to diuretic, ethacrynic acid, in humans with kidney disorder. (GER)

557
Ototoxic effects due to previous administration of antibiotic, (SQ) streptomycin, in 8 humans with pulmonary tuberculosis.
No ototoxic effects due to 1.0 g daily of antibiotic, (SQ) capreomycin (SM),
for long period in same 8 of 38 humans with pulmonary tuberculosis.
Simultaneous administration of antituberculous agent, (SQ) ethambutol (SM),
in 38 humans with pulmonary tuberculosis. (ENG)

560
Ototoxic effects due to antibiotic, streptomycin, in humans with tuberculo-
sis.
Ototoxic effects due to antibiotic, kanamycin, in humans with tuberculosis.
    (AD) Reported 4 to 5 percent incidence in audiometry of ototoxicity from
    streptomycin and kanamycin.
    (AD) Decr in ototoxicity with administration of streptomycin or kanamycin
    in evening before sleeping. (JAP)

569
Slight hearing loss due to 1 g daily in single dose of antibiotic, capreomycin (SM), in 2 of 31 humans with chronic pulmonary tuberculosis.
    (AD) Audiometry and vestibular function tests every 4 weeks and then every
    6 weeks.
    (AD) Cessation of treatment with capreomycin in 4 cases to prevent hearing
    loss.
Simultaneous administration of 25 mg per kg daily in single dose for 12 weeks
and then 15 mg per kg of antituberculous agent, ethambutol (SM), in 31 humans
with chronic pulmonary tuberculosis.
Simultaneous oral administration of 1 other antituberculous agent (SM), in 31
humans with chronic pulmonary tuberculosis. (ENG)

591
Hearing loss due to antibiotic, capreomycin, for long period in 2 of 28
humans with tuberculosis.
    (AD) Results of 1 study of effects of capreomycin.
No ototoxic effects due to antibiotic, (SQ) capreomycin, for 1 to 24 months
in 16 humans with tuberculosis.
    (AD) Results of other study of effects of capreomycin.
Vestibular problems due to previous administration of antibiotic, (SQ) streptomycin, in 8 of 16 humans with tuberculosis.
    (AD) Suggested that less ototoxicity due to capreomycin than to streptomy-
    cin. (ENG)

597
Hearing loss due to salicylates in humans.

Hearing loss due to antimalarial, quinine, in humans.
Hearing loss due to antibiotic, streptomycin, in humans.
Tinnitus due to chemical agent, camphor, in humans.
Tinnitus due to chemical agent, tobacco, in humans.
Tinnitus due to cardiovascular agent, quinidine, in humans.
Tinnitus due to chemical agent, ergot, in humans.
Tinnitus due to chemical agent, alcohol, methyl, in humans.
    (AD) Discussion of toxic effects of drugs. (ENG)

602

Effect on eighth cranial nerve due to antibiotic, streptomycin, in humans.
Effect on eighth cranial nerve due to antibiotic, dihydrostreptomycin, in humans.
    (AD) Comparative study of effect of 2 antibiotics on eighth cranial nerve. (ENG)

610

Possible ototoxic effects due to antibiotic, capreomycin, in humans with tuberculosis of genitourinary system.
Possible hearing loss due to antibiotic, kanamycin, in humans with tuberculosis of genitourinary system.
Possible hearing loss and vestibular problems due to antibiotic, viomycin, in humans with tuberculosis of genitourinary system.
    (AD) Discussion of treatment of tuberculosis of genitourinary system. (GER)

615

Tinnitus, hearing loss, vertigo, and dizziness due to oral administration in tablet of 150 mg daily of antituberculous agent, thiacetazone (CB) (SM), in some of 1002 humans with tuberculosis.
Tinnitus, hearing loss, vertigo, and dizziness due to oral administration in tablet of 300 mg daily of antituberculous agent, isoniazid (CB) (SM), in some of 1002 humans with tuberculosis.
Tinnitus, hearing loss, vertigo, and dizziness due to parenteral administration of 1 g daily of antibiotic, streptomycin (SM), in some of 1002 humans with tuberculosis.
    (AD) Reported 21.4 percent incidence of toxic effects in regimen of thiacetazone, isoniazid, and streptomycin.
    (AD) Suggested that effects of streptomycin potentiated by thiacetazone.
Unspecified ototoxic effects due to oral administration of 300 mg daily of antituberculous agent, isoniazid (SM), in 987 humans with tuberculosis.
Unspecified ototoxic effects due to parenteral administration of 1 g daily of antibiotic, streptomycin (SM), in 987 humans with tuberculosis.
    (AD) Reported 7.8 percent incidence of toxic effects in regimen of isoniazid and streptomycin without thiacetazone. (ENG)

621

Primarily vestibular problems due to antibiotic, streptomycin, in humans.
Primarily hearing loss but also vestibular problems due to antibiotic, dihydrostreptomycin, in humans.
Primarily hearing loss but also vestibular problems due to antibiotic, kanamycin, in humans.
Primarily hearing loss but also vestibular problems due to antibiotic, neomycin, in humans.
Primarily hearing loss but also vestibular problems due to antibiotic, gentamicin, in humans.
Vertigo and ataxia due to antituberculous agent, isoniazid, in humans.
Hearing loss due to salicylate, aspirin, in humans.
Hearing loss and vertigo due to antimalarial, quinine, in humans.
Nystagmus due to barbiturates in humans.
Vestibular problems due to analgesic, morphine, in humans.
Nystagmus due to sedative, alcohol, in humans.
Nystagmus and hearing loss due to chemical agent, carbon monoxide, in humans.
Ototoxic effects due to antineoplastic, nitrogen mustard, in humans.
Ototoxic effects due to chemical agent, aniline, in humans.
Ototoxic effects due to chemical agent, tobacco, in humans.
Nystagmus due to chemical agent, nicotine, in humans.
Vestibular problems due to anticonvulsants in humans.

Vestibular problems due to anesthetics in humans.
Vestibular problems due to diuretics in humans.
   (AD) Inclusion of comprehensive list of ototoxic agents. (SP)

                                                                    627
Sensorineural hearing loss and vestibular problems due to parenteral, oral,
and topical administration of antibiotics in humans with and without kidney
disorder.
Degeneration of cochlea due to parenteral, intratympanic, administration of
antibiotic, neomycin, in animals, guinea pigs.
Transient sensorineural hearing loss due to high doses of salicylates in
humans.
Sensorineural hearing loss due to antimalarial, quinine, in humans.
Sensorineural hearing loss due to chemical agent, tobacco, in humans.
Sensorineural hearing loss due to sedative, alcohol, in humans.
   (AD) Discussion of ototoxicity of various drugs as 1 etiology of sen-
   sorineural hearing loss in adults. (ENG)

                                                                    637
Ototoxic effects due to antibiotic, streptomycin (CB), in humans.
Ototoxic effects due to antibiotic, penicillin (CB), in humans. (GER)

                                                                    641
Possible damage to eighth cranial nerve due to antibiotic, capreomycin, in
humans.
Possible vestibular problems and hearing loss due to antibiotic, gentamicin,
in humans.
Possible delayed transient or permanent hearing loss due to antibiotic,
kanamycin (SM), in humans, in particular with kidney disorders or with simul-
taneous administration of ethacrynic acid.
Possible delayed transient or permanent hearing loss due to diuretic, ethacrynic acid (SM), in humans.
Possible delayed transient or permanent severe hearing loss due to oral,
parenteral, or topical administration of antibiotic, neomycin, in humans.
Possible damage to eighth cranial nerve, primarily hearing loss, due to
antibiotic, paromomycin, in humans.
Possible hearing loss due to antibiotic, rifampicin, in humans.
High risk of damage to eighth cranial nerve, primarily transient or permanent
vestibular problems but also hearing loss, due to antibiotic, streptomycin,
in humans.
Possible damage to eighth cranial nerve, primarily hearing loss, due to high
doses of antibiotic, vancomycin, for long period of more than 10 days in
humans, in particular with kidney disorders.
Risk of damage to eighth cranial nerve, vestibular problems and hearing loss,
due to high doses of antibiotic, viomycin, for long period of more than 10
days in humans, in particular with kidney disorders.
   (AD) Discussion of toxic effects of antibiotics. (ENG)

                                                                    644
Possible vertigo due to antimalarial, amodiaquine (amodiaquine dihydrochloride), in humans with parasitic infections.
Possible sensorineural hearing loss due to antimalarial, chloroquine (chloroquine hydrochloride) (chloroquine phosphate), in humans with parasitic infections.
Possible vertigo and ataxia due to antiparasitic, metronidazole, in humans
with parasitic infections.
Dizziness due to antiparasitic, quinacrine (quinacrine hydrochloride), in
humans with parasitic infections.
Tinnitus due to antimalarial, quinine (quinine dihydrochloride) (quinine
sulfate), in humans with parasitic infections.
Possible vertigo and tinnitus due to antiparasitic, thiabendazole, in humans
with parasitic infections.
Possible tinnitus due to antiparasitic, tryparsamide, in humans with parasitic infections.
   (AD) Discussion of clinical use and toxic effects of drugs used for parasitic infections. (ENG)

653
Possible   ototoxic effects due to antibiotic, kanamycin, in humans with acute
genitourinary system infections.
Possible ototoxic effects due to antibiotic, gentamicin, in humans with acute
genitourinary system infections.
   (AD)   Need for careful consideration in use of kanamycin and gentamicin in
   therapy, in particular in patients with kidney disorders.   (ENG)

656
Possible   permanent severe damage to eighth cranial nerve, primarily vestibular problems but also hearing loss, due to parenteral administration of
antibiotic, streptomycin, in humans with tuberculosis, in particular with
concurrent kidney disorder.
Possible permanent severe damage to eighth cranial nerve due to parenteral
administration of antibiotic, viomycin, in humans with tuberculosis.
Possible permanent severe   damage to eighth cranial nerve due to parenteral
administration of antibiotic, kanamycin, in humans with tuberculosis.
Possible permanent severe   damage to eighth cranial nerve due to parenteral
administration of antibiotic, capreomycin, in humans with tuberculosis.
   (AD) Discussion of primary and secondary drugs used in treatment of tuberculosis. (ENG)

666
Permanent severe and possibly delayed and progressive hearing loss and vestibular problems due to parenteral administration of antibiotic, kanamycin, in
humans, in particular with severe kidney disorders.
Permanent severe and possibly delayed and progressive hearing loss and vestibular problems due to parenteral administration of antibiotic, neomycin, in
humans, in particular with severe kidney disorders.
   (AD) Cochleo-vestibulotoxic effects of kanamycin and neomycin usually dose
   related but occur also after low doses.
   (AD) Higher risk of ototoxic effects due to kanamycin and neomycin in
   older patients.
   (AD) Need for audiometry 2 times a week with administration of antibiotics
   for more than 7 days.
   (AD) Recommended adult dose of 1.5 g daily for not more than 1 week and
   lower doses in patients with kidney disorder and dehydration.
   (AD) Suggested use of kanamycin and neomycin for only severe infections.
   (AD) Kanamycin reported less toxic than neomycin.
Hearing loss due to oral administration of antibiotic, neomycin, in humans.
   (ENG)

670
Possible   vestibular problems due to parenteral administration of antibiotic,
gentamicin, in humans.
Damage to eighth cranial nerve, primarily hearing loss, usually permanent,
due to parenteral administration of high doses of antibiotic, kanamycin, for
more than 10 days in humans, in particular with kidney disorders.
Damage to eighth cranial nerve, primarily hearing loss, usually permanent,
due to parenteral administration of high doses of antibiotic, neomycin, for
more than 10 days in humans, in particular with kidney disorders.
Possible damage to eighth cranial nerve, primarily hearing loss, due to
parenteral administration of antibiotic, paromomycin, in humans.
Transient or permanent vestibular problems due to parenteral administration
of antibiotic, streptomycin, in humans.
Permanent severe hearing loss due to parenteral administration of antibiotic,
dihydrostreptomycin, in humans.
Damage to eighth cranial nerve, primarily hearing loss, due to parenteral
administration of high doses of antibiotic, vancomycin, for more than 10 days
in humans, in particular with kidney disorders.
Damage to eighth cranial nerve, vestibular problems and hearing loss, due to
parenteral administration of high doses of antibiotic, viomycin, for more
than 10 days in humans, in particular with kidney disorders.
   (AD) Discussion of toxic effects of antibiotics.   (ENG)

672
Possible sensorineural hearing loss due to parenteral administration of
antibiotic, kanamycin, in humans with kidney disorders.
   (AD) Need for decr in dosage and 3 to 4 days interval between doses in

patients with kidney disorders.
Possible vestibular problems and hearing loss due to parenteral administration of antibiotic, streptomycin, in humans with kidney disorders.
   (AD) Need for decr in dosage and 3 to 4 days interval between doses in patients with kidney disorders.
Possible vestibular problems due to parenteral administration of antibiotic, gentamicin, in humans with kidney disorders.
   (AD) Need for decr in dosage and unknown period between doses in patients with kidney disorders.
Possible hearing loss due to parenteral administration of antibiotic, vancomycin, in humans with kidney disorders.
   (AD) Need for decr in dosage and 9 days interval between doses in patients with kidney disorders.
   (AD) Report on use of antibiotics in patients with kidney disorders.
   (AD) Need for total initial dose followed by 50 percent of initial dose at recommended intervals.
   (AD) Change in dosage based on serum half-life of antibiotic.
   (AD) Literature review of effect of antibiotics in patients with kidney disorders. (ENG)

676

Vestibular problems due to antibiotic, streptomycin, in humans.
   (AD) Ototoxic effects of streptomycin particularly with high doses, long period of treatment, concurrent kidney disorders, and in older patients.
Hearing loss due to antibiotic, dihydrostreptomycin, in humans.
Hearing loss due to antibiotic, viomycin, in humans.
   (AD) Discussion of toxic effects of various antibiotics.
   (AD) Comment that effect of some inhibitors on ototoxicity not known definitely. (FR)

694

Vertigo and tinnitus due to oral administration in 3 tablets of 750 mg daily of anti-inflammatory agent, (SQ) monophenylbutazone, for 5 days in 1 of 10 humans, male, with rheumatoid arthritis.
Previous oral administration in 3 tablets of 840 mg daily of salicylate, (SQ) acetylsalicylic acid, for 2 weeks in 1 of 10 humans, male, with rheumatoid arthritis. (ENG)

698

Hearing loss, after 3 months in most cases, due to parenteral administration of 0.5 g twice daily for 7 days a week of antibiotic, kanamycin, in 29 (39 percent) of 75 humans with pulmonary tuberculosis.
Damage to eighth cranial nerve due to parenteral administration of 1 g twice daily for 2 days a week of antibiotic, kanamycin, for more than 12 months in 5 (7 percent) of 64 humans with pulmonary tuberculosis.
   (AD) Low incidence of ototoxic effects reported in study possibly due to administration of kanamycin only 2 days a week.
Damage to eighth cranial nerve due to parenteral administration of 15 mg per kg daily of antibiotic, kanamycin, in 4 (6 percent) of 65 humans with pulmonary tuberculosis and with previous hearing loss.
Hearing loss due to parenteral administration of 15 to 20 mg per kg for 5 days a week of antibiotic, (SQ) kanamycin, in 19 (22 percent) of 82 humans with pulmonary tuberculosis and with previous hearing loss in 10 cases.
   (AD) Hearing loss confirmed by audiometry.
   (AD) Ototoxic effects in patients 50 years or over age in 15 of 19 cases.
Previous administration of antibiotic, (SQ) streptomycin, for long period in 82 humans with pulmonary tuberculosis.
Previous administration of antibiotic, (SQ) viomycin, in 10 of 82 humans with pulmonary tuberculosis.
   (AD) Discussion of ototoxic effects of kanamycin reported in 4 studies.
   (AD) Significant factors in kanamycin ototoxicity reported to be age over 50 years, high daily dose of more than 20 mg per kg, high serum level of more than 25 mcg per ml, concurrent kidney disorders, and previous hearing loss. (ENG)

706

Ototoxic effects due to chemical agents and heavy metals in humans.
   (AD) Literature review of ototoxic effects of nicotine, carbon monoxide,

carbon tetrachloride, mercury, arsenic, and lead.
Cochleo-vestibulotoxic effects, functional and structural, due to antibiotics in humans.
   (AD) Literature review of ototoxicity of streptomycin, dihydrostreptomycin, neomycin, kanamycin, gentamicin, capreomycin, rifampicin, viomycin, isoniazid, aminosidine, and framycetin.
Hearing loss due to salicylates in humans.
Hearing loss due to antimalarial, quinine, in humans.
Hearing loss due to diuretic, ethacrynic acid, in humans.
   (AD) Literature review of effects of various ototoxic agents. (IT)

708

Vertigo due to oral administration in capsules of 75 mg in 2 capsules 3 times daily of anti-inflammatory agent, indomethacin, in 2 of 18 humans during treatment for arthritis.
Vertigo due to oral administration in capsules of 75 mg in 2 capsules 3 times daily of anti-inflammatory agent, indomethacin, for 4 weeks in 1 of 7 humans after treatment for arthritis.
Vertigo due to oral administration in capsules of 1500 mg daily in 2 capsules 3 times daily of anti-inflammatory agent, mefenamic acid, for 4 weeks in 1 of 39 humans after treatment for arthritis. (ENG)

731

Possible damage to eighth cranial nerve, vestibular problems, due to antibiotic, streptomycin, in humans with gram-negative bacilli.
Possible damage to eighth cranial nerve, hearing loss, due to antibiotic, kanamycin, in humans with gram-negative bacilli.
Possible damage to eighth cranial nerve, hearing loss, due to antibiotic, neomycin, in humans with gram-negative bacilli.
Possible damage to eighth cranial nerve, vestibular problems, due to antibiotic, gentamicin, in humans with gram-negative bacilli.
Possible ototoxic effects due to antibiotic, vancomycin, in humans with gram-positive cocci.
   (AD) Need to decr dosage of antibiotics in patients with kidney disorders.
   (AD) Discussion of possible toxic effects of antibiotics used in surgery. (ENG)

Fetus, Newborn infant, Infant

410

Damage to organ of Corti of fetus due to antibiotics in humans, female, during pregnancy.
   (AD) Discussion of etiology of damage to organ of Corti in fetus. (FR)

128

Transient tinnitus due to oral administration of 2 tablets every 4 hours or more frequently, to produce serum salicylate level of 92 mg per 100 ml, of salicylate, aspirin, for about 6 days in 1 human, Caucasian, adolescent, 14 years age, female, self treatment for upper respiratory system infection.
Tinnitus and dizziness due to oral administration of about 5 bottles of 100 tablets each, to produce serum salicylate levels of 72 mg per 100 ml after 3 to 4 hours, 59 mg per 100 ml after 6 to 7 hours, 150 mg per 100 ml after 14 to 15 hours, of salicylate, aspirin, in 1 dose in 1 human, Caucasian, adult, 19 years age, female, suicide.
Loss of equilibrium due to oral administration of 62.5 mg per teaspoon of colic medicine of salicylate in 1 human, Caucasian, infant, 3 months age, male, with colic.
   (AD) Low serum salicylate level in infant.
   (AD) Discussion of 3 case reports of salicylate ototoxicity. (ENG)

732

Hearing loss and total degeneration of organ of Corti and moderate degeneration of spiral ganglion and nerve process in fetus due to oral ingestion of 250 mg daily of antimalarial, chloroquine (chloroquine phosphate), in humans, female, during pregnancy.
   (AD) Histopathological study of inner ear after death. (ENG)

383

Nystagmus and cochlear impairment due to high doses of anticonvulsant, di-
phenylhydantoin, in humans, infant and child.
   (AD) Literature review of toxic risks of antibiotics and other drugs.
   (GER)

580

No observed ototoxic effects in follow up study of 10 months due to parenteral, intramuscular, administration of 4 or 5 mg per kg daily in 2 equal
doses at 12 hour intervals, to produce blood levels of 4.9 mcg per ml or
less, of antibiotic, gentamicin, for 1 to 31 days in 16 humans, newborn
infant, 0 to 22 days age, less than 2500 g weight in 8 patients, with infections.
No observed ototoxic effects due to parenteral, intravenous and intraventricular, administration of 1.6 mg per kg of antibiotic, gentamicin, in 1 human,
newborn infant, low birth weight, with infection.
   (AD) Responses of newborn infants to sound monitored. (ENG)

581

No hearing loss detected due to parenteral, intrathecal (SM), administration
of 1 mg daily of antibiotic, gentamicin, in 13 humans, infant.
No hearing loss detected due to parenteral, intramuscular (SM), administration of 2 mg per kg daily of antibiotic, gentamicin, in 13 humans, infant.
   (AD) Evaluation of cochlear function difficult in infants but no hearing
   loss detected after gentamicin therapy. (ENG)

583

No observed ototoxic effects but possible damage to inner ear due to parenteral, intramuscular, administration of 3.0 or 5.0 mg per kg daily, to produce serum levels as high as 7.8 mcg per ml, of antibiotic, gentamicin, for 6
to 7 days in 45 humans, newborn infant, 1.4 to 21 days average age, low birth
weight, with infections.
   (AD) Measurement of blood levels at 0.5, 1, 4, 8, and 12 hours after first
   injection and on third day.
   (AD) Follow up studies with audiology planned to determine if ototoxic
   effects resulted from gentamicin therapy. (ENG)

584

No observed ototoxic effects due to parenteral, intramuscular, administration
of 2.5 mg per kg every 12 hours or 1.7 mg per kg every 8 hours, daily total
of 5 mg per kg, to produce blood levels of 6 mcg per ml or less, of antibiotic, gentamicin, for 10 days in 60 humans, infant, male and female, with
genitourinary system infections.
   (AD) Determination of blood levels at 1, 2, 4, and 8 hours after first
   injection and at 12 hours in group with administration of gentamicin every
   12 hours.
   (AD) Blood levels higher and for longer duration in group with administration every 12 hours.
   (AD) Follow up studies with audiograms planned to determine if ototoxic
   effects resulted from gentamicin therapy. (ENG)

586

Mild sensorineural hearing loss due to parenteral administration of 4 mg per
kg every 24 hours in 4 divided doses, total doses of 1000 and 7788 mg, of
antibiotic, gentamicin (gentamicin sulfate), for 25 to 138 days in 1 of 10
humans with infection secondary to burns.
   (AD) Audiology in 10 patients with therapy of long duration confirmed
   hearing loss in 1 patient.
No reported ototoxic effects due to parenteral (SM) administration of 4 mg
per kg every 24 hours in 4 divided doses of antibiotic, gentamicin (gentamicin sulfate), for several days to over 30 days in other 85 humans, newborn
infant, infant, child, and adolescent, 0 to 16 years age, with infection
secondary to burns.
Simultaneous topical, direct site (SM), administration in cream of 0.1 percent of antibiotic, gentamicin (gentamicin sulfate), in some of 95 humans,
newborn infant, infant, child, and adolescent, 0 to 16 years age, with infection secondary to burns. (ENG)

651
No vestibular problems due to 4 to 6 mg per kg daily of antibiotic, gentami-
cin, in 100 humans, infant, 3 to 12 months age, with various severe infec-
tions.
   (AD)   Vestibular function tests used to determine vestibulotoxic effects.
   (ENG)

229
Auditory system problems due to parenteral, intramuscular, administration of
high doses of antibiotic, kanamycin, for long period in humans, infant, for
infections.
   (AD)   Recommended kanamycin dosage for infants of 7.5 mg per kg daily in
   divided doses every 12 hours by intramuscular administration for 12 days
   at most.   (ENG)

241
Risk of damage to organ of Corti and hearing loss due to antibiotic, kanamy-
cin, in humans, infant.
   (AD) Study of dose response relationships.
   (AD) Recommended dose of 15 mg per kg daily every 12 hours for infants.
   (ENG)

287
Cochlear impairment in fetus due to antibiotic, kanamycin, in humans, female,
treated during pregnancy.
   (AD)   Discussion of cochleotoxic effects of kanamycin in newborn infants
   and infants.   (JAP)

307
No sensorineural hearing loss due to unspecified method of administration of
5 to 21 mg per kg daily, total doses of 30 to 450 mg, of antibiotic, kanamycin, for 3 to 11 days in 20 humans, infant and child, 1 to 4 years age,
treated when newborn infant for various infections.
   (CT)   Study of 7 children, control group, treated with other antibiotics
   during neonatal period for similar infections.
   (AD)   Use of pure tone audiometry or clinical evaluation only to determine
   hearing loss.
   (AD)   Study to determine cochleotoxic effects of kanamycin when used in
   treatment of newborn infants.   (ENG)

391
Hearing loss in 15 fetuses due to parenteral, intramuscular, administration
of 200 mg per kg daily of antibiotic, kanamycin, for 15 days in animals,
rats, Wistar strain, female, about 150 g weight, during pregnancy.
   (AD) Test of Preyer reflex of rats, newborn infant, 30 days after birth.
No hearing loss due to 20 mg per kg daily of antibiotic, kanamycin, for 1 to
5 days in 15 humans, newborn infant.
   (CT)   EEG in newborn infants, before and about 1 month after kanamycin
   administration.
No hearing loss in fetuses due to antibiotic, kanamycin, in humans, female,
treated for pulmonary tuberculosis during pregnancy.
   (AD)   Follow up study for 3 years after birth showed no hearing loss in
   children.
   (AD) Discussion of clinical and experimental studies on effects of kanamycin.
Hearing loss due to range of 30 to 100 mg per kg daily of antibiotic, kanamycin, for range of 3 to 46 days in 9 of 391 humans, newborn infant.
No hearing loss due to less than 60 mg per kg daily of antibiotic, kanamycin,
for less than 11 days in 382 humans, newborn infant.
   (AD)   Discussion of reports from 100 hospitals in Japan on effects of
   kanamycin in newborn infants.
   (AD)   Relationship between cochleotoxic effects of kanamycin and daily
   dosage and duration of treatment.   (ENG)

617
Hearing loss observed after several years possibly due to high doses, 125 mg
per kg daily, total of 10.75 g, of antibiotic, kanamycin, for total of 43
days in 1 human, child, treated after surgery for congenital intestinal
atresia when newborn infant.

(AD) Hearing loss possibly congenital and not due to kanamycin therapy.
Bilateral hearing loss detected after 8 to 10 years but no subjective symp-
toms due to 100 mg per kg daily of antibiotic, kanamycin, for 8 to 14 days in
1 of 51 humans, child, treated for disorder when infant.
   (AD) Study with audiometry of effects of kanamycin used in treatment of 51
   newborn infants and infants.
   (CT) Study of 43 children, control group, without kanamycin therapy.
   (AD) Suggested that high doses of kanamycin not be used.
   (AD) Suggested that less ototoxic effects due to kanamycin in infants and
   children than in adults. (ENG)

208

Hearing loss due to oral ingestion, in contaminated fish, of heavy metal,
mercury (organic methyl mercury), in humans.
   (AD) Recommended international limit of 0.5 ppm of mercury (organic methyl
   mercury) for humans.
   (AD) Reported high levels of mercury (organic methyl mercury) in fetuses.
   (ENG)

445

No specified ototoxic effects due to topical administration in (SQ) ointment
of sufficient dose, in 10 percent ammoniated ointment, to produce urine level
of 80 mcg per 100 mg of heavy metal, mercury, in 1 human, infant, 11 months
age, male, with skin rash.
Dizziness due to topical route, (SQ) inhalation, of about 0.17 mg per m, for
about 8 hours every night, of vapor concentration, sufficient to produce
urine level of 100 mcg per liter, of heavy metal, mercury, for long period in
1 human, child, 11 years age, male. (ENG)

254

Hearing loss due to antibiotic, neomycin, in humans, infant.
   (AD) Routine use of neomycin for gastroenteritis in infants not recommended. (ENG)

385

Possible hearing loss due to oral administration of antibiotic, neomycin, in
humans, infant, with enteritis.
   (AD) Literature review of possible toxic effects of antibiotics in treatment of enteritis. (GER)

352

Severe hearing loss due to ototoxic drugs in humans, newborn infant.
   (AD) Comment on previous report on ototoxicity in premature infants.
   (AD) Discussion of decr in congenital hearing loss and prelingual hearing
   loss due to ototoxic drugs and other etiologic factors. (ENG)

505

Congenital hearing loss due to ototoxic drugs in humans, newborn infant.
   (AD) Discussion of etiology of congenital hearing loss. (ENG)

717

Hearing loss in fetus due to ototoxic drugs in humans treated during pregnancy.
   (AD) Discussion of etiology of hearing loss in risk children. (GER)

388

Hearing loss in 2 fetuses, twin, male, due to oral ingestion of high doses of
antimalarial, quinine, for unspecified period in 1 human, female, at end of
first trimester of pregnancy to induce abortion.
   (AD) No visual perception defect in twins due to ingestion of quinine by
   mother during pregnancy.
   (AD) Suggested vascular or neural mechanism of ototoxic effects of
   quinine. (ENG)

067

High frequency hearing loss in 11.4 percent of fetuses due to 10 g to more
than 100 g of antibiotic, streptomycin, in 44 humans, female, treated for
tuberculosis during pregnancy.

(AD) Hearing loss confirmed by audiogram.
(AD) Damage most often due to streptomycin treatment during first trimester.   (GER)

490

No hearing loss due to average dose of 36.8 mg per kg daily, average total
dose of 118.9 mg per kg, of antibiotic, streptomycin (streptomycin sulfate),
for short period, average of 3.2 days, in 98 humans, child, 7 and 8 years
age, female and male, treated when newborn infants.
   (AD) Follow up study with audiometry of children treated in neonatal
   period with streptomycin.
   (CT) Study of 102 children, control group, not treated in neonatal period
   with ototoxic drugs.
   (AD) Sensorineural hearing loss detected in 3 of 98 children treated with
   streptomycin not attributed to antibiotic. (ENG)

500

Sensorineural hearing loss due to antibiotic, streptomycin, in humans, newborn infant.
   (AD) Discussion of etiology of hearing loss in children. (ENG)

542

Deaf-mutism in fetus due to antibiotic, streptomycin, in human, female,
treated during pregnancy.
   (AD) Case report of congenital hearing loss due to streptomycin therapy in
   mother during pregnancy. (ENG)

661

Hearing loss in fetus due to sedative, thalidomide, in humans, female,
treated during pregnancy. (GER)

695

Hearing loss in fetus due to sedative, thalidomide, in humans, female,
treated during pregnancy.
   (AD) Congenital hearing loss in 5 of 34 humans, child, of mothers treated
   with thalidomide during pregnancy. (ENG)

012

Permanent sensorineural hearing loss due to parenteral, intramuscular, administration of high doses, about 100 mg per kg daily, total of more than 6 g
of antibiotic, (SQ) neomycin (neomycin sulfate), for 7 days in 1 human,
Caucasian, infant, 13 months age.
Unspecified effects due to parenteral, intramuscular, administration of about
12 mg per kg daily recommended dosage, total of 20 mg, of antibiotic, (SQ)
kanamycin (kanamycin sulfate), for less than 24 hours in 1 human, Caucasian,
infant, 13 months age.
   (CT) Normal response to acoustic stimulus before administration of antibiotics.
   (AD) Suggested that ototoxicity of neomycin not potentiated by administration of kanamycin in this case. (ENG)

019

Progressive severe sensorineural hearing loss and tinnitus due to unspecified
method of administration of 0.5 g twice daily, total of 16 g, of antibiotic,
kanamycin, for 16 days in 1 human, Caucasian, adult, 25 years age, male, with
kidney disorder and treated with peritoneal dialysis.
   (AD) Audiograms showed hearing loss and recruitment test showed reversed
   recruitment.
Severe sensorineural hearing loss due to unspecified method of administration
of 0.5 g daily for 40 days and then 0.5 g 3 times a week for 3 weeks of
antibiotic, streptomycin, for total period of about 9 weeks in 1 human,
Negro, child, 9 years age, male, with pulmonary tuberculosis and kidney
disorder.
   (AD) No record of hearing loss before treatment with streptomycin.
Delayed severe bilateral high frequency hearing loss due to unspecified
method of administration of 0.5 g daily for 8 months and then 0.5 g every 3
days for 4 months, followed by a break of 3.5 months, and then 0.5 g every 3
days for 1.5 months, total of 153 g of antibiotic, dihydrostreptomycin, for

total period of about 13.5 months in 1 human, Negro, infant, 16 months age, female, with tuberculosis.

(AD) Hearing loss detected at 13 years age.

Hearing loss and tinnitus due to unspecified method of administration of 1 g daily of antibiotic, streptomycin, for 10 weeks and possibly for a longer period after discharge in 1 human, Negro, adult, 23 years age, male, treated for infection in tuberculosis hospital.

(AD) Hearing loss detected 1 month after treatment with streptomycin.

Progressive severe sensorineural hearing loss due to unspecified method of administration of 0.5 g 3 times a week, total of 61 g of antibiotic, streptomycin, for about 10 months in 1 human, Negro, child, 9 years age, female, with pulmonary tuberculosis.

(AD) Discussion of 5 case reports. (ENG)

087

High frequency hearing loss and tinnitus due to antibiotics in humans, particularly infant and aged, and humans with kidney disorder.

Degeneration in hair cells of organ of Corti due to antibiotics in humans.

Vertigo and unsteady gait due to antibiotic, streptomycin, in humans.

Bilateral damage to vestibular apparatus due to antibiotic, streptomycin, in humans.

(AD) Literature review of physiological and structural cochleo-vestibulo-toxic effects of antibiotics.

(AD) Degree of damage determined by dosage and duration of dosage of antibiotics. (ENG)

088

Ototoxic effects in fetus due to unspecified method of administration of unspecified doses of antibiotic, streptomycin, for long period in humans, female, treated for tuberculosis during pregnancy.

Ototoxic effects in fetus due to unspecified method of administration of unspecified doses of antibiotic, dihydrostreptomycin, for long period in humans, female, treated for tuberculosis during pregnancy. (ENG)

116

Moderate unilateral sensorineural hearing loss in 1 of 36 fetuses due to total of 13 g of antibiotic, dihydrostreptomycin, in 33 humans, female, treated during pregnancy for tuberculosis.

(AD) Child not treated with dihydrostreptomycin or streptomycin.

Sensorineural hearing loss due to 1 g daily for the first 30 days and then 1 g twice a week of antibiotic, dihydrostreptomycin (CB), in 8 (24 percent) of 33 humans, female, treated during pregnancy for tuberculosis.

Sensorineural hearing loss due to 1 g daily for the first 30 days and then 1 g twice a week of antibiotic, streptomycin (CB), in 8 (24 percent) of 33 humans, female, treated during pregnancy for tuberculosis.

Vestibular problems due to antibiotic, (SQ) dihydrostreptomycin, in 1 of 33 humans, female, treated during pregnancy for tuberculosis and chronic pyelonephritis.

Vestibular problems due to antibiotic, (SQ) streptomycin, in 1 of 33 humans, female, treated during pregnancy for tuberculosis and chronic pyelonephritis.

(AD) Case histories, audiometry, and vestibular function tests for children and adults. (ENG)

156

Sensorineural hearing loss due to unspecified method of administration of high doses of antibiotic, streptomycin (SM), in 7 humans, infant and child, with tuberculous meningitis.

Simultaneous administration of unspecified doses of antituberculous agent, PAS (SM), in 7 humans, infant and child, with tuberculous meningitis.

Simultaneous administration of unspecified doses of antituberculous agent, isoniazid (SM), in 7 humans, infant and child, with tuberculous meningitis.

Sensorineural hearing loss due to unspecified method of administration of high doses of antibiotic, viomycin, in 7 humans, infant and child, with tuberculous meningitis.

(AD) Cochleotoxic effect due to antibiotic therapy or infection. (ENG)

164

Ototoxic effects not determined due to parenteral, intramuscular and intra-

thecal, administration of 1.5 mg per kg every 8 to 12 hours, to produce peak
serum levels of 2.5 to 5.0 mcg per ml, of antibiotic, (SQ) gentamicin, for 9
to 13 days in 5 humans, newborn infant, with infections.
Ototoxic effects not determined due to parenteral, intramuscular, administration of 7.5 mg per kg every 12 hours of antibiotic, (SQ) kanamycin, for 7 to
17 days in 3 of 5 humans, newborn infant, with infections.
  (AD) No follow up studies of gentamicin over long period to determine
  ototoxic effects.
  (AD) Need for audiometry and vestibular function tests after several
  months to determine ototoxic effects.
  (AD) Study of clinical pharmacology of gentamicin. (ENG)

188
Possible hearing loss due to antibiotics in humans, child, treated when
newborn infant.
  (AD) Reported that 23 percent of 46 children with idiopathic hearing loss
  treated with antibiotics in neonatal period.
  (CT) Reported that 2 percent of 54 children with normal hearing treated
  with antibiotics in neonatal period.
Possible hearing loss in fetus due to salicylate, aspirin, in humans, female,
during pregnancy.
  (AD) Ingestion of salicylate, aspirin, during pregnancy by mothers of 2
  percent of total of 118 children with hearing loss.
  (CT) Ingestion of salicylate, aspirin, during pregnancy by mothers of 0 of
  54 children with normal hearing.
  (AD) Study of etiology of hearing loss in children. (ENG)

236
Bilateral high frequency hearing loss due to parenteral, intramuscular,
administration of high dose, 90 mg per kg daily, total of 99.2 g, of antibiotic, kanamycin, for 62 days in 1 human, child, with miliary tuberculosis.
High frequency hearing loss due to parenteral, intramuscular, administration
of high dose, 25 mg per kg daily, total of 22.2 g, of antibiotic, kanamycin,
for 148 days in 1 human, child, with miliary tuberculosis.
Permanent severe sensorineural hearing loss due to parenteral, intramuscular,
administration of high doses of antibiotic, kanamycin, in 1 human, child,
with multiple infections.
Progressive sensorineural hearing loss due to oral administration of antibiotic, neomycin, for 11 months in 1 human, child, 11.5 years age, male, with
severe ulcerative ileocolitis.
  (AD) Hearing loss confirmed by audiogram.
  (AD) Discussion of 4 case reports of ototoxic effects due to kanamycin or
  neomycin.
  (AD) Suggested that risk of kanamycin ototoxicity less in children than in
  adults.
Sensorineural hearing loss due to 10 to 100 mg per kg daily of antibiotic,
kanamycin, for 5 to 95 days in 5 of 30 humans, child and infant, with infections.
  (CT) Study of 30 children and infants, control group, not treated with
  kanamycin.
  (AD) Suggested that cochleotoxic effects related to total dose of kanamycin.
  (AD) Report on studies made during 8 years of clinical use of kanamycin.
  (ENG)

237
Hearing loss due to parenteral, intramuscular, administration of 15 mg per kg
daily of antibiotic, kanamycin, for 6 to 10 days in 5.1 percent of 143 humans, child, treated when newborn infant for infection.
Hearing loss due to parenteral, intramuscular, administration of 40 mg per kg
daily of antibiotic, streptomycin, for 6 to 12 days in 5.6 percent of 93
humans, child, treated when newborn infant for infection.
  (CT) Hearing loss in 4.4 percent of 170 children, control group, without
  antibiotic therapy.
  (AD) Hearing loss confirmed by audiogram.
  (AD) Suggested low kanamycin ototoxicity in newborn infants with use of
  recommended dosage. (ENG)

Vestibular problems due to antibiotic, streptomycin, in humans.
Severe cochlear impairment due to antibiotic, dihydrostreptomycin, in humans.
Loss of hair cells in organ of Corti and hearing loss due to antibiotics, aminoglycoside, in humans.
Hearing loss in fetus due to antimalarial, quinine, in humans, female, treated during pregnancy.
Transient hearing loss due to high doses of salicylate, aspirin, for long period in humans.
  (AD) Discussion of possible cochleo-vestibulotoxic effects of ototoxic drugs.
  (AD) Ototoxic effects related to concurrent disorders, dosage, duration of treatment, and age of individuals. (ENG)

Hearing loss due to antibiotic, streptomycin, in 120 of 150 humans, child, 2 to 4 years age, most treated when newborn infant or infant for different disorders.
Hearing loss due to antibiotic, streptomycin (SM), in 30 of 150 humans, child, 2 to 4 years age, most treated when newborn infant or infant for different disorders.
Hearing loss due to antibiotic, neomycin (SM), in 30 of 150 humans, child, 2 to 4 years age, most treated when newborn infant or infant for different disorders.
Hearing loss due to other antibiotics (SM) in 30 of 150 humans, child, 2 to 4 years age, most treated when newborn infant or infant for different disorders.
  (AD) Hearing loss determined by play audiometry.
  (AD) No relationship between hearing loss and dosage or duration of treatment with antibiotics.
  (AD) No improvement in hearing after 1 to 2 years. (RUS)

No hearing loss but tinnitus due to parenteral, intramuscular, administration of range of 0.05 to 1.0 g daily according to age of antibiotic, kanamycin, for short period in 4 of 125 humans, infant, child, and adult, with acute otorhinolaryngological infections.
  (AD) Audiograms showed no hearing loss.
Hearing loss, subjective in 1 case and latent in others, but no vestibular problems due to 1.0 g daily 2 times a week of antibiotic, (SQ) kanamycin, for long period in 15 of 66 humans, adolescent and adult, 15 to 55 years age, with pulmonary tuberculosis and with previous streptomycin treatment.
  (CT) Audiogram before and during treatment with kanamycin.
Hearing loss due to previous administration of antibiotic, (SQ) streptomycin, in 31 of 272 humans.
Sensorineural hearing loss due to previous administration of total of 600 g of antibiotic, (SQ) streptomycin, in 1 human, adult, 27 years age.
More severe sensorineural hearing loss, subjective, due to total of 136 g of antibiotic, (SQ) kanamycin, in 1 human, adult, 27 years age.
  (AD) Case report of hearing loss due to streptomycin potentiated by treatment with kanamycin.
Hearing loss, latent, and tinnitus, but no vestibular problems due to total of over 20 g to over 300 g of antibiotic, kanamycin, for long period in 10 of 70 humans with pulmonary tuberculosis and no previous chemotherapy.
  (CT) Audiogram before and during treatment with kanamycin.
  (AD) Clinical studies of effects of treatment with kanamycin for short and long periods.
Vestibular problems after 10 to 12 days due to parenteral administration of 100 mg per kg daily of antibiotic, streptomycin, in 3 animals, cats, 2 kg weight.
Slight vestibular problems after 30 days due to 300 mg per kg daily of antibiotic, kanamycin, in 3 animals, cats, 2 kg weight.
Decr in cochlear microphonic due to 200 mg per kg daily of antibiotic, streptomycin, in 11 injections in animals, cats.
Slight decr in cochlear microphonic due to 300 mg per kg daily of antibiotic, kanamycin, in 11 to 60 injections in animals, cats.
  (AD) Comparative experimental studies of cochleo-vestibulotoxic effects of kanamycin and streptomycin in cats.

(AD) Different effects of 2 aminoglycoside antibiotics on vestibular
function but similar effects on cochlear function.   (ENG)

434

Slight ototoxic effects due to range of doses of antibiotic, streptomycin, in
8 of 40 humans, female, treated for tuberculosis during pregnancy.
Slight ototoxic effects due to range of doses of antibiotic, dihydrostreptomycin, in 2 of 40 humans, female, treated for tuberculosis during pregnancy.
Vestibular problems and sensorineural hearing loss in mother and vestibular
problems in fetus due to total of 27 g of antibiotic, streptomycin (CB), for
2.5 months in 1 human, adult, 28 years age, female, treated for pulmonary
tuberculosis at end of pregnancy.
Vestibular problems and sensorineural hearing loss in mother and vestibular
problems in fetus due to total of 27 g of antibiotic, dihydrostreptomycin
(CB), for 2.5 months in 1 human, adult, 28 years age, female, treated for
pulmonary tuberculosis at end of pregnancy.
   (AD) Pure tone audiometry and vestibular function tests in child, female,
at 10 years age.
Mixed hearing loss in mother and severe sensorineural hearing loss and vestibular problems in fetus due to total of 28 g of antibiotic, (SQ) dihydrostreptomycin, for 2.5 months in 1 human, adult, 22 years age, female, treated for
tuberculosis at beginning of pregnancy.
Mixed hearing loss in mother and severe sensorineural hearing loss and vestibular problems in fetus due to total of 28 g of antibiotic, (SQ) streptomycin, for 2.5 months in 1 human, adult, 22 years age, female, treated for
tuberculosis at beginning of pregnancy.
   (AD) Pure tone audiometry and vestibular function tests in child, female,
at 10 years age. (ENG)

589

Dizziness during or after 5 or 6 injections but no evidence of hearing loss
due to parenteral, intramuscular and then intravenous (SM), administration of
7 mg per kg total daily, not exceeding 180 mg total dose every 24 hours, of
antibiotic, (SQ) gentamicin, for as long as 30 days in 5 of 80 humans, infant, child, and adult, 8 months to 36 years age, with cystic fibrosis and
severe pulmonary infection.
   (AD) Audiology in 40 of 80 patients showed no evidence of hearing loss.
   (AD) Dizziness possibly due to rapid administration of gentamicin.
High frequency hearing loss before gentamicin therapy possibly due to previous administration of (SQ) ototoxic drugs in some of 80 humans, infant,
child, and adult, 8 months to 36 years age, with cystic fibrosis and severe
pulmonary infection.
Dizziness due to topical administration by inhalation (SM) of 16 to 20 mg up
to 4 times a day, in 2 ml of 0.125 percent phenylephrine hydrochloride and
propylene glycol, of antibiotic, (SQ) gentamicin (CB), in some of 80 humans,
infant, child, and adult, 8 months to 36 years age, with cystic fibrosis and
severe pulmonary infection.
Dizziness due to topical administration by inhalation (SM) of 16 to 20 mg up
to 4 times a day, in 2 ml of 0.125 percent phenylephrine hydrochloride and
propylene glycol, of antibiotic, (SQ) neomycin (CB), in some of 80 humans,
infant, child, and adult, 8 months to 36 years age, with cystic fibrosis and
severe pulmonary infection.   (ENG)

Child, Adolescent

128

Transient tinnitus due to oral administration of 2 tablets every 4 hours or
more frequently, to produce serum salicylate level of 92 mg per 100 ml, of
salicylate, aspirin, for about 6 days in 1 human, Caucasian, adolescent, 14
years age, female, self treatment for upper respiratory system infection.
Tinnitus and dizziness due to oral administration of about 5 bottles of 100
tablets each, to produce serum salicylate levels of 72 mg per 100 ml after 3
to 4 hours, 59 mg per 100 ml after 6 to 7 hours, 150 mg per 100 ml after 14
to 15 hours, of salicylate, aspirin, in 1 dose in 1 human, Caucasian, adult,
19 years age, female, suicide.
Loss of equilibrium due to oral administration of 62.5 mg per teaspoon of
colic medicine of salicylate in 1 human, Caucasian, infant, 3 months age,

male, with colic.
   (AD) Low serum salicylate level in infant.
   (AD) Discussion of 3 case reports of salicylate ototoxicity. (ENG)

                                                                    649
Transient tinnitus, hearing loss, or dizziness due to oral administration in
tablets of 1.4 g, in 4 tablets, in 3 initial doses at 7 hour intervals and
then daily, to produce high serum levels of 20.5 to 28.0 mg per 100 ml, of
salicylate, aspirin, for 2 to 3 weeks in 9 of 20 humans, adolescent, adult,
and aged, 15 to 70 years age, female and male, with bone and joint disorders.
   (AD) Report on use of new sustained release aspirin in treatment of bone
   and joint disorders. (ENG)

                                                                    220
Significant effect on auditory time perception due to parenteral administration of 0.75 cc, in 500 cc normal saline, of 95 percent solution of sedative,
alcohol, ethyl, in humans, adolescent and adult, 18 to 38 years age, male and
female.
   (CT) Same method using 500 cc of normal saline in subjects, control group.
   (ENG)

                                                                    032
Progressive permanent sensorineural hearing loss due to topical administration of unspecified doses of antibiotics for long period in 1 human, child, 6
years age, female, with severe burns on 80 percent of body. (ENG)

                                                                    099
Hearing loss due to antibiotics in humans, adult and child, male and female,
with kidney disorder. (HUN)

                                                                    202
Risk of cochleo-vestibulotoxic effects due to antibiotics, aminoglycoside, in
humans, child, treated for tuberculosis and in particular with kidney disor-
ders.
   (AD) Good prognosis for vestibular problems in children.
   (AD) Need for early detection of hearing loss in children.
   (AD) Comment on maximum doses of antibiotics. (FR)

                                                                    521
Hearing loss due to antibiotics in humans, child, with infections.
   (AD) Analysis of ototoxic effects due to antibiotics. (RUS)

                                                                    224
Slight sensorineural hearing loss due to topical route, inhalation, of large
amount, to produce high carboxyhemoglobin level of 36 percent 1.5 days after
exposure, of chemical agent, carbon monoxide, in 1 human, adult, 21 years
age, male.
Moderate bilateral sensorineural hearing loss due to topical route, inhalation, of large amount, to produce high carboxyhemoglobin level of 48 percent
1.5 days after exposure, of chemical agent, carbon monoxide, in 1 human,
adolescent, 18 years age, male. (ENG)

                                                                    551
Sensorineural hearing loss due to parenteral administration of range of
doses, 3, 15, 25, and 40 g, of antibiotic, dihydrostreptomycin, in humans,
adult and child, range of ages, male and female, in 4 families.
   (AD) Study of familial incidence of dihydrostreptomycin hearing loss and
   hereditary susceptibility of cochlea.
   (AD) Suggested that administration of dihydrostreptomycin in humans with
   hereditary susceptibility of cochlea results in hearing loss. (ENG)

                                                                    383
Nystagmus and cochlear impairment due to high doses of anticonvulsant, di-
phenylhydantoin, in humans, infant and child.
   (AD) Literature review of toxic risks of antibiotics and other drugs.
   (GER)

Possible ataxia due to high doses to produce blood level of 3 mg per 100 ml
or more of anticonvulsant, diphenylhydantoin, in humans, child and adult,
with epilepsy.
Possible nystagmus due to doses to produce blood level of more than 2 mg per
100 ml of anticonvulsant, diphenylhydantoin, in humans, child and adult, with
epilepsy. (ENG)

671

Nystagmus due to anticonvulsant, diphenylhydantoin, in humans, child and
adult, male and female, with epilepsy. (FIN)

625

No ototoxic effects due to oral administration of range of 40 mg daily to 8
mg twice a day, dosage increased at intervals until maximum diuretic response, of diuretic, furosemide, for range of 1 to over 45 weeks in 14 humans,
adolescent, adult, and aged, 18 to 74 years age, male and female, with kidney
disorder. (ENG)

081

Dizziness, tinnitus, and high frequency hearing loss due to parenteral,
intramuscular, administration of 40 mg daily, total of 1470 mg intermittently, of antibiotic, gentamicin, in 74 days in 1 human, adolescent, 15 years
age, male, with kidney disorder.
    (AD) Hearing loss confirmed by audiogram.
    (AD) Loss of hair and visual perception defect due to gentamicin treat-
    ment. (ENG)

431

No vestibular problems or hearing loss due to parenteral, intravenous, administration for 30 to 45 minutes of high doses, 4 to 5 mg per kg daily,
diluted in 30 to 50 cc of sterile water, to produce blood levels of 6.25 mcg
per ml or less, of antibiotic, gentamicin (gentamicin sulfate), for total of
20 days in 1 human, adolescent, 13 years age, with cystic fibrosis.
No vestibular problems or hearing loss due to parenteral, intravenous, administration for 30 to 45 minutes of high doses, 4 to 5 mg per kg daily,
diluted in 30 to 50 cc of sterile water, to produce blood levels of 6.25 mcg
per ml or less of antibiotic, gentamicin (SM) (gentamicin sulfate), for range
of 2 to 13 days in 4 humans, adolescent and child, 2 to 13 years age, with
cystic fibrosis.
Simultaneous parenteral, intravenous, administration of high doses, 100 to
600 mg per kg every 4 hours, of antibiotic, carbenicillin (SM) (disodium
carbenicillin), for range of 2 to 19 days in 4 humans, adolescent and child,
2 to 13 years age, with cystic fibrosis.
    (CT) Audiograms and vestibular function tests before and after treatment
    with gentamicin.
    (AD) Comment on high doses of gentamicin without toxicity. (ENG)

451

No eighth cranial nerve toxicity due to 80 mg every 6 or 8 hours, and lower
dosage in humans with kidney disorder, to produce serum levels of 5 to 8 mcg
per ml of antibiotic, gentamicin, in 104 humans, adult, aged, and child, 2 to
80 years age, with various infections.
    (AD) Suggested that prevention of ototoxicity due to daily assays of serum
    levels. (ENG)

578

No clinical evidence of ototoxic effects due to high doses, 3 to 6 mg per kg
daily, of antibiotic, gentamicin, in 53 humans, child, adolescent, adult, and
aged, 10 to 84 years age, male and female, with bacteremia due to gram-negative bacilli and with kidney disorder in 14 cases.
    (AD) Monitored for clinical symptoms of ototoxic effects.
    (AD) No audiology or vestibular function tests to determine ototoxic
    effects. (ENG)

579

No clinical evidence of ototoxic effects due to parenteral, intravenous,
administration of 1.5 to 6 mg per kg daily, average of 3 mg per kg daily, of
antibiotic, gentamicin, for as long as 36 days in 25 humans, child and adole-

scent, 2.5 to 15 years age, with acute leukemia and infections.
   (AD) No audiology or vestibular function tests used to determine ototoxic
   effects. (ENG)

582

No observed ototoxic effects due to 2 mg per kg daily of antibiotic, gentamicin, for 5 to 10 days in over 100 humans, child, with genitourinary system
infections.
   (AD) Patients observed for evidence of ototoxicity. (ENG)

585

High frequency hearing loss due to parenteral, intramuscular, administration
of 3.0 mg per kg daily or less of antibiotic, (SQ) gentamicin (gentamicin
sulfate), for several days in 1 of 215 humans, child, with genitourinary
system infection.
High frequency hearing loss due to previous administration of (SQ) other
antibiotics in 1 of 215 humans, child, with genitourinary system infection.
   (AD) Clinical evaluation of effect of gentamicin on eighth cranial nerve
   in patients and audiometry and vestibular function tests when indicated.
   (ENG)

586

Mild sensorineural hearing loss due to parenteral administration of 4 mg per
kg every 24 hours in 4 divided doses, total doses of 1000 and 7788 mg, of
antibiotic, gentamicin (gentamicin sulfate), for 25 to 138 days in 1 of 10
humans with infection secondary to burns.
   (AD) Audiology in 10 patients with therapy of long duration confirmed
   hearing loss in 1 patient.
No reported ototoxic effects due to parenteral (SM) administration of 4 mg
per kg every 24 hours in 4 divided doses of antibiotic, gentamicin (gentamicin sulfate), for several days to over 30 days in other 85 humans, newborn
infant, infant, child, and adolescent, 0 to 16 years age, with infection
secondary to burns.
Simultaneous topical, direct site (SM), administration in cream of 0.1 percent of antibiotic, gentamicin (gentamicin sulfate), in some of 95 humans,
newborn infant, infant, child, and adolescent, 0 to 16 years age, with infection secondary to burns. (ENG)

588

No observed ototoxic effects due to parenteral, intramuscular, administration
of range of 1.36 to 7.00 mg per kg daily, in 6 dosage regimens, to produce
blood levels of 10.5 to 18.5 mcg per ml in 8 patients tested, of antibiotic,
gentamicin, for short period in 160 humans, Filipino, adolescent and adult,
15 to 62 years age, male, 78 to 168 lb weight, with venereal disease.
   (AD) Clinical evaluation of vestibular function and cochlear function
   after gentamicin therapy. (ENG)

652

No vestibular problems or hearing loss observed due to parenteral, intravenous, administration of 1 mg per kg initial dose, and then 0.75 mg per kg
every 6 hours, in 200 ml dextrose solution over 2 hour period, of antibiotic,
gentamicin (SM), for 2 weeks minimum or for 5 days after cessation of fever,
whichever longer, in 23 humans, adolescent, adult, and aged, 13 to 68 years
age, with acute leukemia or metastatic cancer and with previous treatment
with other antibiotics in some.
   (AD) No vestibular function tests or audiometry used to determine if
   ototoxic effects.
Simultaneous parenteral, intravenous, administration of 4 g every 4 hours of
antibiotic, carbenicillin (SM), for 2 weeks minimum or for 5 days after
cessation of fever, whichever longer, in 23 humans, adolescent, adult, and
aged, 13 to 68 years age, with acute leukemia or metastatic cancer and with
previous treatment with other antibiotics in some. (ENG)

131

Severe sensorineural hearing loss due to antibiotic, kanamycin, in humans,
adult and child, female and male.
   (AD) Hearing loss confirmed by audiometry. (JAP)

307

No sensorineural hearing loss due to unspecified method of administration of 5 to 21 mg per kg daily, total doses of 30 to 450 mg, of antibiotic, kanamycin, for 3 to 11 days in 20 humans, infant and child, 1 to 4 years age, treated when newborn infant for various infections.
   (CT) Study of 7 children, control group, treated with other antibiotics during neonatal period for similar infections.
   (AD) Use of pure tone audiometry or clinical evaluation only to determine hearing loss.
   (AD) Study to determine cochleotoxic effects of kanamycin when used in treatment of newborn infants. (ENG)

617

Hearing loss observed after several years possibly due to high doses, 125 mg per kg daily, total of 10.75 g, of antibiotic, kanamycin, for total of 43 days in 1 human, child, treated after surgery for congenital intestinal atresia when newborn infant.
   (AD) Hearing loss possibly congenital and not due to kanamycin therapy.
Bilateral hearing loss detected after 8 to 10 years but no subjective symptoms due to 100 mg per kg daily of antibiotic, kanamycin, for 8 to 14 days in 1 of 51 humans, child, treated for disorder when infant.
   (AD) Study with audiometry of effects of kanamycin used in treatment of 51 newborn infants and infants.
   (CT) Study of 43 children, control group, without kanamycin therapy.
   (AD) Suggested that high doses of kanamycin not be used.
   (AD) Suggested that less ototoxic effects due to kanamycin in infants and children than in adults. (ENG)

445

No specified ototoxic effects due to topical administration in (SQ) ointment of sufficient dose, in 10 percent ammoniated ointment, to produce urine level of 80 mcg per 100 mg of heavy metal, mercury, in 1 human, infant, 11 months age, male, with skin rash.
Dizziness due to topical route, (SQ) inhalation, of about 0.17 mg per m, for about 8 hours every night, of vapor concentration, sufficient to produce urine level of 100 mcg per liter, of heavy metal, mercury, for long period in 1 human, child, 11 years age, male. (ENG)

465

Hearing loss, nystagmus, and vertigo due to heavy metal, mercury, organic, in humans, adolescent, adult, and aged.
   (AD) Auditory system problems confirmed by audiology and vestibular function tests. (JAP)

696

Dizziness due to heavy metal, mercury (inorganic mercury), in 1 month to 38 years exposure in 1 of 154 humans, adolescent and adult, 18 to 62 years age, during work in industry.
   (AD) Report on 10 years study of exposure to mercury (inorganic mercury). (ENG)

001

Permanent bilateral high frequency hearing loss due to topical administration by irrigation of joint cavity of left knee with 50 cc of 10 percent solution of antibiotic, neomycin, for every 3 hours for 3 days and every 6 hours for 5 days in 1 human, child, 6 years age, male, 56 lb weight.
   (CT) Pretreatment audiogram showed normal bilateral hearing sensitivity. (ENG)

004

Bilateral sensorineural hearing loss due to oral administration of total of 600 g of antibiotic, neomycin, in 300 days in 1 human, child, 11 years age, male, with chronic colitis.
   (AD) Literature review showed 4 other case reports of hearing loss due to oral administration of neomycin. (ENG)

238

Sensorineural hearing loss due to oral administration of 50 to 100 mg per kg

of antibiotic, neomycin, in 9 of 17 humans, child, 2.5 to 7 years age, with
dyspepsia.
  (AD) Hearing loss determined by audiometry. (FR)

717
Hearing loss in fetus due to ototoxic drugs in humans treated during pregnan-
cy.
  (AD) Discussion of etiology of hearing loss in risk children. (GER)

366
Possible auditory system problems due to cardiovascular agent, quinidine, in
humans.
No ototoxic effects due to 2.40 to 9.00 g of cardiovascular agent, quinidine,
in 150 humans, adolescent and adult, male and female, with auricular fibril-
lation.
  (AD) Other toxic effects in 46 of 150 humans but no ototoxic effects
  reported. (SP)

174
Transient high frequency hearing loss and tinnitus after 4 hours due to oral
administration of 1 g daily of antidiabetic, (SQ) R 94, for 28 days at most
in 26 humans, adolescent and adult, 15 to 55 years age, male, with moderate
to severe diabetes.
Incr in high frequency hearing loss due to oral administration of 1 g of
antidiabetic, (SQ) R 94, for 7 days after onset of hearing loss in 9 of 26
humans, adolescent and adult, 15 to 55 years age, male, with moderate to
severe diabetes.
Decr and complete reversal of hearing loss due to oral administration of 1 g
of antidiabetic, (SQ) R 94 (IB), in 15 of 26 humans, adolescent and adult, 15
to 55 years age, male, with moderate to severe diabetes, with administration
of 100 and 200 mg of nicotinic acid.
  (AD) Reversal of hearing loss after cessation of treatment with R 94 or
  with administration of nicotinic acid.
  (CT) Use of subjects with no recent treatment with ototoxic drugs.
  (CT) Audiometry, pretreatment and 4 hours after every daily dose.
  (AD) Vestibular function tests normal. (ENG)

014
No permanent sensorineural hearing loss or damage to cochlea or vestibular
apparatus due to 20 to 30 mg per kg daily, total of 2 to 39 g, of antibiotic,
streptomycin, for 6 months to 5 years in 205 humans, child and adolescent,
range of 6 to 14 years age, with various disorders. (POL)

040
Sensorineural hearing loss due to parenteral, intramuscular, administration
of 1 g twice a week of antibiotic, streptomycin (streptomycin sulfate), for
335 days in 1 human, adult, 63 years age, male, with bone tuberculosis.
  (AD) Pretreatment hearing loss reported.
Sensorineural hearing loss due to parenteral, intramuscular, administration
of 0.5 g twice a week of antibiotic, streptomycin (streptomycin sulfate), for
333 days in 1 human, child, 3 years age, with bone tuberculosis. (ENG)

071
Cochleo-vestibulotoxic effects due to antibiotic, streptomycin (SM) (streptomycin sulfate), in 65.5 percent of 553 humans, child and adolescent, 3 to
15 years age, with pulmonary tuberculosis.
Simultaneous administration of other unspecified antituberculous agents (SM)
in 553 humans, child and adolescent, 3 to 15 years age, with pulmonary tuberculosis.
  (CT) No cochleo-vestibulotoxic effects in 113 humans, child and adolescent, control group, not treated with streptomycin.
  (AD) Analysis by audiometry of ototoxic effects of streptomycin in children and adolescents. (SER)

133
Sensorineural hearing loss due to antibiotic, streptomycin, in 6 of 420
humans, child, with suppurative meningitis. (RUS)

200

Moderate to profound sensorineural hearing loss, possibly due to 25 mg per kg
every 12 hours of antibiotic, streptomycin (streptomycin sulfate), in 8 doses
in 16 of 17 humans, child, about 4 years age, treated in neonatal period for
hemolytic disease or hyperbilirubinemia.
   (AD) Hearing loss determined by pure tone audiometry using play audiometry
   methods.
   (AD) Reported that not possible to determine role of streptomycin independent of high bilirubin level in hearing loss of 16 children.   (ENG)

243

Hearing loss and vestibular problems due to 1.5 g of antibiotic, streptomycin
(streptomycin pantothenate), in 1 human, child, male.
   (AD)   Literature review of pharmacology and toxicology of aminoglycoside
   antibiotics,   streptomycin,   dihydrostreptomycin, kanamycin, and neomycin.
   (GER)

271

Sensorineural hearing loss due to antibiotic, streptomycin, in humans, child.
   (AD) Statistical analysis of etiology and occurrence of sensorineural
   hearing loss in children.   (JAP)

347

Delayed hearing loss at 2 different times due to 15 g each time of antibiotic, streptomycin, in 1 human, child, male, treated at 8 years age for rheumatism and at 13 years age for pneumonia.
   (AD) Similar audiograms after 2 periods of treatment.
Delayed hearing loss due to 6 and 8 g of antibiotic, streptomycin, in 2
humans, adult and child, female, mother and daughter.
Delayed hearing loss due to 6 and 5 g of antibiotic, streptomycin, in 2
humans, adult, 34 and 36 years age, female, sisters.
Delayed hearing loss due to 10 and 8 g of antibiotic, streptomycin, in 2
humans, adult, 23 and 24 years age, female, sisters.
Sensorineural hearing loss due to 10 and 4 g of antibiotic, streptomycin, in
3 humans, female, sisters.
Delayed hearing loss due to low doses of antibiotic, streptomycin, in 3
humans, adult and child, 50, 26, and 8 years age, female, mother, daughter,
and granddaughter.
   (AD) Suggested familial and constitutional predisposition in streptomycin
   ototoxicity.   (FR)

403

Risk of damage to function of eighth cranial nerve due to antibiotic, streptomycin, for long period in humans, adult and child, with tuberculous meningitis.
   (AD)   Need for tests of function of eighth cranial nerve with clinical use
   of streptomycin.
   (AD) Literature review of treatment of infections of CNS.   (ENG)

452

Hearing loss due to 0.5 g daily, total of 30 to 50 g, of antibiotic, streptomycin, in some of 187 humans, child, adolescent, and adult, 12 to 20 years
age, with tuberculosis.
   (AD) Audiogram confirmed hearing loss.
   (AD) Inclusion of 3 case reports.   (HUN)

490

No hearing loss due to average dose of 36.8 mg per kg daily, average total
dose of 118.9 mg per kg, of antibiotic, streptomycin (streptomycin sulfate),
for short period, average of 3.2 days, in 98 humans, child, 7 and 8 years
age, female and male, treated when newborn infants.
   (AD) Follow up study with audiometry of children treated in neonatal
   period with streptomycin.
   (CT) Study of 102 children, control group, not treated in neonatal period
   with ototoxic drugs.
   (AD) Sensorineural hearing loss detected in 3 of 98 children treated with
   streptomycin not attributed to antibiotic.   (ENG)

534

Dizziness within 6 weeks due to parenteral, intramuscular, administration of
0.75 g daily of antibiotic, streptomycin, in 8 (31 percent) of 27 humans,
child, adult, and aged, 12 to 76 years age, female and male, 34 to 89 kg
weight, with tuberculosis.
   (AD) Use of vestibular function tests in patients reporting dizziness.
   (AD) Study showed significant relationship between higher 24 hour serum
   levels and dizziness.
   (AD) Suggested decr in dosage when serum streptomycin more than 3 mcg per
   ml at 24 hours.
   (AD) More risk of vestibulotoxic effects due to streptomycin in patients
   over 45 years age. (ENG)

695

Hearing loss in fetus due to sedative, thalidomide, in humans, female,
treated during pregnancy.
   (AD) Congenital hearing loss in 5 of 34 humans, child, of mothers treated
   with thalidomide during pregnancy. (ENG)

598

Vertigo or tinnitus due to oral administration in tablets of 1 to 3 tablets
of 200 mg each, total of 200 to 600 mg, of antimalarial, 16-126 RP, in 1 dose
in 3 of 20 humans, African, child, 4 or less to over 9 years age, with malaria.
Vertigo due to oral administration in tablets of 2 to 6 tablets of 200 mg
each, total of 400 to 1200 mg, of antimalarial, 16-126 RP, for 2 days in 1 of
15 humans, African, child, 4 or less to over 9 years age, with malaria. (FR)

019

Progressive severe sensorineural hearing loss and tinnitus due to unspecified
method of administration of 0.5 g twice daily, total of 16 g, of antibiotic,
kanamycin, for 16 days in 1 human, Caucasian, adult, 25 years age, male, with
kidney disorder and treated with peritoneal dialysis.
   (AD) Audiograms showed hearing loss and recruitment test showed reversed
   recruitment.
Severe sensorineural hearing loss due to unspecified method of administration
of 0.5 g daily for 40 days and then 0.5 g 3 times a week for 3 weeks of
antibiotic, streptomycin, for total period of about 9 weeks in 1 human,
Negro, child, 9 years age, male, with pulmonary tuberculosis and kidney
disorder.
   (AD) No record of hearing loss before treatment with streptomycin.
Delayed severe bilateral high frequency hearing loss due to unspecified
method of administration of 0.5 g daily for 8 months and then 0.5 g every 3
days for 4 months, followed by a break of 3.5 months, and then 0.5 g every 3
days for 1.5 months, total of 153 g of antibiotic, dihydrostreptomycin, for
total period of about 13.5 months in 1 human, Negro, infant, 16 months age,
female, with tuberculosis.
   (AD) Hearing loss detected at 13 years age.
Hearing loss and tinnitus due to unspecified method of administration of 1 g
daily of antibiotic, streptomycin, for 10 weeks and possibly for a longer
period after discharge in 1 human, Negro, adult, 23 years age, male, treated
for infection in tuberculosis hospital.
   (AD) Hearing loss detected 1 month after treatment with streptomycin.
Progressive severe sensorineural hearing loss due to unspecified method of
administration of 0.5 g 3 times a week, total of 61 g of antibiotic, streptomycin, for about 10 months in 1 human, Negro, child, 9 years age, female,
with pulmonary tuberculosis.
   (AD) Discussion of 5 case reports. (ENG)

063

Progressive permanent bilateral sensorineural hearing loss due to topical
administration by irrigation of wound with 1000 ml of 1 percent solution (6.5
g) of antibiotic, neomycin (CB) (neomycin sulfate), in 1 administration in 1
human, Caucasian, adolescent, 18 years age, male, with gunshot wound of
abdomen.
   (AD) Hearing loss reported 21 days after treatment.
Progressive permanent bilateral sensorineural hearing loss due to topical
administration by irrigation of wound with 1000 ml of 0.1 percent solution

(650 mg) of antibiotic, polymyxin B (CB) (polymyxin B sulfate), in 1 administration in 1 human, Caucasian, adolescent, 18 years age, male, with gunshot
wound of abdomen.
  (AD) Study reported that ototoxic effects only due to neomycin.
  (AD) Hemodialysis 24 hours after treatment for prevention of hearing loss
  not satisfactory.
Progressive permanent bilateral sensorineural hearing loss due to topical
administration by irrigation of wound with high doses of 1 percent solution
of antibiotic, (SQ) neomycin, for 22 days in 1 human, Caucasian, adult, 20
years age, male, with gunshot wounds.
  (AD) Hearing loss reported after 19 days of treatment.
Previous administration of unspecified dose of antibiotic, (SQ) streptomycin,
for 6 days in 1 human, Caucasian, adult, 20 years age, male, with gunshot
wounds.
Progressive permanent bilateral sensorineural hearing loss due to topical
administration by irrigation of wound with total of 4000 ml of 1 percent
solution of antibiotic, neomycin (CB) (neomycin sulfate), in 4 days in 1
human, Caucasian, adult, 39 years age, male, with wounds.
  (AD) Hearing loss reported within 5 days.
Progressive permanent bilateral sensorineural hearing loss due to topical
administration by irrigation of wound with total of 4000 ml of 0.1 percent
solution of antibiotic, polymyxin B (CB) (polymyxin B sulfate), in 4 days in
1 human, Caucasian, adult, 39 years age, male, with wounds.
  (AD) Discussion of 3 case reports of hearing loss due to topical administration of antibiotics. (ENG)

                                                                       073
Permanent hearing loss due to 10 to 35 mg per kg daily or twice daily of
antibiotic, dihydrostreptomycin, in 23(26.4 percent) of 87 humans, child,
with pulmonary and meningeal tuberculosis.
Permanent hearing loss due to 15 to 35 mg per kg daily or twice daily of
antibiotic, streptomycin, in 1(5.2 percent)of 19 humans, child, with pulmonary and meningeal tuberculosis.
  (AD) More ototoxic effects with 1 dose per day than with 2 doses per day.
Permanent hearing loss due to 15 to 20 mg per kg daily or twice daily of
antibiotic, dihydrostreptomycin (CB), in 4(18.6 percent) of 46 humans, child,
with pulmonary and meningeal tuberculosis.
Permanent hearing loss due to 15 to 20 mg per kg daily or twice daily of
antibiotic, streptomycin (CB), in 4(18.6 percent) of 46 humans, child, with
pulmonary and meningeal tuberculosis.
  (CT) No hearing loss in 14 children, control group, treated with PAS and
  isoniazid.
  (AD) Need to confirm hearing loss with audiometry discussed. (SER)

                                                                       080
Hearing loss and vertigo due to parenteral administration of antibiotic,
streptomycin, in humans, child and adult, with normal kidney function and
with kidney disorder.
  (AD) Suggested use for severe infections only.
Delayed permanent hearing loss due to antibiotic, dihydrostreptomycin, in
humans.
  (AD) High risk of ototoxic effects with clinical use.
Hearing loss due to oral administration of antibiotic, paromomycin, in hu-
mans.
Progressive permanent hearing loss and tinnitus due to parenteral administra-
tion of antibiotic, kanamycin, in humans.
Progressive permanent hearing loss and tinnitus due to parenteral and topical
administration of antibiotic, neomycin, in humans.
  (AD) Need for careful consideration in use of paromomycin, kanamycin, and
  neomycin due to potential ototoxicity.
  (AD) Discussion of ototoxic effects of 5 antibiotics. (ENG)

                                                                       116
Moderate unilateral sensorineural hearing loss in 1 of 36 fetuses due to
total of 13 g of antibiotic, dihydrostreptomycin, in 33 humans, female,
treated during pregnancy for tuberculosis.
  (AD) Child not treated with dihydrostreptomycin or streptomycin.
Sensorineural hearing loss due to 1 g daily for the first 30 days and then 1

g twice a week of antibiotic, dihydrostreptomycin (CB), in 8(24 percent)of 33 humans, female, treated during pregnancy for tuberculosis.
Sensorineural hearing loss due to 1 g daily for the first 30 days and then 1 g twice a week of antibiotic, streptomycin (CB), in 8(24 percent)of 33 humans, female, treated during pregnancy for tuberculosis.
Vestibular problems due to antibiotic, (SQ) dihydrostreptomycin, in 1 of 33 humans, female, treated during pregnancy for tuberculosis and chronic pyelonephritis.
Vestibular problems due to antibiotic, (SQ) streptomycin, in 1 of 33 humans, female, treated during pregnancy for tuberculosis and chronic pyelonephritis.
    (AD) Case histories, audiometry, and vestibular function tests for children and adults. (ENG)

                                                                          156
Sensorineural hearing loss due to unspecified method of administration of high doses of antibiotic, streptomycin (SM), in 7 humans, infant and child, with tuberculous meningitis.
Simultaneous administration of unspecified doses of antituberculous agent, PAS (SM), in 7 humans, infant and child, with tuberculous meningitis.
Simultaneous administration of unspecified doses of antituberculous agent, isoniazid (SM), in 7 humans, infant and child, with tuberculous meningitis.
Sensorineural hearing loss due to unspecified method of administration of high doses of antibiotic, viomycin, in 7 humans, infant and child, with tuberculous meningitis.
    (AD) Cochleotoxic effect due to antibiotic therapy or infection. (ENG)

                                                                          179
Progressive high frequency hearing loss and tinnitus due to 1 g daily of antibiotic, kanamycin, in 3 humans, adolescent and adult, male, with tuberculosis and with previous treatment with ototoxic drugs but with no report of toxic effects.
Less severe sensorineural hearing loss and no tinnitus due to 1 g 5 times a week of antibiotic, kanamycin, in 1 human, male, with tuberculosis and with previous treatment with ototoxic drugs.
Sensorineural hearing loss and tinnitus due to 6 g of antibiotic, kanamycin (SM), in 1 human, male, with tuberculosis and with previous treatment with ototoxic drugs.
Sensorineural hearing loss and tinnitus due to parenteral administration of 1000 mg per day of antibiotic, streptomycin (SM), in 1 human, male, with tuberculosis and with previous treatment with ototoxic drugs.
No high frequency hearing loss due to parenteral administration of 1 g daily of antibiotic, streptomycin, in 1 human, female, with tuberculosis and with previous treatment with ototoxic drugs.
High frequency hearing loss but no tinnitus due to 750 mg daily of antibiotic, streptomycin, in 1 human, female, with tuberculosis and with previous treatment with ototoxic drugs.
Simultaneous administration of range of doses of other antituberculous agents (SM) in total of 7 humans, adolescent and adult, 13 to 49 years age, male and female, with tuberculosis and with previous treatment with ototoxic drugs.
    (AD) Study using high frequency audiometry and conventional audiometry.
    (CT) Pretreatment audiograms obtained. (ENG)

                                                                          188
Possible hearing loss due to antibiotics in humans, child, treated when newborn infant.
    (AD) Reported that 23 percent of 46 children with idiopathic hearing loss treated with antibiotics in neonatal period.
    (CT) Reported that 2 percent of 54 children with normal hearing treated with antibiotics in neonatal period.
Possible hearing loss in fetus due to salicylate, aspirin, in humans, female, during pregnancy.
    (AD) Ingestion of salicylate, aspirin, during pregnancy by mothers of 2 percent of total of 118 children with hearing loss.
    (CT) Ingestion of salicylate, aspirin, during pregnancy by mothers of 0 of 54 children with normal hearing.
    (AD) Study of etiology of hearing loss in children. (ENG)

192

Sensorineural hearing loss, dizziness, vertigo, and nystagmus due to topical, cutaneous, administration in ointment of 0.3 percent concentration of antibiotic, (SQ) neomycin, for 5 months in 1 human, Caucasian, child, 9 years age, with dermatomyositis.

Sensorineural hearing loss, dizziness, vertigo, and nystagmus due to topical, cutaneous, administration in ointment of 1 percent concentration of antibiotic, (SQ) neomycin (CB), for 2 months in 1 human, Caucasian, child, 9 years age, with dermatomyositis.

Sensorineural hearing loss, dizziness, vertigo, and nystagmus due to topical, cutaneous, administration in ointment of 11 percent concentration of chemical agent, (SQ) dimethyl sulfoxide (CB), for 2 months in 1 human, Caucasian, child, 9 years age, with dermatomyositis.

   (AD) Potentiation of cochleo-vestibulotoxic effects of neomycin as result of incr cutaneous absorption due to dimethyl sulfoxide.
   (AD) Hearing loss confirmed by audiogram. (ENG)

196

Sensorineural hearing loss due to unspecified doses of antibiotic, streptomycin, in 8.9 percent of 2917 humans, child, adolescent, and adult, 10 to 34 years age, with pulmonary tuberculosis.

Sensorineural hearing loss due to unspecified doses of antibiotic, streptomycin (SM), in high percent of 608 humans, child, adolescent, and adult, 10 to 34 years age, with pulmonary tuberculosis.

Sensorineural hearing loss due to unspecified doses of antibiotic, kanamycin (SM), in high percent of 608 humans, child, adolescent, and adult, 10 to 34 years age, with pulmonary tuberculosis.

   (CT) Study of 314 humans, control group, without pulmonary tuberculosis.
   (CT) No subjective hearing loss before treatment with antibiotics.
   (CT) Hearing loss after antibiotic treatment confirmed by audiometry.
   (AD) Statistical analysis of 3525 cases with antibiotic therapy.
   (AD) Highest incidence of hearing loss in 30 to 34 years age group.
   (AD) Higher incidence of severe hearing loss in group treated with two antibiotics than in group treated with streptomycin only. (ENG)

227

Bilateral tinnitus and sudden deafness possibly due to cardiovascular agent, (SQ) hexadimethrine bromide, in 1 human, adult, 32 years age, female, with chronic nephritis and treated with hemodialysis.

Previous administration of antituberculous agent, (SQ) PAS, in 1 human, adult, 32 years age, female, with chronic nephritis and treated with hemodialysis.

Previous administration of antituberculous agent, (SQ) isoniazid, in 1 human, adult, 32 years age, female, with chronic nephritis and treated with hemodialysis.

Damage to Reissner's membrane, degeneration of organ of Corti, stria vascularis, and spiral ganglion, and slight changes in vestibular apparatus possibly due to cardiovascular agent, (SQ) hexadimethrine bromide, in 1 human, adult, 32 years age, female, with chronic nephritis and treated with hemodialysis.

Progressive severe sensorineural hearing loss possibly due to cardiovascular agent, hexadimethrine bromide, in 4 humans, adolescent and adult, 17 to 40 years age, with kidney disorders and treated with hemodialysis.

   (AD) Association of hexadimethrine bromide with hearing loss only when used with hemodialysis in treatment of kidney disorder.
   (AD) No hearing loss in group treated with hemodialysis without hexadimethrine bromide. (ENG)

236

Bilateral high frequency hearing loss due to parenteral, intramuscular, administration of high dose, 90 mg per kg daily, total of 99.2 g, of antibiotic, kanamycin, for 62 days in 1 human, child, with miliary tuberculosis.

High frequency hearing loss due to parenteral, intramuscular, administration of high dose, 25 mg per kg daily, total of 22.2 g, of antibiotic, kanamycin, for 148 days in 1 human, child, with miliary tuberculosis.

Permanent severe sensorineural hearing loss due to parenteral, intramuscular, administration of high doses of antibiotic, kanamycin, in 1 human, child, with multiple infections.

Progressive sensorineural hearing loss due to oral administration of antibio-

tic, neomycin, for 11 months in 1 human, child, 11.5 years age, male, with severe ulcerative ileocolitis.
    (AD) Hearing loss confirmed by audiogram.
    (AD) Discussion of 4 case reports of ototoxic effects due to kanamycin or neomycin.
    (AD) Suggested that risk of kanamycin ototoxicity less in children than in adults.
Sensorineural hearing loss due to 10 to 100 mg per kg daily of antibiotic, kanamycin, for 5 to 95 days in 5 of 30 humans, child and infant, with infections.
    (CT) Study of 30 children and infants, control group, not treated with kanamycin.
    (AD) Suggested that cochleotoxic effects related to total dose of kanamycin.
    (AD) Report on studies made during 8 years of clinical use of kanamycin. (ENG)

237

Hearing loss due to parenteral, intramuscular, administration of 15 mg per kg daily of antibiotic, kanamycin, for 6 to 10 days in 5.1 percent of 143 humans, child, treated when newborn infant for infection.
Hearing loss due to parenteral, intramuscular, administration of 40 mg per kg daily of antibiotic, streptomycin, for 6 to 12 days in 5.6 percent of 93 humans, child, treated when newborn infant for infection.
    (CT) Hearing loss in 4.4 percent of 170 children, control group, without antibiotic therapy.
    (AD) Hearing loss confirmed by audiogram.
    (AD) Suggested low kanamycin ototoxicity in newborn infants with use of recommended dosage.   (ENG)

310

Transient decr in vestibular function due to parenteral, intravenous, administration of 2 ml of tranquilizer, droperidol (CB), for 2 minutes in 18 of 21 humans, adolescent and adult, female and male.
Transient decr in vestibular function due to parenteral, intravenous, administration of 2 ml of analgesic, fentanyl (CB) (fentanyl citrate), for 2 minutes in 18 of 21 humans, adolescent and adult, female and male.
    (CT) Caloric tests, pretreatment and posttreatment.   (DAN)

343

No hearing loss but decr in vestibular function, asymptomatic except for dizziness in 1 case, due to 1 g daily of antibiotic, capreomycin (SM), for 4 months or more in 4 of 25 humans, adolescent, adult, and aged, range of 17 to 67 years age, male and female, 80 to 160 lb weight, with pulmonary tuberculosis and with kidney disorder in 2 cases.
Transient dizziness with no objective decr in vestibular function due to 1 g daily of antibiotic, capreomycin (SM), for 4 months or more in 3 of 25 humans, adolescent, adult, and aged, range of 17 to 67 years age, male and female, 80 to 160 lb weight, with pulmonary tuberculosis.
Simultaneous administration of 300 mg daily of antituberculous agent, isoniazid (SM), for 4 months or more in 25 humans, adolescent, adult, and aged, range of 17 to 67 years age, male and female, 80 to 160 lb weight, with pulmonary tuberculosis.
    (CT) Pure tone audiometry, caloric tests, and cupulometry, pretreatment and during treatment with capreomycin.
    (AD) Study of clinical use and cochleo-vestibulotoxic effects of capreomycin.
Hearing loss, asymptomatic in 1 case and symptomatic in 1 case, due to 1 g daily of antibiotic, viomycin, in 2 of 75 humans with pulmonary tuberculosis.
Objective decr in vestibular function due to 1 g daily of antibiotic, viomycin, in 21 of 75 humans with pulmonary tuberculosis.
Hearing loss, asymptomatic, due to 1 g daily of antibiotic, streptomycin, in 2 of 61 humans with pulmonary tuberculosis.
Objective decr in vestibular function due to 1 g daily of antibiotic, streptomycin, in 8 of 61 humans with pulmonary tuberculosis.
    (CT) Audiometry and vestibular function tests, pretreatment and during treatment with viomycin or streptomycin.
    (AD) Results of study on capreomycin comp w results of previous study on

viomycin and streptomycin.   (ENG)

348

No ototoxic effects due to topical administration in ear drops of 3 to 4 ear
drops 3 times daily of fluocinolone acetonide (CB), for 5 to 10 days in 54
humans, child, adolescent, adult, and aged, male and female, with infections
of middle ear and external ear.
No ototoxic effects due to topical administration in ear drops of 3 to 4 ear
drops 3 times daily of antibiotic, polymyxin B (CB), for 5 to 10 days in 54
humans, child, adolescent, adult, and aged, male and female, with infections
of middle ear and external ear.
No ototoxic effects due to topical administration in ear drops of 3 to 4 ear
drops 3 times daily of antibiotic, neomycin (CB) (neomycin sulfate), for 5 to
10 days in 54 humans, child, adolescent, adult, and aged, male and female,
with infections of middle ear and external ear.   (IT)

354

Vestibular problems due to 1 g daily, total doses of 1 to 115 g before onset
of ototoxicity, of antibiotic, streptomycin (SM), for several days to 9
months in 56 of 364 humans, adolescent and adult, 16 to 64 years age, female,
with tuberculosis of genitourinary system.
No specified ototoxic effects due to range of doses of antituberculous agent,
PAS (SM), for several days to 9 months in 13 of 369 humans, adolescent and
adult, 16 to 64 years age, female, with tuberculosis of genitourinary system.
Simultaneous administration of antituberculous agent, isoniazid (SM), in 274
humans, adolescent and adult, 16 to 64 years age, female, with tuberculosis
of genitourinary system.   (ENG)

356

Hearing loss due to antibiotic, streptomycin, in 120 of 150 humans, child, 2
to 4 years age, most treated when newborn infant or infant for different
disorders.
Hearing loss due to antibiotic, streptomycin (SM), in 30 of 150 humans,
child, 2 to 4 years age, most treated when newborn infant or infant for
different disorders.
Hearing loss due to antibiotic, neomycin (SM), in 30 of 150 humans, child, 2
to 4 years age, most treated when newborn infant or infant for different
disorders.
Hearing loss due to other antibiotics (SM) in 30 of 150 humans, child, 2 to 4
years age, most treated when newborn infant or infant for different disorders.
    (AD) Hearing loss determined by play audiometry.
    (AD) No relationship between hearing loss and dosage or duration of treat-
    ment with antibiotics.
    (AD) No improvement in hearing after 1 to 2 years.   (RUS)

362

Hearing loss due to high and low doses of antibiotic, streptomycin, in humans, child and adult, with different disorders and with previous hearing
loss in 2 humans.
Hearing loss due to high doses of antibiotic, neomycin, in humans, child and
adult, with different disorders.
    (AD) Need for daily audiometry and vestibular function tests with adminis-
    tration of aminoglycoside antibiotics.
    (AD) If ototoxic effect observed, need to withdraw ototoxic drug or ad-
    minister vitamins, glucose, dimedrol, calcium chloride, or electrophoresis
    with potassium iodide.   (RUS)

367

Auditory system problems due to oral administration of 150 mg daily of antituberculous agent, thiacetazone (CB), for 12 weeks in 47 of 581 humans,
adolescent and adult, 15 years or over age, male and female, with pulmonary
tuberculosis.
Auditory system problems due to oral administration of 150 mg daily of antituberculous agent, thiacetazone (CB) (IB), for 12 weeks in 39 of 584 humans,
adolescent and adult, 15 years or over age, male and female, with pulmonary
tuberculosis, with administration of vitamins and antihistamine.
Combined oral administration of 300 mg daily of antituberculous agent, i-

soniazid (CB), for 12 weeks in humans, adolescent and adult, 15 years or over age, male and female, with pulmonary tuberculosis.

   (AD) Study of effect of inhibitors on toxicity of drugs in 1 group with drug regimen of thiacetazone and isoniazid in combination.

Auditory system problems due to parenteral administration of 1 g daily of antibiotic, streptomycin (SM), for 12 weeks in 227 of 689 humans, adolescent and adult, 15 years or over age, male and female, with pulmonary tuberculosis.

Auditory system problems due to parenteral administration of 1 g daily of antibiotic, streptomycin (SM) (IB), for 12 weeks in 218 of 707 humans, adolescent and adult, 15 years or over age, male and female, with pulmonary tuberculosis, with administration of vitamins and antihistamine.

Auditory system problems due to simultaneous oral administration of 150 mg daily of antituberculous agent, thiacetazone (SM), for 12 weeks in humans, adolescent and adult, 15 years or over age, male and female, with pulmonary tuberculosis.

Simultaneous oral administration of 300 mg daily of antituberculous agent, isoniazid (SM), for 12 weeks in humans, adolescent and adult, 15 years or over age, male and female, with pulmonary tuberculosis.

   (AD) Study of effect of inhibitors on toxicity of drugs in 1 group with drug regimen of streptomycin, thiacetazone, and isoniazid.

Auditory system problems due to parenteral administration of 1 g daily of antibiotic, streptomycin (SM), for 12 weeks in 109 of 711 humans, adolescent and adult, 15 years or over age, male and female, with pulmonary tuberculosis.

Auditory system problems due to parenteral administration of 1 g daily of antibiotic, streptomycin (SM) (IB), for 12 weeks in 111 of 696 humans, adolescent and adult, 15 years or over age, male and female, with pulmonary tuberculosis, with administration of vitamins and antihistamine.

Simultaneous oral administration of 300 mg daily of antituberculous agent, isoniazid (SM), for 12 weeks in humans, adolescent and adult, 15 years or over age, male and female, with pulmonary tuberculosis.

   (AD) Study of effect of inhibitors on toxicity of drugs in 1 group with drug regimen of streptomycin and isoniazid.

   (AD) Study of effectiveness of inhibitors in prevention of toxic effects of thiacetazone and streptomycin.

   (AD) Study suggested that vitamins and antihistamine not effective in prevention of toxicity. (ENG)

                                                                          384
Usually transient hearing loss and no structural damage to organ of Corti, stria vascularis, and spiral ganglion due to oral or topical administration of salicylates in humans.

Hearing loss due to antimalarial, quinine, in humans.

Usually permanent hearing loss due to antimalarial, chloroquine, in humans.

Transient and permanent hearing loss and possible damage to hair cells of organ of Corti due to diuretic, ethacrynic acid, in humans.

Sensorineural hearing loss due to cardiovascular agent, hexadimethrine bromide, in humans with kidney disorder.

Sensorineural hearing loss and damage to organ of Corti due to topical administration of antineoplastic, nitrogen mustard, in humans.

Sensorineural hearing loss due to high doses of antibiotic, chloramphenicol, in humans.

Primary vestibular problems due to antibiotic, streptomycin, in humans.

Hearing loss due to high doses usually of antibiotic, streptomycin, in humans.

   (AD) Early detection of hearing loss by audiometry prevents permanent damage.

High frequency hearing loss and severe damage to outer hair cells and slight damage to inner hair cells of organ of Corti due to antibiotic, kanamycin, in humans.

Sensorineural hearing loss due to parenteral, oral, and topical administration of antibiotic, neomycin, in humans with or without kidney disorders.

Degeneration of hair cells of organ of Corti and of nerve process due to antibiotics, aminoglycoside, in animals.

   (AD) Literature review of physiological and structural cochleo-vestibulotoxic effects of ototoxic drugs.

   (AD) Discussion of suggested mechanism of ototoxicity and routes of drugs

to inner ear.
Bilateral sensorineural hearing loss due to oral administration of antibiotic, neomycin, in 4 of 8 humans with liver disease.
Bilateral sensorineural hearing loss due to oral administration of range of
doses of antibiotic, neomycin (SM), in 2 of 5 humans with liver disease.
Bilateral sensorineural hearing loss due to diuretics (SM), in 2 of 5 humans
with liver disease.
Transient progression of previous hearing loss due to parenteral, intravenous, administration of diuretic, ethacrynic acid (SM), in 1 injection in 1
of 5 humans with liver disease.
    (CT) Normal cochlear function in 6 humans, control group, with liver
    disease and not treated with neomycin or diuretics.
    (CT) Normal cochlear function in 13 humans, control group, with liver
    disease and treated with diuretics but not with neomycin.
    (AD) Hearing loss confirmed by audiometry.
    (AD) Reported that hearing loss due to neomycin or diuretics in humans
    with liver disease not related to dosage.
    (AD) Clinical study of effects of treatment with neomycin and diuretics in
    humans with liver disease.
Bilateral sensorineural hearing loss and vertigo due to antibiotic, ampicillin, in 1 human, adolescent, 17 years age, female, with tonsillitis.
    (AD) Cited case report.
Severe sensorineural hearing loss and vertigo due to topical administration
in ear drops of antibiotic, framycetin, in 1 human, adult, 42 years age,
male, with previous slight high frequency hearing loss.
    (AD) Cited case report.
Atrophy of hair cells of organ of Corti and hearing loss due to antibiotic,
dihydrostreptomycin, in humans with tuberculous meningitis.
    (AD) Cited study.
Loss of inner hair cells and damage to outer hair cells due to 18 g of antibiotic, neomycin, for 18 days in 1 human.
    (AD) Cited case report. (ENG)

                                                                        392
No hearing loss but tinnitus due to parenteral, intramuscular, administration
of range of 0.05 to 1.0 g daily according to age of antibiotic, kanamycin,
for short period in 4 of 125 humans, infant, child, and adult, with acute
otorhinolaryngological infections.
    (AD) Audiograms showed no hearing loss.
Hearing loss, subjective in 1 case and latent in others, but no vestibular
problems due to 1.0 g daily 2 times a week of antibiotic, (SQ) kanamycin, for
long period in 15 of 66 humans, adolescent and adult, 15 to 55 years age,
with pulmonary tuberculosis and with previous streptomycin treatment.
    (CT) Audiogram before and during treatment with kanamycin.
Hearing loss due to previous administration of antibiotic, (SQ) streptomycin,
in 31 of 272 humans.
Sensorineural hearing loss due to previous administration of total of 600 g
of antibiotic, (SQ) streptomycin, in 1 human, adult, 27 years age.
More severe sensorineural hearing loss, subjective, due to total of 136 g of
antibiotic, (SQ) kanamycin, in 1 human, adult, 27 years age.
    (AD) Case report of hearing loss due to streptomycin potentiated by treat-
    ment with kanamycin.
Hearing loss, latent, and tinnitus, but no vestibular problems due to total
of over 20 g to over 300 g of antibiotic, kanamycin, for long period in 10 of
70 humans with pulmonary tuberculosis and no previous chemotherapy.
    (CT) Audiogram before and during treatment with kanamycin.
    (AD) Clinical studies of effects of treatment with kanamycin for short and
    long periods.
Vestibular problems after 10 to 12 days due to parenteral administration of
100 mg per kg daily of antibiotic, streptomycin, in 3 animals, cats, 2 kg
weight.
Slight vestibular problems after 30 days due to 300 mg per kg daily of antibiotic, kanamycin, in 3 animals, cats, 2 kg weight.
Decr in cochlear microphonic due to 200 mg per kg daily of antibiotic, streptomycin, in 11 injections in animals, cats.
Slight decr in cochlear microphonic due to 300 mg per kg daily of antibiotic,
kanamycin, in 11 to 60 injections in animals, cats.
    (AD) Comparative experimental studies of cochleo-vestibulotoxic effects of

kanamycin and streptomycin in cats.
(AD) Different effects of 2 aminoglycoside antibiotics on vestibular
function but similar effects on cochlear function.   (ENG)

420

Acute hearing loss due to 10 mg on first day and then 60 mg daily for 3 days,
total of 220 mg, of antibiotic, (SQ) gentamicin, in total of 4 days in 1
human, adolescent, 16 years age, with kidney disorder.
   (AD) Hearing loss confirmed by audiogram.
Previous administration of antibiotic, (SQ) colistin, in 1 human, adolescent,
16 years age, with kidney disorder.
Vestibular problems due to 40 mg daily, total of 400 mg, of antibiotic,
gentamicin, in total of 10 days in 1 human, aged, 68 years age, with kidney
disorder. (GER)

434

Slight ototoxic effects due to range of doses of antibiotic, streptomycin, in
8 of 40 humans, female, treated for tuberculosis during pregnancy.
Slight ototoxic effects due to range of doses of antibiotic, dihydrostreptomycin, in 2 of 40 humans, female, treated for tuberculosis during pregnancy.
Vestibular problems and sensorineural hearing loss in mother and vestibular
problems in fetus due to total of 27 g of antibiotic, streptomycin (CB), for
2.5 months in 1 human, adult, 28 years age, female, treated for pulmonary
tuberculosis at end of pregnancy.
Vestibular problems and sensorineural hearing loss in mother and vestibular
problems in fetus due to total of 27 g of antibiotic, dihydrostreptomycin
(CB), for 2.5 months in 1 human, adult, 28 years age, female, treated for
pulmonary tuberculosis at end of pregnancy.
   (AD) Pure tone audiometry and vestibular function tests in child, female,
   at 10 years age.
Mixed hearing loss in mother and severe sensorineural hearing loss and vestibular problems in fetus due to total of 28 g of antibiotic, (SQ) dihydrostreptomycin, for 2.5 months in 1 human, adult, 22 years age, female, treated for
tuberculosis at beginning of pregnancy.
Mixed hearing loss in mother and severe sensorineural hearing loss and vestibular problems in fetus due to total of 28 g of antibiotic, (SQ) streptomycin, for 2.5 months in 1 human, adult, 22 years age, female, treated for
tuberculosis at beginning of pregnancy.
   (AD) Pure tone audiometry and vestibular function tests in child, female,
   at 10 years age. (ENG)

446

Vestibular problems only in 5 and dizziness, tinnitus, and hearing loss in 1
due to parenteral, intramuscular, administration of 1 g daily in single
injection of antibiotic, streptomycin (SM) (streptomycin sulfate), for 6
months only in 6(6 percent) of 65 humans, Negro, adolescent and adult, 15 to
over 55 years age, male and female, 80 to over 140 lb weight, for retreatment
of pulmonary tuberculosis.
Simultaneous oral administration of 15 g of antituberculous agent, PAS (SM)
(sodium PAS), for 1 year in 65 humans, Negro, adolescent and adult, 15 to
over 55 years age, male and female, 80 to over 140 lb weight, for retreatment
of pulmonary tuberculosis.
   (AD) Study of value of regimen of streptomycin, PAS, and pyrazinamide in
   retreatment of pulmonary tuberculosis. (ENG)

447

Dizziness and tinnitus within first 14 weeks due to 150 mg daily in 2 divided
doses of antituberculous agent, thiacetazone (SM), for 26 weeks in 30 of 410
humans, adolescent and adult, 15 to over 55 years age, 30 to over 50 kg
weight, with tuberculosis.
No ototoxic effects due to 300 mg daily in 2 divided doses of antituberculous
agent, isoniazid (SM), for 26 weeks in 30 of 410 humans, adolescent and
adult, 15 to over 55 years age, 30 to over 50 kg weight, with tuberculosis.
   (AD) Study of toxicity of thiacetazone in treatment of tuberculosis.
   (ENG)

537

Dizziness due to oral administration in tablet of 150 mg daily of antituberculous agent, thiacetazone (CB) (SM), in 1 of 147 humans, African, adolescent
and adult, 15 years or more age, with pulmonary tuberculosis and without
previous treatment.
Dizziness due to oral administration in tablet of 300 mg daily of antituberculous agent, isoniazid (CB) (SM), in 1 of 147 humans, African, adolescent
and adult, 15 years or more age, with pulmonary tuberculosis and without
previous treatment.
   (AD) Dizziness in 1 patient due to combined treatment with thiacetazone
   and isoniazid only.
Dizziness due to parenteral, intramuscular, administration of 1 g daily of
antibiotic, streptomycin (SM) (streptomycin sulfate), for first 2 weeks in 1
of 161 humans, African, adolescent and adult, 15 years or more age, with
pulmonary tuberculosis and without previous treatment.
   (AD) Dizziness in 1 patient due to simultaneous treatment with thiacetazone and isoniazid in 1 tablet and intramuscular streptomycin for 2 weeks.
Dizziness due to parenteral, intramuscular, administration of 1 g daily of
antibiotic, streptomycin (SM) (streptomycin sulfate), for first 8 weeks in 10
of 162 humans, African, adolescent and adult, 15 years or more age, with
pulmonary tuberculosis and without previous treatment.
   (AD) Dizziness in 10 patients due to simultaneous treatment with thiacetazone and isoniazid in 1 tablet and intramuscular streptomycin for 8 weeks.
   (AD) Study showed vestibulotoxic effects in total of 12 of 818 patients
   treated for pulmonary tuberculosis. (ENG)

577
No ototoxic effects due to parenteral, intramuscular, administration of 3 to
5 mg per kg daily in 3 or 4 divided doses, average total dose of 3.0 g, of
antibiotic, gentamicin, for 12.7 days average in 41 humans, adolescent,
adult, and aged, 14 to 87 years age, male and female, with genitourinary
system infections primarily and with kidney disorder in 13 cases.
No ototoxic effects due to parenteral, intramuscular, administration of 15 mg
per kg daily in 2 or 3 divided doses, average total dose of 6.6 g, of antibiotic, kanamycin (SM), for 8 days average in 34 humans, adult and aged, 40
to 81 years age, male and female, with genitourinary system infection and
with kidney disorder in 8 cases.
No ototoxic effects due to parenteral, intramuscular or intravenous administration of 1.5 to 2.5 mg per kg daily in 2 to 4 divided doses, average total
dose of 1.0 g, of antibiotic, polymyxin B (SM), for 6 days average in 34
humans, adult and aged, 40 to 81 years age, male and female, with genitourinary system infection and with kidney disorder in 8 cases.
   (AD) Comparative study of effects of 3 antibiotics on infections due to
   gram-negative bacilli. (ENG)

589
Dizziness during or after 5 or 6 injections but no evidence of hearing loss
due to parenteral, intramuscular and then intravenous (SM), administration of
7 mg per kg total daily, not exceeding 180 mg total dose every 24 hours, of
antibiotic, (SQ) gentamicin, for as long as 30 days in 5 of 80 humans, infant, child, and adult, 8 months to 36 years age, with cystic fibrosis and
severe pulmonary infection.
   (AD) Audiology in 40 of 80 patients showed no evidence of hearing loss.
   (AD) Dizziness possibly due to rapid administration of gentamicin.
High frequency hearing loss before gentamicin therapy possibly due to previous administration of (SQ) ototoxic drugs in some of 80 humans, infant,
child, and adult, 8 months to 36 years age, with cystic fibrosis and severe
pulmonary infection.
Dizziness due to topical administration by inhalation (SM) of 16 to 20 mg up
to 4 times a day, in 2 ml of 0.125 percent phenylephrine hydrochloride and
propylene glycol, of antibiotic, (SQ) gentamicin (CB), in some of 80 humans,
infant, child, and adult, 8 months to 36 years age, with cystic fibrosis and
severe pulmonary infection.
Dizziness due to topical administration by inhalation (SM) of 16 to 20 mg up
to 4 times a day, in 2 ml of 0.125 percent phenylephrine hydrochloride and
propylene glycol, of antibiotic, (SQ) neomycin (CB), in some of 80 humans,
infant, child, and adult, 8 months to 36 years age, with cystic fibrosis and
severe pulmonary infection. (ENG)

611
Hearing loss due to range of 0.8 to 15 g of antibiotic, neomycin (SM), in 9
humans, child, adult, and aged, 4 or less to 65 years age, with various
infections.
Simultaneous administration of antibiotic, streptomycin (SM), in 6 humans,
child, adult, and aged, 4 or less to 65 years age, with various infections.
Simultaneous administration of antibiotic, polymyxin (SM), in 1 human, child,
less than 4 years age, with various infections.
   (AD) Hearing loss confirmed by audiograms.
   (AD) Discussion of 9 case reports. (HUN)

628
Hearing loss due to parenteral, intravenous, administration of 1 mg per kg
initial dose and then 0.75 mg per kg every 6 hours, dissolved in 200 ml of 5
percent glucose solution, of antibiotic, (SQ) gentamicin (gentamicin sulfate), in 4 of 60 humans, child, adolescent, adult, and aged, 6 to 76 years
age, with carcinoma, lymphoma, or leukemia and with azotemia in 3 of 4 and
previous hearing loss in 1 of 4.
Hearing loss due to previous administration of diuretic, (SQ) ethacrynic
acid, in 1 of 4 humans with gentamicin hearing loss.
   (AD) Suggested that hearing loss in 1 patient due to both gentamicin and
   ethacrynic acid. (ENG)

685
Total loss of vestibular function but no hearing loss due to total of 840 mg
of antibiotic, gentamicin (SM), in 47 day period in 1 of 181 humans, aged, 70
years age, female, with kidney disorder.
Total loss of vestibular function but no hearing loss due to 2 g of antibiotic, streptomycin (SM), in 47 day period in 1 of 181 humans, aged, 70 years
age, female, with kidney disorder.
Permanent vestibular problems due to 2.56 g of antibiotic, (SQ) gentamicin,
for 18 days in 1 of 181 humans, adult, 39 years age, female, with kidney
disorder.
Vestibular problems due to previous administration of antibiotic, (SQ) streptomycin, in 1 of 181 humans, adult, 39 years age, female, with kidney disorder.
Permanent vestibular problems, with dizziness, due to antibiotic, gentamicin,
in 1 of 181 humans, adult, 38 years age, female, with kidney disorder.
Transient dizziness after 3 days due to antibiotic, gentamicin, in 1 of 181
humans, adolescent, 16 years age, female, with kidney disorder.
   (AD) Serial vestibular function tests and audiometry not conducted in 181
   patients.
Vestibular problems due to parenteral, intramuscular, administration of 1 g
daily of antibiotic, (SQ) streptomycin (SM), in 1 human, adult, 19 years age,
male, with pseudomonas infection.
   (AD) Vestibular problems due to previous streptomycin therapy.
Simultaneous administration of 300 mg daily of antibiotic, (SQ) colistin (SM)
(colistimethate), for 15 days in 1 human, adult, 19 years age, male, with
pseudomonas infection.
Sequential parenteral, intramuscular, administration of 40 mg 3 times a day
of antibiotic, (SQ) gentamicin, for 36 days in 1 human, adult, 19 years age,
male, with pseudomonas infection.
Dizziness after 4 days due to parenteral, intramuscular, administration of 40
mg 4 times a day, total of 2.56 g, of antibiotic, gentamicin, for 16 days in
1 human, adult, 30 years age, female, with kidney disorder.
   (AD) Discussion of 6 case reports of vestibulotoxic effects of gentamicin.
   (ENG)

                              Adult, Aged

594
Transient severe vertigo due to oral administration in tablets of 50 mg per
kg of 500 mg tablets of antiparasitic, A-16612, for 2 days in 1 human, adult,
with schistosomiasis.
Auditory hallucination due to 100 mg per kg daily of antiparasitic, A-16612,
for 3 days in 1 human, adult, with schistosomiasis.
   (AD) Study of chemotherapy of schistosomiasis with new antiparasitic
   agent, A-16612. (ENG)

007

Permanent unilateral sensorineural hearing loss and transient vertigo and tinnitus due to oral administration of range of 0.6 to 0.9 g of salicylate, aspirin, for every 2 hours for 3 days in 1 human, adult, 19 years age, female, with pain after tooth extraction.

   (AD) Literature review showed 2 other case reports of hearing loss due to aspirin. (ENG)

021

Transient bilateral sensorineural hearing loss due to unspecified method of administration of as much as 5.2 g daily of salicylate, acetylsalicylic acid, for unspecified period in 1 human, aged, 76 years age, female, with rheumatoid arthritis.

   (AD) Improvement in hearing after cessation of treatment with acetylsalicylic acid.
   (AD) Suggested that damage to stria vascularis due to presbycusis and not due to acetylsalicylic acid. (ENG)

105

Transient bilateral incr in pure tone threshold but without tone decay and without difference limen and decr in duration of nystagmus and in slow phase velocity of nystagmus due to oral administration of incr doses to about 6 to 8 g per day, until subjective hearing loss observed, of salicylate, aspirin (CB), in 12 humans, adult and aged, range of 23 to 68 years age, with rheumatoid arthritis.
Combined administration of magnesium aluminum hydroxide (CB) in 12 humans, adult and aged, range of 23 to 68 years age, with rheumatoid arthritis.

   (CT) Withdrawal of salicylates before treatment for standardization of salicylate level.
   (CT) Audiometry and vestibular function tests before, during, and after treatment with salicylate.
   (AD) Serum salicylate level determined when subjective hearing loss reported.
Transient sensorineural hearing loss but no damage to hair cells of organ of Corti or to membranous labyrinth due to oral administration of high doses, as high as 7 to 10 g per day, of salicylates for long period in 1 human, Caucasian, adult, 62 years age, female, with previous progressive hearing loss.
Transient sensorineural hearing loss but no damage to organ of Corti, spiral ganglion, or membranous labyrinth due to oral administration of high doses, as high as 5 g per day, of salicylate, aspirin, for 15 years in 1 human, adult, 61 years age, female, with rheumatoid arthritis. (ENG)

128

Transient tinnitus due to oral administration of 2 tablets every 4 hours or more frequently, to produce serum salicylate level of 92 mg per 100 ml, of salicylate, aspirin, for about 6 days in 1 human, Caucasian, adolescent, 14 years age, female, self treatment for upper respiratory system infection.
Tinnitus and dizziness due to oral administration of about 5 bottles of 100 tablets each, to produce serum salicylate levels of 72 mg per 100 ml after 3 to 4 hours, 59 mg per 100 ml after 6 to 7 hours, 150 mg per 100 ml after 14 to 15 hours, of salicylate, aspirin, in 1 dose in 1 human, Caucasian, adult, 19 years age, female, suicide.
Loss of equilibrium due to oral administration of 62.5 mg per teaspoon of colic medicine of salicylate in 1 human, Caucasian, infant, 3 months age, male, with colic.

   (AD) Low serum salicylate level in infant.
   (AD) Discussion of 3 case reports of salicylate ototoxicity. (ENG)

143

Transient unsteady gait and dizziness due to oral administration of high doses, 12 to 30 tablets per day, of salicylate, aspirin, in 1 human, adult, 44 years age, male, self treatment for pain after accident.

   (AD) EEG abnormal for 5 weeks. (ENG)

315

Dysacusis due to oral administration of 9 tablets for 4 days, 6 tablets for 7 days, and 3 tablets for 2 days, each tablet containing 500 mg of salicylate, aspirin (aspirin aluminum), for total of 13 days in 1 of 19 humans, adult, 21

years age, female, with rheumatoid arthritis.
Tinnitus and dysacusis due to oral administration of 6 tablets for 3 days, 12
tablets for 2 days, 8 tablets for 2 days, and 9 tablets for 15 days, each
tablet containing 500 mg of salicylate, aspirin (aspirin aluminum), for total
of 22 days in 1 human, adult, 37 years age, female, with rheumatoid arthritis.
   (AD) Loss of appetite also due to administration of aspirin (aspirin
   aluminum) for 22 days. (ENG)

                                                                          649
Transient tinnitus, hearing loss, or dizziness due to oral administration in
tablets of 1.4 g, in 4 tablets, in 3 initial doses at 7 hour intervals and
then daily, to produce high serum levels of 20.5 to 28.0 mg per 100 ml, of
salicylate, aspirin, for 2 to 3 weeks in 9 of 20 humans, adolescent, adult,
and aged, 15 to 70 years age, female and male, with bone and joint disorders.
   (AD) Report on use of new sustained release aspirin in treatment of bone
   and joint disorders. (ENG)

                                                                          153
Less severe effects on vestibular apparatus due to oral ingestion of 80-proof
and 100-proof concentrations of sedative, alcohol, ethyl, in 4 humans, adult,
27 to 50 years age, male, with bilateral vestibular problems.
   (AD) Same test procedures used in previous study of normal subjects showed
   more severe effects of alcohol on vestibular apparatus.
   (AD) Subjects with vestibular problems less vulnerable to effects of
   alcohol than normal subjects. (ENG)

                                                                          220
Significant effect on auditory time perception due to parenteral administration of 0.75 cc, in 500 cc normal saline, of 95 percent solution of sedative,
alcohol, ethyl, in humans, adolescent and adult, 18 to 38 years age, male and
female.
   (CT) Same method using 500 cc of normal saline in subjects, control group.
   (ENG)

                                                                          262
Possible damage to vestibular apparatus and organ of Corti due to oral ingestion of large amounts of chemical agent, alcohol, ethyl, for long period in 8
humans, adult and aged, 44 to 75 years age, male and female, chronic alcoholics.
   (AD) Report on results of temporal bone study.
   (AD) Previous observations of transient hearing loss and tinnitus during
   alcohol intoxication.
   (AD) Need for more study for interpretation of results. (ENG)

                                                                          463
Nystagmus due to oral ingestion of 50 to 340 cc (0.44 to 2.58 g per kg) of 40
or 45 proof concentration of sedative, alcohol, ethyl, in 20 or 25 minutes in
38 humans, adult, 19 to 42 years age, male and female, 55 to 70 kg weight.
   (AD) Vestibular problems confirmed by vestibular function tests.
   (AD) Discussion of individual differences in responses to ethyl alcohol.
   (FR)

                                                                          252
No cochlear impairment or vestibular problems due to parenteral, intramuscular, administration of average daily dose of 16 mg per kg in 2 doses every 12
hours of antibiotic, aminosidine (aminosidine sulfate), for range of 10 to 30
days in 118 humans, adult, male and female, with disorders.
   (CT) Audiometry and vestibular function tests, pretreatment and posttreatment, immediately after cessation of treatment and 1 month later. (IT)

                                                                          417
No significant effects on threshold at any frequency due to 5 mg of analep-
tic, amphetamine (dextro-amphetamine sulfate), in humans, adult, range of 22
to 38 years age, male and female, with no history of auditory system problem.
   (CT) Audiometry before and 65 minutes after administration of drug.
   (CT) Same method using placebo in 12 subjects, control group.
   (CT) Same method using no drug in 12 subjects, control group.

(AD) Study to determine effects, toxic or therapeutic, of amphetamine on auditory threshold of humans. (ENG)

099

Hearing loss due to antibiotics in humans, adult and child, male and female, with kidney disorder. (HUN)

294

Hearing loss and vestibular problems due to antibiotics in humans, adult, male and female, with chronic kidney disorder. (RUS)

328

Moderate hearing loss, subjective, due to total dose of 100 g of antibiotic, capreomycin (SM), for 31 days or more in 1 of 38 humans, Negro, adult, 63 years age, male, with tuberculosis.
(CT) Audiometry, pretreatment and during treatment.
(AD) Audiometry showed possible hearing loss due to capreomycin.
Simultaneous administration of antituberculous agent, ethionamide (SM), in 1 of 38 humans, Negro, adult, 63 years age, male, with tuberculosis. (ENG)

329

Hearing loss or dizziness due to parenteral, intramuscular, administration of 1 g daily, total doses of 20 to 445 g, of antibiotic, (SQ) capreomycin (SM), for range of 20 days to over 18 months in 5 of 43 humans, adult and aged, 24 to 83 years age, male and female, with pulmonary tuberculosis and with previous treatment with antituberculous agents.
(CT) Audiometry, pretreatment and during treatment.
Simultaneous administration of 500 to 1000 mg daily in single or divided doses of antituberculous agent, (SQ) ethionamide (SM), for range of 20 days to over 18 months in 43 humans, adult and aged, 24 to 83 years age, male and female, with pulmonary tuberculosis and with previous treatment with antituberculous agents.
Previous administration of other (SQ) antituberculous agents in 43 humans, adult and aged, 24 to 83 years age, male and female, with pulmonary tuberculosis. (ENG)

568

Mild ototoxic effects due to 1 g on 6 days a week or 0.75 g when body weight below 50 kg, total of 30 to over 330 g, of antibiotic, capreomycin, for long period in 3 of 82 humans, adult and aged, 21 to 80 years age, male and female, with chronic tuberculosis. (ENG)

665

Transient slight dizziness and equilibrium disorder due to oral administration in tablets of range of less than 600 mg to 1200 mg daily, of anticonvulsant, carbamazepine, for long period in large group of humans, adult and aged, 30 to over 80 years age, male and female, with facial pain.
Severe dizziness due to oral administration in tablets of range of less than 600 mg to 1200 mg daily, of anticonvulsant, carbamazepine, for long period in 2 of 71 humans, adult and aged, 30 to over 80 years age, male and female, with facial pain and with concurrent multiple sclerosis in 1 and cerebral arteriosclerosis in other. (ENG)

180

Bilateral sensorineural hearing loss with partial improvement due to topical route, inhalation, of large amounts, to produce carboxy-hemoglobin level of 25 percent of total hemoglobin, of chemical agent, carbon monoxide, in 1 human, adult, 22 years age, male, with previous high intensity noise exposure.
(AD) Hearing loss confirmed by audiometry but vestibular function tests normal.
(AD) Suggested that audiometric configuration not type due to acoustic trauma. (ENG)

209

Slight incr but no decr in auditory flutter fusion threshold due to topical route, inhalation, of 250 ml in 500 l air, to produce concentration of 10 percent carboxyhemoglobin in blood, of chemical agent, carbon monoxide, for

65 minutes at intervals of 7 days in 8 humans, adult, 23 to 48 years age, male, healthy, 7 without smoking habit.
    (CT) For period before test, 8 subjects had no caffeine, alcohol, drugs, or nicotine.
    (CT) Study with oral administration of 100 mg phenobarbitone and placebo to determine response of same subjects to drug with known effects.
    (AD) Subjects tested with interrupted white noise. (ENG)

                                                                        224
Slight sensorineural hearing loss due to topical route, inhalation, of large amount, to produce high carboxyhemoglobin level of 36 percent 1.5 days after exposure, of chemical agent, carbon monoxide, in 1 human, adult, 21 years age, male.
Moderate bilateral sensorineural hearing loss due to topical route, inhalation, of large amount, to produce high carboxyhemoglobin level of 48 percent 1.5 days after exposure, of chemical agent, carbon monoxide, in 1 human, adolescent, 18 years age, male. (ENG)

                                                                        233
Vestibular problems due to topical route, inhalation, of large amount, to produce average carboxyhemoglobin level of 60 ml per l, of chemical agent, carbon monoxide, in 20 humans, adult, 30 years average age.
    (AD) Vestibular problems determined by vestibular function tests. (FR)

                                                                        472
Vertigo due to topical route, inhalation, of chemical agent, carbon monoxide, in humans, adult. (RUS)

                                                                        299
Transient bilateral sensorineural hearing loss and dizziness due to 25 mg every other day, total of 18 g, of heavy metal, cobalt (cobalt chlorine), in 6 months in 1 human, adult, 35 years age, female, with kidney disorder and anemia.
    (AD) Cochleo-vestibulotoxic effects confirmed by audiometry and caloric tests. (ENG)

                                                                        378
Total unilateral sensorineural hearing loss, tinnitus, and vertigo 7 days after injection due to parenteral, (SQ) intramuscular, administration of 150 mg of (SQ) contraceptive, methoxy progesterone acetate, in 1 injection in 1 human, adult, 26 years age, female.
    (AD) Cochleo-vestibulotoxic effects confirmed by audiometry and vestibular function tests 1 month later.
    (AD) Suggested that ototoxic effects result of obstruction of cochlear artery due to contraceptive.
Dizziness due to previous (SQ) oral administration of other (SQ) contraceptives in 1 human, adult, 26 years age, female. (ENG)

                                                                        379
Sudden deafness, tinnitus, severe vertigo, and objective decr in vestibular function due to oral administration of 2 mg daily of contraceptive, norethindrone (CB), for 3 months in 1 human, adult, 34 years age, female.
Sudden deafness, tinnitus, severe vertigo, and objective decr in vestibular function due to oral administration of 2 mg daily of contraceptive, mestranol (CB), for 3 months in 1 human, adult, 34 years age, female.
    (AD) Cochleo-vestibulotoxic effects confirmed by audiometry and vestibular function tests.
    (AD) Partial improvement in hearing 20 days later.
Severe bilateral sudden deafness, tinnitus, and dizziness due to oral administration of contraceptive, norethindrone (CB), for 2 years in 1 human, adult, 20 years age, female.
Severe bilateral sudden deafness, tinnitus, and dizziness due to oral administration of contraceptive, mestranol (CB), for 2 years in 1 human, adult, 20 years age, female.
    (AD) Audiometry and vestibular function tests 7 days after onset of ototoxic effects.
    (AD) Partial improvement in 1 ear and total recovery in other ear 30 days later.

(AD) Suggested that ototoxic effects resulted from blood coagulation due to contraceptive. (ENG)

402

Pressure in the ears due to contraceptives in 1 human, adult, 33 years age, female.
(AD) Pressure possibly due to obstruction of Eustachian tube.
Possible vertigo, sudden deafness, and distortion of sound due to contraceptives in humans. (ENG)

551

Sensorineural hearing loss due to parenteral administration of range of doses, 3, 15, 25, and 40 g, of antibiotic, dihydrostreptomycin, in humans, adult and child, range of ages, male and female, in 4 families.
(AD) Study of familial incidence of dihydrostreptomycin hearing loss and hereditary susceptibility of cochlea.
(AD) Suggested that administration of dihydrostreptomycin in humans with hereditary susceptibility of cochlea results in hearing loss. (ENG)

160

Tinnitus due to unspecified method of administration of 300 mg daily of anticonvulsant, diphenylhydantoin (diphenylhydantoin sodium), for 2 years in 1 human, aged, 77 years age, female, for dizziness.
(AD) No tinnitus after cessation of treatment with diphenylhydantoin (diphenylhydantoin sodium). (ENG)

654

Possible ataxia due to high doses to produce blood level of 3 mg per 100 ml or more of anticonvulsant, diphenylhydantoin, in humans, child and adult, with epilepsy.
Possible nystagmus due to doses to produce blood level of more than 2 mg per 100 ml of anticonvulsant, diphenylhydantoin, in humans, child and adult, with epilepsy. (ENG)

658

Vertigo due to parenteral, intravenous, administration of 250 mg of anticonvulsant, diphenylhydantoin, in some of 123 humans, adult and aged, male and female, with heart disorders. (GER)

664

Nystagmus due to parenteral, intramuscular or intravenous, administration of 1000 to 1500 mg on first day, and then 400 to 1500 mg on second day, followed by 400 to 600 mg, to produce blood levels of 8.6 to 35.0 mcg per ml, of anticonvulsant, diphenylhydantoin, in 8 of 10 humans, adult and aged, 40 to 65 years age, male and female, 50-94 kg weight, with heart disorders. (ENG)

671

Nystagmus due to anticonvulsant, diphenylhydantoin, in humans, child and adult, male and female, with epilepsy. (FIN)

102

Progressive hearing loss and tinnitus due to diuretic, ethacrynic acid, in 1 human, adult, 48 years age, with kidney disorder.
(AD) Hearing loss confirmed by audiometry.
(AD) Need for audiometry with use of ethacrynic acid in humans with kidney disorder. (FR)

148

Transient sensorineural hearing loss due to diuretic, ethacrynic acid, in 1 human, adult, male. (FIN)

178

Sensorineural hearing loss due to diuretic, ethacrynic acid, in humans, adult, female and male, with kidney disorders. (NOR)

320

Transient hearing loss after 3 days of treatment due to unspecified method of administration of 50 mg twice daily of diuretic, ethacrynic acid, in 1 human,

adult, 56 years age, male, with rheumatic heart disorder and with normal
kidney function. (ENG)

                                                                      503
Transient hearing loss 30 minutes after injection and change in composition
of fluids of cochlea due to parenteral, intravenous, administration of 50 mg
of diuretic, ethacrynic acid, in 1 human, adult, 45 years age, female, with
kidney disorder. (FR)

                                                                      512
Transient bilateral sudden deafness due to parenteral, intravenous, administration of 50 mg of diuretic, (SQ) ethacrynic acid, in 1 human, adult, 42
years age, male, alcoholic, with liver disease.
Previous administration of 25 g of diuretic, (SQ) mannitol, in 1 human,
adult, 42 years age, male, alcoholic, with liver disease. (ENG)

                                                                      603
Tinnitus due to oral administration of 25 mg twice a day, total of 50 mg per
kg, of anti-inflammatory agent, fluorometholone (NSC-33001), for 8 weeks in 1
of 112 humans, adult, 25 years average age, with tumors. (ENG)

                                                                      003
Transient sudden deafness, vertigo, and tinnitus due to parenteral, rapid
intravenous, administration of range of 800 to 3600 mg of diuretic, furosemide, for range of 9 hours to 6 days in 5 humans, adult, 37 to 64 years age,
male and female, with severe kidney disorder. (ENG)

                                                                      072
No reported ototoxic effects due to (SQ) oral administration of incr doses to
maximum of 3 g of diuretic, furosemide, for 10 days in 1 human, Puerto Rican,
adult, 32 years age, male, with kidney disorder.
Transient bilateral sensorineural hearing loss and dizziness due to parenteral, (SQ) intravenous, administration of 200 mg every 2 hours on first day
and 3 doses of 400 mg each on second day, total of 1.2 g, of diuretic, furosemide, for 2 days in 1 human, Puerto Rican, adult, 32 years age, male, with
kidney disorder.
  (AD) Hearing loss not confirmed by audiometry. (ENG)

                                                                      507
Bilateral sensorineural hearing loss and tinnitus due to parenteral, rapid
intravenous, administration of 240 mg of diuretic, furosemide, in 2 injections in 1 human, aged, 67 years age, male, after surgery.
  (AD) Hearing loss confirmed by audiogram. (ENG)

                                                                      625
No ototoxic effects due to oral administration of range of 40 mg daily to 8
mg twice a day, dosage increased at intervals until maximum diuretic response, of diuretic, furosemide, for range of 1 to over 45 weeks in 14 humans,
adolescent, adult, and aged, 18 to 74 years age, male and female, with kidney
disorder. (ENG)

                                                                      190
Sudden deafness and tinnitus due to topical administration of anesthetic,
garrot, in 1 human, adult, 36 years age, female, with previous hearing loss.
  (AD) Need for careful consideration in use of topical garrot in humans
  with history of auditory system problems or vestibular problems. (FR)

                                                                      101
Primary damage to vestibular apparatus but also cochlear impairment due to
parenteral, intramuscular, administration of 40 mg every 8 hours and 80 mg
every 8 hours of antibiotic, gentamicin, in 7 of 16(2 groups of 8) humans,
adult, male and female, with normal kidney function.
Primary damage to vestibular apparatus but also cochlear impairment due to
parenteral, intramuscular, administration of 40 mg daily of antibiotic,
gentamicin, in 7 of 8 humans, adult, male and female, with kidney disorder.
Primary damage to vestibular apparatus but also cochlear impairment due to
parenteral, intravenous, administration of 80 mg of antibiotic, gentamicin,
in 6 of 7 humans, adult, male and female, with chronic kidney disorder and

treated with hemodialysis.
(AD) Comparative study of humans with normal kidney function and with kidney disorder.
(AD) Higher incidence of ototoxic effects due to gentamicin in humans with kidney disorder.
(AD) Cochleo-vestibulotoxic effects confirmed by audiometry and vestibular function tests. (FR)

117

Transient sensorineural hearing loss due to parenteral, intramuscular, administration of 80 mg daily, total of 320 mg, of antibiotic, gentamicin, for 1 to 4 days in 1 of 339 humans, adult, female, with chronic pyelonephritis.
Transient sensorineural hearing loss due to parenteral, intramuscular, administration of 80 mg daily, total of 1200 mg, of antibiotic, gentamicin, for 1 to 15 days in 1 of 339 humans, adult, female.
Transient vestibular problem due to 80 mg daily, total of 560 mg, of antibiotic, gentamicin, for 7 days in 1 of 339 humans, adult, female, with kidney disorder.
(AD) Need for vestibular function tests with use of gentamicin in humans with kidney disorder.
(AD) Report of results of 33 investigations. (ENG)

218

Transient vertigo due to parenteral, intramuscular, administration of 2 x 40 mg of antibiotic, gentamicin, for 15 days in 1 human, adult, 39 years age, 72 kg weight, with diabetes mellitus and chronic pyelonephritis. (GER)

301

Severe vertigo 2 days after cessation of treatment due to topical (SM) administration of 0.1 percent solution of antibiotic, gentamicin, for 4 weeks in 1 human, aged, 65 years age, male, with mild kidney disorder.
Severe vertigo 2 days after cessation of treatment due to parenteral (SM) administration of 40 mg every 6 hours of antibiotic, gentamicin (gentamicin sulfate), for 4 weeks in 1 human, aged, 65 years age, male, with mild kidney disorder.
(CT) Study of gentamicin serum levels in normal subjects and humans treated for pseudomonas infections with recommended dose of gentamicin.
(AD) Case report of vestibulotoxic effect of gentamicin. (ENG)

302

Transient dizziness due to parenteral, intramuscular, administration of 120 mg 2 or 3 times daily of antibiotic, gentamicin, for several weeks in 4 of 23 humans, adult and aged, range of 50 to over 70 years age, male, with bronchial infections and with normal kidney function.
(AD) Vestibulotoxic effect confirmed by caloric tests. (ENG)

451

No eighth cranial nerve toxicity due to 80 mg every 6 or 8 hours, and lower dosage in humans with kidney disorder, to produce serum levels of 5 to 8 mcg per ml of antibiotic, gentamicin, in 104 humans, adult, aged, and child, 2 to 80 years age, with various infections.
(AD) Suggested that prevention of ototoxicity due to daily assays of serum levels. (ENG)

474

Transient dizziness due to parenteral, intramuscular, administration of 80 mg, to produce serum level of 12 mcg per ml, of antibiotic, gentamicin, in 1 injection in 1 human, adult, 62 years age, female, 46.5 kg weight. (ENG)

578

No clinical evidence of ototoxic effects due to high doses, 3 to 6 mg per kg daily, of antibiotic, gentamicin, in 53 humans, child, adolescent, adult, and aged, 10 to 84 years age, male and female, with bacteremia due to gram-negative bacilli and with kidney disorder in 14 cases.
(AD) Monitored for clinical symptoms of ototoxic effects.
(AD) No audiology or vestibular function tests to determine ototoxic effects. (ENG)

588

No observed ototoxic effects due to parenteral, intramuscular, administration
of range of 1.36 to 7.00 mg per kg daily, in 6 dosage regimens, to produce
blood levels of 10.5 to 18.5 mcg per ml in 8 patients tested, of antibiotic,
gentamicin, for short period in 160 humans, Filipino, adolescent and adult,
15 to 62 years age, male, 78 to 168 lb weight, with venereal disease.
(AD) Clinical evaluation of vestibular function and cochlear function
   after gentamicin therapy. (ENG)

595

Bilateral hearing loss due to parenteral, intramuscular, administration of 80
mg daily of antibiotic, gentamicin, in 1 human, adult, 38 years age, male,
with pulmonary infection.
(AD) Hearing loss confirmed by audiogram. (FR)

606

Transient vertigo after 7 days due to doses to produce blood level of 20 mcg
per ml of antibiotic, gentamicin, in 1 human, adult, 53 years age, male, with
kidney disorder and with previous hearing loss due to other aminoglycoside
antibiotics.
Transient vertigo after 5 days due to doses to produce blood level of 10 mcg
per ml of antibiotic, gentamicin, in 1 human, adult, 32 years age, female,
with chronic pyelonephritis.
Transient vertigo and hearing loss after 6 days due to high doses to produce
blood level of 40 mcg per ml of antibiotic, gentamicin, in 1 human, adult, 20
years age, male, with kidney disorder and severe pseudomonas infection.
(CT) Audiometry and vestibular function tests, pretreatment and posttreatment.
(AD) Ototoxic effects in 3 of 58 patients in study.
Unilateral vestibular problem with dizziness due to high daily doses and high
total doses to produce blood levels of 4 to 32 mcg per ml of antibiotic,
gentamicin, in 10 of 40 humans, 7 with kidney disorders.
(CT) Audiometry and vestibular function tests, pretreatment and posttreatment in 5 patients.
(AD) Ototoxic effects in 10 of 40 patients in study.
(AD) Bilateral high frequency hearing loss in 2 patients without pretreatment audiograms possibly not due to gentamicin.
Unilateral tinnitus possibly due to topical, (SQ) direct site, administration
of 40 mg of antibiotic, gentamicin, in 1 human with previous noise induced
hearing loss.
Unilateral tinnitus possibly due to parenteral, (SQ) intramuscular, administration of total of 160 mg of antibiotic, gentamicin, in 1 human with previous noise induced hearing loss.
(AD) Tinnitus, as well as hearing loss, possibly present before administration of gentamicin.
Incr vertigo due to 120 mg daily of antibiotic, gentamicin, in 1 human,
adult, 36 years age, male, with previous vertigo.
(CT) Audiometry and vestibular function tests, pretreatment and posttreatment.
(AD) Ototoxic effects in possibly 2 of 148 patients in study treated with
   topical or parenteral gentamicin.
(AD) Discussion of 3 studies of ototoxic effects of gentamicin. (ENG)

652

No vestibular problems or hearing loss observed due to parenteral, intravenous, administration of 1 mg per kg initial dose, and then 0.75 mg per kg
every 6 hours, in 200 ml dextrose solution over 2 hour period, of antibiotic,
gentamicin (SM), for 2 weeks minimum or for 5 days after cessation of fever,
whichever longer, in 23 humans, adolescent, adult, and aged, 13 to 68 years
age, with acute leukemia or metastatic cancer and with previous treatment
with other antibiotics in some.
(AD) No vestibular function tests or audiometry used to determine if
   ototoxic effects.
Simultaneous parenteral, intravenous, administration of 4 g every 4 hours of
antibiotic, carbenicillin (SM), for 2 weeks minimum or for 5 days after
cessation of fever, whichever longer, in 23 humans, adolescent, adult, and
aged, 13 to 68 years age, with acute leukemia or metastatic cancer and with
previous treatment with other antibiotics in some. (ENG)

702

Permanent total bilateral sensorineural hearing loss 5 days after cessation of treatment but no vestibular problems due to parenteral, intramuscular, administration of total dose of 0.32 g of antibiotic, gentamicin, in 16 single injections in 1 human, adult, 27 years age, male, with severe bilateral kidney disorder.
  (AD) Hearing loss confirmed by audiology. (GER)

360

Transient dizziness due to 0.9 or 0.6 g daily of anti-inflammatory agent, ibuprofen, for 7 or 14 days in 1 of 39 humans, adult, range of ages, male and female, with arthritis.
  (AD) Comparative study of ibuprofen and placebo in treatment of arthritis. (ENG)

668

Possible vertigo due to anti-inflammatory agent, indomethacin, in humans, adult.
  (AD) High incidence of vertigo due to indomethacin reported in studies.
  (AD) Incidence and degree of effect usually dose related. (ENG)

131

Severe sensorineural hearing loss due to antibiotic, kanamycin, in humans, adult and child, female and male.
  (AD) Hearing loss confirmed by audiometry. (JAP)

161

No reported ototoxic effects due to parenteral, intramuscular, administration of 2 g of antibiotic, kanamycin, in 1 injection in 4 humans, adult, 27 to 36 years age, with rectal gonorrhea.
  (AD) Audiogram after treatment with kanamycin within normal range. (ENG)

165

Hearing loss, tinnitus, or vertigo due to parenteral administration of 36.0 mg per kg daily, total of 46.7 g, of antibiotic, kanamycin, for 20.3 average days in 22 of 106 humans, adult, 50.8 years average age.
  (AD) Report on case study from previous study.
  (AD) Literature review of clinical and experimental studies. (ENG)

199

Progressive high frequency hearing loss due to parenteral, intramuscular, administration of 500 mg twice a day of antibiotic, kanamycin, in 1 human, aged, male, with diabetes mellitus, vascular disorder, and osteomyelitis.
  (AD) Hearing loss confirmed by audiogram.
  (AD) Report on clinical use and toxicity of antibiotics. (ENG)

223

Sensorineural hearing loss due to antibiotic, kanamycin, in 1 human, adult, female.
  (AD) Claim of negligence in treatment with kanamycin. (JAP)

267

Degeneration of outer hair cells of organ of Corti and damage to spiral ganglion due to 400 mg per kg daily of antibiotic, kanamycin, for 14 days in animals, guinea pigs.
Permanent histological changes in cochlea due to 100 mg per kg of antibiotic, kanamycin, in animals, guinea pigs.
Damage to organ of Corti of fetuses due to 200 mg per kg of antibiotic, kanamycin, in animals, guinea pigs, treated during pregnancy.
  (AD) Report on previous results of experimentation.
Cochleotoxic effects due to antibiotic, kanamycin, in average of 30 percent of more than 1000 humans, adult.
  (AD) Discussion of relationship between kanamycin ototoxicity and dosage, duration of treatment, age, previous auditory system problems, administration of other ototoxic drugs, kidney function, and individual responses to drug. (ENG)

268

Hearing loss due to antibiotic, kanamycin, in humans, adult.
   (AD) Discussion on incidence of hearing loss due to kanamycin, correlation
   between blood levels and ototoxicity, and relationship between kidney
   function and cochleotoxic effects. (ENG)

309

Bilateral sensorineural hearing loss and tinnitus, tinnitus only, or vertigo
due to parenteral, intramuscular, administration of 1 g daily in 2 doses or
15 mg per kg, total doses of 6 to 9 g, of antibiotic, kanamycin, for 6 to 9
days in 5 of 17 humans, adult and aged, female and male, with genitourinary
system infections and normal kidney function.
Bilateral sensorineural hearing loss, tinnitus, and vertigo due to parenteral, intramuscular, administration of less than normal dosage of antibiotic, kanamycin, for 6 to 9 days in 2 of 17 humans, adult, male and female,
with genitourinary system infections and kidney disorder.
   (CT) Pure tone audiometry, pretreatment, during treatment, and posttreatment.
   (AD) Discussion of case reports.
   (AD) Prospective study to determine clinical effectiveness of kanamycin in
   genitourinary system infections. (ENG)

393

Severe hearing loss due to parenteral administration of 1 to 2 g daily, total
doses of 30, 40, 21, and 4 g, of antibiotic, kanamycin, in 4 humans, adult,
53, 20, 32, and 37 years age, female and male, with kidney disorders.
   (AD) Case reports of cochleotoxic effects of kanamycin in humans with
   kidney disorders. (ENG)

618

Hearing loss due to parenteral, intramuscular, administration of 2 g in 2
doses, twice weekly, of antibiotic, kanamycin, in 7(1.1 percent) of 608
humans with pulmonary tuberculosis.
   (AD) Relationship between hearing loss and total dosage of kanamycin.
No hearing loss due to parenteral, intravenous, administration of 1 g twice
weekly, dissolved in 300 ml of saline solution, of antibiotic, kanamycin, for
long period in 1 human, adult, 40 years age, male, with pulmonary tuberculosis.
   (AD) Cochlear function monitored by audiometry during therapy.
   (AD) Higher blood levels of kanamycin with intravenous route than with
   intramuscular route. (ENG)

692

Bilateral sensorineural hearing loss possibly due to topical, direct site,
administration in vertebral canal of 500 mg, in 2 cc water, of antibiotic,
kanamycin (kanamycin sulfate), in 1 dose in 1 human, aged, 67 years age,
male, with previous hearing loss, during surgery for lumbar disc.
   (AD) Case report of hearing loss possibly due to kanamycin.
   (AD) Hearing loss confirmed by audiometry.
   (AD) Neurotoxic effects resulted from kanamycin administration. (ENG)

078

Transient acute vertigo and nystagmus due to sufficient doses to produce 122
mcg per 100 ml blood level and 115 mcg per 24 hours urine level of heavy
metal, lead, in 1 human, adult, 55 years age, male.
Transient acute vertigo and nystagmus due to oral ingestion of total of about
0.606 to 1.15 mg daily of heavy metal, lead, in 1 human, adult, 41 years age,
male. (ENG)

691

Vertigo due to oral administration in tablets of 300 to 2400 mg daily of
heavy metal, lithium (lithium carbonate), for 1 to 30 months in some of 91
humans, adult and aged, 20 to 73 years age, male and female, with psychologi-
cal disorders. (ENG)

465

Hearing loss, nystagmus, and vertigo due to heavy metal, mercury, organic, in
humans, adolescent, adult, and aged.
   (AD) Auditory system problems confirmed by audiology and vestibular func-

tion tests.   (JAP)

                                                                    696
Dizziness due   to heavy metal, mercury (inorganic mercury), in 1 month to 38
years exposure in 1 of 154 humans, adolescent and adult, 18 to 62 years age,
during work in industry.
   (AD)   Report on 10 years study of exposure to mercury (inorganic mercury).
   (ENG)

                                                                    104
Hearing loss due to 1.5 g daily, total of 12 g, of antibiotic, neomycin, in 1
human, aged, 90 years age.
   (AD) Cochleotoxic effect due to negligence of physician.   (SW)

                                                                    150
Total sensorineural hearing loss due to topical administration by irrigation
of mediastinum with 2400 ml per 24 hours, total of 72 g, of 0.3 percent
solution of antibiotic, neomycin, for 11 days in 1 human, adult, 60 years
age, male, with purulent mediastinitis.
   (AD) High serum neomycin concentrations decr by hemodialysis.   (ENG)

                                                                    231
No hearing loss due to 8 g and then 12 g daily of antibiotic, neomycin
(neomycin sulfate), for total of 19 months in 1 human, adult, 48 years age,
male, chronic alcoholic, treated for infections.   (ENG)

                                                                    498
Severe hearing loss 8 days after first dose due to oral administration of 7 g
on first day followed by 4 g on second day, total dose of 11 g, of antibio-
tic, neomycin, for total of 2 days in 1 human, adult, 45 years age, female,
treated before surgery.
   (AD) Case report of severe hearing loss due to neomycin therapy.
   (AD) Hearing clinically normal before neomycin treatment.
   (AD) Audiometry 1.5 years later confirmed auditory system problem.   (ENG)

                                                                    138
Sensorineural hearing loss due to antiparasitic, oil of chenopodium, in 1
human, adult, 56 years age, male.
   (AD) Hearing loss confirmed by audiograms.   (POL)

                                                                    292
Cochlear   impairment due to parenteral, intramuscular, administration of 1.2,
10, or 1 ml of antibiotic, penicillin (procaine penicillin G), in humans,
adult, with various infections.
   (AD) Discussion of 3 case reports.   (SL)

                                                                    682
Possible dizziness and ataxia due to high blood levels of over 5 mcg per ml
of antibiotic, polymyxin B, in humans, adult.
   (AD) Discussion of clinical pharmacology, dosage, toxic effects, and use
   in therapy of polymyxins.   (ENG)

                                                                    552
Tinnitus within several hours due to 10 mg twice daily of cardiovascular
agent, propranolol, for 4 days in 1 human, adult, 56 years age, female, with
mild hypertension.
   (AD) Case report of tinnitus for duration of dosage of 10 mg twice daily
   of propranolol.
   (AD) Cessation of tinnitus after decr in dosage to 10 mg daily of propranolol.   (ENG)

                                                                    366
Possible auditory system problems due to cardiovascular agent, quinidine, in
humans.
No ototoxic effects due to 2.40 to 9.00 g of cardiovascular agent, quinidine,
in 150 humans, adolescent and adult, male and female, with auricular fibril-
lation.
   (AD) Other toxic effects in 46 of 150 humans but no ototoxic effects

reported. (SP)

239

Transient sensorineural hearing loss due to oral ingestion in tablets of 3 to 5 g (10 to 15 tablets) of antimalarial, quinine, in 1 human, adult, 26 years age, male, with alcohol intoxication.
(AD) Case of attempted suicide.
(AD) Hearing loss confirmed by audiogram. (GER)

607

Transient tinnitus and hearing loss after 2 hours due to oral ingestion of 6 g of antimalarial, quinine (quinine sulfate), in 1 dose in 1 human, adult, 26 years age, female, in suicide attempt.
Transient tinnitus and sensorineural hearing loss within 5 hours due to oral ingestion of 12 g, to produce serum level of 9.2 mg per l, of antimalarial, quinine (quinine sulfate), in 1 human, adult, 24 years age, female, during pregnancy in attempt to induce abortion. (ENG)

174

Transient high frequency hearing loss and tinnitus after 4 hours due to oral administration of 1 g daily of antidiabetic, (SQ) R94, for 28 days at most in 26 humans, adolescent and adult, 15 to 55 years age, male, with moderate to severe diabetes.
Incr in high frequency hearing loss due to oral administration of 1 g of antidiabetic, (SQ) R94, for 7 days after onset of hearing loss in 9 of 26 humans, adolescent and adult, 15 to 55 years age, male, with moderate to severe diabetes.
Decr and complete reversal of hearing loss due to oral administration of 1 g of antidiabetic, (SQ) R94 (IB), in 15 of 26 humans, adolescent and adult, 15 to 55 years age, male, with moderate to severe diabetes, with administration of 100 and 200 mg of nicotinic acid.
(AD) Reversal of hearing loss after cessation of treatment with R94 or with administration of nicotinic acid.
(CT) Use of subjects with no recent treatment with ototoxic drugs.
(CT) Audiometry, pretreatment and 4 hours after every daily dose.
(AD) Vestibular function tests normal. (ENG)

626

Transient hearing loss during therapy due to 300 mg 3 times a day of antibiotic, rifampicin, for 14 days in 2 of 27 humans, adult and aged, 20 to 79 years age, female and male, with genitourinary system infections. (ENG)

024

Suppression of semicircular canal function due to parenteral administration of range of 22.5 to 54 g, total doses, of antibiotic, streptomycin (streptomycin sulfate), for range of 7.5 to 26 days in 4 humans, adult, male and female, treated for Meniere's disease.
(AD) Use of ototoxic effect of streptomycin in treatment of Meniere's disease. (ENG)

040

Sensorineural hearing loss due to parenteral, intramuscular, administration of 1 g twice a week of antibiotic, streptomycin (streptomycin sulfate), for 335 days in 1 human, adult, 63 years age, male, with bone tuberculosis.
(AD) Pretreatment hearing loss reported.
Sensorineural hearing loss due to parenteral, intramuscular, administration of 0.5 g twice a week of antibiotic, streptomycin (streptomycin sulfate), for 333 days in 1 human, child, 3 years age, with bone tuberculosis. (ENG)

211

Severe and slight vertigo due to total of 29 to 57 g of antibiotic, streptomycin, for long period in 14 of 180 humans, adult, 50 years or less age, male, with pneumoconiosis. (ENG)

347

Delayed hearing loss at 2 different times due to 15 g each time of antibiotic, streptomycin, in 1 human, child, male, treated at 8 years age for rheumatism and at 13 years age for pneumonia.

(AD) Similar audiograms after 2 periods of treatment.
Delayed hearing loss due to 6 and 8 g of antibiotic, streptomycin, in 2 humans, adult and child, female, mother and daughter.
Delayed hearing loss due to 6 and 5 g of antibiotic, streptomycin, in 2 humans, adult, 34 and 36 years age, female, sisters.
Delayed hearing loss due to 10 and 8 g of antibiotic, streptomycin, in 2 humans, adult, 23 and 24 years age, female, sisters.
Sensorineural hearing loss due to 10 and 4 g of antibiotic, streptomycin, in 3 humans, female, sisters.
Delayed hearing loss due to low doses of antibiotic, streptomycin, in 3 humans, adult and child, 50, 26, and 8 years age, female, mother, daughter, and granddaughter.
   (AD) Suggested familial and constitutional predisposition in streptomycin ototoxicity. (FR)

                                                                       399
Risk of vestibular problems due to antibiotic, streptomycin, in humans, adult, with tuberculous meningitis.
   (AD) Report on treatment of meningitis and possible toxic effects of drugs used. (GER)

                                                                       403
Risk of damage to function of eighth cranial nerve due to antibiotic, streptomycin, for long period in humans, adult and child, with tuberculous meningitis.
   (AD) Need for tests of function of eighth cranial nerve with clinical use of streptomycin.
   (AD) Literature review of treatment of infections of CNS. (ENG)

                                                                       421
Damage to cochlear function and vestibular function due to antibiotic, streptomycin, in humans, adult, with tuberculosis. (RUS)

                                                                       449
Vertigo due to antibiotic, streptomycin, in 1 human, adult, female. (JAP)

                                                                       452
Hearing loss due to 0.5 g daily, total of 30 to 50 g, of antibiotic, streptomycin, in some of 187 humans, child, adolescent, and adult, 12 to 20 years age, with tuberculosis.
   (AD) Audiogram confirmed hearing loss.
   (AD) Inclusion of 3 case reports. (HUN)

                                                                       453
Damage to vestibular function due to antibiotic, streptomycin, in 2 humans, adult, 20 and 60 years age, male, with tuberculosis.
   (AD) Vestibular problem confirmed by vestibular function tests.
   (AD) Discussion of restoration of vestibular function after damage due to streptomycin therapy. (GER)

                                                                       534
Dizziness within 6 weeks due to parenteral, intramuscular, administration of 0.75 g daily of antibiotic, streptomycin, in 8 (31 percent) of 27 humans, child, adult, and aged, 12 to 76 years age, female and male, 34 to 89 kg weight, with tuberculosis.
   (AD) Use of vestibular function tests in patients reporting dizziness.
   (AD) Study showed significant relationship between higher 24 hour serum levels and dizziness.
   (AD) Suggested decr in dosage when serum streptomycin more than 3 mcg per ml at 24 hours.
   (AD) More risk of vestibulotoxic effects due to streptomycin in patients over 45 years age. (ENG)

                                                                       416
Delayed unilateral sensorineural hearing loss and vestibular problems detected 22 years after treatment due to heavy metal, thorium dioxide, in 1 human, adult, 36 years age when treated, female, during roentgenography.
Delayed tinnitus, unilateral sensorineural hearing loss, and damage to vesti-

bular function detected 21 years after treatment due to heavy metal, thorium
dioxide, in 1 human, adult, 36 years age when treated, male, during roentgenography.
   (AD) Cochleo-vestibulotoxic effects of thorium dioxide confirmed by audiology and vestibular function tests.
   (AD) Case reports of delayed ototoxic effects of thorium dioxide. (ENG)

                                                                         010
Permanent sensorineural hearing loss due to parenteral, intramuscular, administration of low doses, less than 2 g, of antibiotic, (SQ) kanamycin
(kanamycin sulfate), for short period in 5 humans, adult, range of 33 to 47
years age, range of 90 to 177 lb weight, with kidney disorder.
Permanent sensorineural hearing loss due to parenteral, intramuscular, administration of low doses, less than 2 g, of antibiotic, (SQ) streptomycin,
for short period in 5 humans, adult, range of 33 to 47 years age, range of 90
to 177 lb weight, with kidney disorder.
Permanent sensorineural hearing loss due to parenteral, intramuscular, administration of low doses, less than 2 g, of antibiotic, (SQ) neomycin, for
short period in 5 humans, adult, range of 33 to 47 years age, range of 90 to
177 lb weight, with kidney disorder.
Permanent sensorineural hearing loss due to parenteral, intramuscular, administration of low doses, less than 2 g, of diuretic, (SQ) ethacrynic acid,
for short period in 5 humans, adult, range of 33 to 47 years age, range of 90
to 177 lb weight, with kidney disorder.
   (AD) Study of cochleotoxic effects of kanamycin with other antibiotics and
   with ethacrynic acid. (ENG)

                                                                         016
Progressive bilateral sensorineural hearing loss and vertigo due to unspecified method of administration of total of 3 g of antibiotic, (SQ) streptomycin (SM), for unspecified period in 1 human, Caucasian, adult, 32 years age,
male, with kidney disorder and on intermittent hemodialysis.
Progressive bilateral sensorineural hearing loss and vertigo due to unspecified method of administration of antibiotic, (SQ) colistin (SM), for unspecified period in 1 human, Caucasian, adult, 32 years age, male, with kidney
disorder and on intermittent hemodialysis.
Permanent sensorineural hearing loss due to parenteral, intravenous, administration of 1.6 mg per kg 2 times daily, total of 500 mg of antibiotic, (SQ)
gentamicin, for unspecified period in 1 human, Caucasian, adult, 32 years
age, male, with kidney disorder and on intermittent hemodialysis.
No definite ototoxic effects reported due to unspecified method of administration of 1 g every 2 weeks, total of 12 g, of antibiotic, (SQ) vancomycin,
for about 6 months in 1 human, Caucasian, adult, 32 years age, male, with
kidney disorder and on intermittent hemodialysis.
   (AD) Hearing loss due to streptomycin and colistin potentiated by gentamicin. (ENG)

                                                                         018
Hearing loss due to parenteral administration of low doses, 1 g daily, of
antibiotic, (SQ) streptomycin, in 3 injections in 1 human, adult, 22 years
age, male, with pulmonary tuberculosis.
Unspecified effects due to previous administration of 3 unspecified doses of
antimalarial, (SQ) quinine, in 1 human, adult, 22 years age, male, with
pulmonary tuberculosis. (ENG)

                                                                         019
Progressive severe sensorineural hearing loss and tinnitus due to unspecified
method of administration of 0.5 g twice daily, total of 16 g, of antibiotic,
kanamycin, for 16 days in 1 human, Caucasian, adult, 25 years age, male, with
kidney disorder and treated with peritoneal dialysis.
   (AD) Audiograms showed hearing loss and recruitment test showed reversed
   recruitment.
Severe sensorineural hearing loss due to unspecified method of administration
of 0.5 g daily for 40 days and then 0.5 g 3 times a week for 3 weeks of
antibiotic, streptomycin, for total period of about 9 weeks in 1 human,
Negro, child, 9 years age, male, with pulmonary tuberculosis and kidney
disorder.
   (AD) No record of hearing loss before treatment with streptomycin.

Delayed severe bilateral high frequency hearing loss due to unspecified
method of administration of 0.5 g daily for 8 months and then 0.5 g every 3
days for 4 months, followed by a break of 3.5 months, and then 0.5 g every 3
days for 1.5 months, total of 153 g of antibiotic, dihydrostreptomycin, for
total period of about 13.5 months in 1 human, Negro, infant, 16 months age,
female, with tuberculosis.
    (AD) Hearing loss detected at 13 years age.
Hearing loss and tinnitus due to unspecified method of administration of 1 g
daily of antibiotic, streptomycin, for 10 weeks and possibly for a longer
period after discharge in 1 human, Negro, adult, 23 years age, male, treated
for infection in tuberculosis hospital.
    (AD) Hearing loss detected 1 month after treatment with streptomycin.
Progressive severe sensorineural hearing loss due to unspecified method of
administration of 0.5 g 3 times a week, total of 61 g of antibiotic, streptomycin, for about 10 months in 1 human, Negro, child, 9 years age, female,
with pulmonary tuberculosis.
    (AD) Discussion of 5 case reports. (ENG)

                                                                        027
Progressive bilateral high frequency hearing loss and tinnitus due to topical
administration by irrigation of wound with 80 ml every 4 hours for 2 weeks
and then 40 ml every 4 hours of 0.5 percent solution of antibiotic, (SQ)
neomycin (SM), in 1 human, adult, 24 years age, male, paraplegic, with infection of ulcer of left hip.
Progressive bilateral high frequency hearing loss and tinnitus due to topical
administration by irrigation of wound with 80 ml every 4 hours for 2 weeks
and then 40 ml every 4 hours of 0.1 percent solution of antibiotic, (SQ)
polymyxin B (SM), in 1 human, adult, 24 years age, male, paraplegic, with
infection of ulcer of left hip.
No reported ototoxic effects due to unspecified method of administration of 1
g daily of antibiotic, (SQ) streptomycin, for 5 days in 1 human, adult, 24
years age, male, paraplegic, with infection of ulcer of left hip. (ENG)

                                                                        028
Bilateral sensorineural hearing loss and tinnitus due to parenteral, intravenous, administration of 100 mg of diuretic, ethacrynic acid (SM), in 2
doses in 1 human, adult, 24 years age, male, with kidney disorder.
Bilateral sensorineural hearing loss and tinnitus due to parenteral, intravenous, administration of 4 g of antibiotic, streptomycin (SM), for 5 days in
1 human, adult, 24 years age, male, with kidney disorder.
Bilateral sensorineural hearing loss due to parenteral, intravenous, administration of 500 mg of diuretic, ethacrynic acid (SM), for 4 days in 1 human,
adult, 35 years age, female, with kidney disorder.
Bilateral sensorineural hearing loss due to parenteral, intravenous, administration of 1.5 g of antibiotic, streptomycin (SM), for 4 days in 1 human,
adult, 35 years age, female, with kidney disorder.
Permanent hearing loss due to parenteral, intravenous, administration of 200
mg of diuretic, ethacrynic acid, in humans. (ENG)

                                                                        038
Bilateral sensorineural hearing loss due to oral administration of 200 mg
twice a day of diuretic, (SQ) ethacrynic acid, for several weeks in 1 human,
adult, 40 years age, female, with kidney disorder.
Previous oral administration of 40 mg daily of diuretic, (SQ) furosemide
(SM), for unspecified period in 1 human, adult, 40 years age, female, with
kidney disorder.
Previous oral administration of 500 mg daily of diuretic, (SQ) chlorothiazide
(SM), for unspecified period in 1 human, adult, 40 years age, female, with
kidney disorder.
Sensorineural hearing loss and unsteady gait due to parenteral, intravenous,
administration of 200 mg of diuretic, (SQ) ethacrynic acid (SM), for unspeci-
fied period in 1 human, adult, 20 years age, female, with kidney disorder.
Simultaneous parenteral, intravenous, administration of 25 g of diuretic,
(SQ) mannitol (SM), for unspecified period in 1 human, adult, 20 years age,
female, with kidney disorder.
Previous administration of unspecified dose of chemical agent, (SQ) carbon
tetrachloride, for unspecified period in 1 human, adult, 20 years age, female, with kidney disorder.

Transient sensorineural hearing loss due to parenteral, intravenous, administration of 800 mg daily of diuretic, ethacrynic acid (SM), for unspecified
period in 1 human, adult, 25 years age, female, with chronic kidney disorder.
Simultaneous administration of unspecified doses of diuretic, chlorothiazide
(SM), for unspecified period in 1 human, adult, 25 years age, female, with
chronic kidney disorder.
Simultaneous administration of unspecified doses of diuretic, mannitol (SM),
for unspecified period in 1 human, adult, 25 years age, female, with chronic
kidney disorder.
Transient sensorineural hearing loss and dizziness due to parenteral, (SQ)
intravenous, administration of unspecified doses of diuretic, ethacrynic
acid, for unspecified period in 1 human, adult, 52 years age, female, with
kidney disorder.
Transient sensorineural hearing loss and dizziness due to (SQ) oral administration of 300 mg of diuretic, ethacrynic acid, for unspecified period in 1
human, adult, 52 years age, female, with kidney disorder.
Sensorineural hearing loss due to oral administration of 20 mg 3 times daily
of diuretic, ethacrynic acid, for 3 days in 1 human, adult, 28 years age,
male, with kidney disorder.
   (AD) Discussion of 5 case reports of ototoxic effects due to treatment
   with ethacrynic acid. (ENG)

                                                                          042
Transient bilateral sensorineural hearing loss due to parenteral, intravenous, administration of 50 mg of diuretic, (SQ) ethacrynic acid, in 1
injection in 1 human, adult, 45 years age, female, with lymphosarcoma and
with normal kidney function.
   (AD) Hearing loss reported 15 minutes after treatment with ethacrynic
   acid.
Previous parenteral, intramuscular, administration of 60 mg every 6 hours of
antibiotic, (SQ) gentamicin (gentamicin sulfate), for unspecified period in 1
human, adult, 45 years age, female, with lymphosarcoma and with normal kidney
function.
Bilateral sensorineural hearing loss due to parenteral, intravenous, administration of 100 mg of diuretic, (SQ) ethacrynic acid, in 2 injections of 50 mg
each 6 hours apart in 1 human, adult, 64 years age, female, with acute leukemia and with normal kidney function.
   (AD) Histological study after death showed no damage to inner ear.
Previous unspecified method of administration of unspecified dose of antibiotic, (SQ) polymyxin B (polymyxin B sulfate), in 1 human, adult, 64 years age,
female, with acute leukemia and with normal kidney function.
Previous parenteral, intramuscular, administration of 0.5 g every 12 hours of
antibiotic, (SQ) kanamycin (kanamycin sulfate), for unspecified period in 1
human, adult, 64 years age, female, with acute leukemia and with normal
kidney function.
   (AD) Suggested that hearing loss due to combined action of ethacrynic acid
   and antibiotics. (ENG)

                                                                          051
Progressive permanent sensorineural hearing loss and tinnitus due to topical
administration to joint of left knee and parenteral, intramuscular, administration of high doses, total of 42.5 g, of antibiotic, (SQ) neomycin, for
long period, 19 days, in 1 human, adult, with infection of left knee.
Previous administration of high doses of antibiotic, (SQ) chloramphenicol,
for unspecified period in 1 human, adult, with infection of left knee.
   (AD) Report of case in court with claim of negligence for administration
   of high doses of neomycin that resulted in hearing loss. (ENG)

                                                                          055
Transient bilateral sensorineural hearing loss and tinnitus due to parenteral, intravenous, administration of 100 mg of diuretic, (SQ) ethacrynic
acid, in 1 injection in 1 human, adult, 64 years age, male, with kidney
disorder.
   (CT) Pretreatment audiology showed no auditory system problems.
   (AD) Hearing loss 5 minutes after administration of ethacrynic acid.
Previous parenteral, intravenous, administration of unspecified doses of
diuretic, (SQ) furosemide, for unspecified period in 1 human, adult, 64 years
age, male, with kidney disorder. (ENG)

059
Bilateral sensorineural hearing loss due to oral administration of 0 to 12 g daily, total of 2500 g, of antibiotic, neomycin, for 16 months in 1 human, Caucasian, adult, 49 years age, female, chronic alcoholic, with hepatic encephalopathy and normal kidney function.
Bilateral sensorineural hearing loss due to oral administration of 0 to 4 g daily, total of 800 g, of antibiotic, (SQ) neomycin, for 21 months in 1 human, Caucasian, adult, 47 years age, female, chronic alcoholic, with hepatic encephalopathy and normal kidney function.
More severe sensorineural hearing loss due to oral administration of 6 g daily, total of 111 g, of antibiotic, (SQ) paromomycin, for 9 months in 1 human, Caucasian, adult, 47 years age, female, chronic alcoholic, with hepatic encephalopathy and normal kidney function.
Sensorineural hearing loss due to oral administration of 0 to 12 g daily, total of 1500 g, of antibiotic, neomycin, for 11 months in 1 human, Caucasian, adult, 39 years age, female, chronic alcoholic, with hepatic encephalopathy and some kidney disorder.
Sensorineural hearing loss in right ear due to oral administration of 3 to 4 g daily, total of 500 g, of antibiotic, (SQ) neomycin, for 8 months in 1 human, Caucasian, aged, 66 years age, female, with hepatic encephalopathy and kidney disorder.
    (AD) Tinnitus and sudden deafness in left ear 27 years earlier.
Sensorineural hearing loss in right ear due to oral administration of total of 240 g of antibiotic, (SQ) paromomycin, for long period in 1 human, Caucasian, aged, 66 years age, female, with hepatic encephalopathy and kidney disorder.
Sequential administration of unspecified doses of diuretic, (SQ) furosemide, for unspecified period in 1 human, Caucasian, aged, 66 years age, female, with hepatic encephalopathy and kidney disorder.
Bilateral sensorineural hearing loss due to oral administration of 0 to 12 g daily, total of 1000 to 1500 g, of antibiotic, (SQ) neomycin, for 28 months in 1 human, Caucasian, adult, 60 years age, male, chronic alcoholic, with hepatic encephalopathy and kidney disorder.
Bilateral sensorineural hearing loss due to oral administration of total of 300 g of antibiotic, (SQ) paromomycin, for long period in 1 human, Caucasian, adult, 60 years age, male, chronic alcoholic, with hepatic encephalopathy and kidney disorder.
Sequential administration of unspecified doses of (SQ) diuretics for unspecified period in 1 human, Caucasian, adult, 60 years age, male, chronic alcoholic, with hepatic encephalopathy and kidney disorder.
    (AD) Discussion of 5 case reports of hearing loss due to antibiotic therapy.
    (AD) Audiograms confirmed hearing loss in all cases. (ENG)

063
Progressive permanent bilateral sensorineural hearing loss due to topical administration by irrigation of wound with 1000 ml of 1 percent solution (6.5 g) of antibiotic, neomycin (CB) (neomycin sulfate), in 1 administration in 1 human, Caucasian, adolescent, 18 years age, male, with gunshot wound of abdomen.
    (AD) Hearing loss reported 21 days after treatment.
Progressive permanent bilateral sensorineural hearing loss due to topical administration by irrigation of wound with 1000 ml of 0.1 percent solution (650 mg) of antibiotic, polymyxin B (CB) (polymyxin B sulfate), in 1 administration in 1 human, Caucasian, adolescent, 18 years age, male, with gunshot wound of abdomen.
    (AD) Study reported that ototoxic effects only due to neomycin.
    (AD) Hemodialysis 24 hours after treatment for prevention of hearing loss not satisfactory.
Progressive permanent bilateral sensorineural hearing loss due to topical administration by irrigation of wound with high doses of 1 percent solution of antibiotic, (SQ) neomycin, for 22 days in 1 human, Caucasian, adult, 20 years age, male, with gunshot wounds.
    (AD) Hearing loss reported after 19 days of treatment.
Previous administration of unspecified dose of antibiotic, (SQ) streptomycin, for 6 days in 1 human, Caucasian, adult, 20 years age, male, with gunshot wounds.
Progressive permanent bilateral sensorineural hearing loss due to topical

administration by irrigation of wound with total of 4000 ml of 1 percent
solution of antibiotic, neomycin (CB) (neomycin sulfate), in 4 days in 1
human, Caucasian, adult, 39 years age, male, with wounds.
  (AD) Hearing loss reported within 5 days.
Progressive permanent bilateral sensorineural hearing loss due to topical
administration by irrigation of wound with total of 4000 ml of 0.1 percent
solution of antibiotic, polymyxin B (CB) (polymyxin B sulfate), in 4 days in
1 human, Caucasian, adult, 39 years age, male, with wounds.
    (AD) Discussion of 3 case reports of hearing loss due to topical adminis-
    tration of antibiotics. (ENG)

                                                                      076
Ototoxic effects due to parenteral, intramuscular, administration of 1 g
daily of antibiotic, capreomycin (SM), for 9 months in 4 of 65 humans, adult
and aged, range of 20 to 70 years age, male and female, with pulmonary tuberculosis.
Simultaneous administration of ethambutol (SM) in 65 humans, adult and aged,
range of 20 to 70 years age, male and female, with pulmonary tuberculosis.
Simultaneous administration of antibiotic, rifampicin (SM), in 65 humans,
adult and aged, range of 20 to 70 years age, male and female, with pulmonary
tuberculosis. (ENG)

                                                                      080
Hearing loss and vertigo due to parenteral administration of antibiotic,
streptomycin, in humans, child and adult, with normal kidney function and
with kidney disorder.
  (AD) Suggested use for severe infections only.
Delayed permanent hearing loss due to antibiotic, dihydrostreptomycin, in
humans.
  (AD) High risk of ototoxic effects with clinical use.
Hearing loss due to oral administration of antibiotic, paromomycin, in hu-
mans.
Progressive permanent hearing loss and tinnitus due to parenteral administra-
tion of antibiotic, kanamycin, in humans.
Progressive permanent hearing loss and tinnitus due to parenteral and topical
administration of antibiotic, neomycin, in humans.
  (AD) Need for careful consideration in use of paromomycin, kanamycin, and
  neomycin due to potential ototoxicity.
  (AD) Discussion of ototoxic effects of 5 antibiotics. (ENG)

                                                                      087
High frequency hearing loss and tinnitus due to antibiotics in humans, parti-
cularly infant and aged, and humans with kidney disorder.
Degeneration in hair cells of organ of Corti due to antibiotics in humans.
Vertigo and unsteady gait due to antibiotic, streptomycin, in humans.
Bilateral damage to vestibular apparatus due to antibiotic, streptomycin, in
humans.
  (AD) Literature review of physiological and structural cochleo-vestibulo-
  toxic effects of antibiotics.
  (AD) Degree of damage determined by dosage and duration of dosage of
  antibiotics. (ENG)

                                                                      089
Sudden deafness due to parenteral, intravenous, administration of 100 mg, in
100 ml saline solution, of diuretic, (SQ) ethacrynic acid, in 1 injection in
1 human, adult, 42 years age, female, quadriplegic, with kidney disorder.
Previous administration of unspecified dose of antibiotic, (SQ) chloramphenicol, for unspecified period in 1 human, adult, 42 years age, female, quadriplegic, with kidney disorder.
Previous administration of 1 g of antibiotic, (SQ) kanamycin, for unspecified
period in 1 human, adult, 42 years age, female, quadriplegic, with kidney
disorder and genitourinary system infection. (ENG)

                                                                      090
Tinnitus and vertigo due to unspecified method of administration of 0.75 g
daily of antibiotic, (SQ) streptomycin (SM), for 5 weeks in 1 human, adult,
38 years age, female, with pulmonary tuberculosis.
Simultaneous administration of antituberculous agent, (SQ) PAS (SM), in 1

human, adult, 38 years age, female, with pulmonary tuberculosis.
Simultaneous administration of antituberculous agent, (SQ) isoniazid (SM), in
1 human, adult, 38 years age, female, with pulmonary tuberculosis.
No reported ototoxic effects due to unspecified method of administration of
150 mg daily of antituberculous agent, (SQ) thiacetazone, for 11 months in 1
human, adult, 38 years age, female, with pulmonary tuberculosis.
    (AD) Hemolytic disease due to treatment with thiacetazone. (ENG)

103

Cochleo-vestibulotoxic effects due to range of less than 50 g to 300 g of
antibiotic, streptomycin (SM) (streptomycin sulfate), for 6 to 8 months in
humans, adult, with tuberculous meningitis.
Simultaneous administration of antituberculous agent, PAS (SM), in humans,
adult, with tuberculous meningitis.
Simultaneous administration of antituberculous agent, isoniazid (SM), in
humans, adult, with tuberculous meningitis.
    (AD) Follow up study after average of 7 years.   (GER)

118

Nystagmus and unsteady gait due to unspecified doses of antibiotics (SM) in 1
human, adult, 47 years age, male, with epilepsy.
Simultaneous administration of anticonvulsant, primidone (SM), in 1 human,
adult, 47 years age, male, with epilepsy.
Simultaneous administration of antihistamine, dimenhydrinate (SM), in 1
human, adult, 47 years age, male, with epilepsy. (ENG)

140

Total bilateral sensorineural hearing loss due to 40 mg daily, total of 1.80
g, of antibiotic, gentamicin, for 45 days in 1 human, aged, 69 years age,
female, with kidney disorder.
    (AD) Hearing loss confirmed by audiogram.
Sensorineural hearing loss due to parenteral administration of 40 mg in 2
injections daily, total of 480 mg, of antibiotic, gentamicin (SM), in 1
human, aged, 65 years age, male.
Simultaneous administration of antibiotic, transcycline (SM), in 1 human,
aged, 65 years age, male.
Simultaneous administration of antibiotic, colistin (SM) (colistimethate), in
1 human, aged, 65 years age, male.
Sensorineural hearing loss due to 40 mg daily, total of 0.84 g, of antibiotic, gentamicin, for 21 days in 1 human, adult, 50 years age, male, with
normal kidney function.
    (AD) Hearing loss confirmed by audiogram.
    (AD) Discussion of 3 case reports of gentamicin ototoxicity. (FR)

141

Total bilateral sensorineural hearing loss, tinnitus, and vestibular problems
due to 120 mg daily, total of 1.2 g, of antibiotic, gentamicin (SM), for 10
days in 1 human, adult, 22 years age, female, 46 kg weight, with purulent
pleurisy after surgery.
Total bilateral sensorineural hearing loss, tinnitus, and vestibular problems
due to 1 g every 2 days, total of 9 g, of antibiotic, kanamycin (SM), for 18
days in 1 human, adult, 22 years age, female, 46 kg weight, with purulent
pleurisy after surgery.
Total bilateral sensorineural hearing loss and vestibular problems due to
high doses, 160 mg daily, of antibiotic, gentamicin, for long period, 47
days, in 1 human, adult, 35 years age, with pleurisy.
Total bilateral sensorineural hearing loss and vestibular problems due to 1 g
every 2 days of antibiotic, kanamycin, for 26 days in 1 human, adult, 35
years age, with pleurisy.
Total bilateral sensorineural hearing loss and vestibular problems due to 160
mg daily of antibiotic, gentamicin (SM), for 12 days in 1 human, adult, 35
years age, with pleurisy.
Total bilateral sensorineural hearing loss and vestibular problems due to 1 g
every 2 days of antibiotic, kanamycin (SM), for 12 days in 1 human, adult, 35
years age, with pleurisy.
    (AD) Hearing loss confirmed by audiogram.
    (AD) Discussion of 2 case reports of gentamicin ototoxicity. (FR)

158

No reported ototoxic effects due to 5 g of antibiotic, (SQ) streptomycin, in 1 human, adult, 63 years age, male, with bronchopleural fistula and staphylococcal empyema.
Progressive total bilateral sensorineural hearing loss due to topical administration by irrigation of empyema cavity with (SQ) 1200 ml of 1 percent solution of antibiotic, (SQ) neomycin, for 10 days, total of 33 irrigations, in 1 human, adult, 63 years age, male, with bronchopleural fistula and staphylococcal empyema.
Progressive total bilateral sensorineural hearing loss due to topical administration by irrigation of empyema cavity with (SQ) 700 ml of 1 percent solution, total of 403 g in all, of antibiotic, (SQ) neomycin, in 1 administration in 1 human, adult, 63 years age, male, at time of surgery to close cavity.
Sequential parenteral, intramuscular, administration of total of 4 g of antibiotic, (SQ) streptomycin (streptomycin sulfate), for 4 to 5 days in 1 human, adult, 63 years age, male, after closure of empyema cavity.
(AD) No hearing loss before closure of cavity.
(AD) Hearing loss confirmed by audiogram but no vestibular problems detected by vestibular function tests.
(AD) Suggested that hearing loss due to neomycin only and not to streptomycin. (ENG)

179

Progressive high frequency hearing loss and tinnitus due to 1 g daily of antibiotic, kanamycin, in 3 humans, adolescent and adult, male, with tuberculosis and with previous treatment with ototoxic drugs but with no report of toxic effects.
Less severe sensorineural hearing loss and no tinnitus due to 1 g 5 times a week of antibiotic, kanamycin, in 1 human, male, with tuberculosis and with previous treatment with ototoxic drugs.
Sensorineural hearing loss and tinnitus due to 6 g of antibiotic, kanamycin (SM), in 1 human, male, with tuberculosis and with previous treatment with ototoxic drugs.
Sensorineural hearing loss and tinnitus due to parenteral administration of 1000 mg per day of antibiotic, streptomycin (SM), in 1 human, male, with tuberculosis and with previous treatment with ototoxic drugs.
No high frequency hearing loss due to parenteral administration of 1 g daily of antibiotic, streptomycin, in 1 human, female, with tuberculosis and with previous treatment with ototoxic drugs.
High frequency hearing loss but no tinnitus due to 750 mg daily of antibiotic, streptomycin, in 1 human, female, with tuberculosis and with previous treatment with ototoxic drugs.
Simultaneous administration of range of doses of other antituberculous agents (SM) in total of 7 humans, adolescent and adult, 13 to 49 years age, male and female, with tuberculosis and with previous treatment with ototoxic drugs.
(AD) Study using high frequency audiometry and conventional audiometry.
(CT) Pretreatment audiograms obtained. (ENG)

196

Sensorineural hearing loss due to unspecified doses of antibiotic, streptomycin, in 8.9 percent of 2917 humans, child, adolescent, and adult, 10 to 34 years age, with pulmonary tuberculosis.
Sensorineural hearing loss due to unspecified doses of antibiotic, streptomycin (SM), in high percent of 608 humans, child, adolescent, and adult, 10 to 34 years age, with pulmonary tuberculosis.
Sensorineural hearing loss due to unspecified doses of antibiotic, kanamycin (SM), in high percent of 608 humans, child, adolescent, and adult, 10 to 34 years age, with pulmonary tuberculosis.
(CT) Study of 314 humans, control group, without pulmonary tuberculosis.
(CT) No subjective hearing loss before treatment with antibiotics.
(CT) Hearing loss after antibiotic treatment confirmed by audiometry.
(AD) Statistical analysis of 3525 cases with antibiotic therapy.
(AD) Highest incidence of hearing loss in 30 to 34 years age group.
(AD) Higher incidence of severe hearing loss in group treated with two antibiotics than in group treated with streptomycin only. (ENG)

Transient bilateral sensorineural hearing loss due to oral administration of
50 mg every 6 hours of diuretic, ethacrynic acid, for 4 days initially and
then again 2 weeks later for 2 days in 1 human, Negro, adult, 55 years age,
female, with diabetes mellitus and kidney disorder.
  (AD) Hearing loss confirmed by audiogram.
Transient sensorineural hearing loss and tinnitus due to (SQ) oral and parenteral, (SQ) intravenous, administration of 300,300,400, and 500 mg of diuretic, ethacrynic acid, in 4 doses in 1 human, Caucasian, adult, 40 years age,
female, with chronic kidney disorder.
No auditory system problems due to parenteral, intravenous, administration of
(SQ) unspecified doses of diuretic, (SQ) ethacrynic acid, in (SQ) 3 injections in 1 human, Caucasian, adult, 20 years age, female, with kidney disorder.
Transient severe bilateral tinnitus, sensorineural hearing loss, and bilateral nystagmus due to parenteral, intravenous, administration of (SQ) 50 and
100 mg of diuretic, (SQ) ethacrynic acid, in (SQ) 2 injections in 1 human,
Caucasian, adult, 20 years age, female, with kidney disorder.
Previous administration, 2 days before onset of ototoxic effects, of antibiotic, (SQ) colistin (sodium colistimethate), in 1 injection in 1 human, Caucasian, adult, 20 years age, female, with kidney disorder.
Transient sensorineural hearing loss within 12 hours of first dose due to
oral administration of 50 mg of diuretic, ethacrynic acid, in 4 doses in 1
human, Caucasian, aged, 76 years age, male, with kidney disorder and with
previous moderate hearing loss due to otosclerosis.
Severe tinnitus within 1 hour of first dose and sensorineural hearing loss
within 1 half hour of second dose due to parenteral, intravenous, administration of 50 and 100 mg of diuretic, (SQ) ethacrynic acid, in 2 injections in 1
human, Caucasian, adult, 57 years age, female, with leukemia and kidney
disorder.
Administration about 1 week previously of antibiotic, (SQ) streptomycin, in 1
human, Caucasian, adult, 57 years age, female, with leukemia and kidney
disorder, for pneumonitis.
Administration about 1 week previously of antibiotic, (SQ) colistin (sodium
colistimethate), in 1 human, Caucasian, adult, 57 years age, female, with
leukemia and kidney disorder, for pneumonitis.
  (AD) Discussion of 5 case reports of transient hearing loss due to treatment with ethacrynic acid. (ENG)

                                                                       227
Bilateral tinnitus and sudden deafness possibly due to cardiovascular agent,
(SQ) hexadimethrine bromide, in 1 human, adult, 32 years age, female, with
chronic nephritis and treated with hemodialysis.
Previous administration of antituberculous agent, (SQ) PAS, in 1 human,
adult, 32 years age, female, with chronic nephritis and treated with hemodialysis.
Previous administration of antituberculous agent, (SQ) isoniazid, in 1 human,
adult, 32 years age, female, with chronic nephritis and treated with hemodialysis.
Damage to Reissner's membrane, degeneration of organ of Corti, stria vascularis, and spiral ganglion, and slight changes in vestibular apparatus possibly due to cardiovascular agent, (SQ) hexadimethrine bromide, in 1 human,
adult, 32 years age, female, with chronic nephritis and treated with hemodialysis.
Progressive severe sensorineural hearing loss possibly due to cardiovascular
agent, hexadimethrine bromide, in 4 humans, adolescent and adult, 17 to 40
years age, with kidney disorders and treated with hemodialysis.
  (AD) Association of hexadimethrine bromide with hearing loss only when
  used with hemodialysis in treatment of kidney disorder.
  (AD) No hearing loss in group treated with hemodialysis without hexadimethrine bromide. (ENG)

                                                                       250
Damage to vestibular apparatus due to more than 1 g daily of antibiotic,
streptomycin, for 60 to 120 days in 25 percent of humans.
Dizziness 5 days after cessation of treatment due to parenteral, intramuscular, administration of 1 g every 12 hours of antibiotic, streptomycin (SM),
for 9 days in 1 human, adult, 44 years age, female, with peritonitis.
Simultaneous parenteral, intravenous, administration of 600 mg every 18 hours

of antibiotic, lincomycin (SM), for 9 days in 1 human, adult, 44 years age, female, with peritonitis.
   (AD) Case report of vestibular problem due to streptomycin.
Damage to cochlea due to antibiotic, dihydrostreptomycin, for more than 1 week in 4 to 15 percent of humans.
Sensorineural hearing loss and damage to organ of Corti due to antibiotic, kanamycin, in humans.
Sensorineural hearing loss and damage to organ of Corti due to antibiotic, vancomycin, in humans.
   (AD) Discussion of cochleo-vestibulotoxic effects due to antibiotic thera-
   py in surgery. (ENG)

                                                                          255
Slight hearing loss and vertigo due to parenteral, intramuscular, administration of 1 g every 24 hours of antibiotic, capreomycin (SM), for range of 5 to
12 months in 4 of 21 humans, adult, with pulmonary tuberculosis and without
pretreatment audiometric changes.
Slight and severe hearing loss and vertigo due to parenteral, intramuscular,
administration of 1 g every 24 hours of antibiotic, capreomycin (SM), for
range of 5 to 12 months in 12 of 40 humans, adult, with pulmonary tuberculosis and with pretreatment audiometric changes.
Simultaneous administration of antituberculous agent, ethambutol (SM), in all
of 61 humans, adult, with pulmonary tuberculosis.
   (AD) Treatment with capreomycin discontinued in 4 humans with severe
   ototoxic effects.
   (AD) Audiometry every 4 weeks during treatment. (ENG)

                                                                          280
High frequency hearing loss 3 weeks after beginning of therapy due to oral
administration of 20 mg daily, then 60 mg daily for 1 week, with interval of
1 week, and then 30 mg daily for 12 days of cardiovascular agent, (SQ) propranolol, for total of 19 days in 1 human, aged, 68 years age, female, with
heart disorder, arteriosclerosis.
   (AD) Sensorineural hearing loss confirmed by audiometry.
   (AD) Some improvement in hearing sensitivity during 6 months after cessation of drug.
No reported ototoxic effects due to unspecified method of administration
about 2 years previously of unspecified dose of cardiovascular agent, (SQ)
quinidine, for unspecified period in 1 human, aged, 68 years age, female,
with heart disorder, arteriosclerosis.
   (AD) Effects on gastrointestinal system and skin rash due to quinidine.
   (AD) Patient had history of toxic effects of drugs.
   (AD) Suggested that possible previous hearing loss made more severe by
   propranolol. (ENG)

                                                                          303
Transient sensorineural hearing loss and tinnitus due to unspecified method
of administration of 300 mg of diuretic, (SQ) ethacrynic acid (SM), for first
24 hours in 1 human, adult, 22 years age, female, with preeclampsia during
pregnancy.
Transient sensorineural hearing loss and tinnitus due to unspecified method
of administration of 180 mg of diuretic, (SQ) furosemide (SM), for first 24
hours in 1 human, adult, 22 years age, female, with preeclampsia during
pregnancy.
Transient sensorineural hearing loss and tinnitus due to unspecified method
of administration of 100 mg of diuretic, (SQ) ethacrynic acid (SM), for 5
days in 1 human, adult, 22 years age, female, with preeclampsia during pregnancy.
Transient sensorineural hearing loss and tinnitus due to unspecified method
of administration of 80 mg of diuretic, (SQ) furosemide (SM), for 5 days in 1
human, adult, 22 years age, female, with preeclampsia during pregnancy.
   (AD) Cochleotoxic effects confirmed by audiology. (ENG)

                                                                          305
Dizziness, vertigo, tinnitus, and hearing loss due to oral administration of
50, 100, 150, and then 200 mg, incr daily doses each week, of anti-inflammatory agent, indomethacin, for 4 weeks in 7 of 24 humans, adult and aged,
range of 23 to 69 years age, male and female, with rheumatoid arthritis.

Dizziness, vertigo, tinnitus, and hearing loss due to oral administration of
1.6, 3.2, 4.8, and then 6.4 g, incr daily doses each week, of salicylate,
acetylsalicylic acid, for 4 weeks in 18 of 24 humans, adult and aged, range
of 23 to 69 years age, male and female, with rheumatoid arthritis.
   (AD) Comparative study of effectiveness of indomethacin and acetylsalicylic acid in treatment of rheumatoid arthritis. (ENG)

                                                                          310
Transient decr in vestibular function due to parenteral, intravenous, administration of 2 ml of tranquilizer, droperidol (CB), for 2 minutes in 18 of 21
humans, adolescent and adult, female and male.
Transient decr in vestibular function due to parenteral, intravenous, administration of 2 ml of analgesic, fentanyl (CB) (fentanyl citrate), for 2
minutes in 18 of 21 humans, adolescent and adult, female and male.
   (CT) Caloric tests, pretreatment and posttreatment. (DAN)

                                                                          316
Possible vestibular problems and cochlear impairment due to more than recommended dose of 15 to 30 mg per kg daily of antibiotic, streptomycin, for long
period in humans.
Hearing loss due to parenteral, intramuscular, administration of total doses
of 5 to 6 g of antibiotic, kanamycin, in humans, adult, with kidney disorder.
Possible hearing loss due to parenteral, topical, or oral administration of
high doses of antibiotic, neomycin, for long period in humans.
Possible hearing loss due to high doses of antibiotic, framycetin, for long
period in humans.
Possible hearing loss due to antibiotic, vancomycin, in humans.
Possible hearing loss and vestibular problems due to antibiotic, viomycin, in
humans.
   (AD) High risk of ototoxicity with simultaneous administration of viomycin
   and streptomycin.
Possible vestibular problems due to antibiotic, gentamicin, in humans.
   (AD) Administration of gentamicin not recommended for newborn infants, for
   humans during pregnancy, and for humans treated with other ototoxic drugs.
Ataxia and hearing loss due to antibiotic, colistin, in humans.
   (AD) Literature review on ototoxic antibiotics.
   (AD) Results of studies on use of pantothenate salt of some antibiotics
   for decr in ototoxicity not clear.
   (AD) Suggested effect of ototoxic antibiotics on breakdown of glucose on
   which hair cells of inner ear depend for energy. (ENG)

                                                                          322
Cochleo-vestibulotoxic effects due to parenteral, intramuscular, administra-
tion of 1 g daily and then 1 g every other day of antibiotic, (SQ) capreomycin (SM), for 6 months in 3 of 36 humans, adult and aged, range of 20 to 80
years age, male and female, with pulmonary tuberculosis.
   (AD) Ototoxic effects confirmed by audiogram.
Simultaneous administration of 600 mg daily of antibiotic, (SQ) rifampicin
(SM), for 6 months in 36 humans, adult and aged, range of 20 to 80 years age,
male and female, with pulmonary tuberculosis.
Simultaneous administration of 25 mg per kg daily and then 15 mg per kg daily
of antituberculous agent, (SQ) ethambutol (SM), for 6 months in 36 humans,
adult and aged, range of 20 to 80 years age, male and female, with pulmonary
tuberculosis.
Cochleo-vestibulotoxic effects due to previous administration of (SQ) antibiotics, aminoglycoside, in 36 humans, adult and aged, range of 20 to 80
years age, male and female, with pulmonary tuberculosis.
   (AD) Therapy with antibiotics not satisfactory. (FR)

                                                                          323
Progressive severe bilateral sensorineural hearing loss and vestibular problems due to parenteral administration of 1 g twice weekly of antibiotic, (SQ)
viomycin (viomycin pantothenate), for total of 10 weeks in 1 human, adult, 59
years age, female, with pulmonary tuberculosis and kidney disorder.
   (AD) Cochleo-vestibulotoxic effects confirmed by audiometry at different
   periods during and after treatment and by caloric test.
Previous administration of antibiotic, (SQ) chloramphenicol, in 1 human,
adult, 59 years age, female, for infection before diagnosis of tuberculosis.

488Adult, Aged (Multiple agents)

Possible but not reported auditory system problems due to previous parenteral administration of 0.5 g twice daily of antibiotic, (SQ) streptomycin, for 1 week in 1 human, adult, 59 years age, female, for infection before diagnosis of tuberculosis.

(AD) Suggested that possible previous ototoxic effects of streptomycin potentiated by viomycin (viomycin pantothenate).

Previous administration of antituberculous agent, (SQ) PAS, in 1 human, adult, 59 years age, female, with pulmonary tuberculosis and kidney disorder. (ENG)

325

High frequency hearing loss due to parenteral, intramuscular, administration of total of 15 mg per kg in 2 doses 5 times a week of antibiotic, (SQ) capreomycin (SM), for 37 and 45 days in 2 of 70 humans, adult, 35 and 64 years age, with pulmonary tuberculosis and with previous treatment with other ototoxic drugs.

Transient vertigo due to parenteral, intramuscular, administration of total of 15 mg per kg in 2 doses 5 times a week of antibiotic, (SQ) capreomycin (SM), for 5, 25, and 94 days in 3 of 70 humans, adult, 39, 61, and 62 years age, with pulmonary tuberculosis and with previous treatment with streptomycin.

Simultaneous administration of other (SQ) antituberculous agents (SM), in 70 humans, adult, male and female, with pulmonary tuberculosis.

Possible ototoxic effects due to previous administration of antibiotic, (SQ) streptomycin, in 3 of 70 humans, adult, 39, 61, and 62 years age, with pulmonary tuberculosis. (ENG)

327

More severe hearing loss due to parenteral, intramuscular, administration of 1 g daily of antibiotic, (SQ) capreomycin (SM), for long period in 1 of 32 humans, male, with pulmonary tuberculosis and with previous antibiotic therapy.

Hearing loss before capreomycin treatment due to (SQ) antibiotics, aminoglycoside, in 1 of 32 humans, male, with pulmonary tuberculosis.

(AD) Hearing loss confirmed by audiogram.

Tinnitus due to parenteral, intramuscular, administration of 1 g daily of antibiotic, (SQ) capreomycin (SM), for long period in 3 of 32 humans with pulmonary tuberculosis.

Simultaneous administration of other (SQ) antituberculous agents (SM), in 32 humans, adult and aged, 20 to 69 years age, male and female, with pulmonary tuberculosis.

Previous administration of antituberculous agent, (SQ) PAS, in 32 humans, adult and aged, 20 to 69 years age, male and female, with pulmonary tuberculosis. (ENG)

343

No hearing loss but decr in vestibular function, asymptomatic except for dizziness in 1 case, due to 1 g daily of antibiotic, capreomycin (SM), for 4 months or more in 4 of 25 humans, adolescent, adult, and aged, range of 17 to 67 years age, male and female, 80 to 160 lb weight, with pulmonary tuberculosis and with kidney disorder in 2 cases.

Transient dizziness with no objective decr in vestibular function due to 1 g daily of antibiotic, capreomycin (SM), for 4 months or more in 3 of 25 humans, adolescent, adult, and aged, range of 17 to 67 years age, male and female, 80 to 160 lb weight, with pulmonary tuberculosis.

Simultaneous administration of 300 mg daily of antituberculous agent, isoniazid (SM), for 4 months or more in 25 humans, adolescent, adult, and aged, range of 17 to 67 years age, male and female, 80 to 160 lb weight, with pulmonary tuberculosis.

(CT) Pure tone audiometry, caloric tests, and cupulometry, pretreatment and during treatment with capreomycin.

(AD) Study of clinical use and cochleo-vestibulotoxic effects of capreomycin.

Hearing loss, asymptomatic in 1 case and symptomatic in 1 case, due to 1 g daily of antibiotic, viomycin, in 2 of 75 humans with pulmonary tuberculosis.

Objective decr in vestibular function due to 1 g daily of antibiotic, viomycin, in 21 of 75 humans with pulmonary tuberculosis.

Hearing loss, asymptomatic, due to 1 g daily of antibiotic, streptomycin, in

2 of 61 humans with pulmonary tuberculosis.
Objective decr in vestibular function due to 1 g daily of antibiotic, streptomycin, in 8 of 61 humans with pulmonary tuberculosis.
   (CT) Audiometry and vestibular function tests, pretreatment and during
   treatment with viomycin or streptomycin.
   (AD) Results of study on capreomycin comp w results of previous study on
   viomycin and streptomycin.   (ENG)

348

No ototoxic effects due to topical administration in ear drops of 3 to 4 ear
drops 3 times daily of fluocinolone acetonide (CB), for 5 to 10 days in 54
humans, child, adolescent, adult, and aged, male and female, with infections
of middle ear and external ear.
No ototoxic effects due to topical administration in ear drops of 3 to 4 ear
drops 3 times daily of antibiotic, polymyxin B (CB), for 5 to 10 days in 54
humans, child, adolescent, adult, and aged, male and female, with infections
of middle ear and external ear.
No ototoxic effects due to topical administration in ear drops of 3 to 4 ear
drops 3 times daily of antibiotic, neomycin (CB) (neomycin sulfate), for 5 to
10 days in 54 humans, child, adolescent, adult, and aged, male and female,
with infections of middle ear and external ear.   (IT)

353

Dizziness due to oral administration of 600 mg of analgesic, clonixin, in 1
dose in 2 of 24 humans, adult and aged, 21 to 68 years age, male and female,
126 to 210 lb weight, treated after surgery.
Hearing loss due to parenteral, intramuscular, administration of 6 mg of
analgesic, morphine (morphine sulfate), in 1 dose in 1 of 24 humans, adult
and aged, 21 to 68 years age, male and female, 126 to 210 lb weight, treated
after surgery.
   (AD) Comparative study of effectiveness of oral clonixin and parenteral
   morphine in treatment after surgery.   (ENG)

354

Vestibular problems due to 1 g daily, total doses of 1 to 115 g before onset
of ototoxicity, of antibiotic, streptomycin (SM), for several days to 9
months in 56 of 364 humans, adolescent and adult, 16 to 64 years age, female,
with tuberculosis of genitourinary system.
No specified ototoxic effects due to range of doses of antituberculous agent,
PAS (SM), for several days to 9 months in 13 of 369 humans, adolescent and
adult, 16 to 64 years age, female, with tuberculosis of genitourinary system.
Simultaneous administration of antituberculous agent, isoniazid (SM), in 274
humans, adolescent and adult, 16 to 64 years age, female, with tuberculosis
of genitourinary system.   (ENG)

355

Tinnitus and hearing loss due to previous oral administration of (SQ) 4.5 g
daily of salicylate, (SQ) aspirin, in 4 of 6 humans with rheumatoid arthritis.
Tinnitus and hearing loss due to oral administration of (SQ) 3.6 g daily of
salicylate, (SQ) aspirin, for short period, 2 weeks, in 1 of 6 humans with
rheumatoid arthritis.
No ototoxic effects due to oral administration of 0.3, 0.6, and 0.9 g daily
of anti-inflammatory agent, (SQ) ibuprofen, for short period, 2 weeks, in 6
humans with rheumatoid arthritis.
No ototoxic effects due to range of 200 to 1200 mg daily, average of 600 mg
daily, of anti-inflammatory agent, ibuprofen, for long period, 3 months to
over 12 months, in 27 humans, adult, 60.6 years average age, male and female,
with rheumatoid arthritis.
   (AD) Comparative study of effectiveness of aspirin and ibuprofen in treatment of rheumatoid arthritis.   (ENG)

359

Hearing loss due to oral administration of 400, 600, or 800 mg of anti-inflammatory agent, ibuprofen, for 2 weeks in 2 of 30 humans, adult and aged, 30
to 79 years age, female and male, with rheumatoid arthritis.
Unspecified ototoxic effects due to oral administration of 2.4, 3.6, or 4.8 g
daily of salicylate, aspirin, for 2 weeks in 18 of 30 humans, adult and aged,

30 to 79 years age, female and male, with rheumatoid arthritis.
   (AD) Comparative study of ibuprofen, aspirin, and placebo in treatment of
   rheumatoid arthritis.   (ENG)

                                                                          361
Transient dizziness and tinnitus due to oral administration of 750 mg daily
of anti-inflammatory agent, ibuprofen, for 5 days in 1 of 9 humans, adult and
aged, 37 to 67 years age, male and female, with rheumatoid arthritis.
   (AD) Ibuprofen therapy discontinued after 5 days.
Hearing loss and tinnitus due to oral administration of 5 g daily of salicylate, aspirin, for 1 week in 3 of 9 humans, adult and aged, 37 to 67 years
age, male and female, with rheumatoid arthritis.
   (AD) Comparative study of ibuprofen, aspirin, and prednisolone in treatment of rheumatoid arthritis.   (ENG)

                                                                          362
Hearing loss due to high and low doses of antibiotic, streptomycin, in humans, child and adult, with different disorders and with previous hearing
loss in 2 humans.
Hearing loss due to high doses of antibiotic, neomycin, in humans, child and
adult, with different disorders.
   (AD) Need for daily audiometry and vestibular function tests with administration of aminoglycoside antibiotics.
   (AD) If ototoxic effect observed, need to withdraw ototoxic drug or ad-
   minister vitamins, glucose, dimedrol, calcium chloride, or electrophoresis
   with potassium iodide.   (RUS)

                                                                          367
Auditory system problems due to oral administration of 150 mg daily of antituberculous agent, thiacetazone (CB), for 12 weeks in 47 of 581 humans,
adolescent and adult, 15 years or over age, male and female, with pulmonary
tuberculosis.
Auditory system problems due to oral administration of 150 mg daily of antituberculous agent, thiacetazone (CB) (IB), for 12 weeks in 39 of 584 humans,
adolescent and adult, 15 years or over age, male and female, with pulmonary
tuberculosis, with administration of vitamins and antihistamine.
Combined oral administration of 300 mg daily of antituberculous agent, i-
soniazid (CB), for 12 weeks in humans, adolescent and adult, 15 years or over
age, male and female, with pulmonary tuberculosis.
   (AD) Study of effect of inhibitors on toxicity of drugs in 1 group with
   drug regimen of thiacetazone and isoniazid in combination.
Auditory system problems due to parenteral administration of 1 g daily of
antibiotic, streptomycin (SM), for 12 weeks in 227 of 689 humans, adolescent
and adult, 15 years or over age, male and female, with pulmonary tuberculosis.
Auditory system problems due to parenteral administration of 1 g daily of
antibiotic, streptomycin (SM) (IB), for 12 weeks in 218 of 707 humans, adolescent and adult, 15 years or over age, male and female, with pulmonary tuberculosis, with administration of vitamins and antihistamine.
Auditory system problems due to simultaneous oral administration of 150 mg
daily of antituberculous agent, thiacetazone (SM), for 12 weeks in humans,
adolescent and adult, 15 years or over age, male and female, with pulmonary
tuberculosis.
Simultaneous oral administration of 300 mg daily of antituberculous agent,
isoniazid (SM), for 12 weeks in humans, adolescent and adult, 15 years or
over age, male and female, with pulmonary tuberculosis.
   (AD) Study of effect of inhibitors on toxicity of drugs in 1 group with
   drug regimen of streptomycin, thiacetazone, and isoniazid.
Auditory system problems due to parenteral administration of 1 g daily of
antibiotic, streptomycin (SM), for 12 weeks in 109 of 711 humans, adolescent
and adult, 15 years or over age, male and female, with pulmonary tuberculosis.
Auditory system problems due to parenteral administration of 1 g daily of
antibiotic, streptomycin (SM) (IB), for 12 weeks in 111 of 696 humans, adolescent and adult, 15 years or over age, male and female, with pulmonary tuberculosis, with administration of vitamins and antihistamine.
Simultaneous oral administration of 300 mg daily of antituberculous agent,
isoniazid (SM), for 12 weeks in humans, adolescent and adult, 15 years or

over age, male and female, with pulmonary tuberculosis.
 (AD) Study of effect of inhibitors on toxicity of drugs in 1 group with
 drug regimen of streptomycin and isoniazid.
 (AD) Study of effectiveness of inhibitors in prevention of toxic effects
 of thiacetazone and streptomycin.
 (AD) Study suggested that vitamins and antihistamine not effective in
 prevention of toxicity. (ENG)

                                                                        373
Possible progressive sensorineural hearing loss due to antibiotics, aminogly-
coside, in humans.
Possible transient hearing loss due to high doses of salicylate, aspirin, in
humans.
Possible transient hearing loss due to high doses of antimalarial, quinine,
in humans.
Possible hearing loss due to diuretic, ethacrynic acid, in humans.
Bilateral sudden deafness due to antibiotic, kanamycin, in 4 humans, adult,
34 years average age, male and female.
 (AD) Hearing loss due to ototoxic drugs usually progressive.
 (AD) Sudden deafness due to ototoxic drugs possible in some cases, as in
 humans with kidney disorder.
 (AD) Literature review on etiology of sudden deafness. (ENG)

                                                                        384
Usually transient hearing loss and no structural damage to organ of Corti,
stria vascularis, and spiral ganglion due to oral or topical administration
of salicylates in humans.
Hearing loss due to antimalarial, quinine, in humans.
Usually permanent hearing loss due to antimalarial, chloroquine, in humans.
Transient and permanent hearing loss and possible damage to hair cells of
organ of Corti due to diuretic, ethacrynic acid, in humans.
Sensorineural hearing loss due to cardiovascular agent, hexadimethrine
bromide, in humans with kidney disorder.
Sensorineural hearing loss and damage to organ of Corti due to topical ad-
ministration of antineoplastic, nitrogen mustard, in humans.
Sensorineural hearing loss due to high doses of antibiotic, chloramphenicol,
in humans.
Primary vestibular problems due to antibiotic, streptomycin, in humans.
Hearing loss due to high doses usually of antibiotic, streptomycin, in humans.
 (AD) Early detection of hearing loss by audiometry prevents permanent
 damage.
High frequency hearing loss and severe damage to outer hair cells and slight
damage to inner hair cells of organ of Corti due to antibiotic, kanamycin, in
humans.
Sensorineural hearing loss due to parenteral, oral, and topical administration of antibiotic, neomycin, in humans with or without kidney disorders.
Degeneration of hair cells of organ of Corti and of nerve process due to
antibiotics, aminoglycoside, in animals.
 (AD) Literature review of physiological and structural cochleo-vestibulotoxic effects of ototoxic drugs.
 (AD) Discussion of suggested mechanism of ototoxicity and routes of drugs
 to inner ear.
Bilateral sensorineural hearing loss due to oral administration of antibiotic, neomycin, in 4 of 8 humans with liver disease.
Bilateral sensorineural hearing loss due to oral administration of range of
doses of antibiotic, neomycin (SM), in 2 of 5 humans with liver disease.
Bilateral sensorineural hearing loss due to diuretics (SM), in 2 of 5 humans
with liver disease.
Transient progression of previous hearing loss due to parenteral, intravenous, administration of diuretic, ethacrynic acid (SM), in 1 injection in 1
of 5 humans with liver disease.
 (CT) Normal cochlear function in 6 humans, control group, with liver
 disease and not treated with neomycin or diuretics.
 (CT) Normal cochlear function in 13 humans, control group, with liver
 disease and treated with diuretics but not with neomycin.
 (AD) Hearing loss confirmed by audiometry.
 (AD) Reported that hearing loss due to neomycin or diuretics in humans

with liver disease not related to dosage.

(AD) Clinical study of effects of treatment with neomycin and diuretics in humans with liver disease.

Bilateral sensorineural hearing loss and vertigo due to antibiotic, ampicillin, in 1 human, adolescent, 17 years age, female, with tonsillitis.

(AD) Cited case report.

Severe sensorineural hearing loss and vertigo due to topical administration in ear drops of antibiotic, framycetin, in 1 human, adult, 42 years age, male, with previous slight high frequency hearing loss.

(AD) Cited case report.

Atrophy of hair cells of organ of Corti and hearing loss due to antibiotic, dihydrostreptomycin, in humans with tuberculous meningitis.

(AD) Cited study.

Loss of inner hair cells and damage to outer hair cells due to 18 g of antibiotic, neomycin, for 18 days in 1 human.

(AD) Cited case report. (ENG)

392

No hearing loss but tinnitus due to parenteral, intramuscular, administration of range of 0.05 to 1.0 g daily according to age of antibiotic, kanamycin, for short period in 4 of 125 humans, infant, child, and adult, with acute otorhinolaryngological infections.

(AD) Audiograms showed no hearing loss.

Hearing loss, subjective in 1 case and latent in others, but no vestibular problems due to 1.0 g daily 2 times a week of antibiotic, (SQ) kanamycin, for long period in 15 of 66 humans, adolescent and adult, 15 to 55 years age, with pulmonary tuberculosis and with previous streptomycin treatment.

(CT) Audiogram before and during treatment with kanamycin.

Hearing loss due to previous administration of antibiotic, (SQ) streptomycin, in 31 of 272 humans.

Sensorineural hearing loss due to previous administration of total of 600 g of antibiotic, (SQ) streptomycin, in 1 human, adult, 27 years age.

More severe sensorineural hearing loss, subjective, due to total of 136 g of antibiotic, (SQ) kanamycin, in 1 human, adult, 27 years age.

(AD) Case report of hearing loss due to streptomycin potentiated by treatment with kanamycin.

Hearing loss, latent, and tinnitus, but no vestibular problems due to total of over 20 g to over 300 g of antibiotic, kanamycin, for long period in 10 of 70 humans with pulmonary tuberculosis and no previous chemotherapy.

(CT) Audiogram before and during treatment with kanamycin.

(AD) Clinical studies of effects of treatment with kanamycin for short and long periods.

Vestibular problems after 10 to 12 days due to parenteral administration of 100 mg per kg daily of antibiotic, streptomycin, in 3 animals, cats, 2 kg weight.

Slight vestibular problems after 30 days due to 300 mg per kg daily of antibiotic, kanamycin, in 3 animals, cats, 2 kg weight.

Decr in cochlear microphonic due to 200 mg per kg daily of antibiotic, streptomycin, in 11 injections in animals, cats.

Slight decr in cochlear microphonic due to 300 mg per kg daily of antibiotic, kanamycin, in 11 to 60 injections in animals, cats.

(AD) Comparative experimental studies of cochleo-vestibulotoxic effects of kanamycin and streptomycin in cats.

(AD) Different effects of 2 aminoglycoside antibiotics on vestibular function but similar effects on cochlear function. (ENG)

413

Decr in threshold of detection of acoustic stimuli of shorter duration than 16 msec due to 0.4 g of analeptic, caffeine, in humans, adult, and animals.

Decr in threshold of detection of acoustic stimuli of longer duration than 16 msec due to 0.015 to 0.02 g of analeptic, amphetamine, in humans, adult, and animals. (RUS)

414

Transient hearing loss in short time after injection due to parenteral, intravenous, administration of (SQ) high doses, 500 mg each dose, of diuretic, (SQ) furosemide, in (SQ) total of 2 doses, each for duration of 3 minutes, on consecutive days in 1 human, adult, 49 years age, female, with

chronic kidney disorder.
    (AD) No observed hearing loss before treatment with furosemide.
    (AD) Normal hearing within 4 hours.
No hearing loss due to parenteral, intravenous, administration of (SQ) 240 mg
of diuretic, (SQ) furosemide, in (SQ) 1 dose for duration of 5 minutes in 1
human, adult, 49 years age, female, with chronic kidney disorder.
    (AD) Suggested that cochleotoxic effect of furosemide is dose related.
    (AD) Different individual responses to furosemide suggest other factors in
    ototoxic effects.
Previous administration of antibiotic, (SQ) nalidixic acid, in 1 human,
adult, 49 years age, female, with chronic kidney disorder. (ENG)

                                                                      420
Acute hearing loss due to 10 mg on first day and then 60 mg daily for 3 days,
total of 220 mg, of antibiotic, (SQ) gentamicin, in total of 4 days in 1
human, adolescent, 16 years age, with kidney disorder.
    (AD) Hearing loss confirmed by audiogram.
Previous administration of antibiotic, (SQ) colistin, in 1 human, adolescent,
16 years age, with kidney disorder.
Vestibular problems due to 40 mg daily, total of 400 mg, of antibiotic,
gentamicin, in total of 10 days in 1 human, aged, 68 years age, with kidney
disorder. (GER)

                                                                      423
More severe and more rapid progression of presbycusis due to antimalarial,
quinine, in humans, adult and aged.
More severe and more rapid progression of presbycusis due to antibiotics,
aminoglycoside, in humans, adult and aged.
More severe and more rapid progression of presbycusis due to salicylate,
aspirin, in humans, adult and aged.
More severe and more rapid progression of presbycusis due to chemical agent,
carbon monoxide, in humans, adult and aged.
    (AD) Discussion of factors resulting in more severe and more rapid pro-
    gression of presbycusis. (FR)

                                                                      434
Slight ototoxic effects due to range of doses of antibiotic, streptomycin, in
8 of 40 humans, female, treated for tuberculosis during pregnancy.
Slight ototoxic effects due to range of doses of antibiotic, dihydrostreptomycin, in 2 of 40 humans, female, treated for tuberculosis during pregnancy.
Vestibular problems and sensorineural hearing loss in mother and vestibular
problems in fetus due to total of 27 g of antibiotic, streptomycin (CB), for
2.5 months in 1 human, adult, 28 years age, female, treated for pulmonary
tuberculosis at end of pregnancy.
Vestibular problems and sensorineural hearing loss in mother and vestibular
problems in fetus due to total of 27 g of antibiotic, dihydrostreptomycin
(CB), for 2.5 months in 1 human, adult, 28 years age, female, treated for
pulmonary tuberculosis at end of pregnancy.
    (AD) Pure tone audiometry and vestibular function tests in child, female,
    at 10 years age.
Mixed hearing loss in mother and severe sensorineural hearing loss and vestibular problems in fetus due to total of 28 g of antibiotic, (SQ) dihydrostreptomycin, for 2.5 months in 1 human, adult, 22 years age, female, treated for
tuberculosis at beginning of pregnancy.
Mixed hearing loss in mother and severe sensorineural hearing loss and vestibular problems in fetus due to total of 28 g of antibiotic, (SQ) streptomycin, for 2.5 months in 1 human, adult, 22 years age, female, treated for
tuberculosis at beginning of pregnancy.
    (AD) Pure tone audiometry and vestibular function tests in child, female,
    at 10 years age. (ENG)

                                                                      446
Vestibular problems only in 5 and dizziness, tinnitus, and hearing loss in 1
due to parenteral, intramuscular, administration of 1 g daily in single
injection of antibiotic, streptomycin (SM) (streptomycin sulfate), for 6
months only in 6 (6 percent) of 65 humans, Negro, adolescent and adult, 15 to
over 55 years age, male and female, 80 to over 140 lb weight, for retreatment

ot pulmonary tuberculosis.
Simultaneous oral administration of 15 g of antituberculous agent, PAS (SM)
(sodium PAS), for 1 year in 65 humans, Negro, adolescent and adult, 15 to
over 55 years age, male and female, 80 to over 140 lb weight, for retreatment
of pulmonary tuberculosis.
  (AD) Study of value of regimen of streptomycin, PAS, and pyrazinamide in
  retreatment of pulmonary tuberculosis. (ENG)

447

Dizziness and tinnitus within first 14 weeks due to 150 mg daily in 2 divided
doses of antituberculous agent, thiacetazone (SM), for 26 weeks in 30 of 410
humans, adolescent and adult, 15 to over 55 years age, 30 to over 50 kg
weight, with tuberculosis.
No ototoxic effects due to 300 mg daily in 2 divided doses of antituberculous
agent, isoniazid (SM), for 26 weeks in 30 of 410 humans, adolescent and
adult, 15 to over 55 years age, 30 to over 50 kg weight, with tuberculosis.
  (AD) Study of toxicity of thiacetazone in treatment of tuberculosis.
  (ENG)

457

Tinnitus and progressive sensorineural hearing loss due to parenteral, intramuscular, administration of antibiotic, (SQ) streptomycin, for 10 days in 1
human, adult, 38 years age, female, with infections and later development of
kidney disorder.
Tinnitus and progressive sensorineural hearing loss due to 13.2 g of antibiotic, (SQ) kanamycin, for 11 days in 1 human, adult, 38 years age, female,
with infections and kidney disorder.
Hearing loss due to antimalarial, (SQ) quinine, in 1 human, adult, 20 years
age, male, with various infections and later development of kidney disorder.
Hearing loss due to 400 mg 2 times daily, total dose of 6.5 g, of antibiotic,
(SQ) kanamycin (SM), for 8 days in 1 human, adult, 20 years age, male, with
various infections and later development of kidney disorder.
Hearing loss due to 150 mg 2 times daily, total dose of 2400 mg, of antibiotic, (SQ) colistin (SM), for 8 days in 1 human, adult, 20 years age, male,
with various infections and later development of kidney disorder.
Tinnitus, total bilateral hearing loss, and vestibular problems due to parenteral, intramuscular, administration of 4.0 g daily, total of 21 g, of antibiotic, (SQ) kanamycin (SM), for 5 days in 1 human, adult, 20 years age,
male, with infections and kidney disorder.
Tinnitus, total bilateral hearing loss, and vestibular problems due to 0.6 g
daily, total dose of 1.3 g, of antibiotic, (SQ) colistin (SM), for 2 days in
1 human, adult, 20 years age, male, with infections and kidney disorder.
Tinnitus, total bilateral hearing loss, and vestibular problems due to 2 g
and then 8 g per 24 hours in divided doses, total dose of 26.5 g, of antibiotic, (SQ) chloramphenicol, for 9 days in 1 human, adult, 20 years age, male,
with infections and kidney disorder.
Bilateral hearing loss due to 1 g daily of antibiotic, actinomycin (SM), for
5 days in 1 human, adult, 62 years age, male, with infections and kidney
disorder.
Bilateral hearing loss due to unknown dose of antibiotic, kanamycin (SM), for
5 days in 1 human, adult, 62 years age, male, with infections and kidney
disorder.
Bilateral hearing loss and vestibular problems due to parenteral administration of high doses of antibiotic, (SQ) neomycin, for total of 21 days in 1
human, adult, 25 years age, male, with infection from wound.
Previous administration of unspecified doses of antibiotic, (SQ) streptomycin, in 1 human, adult, 25 years age, male, with infection from wound.
Later administration of antibiotic, (SQ) chloramphenicol, in 1 human, adult,
25 years age, male, with infection from wound.
Tinnitus and rapidly progressive bilateral hearing loss due to parenteral,
intramuscular, administration of 0.5 g every 12 hours of antibiotic, (SQ)
streptomycin, for 5 days in 1 human, adult, 21 years age, male, with infection from wound.
Tinnitus and rapidly progressive bilateral hearing loss due to parenteral,
intramuscular, administration of 200 mg daily, total of 6.8 g, of antibiotic,
(SQ) colistin (SM), in 1 human, adult, 21 years age, male, with infection
from wound.
Tinnitus and rapidly progressive bilateral hearing loss due to parenteral

administration of unspecified doses of antibiotic, (SQ) neomycin (SM), for about 35 days in 1 human, adult, 21 years age, male, with infection from wound.
Tinnitus and progressive bilateral hearing loss due to parenteral administration of 2 l per 24 hours of 1 percent solution of antibiotic, (SQ) neomycin, for 10 days in 1 human, adult, 26 years age, male, with infection from wound.
  (AD) Hearing loss confirmed by audiometry.
Previous administration of 500 mg four times a day of antibiotic, (SQ) ampicillin, in 1 human, adult, 26 years age, male, with infection from wound.
Bilateral sudden deafness due to administration in dialysis fluid of less than 150 mg of antibiotic, neomycin (SM), in 1 human, adult, 44 years age, female, with kidney disorder.
Bilateral sudden deafness due to 50 mg of diuretic, ethacrynic acid (SM), in 1 human, adult, 44 years age, female, with kidney disorder.
  (AD) Hearing loss confirmed by audiology.
Tinnitus and progressive bilateral hearing loss beginning after 8 days of treatment due to parenteral administration of 1 l every 4 hours for 3 days and then every 8 hours for 10 days of 1 percent solution of antibiotic, neomycin, in 1 human, adult, 20 years age, male, with infection from wound.
  (AD) Hearing loss confirmed by audiology.
Tinnitus and bilateral sensorineural hearing loss due to parenteral, intramuscular, administration of 1 g and then 0.5 g every 12 hours of antibiotic, streptomycin (SM), for 15 days in 1 human, adult, 23 years age, male, with infection from wound.
Tinnitus and bilateral sensorineural hearing loss due to topical administration by irrigation of 1 percent solution every 12 hours of antibiotic, neomycin (SM), for 14 days in 1 human, adult, 23 years age, male, with infection from wound.
  (AD) Hearing loss confirmed by audiometry.
  (AD) Discussion of 10 case reports. (ENG)

511
Transient severe sudden deafness due to 1 g of diuretic, (SQ) furosemide, in 1 human, Korean, adult, 26 years age, female, with lupus erythematosus.
Transient severe sudden deafness due to administration 2 months later of 100 mg of diuretic, (SQ) ethacrynic acid, in 1 human, Korean, adult, 26 years age, female, with lupus erythematosus.
  (AD) Suggested that cochleotoxic effects related to potent diuretic action. (ENG)

519
Dizziness but no other ototoxic effects due to parenteral, intramuscular, administration of 1 g daily in single dose of antibiotic, capreomycin (SM), for long period in 1 of 33 humans, adult and aged, 21 to over 70 years age, with pulmonary tuberculosis of long duration and with previous treatment with other drugs.
Simultaneous oral administration of 25 mg per kg during first 60 days and then 15 mg per kg of antituberculous agent, ethambutol (SM), in 1 of 33 humans, adult and aged, 21 to over 70 years age, with pulmonary tuberculosis of long duration and with previous treatment with other drugs.
Simultaneous administration of 600 mg of antibiotic, rifampicin (SM), in 1 of 33 humans, adult and aged, 21 to over 70 years age, with pulmonary tuberculosis of long duration and with previous treatment with other drugs.
  (AD) Otoneurology tests every 4 to 8 weeks. (ENG)

535
Dizziness due to parenteral administration of 0.75 g on 6 days a week for 3 months and then 1 g on 2 days a week with intervals of 2 to 3 days for 15 months of antibiotic, streptomycin (SM), for total of 18 months in 2 of 80 humans, adult, range of ages, female and male, 16 to 92 kg weight, with pulmonary tuberculosis.
Dizziness due to 300 mg on 6 days a week for 3 months and then 600 mg on 2 days a week with intervals of 2 to 3 days for 15 months of antituberculous agent, isoniazid (SM), for total of 18 months in 1 of 80 humans, adult, range of ages, female and male, 16 to 92 kg weight, with pulmonary tuberculosis.
Simultaneous administration of 12 g on 6 days a week of antituberculous agent, PAS (SM), for 3 months in 80 humans, adult, range of ages, female and male, 16 to 92 kg weight, with pulmonary tuberculosis. (ENG)

536

Damage to eighth cranial nerve and vertigo due to 1 g or 0.75 g daily of antibiotic, streptomycin (SM), for about 3 months usually in less than 55 of 181 humans, adult and aged, primarily 50 years or over age, male and female, with pulmonary tuberculosis.
Simultaneous administration of 300 mg daily of antituberculous agent, isoniazid (SM), for 18 months to 2 years usually in 181 humans, adult and aged, primarily 50 years or over age, male and female, with pulmonary tuberculosis.
Simultaneous administration of 12 g daily of antituberculous agent, PAS (SM), for 18 months to 2 years usually in 181 humans, adult and aged, primarily 50 years or over age, male and female, with pulmonary tuberculosis. (ENG)

537

Dizziness due to oral administration in tablet of 150 mg daily of antituberculous agent, thiacetazone (CB) (SM), in 1 of 147 humans, African, adolescent and adult, 15 years or more age, with pulmonary tuberculosis and without previous treatment.
Dizziness due to oral administration in tablet of 300 mg daily of antituberculous agent, isoniazid (CB) (SM), in 1 of 147 humans, African, adolescent and adult, 15 years or more age, with pulmonary tuberculosis and without previous treatment.
   (AD) Dizziness in 1 patient due to combined treatment with thiacetazone and isoniazid only.
Dizziness due to parenteral, intramuscular, administration of 1 g daily of antibiotic, streptomycin (SM) (streptomycin sulfate), for first 2 weeks in 1 of 161 humans, African, adolescent and adult, 15 years or more age, with pulmonary tuberculosis and without previous treatment.
   (AD) Dizziness in 1 patient due to simultaneous treatment with thiacetazone and isoniazid in 1 tablet and intramuscular streptomycin for 2 weeks.
Dizziness due to parenteral, intramuscular, administration of 1 g daily of antibiotic, streptomycin (SM) (streptomycin sulfate), for first 8 weeks in 10 of 162 humans, African, adolescent and adult, 15 years or more age, with pulmonary tuberculosis and without previous treatment.
   (AD) Dizziness in 10 patients due to simultaneous treatment with thiacetazone and isoniazid in 1 tablet and intramuscular streptomycin for 8 weeks.
   (AD) Study showed vestibulotoxic effects in total of 12 of 818 patients treated for pulmonary tuberculosis. (ENG)

547

Bilateral sensorineural hearing loss within 20 minutes but normal vestibular function due to parenteral, intravenous, administration of 50 mg of diuretic, ethacrynic acid (SM), in 1 injection in 1 human, adult, 53 years age, female, with kidney disorder.
   (AD) Hearing loss confirmed by audiogram.
   (AD) Vestibular function tests showed normal vestibular function.
Simultaneous oral administration of 18 g of antibiotic, neomycin (SM), in 7 days in 1 human, adult, 53 years age, female, with kidney disorder.
Severe destruction of outer hair cells of organ of Corti in basal coil of cochlea due to parenteral, intravenous, administration of 50 mg of diuretic, ethacrynic acid (SM), in 1 injection in 1 human, adult, 53 years age, female, with kidney disorder.
   (AD) Suggested that damage to hair cells possibly due to neomycin also.
   (AD) Suggested possible permanent hearing loss as result of ethacrynic acid treatment in patients with kidney disorders.
Transient and permanent total hearing loss within 15 minutes due to parenteral administration of diuretic, ethacrynic acid, in animals, cats. (ENG)

558

Severe hearing loss due to antibiotic, kanamycin (SM), in 1 human, adult, 44 years age, female, with basilar meningitis.
Simultaneous administration of 1 g daily of antituberculous agent, ethambutol (SM), in 1 human, adult, 44 years age, female, with basilar meningitis. (ENG)

564

Hearing loss due to antibiotic, kanamycin (SM), for long period in 3 of 4 humans, adult, range of ages, male and female, during retreatment for pulmonary tuberculosis.

Simultaneous administration of 25 mg per kg for 2 months and then 15 mg per kg of antituberculous agent, ethambutol (SM), in 4 humans, adult, range of ages, male and female, during retreatment for pulmonary tuberculosis.
   (CT) Treatment with ethambutol and 2 other antituberculous agents in humans, control group. (ENG)

570

Transient slight hearing loss due to parenteral, intramuscular, administration of 1 g daily, maximum dose of 90 g, of antibiotic, capreomycin (SM), in 1 of 16 humans with chronic tuberculosis of genitourinary system.
Simultaneous administration of 2 other antituberculous agents (SM), in 16 humans with chronic tuberculosis of genitourinary system.
Hearing loss due to 1 g daily average dose of antibiotic, capreomycin (SM), for long period in 1 of 20 humans, adult, male and female, with chronic tuberculosis, and 5 also alcoholics.
Simultaneous administration of other antituberculous agents (SM), in 20 humans, adult, male and female, with chronic tuberculosis, and 5 also alcoholics.
   (AD) Discussion of various reports of auditory system problems due to capreomycin therapy. (ENG)

577

No ototoxic effects due to parenteral, intramuscular, administration of 3 to 5 mg per kg daily in 3 or 4 divided doses, average total dose of 3.0 g, of antibiotic, gentamicin, for 12.7 days average in 41 humans, adolescent, adult, and aged, 14 to 87 years age, male and female, with genitourinary system infections primarily and with kidney disorder in 13 cases.
No ototoxic effects due to parenteral, intramuscular, administration of 15 mg per kg daily in 2 or 3 divided doses, average total dose of 6.6 g, of antibiotic, kanamycin (SM), for 8 days average in 34 humans, adult and aged, 40 to 81 years age, male and female, with genitourinary system infection and with kidney disorder in 8 cases.
No ototoxic effects due to parenteral, intramuscular or intravenous administration of 1.5 to 2.5 mg per kg daily in 2 to 4 divided doses, average total dose of 1.0 g, of antibiotic, polymyxin B (SM), for 6 days average in 34 humans, adult and aged, 40 to 81 years age, male and female, with genitourinary system infection and with kidney disorder in 8 cases.
   (AD) Comparative study of effects of 3 antibiotics on infections due to gram-negative bacilli. (ENG)

589

Dizziness during or after 5 or 6 injections but no evidence of hearing loss due to parenteral, intramuscular and then intravenous (SM), administration of 7 mg per kg total daily, not exceeding 180 mg total dose every 24 hours, of antibiotic, (SQ) gentamicin, for as long as 30 days in 5 of 80 humans, infant, child, and adult, 8 months to 36 years age, with cystic fibrosis and severe pulmonary infection.
   (AD) Audiology in 40 of 80 patients showed no evidence of hearing loss.
   (AD) Dizziness possibly due to rapid administration of gentamicin.
High frequency hearing loss before gentamicin therapy possibly due to previous administration of (SQ) ototoxic drugs in some of 80 humans, infant, child, and adult, 8 months to 36 years age, with cystic fibrosis and severe pulmonary infection.
Dizziness due to topical administration by inhalation (SM) of 16 to 20 mg up to 4 times a day, in 2 ml of 0.125 percent phenylephrine hydrochloride and propylene glycol, of antibiotic, (SQ) gentamicin (CB), in some of 80 humans, infant, child, and adult, 8 months to 36 years age, with cystic fibrosis and severe pulmonary infection.
Dizziness due to topical administration by inhalation (SM) of 16 to 20 mg up to 4 times a day, in 2 ml of 0.125 percent phenylephrine hydrochloride and propylene glycol, of antibiotic, (SQ) neomycin (CB), in some of 80 humans, infant, child, and adult, 8 months to 36 years age, with cystic fibrosis and severe pulmonary infection. (ENG)

593

Vestibular problems due to 1 g in 24 hours of antibiotic, (SQ) streptomycin (SM), in 1 human, adult, 32 years age, female, with tuberculosis.
Vestibular problems due to 450 mg of antituberculous agent, (SQ) isoniazid

(SM), in 1 human, adult, 32 years age, female, with tuberculosis.
Vestibular problems due to oral administration in tablets of 0.10 g of anti-
convulsant, (SQ) diphenylhydantoin, in 1 human, adult, 32 years age, female,
with tuberculosis.
Vestibular problems due to oral administration in tablets of 3 tablets of
0.10 g each daily of anticonvulsant, (SQ) diphenylhydantoin (SM), in 1 human,
adult, 49 years age, female, with tuberculosis.
Vestibular problems due to 300 mg of antituberculous agent, (SQ) isoniazid
(SM), in 1 human, adult, 49 years age, female, with tuberculosis.
Simultaneous administration of 500 cm of antituberculous agent, (SQ) PAS
(SM), in 1 human, adult, 49 years age, female, with tuberculosis.
   (AD) Report of vestibulotoxic effects in 2 patients due to diphenylhydan-
   toin with isoniazid or streptomycin. (FR)

604

Decr in middle ear muscle reflex due to oral administration of amount to
produce blood levels of 0.02 to 0.15 percent of sedative, alcohol, ethyl, in
9 humans, adult, 21 to 24 years age, with normal pure tone audiograms.
Decr in middle ear muscle reflex due to oral administration of 1.5 to 4.3 mg
per kg of sedative, pentobarbital (pentobarbital sodium), in 6 humans, adult,
21 to 24 years age, with normal pure tone audiograms.
   (AD) More risk of noise induced hearing loss due to decr in middle ear
   muscle reflex. (ENG)

611

Hearing loss due to range of 0.8 to 15 g of antibiotic, neomycin (SM), in 9
humans, child, adult, and aged, 4 or less to 65 years age, with various
infections.
Simultaneous administration of antibiotic, streptomycin (SM), in 6 humans,
child, adult, and aged, 4 or less to 65 years age, with various infections.
Simultaneous administration of antibiotic, polymyxin (SM), in 1 human, child,
less than 4 years age, with various infections.
   (AD) Hearing loss confirmed by audiograms.
   (AD) Discussion of 9 case reports. (HUN)

614

Vertigo due to parenteral administration of 0.5 g twice daily of antibiotic,
streptomycin (SM), for 7 days in 3 of 59 humans, aged, 70 years or over age,
with chronic bronchitis.
Simultaneous administration of 3,000,000 units twice daily of antibiotic,
penicillin (SM), for 14 days in 3 of 59 humans, aged, 70 years or over age,
with chronic bronchitis. (ENG)

619

Tinnitus in 7 cases and vertigo in 2 cases due to 1 g twice weekly of antibiotic, streptomycin (SM), in total of 9 of 190 humans, Japanese, adult, 20
to 61 years age, male and female, with pulmonary tuberculosis and without
previous chemotherapy.
Tinnitus in 7 cases and vertigo in 2 cases due to about 7.5 mg per kg in
single dose daily of antituberculous agent, isoniazid (SM), in total of 9 of
190 humans, Japanese, adult, 20 to 61 years age, male and female, with pulmonary tuberculosis and without previous chemotherapy.
Simultaneous administration of 10 g daily in 3 divided doses of antituberculous agent, PAS (SM), in 190 humans, Japanese, adult, 20 to 61 years age,
male and female, with pulmonary tuberculosis and without previous chemotherapy.
Tinnitus in 3 cases and hearing loss in 2 cases due to 1 g twice weekly of
antibiotic, streptomycin (SM), in total of 5 of 160 humans, Japanese, adult,
20 to 61 years age, male and female, with pulmonary tuberculosis and without
previous chemotherapy.
Tinnitus in 3 cases and hearing loss in 2 cases due to 18 mg per kg in 3
divided doses of antituberculous agent, isoniazid (SM), in total of 5 of 160
humans, Japanese, adult, 20 to 61 years age, male and female, with pulmonary
tuberculosis and without previous chemotherapy.
Simultaneous administration of 10 g daily in 3 divided doses of antituberculous agent, PAS (SM), in 160 humans, Japanese, adult, 20 to 61 years age,
male and female, with pulmonary tuberculosis and without previous chemotherapy.

(AD) Similar ototoxic effects in both drug regimens.   (ENG)

628

Hearing loss due to parenteral, intravenous, administration of 1 mg per kg
initial dose and then 0.75 mg per kg every 6 hours, dissolved in 200 ml of 5
percent glucose solution, of antibiotic, (SQ) gentamicin (gentamicin sulfate), in 4 of 60 humans, child, adolescent, adult, and aged, 6 to 76 years
age, with carcinoma, lymphoma, or leukemia and with azotemia in 3 of 4 and
previous hearing loss in 1 of 4.
Hearing loss due to previous administration of diuretic, (SQ) ethacrynic
acid, in 1 of 4 humans with gentamicin hearing loss.
   (AD) Suggested that hearing loss in 1 patient due to both gentamicin and
   ethacrynic acid. (ENG)

674

No ototoxic effects due to parenteral, intramuscular, administration of 1 g
twice daily for 1 to 2 days, followed by 1 g daily for 8 to 10 days, with
reduced doses in patients with kidney disorder, of antibiotic, kanamycin
(SM), for total of about 9 to 12 days in 28 humans, adult and aged, 26 to 80
years age, male and female, with severe infections due to gram-negative
bacilli, with bacteremia in 16 cases and kidney disorder in 8 cases.
Simultaneous administration of antibiotic, chloramphenicol (SM), in most of
16 humans with bacteremia.
   (AD) Use of kanamycin without ototoxic effects in patients with kidney
   disorders due to decr in dosage and tests of serum levels of antibiotic.
   (ENG)

685

Total loss of vestibular function but no hearing loss due to total of 840 mg
of antibiotic, gentamicin (SM), in 47 day period in 1 of 181 humans, aged, 70
years age, female, with kidney disorder.
Total loss of vestibular function but no hearing loss due to 2 g of antibiotic, streptomycin (SM), in 47 day period in 1 of 181 humans, aged, 70 years
age, female, with kidney disorder.
Permanent vestibular problems due to 2.56 g of antibiotic, (SQ) gentamicin,
for 18 days in 1 of 181 humans, adult, 39 years age, female, with kidney
disorder.
Vestibular problems due to previous administration of antibiotic, (SQ) streptomycin, in 1 of 181 humans, adult, 39 years age, female, with kidney disorder.
Permanent vestibular problems, with dizziness, due to antibiotic, gentamicin,
in 1 of 181 humans, adult, 38 years age, female, with kidney disorder.
Transient dizziness after 3 days due to antibiotic, gentamicin, in 1 of 181
humans, adolescent, 16 years age, female, with kidney disorder.
   (AD) Serial vestibular function tests and audiometry not conducted in 181
   patients.
Vestibular problems due to parenteral, intramuscular, administration of 1 g
daily of antibiotic, (SQ) streptomycin (SM), in 1 human, adult, 19 years age,
male, with pseudomonas infection.
   (AD) Vestibular problems due to previous streptomycin therapy.
Simultaneous administration of 300 mg daily of antibiotic, (SQ) colistin (SM)
(colistimethate), for 15 days in 1 human, adult, 19 years age, male, with
pseudomonas infection.
Sequential parenteral, intramuscular, administration of 40 mg 3 times a day
of antibiotic, (SQ) gentamicin, for 36 days in 1 human, adult, 19 years age,
male, with pseudomonas infection.
Dizziness after 4 days due to parenteral, intramuscular, administration of 40
mg 4 times a day, total of 2.56 g, of antibiotic, gentamicin, for 16 days in
1 human, adult, 30 years age, female, with kidney disorder.
   (AD) Discussion of 6 case reports of vestibulotoxic effects of gentamicin.
   (ENG)

700

Dizziness or vertigo, during first 3 months in 7 cases and after 3 to 6
months in 5 cases, due to 1 g daily for first 3 months, and then 1 g 3 times
a week for second 3 months in patients 50 years age or less, or 1 g 3 times a
week for 6 months in patients over 50 years age, of antibiotic, streptomycin
(SM) (streptomycin sulfate), for 6 months in 12 (20 percent) of 59 humans,

adult and aged, 55 years or more age in most cases, male, with chronic pulmonary tuberculosis and pneumoconiosis.
   (AD) Reported 20 percent incidence of streptomycin ototoxicity in first
   year of therapy.
Incr hearing loss reported after 6 months due to 1 g daily for first 3
months, and then 1 g 3 times a week for second 3 months in patients 50 years
age or less, or 1 g 3 times a week for 6 months in patients over 50 years
age, of antibiotic, streptomycin (SM) (streptomycin sulfate), for 6 months in
1 of 59 humans, adult and aged, 55 years or more age in most cases, male,
with chronic pulmonary tuberculosis and pneumoconiosis and with previous
hearing loss.
   (AD) Reported 1 case of hearing loss due to streptomycin in first year of
   therapy.
Dizziness and tinnitus after 14 months due to 1 g daily for first 3 months,
and then 1 g 3 times a week for second 3 months in patients 50 years age or
less, or 1 g 3 times a week for 6 months in patients over 50 years age, of
antibiotic, streptomycin (SM) (streptomycin sulfate), for 6 months in 1 of 31
humans, male, with chronic pulmonary tuberculosis and pneumoconiosis.
   (AD) Reported 1 case with ototoxic effects within 18 months of therapy.
Simultaneous oral administration in cachets of 333 mg daily of antituberculous agent, isoniazid (SM) (CB), for 18 months or more in 59 humans, male,
with chronic pulmonary tuberculosis and pneumoconiosis.
Simultaneous oral administration in cachets of 15 g daily of antituberculous
agent, PAS (SM) (CB) (sodium PAS), for 18 months or more in 59 humans, male,
with chronic pulmonary tuberculosis and pneumoconiosis. (ENG)

                              ANIMALS

                                                                         506
Damage to hair cells of vestibular apparatus and cochlea due to antibiotics
in humans and animals.
   (AD) Discussion of relationship between elimination of drugs and damage to
   ear.
   (AD) Need for careful consideration in use of aminoglycoside antibiotics.
   (ENG)

                                                                         704
Functional damage to cochlea evident before changes in structure due to
antibiotics in animals.
   (AD) Need for correlation of various methods, morphological, electrophy-
   siological, and biochemical, in study of function of inner ear.
   (AD) Literature review of various methods of study of auditory system.
   (ENG)

                                                                         590
Ototoxic effects due to antibiotic, capreomycin, in animals.
   (AD) In vivo and in vitro studies of capreomycin. (IT)

                                                                         436
Hearing loss and damage to organ of Corti due to topical route, inhalation,
of chemical agent, carbon monoxide, in animals. (GER)

                                                                         540
Effect on cells of cochlea due to antineoplastic, nitrogen mustard, in animals. (JAP)

                                                                         235
Effect on hair cells of vestibular apparatus and organ of Corti due to ototo-
xic drugs in humans and animals.
   (AD) Suggested role of hair cells of vestibular apparatus and organ of
   Corti as sensory meters with relative resistance to drugs.
   (AD) Literature review of effects of drugs on sensory endings. (ENG)

                                                                         336
Damage to type 1 hair cells of vestibular apparatus and vestibular problems
due to topical administration to middle ear of antibiotic, streptomycin, in 1
injection in animals.
   (AD) Destruction of hair cells and ototoxicity result of effect of strep-

tomycin on protein synthesis of cells.   (FR)

375
Possible hearing loss due to antibiotic, streptomycin, in humans.
   (AD) Discussion of value of experimentation with animals to determine use
   and effects of drugs in humans.
   (AD) Possible to determine total hearing loss due to drugs in dogs and
   monkeys but more difficult to determine partial hearing loss in animals.
   (AD) Possible that high doses of drugs used in experimentation help to
   determine effects in therapeutic doses.   (ENG)

480
Changes in acid phosphatase activity of vestibular apparatus due to antibiotic, streptomycin (streptomycin sulfate), in animals.
   (AD) Study using electron microscopy of acid phosphatase activity of
   vestibular apparatus.   (JAP)

015
Damage to cells of ampulla due to range of doses of antibiotic, viomycin, in
animals.
   (AD) Electron microscopic study of effects of viomycin on vestibular
   apparatus.   (JAP)

346
Temporary inhibition of oxygen consumption at level of mitochondria of cen-
tral vestibular nuclei due to antibiotic, streptomycin, in animals.
Temporary inhibition of oxygen consumption at level of mitochondria of cen-
tral vestibular nuclei due to antibiotic, rifampicin, in animals.
   (AD) Discussion of chronic and acute vestibular toxicity.   (ENG)

384
Usually transient hearing loss and no structural damage to organ of Corti,
stria vascularis, and spiral ganglion due to oral or topical administration
of salicylates in humans.
Hearing loss due to antimalarial, quinine, in humans.
Usually permanent hearing loss due to antimalarial, chloroquine, in humans.
Transient and permanent hearing loss and possible damage to hair cells of
organ of Corti due to diuretic, ethacrynic acid, in humans.
Sensorineural hearing loss due to cardiovascular agent, hexadimethrine
bromide, in humans with kidney disorder.
Sensorineural hearing loss and damage to organ of Corti due to topical ad-
ministration of antineoplastic, nitrogen mustard, in humans.
Sensorineural hearing loss due to high doses of antibiotic, chloramphenicol,
in humans.
Primary vestibular problems due to antibiotic, streptomycin, in humans.
Hearing loss due to high doses usually of antibiotic, streptomycin, in humans.
   (AD) Early detection of hearing loss by audiometry prevents permanent
   damage.
High frequency hearing loss and severe damage to outer hair cells and slight
damage to inner hair cells of organ of Corti due to antibiotic, kanamycin, in
humans.
Sensorineural hearing loss due to parenteral, oral, and topical administration of antibiotic, neomycin, in humans with or without kidney disorders.
Degeneration of hair cells of organ of Corti and of nerve process due to
antibiotics, aminoglycoside, in animals.
   (AD) Literature review of physiological and structural cochleo-vestibulotoxic effects of ototoxic drugs.
   (AD) Discussion of suggested mechanism of ototoxicity and routes of drugs
   to inner ear.
Bilateral sensorineural hearing loss due to oral administration of antibiotic, neomycin, in 4 of 8 humans with liver disease.
Bilateral sensorineural hearing loss due to oral administration of range of
doses of antibiotic, neomycin (SM), in 2 of 5 humans with liver disease.
Bilateral sensorineural hearing loss due to diuretics (SM), in 2 of 5 humans
with liver disease.
Transient progression of previous hearing loss due to parenteral, intravenous, administration of diuretic, ethacrynic acid (SM), in 1 injection in 1

of 5 humans with liver disease.
   (CT)   Normal cochlear function in 6 humans, control group, with liver
disease and not treated with neomycin or diuretics.
   (CT)   Normal cochlear function in 13 humans, control group, with liver
disease and treated with diuretics but not with neomycin.
   (AD) Hearing loss confirmed by audiometry.
   (AD)   Reported that hearing loss due to neomycin or diuretics in humans
with liver disease not related to dosage.
   (AD) Clinical study of effects of treatment with neomycin and diuretics in
humans with liver disease.
Bilateral sensorineural hearing loss and vertigo due to antibiotic, ampicil-
lin, in 1 human, adolescent, 17 years age, female, with tonsillitis.
   (AD) Cited case report.
Severe sensorineural hearing loss and vertigo due to topical administration
in ear drops of antibiotic, framycetin, in 1 human, adult, 42 years age,
male, with previous slight high frequency hearing loss.
   (AD) Cited case report.
Atrophy of hair cells of organ of Corti and hearing loss due to antibiotic,
dihydrostreptomycin, in humans with tuberculous meningitis.
   (AD) Cited study.
Loss of inner hair cells and damage to outer hair cells due to 18 g of anti-
biotic, neomycin, for 18 days in 1 human.
   (AD) Cited case report. (ENG)

413
Decr in threshold of detection of acoustic stimuli of shorter duration than
16 msec due to 0.4 g of analeptic, caffeine, in humans, adult, and animals.
Decr in threshold of detection of acoustic stimuli of longer duration than 16
msec due to 0.015 to 0.02 g of analeptic, amphetamine, in humans, adult, and
animals. (RUS)

444
Changes in cochlear function and vestibular function due to analeptic, caf-
feine, in animals and humans.
Changes in cochlear function and vestibular function due to analeptic, amphe-
tamine, in animals and humans.
Changes in cochlear function and vestibular function due to sedatives and
tranquilizers in animals and humans.
   (AD) Suggested mechanism of action of drugs.
   (AD) Literature review of ototoxic effects of drugs. (IT)

455
Damage to sensory epithelia of vestibular apparatus due to 250 mg per kg of
antibiotic, streptomycin, in animals.
Damage to sensory epithelia of vestibular apparatus due to 250 mg per kg of
antibiotic, kanamycin, in animals. (JAP)

MAMMALS

Cat

527
Decr in vestibular neurons due to parenteral, slow intravenous, administration of low doses, corresponding to 0.6 g per kg of 100 percent alcohol, of
diluted 30 percent concentration of sedative, alcohol, ethyl, in 1 injection
in animals, cats, adult, male and female, 3.0 kg weight.
   (AD) Suggested susceptibility of vestibular neurons to direct effects of
   alcohol.
   (AD) Suggested that clinical alcoholic intoxication, with nystagmus, due
   to direct action of alcohol on vestibular neurons. (ENG)

330
Hearing loss due to parenteral, intramuscular, administration of 31 mg per kg
or 62 mg per kg daily of antibiotic, capreomycin (capreomycin disulfate), for
more than 1000 days in 4 animals, dogs, male and female.
Hearing loss due to parenteral, subcutaneous, administration of 13 mg per kg
or 130 mg per kg daily of antibiotic, capreomycin (capreomycin tetrahydroch-
loride), for 91 days in 2 animals, cats, male.

(AD) Hearing loss determined by response of animals to reproducible sound. (ENG)

555

Cochlear impairment due to parenteral, intramuscular, administration of 100 mg per kg 3 times per week or 25 or 50 mg per kg daily of antibiotic, capreomycin, for 2 years in several animals, dogs.
Vestibular problems due to parenteral, subcutaneous, administration of 125 mg per kg daily of antibiotic, capreomycin, for 84 days in several animals, cats.
   (AD) Discussion of chemistry of capreomycin, results of in vitro and in vivo studies, and toxicity of capreomycin in animals. (ENG)

344

No significant change in perrotatory neuronal response of medial vestibular nucleus due to parenteral, intravenous, administration of 2, 8, or 20 mg per kg of antihistamine, dimenhydrinate, in animals, cats, adult, 2.5 kg average weight.
Significant decr in perrotatory neuronal response of medial vestibular nucleus due to parenteral, intravenous, administration of 0.4 mg per kg of diazepan in animals, cat s, adult, 2.5 kg average weight.
   (CT) Same method using 1 ml Ringer's solution in cats, control group, showed no significant changes.
   (AD) Possible peripheral or central location, or both, of action of dimenhydrinate.
   (AD) Study to determine if changes in perrotatory response of medial vestibular nucleus is result of action on vestibular apparatus.
   (AD) Suggest that endorgan not location of action of dimenhydrinate. (ENG)

134

Decr in threshold shift of 20 db and damage to outer hair cells and inner hair cells of organ of Corti due to topical administration to external auditory meatus of 50 percent solution of chemical agent, dimethyl sulfoxide, for 21 days in 7 animals, cats.
Damage to 40 percent of eighth cranial nerve action potential due to topical administration to external auditory meatus of chemical agent, dimethyl sulfoxide, for 6 hours in 4 animals, cats.
Damage to 60 percent of eighth cranial nerve action potential due to topical administration to middle ear of chemical agent, dimethyl sulfoxide, for 6 hours in 4 animals, cats.
   (CT) Control group of 4 cats used.
   (AD) Suggested that dimethyl sulfoxide new ototoxic drug. (GER)

405

Decr in cochlear potentials due to parenteral, intravenous, administration of total dose of 5 to 35 mg per kg of solution of chemical agent, dinitrophenol, in several doses in animals, cats, young, 1.0 to 1.8 kg weight, normal.
   (AD) Use of various intensities of test tone of 2 kcps.
More decr in cochlear potentials due to topical administration to round window of 1 drop at a time of 3 concentrations, in order of increasing concentration, of chemical agent, dinitrophenol, in animals, cats, young, 1.0 to 1.8 kg weight, normal.
   (AD) Use of various intensities of test tone of 2 kcps.
   (CT) Measurement of cochlear potentials before and after administration of chemical agent, dinitrophenol.
   (CT) Measurement of cochlear potentials for longer than usual before administration of chemical agent, dinitrophenol, in some animals, control group.
   (CT) Higher frequency test tone of 5 kcps used in some animals, control group.
   (CT) Same method with administration of intravenous 2 percent solution of sodium bicarbonate with chemical agent, dinitrophenol, in cats, control group, resulted in no decr in cochlear potentials. (ENG)

406

Incr in cochlear potentials due to parenteral, intravenous, administration of 1 dose of 10 mg per kg and then doses of 5 mg per kg of chemical agent,

dinitrophenol, in total of 5 doses in animals, cats, with acoustic trauma.
    (AD) Use of low intensity test tone of 2 kcps.
Decr in cochlear potentials due to topical administration to round window of
1 drop at a time of various concentrations of chemical agent, dinitrophenol,
in animals, cats, with acoustic trauma.
    (AD) Use of low intensity test tone of 2 kcps.
    (AD) No consistent difference in effect on cochlear potentials of topical
    administration of chemical agent, dinitrophenol, in cats with and without
    acoustic trauma.
Decr in cochlear potentials due to parenteral, intravenous, administration of
1 dose of 5 mg per kg, followed by 1 dose of 10 mg per kg, followed by other
doses of 5 mg per kg of chemical agent, dinitrophenol, in total of 4 doses in
animals, cats, with acoustic trauma.
    (AD) Use of high intensity test tone of 2 kcps.
    (CT) Measurement of cochlear potentials for longer than usual before
    administration of chemical agent, dinitrophenol, in some animals, control
    group.
    (CT) Same method with administration of intravenous 2 percent solution of
    sodium bicarbonate with chemical agent, dinitrophenol, in cats, control
    group. (ENG)

                                                                         144
Moderate bilateral sensorineural hearing loss within 20 minutes and damage to
outer hair cells of organ of Corti due to unspecified method of administration of 50 mg of diuretic, ethacrynic acid, in 1 dose in humans with kidney
disorder.
    (AD) Hearing loss confirmed by audiogram.
Sensorineural hearing loss within 15 minutes due to unspecified method of
administration of 20 to 30 mg per kg daily of diuretic, ethacrynic acid, in
20 animals, cats.
    (AD) Ethacrynic acid not recommended for clinical use in humans with
    kidney disorders. (ENG)

                                                                         093
Cochleo-vestibulotoxic effects due to parenteral administration of 50 to 100
mg per kg daily of antibiotic, gentamicin (gentamicin sulfate), for 20 days
in humans and animals, cats and guinea pigs.
    (AD) Literature review showed ototoxic effects of gentamicin in 2.8 per-
    cent of cases reported. (ENG)

                                                                         574
Ataxia due to parenteral, subcutaneous, administration of 20, 40, or 60 mg
per kg daily, dissolved in distilled water in volume of 0.5 ml per kg, of
antibiotic, gentamicin (gentamicin sulfate), for 10 to 70 days in animals,
cats, male, 2.5 to 5.0 kg weight.
    (AD) Tests to determine ataxia conducted.
    (AD) Relationship between onset of ataxia and dosage.
Permanent ataxia due to parenteral, subcutaneous, administration of 40 mg per
kg daily of antibiotic, gentamicin (gentamicin sulfate), for 16, 18, or 19
days, followed by a rest for 29 to 32 days, and then 19 to 20 days more in 3
animals, cats.
    (AD) Ataxia persisted during period without gentamicin treatment.
Ataxia due to parenteral, subcutaneous, administration of 20, 40, or 60 mg
per kg daily, total doses of 600 to about 900 mg per kg, of antibiotic,
gentamicin (gentamicin sulfate), in animals, cats.
    (AD) Occurrence of ataxia after smaller average total dose at lower dosage
    levels than at higher levels.
    (AD) Inverse relationship between onset of ataxia and total dosage sug-
    gests that duration of treatment possibly significant factor at dosage
    levels studied.
Ataxia after 25 days due to parenteral, subcutaneous, administration of 40 mg
per kg daily of antibiotic, gentamicin (gentamicin sulfate), for 5 days in 5
animals, cats.
Ataxia after 18 days due to parenteral, subcutaneous, administration of 40 mg
per kg daily of antibiotic, gentamicin (gentamicin sulfate), for 7 days in 5
animals, cats.
    (AD) Results of experiment suggest significance of total dosage and dura-
    tion of treatment.

Ataxia after 17 days due to parenteral, subcutaneous, administration of 40 mg per kg 1 time daily, average total of 680 mg per kg, of antibiotic, gentamicin (gentamicin sulfate), in 6 animals, cats.

Ataxia after 19.4 days due to parenteral, subcutaneous, administration of 20 mg per kg twice daily, average total of 776 mg per kg of antibiotic, gentamicin (gentamicin sulfate), in 5 animals, cats.

(AD) Average total dose to produce ataxia higher with 2 doses daily than with single daily dose.

Ataxia after 16 days due to parenteral, (SQ) subcutaneous, administration of 40 mg per kg daily, to produce blood levels of 100 mcg per ml 30 minutes after treatment, of antibiotic, gentamicin (gentamicin sulfate), in 1 dose in 2 animals, cats.

(AD) Rapid decr in blood levels 24 hours after treatment.

Ataxia after 16 days due to parenteral, (SQ) intraarterial, administration of 40 mg per kg daily of antibiotic, gentamicin (gentamicin sulfate), in 2 animals, cats.

(AD) Blood levels monitored daily.

(AD) Peak blood levels with intraarterial administration 2 to 6 times as high as with subcutaneous route and decr rapidly to less than 1 mcg per ml 24 hours after treatment.

(AD) Decr in kidney function at time of occurrence of ataxia.

(AD) Report on various experiments in study of factors in effect of gentamicin on vestibular function in cats.

(AD) Suggested that total dosage and duration of treatment possibly more significant factors than peak blood levels with reference to time of onset of ataxia at dosage levels studied. (ENG)

605

Decr in ototoxic effects due to parenteral, subcutaneous, administration of high doses of antibiotic, gentamicin (IB) (gentamicin sulfate), in acute intoxication in 20 animals, mice, male, 20 g weight, with simultaneous subcutaneous administration of calcium chloride.

(CT) Same method using 8 mg of calcium chloride in mice, control group, showed no ototoxic effects.

(CT) Same method using 12.5 mg of gentamicin (gentamicin sulfate) in mice, control group, showed ototoxic effects.

Decr in ototoxic effects due to parenteral, subcutaneous or intravenous, administration of 25 mg per ml solution of antibiotic, gentamicin (IB) (gentamicin sulfate), in acute intoxication in animals, mice, male, 20 g weight, with combined administration of 1, 2, 4, 8, 16, or 32 mg per ml concentrations of calcium chloride.

Decr in ototoxic effects due to parenteral, subcutaneous, administration of antibiotic, gentamicin (IB) (gentamicin hydrochloride), in acute intoxication in animals, mice, male, 20 g weight, with combined administration of complex of calcium chloride.

(AD) Decr in ototoxic effects in mice to less than 0.2 of effects of gentamicin (gentamicin hydrochloride) and to less than 0.5 of effects of gentamicin (gentamicin sulfate) due to calcium chloride.

Ataxia and equilibrium disorder due to parenteral, subcutaneous, administration of 60 and 120 mg per kg 1 time daily of antibiotic, gentamicin (gentamicin sulfate), in chronic intoxication in 20 animals, cats, male and female.

(CT) Same method using saline in cats, control group.

Ataxia and equilibrium disorder due to parenteral, subcutaneous, administration of 60 and 120 mg per kg 1 time daily of antibiotic, gentamicin (IB) (gentamicin hydrochloride), in chronic intoxication in 20 animals, cats, male and female, with administration of complex of calcium chloride.

(AD) No decr in ototoxicity due to calcium chloride in cats. (ENG)

086

Damage to organ of Corti due to parenteral, subcutaneous, administration of 150 mg per kg and 250 mg per kg of antibiotic, kanamycin, in 10 days in animals, cats.

(AD) Comparative study of ototoxicity of 4 compounds of kanamycin. (GER)

096

Loss of outer hair cells and inner hair cells and damage to reticular membrane of organ of Corti due to parenteral, intraperitoneal (SM), administration of 400 mg per kg (SM) of antibiotic, kanamycin (kanamycin sulfate), in 5

days in animals, 15 cats, adult, 2.5 kg weight, and 30 guinea pigs, young, 300 g weight.
Simultaneous topical (SM) administration to middle ear cavity of 0.6 ml of 20 percent solution (SM) of antibiotic, kanamycin (kanamycin sulfate), for '1 day in animals, 15 cats, adult, 2.5 kg weight, and 30 guinea pigs, young, 300 g weight.
   (AD) Study of repair pattern in reticular membrane after loss of hair cells. (ENG)

147
Protection from ototoxic effects on inner ear due to antibiotic, kanamycin (IB), in animals, cats, with administration of vitamin B.
   (AD) Preliminary study. (SP)

727
Decr in cochleotoxic effects due to parenteral, subcutaneous, administration of antibiotic, kanamycin (IB), in animals, cats, with administration of pantothenic acid.
   (AD) Electrophysiological study of effect of pantothenic acid on kanamycin ototoxicity in cats. (GER)

376
High concentration of drug in fluids of ear for long period due to parenteral, intravenous, administration of 15000 units per kg of antibiotic, neomycin, in 22 animals, cats.
   (AD) Comparative study of neomycin level in fluids of ear and in other biological fluids. (RUS)

048
Severe sensorineural hearing loss and loss of hair cells of organ of Corti in basal and middle coils of cochlea due to parenteral, intravenous, administration of high doses, 1.0 mg per kg, of antineoplastic, nitrogen mustard, in 1 injection in animals, cats, conditioned. (ENG)

291
Cochlear impairment due to 5.0 g of antimalarial, quinine (quinine hydrochloride), in humans.
Cochlear impairment due to antimalarial, quinine (quinine hydrochloride), in animals, cats and rabbits.
   (AD) Comparative animal studies and clinical case reports.
   (AD) Study of ocular toxicity with comment on ototoxicity. (GER)

189
Threshold shift due to parenteral, intraperitoneal, administration of 300 mg per kg of salicylate, sodium salicylate, in 1 dose in 4 animals, cats.
Small threshold shift of about 3 decibels due to parenteral, intraperitoneal, administration of 125 mg per kg daily of salicylate, sodium salicylate, for total of 28 injections in 4 animals, cats.
Threshold shift due to parenteral, intraperitoneal, administration of (SQ) 300 mg per kg of salicylate, sodium salicylate, in (SQ) 1 dose in 6 animals, guinea pigs.
Small threshold shift of about 4 decibels due to parenteral, intraperitoneal, administration of (SQ) 150,225, or 300 mg per kg daily of salicylate, sodium salicylate, for (SQ) total of 10 injections in 6 animals, guinea pigs. (ENG)

205
Changes in biochemical composition of endolymph and perilymph due to parenteral, intraperitoneal, administration of 350 mg per kg of salicylate, sodium salicylate, in 1 injection in 6 animals, cats.
   (CT) Same method using 10 ml saline solution in 3 cats, control group.
Decr in cochlear microphonic and neural potential due to parenteral, intraperitoneal, administration of 350 mg per kg of salicylate, sodium salicylate, in 1 injection in 7 animals, cats.
   (CT) Baseline cochlear microphonic and neural potential obtained.
   (AD) Suggested that hearing loss in salicylate intoxication due to biochemical changes in cochlea. (ENG)

110

Nystagmus and other vestibular problems due to topical administration to
bulla of 0.5 g of antibiotic, streptomycin, in 1 injection in cats.
(AD) Suggested route of streptomycin in cat from bulla by way of large
membrane of round window to inner ear.
Changes in chromatin in hair cells, type 1, of maculae due to topical administration to bulla of 0.5 g of antibiotic, streptomycin, in 1 injection in
cats.
(AD) Suggested that destruction of hair cells due to changes in protein
metabolism as result of action of streptomycin. (ENG)

253

Severe vestibular problems, as nystagmus, after 3 to 6 hours due to topical
administration to middle ear and parenteral administration of high doses of
antibiotic, streptomycin, for range of 1 to 7 days in 28 animals, cats.
Decr in ribosomes of cytoplasm of type 1 hair cells of vestibular apparatus
due to topical administration to middle ear and parenteral administration of
high doses of antibiotic, streptomycin, for range of 1 to 7 days in 28 animals, cats.
(CT) Study of cats, control group.
(AD) Suggested that primary location of action of streptomycin is protein
synthesis of cells. (GER)

380

Unilateral loss of vestibular function and no ataxia due to parenteral administration, infusion into carotid artery, of 150 cc in Ringer's Lactate
every 24 hours, total dose of 0.84 to 1.5 g per kg, of antibiotic, streptomycin (streptomycin sulfate), for 3 to 10 days in 5 animals, cat s, adult, 1.9
to 3.1 kg weight.
Bilateral loss of vestibular function with ataxia and destruction of hair
cells of crista ampullaris and semicircular canal due to parenteral administration, infusion into carotid artery, of 150 cc in Ringer's Lactate every 24
hours, total dose of 1.2 to 2.5 g per kg, of antibiotic, streptomycin (streptomycin sulfate), for 6 to 12 days in 5 animals, cats, adult, 2.3 to 5.1 kg
weight.
No hearing loss and no damage to hair cells of organ of Corti due to parenteral administration, infusion into carotid artery, of 150 cc in Ringer's
Lactate every 24 hours, total dose of 0.84 to 2.5 g per kg, of antibiotic,
streptomycin (streptomycin sulfate), for 3 to 12 days in 10 animals, cats,
adult, 1.9 to 5.1 kg weight.
Decr in cochlear microphonic but no damage to hair cells of organ of Corti
due to parenteral administration, infusion into carotid artery, of 150 cc in
Ringer's Lactate every 24 hours, total dose of 1.0 g per kg, of antibiotic,
streptomycin (streptomycin sulfate), for 4 days in 1 animal, cat, adult, 3.0
kg weight.
(CT) Measurement of cochlear function and vestibular function before and
after infusion of streptomycin.
(AD) Type of loss of vestibular function due to total dosage of streptomycin and duration of administration.
(AD) Unilateral destruction of vestibular function without cochlear impairment is goal in treatment of Meniere's disease. (ENG)

047

Range of degree of damage to crista ampullaris and macula due to parenteral,
intramuscular, administration of 150 mg per kg daily of antibiotic, viomycin
(viomycin sulfate), for about 2 to 3 weeks in 3 animals, squirrel monkeys.
Range of degree of damage to crista ampullaris and macula due to parenteral,
intramuscular, administration of 200 to 300 mg per kg daily of antibiotic,
viomycin (viomycin sulfate), for about 2 to 3 weeks in 3 animals, cats.
More severe damage to crista ampullaris and macula due to topical administration in solution of range of 113 mg per ml to 500 mg per ml solution of
antibiotic, viomycin (viomycin sulfate), in 1 or 2 doses in 9 animals, cats.
(CT) Control group of 2 monkeys and 2 cats used. (ENG)

005

Transient primary decr in cochlear microphonic and action potential due to
parenteral, intravenous, administration of 10 mg per kg of diuretic, ethacrynic acid, in 1 injection in 20 animals, cats, adult.
Transient primary decr in cochlear microphonic and action potential due to

parenteral, intravenous, administration of 10 mg per kg of diuretic, furosemide, in 1 injection in 20 animals, cats, adult.
Delayed severe secondary decr in cochlear microphonic and action potential
due to parenteral, intravenous, administration of more than 10 mg per kg of
diuretic, ethacrynic acid, in animals, cats.
    (CT) Same method using 50 mg per kg and 100 mg per kg of diuretic, chloro-
    thiazide, in cats, control group, showed no ototoxic effect.
Degeneration of outer hair cells of organ of Corti in basal and middle coils
of cochlea due to parenteral, intravenous, administration of 30 mg per kg of
diuretic, ethacrynic acid, in 1 injection in 2 animals, cats.
Degeneration of outer hair cells of organ of Corti due to parenteral, intramuscular, administration of 15 mg per kg of diuretic, ethacrynic acid, for 2
weeks in 1 animal, cat. (ENG)

                                                                          020
Effect on function of inner ear due to parenteral, subcutaneous, administration of high doses, range of 30 to 75 mg per kg of antibiotic, gentamicin,
for about 8 to 20 days in 11 animals, cats.
    (AD) Preliminary study of dosage levels.
Damage to semicircular canal, membranous labyrinth, and outer hair cells and
inner hair cells of the cochlea due to parenteral, subcutaneous, administration of high doses, range of 30 to 75 mg per kg of antibiotic, gentamicin,
for about 8 to 20 days in 11 animals, cats, with kidney damage resulting from
gentamicin.
    (AD) Preliminary study of dosage levels.
Partial hearing loss due to parenteral, subcutaneous, administration of 20 mg
per kg of antibiotic, gentamicin, for 14 days in 1 out of 15 animals, cats.
Complete degeneration of outer hair cells of organ of Corti due to parenteral, subcutaneous, administration of 20 mg per kg of antibiotic, gentamicin, for 14 days in 1 out of 15 animals, cats.
Range of degree of damage, transient and permanent, to vestibular apparatus
due to parenteral, subcutaneous, administration of 20 mg per kg of antibiotic, gentamicin, for 14 days in 15 animals, cats.
Complete damage to vestibular apparatus due to parenteral, subcutaneous,
administration of 200 mg per kg of antibiotic, streptomycin, for 9 days in
animals, cats.
Higher incidence and earlier symptoms of ototoxic effects due to parenteral,
subcutaneous, administration of 20 mg per kg of antibiotic, gentamicin, for
14 days in 66.6 percent of 15 animals, cats, with kidney damage than in cats
with normal kidney function.
    (AD) Study of correlation of functional and histological effects of genta-
    micin.
    (AD) Comparative study of effect on vestibular apparatus of gentamicin and
    streptomycin. (ENG)

                                                                          130
Decr in cochlear microphonic and neural potentials and incr in sodium and
glucose of endolymph due to parenteral, intravenous, administration of 30 to
60 mg per kg, in saline solution, of diuretic, ethacrynic acid, for 5 minute
period in animals, cats.
Changes in stria vascularis and damage to outer hair cells of organ of Corti
due to parenteral, intravenous, administration of 30 to 60 mg per kg, in
saline solution, of diuretic, ethacrynic acid, for 5 minute period in animals, cats.
No change in cochlear microphonic, no incr in endolymph glucose, and normal
endolymph chemical composition due to parenteral, intravenous, administration
of 50 mg per kg, in saline solution, of diuretic, acetazolamide, for 5 minute
period in animals, cats.
Slow decr in cochlear microphonic and neural potentials due to parenteral,
intravenous, administration of 200 mg per kg, in saline solution, of diuretic, acetazolamide, for 5 minute period in animals, cats.
    (CT) Same method using 7 cc per kg of saline solution in 14 cats, control
    group.
    (AD) Clinical significance of study of acetazolamide not determined due to
    lack of reports of hearing loss with use of drug.
Severe decr in cochlear microphonic and neural potentials but no changes in
electrolyte concentrations of endolymph or perilymph due to parenteral,
intravenous, administration of 30 mg per kg daily of diuretic, ethacrynic

acid, for 3 to 4 days in 3 animals, cats.
    (AD) Results of study suggest severe hearing loss.
Edema of stria vascularis and damage to outer hair cells of organ of Corti
but normal chemical composition of endolymph and perilymph due to parenteral,
intraperitoneal, administration of 30 mg per kg of diuretic, ethacrynic acid,
in 1 dose in 9 animals, cats.
    (AD) Study of effect of diuretics on chemical composition of fluids of
    inner ear and relationship to cochlear microphonic and histopathology of
    temporal bone. (ENG)

185

Ataxia, damage to hair cells of macula, and damage to hair cells of organ of
Corti due to parenteral, subcutaneous, administration of 10 to 80 mg per kg
daily of antibiotic, gentamicin (gentamicin sulfate), for 19 to 120 days in
animals, cats.
Ataxia due to 100 and 200 mg per kg daily of antibiotic, streptomycin (streptomycin sulfate), for 8 to 40 days in animals, cats.
Loss of Preyer reflex, decr in cochlear potential and eighth cranial nerve
action potential, and loss of outer hair cells of organ of Corti due to 80 to
200 mg per kg daily of antibiotic, gentamicin (gentamicin sulfate), in animals, guinea pigs.
Damage to cochlea due to 100 and 200 mg per kg of antibiotic, kanamycin
(kanamycin sulfate), in animals, guinea pigs.
    (AD) Comparative study of ototoxicity of gentamicin and other aminoglyco-
    side antibiotics.
    (AD) Study suggested low risk of ototoxicity when gentamicin used in
    recommended clinical dose of 1 to 3 mg per kg. (ENG)

283

Effect on action potentials and cochlear microphonic and on vestibular apparatus due to range of doses of antibiotic, streptomycin, for range of
periods in animals, cats.
Effect on action potentials and cochlear microphonic and on vestibular apparatus due to range of doses of antibiotic, kanamycin, for range of periods
in animals, cats. (IT)

288

Changes in cochlear microphonic due to parenteral, intramuscular, administration of 300 mg per kg daily of antibiotic, kanamycin, in animals, cats.
Changes in cochlear microphonic due to parenteral, intramuscular, administration of 200 and 100 mg per kg daily of antibiotic, streptomycin, in animals,
cats.
Hearing loss due to 300 mg per kg daily of antibiotic, kanamycin, in humans.
Hearing loss due to range of 50 to 200 mg per kg daily of antibiotic, streptomycin, in humans.
    (CT) Study of subjects, control group, not treated with aminoglycoside
    antibiotics.
    (AD) Hearing loss confirmed by audiogram. (JAP)

324

Ataxia, vestibular problems with improvement in some, and damage to hair
cells of vestibular apparatus due to parenteral, subcutaneous, administration
of 20 mg per kg of antibiotic, gentamicin (gentamicin sulfate), for 19 days
maximum for acute intoxication and 14 days for chronic intoxication in 15
animals, cats.
Hearing loss and damage to hair cells of cochlea due to parenteral, subcutaneous, administration of 20 mg per kg of antibiotic, gentamicin (gentamicin
sulfate), for 19 days maximum for acute intoxication and 14 days for chronic
intoxication in 1 of 15 animals, cats.
    (AD) Preliminary study to determine minimum toxic level of gentamicin by
    parenteral route made previously.
    (AD) Cochleo-vestibulotoxic effects determined by audiometry and vestibu-
    lar function tests.
Permanent severe vestibular problems and damage to hair cells of vestibular
apparatus due to parenteral, subcutaneous, administration of 200 mg per kg of
antibiotic, streptomycin (streptomycin sulfate), in 3 animals, cats.
Hearing loss and damage to hair cells of cochlea due to parenteral, subcutaneous, administration of 200 mg per kg of antibiotic, streptomycin (strep-

tomycin sulfate), in 2 of 3 animals, cats.
Ataxia, vestibular problems, and damage to hair cells of vestibular apparatus
due to topical administration to bulla in solution of 6 percent concentration
in water of antibiotic, gentamicin (gentamicin sulfate), for 19 days in 1
animal, cat.
Ataxia, vestibular problems, and more severe damage to hair cells of vestibular apparatus due to topical administration to bulla in solution of 6 percent
concentration in Monex of antibiotic, gentamicin (gentamicin sulfate), for 5
days in 3 animals, cats.
    (CT) Same method using water or Monex without gentamicin in 11 cats,
    control group, showed no ototoxic effects.
    (AD) Preliminary study to determine concentration of gentamicin for topi-
    cal route made previously.
Vestibular problems due to topical administration to bulla in solution of 6
percent concentration in water of antibiotic, neomycin, for 31 days in 2
animals, cats.
    (AD) Comparative study of effects of gentamicin and other aminoglycoside
    antibiotics.
    (AD) Ototoxicity of gentamicin dose related. (ENG)

                                                                        345
Transient hearing loss and vestibular problem due to salicylate, aspirin, in
humans.
Decr in cochlear microphonic and action potential and decr in malic dehydrogenase in endolymph and perilymph due to salicylate, aspirin, in humans.
    (AD) Suggested that cochleo-vestibulotoxic effects of salicylates due to
    electrophysiological and biochemical changes and not structural changes.
Primary distribution in stria vascularis and spiral ligament due to salicylate, aspirin, in humans.
    (AD) Possible but not definite location of toxic activity of aspirin.
High concentration in inner ear after 5 to 7 hours due to parenteral, intraperitoneal, administration of salicylate, sodium salicylate, in animals,
cats.
    (AD) Report on clinical use and ototoxic effects of aspirin. (ENG)

                                                                        392
No hearing loss but tinnitus due to parenteral, intramuscular, administration
of range of 0.05 to 1.0 g daily according to age of antibiotic, kanamycin,
for short period in 4 of 125 humans, infant, child, and adult, with acute
otorhinolaryngological infections.
    (AD) Audiograms showed no hearing loss.
Hearing loss, subjective in 1 case and latent in others, but no vestibular
problems due to 1.0 g daily 2 times a week of antibiotic, (SQ) kanamycin, for
long period in 15 of 66 humans, adolescent and adult, 15 to 55 years age,
with pulmonary tuberculosis and with previous streptomycin treatment.
    (CT) Audiogram before and during treatment with kanamycin.
Hearing loss due to previous administration of antibiotic, (SQ) streptomycin,
in 31 of 272 humans.
Sensorineural hearing loss due to previous administration of total of 600 g
of antibiotic, (SQ) streptomycin, in 1 human, adult, 27 years age.
More severe sensorineural hearing loss, subjective, due to total of 136 g of
antibiotic, (SQ) kanamycin, in 1 human, adult, 27 years age.
    (AD) Case report of hearing loss due to streptomycin potentiated by treat-
    ment with kanamycin.
Hearing loss, latent, and tinnitus, but no vestibular problems due to total
of over 20 g to over 300 g of antibiotic, kanamycin, for long period in 10 of
70 humans with pulmonary tuberculosis and no previous chemotherapy.
    (CT) Audiogram before and during treatment with kanamycin.
    (AD) Clinical studies of effects of treatment with kanamycin for short and
    long periods.
Vestibular problems after 10 to 12 days due to parenteral administration of
100 mg per kg daily of antibiotic, streptomycin, in 3 animals, cats, 2 kg
weight.
Slight vestibular problems after 30 days due to 300 mg per kg daily of antibiotic, kanamycin, in 3 animals, cats, 2 kg weight.
Decr in cochlear microphonic due to 200 mg per kg daily of antibiotic, streptomycin, in 11 injections in animals, cats.
Slight decr in cochlear microphonic due to 300 mg per kg daily of antibiotic,

kanamycin, in 11 to 60 injections in animals, cats.
    (AD) Comparative experimental studies of cochleo-vestibulotoxic effects of kanamycin and streptomycin in cats.
    (AD) Different effects of 2 aminoglycoside antibiotics on vestibular function but similar effects on cochlear function.   (ENG)

468

Complete inhibition of acetylcholine induced decr in cochlear potential due to parenteral, intravenous, administration of 1.0 mg of antibiotic, streptomycin (streptomycin sulfate), in 1 injection in 5 animals, cats, male and female, 1.5 to 2.8 kg weight, with injection of acetylcholine.
Minimum inhibition of acetylcholine induced decr in cochlear potential due to parenteral, intravenous, administration of 1.0 mg of antibiotic, dihydrostreptomycin (dihydrostreptomycin sulfate), in 1 injection in 5 animals, cats, male and female, 1.5 to 2.8 kg weight, with injection of acetylcholine.
Complete inhibition of acetylcholine induced decr in cochlear potential due to parenteral, intravenous, administration of 1.0 mg of antibiotic, kanamycin (kanamycin sulfate), in 1 injection in 5 animals, cats, male and female, 1.5 to 2.8 kg weight, with injection of acetylcholine.
Complete inhibition of acetylcholine induced decr in cochlear potential due to parenteral, intravenous, administration of 1.0 mg of antibiotic, neomycin (neomycin sulfate), in 1 injection in 5 animals, cats, male and female, 1.5 to 2.8 kg weight, with injection of acetylcholine.
Acute inhibition of acetylcholine induced decr in cochlear potential due to parenteral, intravenous, administration of 1.0 mg of antimalarial, quinine (quinine hydrochloride), in 1 injection in 5 animals, cats, male and female, 1.5 to 2.8 kg weight, with injection of acetylcholine.
    (CT) Injections of 0.1 ml isotonic saline in cats, control group.
Inhibition of acetylcholine induced decr in cochlear potential due to parenteral, subcutaneous, administration of 300 mg per kg daily of antibiotic, streptomycin, for 7 to 9 days in 10 animals, cats.
Inhibition of acetylcholine induced decr in cochlear potential due to parenteral, subcutaneous, administration of 100 mg per kg daily of antibiotic, neomycin, for 7 to 9 days in 10 animals, cats.
    (CT) Study of 7 cats, control group, not treated with antibiotics.
    (AD) Study of effect of acetylcholine on cochlear potential after acute and chronic administration of ototoxic drugs.
    (AD) Suggested relationship between change in acetylcholine activity and ototoxic drugs.
    (AD) Suggested that ototoxicity partially due to disruption of efferent effect on cochlea. (ENG)

547

Bilateral sensorineural hearing loss within 20 minutes but normal vestibular function due to parenteral, intravenous, administration of 50 mg of diuretic, ethacrynic acid (SM), in 1 injection in 1 human, adult, 53 years age, female, with kidney disorder.
    (AD) Hearing loss confirmed by audiogram.
    (AD) Vestibular function tests showed normal vestibular function.
Simultaneous oral administration of 18 g of antibiotic, neomycin (SM), in 7 days in 1 human, adult, 53 years age, female, with kidney disorder.
Severe destruction of outer hair cells of organ of Corti in basal coil of cochlea due to parenteral, intravenous, administration of 50 mg of diuretic, ethacrynic acid (SM), in 1 injection in 1 human, adult, 53 years age, female, with kidney disorder.
    (AD) Suggested that damage to hair cells possibly due to neomycin also.
    (AD) Suggested possible permanent hearing loss as result of ethacrynic acid treatment in patients with kidney disorders.
Transient and permanent total hearing loss within 15 minutes due to parenteral administration of diuretic, ethacrynic acid, in animals, cats. (ENG)

576

Progressive ataxia beginning after 4 days of treatment due to topical administration to bulla of 0.4 ml daily of aqueous solution of 10 percent concentration, to produce blood level of 7 mcg per ml, of antibiotic, gentamicin, for 19 days maximum in 1 of 2 animals, cats.
Minimal transient ataxia beginning after 10 to 18 days of treatment and moderate damage to cristae and maculae but normal cochlea due to topical

administration to bulla of 0.4 ml daily of aqueous solution of 3 percent
concentration, to produce blood levels of less than 0.5 mcg per ml, of antibiotic, gentamicin, for 19 days maximum in 1 of 3 animals, cats.

(AD) Preliminary studies of topical gentamicin in cats.

(AD) Not possible to obtain audiograms due to administration of gentamicin
in middle ear so evaluation of cochlear function depended on histological
study of cochlea.

(AD) Evaluation of vestibular function with vestibular function tests.
Ataxia beginning after 12 days of treatment, decr in duration of rotatory
nystagmus, change in ENG, and loss of hair cells of cristae and of organ of
Corti in basal coil of cochlea due to topical administration to bulla of 0.4
ml daily of aqueous solution of 6 percent concentration of antibiotic, gentamicin, for 19 days maximum in 4 animals, cats.
No clinical vestibular problems and no significant change in duration of
rotatory nystagmus and in ENG but degeneration of cochlea and spiral ganglion
and changes in saccule due to topical administration to bulla of 0.4 ml daily
of aqueous solution of 3 percent concentration of antibiotic, gentamicin, for
30 days maximum in 5 animals, cats.

(AD) Direct relationship between onset of ataxia and concentration of
gentamicin solution.

(AD) Correlation between duration of rotatory nystagmus and ataxia.

(AD) Topical gentamicin most toxic to cochlea and saccule.

(AD) Need to monitor clinical use of gentamicin with audiology.
No clinical vestibular problems, transient decr in duration of rotatory
nystagmus, transient bilateral decr in ENG, and loss of hair cells of organ
of Corti in basal coil of cochlea but normal vestibular apparatus due to
topical administration to bulla of 0.4 ml daily of solution of 6 percent
concentration of antibiotic, neomycin, for 30 days maximum in 2 animals,
cats.

(AD) Comparative study of effects of topical gentamicin and neomycin.

(CT) Same methods using 0.4 ml distilled water for 30 days in 7 cats,
control group, showed no clinical vestibular problems and no histological
changes. (ENG)

Dog

330

Hearing loss due to parenteral, intramuscular, administration of 31 mg per kg
or 62 mg per kg daily of antibiotic, capreomycin (capreomycin disulfate), for
more than 1000 days in 4 animals, dogs, male and female.
Hearing loss due to parenteral, subcutaneous, administration of 13 mg per kg
or 130 mg per kg daily of antibiotic, capreomycin (capreomycin tetrahydroch-
loride), for 91 days in 2 animals, cats, male.

(AD) Hearing loss determined by response of animals to reproducible sound.
(ENG)

555

Cochlear impairment due to parenteral, intramuscular, administration of 100
mg per kg 3 times per week or 25 or 50 mg per kg daily of antibiotic, capreomycin, for 2 years in several animals, dogs.
Vestibular problems due to parenteral, subcutaneous, administration of 125 mg
per kg daily of antibiotic, capreomycin, for 84 days in several animals,
cats.

(AD) Discussion of chemistry of capreomycin, results of in vitro and in
vivo studies, and toxicity of capreomycin in animals. (ENG)

339

Decr in potassium concentration and incr in sodium concentration of endolymph
within 10 minutes of treatment but no change in perilymph due to parenteral,
intravenous, administration of 1 to 5 mg per kg of diuretic, ethacrynic acid,
in 1 injection in 6 animals, dogs, young.

(CT) Study of potassium and sodium concentrations of endolymph and perilymph before injection of ethacrynic acid. (ENG)

398

Effect on auditory threshold due to parenteral, subcutaneous, administration
of ototoxic drugs in 4 animals, dogs, 1 to 2 years age, 7 to 10 kg weight,
conditioned.

(CT) Determined standard deviation of auditory threshold in dogs by measurement of changes without administration of drugs.
(CT) Measurement of auditory threshold before and after administration of
drugs. (ENG)

484

No observed ototoxic effects in fetuses due to parenteral, intramuscular,
administration of 15, 30, or 50 mg per kg in 1 injection daily of antimalarial, quinine, for 30 days in 3 groups of 12 animals, dogs, during pregnancy.
(CT) Study of 7 dogs, control group, not treated with quinine.
(AD) Study of effects of quinine on fetuses of animals. (FR)

Guinea pig

526

Decr in perilymph activity and slower permeation of NA-24 sodium isotope into
perilymph due to parenteral, intraperitoneal, administration of doses, corresponding to 1.4 g of 100 percent alcohol per 1 kg body weight, of 10 percent
concentration of sedative, alcohol, ethyl, in 1 injection in 40 animals,
guinea pigs, adult, with intraperitoneal administration of NA-24 sodium
isotope.
(CT) Same method with administration of NA-24 sodium isotope only in 13
guinea pigs, control group. (ENG)

721

Decr in eighth cranial nerve action potential and change in Preyer reflex
threshold due to parenteral, subcutaneous, administration of 2 or 3 to 20 mg
per kg of anticonvulsant, amino-oxyacetic acid, in animals, guinea pigs.
(CT) Same method using saline in guinea pigs, control group, showed no
change in reflex threshold.
(AD) Changes in Preyer reflex threshold in part due to effects on auditory
pathway. (ENG)

247

No ototoxic effects due to parenteral, subcutaneous, administration of low
doses used in therapy, 20 mg per kg daily in 2 doses every 12 hours, of
antibiotic, aminosidine (aminosidine sulfate), for 60 days in 20 animals,
guinea pigs, adult, 300 g average weight.
(CT) Study of 5 guinea pigs, control group.
(CT) Test for Preyer reflex and vestibular function tests, pretreatment
and during treatment.
(AD) Previous studies showed ototoxic effects of high doses of aminosidine
in animals.
(AD) Suggested clinical use of aminosidine in low doses for short periods.
(IT)

251

Damage to organ of Corti and crista ampullaris due to parenteral, subcutaneous, administration of 200 or 400 mg per kg daily in 3 doses every 8
hours of antibiotic, aminosidine (aminosidine sulfate), for 30 days in 2
groups of 16 animals, guinea pigs, 300 g weight.
Less damage to organ of Corti and crista ampullaris due to parenteral, subcutaneous, administration of 50 or 100 mg per kg daily in 3 doses every 8 hours
of antibiotic, aminosidine (aminosidine sulfate), for 30 days in 2 groups of
16 animals, guinea pigs, 300 g weight.
(CT) Study of 8 guinea pigs, control group.
(CT) Observation of function of cochlea and vestibular apparatus, pretreatment and during treatment. (IT)

065

Prevention of destruction of organ of Corti due to low doses of antibiotics
(IB) in animals, guinea pigs, with administration of vitamin B and amino
acids.
(AD) Need for histological studies to determine method for prevention of
ototoxicity. (FR)

240

Ototoxic effects due to topical administration to inner ear of antibiotics, aminoglycoside, in 200 animals, guinea pigs, 250 g weight, with positive Preyer reflex.
   (CT) Study of guinea pigs, control group.
   (AD) Comparative study of ototoxicity of aminoglycoside antibiotics. (GER)

260

High antibiotic levels in perilymph due to topical administration to inner ear of antibiotics in animals, guinea pigs.
   (AD) Antibiotic levels in perilymph due to topical administration comp w levels due to intramuscular administration.
   (AD) Neomycin levels due to topical route higher than levels due to intramuscular route. (GER)

458

Damage to cochlear function and vestibular function and structural damage to cochlea and vestibular apparatus due to antibiotics in animals, guinea pigs.
   (AD) Use of Preyer reflex, vestibular function tests, and measurement of cochlear microphonics to determine ototoxic effects of antibiotics on function of inner ear.
   (AD) Histological study to determine structural damage to inner ear. (ENG)

462

Damage to hair cells of organ of Corti, stria vascularis, nerve process, spiral ganglion, limbus, and cochlear wall due to antibiotics in animals, guinea pigs.
   (AD) Ototoxic effects result of retention of antibiotics in inner ear longer than in blood due to slower elimination.
   (AD) More active cells of cochlea more sensitive to ototoxic antibiotics.
   (AD) Neomycin most ototoxic, followed by kanamycin, viomycin, streptomycin, and capreomycin.
   (AD) Study of effect of inhibitors, nialamide, pantothenic acid, methylated compounds, and vitamin B on ototoxicity of antibiotics.
   (AD) Electrophysiological and histological study of cochleo-vestibulotoxic effects of antibiotics in guinea pig. (ENG)

713

Inhibition of oxygen consumption of cochlea due to antibiotics in animals, guinea pigs.
   (AD) In vitro study using microrespirometer of effect of antibiotics on oxygen consumption in guinea pig cochlea. (JAP)

510

Changes in metabolism of inner ear due to heavy metal, arsenic, for chronic intoxication in animals, guinea pigs. (GER)

002

Damage to organ of Corti and stria vascularis due to topical administration to round window of 16 mg of 1.44M solution and 8 mg of 0.72M solution of antibiotic, chloramphenicol (chloramphenicol succinate), for 30 minutes in 11 animals, guinea pigs, adult, for each solution.
   (CT) Same method using 1.44M solution of sodium (sodium succinate) in 8 guinea pigs, control group, showed no histological damage. (ENG)

069

Progressive decr in cochlear response due to topical administration by insufflation to round window in powder of 8 mg (only 0.5 mg actually fell on round window) of antibiotic, chloramphenicol, in 1 administration in 8 animals, guinea pigs, 459 to 996 g weight.
   (CT) Same method using saline in 2 guinea pigs, control group.
   (AD) Measurement of cochlear response at 15 minutes and 1, 5, and 20 hours after insufflation. (ENG)

258

Cessation of blood flow in some capillaries of basilar membrane due to parenteral, intraperitoneal, administration of 125 mg of antimalarial, quinine

(quinine dihydrochloride), in 1 dose in animals, guinea pigs, 500 g weight.
Transient cessation of blood flow in some capillaries of basilar membrane due
to parenteral, intraperitoneal, administration of 62.5 mg per dose, total of
125 mg, of antimalarial, quinine (quinine dihydrochloride), in gradual doses
in animals, guinea pigs, 500 g weight.
  (CT) Study of guinea pigs, control group.
  (AD) Transient hearing loss due to quinine (quinine dihydrochloride) known
  from previous studies.
  (AD) Drugs known to produce hearing loss also produce cessation of blood
  flow in capillaries of basilar membrane. (ENG)

                                                                       571
No significant effect on vestibular apparatus due to oral administration of
50 or 150 mg per kg daily, total of 1.55 and 4.65 g per kg, of antibiotic,
rifampicin, for 5 weeks in 2 groups of 7 animals, rabbits, male.
  (CT) Same method using 1 percent carboxymethyl-cellulose in rabbits,
  control group.
  (AD) Measurement of horizontal nystagmus 2, 3, 4, and 5 weeks after beginning of treatment.
No accumulation in perilymph due to oral administration of 100 mg per kg of
antibiotic, rifampicin, for 1 dose in animals, guinea pigs.
  (AD) Determination of rifampicin concentration in perilymph and blood
  after 2, 6, and 24 hours.
  (AD) Study of vestibulotoxic effects and retention in inner ear of rifampicin. (ENG)

                                                                       448
Significant decr in ATP levels of Reissner's membrane but no change in P-
creatine due to parenteral, intraperitoneal, administration of high doses,
400 mg per kg, of salicylate in animals, guinea pigs, young, about 200 g
weight.
Incr in ATP of cochlear nerve and incr in P-creatine of stria vascularis due
to parenteral, intraperitoneal, administration of high doses, 400 mg per kg,
of salicylate in animals, guinea pigs, young, 200 g weight.
  (CT) Same method using 0.9 percent saline in 3 guinea pigs, control group.
  (AD) Suggested that ototoxicity of salicylate possibly due to impairment
  of energy metabolism of Reissner's membrane. (ENG)

                                                                       686
Decr in ATP and p-creatine of organ of Corti, spiral ganglion, cochlear
nerve, stria vascularis, and Reissner's membrane only after 3 days of exposure due to range of doses of salicylate in animals, guinea pigs.
  (AD) Results of study suggest that ototoxicity of salicylates not due to
  impairment of energy metabolism of cochlea. (ENG)

                                                                       168
Appearance of salicylate in blood vessels of stria vascularis and spiral
ligament after 15 minutes due to parenteral, intravenous and intraperitoneal,
administration of 6.6 to 49.5 mc per kg, tritium-labelled solution, of salicylate, salicylic acid, in 5 animals, guinea pigs, albino, adult, 300 to 320
g weight.
Concentration of salicylate in stria vascularis and spiral ligament and
diffusion into organ of Corti and Rosenthal's canal after 1 hour due to
parenteral, intravenous and intraperitoneal, administration of 6.6 to 49.5 mc
per kg, tritium-labelled solution, of salicylate, salicylic acid, in 5 animals, guinea pigs, albino, adult, 300 to 320 g weight.
Small amount of salicylate after 6 hours and no salicylate after 13 hours in
cochlea due to parenteral, intravenous and intraperitoneal, administration of
6.6 to 49.5 mc per kg, tritium-labelled solution, of salicylate, salicylic
acid, in 5 animals, guinea pigs, albino, adult, 300 to 320 g weight.
  (AD) Autoradiographical study to determine mechanism of salicylate ototoxicity by localization of tritiated salicylate in cochlea of guinea pigs.
  (AD) Salicylate levels in cochlea due to vascular route and diffusion into
  cochlear duct and not due to accumulation in specific areas. (ENG)

                                                                       082
Transient threshold shift due to parenteral, intraperitoneal, administration
of 300 mg per kg (equivalent to 65 aspirin tablets for 70 kg man), in saline

solution, of salicylate, sodium salicylate, in 1 injection in animals, guinea pigs.
   (CT) Electrophysiological measurement of hearing sensitivity before and after salicylate injection.
Transient threshold shift due to parenteral, intraperitoneal, administration of 100 to 250 mg per kg of salicylate, sodium salicylate, in animals, guinea pigs, conditioned. (ENG)

                                                                        166
Decr in succinic dehydrogenase concentration, in particular in stria vascularis and outer hair cells of organ of Corti, and decr in esterases and sulfhydryl compounds due to parenteral, subcutaneous, administration of 100 mg per kg daily, in 2 ml distilled water, of salicylate, sodium salicylate, for 28 days in animals, guinea pigs.
   (CT) Study of guinea pigs, control group, not treated with sodium salicylate.
   (AD) Report on relationship between changes in metabolism in inner ear due to sodium salicylate and auditory system problems. (GER)

                                                                        189
Threshold shift due to parenteral, intraperitoneal, administration of 300 mg per kg of salicylate, sodium salicylate, in 1 dose in 4 animals, cats.
Small threshold shift of about 3 decibels due to parenteral, intraperitoneal, administration of 125 mg per kg daily of salicylate, sodium salicylate, for total of 28 injections in 4 animals, cats.
Threshold shift due to parenteral, intraperitoneal, administration of (SQ) 300 mg per kg of salicylate, sodium salicylate, in (SQ) 1 dose in 6 animals, guinea pigs.
Small threshold shift of about 4 decibels due to parenteral, intraperitoneal, administration of (SQ) 150,225, or 300 mg per kg daily of salicylate, sodium salicylate, for (SQ) total of 10 injections in 6 animals, guinea pigs. (ENG)

                                                                        023
No degeneration in inner hair cells and outer hair cells of organ of Corti due to parenteral, intramuscular, administration of 200 mg per kg daily of antibiotic, streptomycin (streptomycin sulfate), for 10 days in 15 animals, guinea pigs, 150 to 200 g weight.
   (CT) Study of 5 guinea pigs, control group.
Changes in succinic dehydrogenase activity in hair cells of organ of Corti due to parenteral, intramuscular, administration of 200 mg per kg daily of antibiotic, streptomycin (streptomycin sulfate), for 10 days in 15 animals, guinea pigs, 150 to 200 g weight.
   (CT) Study of 10 guinea pigs, control group.
   (AD) Difference between inner hair cells and outer hair cells discussed. (ENG)

                                                                        029
Concentration of streptomycin in blood and perilymph due to 250, 50, 25, and 15 mg per kg of antibiotic, streptomycin (streptomycin sulfate), in 4 injections in 325 animals, guinea pigs.
Concentration of streptomycin in blood and perilymph due to 250, 50, 25, and 15 mg per kg of antibiotic, streptomycin (IB) (streptomycin sulfate), in 4 injections in 325 animals, guinea pigs, with administration of ozothin.
   (AD) Protective action of ozothin not dependable. (GER)

                                                                        031
Damage to cochlea due to antibiotic, streptomycin, in animals, guinea pigs.
   (AD) Study of RNA and protein in cochlea for evaluation of streptomycin ototoxicity. (GER)

                                                                        092
Decr of enzyme activity in vestibular apparatus due to topical administration to bulla of 0.2 cc of 50 percent solution of antibiotic, streptomycin, in 10 animals, guinea pigs. (GER)

                                                                        111
Damage to organ ofCorti and vestibular apparatus due to antibiotic, streptomycin, in humans and animals, guinea pigs.

(AD) Comparative study of ototoxic effects of streptomycin in humans and animals. (GER)

112

Permanent inhibition of cochlear microphonic due to parenteral administration of high doses of antibiotic, streptomycin, in animals, guinea pigs and rabbits.
Rapid decr in cochlear potentials due to lower doses of antibiotic, streptomycin, in animals, guinea pigs and rabbits, sensitized with horse serum.
   (AD) Study to show pathogenesis of cochlear neuritis in association with streptomycin treatment. (RUS)

212

Changes in hair cells of vestibular apparatus due to 250 mg per kg daily of antibiotic, streptomycin (streptomycin sulfate), for 10 or 20 days in 9 animals, guinea pigs, 140 to 300 g weight.
Decr in damage to cochlea due to 250 mg per kg daily of antibiotic, streptomycin (IB) (streptomycin sulfate), for 10 or 15 days in 10 animals, guinea pigs, 140 to 300 g weight, with intramuscular administration of 1.25 ml per kg daily of ozothin.
   (CT) Study of 10 guinea pigs, control group, 5 normal and 5 with parenteral administration of 2.5 ml per kg daily of ozothin for 10 days.
   (AD) Study not show decr in streptomycin damage to vestibular apparatus with administration of ozothin. (GER)

216

Damage to hair cells and decr in excitation of vestibular apparatus due to parenteral, intramuscular, administration of 250 mg per kg of antibiotic, streptomycin (streptomycin sulfate), for 10 and 30 days in animals, guinea pigs.
Damage to hair cells and decr in excitation of vestibular apparatus due to parenteral, intramuscular, administration of 250 mg per kg of antibiotic, streptomycin (IB) (streptomycin sulfate), for 10 and 30 days in animals, guinea pigs, with intramuscular administration of 1.25 ml per kg of ozothin.
   (CT) Study of 14 guinea pigs, control group, with 1.25 ml per kg or 2.5 ml per kg daily of ozothin.
   (AD) No decr in streptomycin damage to hair cells of vestibular apparatus with administration of ozothin.
   (AD) Evaluation of damage with cytovestibulogram and caloric test.
   (AD) Vestibulotoxic effects depend on total dosage of streptomycin used. (GER)

259

Damage to hair cells of organ of Corti and decr in action potentials due to parenteral, intramuscular, administration of 250 mg per kg, in distilled water, of antibiotic, streptomycin (streptomycin sulfate), in 10 doses in 1 group of total of over 100 animals, guinea pigs, 200 g average weight.
Normal hair cells of organ of Corti and no decr in action potentials due to parenteral, intramuscular, administration of 250 mg per kg of antibiotic, streptomycin (IB) (streptomycin sulfate), in 10 doses in 1 group of total of over 100 animals, guinea pigs, 200 g average weight, with administration of 1.2 ml of ozothin.
   (CT) Study of guinea pigs, control group.
   (AD) Significant decr in ototoxicity of streptomycin due to administration of ozothin. (ENG)

364

Damage to organ of Corti, spiral ganglion, and cochlear nuclei of medulla oblongata 15 days after beginning of treatment due to 100 mg per kg of antibiotic, streptomycin, in 38 animals, guinea pigs.
Decr in damage to spiral ganglion and cochlear nuclei of medulla oblongata due to 100 mg per kg of antibiotic, streptomycin (IB), in 8 of 18 animals, guinea pigs, with simultaneous administration of 2 ml of 5 percent unitiol for 30 to 60 days.
Decr in hearing loss due to ototoxic drugs (IB) in 3 of 25 humans with administration of unitiol.
No hearing loss due to antibiotic, streptomycin (IB), in 25 humans with pulmonary tuberculosis with administration of unitiol.

(AD) Study of effect of inhibitor, unitiol, on streptomycin ototoxicity.
(RUS)

395
Damage first to outer hair cells of organ of Corti in basal coil of cochlea
due to high doses of antibiotics, aminoglycoside, in animals, guinea pigs.
(AD) Same damage due to x-ray radiation.
Primary damage to central areas of crista ampullaris, crista neglecta, and
macula due to antibiotics, aminoglycoside, in animals, guinea pigs.
(AD) Damage to peripheral areas of crista ampullaris, crista neglecta, and
macula due to x-ray radiation.
Disturbance of protein synthesis due to topical administration to bulla of
antibiotic, streptomycin, in animals, guinea pigs.
(AD) Similar electron microscopy findings for streptomycin administration
to bulla and for x-ray radiation.
(AD) Cochleo-vestibulotoxic effects due to x-ray radiation comp w effects
due to antibiotics. (ENG)

425
Decr in ototoxic effect on organ of Corti and crista ampullaris due to topical administration to bulla of 0.2 ccm of 50 percent solution of antibiotic,
streptomycin (IB) (streptomycin sulfate), in 10 animals, guinea pigs with
intramuscular administration of 1 ml per 100 g ozothin.
(AD) Histochemical study of effect of ozothin on ototoxicity of streptomycin in guinea pigs. (GER)

266
Effect on enzymes of cochlea and vestibular apparatus due to topical adminis-
tration to bulla of 0.2 ml of 2 percent solution of anesthetic, tetracaine
(tetracaine hydrochloride), in animals, guinea pigs.
(CT) Study of guinea pigs, control group, not treated with tetracaine.
(GER)

389
Damage to epithelial cells of round window due to 1 percent solution of
anesthetic, tetracaine, in animals, guinea pigs, 250 to 500 g weight. (GER)

049
Hearing loss and damage to hair cells of organ of Corti due to parenteral,
(SQ) intraperitoneal, administration of 200 mg per kg daily of antibiotic,
tobramycin (nebramycin (factor 6)), for 6 days in 13 animals, guinea pigs,
220 to 260 g weight.
Hearing loss and damage to hair cells of organ of Corti due to parenteral,
(SQ) subcutaneous, administration of 150 mg per kg daily of antibiotic,
tobramycin (nebramycin (factor 6)), for 6 weeks in 13 animals, guinea pigs,
220 to 260 g weight.
(CT) Control group of 5 guinea pigs used.
(AD) Loss of Preyer reflex showed hearing loss. (ENG)

006
Range of degrees of degeneration of endorgan of organ of Corti due to parenteral, intratympanic, administration of range of 1 to 100 mg per ml concentration of antibiotic, neomycin, in 1 injection in animals, guinea pigs,
young, 250 g average weight.
Range of degrees of degeneration of endorgan of organ of Corti due to parenteral, intratympanic, administration of range of 1 to 100 mg per ml concentration of antibiotic, polymyxin B, in 1 injection in animals, guinea pigs,
young, 250 g average weight.
Range of degrees of degeneration of endorgan of organ of Corti due to parenteral, intratympanic, administration of range of 1 to 100 mg per ml concentration of antibiotic, colistin, in 1 injection in animals, guinea pigs,
young, 250 g average weight.
(CT) Same method using comparable concentration of saline solution or
solution of glucose or sodium G penicillin in guinea pigs, control group,
showed no histological damage.
Degeneration of endorgan of organ of Corti due to topical administration to
ear canal of range of 5 to 100 mg per ml 1 time daily of antibiotic, neomycin, for 8 to 25 days in 14 animals, guinea pigs. (ENG)

009

Delayed permanent sensorineural hearing loss and damage to outer hair cells
of basal and middle coils of cochlea due to unspecified doses of antibiotic,
dihydrostreptomycin, in humans.
Vertigo and dizziness due to unspecified method of administration of 2 to 3 g
daily of antibiotic, streptomycin (streptomycin sulfate), for 30 to 50 days
in humans with tuberculosis.
Hearing loss due to unspecified method of administration of high doses of
antibiotic, streptomycin (streptomycin sulfate), for long period in humans.
Gradual high frequency hearing loss and tinnitus and degeneration of hair
cells of organ of Corti in basal coil of cochlea due to unspecified doses of
antibiotic, kanamycin, in humans.
Delayed severe high frequency hearing loss due to parenteral, oral, or topical administration by inhalation of unspecified doses of antibiotic, neomycin, for unspecified period in humans with kidney disorder.
Complete degeneration of inner hair cells due to unspecified method of administration of 18 g of antibiotic, neomycin, for unspecified period in
humans with bacterial endocarditis.
Lesions in organ of Corti due to parenteral administration of unspecified
doses of antibiotic, polymyxin B, for unspecified period in animals, guinea
pigs.
Sensorineural hearing loss due to parenteral, intravenous, administration of
80 to 95 mg per ml of antibiotic, vancomycin, for unspecified period in
humans with kidney disorder.
  (AD) Sensorineural hearing loss and vestibular problems due to 6 antibiotics in humans and animals, guinea pigs.
  (AD) Literature review of ototoxic effects of antibiotics. (ENG)

045

Progressive degeneration of endorgan of cochlea due to low doses of antibiotic, dihydrostreptomycin, in animals, guinea pigs.
Progressive degeneration of endorgan of cochlea due to low doses of antibiotic, neomycin, in animals, guinea pigs. (JAP)

074

Decr in cochlear microphonic due to topical administration to round window of
range of 210 to 680 g of antibiotic, streptomycin, in animals, guinea pigs.
Decr in cochlear microphonic due to topical administration to round window of
range of 210 to 680 g of antibiotic, kanamycin, in animals, guinea pigs.
No decr in cochlear microphonic due to topical administration to round window
of range of 210 to 680 g of antibiotic, neomycin, in animals, guinea pigs.
(POL)

084

Decr in damage to organ of Corti due to topical administration of antibiotic,
kanamycin (IB), in animals, guinea pigs, 300 to 500 g weight, with intravenous administration of cytochrome C.
Decr in damage to organ of Corti due to topical administration of antibiotic,
streptomycin (IB) (streptomycin sulfate), in animals, guinea pigs, 300 to 500
g weight, with intravenous administration of cytochrome C. (POL)

109

Damage to hair cells in organ of Corti due to topical administration of 300
mg per kg of antibiotic, kanamycin, in 14 injections in animals, guinea pigs.
Severe degeneration of hair cells of organ of Corti and membranous labyrinth
due to topical administration to middle ear of low doses of antibiotics in
animals, guinea pigs.
  (AD) Report on studies of several years on cochleo-vestibulotoxic effects
  due to antibiotics. (ENG)

139

Cochleotoxic effects due to antibiotic, kanamycin, in humans and animals,
guinea pigs.
Cochleotoxic effects due to antibiotic, streptomycin, in humans and animals,
guinea pigs.
  (AD) Literature review of mechanism of action of ototoxic antibiotics.
  (POL)

181

Decr in succinic dehydrogenase in outer hair cells of organ of Corti due to parenteral, intratympanic, administration of 200 mg per ml solution of antibiotic, kanamycin (kanamycin sulfate), in animals, guinea pigs, adult.
Decr in succinic dehydrogenase in outer hair cells of organ of Corti due to parenteral, intratympanic, administration of 200 mg per ml solution of antibiotic, dihydrostreptomycin (dihydrostreptomycin sulfate), in animals, guinea pigs, adult.
Decr in succinic dehydrogenase in outer hair cells of organ of Corti due to parenteral, intratympanic, administration of 200 mg per ml solution of antibiotic, chloramphenicol (chloramphenicol succinate), in animals, guinea pigs, adult.
  (AD) Same type of damage to organ of Corti due to all 3 antibiotics.
Severe decr in succinic dehydrogenase in organ of Corti, in particular in outer hair cells, and atrophy of outer hair cells due to saturated solution of antimalarial, quinine (quinine hydrochloride), in animals, guinea pigs.
Complete degeneration of organ of Corti due to saturated solution of antimalarial, quinine (quinine hydrochloride), in animals, guinea pigs.
  (AD) Damage to organ of Corti more severe due to quinine than to antibiotics.
  (AD) Activity of succinic dehydrogenase often higher in outer hair cells.
  (AD) Possible that damage to outer hair cells due to higher rate of metabolism. (ENG)

183

Inhibition of oxygen consumption of cochlea due to 0.04 mg of antibiotic, chloramphenicol (chloramphenicol sodium succinate), in animals, guinea pigs, adult, 300 g weight, with normal Preyer reflex.
More inhibition of oxygen consumption of cochlea due to 0.04 mg of antibiotic, kanamycin (kanamycin sulfate), in animals, guinea pigs, adult, 300 g weight, with normal Preyer reflex.
  (CT) Study of oxygen consumption in normal cochlea.
  (AD) Measurement of oxygen consumption with differential type of microrespirometer.
  (AD) In vitro study.
No detected change in Preyer reflex due to parenteral, intracutaneous, administration of 400 mg per kg of antibiotic, chloramphenicol, for 20 days in animals, guinea pigs.
  (AD) In vivo study.
  (AD) Results with chloramphenicol in vivo not same as results in vitro. (ENG)

184

Incr in ATP hydrolyzing system in stria vascularis and spiral ligament and incr in ATP activity in membranous labyrinth due to parenteral, intraperitoneal, administration of 400 mg per kg 5 days a week of antibiotic, kanamycin (kanamycin sulfate), for 20 days in animals, guinea pigs, adult, with normal pinna reflex.
Incr in ATP hydrolyzing system in stria vascularis and spiral ligament due to parenteral, intraperitoneal, administration of 400 mg per kg 5 days a week of antibiotic, streptomycin (streptomycin sulfate), for 20 days in animals, guinea pigs, adult, with normal pinna reflex.
Decr in ATP hydrolyzing system in stria vascularis and spiral ligament and decr in ATP activity in membranous labyrinth due to parenteral, intraperitoneal, administration of 400 mg per kg 5 days a week of antibiotic, dihydrostreptomycin (dihydrostreptomycin sulfate), for 20 days in animals, guinea pigs, adult, with normal pinna reflex.
  (CT) Study of normal activity of ATP hydrolyzing system. (ENG)

185

Ataxia, damage to hair cells of macula, and damage to hair cells of organ of Corti due to parenteral, subcutaneous, administration of 10 to 80 mg per kg daily of antibiotic, gentamicin (gentamicin sulfate), for 19 to 120 days in animals, cats.
Ataxia due to 100 and 200 mg per kg daily of antibiotic, streptomycin (streptomycin sulfate), for 8 to 40 days in animals, cats.
Loss of Preyer reflex, decr in cochlear potential and eighth cranial nerve action potential, and loss of outer hair cells of organ of Corti due to 80 to

200 mg per kg daily of antibiotic, gentamicin (gentamicin sulfate), in animals, guinea pigs.
Damage to cochlea due to 100 and 200 mg per kg of antibiotic, kanamycin
(kanamycin sulfate), in animals, guinea pigs.
   (AD) Comparative study of ototoxicity of gentamicin and other aminoglycoside antibiotics.
   (AD) Study suggested low risk of ototoxicity when gentamicin used in
   recommended clinical dose of 1 to 3 mg per kg. (ENG)

197

Progressive degeneration of organ of Corti beginning at base of cochlea due
to antibiotic, neomycin, in animals, guinea pigs.
Progressive degeneration of organ of Corti beginning at base of cochlea due
to antibiotic, kanamycin, in animals, guinea pigs.
Progressive degeneration of organ of Corti beginning at base of cochlea due
to antibiotic, framycetin, in animals, guinea pigs.
No damage to hair cells of organ of Corti due to parenteral administration of
high doses of antibiotic, dihydrostreptomycin, for long periods in animals,
guinea pigs.
   (AD) Surface specimen technique used in study of organ of Corti.
   (AD) Damage to organ of Corti due to ototoxic drugs different from that
   due to noise. (ENG)

226

Changes in hair cells of inner ear but no damage to stria vascularis due to
parenteral, intramuscular, administration of 300 mg per kg of antibiotic,
streptomycin (streptomycin sulfate), in animals, guinea pigs.
Damage to hair cells, then complete degeneration of organ of Corti, and
degeneration of spiral ganglion due to parenteral, intramuscular, administration of 200 or 300 mg per kg daily of antibiotic, kanamycin (kanamycin sulfate), for range of 7 to 29 injections in 28 animals, guinea pigs.
   (AD) Studies using electron microscopy and light microscopy.
   (AD) Study of transport in cochlea.
   (AD) Suggested that debris from degeneration in cochlea removed by Claudius cells and Reissner's membrane. (ENG)

232

Degeneration of hair cells of vestibular apparatus due to parenteral administration of antibiotic, kanamycin, in animals, guinea pigs.
Degeneration of hair cells of vestibular apparatus due to administration to
middle ear of antibiotic, streptomycin, in animals, guinea pigs.
   (AD) Study using surface specimen technique. (ENG)

245

Degeneration of outer hair cells of organ of Corti and changes in supporting
cells due to 400 mg per kg daily of antibiotic, kanamycin, for 14 days in
animals, guinea pigs.
Degeneration of organ of Corti due to 400 mg per kg daily of antibiotic,
dihydrostreptomycin, for 14 days in animals, guinea pigs.
   (AD) Comparative study of cochleotoxic effects of kanamycin and dihydrostreptomycin. (FR)

261

Nystagmus, ataxia, and loss of pinna reflex after 4 to 5 hours due to parenteral, intratympanic, administration of 5 to 20 mg, in 0.1 ml Ringer's solution, of antibiotic, streptomycin (streptomycin sulfate), in 1 ear of 15
animals, guinea pigs, pigmented, 250 to 350 g weight, with normal pinna
reflex.
   (CT) Use of other ear of 15 guinea pigs, control group.
No detected vestibular problems due to parenteral administration of 300 mg
per kg daily of antibiotic, kanamycin (kanamycin sulfate), for 8 to 15 days
in 5 animals, guinea pigs, pigmented, 250 to 350 g weight, with normal pinna
reflex.
Degeneration of hair cells of vestibular apparatus and organ of Corti due to
parenteral, intratympanic, administration of 5 to 20 mg, in 0.1 ml Ringer's
solution, of antibiotic, streptomycin (streptomycin sulfate), in all 15
animals, guinea pigs, pigmented, 250 to 350 g weight, with normal pinna
reflex.

(AD)   Suggested relationship between histological changes and streptomycin
dosage.
Degeneration of hair cells of vestibular apparatus and organ of Corti due to
parenteral   administration   of   300   mg per kg daily of antibiotic, kanamycin
(kanamycin sulfate),   for 8 to 15 days in 4 out of 5 animals, guinea pigs,
pigmented, 250 to 350 g weight, with normal pinna reflex.
   (AD) Same pattern of degeneration in vestibular apparatus due to streptomycin and kanamycin.
   (AD) Hair cells of vestibular apparatus more sensitive to streptomycin and
hair cells of organ of Corti more sensitive to kanamycin.   (ENG)

                                                                          275
Loss of some hair cells of crista ampullaris with replacement by supporting
cells due to parenteral, intraperitoneal, administration of 250 mg per kg
every other day of antibiotic, streptomycin (streptomycin sulfate), for 8
weeks in 1 group of 48 animals, guinea pigs, pigmented, young, 300 g average
weight.
Loss of some hair cells of crista ampullaris with replacement by supporting
cells due to parenteral, intraperitoneal, administration of 250 mg per kg
every other day of antibiotic, kanamycin (kanamycin sulfate), for 8 weeks in
1 group of 48 animals, guinea pigs, pigmented, young, 300 g average weight.
Loss of some hair cells of crista ampullaris with replacement by supporting
cells due to topical administration to middle ear of 0.6 ml of 250 mg per kg
of antibiotic, streptomycin (streptomycin sulfate), for 3 times with interval
of 1 week in 1 group of 48 animals, guinea pigs, pigmented, young, 300 g
average weight.
Loss of some hair cells of crista ampullaris with replacement by supporting
cells due to topical administration to middle ear of 0.6 ml of 250 mg per kg
of antibiotic, kanamycin (kanamycin sulfate), for 3 times with interval of 1
week in 1 group of 48 animals, guinea pigs, pigmented, young, 300 g average
weight.
   (AD) Degeneration of hair cells of crista ampullaris most severe in group
with topical administration of streptomycin to middle ear.
   (AD) Degeneration of hair cells of crista ampullaris least severe in group
with intraperitoneal administration of kanamycin. (ENG)

                                                                          276
Decr in vestibular responses due to parenteral, intramuscular, administration
of 250 mg per kg of antibiotic, streptomycin (streptomycin sulfate), in 10 or
25 injections in 13 animals, guinea pigs, 250 to 300 g weight.
Decr in vestibular responses for several hours due to parenteral, intraperitoneal, administration of 1.5, 3.0, or 4.5 mg of analeptic, dimorpholamine,
in 17 animals, guinea pigs, 250 to 300 g weight. (GER)

                                                                          278
Histochemical changes in cochlea due to parenteral administration of 15 mg
per kg daily of diuretic, furosemide, for 8 to 14 days in animals, guinea
pigs, 300 g weight.
Histochemical changes in cochlea due to parenteral administration of 8 mg per
kg daily of diuretic, acetazolamide, for 8 to 14 days in animals, guinea
pigs, 300 g weight. (GER)

                                                                          282
Limited effects on blood vessels of stria vascularis and spiral prominence
due to 300 mg per kg daily of antibiotic, kanamycin, for 4 to 9 days in
animals, guinea pigs.
Limited effects on blood vessels of stria vascularis and spiral prominence
due to 30 mg per kg daily of antibiotic, dihydrostreptomycin, for 4 to 9 days
in animals, guinea pigs.
Limited effects on blood vessels of stria vascularis and spiral prominence
due to 30 mg per kg daily of antibiotic, chloramphenicol, for 4 to 9 days in
animals, guinea pigs.
   (CT) Study of guinea pigs, control group. (JAP)

                                                                          314
Loss of enzymes, succinic dehydrogenase and DPN diaphorase, in outer hair
cells of organ of Corti but usually no enzyme loss in inner hair cells due to
topical administration to bulla of 200 mg per ml of antibiotic, kanamycin

(kanamycin sulfate), in 1 injection in animals, guinea pigs.
Loss of enzymes, succinic dehydrogenase and DPN diaphorase, in outer hair
cells of organ of Corti but usually no enzyme loss in inner hair cells due to
topical administration to bulla of 200 mg per ml of antibiotic, dihydrostreptomycin (dihydrostreptomycin sulfate), in 1 injection in animals, guinea
pigs.
Loss of enzymes, succinic dehydrogenase and DPN diaphorase, in outer hair
cells of organ of Corti but usually no enzyme loss in inner hair cells due to
topical administration to bulla of 200 mg per ml of antibiotic, chloramagheni-
col (chloramphenicol succinate), in 1 injection in animals, guinea pigs.
More severe effects on enzymes, succinic hydrogenase and DPN diaphorase, in
outer hair cells of organ of Corti due to topical administration to bulla of
saturated solution of antimalarial, quinine (quinine hydrochloride), in 1
injection in animals, guinea pigs.
    (CT) Activity of succinic dehydrogenase often higher in outer hair cells
    than in inner hair cells of organ of Corti in guinea pigs, control group.
    (AD) Suggested correlation between cochleotoxic effects of drugs and
    metabolic activity of hair cells. (ENG)

338

No loss of pinna reflex and no significant histological changes due to parenteral, subcutaneous, administration of 400 mg per kg daily in 1 injection of
antibiotic, dihydrostreptomycin, for 8 to 37 injections in 8 animals, guinea
pigs, young, 200 to 290 g weight.
Hearing loss after 64 injections and moderate damage to hair cells of cochlea
due to parenteral, subcutaneous, administration of 600 mg per kg daily, total
dose of 38.4 g, of antibiotic, dihydrostreptomycin, for 9 to 64 injections in
1 of 5 animals, guinea pigs, young, 200 to 290 g weight.
No loss of pinna reflex and no significant histological changes due to 50 mg
per kg daily of antibiotic, kanamycin, for 64 injections in 10 animals,
guinea pigs.
    (CT) Test of pinna reflex, pretreatment and daily during treatment with
    antibiotics.
    (AD) Suggested relationship between degree of kanamycin damage to cochlea
    and daily dose rather than total dose. (ENG)

374

Decr in cochlear microphonic due to 4-300 mg per percent of solution of
diuretic, furosemide, in animals, guinea pigs.
Decr in cochlear microphonic due to 2-200 mg per percent of solution of
diuretic, ethacrynic acid, in animals, guinea pigs. (GER)

430

Permanent hearing loss, partial or total, due to parenteral, intramuscular,
administration of 200,000 units per kg daily of antibiotic, streptomycin, for
30 days in animals, guinea pigs.
Permanent hearing loss, partial or total, due to parenteral, intramuscular,
administration of 150,000 units per kg daily of antibiotic, colistin (colistin sulfate), for 7 to 21 days in animals, guinea pigs. (RUS)

432

Damage to sensory epithelia of macula utriculi and macula sacculi due to
parenteral, intraperitoneal, administration of 250 mg per kg every other day
of antibiotic, streptomycin (streptomycin sulfate), for 8 weeks in 12 animals, guinea pigs, pigmented, young, about 300 g weight.
Least severe damage to sensory epithelia of macula utriculi and macula sacculi due to parenteral, intraperitoneal, administration of 250 mg per kg every
day of antibiotic, kanamycin (kanamycin sulfate), for 8 weeks in 12 animals,
guinea pigs, pigmented, young, about 300 g weight.
Most severe damage to sensory epithelia of macula utriculi and macula sacculi
due to topical administration to middle ear cavity through tympanic membrane
of about 0.6 ml of concentration of 250 mg per kg of antibiotic, streptomycin
(streptomycin sulfate), in 8 injections, with interval of 1 week between
injections, in 12 animals, guinea pigs, pigmented, young, about 300 g weight.
Damage to sensory epithelia of macula utriculi and macula sacculi due to
topical administration to middle ear cavity through tympanic membrane of
about 0.6 ml of concentration of 250 mg per kg of antibiotic, kanamycin
(kanamycin sulfate), in 8 injections, with interval of 1 week between injec-

tions, in 12 animals, guinea pigs, pigmented, young, about 300 g weight.
  (AD) More damage to vestibular apparatus due to topical administration
than due to parenteral administration of antibiotics.
  (AD) More loss of hair cells in sensory epithelium of macula utriculi than
in that of macula sacculi.
  (AD) Type 1 hair cells more vulnerable to aminoglycoside antibiotics than
type 2 hair cells.
  (AD) Comment on morphological and phylogenetical vulnerability of hair
cells.
  (AD) Replacement of hair cells of vestibular apparatus by supporting
cells. (ENG)

                                                                    437
Hearing loss and damage to cochlea due to antibiotic, neomycin, in animals,
guinea pigs and monkeys, and humans.
Hearing loss and damage to cochlea due to antibiotic, streptomycin, in animals, guinea pigs and monkeys, and humans.
  (AD) Discussion of findings on decr of ototoxicity of aminoglycoside
antibiotics. (GER)

                                                                    443
Decr in summating potential and threshold shift due to topical administration
to round window of 2 percent solution of anesthetic, tetracaine, in animals,
guinea pigs.
Decr in summating potential and threshold shift due to topical administration
to round window of 4 percent solution of anesthetic, lidocaine, in animals,
guinea pigs.
  (AD) More changes in summating potential and threshold due to tetracaine
than to lidocaine.
  (AD) Partial recovery of summating potential after 60 minutes in guinea
pigs treated with lidocaine. (GER)

                                                                    460
No significant decr in cochlear microphonics due to parenteral, subcutaneous,
administration of 100 mg per kg daily for 5 days a week, total dose of 7.5 g
per kg, of antibiotic, streptomycin (streptomycin sulfate), for 75 days in
animals, guinea pigs.
Statistically significant decr in cochlear microphonics at 1 of 18 points
examined, damage to hair cells of organ of Corti, slight damage to stria
vascularis and spiral ganglion, damage to macula utriculi and cristae, slight
damage to macula sacculi, and vestibular problems due to parenteral, subcutaneous, administration of 200 mg per kg daily, then 400 mg per kg, followed
by return to 200 mg per kg, total dose of 15 g per kg, of antibiotic, streptomycin (streptomycin sulfate), for 58 days in animals, guinea pigs.
  (AD) Vestibular problems confirmed by vestibular function tests.
No significant decr in cochlear microphonics due to parenteral, subcutaneous,
administration of 100 mg per kg daily for 5 days a week, total dose of 7.5 g
per kg, of antibiotic, viomycin (viomycin sulfate), for 75 days in animals,
guinea pigs.
Significant decr in cochlear microphonics, damage to hair cells of organ of
Corti and to stria vascularis, slight damage to spiral ganglion, and slight
damage to macula utriculi and crista ampullaris due to parenteral, subcutaneous, administration of 200 mg per kg daily for 5 days a week, then 400 mg
per kg, total dose of 15 g per kg, of antibiotic, viomycin (viomycin sulfate), for total of 67 days in animals, guinea pigs.
  (AD) Most toxicity for cochlear microphonics in guinea pig due to viomycin.
No significant decr in cochlear microphonics due to parenteral, subcutaneous,
administration of 100 mg per kg daily for 5 days each week, total dose of 7.5
g per kg, of antibiotic, capreomycin (capreomycin sulfate), for 75 days in
animals, guinea pigs.
No significant decr in cochlear microphonics, slight damage to outer hair
cells of organ of Corti and to stria vascularis, and no damage to vestibular
apparatus due to parenteral, subcutaneous, administration of 200 mg per kg
daily for 5 days a week, then 400 mg per kg, total dose of 15 g per kg, of
antibiotic, capreomycin (capreomycin sulfate), for total of 67 days in animals, guinea pigs.
  (CT) Same method using subcutaneous administration of 0.25 cc daily of

isotonic saline in guinea pigs, control group.
(AD) Least toxicity for inner ear of guinea pig due to capreomycin.
(AD) Study of functional and structural cochleo-vestibulotoxic effects of
streptomycin, viomycin, and capreomycin.
(AD) Statistical analysis of results. (ENG)

477
Significant decr in oxygen consumption of cochlea due to high doses of anti-
biotic, kanamycin, in animals, guinea pigs.
Significant decr in oxygen consumption of cochlea due to high doses of antibiotic, streptomycin, in animals, guinea pigs.
Incr followed by significant decr in oxygen consumption of cochlea due to
high doses of antibiotic, dihydrostreptomycin, in animals, guinea pigs.
(CT) Determination of oxygen consumption of guinea pigs, control group,
not treated with ototoxic drugs.
(AD) Suggested that ototoxicity of aminoglycoside antibiotics due to
inhibition of respiratory enzymes of cells of inner ear. (ENG)

482
Decr in cochlear function and vestibular function due to parenteral, intramuscular, administration of 50 to 100 mg per kg of antibiotic, streptomycin
(streptomycin sulfate), for 35 days in animals, guinea pigs, pigmented, 400
to 500 g weight.
(AD) More ototoxic effects with higher dosage.
Decr in cochlear function with both doses but decr in vestibular function
with only higher dose due to parenteral, intramuscular, administration of 50
to 100 mg per kg of antibiotic, dihydrostreptomycin (dihydrostreptomycin
sulfate), for 35 days in animals, guinea pigs, pigmented, 400 to 500 g
weight.
(AD) More decr in cochlear function with higher dosage.
Decr in cochlear function in all animals but decr in vestibular function in 2
groups only due to parenteral, intramuscular, administration of 50 to 100 mg
per kg of antibiotic, kanamycin, for 35 days in animals, guinea pigs, pigmented, 400 to 500 g weight.
(AD) More decr in cochlear function with higher dosage.
Decr in cochlear function due to parenteral, intramuscular, administration of
20 mg per kg of diuretic, ethacrynic acid, for 35 days in animals, guinea
pigs, pigmented, 400 to 500 g weight.
(CT) Study of guinea pigs, control group, not treated with ototoxic drugs.
Decr in ototoxic effects due to parenteral, intramuscular, administration of
100 mg per kg of antibiotic, streptomycin (IB) (streptomycin sulfate), for 35
days in animals, guinea pigs, pigmented, 400 to 500 g weight, with administration of 1 mg per kg of various inhibitors.
Decr in ototoxic effects due to parenteral, intramuscular, administration of
100 mg per kg of antibiotic, dihydrostreptomycin (IB) (dihydrostreptomycin
sulfate), for 35 days in animals, guinea pigs, pigmented, 400 to 500 g
weight, with administration of 1 mg per kg of various inhibitors.
Decr in ototoxic effects due to parenteral, intramuscular, administration of
100 mg per kg of antibiotic, kanamycin (IB), for 35 days in animals, guinea
pigs, pigmented, 400 to 500 g weight, with administration of 1 mg per kg of
various inhibitors.
Decr in ototoxic effects due to parenteral, intramuscular, administration of
20 mg per kg of diuretic, ethacrynic acid (IB), for 35 days in animals,
guinea pigs, pigmented, 400 to 500 g weight, with administration of 1 mg per
kg of various inhibitors.
(AD) Measurement of Preyer reflex and vestibular function tests.
Ototoxic effects, functional and structural, due to parenteral, intraperitoneal, administration of 100 mg per kg of antibiotic, streptomycin (streptomycin sulfate), for 50 days in animals, mice, male, 18 to 22 g weight.
No ototoxic effects due to parenteral, intraperitoneal, administration of 100
mg per kg of antibiotic, dihydrostreptomycin (dihydrostreptomycin sulfate),
for 50 days in animals, mice, male, 18 to 22 g weight.
Ototoxic effects, functional and structural, due to parenteral, intraperitoneal, administration of 100 mg per kg of antibiotic, kanamycin, for 50 days
in animals, mice, male, 18 to 22 g weight.
(CT) Study of mice, control group, not treated with ototoxic drugs.
No ototoxic effects due to parenteral, intraperitoneal, administration of 100
mg per kg of antibiotic, streptomycin (IB) (streptomycin sulfate), for 50

days in animals, mice, male, 18 to 22 g weight, with administration of 1 mg
per kg of vitamin B.
No ototoxic effects due to parenteral, intraperitoneal, administration of 100
mg per kg of antibiotic, dihydrostreptomycin (IB) (dihydrostreptomycin sulfate), for 50 days in animals, mice, male, 18 to 22 g weight, with administration of 1 mg per kg of vitamin B.
No ototoxic effects due to parenteral, intraperitoneal, administration of 100
mg per kg of antibiotic, kanamycin (IB), for 50 days in animals, mice, male,
18 to 22 g weight, with administration of vitamin B.
   (AD) More ototoxic effects of aminoglycoside antibiotics in guinea pigs
   than in mice.
   (AD) Ototoxic effects of diuretic in guinea pigs. (IT)

485
High concentration in fluids of inner ear and ototoxic effects due to 250 mg
per kg of antibiotic, streptomycin, in animals, guinea pigs.
High concentration in fluids of inner ear and ototoxic effects due to 250 mg
per kg of antibiotic, kanamycin, in animals, guinea pigs.
Higher concentration in fluids of inner ear and more severe ototoxic effects
due to 250 mg per kg of antibiotic, dihydrostreptomycin, in animals, guinea
pigs.
Higher concentration in fluids of inner ear and more severe ototoxic effects
due to 100 mg per kg of antibiotic, neomycin, in animals, guinea pigs.
   (AD) High concentration of aminoglycoside antibiotics in fluids of inner
   ear due to low doses as well as high doses.
   (AD) Ototoxic effect of aminoglycoside antibiotics due to retention of
   high concentrations in inner ear for long period and slow elimination of
   drugs.
Significant decr in concentration in fluids of inner ear and in serum and
decr in ototoxicity due to 250 mg per kg or 100 mg per kg of antibiotics
(IB), aminoglycoside, in animals, guinea pigs, with administration of ozothin.
Decr in concentration in fluids of inner ear and decr in ototoxicity due to
250 mg per kg or 100 mg per kg of antibiotics (IB), aminoglycoside, in animals, guinea pigs, with administration of pantothenic acid. (GER)

486
Incr in ATP activity of stria vascularis and spiral ligament but no pattern
of enzyme changes observed in membranous labyrinth due to 400 mg per kg daily
of antibiotic, kanamycin, for 3 weeks in animals, guinea pigs.
Incr in ATP activity of stria vascularis and spiral ligament but no pattern
of enzyme changes observed in membranous labyrinth due to 400 mg per kg daily
of antibiotic, streptomycin, for 3 weeks in animals, guinea pigs.
Decr in ATP activity of stria vascularis and spiral ligament but no pattern
of enzyme changes observed in membranous labyrinth due to 400 mg per kg daily
of antibiotic, dihydrostreptomycin, for 3 weeks in animals, guinea pigs.
   (CT) Study of guinea pigs, control group, not treated with aminoglycoside
   antibiotics.
   (AD) Study of effects of ototoxic drugs on ATP activity of inner ear of
   guinea pigs. (JAP)

495
Ototoxic effects due to parenteral, intramuscular, administration of 100 mg
per kg of antibiotic, neomycin (neomycin sulfate), in 10 injections in 10
animals, guinea pigs.
Significant decr in ototoxic effects due to parenteral, intramuscular, administration of 100 mg per kg of antibiotic, neomycin (IB) (neomycin sulfate), in 10 injections in 10 animals, guinea pigs, with combined administration of 1.2 ml per kg of ozothin.
Ototoxic effects due to parenteral, intramuscular, administration of 250 mg
per kg of antibiotic, streptomycin (streptomycin sulfate), in 10 injections
in animals, guinea pigs.
Decr in ototoxic effects due to parenteral, intramuscular, administration of
250 mg per kg of antibiotic, streptomycin (IB) (streptomycin sulfate), in 10
injections in 15 animals, guinea pigs, with combined administration of 1.2 ml
per kg of ozothin.
No ototoxic effects due to parenteral, intramuscular, administration of 250
mg per kg of antibiotic, streptomycin (IB) (streptomycin sulfate), in 10

injections in 6 animals, guinea pigs, with previous intramuscular administration of 1.2 ml per kg of ozothin.
   (CT) Study of 12 guinea pigs, control group.
   (AD) Electrophysiological study of effects of ozothin on ototoxicity of
   aminoglycoside antibiotics. (GER)

520

Decr in time of latency with incr in intensity of acoustic stimuli due to
parenteral, intraperitoneal, administration of 80 mg per kg daily, total of
480 mg, of antibiotic, cephalothin (cephalothin sodium), for 15 days in 10
animals, guinea pigs, albino.
Decr in time of latency with incr in intensity of acoustic stimuli due to
parenteral, intraperitoneal, administration of 20 mg per kg daily, total of
120 mg, of antibiotic, lincomycin (lincomycin chloride), for 15 days in 10
animals, guinea pigs, albino.
Decr in time of latency with incr in intensity of acoustic stimuli due to
parenteral, intraperitoneal, administration of 50 mg per kg daily, total of
300 mg, of antibiotic, cephaloridine, for 15 days in 10 animals, guinea pigs,
albino.
   (CT) Study of guinea pigs, control group, not treated with antibiotics.
   (AD) Study of response of guinea pigs to acoustic stimuli after treatment
   with antibiotics. (IT)

550

Decr in cochlear potentials due to parenteral, intraperitoneal, administration of 15 mg per kg of anesthetics (CB) in 2 groups of 15 animals, guinea
pigs, pigmented and albino, 300 g weight.
Decr in cochlear potentials due to parenteral, intraperitoneal, administration of 15 mg per kg of sedative, barbiturate (CB) in 2 groups of 15 animals,
guinea pigs, pigmented and albino, 300 g weight. (IT)

565

Inhibition of oxygen consumption of cochlea due to 0.04 M of antibiotic,
kanamycin (kanamycin sulfate), in animals, guinea pigs, adult, 300 g weight,
with normal Preyer reflex.
Inhibition of oxygen consumption of cochlea due to 0.04 M of antibiotic,
chloramphenicol (chloramphenicol sodium succinate), in animals, guinea pigs,
adult, 300 g weight, with normal Preyer reflex.
   (AD) Less inhibition of oxygen consumption by chloramphenicol than by
   kanamycin.
Incr inhibition of oxygen consumption of cochlea due to 0.04 M of antibiotic,
kanamycin (SM) (kanamycin sulfate), in animals, guinea pigs, adult, 300 g
weight, with normal Preyer reflex.
Incr inhibition of oxygen consumption of cochlea due to 0.04 M of antibiotic,
chloramphenicol (SM) (chloramphenicol sodium succinate), in animals, guinea
pigs, adult, 300 g weight, with normal Preyer reflex.
   (CT) Measurement of oxygen consumption of normal cochlea without administration of ototoxic drugs.
   (AD) In vitro study using microrespirometer of effect of interaction of
   kanamycin and chloramphenicol on oxygen consumption in guinea pig cochlea.
   (AD) Potentiation of inhibition of oxygen consumption of cochlea with
   simultaneous administration of kanamycin and chloramphenicol.
   (AD) Suggested risk of ototoxicity in clinical use of kanamycin and
   chloramphenicol. (ENG)

566

Gradual decr in cochlear microphonics and decr in endocochlear potentials,
but not significant, due to salicylate, acetylsalicylic acid, in animals,
guinea pigs, 250 to 400 g weight.
Severe decr in cochlear potentials due to 2.0 mM of chemical agent, cyanide
(potassium cyanide), in animals, guinea pigs, 250 to 400 g weight.
   (AD) Study of effects of various agents on cochlear potentials. (ENG)

613

Significant decr in cochlear microphonic due to topical administration to
round window of 10 percent concentration of anesthetic, cocaine, in 15
minutes in animals, guinea pigs, 400 to 600 g weight.
Less, but permanent, decr in cochlear microphonic due to topical administra-

tion to round window of 2 percent concentration of anesthetic, tetracaine, in
15 minutes in animals, guinea pigs, 400 to 600 g weight.
  (AD) Need for careful consideration in use of topical anesthetic within
  middle ear.
  (AD) Suggested that cocaine not be used within middle ear. (GER)

                                                                       627
Sensorineural hearing loss and vestibular problems due to parenteral, oral,
and topical administration of antibiotics in humans with and without kidney
disorder.
Degeneration of cochlea due to parenteral, intratympanic, administration of
antibiotic, neomycin, in animals, guinea pigs.
Transient sensorineural hearing loss due to high doses of salicylates in
humans.
Sensorineural hearing loss due to antimalarial, quinine, in humans.
Sensorineural hearing loss due to chemical agent, tobacco, in humans.
Sensorineural hearing loss due to sedative, alcohol, in humans.
  (AD) Discussion of ototoxicity of various drugs as 1 etiology of sen-
  sorineural hearing loss in adults. (ENG)

                                                                       715
Loss of outer hair cells of organ of Corti in lower part of first coil of
cochlea due to parenteral, intramuscular, administration of 400 mg per kg of
antibiotic, capreomycin, for 28 days in 40 percent of 10 animals, guinea
pigs, albino, 300 g weight.
Severe loss of outer hair cells of organ of Corti from lower part of basal
coil to upper coil of cochlea due to parenteral, intramuscular, administration of 400 mg per kg of antibiotic, kanamycin, for 28 days in 100 percent of
11 animals, guinea pigs, albino, 300 g weight.
  (CT) Test of Preyer reflex before, during, and after administration of
  antibiotics.
  (AD) Study suggested that capreomycin less ototoxic than kanamycin in
  guinea pigs.
  (AD) No observed damage to vestibular apparatus. (JAP)

                              Mice

                                                                       142
No toxic effects on eighth cranial nerve due to antibiotic, modified dihydrostreptomycin, in animals, guinea pigs and mice.
  (AD) Decr in antibiotic action and toxicity due to modification of quanidine group of dihydrostreptomycin molecule.
  (AD) Study of effect of chemical modification of dihydrostreptomycin
  molecule on biological activity and toxic effects of antibiotic. (RUS)

                                                                       187
Unspecified ototoxic effects due to parenteral, intravenous, intramuscular,
and intraperitoneal, administration of 0.9 percent sodium chloride solution
of antibiotics, aminoglycoside, in animals, mice, albino, adult, male and
female, 15 to 30 g weight.
  (CT) Same method using 0.9 percent sodium chloride solution in mice,
  control group.
  (AD) Comment on relationship of study to ototoxicity of antibiotics.
Risk of ototoxic effects due to antibiotic, dihydrostreptomycin, in chronic
intoxication in humans. (ENG)

                                                                       605
Decr in ototoxic effects due to parenteral, subcutaneous, administration of
high doses of antibiotic, gentamicin (IB) (gentamicin sulfate), in acute
intoxication in 20 animals, mice, male, 20 g weight, with simultaneous subcutaneous administration of calcium chloride.
  (CT) Same method using 8 mg of calcium chloride in mice, control group,
  showed no ototoxic effects.
  (CT) Same method using 12.5 mg of gentamicin (gentamicin sulfate) in mice,
  control group, showed ototoxic effects.
Decr in ototoxic effects due to parenteral, subcutaneous or intravenous,
administration of 25 mg per ml solution of antibiotic, gentamicin (IB) (gentamicin sulfate), in acute intoxication in animals, mice, male, 20 g weight,

with combined administration of 1, 2, 4, 8, 16, or 32 mg per ml concentrations of calcium chloride.
Decr in ototoxic effects due to parenteral, subcutaneous, administration of
antibiotic, gentamicin (IB) (gentamicin hydrochloride), in acute intoxication
in animals, mice, male, 20 g weight, with combined administration of complex
of calcium chloride.
   (AD) Decr in ototoxic effects in mice to less than 0.2 of effects of
   gentamicin (gentamicin hydrochloride) and to less than 0.5 of effects of
   gentamicin (gentamicin sulfate) due to calcium chloride.
Ataxia and equilibrium disorder due to parenteral, subcutaneous, administration of 60 and 120 mg per kg 1 time daily of antibiotic, gentamicin (gentamicin sulfate), in chronic intoxication in 20 animals, cats, male and female.
   (CT) Same method using saline in cats, control group.
Ataxia and equilibrium disorder due to parenteral, subcutaneous, administration of 60 and 120 mg per kg 1 time daily of antibiotic, gentamicin (IB)
(gentamicin hydrochloride), in chronic intoxication in 20 animals, cats, male
and female, with administration of complex of calcium chloride.
   (AD) No decr in ototoxicity due to calcium chloride in cats. (ENG)

                                                                      525

No loss of Preyer reflex and no structural changes in organ of Corti and
stria vascularis due to parenteral, intraperitoneal, administration of 3 to 5
mg per kg, in aqueous solution, of antineoplastic, mechlorethamine, for 5
days to 5 weeks in animals, 8 guinea pigs, adult, 300 to 400 g weight, and 6
mice, adult, 25 to 35 g weight, with normal Preyer reflex.
Loss of Preyer reflex and severe destruction of outer hair cells of organ of
Corti in basal and middle coils of cochlea but little or no change in stria
vascularis, spiral ganglion, and cochlear nerve due to parenteral, intraperitoneal, administration of 10 to 30 mg per kg, in aqueous solution, of antineoplastic, mechlorethamine, for 1 day to 5 weeks in animals, 7 guinea
pigs, adult, 300 to 400 g weight, and 19 mice, adult, 25 to 35 g weight, with
normal Preyer reflex.
   (CT) Same method using same volume of Ringer's solution in 5 animals,
   control group.
   (AD) Electron microscopic study of degeneration of cochlea in mechlorethamine intoxicated animals and in animals with congenital hearing loss to
   determine the mechanism of degeneration.
   (AD) Suggested possible effect on protein synthesis in hair cells of organ
   of Corti in early stages of mechlorethamine ototoxicity. (ENG)

                                                                      719

Progressive severe degeneration primarily in organ of Corti beginning after
24 hours but also damage to spiral ganglion and effect on cochlear function
due to parenteral, intraperitoneal, administration of 10 or 20 mg per kg of
chemical agent, 6-aminonicotinic acid, in animals, mice, audiogenic seizure-
susceptible.
Decr in ototoxic effects due to parenteral, intraperitoneal, administration
of 10 mg per kg of chemical agent, 6-aminonicotinic acid, in animals, mice,
audiogenic seizure-susceptible, with administration 5 minutes previously of
10 mg per kg of nicotinamide. (ENG)

                                                                      720

Damage to cochlear function and progressive severe degeneration in cochlear
duct, beginning after 24 hours in spiral ligament, with severe damage to
organ of Corti, and with later atrophy of spiral ganglion due to parenteral,
intraperitoneal, administration of 20 mg per kg, in concentration of 2 mg per
ml sterile water, of chemical agent, 6-aminonicotinic acid, in 1 injection in
9 animals, mice, male, audiogenic seizure-susceptible.
   (CT) Same method using water in 3 mice, control group.
   (CT) Same method using 2 mice, chronic control group, not treated.
Damage to cochlear function and degeneration in cochlea due to parenteral,
intraperitoneal, administration of 20 mg per kg of chemical agent, 6-aminoni-
cotinic acid, in 6 animals, mice, not audiogenic seizure-susceptible.
   (CT) Same method using water in 2 mice, control group, showed no histological changes. (ENG)

                                                                      730

Damage to cochlear function due to parenteral, intraperitoneal, administra-

tion of 20, 10, or 5 mg per kg, in concentration of 2 mg per ml of sterile
distilled water, of chemical agent, 6-aminonicotinic acid, in 1 injection in
18 animals, mice, about 30 days age, male, audiogenic seizure-susceptible.
   (AD) More severe hearing loss in mice with higher doses of 6-aminonico-
   tinic acid.
No damage to cochlear function due to parenteral, intraperitoneal, administration of 1 mg per kg, in concentration of 2 mg per ml of sterile distilled
water, of chemical agent, 6-aminonicotinic acid, in 1 injection in 4 animals,
mice, about 30 days age, male, audiogenic seizure-susceptible.
   (CT) Same method using intraperitoneal administration of same amount of
   water in 8 mice, control group, showed no damage to cochlear function.
   (ENG)

                                                                        482
Decr in cochlear function and vestibular function due to parenteral, intramuscular, administration of 50 to 100 mg per kg of antibiotic, streptomycin
(streptomycin sulfate), for 35 days in animals, guinea pigs, pigmented, 400
to 500 g weight.
   (AD) More ototoxic effects with higher dosage.
Decr in cochlear function with both doses but decr in vestibular function
with only higher dose due to parenteral, intramuscular, administration of 50
to 100 mg per kg of antibiotic, dihydrostreptomycin (dihydrostreptomycin
sulfate), for 35 days in animals, guinea pigs, pigmented, 400 to 500 g
weight.
   (AD) More decr in cochlear function with higher dosage.
Decr in cochlear function in all animals but decr in vestibular function in 2
groups only due to parenteral, intramuscular, administration of 50 to 100 mg
per kg of antibiotic, kanamycin, for 35 days in animals, guinea pigs, pigmented, 400 to 500 g weight.
   (AD) More decr in cochlear function with higher dosage.
Decr in cochlear function due to parenteral, intramuscular, administration of
20 mg per kg of diuretic, ethacrynic acid, for 35 days in animals, guinea
pigs, pigmented, 400 to 500 g weight.
   (CT) Study of guinea pigs, control group, not treated with ototoxic drugs.
Decr in ototoxic effects due to parenteral, intramuscular, administration of
100 mg per kg of antibiotic, streptomycin (IB) (streptomycin sulfate), for 35
days in animals, guinea pigs, pigmented, 400 to 500 g weight, with administration of 1 mg per kg of various inhibitors.
Decr in ototoxic effects due to parenteral, intramuscular, administration of
100 mg per kg of antibiotic, dihydrostreptomycin (IB) (dihydrostreptomycin
sulfate), for 35 days in animals, guinea pigs, pigmented, 400 to 500 g
weight, with administration of 1 mg per kg of various inhibitors.
Decr in ototoxic effects due to parenteral, intramuscular, administration of
100 mg per kg of antibiotic, kanamycin (IB), for 35 days in animals, guinea
pigs, pigmented, 400 to 500 g weight, with administration of 1 mg per kg of
various inhibitors.
Decr in ototoxic effects due to parenteral, intramuscular, administration of
20 mg per kg of diuretic, ethacrynic acid (IB), for 35 days in animals,
guinea pigs, pigmented, 400 to 500 g weight, with administration of 1 mg per
kg of various inhibitors.
   (AD) Measurement of Preyer reflex and vestibular function tests.
Ototoxic effects, functional and structural, due to parenteral, intraperitoneal, administration of 100 mg per kg of antibiotic, streptomycin (streptomycin sulfate), for 50 days in animals, mice, male, 18 to 22 g weight.
No ototoxic effects due to parenteral, intraperitoneal, administration of 100
mg per kg of antibiotic, dihydrostreptomycin (dihydrostreptomycin sulfate),
for 50 days in animals, mice, male, 18 to 22 g weight.
Ototoxic effects, functional and structural, due to parenteral, intraperitoneal, administration of 100 mg per kg of antibiotic, kanamycin, for 50 days
in animals, mice, male, 18 to 22 g weight.
   (CT) Study of mice, control group, not treated with ototoxic drugs.
No ototoxic effects due to parenteral, intraperitoneal, administration of 100
mg per kg of antibiotic, streptomycin (IB) (streptomycin sulfate), for 50
days in animals, mice, male, 18 to 22 g weight, with administration of 1 mg
per kg of vitamin B.
No ototoxic effects due to parenteral, intraperitoneal, administration of 100
mg per kg of antibiotic, dihydrostreptomycin (IB) (dihydrostreptomycin sulfate), for 50 days in animals, mice, male, 18 to 22 g weight, with adminis-

tration of 1 mg per kg of vitamin B.
No ototoxic effects due to parenteral, intraperitoneal, administration of 100
mg per kg of antibiotic, kanamycin (IB), for 50 days in animals, mice, male,
18 to 22 g weight, with administration of vitamin B.
  (AD) More ototoxic effects of aminoglycoside antibiotics in guinea pigs
  than in mice.
  (AD) Ototoxic effects of diuretic in guinea pigs. (IT)

Monkey, Squirrel monkey

                                                                         573
Bilateral vestibular problems, ataxia, and damage to hair cells of organ of
Corti in basal coil of cochlea and of cristae and maculae due to parenteral,
intramuscular, administration of 80 or 50 mg per kg on 5 days a week of
antibiotic, gentamicin, in 5 animals, squirrel monkeys, Saimiri sciureus,
about 2 years age, male and female.
Loss of equilibrium, ataxia, damage to hair cells of cristae and maculae, and
some degeneration of nerve process near hair cells due to parenteral, subcutaneous, administration of 60, 30, or 20 mg per kg on 7 days a week of antibiotic, gentamicin, in 7 animals, squirrel monkeys, Saimiri sciureus, about 2
years age, male and female.
  (AD) Type 1 hair cells of cristae and maculae more vulnerable to gentamicin than type 2 hair cells.
  (CT) Squirrel monkey rail method and test of nystagmus, pretreatment and
  posttreatment.
  (AD) Earlier onset of equilibrium disorders with high daily doses than
  with low daily doses.
  (AD) Total doses before onset of ataxia slightly more in group with high
  daily doses.
  (AD) Less ototoxic effects and slower onset with administration of gentamicin 5 days a week than 7 days a week.
  (AD) Lower doses in group with injections 7 days a week resulted in more
  severe and earlier onset of loss of equilibrium.
  (AD) Damage to vestibular apparatus slightly more severe in animals with
  higher daily doses.
  (AD) Correlation between equilibrium test and electron microscopic findings. (ENG)

                                                                         155
Suppression of function of semicircular canal due to parenteral, intramuscular, administration of range of 1100 to 4600 mg total doses of antibiotic,
streptomycin (streptomycin sulfate), for 16 to 23 doses in 8 animals, squirrel monkeys, with normal semicircular canal function.
  (CT) Vestibular function tests used to confirm pretreatment normal function of semicircular canal.
Moderate to severe damage to hair cells of cristae and organ of Corti and
some changes in spiral ganglion and maculae due to parenteral, intramuscular,
administration of range of 1100 to 4600 mg total doses of antibiotic, streptomycin (streptomycin sulfate), for 16 to 23 doses in 8 animals, squirrel
monkeys, with normal semicircular canal function.
  (AD) Report on 8 case studies to show clinical and pathological correlations. (ENG)

                                                                         456
Damage to type 1 hair cells of cristae and macula utriculi, no significant
changes in macula sacculi, and no changes in type 2 hair cells of vestibular
apparatus due to parenteral, intramuscular, administration of 200 mg per kg
daily, total doses of 1600 to 3800 mg per kg, of antibiotic, streptomycin
(streptomycin sulfate), for range of 10 to 26 days, until decline in caloric
threshold values of 2 to 10 degrees C, in 4 animals, squirrel monkeys, 500 to
600 g weight.
Severe damage to type 1 and 2 hair cells of cristae, loss of type 1 hair
cells of macula utriculi, and slight changes in macula sacculi due to parenteral, intramuscular, administration of 200 mg per kg daily, total doses of
2000 and 2600 mg per kg, of antibiotic, streptomycin (streptomycin sulfate),
for 14 and 18 days, until complete suppression of vestibular function, in 2
animals, squirrel monkeys, 500 to 600 g weight.
  (AD) Damage to vestibular function determined by vestibular function

tests.
(AD) Relative mild damage in early period of intoxication result of low
concentration of streptomycin in endolymph due to intramuscular route.
(AD) Suggested mechanism of streptomycin action is damage to enzyme system, damage to cytoplasmic membrane, and inhibition of protein synthesis
and ribosome function. (ENG)

047

Range of degree of damage to crista ampullaris and macula due to parenteral,
intramuscular, administration of 150 mg per kg daily of antibiotic, viomycin
(viomycin sulfate), for about 2 to 3 weeks in 3 animals, squirrel monkeys.
Range of degree of damage to crista ampullaris and macula due to parenteral,
intramuscular, administration of 200 to 300 mg per kg daily of antibiotic,
viomycin (viomycin sulfate), for about 2 to 3 weeks in 3 animals, cats.
More severe damage to crista ampullaris and macula due to topical administration in solution of range of 113 mg per ml to 500 mg per ml solution of
antibiotic, viomycin (viomycin sulfate), in 1 or 2 doses in 9 animals, cats.
   (CT) Control group of 2 monkeys and 2 cats used. (ENG)

169

Progressive sensorineural hearing loss, complete range of degrees of damage
to organ of Corti, and degeneration in cochlear nuclei due to parenteral,
intramuscular, administration of 15 to 100 mg per kg daily of antibiotic,
kanamycin (kanamycin sulfate), for 28 to 180 days in 3 animals, monkeys,
young, 2 to 6 years age, male and female, 3 to 9 kg weight, conditioned.
High frequency hearing loss and damage to organ of Corti due to parenteral,
intramuscular, administration of 100 mg per kg daily of antibiotic, neomycin
(neomycin sulfate), for 5 days in 1 animal, monkey, young, conditioned.
Delayed severe sensorineural hearing loss after 2 months and severe damage to
organ of Corti due to parenteral, intramuscular, administration of 50 mg per
kg of antibiotic, neomycin (neomycin sulfate), for 15 days in 1 animal,
monkey, young, conditioned.
   (CT) Pretreatment hearing baseline determined.
   (AD) Study showed correlation of measurement of hearing loss and histopathology of cochlea in same subject.
   (AD) Cochleograms made to show patterns of cell loss.
   (AD) Reported that neomycin more ototoxic than kanamycin. (ENG)

437

Hearing loss and damage to cochlea due to antibiotic, neomycin, in animals,
guinea pigs and monkeys, and humans.
Hearing loss and damage to cochlea due to antibiotic, streptomycin, in animals, guinea pigs and monkeys, and humans.
   (AD) Discussion of findings on decr of ototoxicity of aminoglycoside
   antibiotics. (GER)

Rabbit

033

Damage to organ of Corti due to topical route, inhalation, of chemical agent,
carbon monoxide, in 40 exposures in 5 animals, rabbits. (GER)

044

Change in cochlear response and damage to hair cells of organ of Corti due to
100 mg per kg daily of antibiotic, dihydrostreptomycin, in animals, rabbits.
Change in cochlear response and damage to stria vascularis due to 250 mg per
kg daily and 500 mg per kg daily of antibiotic, dihydrostreptomycin, in 2
other groups of animals, rabbits. (JAP)

146

Cochleotoxic effects due to antibiotic, kanamycin, in chronic intoxication in
animals, rabbits.
   (AD) Electrophysiological study of ototoxicity of kanamycin. (JAP)

242

Variations in decr in cochlear microphonic due to parenteral, intraperitoneal, administration of 100 mg per kg of antibiotic, kanamycin, for period
until measurement of cochlear microphonic not possible in 12 animals, rab-

bits, adult, normal.

Changes in outer hair cells and supporting cells, in particular in basal coil of cochlea, and slight damage to inner hair cells of organ of Corti due to parenteral, intraperitoneal, administration of 100 mg per kg of antibiotic, kanamycin, for period until measurement of cochlear microphonic not possible in 12 animals, rabbits, adult, normal.

(AD) Serial observations on beginning and progression of cochleotoxic effects of kanamycin by daily measurement of cochlear microphonic and study of correlations between electrophysiological and histopathological changes.

(AD) Variations in response of cochlea to kanamycin but correlation between electrophysiological and histopathological changes. (ENG)

337

Shifts in cochlear microphonic and action potential thresholds and loss of Preyer reflex due to parenteral, subcutaneous, administration of 400 mg per kg daily of antibiotic, kanamycin, for 10, 14, or 20 days in 3 groups of animals, guinea pigs, adult, male.

(CT) Study of guinea pigs, control group.

(AD) Correlation between duration of dosage and decr in function.

(AD) Study of guinea pigs showed individual responses to kanamycin.

Shifts in cochlear microphonic and action potential thresholds and loss of Preyer reflex due to parenteral, subcutaneous, administration of 400 mg per kg daily of antibiotic, kanamycin, for 10, 14, or 20 days in 3 groups of animals, rats, adult, male.

(CT) Study of rats, control group.

(AD) Results of study of rats showed high degree of individual response to kanamycin or technical difficulty in recording from round window of rat.

Shifts in cochlear microphonic and action potential thresholds and loss of Preyer reflex due to parenteral, subcutaneous, administration of 400 mg per kg daily of antibiotic, kanamycin, for 10, 14, or 20 days in 3 groups of animals, rabbits, adult, male.

(CT) Study of rabbits, control group.

(AD) Similarity between cochlear impairment of rabbit and hearing loss in humans due to kanamycin.

Destruction of hair cells of organ of Corti in all coils of cochlea and damage to stria vascularis and spiral ganglion due to unspecified method of administration of 200 mg per kg of antibiotic, kanamycin, for 20 days in animals, guinea pigs.

(AD) Difference in pattern and degree of cochlear impairment in different species of animals.

(AD) Suggested that physiological changes precede histological changes and so show more clearly the ototoxic effects of the drug. (ENG)

349

Effect on hearing loss due to antibiotic, kanamycin (IB), in animals, rabbits, with administration of vitamin B derivatives.

(AD) Study of effects of vitamin B derivatives on cochleotoxic effects of kanamycin. (JAP)

635

Effect on cochlear impairment due to antibiotic, kanamycin (IB), in animals, rabbits, with administration of derivative of thiamine. (JAP)

291

Cochlear impairment due to 5.0 g of antimalarial, quinine (quinine hydrochloride), in humans.

Cochlear impairment due to antimalarial, quinine (quinine hydrochloride), in animals, cats and rabbits.

(AD) Comparative animal studies and clinical case reports.

(AD) Study of ocular toxicity with comment on ototoxicity. (GER)

571

No significant effect on vestibular apparatus due to oral administration of 50 or 150 mg per kg daily, total of 1.55 and 4.65 g per kg, of antibiotic, rifampicin, for 5 weeks in 2 groups of 7 animals, rabbits, male.

(CT) Same method using 1 percent carboxymethyl-cellulose in rabbits, control group.

(AD) Measurement of horizontal nystagmus 2, 3, 4, and 5 weeks after beginning of treatment.
No accumulation in perilymph due to oral administration of 100 mg per kg of
antibiotic, rifampicin, for 1 dose in animals, guinea pigs.
(AD) Determination of rifampicin concentration in perilymph and blood
after 2, 6, and 24 hours.
(AD) Study of vestibulotoxic effects and retention in inner ear of rifampicin. (ENG)

112

Permanent inhibition of cochlear microphonic due to parenteral administration
of high doses of antibiotic, streptomycin, in animals, guinea pigs and rabbits.
Rapid decr in cochlear potentials due to lower doses of antibiotic, streptomycin, in animals, guinea pigs and rabbits, sensitized with horse serum.
(AD) Study to show pathogenesis of cochlear neuritis in association with
streptomycin treatment. (RUS)

703

No nystagmus due to parenteral, intramuscular, administration of 0.150 mg of
analgesic, fentanyl, in 5 animals, rabbits, 2.5 to 3 kg weight.
Positional nystagmus within 15 to 30 minutes due to parenteral administration
of 4 ml per kg of 96 percent solution of sedative, alcohol, in 8 animals,
rabbits, 2.5 to 3 kg weight.
Positional nystagmus within 15 to 30 minutes due to parenteral administration
of 4 ml per kg of 96 percent solution of sedative, (SQ) alcohol, in 11 animals, rabbits, 2.5 to 3 kg weight.
Partial or total suppression of positional nystagmus due to parenteral,
intramuscular, administration of 0.150 mg of analgesic, (SQ) fentanyl, in 6
of 11 animals, rabbits, 2.5 to 3 kg weight.
Decr in positional nystagmus due to parenteral, intramuscular, administration
of 0.08 to 0.10 mg of analgesic, (SQ) fentanyl, in 5 of 11 animals, rabbits,
2.5 to 3 kg weight. (IT)

Rat

337

Shifts in cochlear microphonic and action potential thresholds and loss of
Preyer reflex due to parenteral, subcutaneous, administration of 400 mg per
kg daily of antibiotic, kanamycin, for 10, 14, or 20 days in 3 groups of
animals, guinea pigs, adult, male.
(CT) Study of guinea pigs, control group.
(AD) Correlation between duration of dosage and decr in function.
(AD) Study of guinea pigs showed individual responses to kanamycin.
Shifts in cochlear microphonic and action potential thresholds and loss of
Preyer reflex due to parenteral, subcutaneous, administration of 400 mg per
kg daily of antibiotic, kanamycin, for 10, 14, or 20 days in 3 groups of
animals, rats, adult, male.
(CT) Study of rats, control group.
(AD) Results of study of rats showed high degree of individual response to
kanamycin or technical difficulty in recording from round window of rat.
Shifts in cochlear microphonic and action potential thresholds and loss of
Preyer reflex due to parenteral, subcutaneous, administration of 400 mg per
kg daily of antibiotic, kanamycin, for 10, 14, or 20 days in 3 groups of
animals, rabbits, adult, male.
(CT) Study of rabbits, control group.
(AD) Similarity between cochlear impairment of rabbit and hearing loss in
humans due to kanamycin.
Destruction of hair cells of organ of Corti in all coils of cochlea and
damage to stria vascularis and spiral ganglion due to unspecified method of
administration of 200 mg per kg of antibiotic, kanamycin, for 20 days in
animals, guinea pigs.
(AD) Difference in pattern and degree of cochlear impairment in different
species of animals.
(AD) Suggested that physiological changes precede histological changes and
so show more clearly the ototoxic effects of the drug. (ENG)

Hearing loss in 15 fetuses due to parenteral, intramuscular, administration
of 200 mg per kg daily of antibiotic, kanamycin, for 15 days in animals,
rats, Wistar strain, female, about 150 g weight, during pregnancy.
   (AD) Test of Preyer reflex of rats, newborn infant, 30 days after birth.
No hearing loss due to 20 mg per kg daily of antibiotic, kanamycin, for 1 to
5 days in 15 humans, newborn infant.
   (CT) EEG in newborn infants, before and about 1 month after kanamycin
   administration.
No hearing loss in fetuses due to antibiotic, kanamycin, in humans, female,
treated for pulmonary tuberculosis during pregnancy.
   (AD) Follow up study for 3 years after birth showed no hearing loss in
   children.
   (AD) Discussion of clinical and experimental studies on effects of kanamycin.
Hearing loss due to range of 30 to 100 mg per kg daily of antibiotic, kanamycin, for range of 3 to 46 days in 9 of 391 humans, newborn infant.
No hearing loss due to less than 60 mg per kg daily of antibiotic, kanamycin,
for less than 11 days in 382 humans, newborn infant.
   (AD) Discussion of reports from 100 hospitals in Japan on effects of
   kanamycin in newborn infants.
   (AD) Relationship between cochleotoxic effects of kanamycin and daily
   dosage and duration of treatment.   (ENG)

722

Effect on reaction time to acoustic stimuli due to parenteral, intraperitoneal, administration of 0.16 and 0.04 mg per kg of chemical agent, lysergide, in 3 animals, rats, albino, about 120 days age, male, 300 g weight.
   (CT) Same method using 0.05 cc saline in rats, control group.   (ENG)

334

Effect on organ of Corti of fetuses due to parenteral, intraperitoneal,
administration of daily doses of antibiotic, streptomycin, in animals, rats,
female, during pregnancy.
Effect on organ of Corti of fetuses due to parenteral, intraperitoneal,
administration of daily doses of antibiotic, dihydrostreptomycin, in animals,
rats, female, during pregnancy.
   (AD) Determined concentration of antibiotic in blood of fetus.   (GER)

529

Total loss of Preyer reflex within several days but no vestibular problems
due to parenteral, subcutaneous, administration of range of high doses to
more than 1000 mg per kg daily of antibiotic, kanamycin (kanamycin sulfate),
in animals, rats, Wistar, albino, female, 50 g weight.
   (AD) Linear relationship between hearing loss and kanamycin dosage.
Loss of Preyer reflex but no vestibular problems due to parenteral, subcutaneous, administration of range of high doses to more than 600 mg per kg
daily of antibiotic, neomycin, in animals, rats, Wistar, albino, female, 50 g
weight.
   (AD) Linear relationship between hearing loss and neomycin dosage.
   (AD) Hearing loss observed with lower doses of neomycin than kanamycin.
Moderate to severe vestibular problems but cochlear impairment in only 1 case
due to parenteral, subcutaneous, administration of high doses, 471, 583, 720,
887, and 1089 mg per kg daily, of antibiotic, streptomycin (streptomycin
sulfate), in animals, rats, Wistar, albino, female, 50 g weight.
   (AD) Linear realtionship between vestibular problems and streptomycin
   dosage.
Transient moderate to severe vestibular problems but cochlear impairment in
only 1 case due to parenteral, subcutaneous, administration of high doses,
765, 940, 1151, and 1377 mg per kg daily, of antibiotic, dihydrostreptomycin
(dihydrostreptomycin sulfate), in 40 animals, rats, Wistar, albino, female,
50 g weight.
   (CT) Same method using saline in 30 rats, control group, showed no cochleo-vestibulotoxic effects.
Hearing loss due to parenteral, subcutaneous, administration of 500 mg per kg
daily of antibiotic, kanamycin (SM), in animals, rats, Wistar, albino, female, 50 g weight.
Hearing loss due to parenteral, subcutaneous, administration of range of
doses of antibiotic, neomycin (SM), in animals, rats, Wistar, albino, female,

50 g weight.
    (AD) Incr in ototoxicity of neomycin due to kanamycin.
Hearing loss but no vestibular problems due to parenteral, subcutaneous,
administration of 500 mg per kg of antibiotic, kanamycin (SM), in animals,
rats, Wistar, albino, female, 50 g weight.
Hearing loss but no vestibular problems due to parenteral, subcutaneous,
administration of 200, 270, 364.5, and 492 mg per kg daily of antibiotic,
streptomycin (SM), in animals, rats, Wistar, albino, female, 50 g weight.
Hearing loss but no vestibular problems due to parenteral, subcutaneous,
administration of 500 mg per kg daily of antibiotic, kanamycin (SM), in
animals, rats, Wistar, albino, female, 50 g weight.
Hearing loss but no vestibular problems due to parenteral, subcutaneous,
administration of 350, 472.5, 637.9, and 861.1 mg per kg daily of antibiotic,
dihydrostreptomycin (SM), in animals, rats, Wistar, albino, female, 50 g
weight.
    (AD) Tests of cochlear function and vestibular function, pretreatment and
    daily during treatment.
    (AD) Comparative study of ototoxic effects of aminoglycoside antibiotics
    in Wistar rats.
    (AD) Report of hearing loss in 321 (43.4 percent) of total of 740 rats in
    study.
    (AD) Suggested that ototoxic effects of kanamycin and neomycin due to
    different mechanisms of action than ototoxic effects of streptomycin and
    dihydrostreptomycin. (ENG)

OTHER ANIMALS

279

Transient inhibition of endorgan of ampulla of semicircular canal due to
range of doses of antibiotics, aminoglycoside, in animals, frogs.
    (CT) Study of frogs, control group.
    (AD) In vitro study of effect of antibiotics on function of ampullar
    endorgan of semicircular canal of frog. (IT)

567

Effect on sensory hair cells in lateral line organ due to concentrations of 1
to 4 ppm, in aquaria containing 15 l of water, of chemical agent, chlorophenothane, for 18 hours at temperature of 22 to 23 degrees C in animals,
clawed toads, Xenopus laevis.
    (AD) Sensory hair cells of lateral line organ of toad comparable to hair
    cells in inner ear of higher vertebrates. (ENG)

563

Effect on cochlear microphonic due to topical administration of chemical
agent, cyanide, in animals, birds.
    (AD) Study of cochlear potentials of various birds. (GER)

636

Inhibition of potentials of endorgan of ampulla of posterior semicircular
canal due to 2.5, 10, or 20 mcg per ml, in Tyrode solution, of antimalarial,
quinine (quinine hydrochloride), in animals, frogs.
    (CT) Study of effect on potentials of Tyrode solution without quinine.
    (AD) Electrophysiological study of effect of quinine on potentials of
    endorgan of ampulla of posterior semicircular canal.
    (AD) Some recovery of potentials after cessation of quinine administra-
    tion.
    (AD) Suggested that toxic effects on endorgan of semicircular canal result
    from administration of quinine. (ENG)

476

Vestibulotoxic effects due to 100 mg per kg of antibiotic, streptomycin, in
animals, pigeons.
Some decr in vestibulotoxic effects due to 100 mg per kg of antibiotic,
streptomycin (IB), for 30 days in animals, pigeons, with administration of
25000 units of vitamin A.
    (AD) Structural damage similar in both groups of pigeons. (POL)

620
Changes of various degrees of intensity in cerebellar vermis, including Purkinje's cell, due to 30 mg per kg, total doses of 600 mg and 1200 mg, of antibiotic, streptomycin, in 2 groups of 24 animals, pigeons. (POL)

285
Transient inhibition of endorgan of ampulla due to range of doses of antibiotic, streptomycin (streptomycin sulfate), in animals, frogs.
Transient inhibition of endorgan of ampulla due to range of doses of antibiotic, dihydrostreptomycin (dihydrostreptomycin sulfate), in animals, frogs.
Transient inhibition of endorgan of ampulla due to range of doses of antibiotic, neomycin (neomycin sulfate), in animals, frogs.
Transient inhibition of endorgan of ampulla due to range of doses of antibiotic, kanamycin (kanamycin sulfate), in animals, frogs.
   (CT) Study of frogs, control group.
   (AD) More inhibition of endorgan of ampulla with streptomycin than with other aminoglycoside antibiotics.
   (AD) Agreement between in vivo and in vitro observations of intensity of action on endorgans of vestibular apparatus.   (ENG)

438
Suppression of microphonic potentials of saccule due to topical, intraluminal, administration of antibiotic, streptomycin, in animals, goldfish.
Suppression of microphonic potentials of saccule due to topical, intraluminal, administration of antibiotic, kanamycin, in animals, goldfish.
Suppression of microphonic potentials of saccule due to topical, intraluminal or extraluminal, administration of 0.5 mg of chemical agent, cyanide, in animals, goldfish.
Suppression of microphonic potentials of saccule due to topical, intraluminal or extraluminal, administration of 0.1 mg of antimalarial, quinine, in animals, goldfish.
Suppression of microphonic potentials of saccule due to topical, intraluminal or extraluminal, administration of 2 mg of anesthetic, procaine, in animals, goldfish.
No effect on microphonic potentials of saccule due to topical administration of salicylates in animals, goldfish.   (ENG)

491
Changes in sensory epithelium of otocyst due to antibiotic, streptomycin, in animals, chickens, embryo.
Changes in sensory epithelium of otocyst due to antibiotic, neomycin, in animals, chickens, embryo.
Changes in sensory epithelium of otocyst due to antibiotic, kanamycin, in animals, chickens, embryo.
   (CT) Study of otocysts of chickens, control group, not treated with aminoglycoside antibiotics.
   (AD) Neomycin and kanamycin more toxic to otocysts of chickens than streptomycin.   (CZ)

562
Decr in microphonic potential of saccule due to topical, intraluminal, administration of antibiotic, streptomycin, in animals, goldfish.
Decr in microphonic potential of saccule due to topical, intraluminal, administration of antibiotic, kanamycin, in animals, goldfish.
Permanent decr in microphonic potential of saccule due to topical, intraluminal or extraluminal, administration of 0.5 mg per ml of chemical agent, cyanide, in animals, goldfish.
Permanent decr in microphonic potential of saccule due to topical, intraluminal or extraluminal, administration of 0.1 mg per ml of antimalarial, quinine, in animals, goldfish.
No effect on microphonic potential of saccule due to salicylate, aspirin, in animals, goldfish.
Some decr in microphonic potential of saccule due to 2 mg per ml of anesthetic, procaine, in animals, goldfish.
   (AD) Study of effects of various agents on microphonic potential of saccule of goldfish.   (JAP)

681
Degrees of inhibition of potential of endorgan of ampulla of posterior semi-

circular canal due to 50, 200, 300, and 500 mcg per cc, in Tyrode solution, of antibiotic, streptomycin (streptomycin sulfate), in animals, frogs.
Degrees of inhibition of potential of endorgan of ampulla of posterior semi-circular canal due to 100, 200, and 500 mcg per cc, in Tyrode solution, of antibiotic, dihydrostreptomycin, in animals, frogs.
    (AD) Recovery of potential after cessation of administration of antibio-tics. (IT)

CITATION SECTION

ABBREVIATIONS USED IN CITATION SECTION

Languages

Bul - Bulgarian
Cz - Czech
Dan - Danish
Dut - Dutch
Eng - English
Fin - Finnish
Fr - French
Ger - German
Hun - Hungarian
It - Italian

Jap - Japanese
Nor - Norwegian
Pol - Polish
Rum - Rumanian
Rus - Russian
Ser - Serbo-Croatian
Sl - Slovene
Sp - Spanish
Sw - Swedish

Types of Papers

Art - article
Rev - review
Clin - clinical

Monogr - monograph
Exp - experimental
Histol - histological

CITATION SECTION

001

Campanelli PA* Grimes E* West ML*
Hearing Loss in a Child Following Neomycin Irrigation.   Report of a Case
    Med Ann DC 35 541-543, Oct 1966
    016 Refs Clin Type Eng

002

Proud GO* Mittelman H* Seiden GD*
Ototoxicity of Topically Applied Chloramphenicol
    Arch Otolaryng (Chicago) 87 (6) 580-587, Jun 1968
    013 Refs Exp Histol Type Eng

003

Schwartz GH* David DS* Riggio RR* Stenzel KH* Rubin AL*
Ototoxicity Induced by Furosemide
    New Eng J Med 282 (25) 1413-1414, Jun 1970
    013 Refs Clin Type Eng

004

Gibson WS,Jr*
Deafness due to Orally Administered Neomycin
    Arch Otolaryng (Chicago) 86 (2) 163-165, Aug 1967
    010 Refs Clin Type Eng

005

Mathog RH* Thomas WG* Hudson WR*
Ototoxicity of New and Potent Diuretics. A Preliminary Study
    Arch Otolaryng (Chicago) 92 (1) 7-13, Jul 1970
    009 Refs Exp Histol Type Eng

006

Kohonen A* Tarkkanen J*
Cochlear Damage from Ototoxic Antibiotics by Intratympanic Application
    Acta Otolaryng (Stockholm) 68 (1-2) 90-97, Jul-Aug 1969
    010 Refs Exp Histol Type Eng

007

Jarvis JF*
A Case of Unilateral Permanent Deafness Following Acetylsalicylic Acid
    J Laryng 80 318-320, 1966
    006 Refs Clin Type Eng

008

Meyers RM*
Ototoxic Effects of Gentamicin
    Arch Otolaryng (Chicago) 92 (2) 160-162, Aug 1970
    001 Refs Clin Type Eng

009

Mc Gee TM*
Ototoxic Antibiotics
    Volta Rev 70 (9) 667-671, Dec 1968
    006 Refs Rev Type Eng

010

Johnson AH* Hamilton CH*

Kanamycin Ototoxicity--Possible Potentiation by Other Drugs
    Southern Med J 63 511-513, May 1970
    015 Refs Clin Type Eng

011

Levkovskii VA* Aberman AA*
(The Ototoxicity of Kanamycin in Tuberculosis Patients)
    In-- Aktual'nye Voprosy Meditsiny Kiev,Zdorovya 1966
    000 Refs Clin Type Rus
    Abstr. (Biol Abstr 49 1723, 1968)

012

De Beukelaer MM* Travis LB* Dodge WF* Guerra FA*
Deafness and Acute Tubular Necrosis Following Parenteral Administration of
Neomycin
    Amer J Dis Child 121 250-252, Mar 1971
    013 Refs Clin Type Eng

013

Despons JL*
(The Treatment of Inflammatory Diseases of the External Auditory Meatus with
the Combination of Polymyxin B, Neomycin and Fluocinolone Acetonide)
    J Med Bordeaux 144 (6) 915-917, 1967
    000 Refs Clin Type Fr
    Abstr. (Excer Med Sect 11 20 665, 1967)

014

Guzy K* Kindracka E* Lewandowska J*
(Impairment of the Organs of Hearing and Equilibrium in Children Treated with
Streptomycin)
    Przegl Lek 23 (5) 436-438, 1967
    000 Refs Clin Type Pol
    Abstr. (Excer Med Sect 11 20 675, 1967)

015

Takenaka B* Hama H* Suzuki M* Kawamoto S* Hirayama M*
(Electron Microscopic Observation on the Effect of Actinomycete Streptomyces
Punicens (Viomycin) in the Vestibular Apparatus)
    J Otolaryng Jap 70 (6) 1124-1127, 1967
    000 Refs Exp Histol Type Jap
    Abstr. (Excer Med Sect 11 20 662, 1967)

016

Stephens SDG*
A Case of Gentamicin Accentuated Hearing Loss
    J Laryng 82 (9) 803-808, Sep 1968
    029 Refs Clin Type Eng

017

Gupta KR* Kakar PK* Misra UC*
Early Detection of Streptomycin Ototoxicity
    J Indian Med Ass 54 184-186, Mar 1 1970
    005 Refs Clin Type Eng

018

Govindaraj M*
Multiple-Drug Reactions in Tuberculosis--An Illustrative Case
    Tubercle 49 416-418, Dec 1968
    002 Refs Clin Type Eng

019

Jarvis JF*
Some Aspects of the Oto-Toxic Antibiotics
    S Afr Med J 42 1016-1019, Oct 5 1968
    013 Refs Clin Type Eng

020

Mc Gee TM* Webster J* Williams M*

Histological and Functional Changes in the Ears of Cats after Subcutaneous
Administration of Gentamicin
    J Infect Dis 119 432-442, Apr-May 1969
    000 Refs Exp Histol Type Eng

021

De Moura LFP* Hayden RC,Jr*
Salicylate Ototoxicity. A Human Temporal Bone Report
    Arch Otolaryng (Chicago) 87 (4) 368-372, Apr 1968
    013 Refs Clin Histol Type Eng

022

Wersall J* Lundquist PG* Bjorkroth B*
Ototoxicity of Gentamicin
    J Infect Dis 119 (4-5) 410-416, Apr-May 1969
    013 Refs Rev Exp Histol Type Eng

023

Gozdzik-Zolnierkiewicz T*
Outer and Inner Hair Cells in Streptomycin Poisoning
    Laryngoscope 79 (1) 125-133, Jan 1969
    021 Refs Exp Histol Type Eng

024

Graybiel A* Schuknecht HF* Fregly AR* Miller EF* Mc Leod ME*
Streptomycin in Meniere's Disease. Long-Term Follow-Up
    Arch Otolaryng (Chicago) 85 156-170, Feb 1967
    021 Refs Clin Type Eng

025

Faltynek L* Vesely C*
(Effect of Neomycin on the Function of the Guinea Pig Cochlea)
    Mschr Ohrenheilk 103 545-547, 1969
    005 Refs Exp Type Ger Trans Summ

026

Bablik L*
(Experimental Studies on the Influence of Alcohol on Normal Hearing)
    Mschr Ohrenheilk 102 305-319, 1968
    029 Refs Exp Type Ger Trans Summ

027

Kelly DR* Nilo ER* Berggren RB*
Deafness after Topical Neomycin Wound Irrigation
    New Eng J Med 280 1338-1339, Jun 12 1969
    008 Refs Clin Type Eng

028

Mathog RH* Klein WJ,Jr*
Ototoxicity of Ethacrynic Acid and Aminoglycoside Antibiotics in Uremia
    New Eng J Med 230 1223-1224, May 29 1969
    015 Refs Clin Type Eng

029

Cada K* Brun JP* Rauch S*
(Streptomycin Concentration with and without Ozothin in the Guinea Pig Blood
and Perilymph)
    Z Laryng Rhinol Otol 47 929-933, Dec 1968
    013 Refs Exp Type Ger Trans Summ

030

Fritsche F*
(Directional Audiometric Studies in a Free Field on Patients with U-shaped
Audiograms)
    Z Laryng Rhinol Otol 48 291-302, Apr 1969
    034 Refs Clin Type Ger Trans Summ

031

Kraus H* Doennig G*
(Cytophotometric RNA and Protein Determination in the Membranous Labyrinth of
Guinea Pigs as a Basis for the Evaluation of Protein Metabolism and Strep-
tomycin Ototoxicity)
    Arch Klin Exp Ohr Nas Kehlkopfheilk 194 551-557, Dec 22 1969
    046 Refs Exp Type Ger Trans Summ

032

Graham WCS*
Survival of a Severely Burned Child with Nerve Deafness from Local Antibiotics
    Panminerva Med 9 (10) 380, Oct 1967
    000 Refs Clin Comment Type Eng

033

Kuttner K*
(On the Pathomorphology of Changes in the Peripheral Organ of Hearing during
Repeated Experimental Carbon Monoxide Intoxication)
    Z Laryng Rhinol Otol 47 779-785, Oct 1968
    322 Refs Exp Type Ger Trans Summ

034

Gozdzik-Zolnierkiewicz T* Moszynski B*
Eighth Nerve in Experimental Lead Poisoning
    Acta Otolaryng (Stockholm) 68 85-89, Jul-Aug 1969
    014 Refs Exp Histol Type Eng

035

Schwartz FD* Pillay VK* Kark RM*
Ethacrynic Acid -- Its Usefulness and Untoward Effects
    Amer Heart J 79 427-428, Mar 1970
    020 Refs Comment Type Eng

036

Anon*
Gentamicin Sulphate
    S Afr Med J 42 1, Jan 6 1968
    010 Refs Comment Type Eng

037

Rempt E*
(Observation on the Course of Ear Damage due to Streptomycin)
    Z Laryng Rhinol Otol 48 519-527, Jul 1969
    016 Refs Clin Type Ger Trans Summ

038

Pillay VK* Schwartz FD* Aimi K* Kark RM*
Transient and Permanent Deafness Following Treatment with Ethacrynic Acid in
Renal Failure
    Lancet 1 77-79, Jan 11 1969
    007 Refs Clin Type Eng

039

Anon*
The Ototoxic Antibiotics in Relation to Iatrogenic Deafness
    Eye Ear Nose Throat Monthly 48 280, May 1969
    000 Refs Comment Type Eng

040

Allen AR* Stevenson AW*
Follow-Up Notes on Articles Previously Published in the Journal. A Ten-Year
Follow-Up of Combined Drug Therapy and Early Fusion in Bone Tuberculosis
    J Bone Joint Surg (Amer) 49 1001-1003, Jul 1967
    000 Refs Clin Type Eng

041

Dayal D* Shanta H*
Some Observations on the Ototoxicity of Thiacetazone

Indian J Tuberc 17 (4) 155-159, 1970
000 Refs Clin Type Eng
Abstr. (Abstr on Hygiene 46 545, 1971)

042

Meriwether WD* Mangi RJ* Serpick AA*
Deafness Following Standard Intravenous Dose of Ethacrynic Acid
    JAMA 216 (5) 795-798, May 3 1971
    012 Refs Clin Type Eng

043

Kaneko Y* Nakagawa T* Tanaka K*
Reissner's Membrane after Kanamycin Administration
    Arch Otolaryng (Chicago) 92 (5) 457-462, Nov 1970
    030 Refs Exp Histol Type Eng

044

Fujita M*
(Histopathological Study on Ototoxicity of Dihydrostreptomycin)
    J Otolaryng Jap 72 1901-1916, Oct 1969
    000 Refs Exp Histol Type Jap
    Abstr. (J Otolaryng Jap Abstr 3 (2) 20, 1969)

045

Ishii Y*
(Early Morphologic Features of the Lesions in the Cochlear Sensory Cells. A
Phase Contrast Microscopic Study)
    J Otolaryng Jap 72 1969
    000 Refs Exp Histol Type Jap
    Abstr. (J Otolaryng Jap Abstr 3 (2) 21-23, 1969)

046

Nakajima R* Watanabe Y* Oda R* Uno M*
(Kanamycin Levels of the Inner Ear of Guinea Pig)
    J Otolaryng Jap 72 748-751, Mar 1969
    000 Refs Exp Type Jap
    Abstr. (J Otolaryng Jap Abstr 3 (1) 5, 1969)

047

Kanda T* Igarashi M*
Ultra-Structural Changes in Vestibular Sensory End Organs after Viomycin
Sulfate Intoxication
    Acta Otolaryng (Stockholm) 68 (6) 474-488, Dec 1969
    020 Refs Exp Histol Type Eng

048

Cummings CW*
Experimental Observations on the Ototoxicity of Nitrogen Mustard
    Laryngoscope 78 (4) 530-538, Apr 1968
    013 Refs Exp Type Eng

049

Brummett RE* Meikle MM* Vernon JA*
Ototoxicity of Tobramycin in Guinea Pigs
    Arch Otolaryng (Chicago) 94 (1) 59-63, Jul 1971
    004 Refs Exp Type Eng

050

Balogh K,Jr* Hiraide F* Ishii D*
Distribution of Radioactive Dihydrostreptomycin in the Cochlea. An Autora-
diographic Study
    Ann Otol 79 (3) 641-652, Jun 1970
    027 Refs Exp Type Eng

051

Fisher TL*
Negligence
    Canad Med Ass J 98 965-966, May 18 1968

000 Refs Clin Comment Type Eng

052
Trimble GX*
Neomycin Ototoxicity -- Dossier and Doses
    New Eng J Med 281 219, Jul 24 1969
    000 Refs Letter Type Eng

053
Jawetz E*
Neomycin Ototoxicity -- Dossier and Doses
    New Eng J Med 281 219, Jul 24 1969
    000 Refs Letter Type Eng

054
Berry YJ*
Ototoxicity of Furosemide
    New Eng J Med 283 434, Aug 20 1970
    000 Refs Letter Type Eng

055
Hanzelik E* Peppercorn M*
Deafness after Ethacrynic Acid
    Lancet 1 416, Feb 22 1969
    000 Refs Letter Clin Type Eng

056
Gruuic M* Popovic J* Putnik DJ* Zegarac D* Martinis U* Praso R* Vanic
D* Milovanovic M* Djuric-Milosavljevic O* Stosic IZ*
(Hearing Damage in Patients Treated by Streptomycin)
    Pluc Bolest Tuberk 21 348-357, Jul-Dec 1969
    020 Refs Clin Type Ser Trans Summ

057
Stepanyan ES* Utkin VV* Kovyazina AI* Gridneva SM*
(Test Use of Dihydrostreptomycin Ascorbinate in Pulmonary Tuberculosis)
    Antibiotiki 11 468-471, May 1966
    007 Refs Clin Type Rus Trans Summ

058
Stupp H* Rauch S* Sous H* Lagler F*
(Experiments on Cause of the Specific Ototoxic Effect of Basic Streptomyces
Antibiotics with Special Consideration of Kanamycin)
    Acta Otolaryng (Stockholm) 61 435-444, May 1966
    028 Refs Exp Type Ger Trans Summ
    Abstr. (Yearb Ear Nose Throat 61-62, 1966-1967)

059
Berk DP* Chalmers T*
Deafness Complicating Antibiotic Therapy of Hepatic Encephalopathy
    Ann Intern Med 73 393-396, Sep 1970
    019 Refs Clin Type Eng

060
Chaffee WG,Jr*
Hazards of Ethacrynic Acid
    JAMA 212 159, Apr 6 1970
    004 Refs Letter Type Eng

061
Merrill JP*
Hazards of Ethacrynic Acid
    JAMA 212 159, Apr 6 1970
    002 Refs Letter Type Eng

062
Donomae I*
The Combined Use of Capreomycin and Ethambutol in Re-Treatment of Pulmonary

Tuberculosis
    Amer Rev Resp Dis 98 699-702, Oct 1968
    018 Refs Clin Type Eng

                                                                   063

Davia JE* Siemsen AW* Anderson RW*
Uremia, Deafness, and Paralysis due to Irrigating Antibiotic Solutions
    Arch Intern Med (Chicago) 125 135-139, Jan 1970
    034 Refs Clin Type Eng

                                                                   064

Anon*
Deafness after Topical Neomycin
    Brit Med J 4 181-182, Oct 25 1969
    007 Refs Comment Type Eng

                                                                   065

Darrouzet J*
Essais de Protection de l'Organe de Corti Contre l'Ototoxicite des Antibioti-
ques. Etude Histologique. Deuxieme Serie Experimentale (Experimental Protection of the Organ of Corti Against the Ototoxicity of Antibiotics. Histological Study 2)
    Rev Laryng 88 (3-4) 188-203, 1967
    008 Refs Exp Histol Type Fr Trans Summ
    Abstr. (Excer Med Sect 11 20 667, 1967)

                                                                   066

Preobrazhenskii BS*
Primenenie Antibiotikov v Otorinolaringologii (The Use of Antibiotics in
Otorhinolaryngology)
    Ref Zh Otd Vyp Farmakol Khimioter Sredstva Toksikol 8.54.628 1967
    000 Refs Art Type Rus
    Abstr. (Biol Abstr 49 1815, 1968)

                                                                   067

Ganguin G* Rempt E*
Streptomycinbehandlung in der Schwangerschaft und ihre Auswirkung auf das
Gehor des Kindes (Streptomycin Treatment during Pregnancy and its Effect on
Hearing of the Children)
    Z Laryng Rhinol Otol 49 (8) 496-503, Aug 1970
    020 Refs Art Type Ger Trans Summ

                                                                   068

Hesling CM*
Treatment with Capreomycin, with Special Reference to Toxic Effects
    Tubercle 50 Suppl 39-41, Mar 1969
    000 Refs Clin Type Eng

                                                                   069

D'Angelo EP* Patterson WC* Morrow RC*
Chloramphenicol -- Topical Application in Middle Ear
    Arch Otolaryng (Chicago) 85 682-684, Jun 1967
    008 Refs Exp Type Eng

                                                                   070

Eivazov AA*
(Effect of Streptomycin on the Vestibular and Auditory Function in Tuberculous Patients)
    Vestn Otorinolaring 30 24-28, May-Jun 1968
    014 Refs Clin Type Rus Trans Summ

                                                                   071

Prazic M* Salaj B* Blazevic M*
(Damages to the Vestibular Apparatus in Children in the Course of Streptomycin Therapy)
    Tuberkuloza 19 387-396, Jul-Aug 1967
    015 Refs Clin Exp Type Ser Trans Summ

072

Vargish T* Benjamin R* Shenkman L*
Deafness from Furosemide
    Ann Intern Med 72 761, May 1970
    001 Refs Letter Clin Type Eng

073

Basicevic V* Topolac R* Camprag DJ*
(Streptomycin Induced Damages of Cochlear Apparatus in Children)
    Tuberkuloza 20 219-224, Jul-Oct 1968
    000 Refs Clin Type Ser Trans Summ

074

Ziemski Z*
(Reactions of the Organ of Corti to Topical Effect of Antibiotics)
    Otolaryng Pol 22 (5) 651-655, 1968
    014 Refs Exp Type Pol Trans Summ

075

Wilson TM*
Capreomycin, Ethambutol and Rifampicin. Clinical Experience in Manchester
    Scand J Resp Dis 69 Suppl 33-42, 1969
    006 Refs Art Clin Type Eng

076

Ware M* Heinivaara O* Elo R* Tala E*
Clinical Experience of the Treatment of Drug-Resistant Pulmonary Tuberculosis
with Rifampicin Combined with Ethambutol and Capreomycin
    Scand J Resp Dis 69 Suppl 59-63, 1969
    003 Refs Clin Type Eng

077

Radenbach KL*
Results of Clinical Studies with Capreomycin, Ethambutol , and Rifampicin in
the Heckeshorn Hospital, Berlin
    Scand J Resp Dis 69 Suppl 43-53, 1969
    016 Refs Clin Type Eng

078

Wilson AT*
Acute Vertigo and the Lead Content of Food and Drink
    Practitioner 200 282-285, Feb 1968
    004 Refs Clin Type Eng

079

Wright I*
Investigation of Ototoxicity of an Antibiotic from Micromonospora Purpurea
(Gentamicin)
    J Path 98 129-136, Jun 1969
    017 Refs Exp Type Eng

080

Simon HJ*
Streptomycin, Kanamycin, Neomycin, and Paromomycin
    Pediat Clin N Amer 15 73-83, Feb 1968
    033 Refs Art Type Eng

081

Yoshioka H* Matsuda I*
Loss of Hair Related to Gentamicin Treatment
    JAMA 211 123, Jan 5 1970
    000 Refs Letter Clin Type Eng

082

Wilpizeski C* Tanaka Y*
Recent Animal Contributions to the Study of Salicylate Ototoxicity
    Delaware Med J 39 90-93, Apr 1967
    004 Refs Exp Type Eng

083

Vanommen RA*
Adverse Effects of Antimicrobial Agents on Major Organ Systems
    Cleveland Clin Quart 37 59-71, Jan 1970
    049 Refs Rev Type Eng

084

Jankowski W* Ziemski Z*
(Protective Agent of Cytochrome C in Local Kanamycin or Streptomycin Toxicity
to the Organ of Corti in Animals)
    Otolaryng Pol 22 (4) 513-518, 1968
    009 Refs Exp Type Pol Trans Summ

085

Erlach A*
(Clinical Studies of Cochleotoxicosis due to Viomycin and Kanamycin during
Tuberculostatic Treatment (A Prophylactic Attempt))
    Mschr Ohrenheilk 102 (11) 624-630, 1968
    014 Refs Clin Type Ger Trans Summ

086

Merkle U* Plattig KH* Keidel UO*
(Histological Studies on the Ototoxic Effect of Kanamycin on the Organ of
Corti in the Cat)
    Z Mikr Anat Forsch 78 441-460, 1968
    040 Refs Exp Histol Type Ger Trans Summ

087

Goldner JC*
Neurotoxicity of Antibiotics
    Minn Med 51 (11) 1629-1632, 1968
    041 Refs Rev Type Eng

088

Goplerud CP* Miller GH*
Drugs in Pregnancy
    Neb St Med J 53 (12) 575-579, 1968
    039 Refs Art Type Eng

089

Ng PS* Conley CE* Ing TS*
Deafness after Ethacrynic Acid
    Lancet 1 673-674, Mar 29 1969
    002 Refs Letter Clin Type Eng

090

Masel MA* Johnston NG*
Haemolytic Anaemia in a Patient Taking Thiacetazone
    Med J Aust 2 (19) 840-843, 1968
    016 Refs Clin Type Eng

091

Stepanyan ES* Gavril'Ev SS* Golytsina LV*
(Comparative Data on the Toxicity of Different Derivatives of Dihydrostreptomycin, Streptomycin, Kanamycin and Florimycin)
    Antibiotiki 12 1105-1109, Dec 1967
    009 Refs Clin Exp Type Rus Trans Summ

092

Von Westernhagen B* Schatzle W*
(Histochemical Studies on the Action of Streptomycin on Enzymes of the Peripheral Vestibular Apparatus)
    Acta Otolaryng (Stockholm) 66 433-443, Nov 1968
    045 Refs Exp Type Ger Trans Summ

093

Falco FG*
Review of Bacteriology and Preclinical Studies and Clinical Pharmacology of

Gentamicin Sulfate
  Ther Umsch Suppl 8-16, Jan 1969
  036 Refs Rev Clin Exp Type Eng

                                                                         094
Watanuki K* Kashiwazaki H* Kawamoto K* Katagiri S*
The Effect of Kanamycin Intoxication on the RNA Metabolism in the Cells of
Reissner's Membrane
  Arch Klin Exp Ohr Nas Kehlkopfheilk 192 (4) 369-375, 1968
  030 Refs Exp Type Eng

                                                                         095
Poole G* Stradling P*
Intermittent Chemotherapy for Tuberculosis in an Urban Community
  Brit Med J 1 (5626) 82-84, 1969
  024 Refs Clin Type Eng

                                                                         096
Watanuki K* Kawamoto K* Katagiri S*
Repair Pattern in the Reticular Lamina of the Organ of Corti after Hair Cell
Loss
  Ann Otol 78 1210-1219, Dec 1969
  031 Refs Exp Histol Type Eng

                                                                         097
Anon*
(A Report About Drug Side Effects. 10)
  Lakartidningen 66 5340-5342, Dec 17 1969
  009 Refs Art Clin Type Sw Trans Summ

                                                                         098
Anon*
(Ototoxicity of Ethacrynic Acid in Patients with Reduced Kidney Function)
  Ugeskr Laeg 132 800, Apr 23 1970
  012 Refs Clin Comment Type Dan Trans Summ

                                                                         099
Halmai T*
(Hazards of Antibiotics in Patients with Impaired Kidney Function)
  Orv Hetil 108 1897-1898, Oct 1 1967
  003 Refs Clin Type Hun Trans Summ

                                                                         100
Schmelcher R*
(Liability of a Ward Physician for Streptomycin Induced Damages)
  Deutsch Med Wschr 92 1988, Oct 27 1967
  005 Refs Clin Comment Type Ger Trans Summ

                                                                         101
Brogard JM* Conraux C* Collard M* Stahl J* Greiner GF* Lavillaureix J*
(Renal and Cochleovestibular Tolerance of Gentamicin. Comparative Study in
Patients with Normal and Impaired Renal Function)
  Therapeutique 46 627-638, Jun-Jul 1970
  000 Refs Clin Type Fr Trans Summ

                                                                         102
Barrillon A* Felix J*
Acide Etacrynique et Troubles Auditifs (Ethacrynic Acid and Auditory Disor-
ders)
  Presse Med 78 (51) 2283, Nov 28 1970
  004 Refs Letter Comment Type Fr

                                                                         103
Bender F*
(Studies and Catamnestic Surveys after Tuberculous Meningitis)
  Prax Pneumol 21 (6) 329-336, Jun 1967
  006 Refs Clin Type Ger Trans Summ

104

Anon*
(Disciplinary Board. Physician Warned--Patient Deaf after Neomycin Therapy)
    Lakartidningen 66 3783, Sep 17 1969
    000 Refs Clin Comment Type Sw Trans Summ

105

Bernstein JM* Weiss AD*
Further Observations on Salicylate Ototoxicity
    J Laryng 81 915-925, Aug 1967
    008 Refs Clin Exp Type Eng

106

Midtvedt T*
(Dihydrostreptomycin)
    T Norsk Laegeforen 90 791, Apr 15 1970
    002 Refs Comment Type Nor Trans Summ

107

Sacquepee R* Masselot Y*
(Preclinical Detection of Toxic Vestibular Disorder by Pendular Electronystagmography)
    Rev Otoneuroophtal 40 49-60, Jan-Feb 1968
    006 Refs Clin Type Fr Trans Summ

108

Darrouzet J*
(Fragilitation of the Cochlea by Other Agents Following Poisoning)
    Acta Otolaryng (Stockholm) 63 Suppl 39-40, 1967
    000 Refs Exp Type Fr

109

Engstrom H*
The Pathological Sensory Cell in the Cochlea
    Acta Otolaryng (Stockholm) 63 Suppl 20-26, 1967
    002 Refs Exp Histol Type Eng

110

Spoendlin H*
Acute Streptomycin Intoxication of the Labyrinth
    Acta Otolaryng (Stockholm) 63 Suppl 26-38, 1967
    008 Refs Exp Histol Type Eng

111

Stupp H*
(Streptomycin Ototoxicosis in Humans)
    Arch Klin Exp Ohr Nas Kehlkopfheilk 194   562-566, Dec 22 1969
    000 Refs Clin Exp Type Ger Trans Summ

112

Sagalovich BM* Krasnov VA*
(Significance of Sensitization of the Organism for the Manifestation of
Ototoxic Action of Streptomycin)
    Vestn Otorinolaring 31 (2) 75-82, Mar-Apr 1969
    033 Refs Exp Type Rus Trans Summ

113

Poulsen J*
Ototoksisk Virkning af Letoploselig Acetylsalicylsyre (The Ototoxic Effect of
Readily Soluble Acetylsalicylic Acid)
    Ugeskr Laeg 132 (51) 2435-2437, Dec 17 1970
    011 Refs Clin Type Dan Trans Summ

114

Schubert K*
(Measurements on the Influence of Alcohol on the Equilibrium System)
    Z Laryng Rhinol Otol 46 825-831, Nov 1967
    010 Refs Clin Type Ger Trans Summ

115

Savary P*
Ototoxicite des Medicaments (The Ototoxicity of Drugs)
   Laval Med 39 (7) 604-605, 1968
   000 Refs Art Type Fr

116

Rasmussen P*
The Ototoxic Effect of Streptomycin and Dihydrostreptomycin on the Foetus
   Scand J Resp Dis 50 (1) 61-67, 1969
   020 Refs Clin Type Eng

117

Shimizu K*
Clinical Experience with Gentamicin in Japan
   J Infect Dis 119 448-452, Apr-May 1969
   000 Refs Clin Type Eng

118

Alberti PW* Black JI*
Iatrogenic Symptoms in Otolaryngology
   J Laryng 82 731-737, Aug 1968
   009 Refs Clin Type Eng

119

Soda   T* Holz E* Stange G*
(Ototoxicity of Gentamicin Sulfate. Electrophysiological and Histological
Results)
   Arzneimittelforschung 18 824-827, Jul 1968
   028 Refs Exp Histol Type Ger Trans Summ

120

Radecki A* Kanwiszer H* Donderowicz A* Krzanowska E*
(Toxic Reactions during Treatment with Viomycin in Pulmonary Tuberculosis)
   Gruzlica 36 (4) 323-327, Apr 1968
   010 Refs Clin Type Pol Trans Summ

121

Bunn PA*
Kanamycin
   Med Clin N Amer 54 (5) 1245-1256, Sep 1970
   029 Refs Rev Type Eng

122

Pyle MM*
Ethambutol and Viomycin
   Med Clin N Amer 54 (5) 1317-1327, Sep 1970
   024 Refs Rev Type Eng

123

Martin WJ* Wellman WE*
Clinically Useful Antimicrobial Agents. Untoward Reactions
   Postgrad Med 42 369-419, Nov 1967
   020 Refs Art Type Eng

124

Schwartz GH*
Ototoxicity of Furosemide
   New Eng J Med 283 434, Aug 20 1970
   000 Refs Letter Comment Type Eng

125

Quick CA* Duvall AJ,3*
Early Changes in the Cochlear Duct from Ethacrynic Acid -- An Electronmicros-
copic Evaluation
   Laryngoscope 80 954-965, Jun 1970
   014 Refs Exp Histol Type Eng

126

Saito H* Daly JF*
Quantitative Analysis of Acid Mucopolysaccharides in the Normal and Kanamycin
Intoxicated Cochlea
    Acta Otolaryng (Stockholm) 71 (1) 22-26, Jan 1971
    013 Refs Exp Type Eng

127

Strauss I*
Konservative Therapie der Nierentuberkulose unter Besonderer Berucksichtigung
der Tuberkulostatikatoleranz bei Verminderter Nierenfunktion (Conservative
Therapy of Renal Tb, with Special Reference to Tuberculostatic Tolerance in
Reduced Renal Function)
    Therapiewoche 19 (2) 81-88, Jan 8 1969
    085 Refs Rev Type Ger Trans Summ

128

Surapathana LO* Prasit F* Campbell RA*
Salicylism Revisited. Unusual Problems in Diagnosis and Management
    Clin Pediat 9 (11) 658-661, Nov 1970
    006 Refs Clin Type Eng

129

Cavalazzi G* Conti A* Aliprandi G*
Primeros Datos Experimentales sobre las Variaciones Ionicas Perilinfaticas
despues del Tratamiento con Farmacos Ototoxicos (Kanamicina) (First Experimental Results of Ionic Perilymphatic Changes after Therapy with Ototoxic
Drugs (Kanamycin))
    Rev Esp Otoneurooftal 27 (156) 96-102, Mar-Apr 1968
    022 Refs Exp Type Sp Trans Summ

130

Silverstein H* Yules RB*
The Effect of Diuretics on Cochlear Potentials and Inner Ear Fluids
    Laryngoscope 81 (6) 873-888, Jun 1971
    014 Refs Exp Histol Type Eng

131

Tachiki T* Honma T* Kawase A*
(Severe Hearing Disorders Caused by Kanamycin)
    J Otolaryng Jap 73 Suppl 982-983, Jul 1970
    000 Refs Clin Type Jap Trans Summ

132

Rauch S*
(Iatrogenic Hearing Impairment)
    Praxis 57 1478-1485, Oct 29 1968
    000 Refs Clin Type Ger Trans Summ

133

Sheidina RB*
(Hearing Disorders Complicating Suppurative Meningitis during Current Methods
of Treatment)
    Zh Nevropat Psikhiat Korsakov 66 349-353, 1966
    011 Refs Clin Type Rus Trans Summ

134

Stange G* Winter H*
Dimethylsulfoxyd--Ein Neues Ototoxisches Pharmakum. Elektrophysiologische
Untersuchungen an der Katze (Dimethylsulfoxyd--A New Ototoxic Substance.
Electrophysiological Results on the Cat)
    Arch Klin Exp Ohr Nas Kehlkopfheilk 197 (3) 208-222, 1970
    053 Refs Exp Type Ger Trans Summ

135

Smith JL*
Dizzy Patient
    Tex Med 65 (1) 58-61, Jan 1969

007 Refs Art Type Eng

136

Hong Kong Anti-Tuberculosis Association and Government Tuberculosis Service*
British Medical Research Council Investigation*
A Controlled Comparison of Thiacetazone (Thioacetazone) plus Isoniazid with
PAS plus Isoniazid in Hong Kong
    Tubercle 49 (3) 243-280, 1968
    025 Refs Clin Type Eng

137

Ovreberg K*
Preliminary Results of the Norwegian Coordinated Therapy Project 1968-1969
    Scand J Resp Dis 69 Suppl 65-68, 1969
    000 Refs Clin Type Eng

138

Kociolek G* Sulkowski W* Starzynski Z* Zolnowski Z*
(Toxic Damage to Hearing during Poisoning with Chenopodium Oil)
    Otolaryng Pol 22 (5) 737-739, 1968
    006 Refs Clin Type Pol Trans Summ

139

Miszke A*
(New Views on the Mechanism of Action of Ototoxic Antibiotics)
    Pol Tyg Lek 23 (6) 199-201, Feb 5 1968
    008 Refs Rev Type Pol Trans Summ

140

Bourdial J* Lallemant Y* Laffolee P* Flieder J*
Gentamycine et Cophose Auriculaire (Gentamycin and Auricular Involvement)
    Ann Otolaryng (Paris) 87 (12) 812-814, Dec 1970
    003 Refs Clin Type Fr

141

Debain JJ* Freyss G* Poulain H*
(Gentamicin and Auricular Toxicity)
    Ann Otolaryng (Paris) 86 (9) 584-588, Sep 1969
    008 Refs Clin Type Fr

142

Lazareva EN* Golubev VN* Veis RA* Shneerson AN*
(On the Question of the Role of Quanidine Groups of Dihydrostreptomycin
Molecules in the Manifestation of Biological Activity and Neurotoxic Action)
    Antibiotiki 11 522-526, Jun 1966
    014 Refs Exp Type Rus Trans Summ

143

Brown GL* Wilson WP*
Salicylate Intoxication and the CNS. With Special Reference to EEG Findings
    Dis Nerv Syst 32 (2) 135-140, Feb 1971
    033 Refs Clin Type Eng

144

Matz GJ* Naunton RF*
Ototoxic Drugs and Poor Renal Function
    JAMA 206 2119, Nov 25 1968
    006 Refs Letter Clin Exp Histol Type Eng

145

Kerr A* Schuknecht HF*
The Spiral Ganglion in Profound Deafness
    Acta Otolaryng (Stockholm) 65 586-598, Jun 1968
    038 Refs Exp Histol Type Eng

146

Otani I*
(Experimental Studies on Chronic Ototoxicity of Kanamycin)

    J Otolaryng Jap 71 688-707, May 1968
    000 Refs Exp Type Jap

147

Ortega I* Smoler J* Vivar G*
(Protection Against Kanamycin Toxicity. Preliminary Report)
    Acta Otorinolaring Iber Amer 18 417-426, 1967
    000 Refs Exp Type Sp Trans Summ

148

Paloheimo JA*
(Transient Deafness-a Rare Complication of Ethacrynic Acid Therapy)
    Duodecim 84 48-50, 1968
    000 Refs Clin Type Fin Trans Summ

149

Anon*
(The Sensory Cell of the Organ of Corti. Conclusion)
    Acta Otolaryng (Stockholm) 63 Suppl 65-71, 1967
    000 Refs Exp Type Fr Trans Summ

150

Gruhl VR*
Renal Failure, Deafness, and Brain Lesions Following Irrigation of the Mediastinum with Neomycin
    Ann Thorac Surg 11 (4) 376-379, Apr 1971
    015 Refs Clin Type Eng

151

Heidland A* Klutsch K* Moormann A* Hennemann H*
(Possibilities and Limitations of High Dosage Diuretic Therapy in Hydropic
Renal Insufficiency)
    Deutsch Med Wschr 94 (31) 1568-1574, Aug 1 1969
    051 Refs Clin Type Ger Trans Summ

152

Klein SW* Sutherland RL* Morch JE*
Hemodynamic Effects of Intravenous Lidocaine in Man
    Canad Med Ass J 99 (10) 472-475, Jul-Sep 1968
    014 Refs Clin Exp Type Eng

153

Fregly AR* Graybiel A*
Acute Alcohol Ataxia in Persons with Loss of Labyrinthine Function
    Acta Otolaryng (Stockholm) 65 468-478, May 1968
    019 Refs Exp Type Eng

154

Gartmann J*
Therapie mit Neuen Tuberkulostatika (Treatment with New Tuberculostatic
Agents)
    Deutsch Med Wschr 93 (47) 2281-2282, Nov-Dec 1968
    005 Refs Rev Type Ger

155

Igarashi M* Mcleod ME* Graybiel A*
Clinical Pathological Correlations in Squirrel Monkeys after Suppression of
Semicircular Canal Function by Streptomycin Sulfate
    Acta Otolaryng (Stockholm) Suppl 214, 1966
    035 Refs Exp Histol Type Eng

156

Vernon M*
Tuberculous Meningitis and Deafness
    J Speech Hear Dis 32 (2) 177-181, May 1967
    014 Refs Clin Type Eng

Friedmann I* Dadswell JV* Bird ES*
Electron-Microscope Studies of the Neuroepithelium of the Inner Ear in Guinea
Pigs Treated with Neomycin
    J Path Bact 92 415-422, Oct 1966
    030 Refs Exp Histol Type Eng

                                                                        158
Myerson M* Knight HF* Gambarini AJ* Curran TL*
Intrapleural Neomycin Causing Ototoxicity
    Ann Thorac Surg 9 483-486, May 1970
    051 Refs Clin Type Eng

                                                                        159
Mibe T*
(Therapeutic Results of Kanendomycin in Infectious Otorhinolaryngological
Diseases and its Effect on the Organ of Hearing)
    J Jap Med Ass 62 537-542, Sep 15 1969
    000 Refs Clin Type Jap Trans Summ

                                                                        160
Frantzen E* Hansen JM* Hansen OE* Kristensen M*
Phenytoin (Dilantin) Intoxication
    Acta Neurol Scand 43 (4) 440-446, 1967
    018 Refs Clin Type Eng

                                                                        161
Fluker JL* Hewitt AB*
Kanamycin in the Treatment of Rectal Gonorrhoea
    Brit J Vener Dis 46 (6) 454-456, Dec 1970
    010 Refs Clin Type Eng

                                                                        162
Hansz J* Styperek J*
(Unilateral Damage of the Acoustic Nerve during Acute Carbon Monoxide Poi-
soning)
    Pol Tyg Lek 23 (38) 1441-1442, Sep 16 1968
    013 Refs Clin Type Pol Trans Summ

                                                                        163
Goralski H* Januszko L*
(Neurological and Psychiatric Syndromes after Carbon Monoxide Poisoning)
    Neurol Neurochir Pol 2 (5) 633-637, Sep-Oct 1968
    035 Refs Rev Type Pol Trans Summ

                                                                        164
Mc Cracken GH,Jr* Jones LG*
Gentamicin in the Neonatal Period
    Amer J Dis Child 120 (6) 524-533, Dec 1970
    020 Refs Clin Type Eng

                                                                        165
Finegold SM*
Toxicity of Kanamycin in Adults
    Ann NY Acad Sci 132 942-956, 1966
    048 Refs Rev Type Eng

                                                                        166
Von Westernhagen B*
(Histochemical Studies of the Effect of Salicylic Acid on the Inner Ear)
    Arch Klin Exp Ohr Nas Kehlkopfheilk 190 86-94, 1968
    041 Refs Exp Type Ger Trans Summ

                                                                        167
Von Westernhagen B*
(Inner Ear Changes in Guinea-Pig after Chronic Mercury Poisoning. A Histoche-
mical Study)
    Arch Klin Exp Ohr Nas Kehlkopfheilk 193 (1) 70-77, 1969
    045 Refs Exp Type Ger Trans Summ

168

Ishii   T* Bernstein   JM* Balogh   K,Jr*
Distribution of Tritium-Labeled Salicylate in the Cochlea. An Autoradiographical Study
    Ann Otol 76 (2) 368-376, Jun 1967
    013 Refs Exp Type Eng

169

Stebbins WC* Miller   JM* Johnsson LG* Hawkins   JE,Jr*
Ototoxic Hearing Loss and Cochlear Pathology in the Monkey
    Ann Otol 78 (5) 1007-1025, Oct 1969
    027 Refs Exp Histol Type Eng

170

Murphy KW*
Deafness after Topical Neomycin
    Brit Med J 2 114, Apr 11 1970
    003 Refs Letter Type Eng

171

Kohonen   A* Jauhiainen T* Tarkkanen   J*
Experimental Deafness Caused by Etachrynic (sic) Acid
    Acta Otolaryng (Stockholm) 70 (3) 187-189, Sep 1970
    006 Refs Exp Histol Type Eng

172

Schrader A*
(Leading Symptom -- Vertigo from the Point of View of the Internist)
    Munchen Med Wschr 108 685-693, Apr 1 1966
    015 Refs Art Type Ger Trans Summ

173

Mizukoshi O* Daly JF*
Oxygen Consumption in Normal and Kanamycin Damaged Cochleae
    Acta Otolaryng (Stockholm) 64 (1) 45-54, Jul 1967
    025 Refs Exp Type Eng

174

De Sa   JV* Bhargava KB*
Study of Experimental Deafness in Human Volunteers with a New Oral Antidiabetic Drug R 94
    Acta Otolaryng (Stockholm) 64 (5-6) 537-542, Dec 1967
    002 Refs Exp Type Eng

175

Mendelsohn M* Mittelman J*
Diuretics and the Cation Content of Guinea Pig Endolymph
    Ann Otol 80 (2) 186-191, Apr 1971
    015 Refs Exp Type Eng

176

Reimann HA*
Infectious Diseases. Annual Review of Significant Publications
    Postgrad Med J 45 (525) 428-445, Jul 1969
    306 Refs Rev Type Eng

177

Majcherska-Matuchniak B* Latkowski B*
(Hearing Behavior in Workers in Chemical Industry Exposed to the Action of
Nitro and Amino-Compounds)
    Otolaryng Pol 22 (2) 301-304, 1968
    010 Refs Clin Type Pol Trans Summ

178

Stenbaek O*
(Hearing Disorders after Treatment with Ethacrynic Acid (Edecrin) in Patients
with Reduced Kidney Function)
    T Norsk Laegeforen 90 34, Jan 1 1970

000 Refs Clin Type Nor Trans Summ

                                                                        179
Jacobson   EJ* Downs   MP* Fletcher   JL*
Clinical Findings in High-Frequency Thresholds during Known Ototoxic Drug
Usage
   J Aud Res 9 (4) 379-385, Oct 1969
   009 Refs Clin Type Eng

                                                                        180
Morris   TM*
Deafness Following Acute Carbon Monoxide Poisoning
   J Laryng 83 (12) 1219-1225, Dec 1969
   002 Refs Clin Type Eng

                                                                        181
Koide   Y* Hata   A* Hando   R*
Vulnerability of the Organ of Corti in Poisoning
   Acta Otolaryng (Stockholm) 61 332-344,   1966
   019 Refs Exp Type Eng

                                                                        182
Horiguti   S* Ebihara   I*
Single Pure Tone Screening Test for Deafness
   Int Audiol 5 (2) 217-220,   1966
   000 Refs Art Type Eng

                                                                        183
Sato   Y*
The Effect of Chloramphenicol upon the Oxygen Consumption of the Membranous
Cochlea
   Laryngoscope 79 (2) 295-305, Feb 1969
   021 Refs Exp Type Eng

                                                                        184
Iinuma   T* Mizukoshi   O* Daly   JF*
Possible Effects of Various Ototoxic Drugs upon the ATP-hydrolyzing System in
the Stria Vascularis and Spiral Ligament of the Guinea Pig
   Laryngoscope 77 (2) 159-170, Feb 1967
   028 Refs Exp Type Eng

                                                                        185
Hawkins   JE,Jr* Johnsson   LG* Aran   JM*
Comparative Tests of Gentamicin Ototoxicity
   J Infect Dis 119 (4-5) 417-426, Apr-May 1969
   020 Refs Exp Type Eng

                                                                        186
Albers   GD* Wilson   WH*
Diplacusis. 2. Etiology
   Arch Otolaryng (Chicago) 87 (6) 604-606, Jun 1968
   010 Refs Art Type Eng

                                                                        187
Nord   NM* Watanabe   F* Parker   RH* Hoeprich   PD*
Comparative Acute Toxicity of Four Drugs. A Study of Neomycin, Gentamicin,
Kanamycin, and Dihydrostreptomycin
   Arch Intern Med (Chicago) 119 493-502, May 1967
   021 Refs Exp Type Eng

                                                                        188
Johnston   PW*
Factors Associated with Deafness in Young Children
   Public Health Rep 82 1019-1024, Nov 1967
   017 Refs Clin Type Eng

                                                                        189
Gold   A* Wilpizeski   CR*

Studies in Auditory Adaptation. 2. Some Effects of Sodium Salicylate on
Evoked Auditory Potentials in Cats
   Laryngoscope 76 674-685, 1966
   002 Refs Exp Type Eng

190

Gaillard J* Dumolard P* Cetre J*
Surdite Brusque apres Anesthesie Loco-Regionale sous Garrot, dite Anesthesie
Canadienne (Sudden Deafness after Loco-Regional Anesthesia with Garrot, a
Canadian Anesthesia)
   J Franc Otorhinolaryng 19 (10) 819-820, 1970
   000 Refs Clin Type Fr

191

Neff TA* Coan BJ*
Incidence of Drug Intolerance to Antituberculosis Chemotherapy
   Dis Chest 56 (1) 10-12, Jul 1969
   011 Refs Clin Type Eng

192

Herd JK* Cramer A* Hoak FC* Norcross BM*
Ototoxicity of Topical Neomycin Augmented by Dimethyl Sulfoxide
   Pediatrics 40 905-907, 1967
   011 Refs Clin Type Eng

193

Cernelc-Dular S*
Ototoksicni Antibiotiki (Ototoxic Antibiotics)
   Zdrav Vestn 39 (6) 227-230, 1970
   021 Refs Art Type Ser Trans Summ

194

Cruz NA* Gananca MM*
(Ototoxic Effect of Nitrogen Mustard)
   Hospital (Rio) 76 (5) 1811-1823, Nov 1969
   011 Refs Clin Type Sp

195

White A*
Gentamicin
   J Indiana Med Ass 63 (5) 436, May 1970
   001 Refs Art Type Eng

196

Suzuki Y* Koga K* Kanzaki J*
Statistical Observations of Dihydrostreptomycin and Kanamycin Ototoxicity
   Int Audiol 5 (2) 162-165, Jun 1966
   000 Refs Clin Type Eng

197

Engstrom H* Ades HW* Bredberg G*
Cytoarchitecture of the Mammalian Organ of Corti
   Int Audiol 5 86-90, 1966
   003 Refs Exp Histol Type Eng

198

East African-British Medical Research Council*
A Comparison of Two Regimens of Streptomycin plus PAS in the Retreatment of
Pulmonary Tuberculosis
   Tubercle 49 70-78, Mar 1968
   027 Refs Clin Type Eng

199

Benner EJ*
The Use and Abuse of Antibiotics--1967
   J Bone Joint Surg (Amer) 49 977-988, Jul 1967
   007 Refs Art Clin Type Eng

200

Keaster J* Hyman CB* Harris I*
Hearing Problems Subsequent to Neonatal Hemolytic Disease or Hyperbilirubinemia
   Amer J Dis Child 117 406-410, Apr 1969
   014 Refs Clin Type Eng

201

Chenebault J*
(Therapeutic Risks during Anti-Infectious Treatment)
   Maroc Med 49 (529) 631-636, 1969
   000 Refs Art Type Fr

202

Guignard J*
(Risks of Anti-Infectious Treatment in Pediatric Practice)
   Maroc Med 49 (529) 637-640, 1969
   008 Refs Art Type Fr

203

Rempt E*
Gehorschaden bei Kanamycinlangzeittherapie (Hearing Damage as a Result of
Kanamycin Treatment)
   Z Laryng Rhinol Otol 49 (8) 504-509, Aug 1970
   027 Refs Clin Type Ger Trans Summ

204

Ishii T* Ishii D* Balogh K,Jr*
Lysosomal Enzymes in the Inner Ears of Kanamycin-Treated Guinea Pigs
   Acta Otolaryng (Stockholm) 65 449-458, May 1968
   041 Refs Exp Type Eng

205

Silverstein H* Bernstein JM* Davies DG*
Salicylate Ototoxicity. A Biochemical and Electrophysiological Study
   Ann Otol 76 (1) 118-128, Mar 1967
   010 Refs Exp Type Eng

206

Schneider WJ* Becker EL*
Acute Transient Hearing Loss after Ethacrynic Acid Therapy
   Arch Intern Med 117 715-717, May 1966
   007 Refs Clin Type Eng

207

Delaude A* Albarede JL*
Les Nouveaux Antituberculeux (New Antituberculous Agents)
   Concours Med 91 (3) 429-435, 1969
   000 Refs Art Type Fr

208

Eyl TB*
Methyl Mercury Poisoning in Fish and Human Beings
   Clin Toxicol 4 (2) 291-296, Jun 1971
   000 Refs Art Type Eng

209

Guest AD* Duncan C* Lawther PJ*
Carbon Monoxide and Phenobarbitone -- A Comparison of Effects on Auditory
Flutter Fusion Threshold and Critical Flicker Fusion Threshold
   Ergonomics 13 (5) 587-594, 1970
   012 Refs Exp Type Eng

210

Wersall J*
Ototoxiska Antibiotika (Ototoxic Antibiotics)
   Lakartidningen 66 Suppl 4 85-92, 1969
   022 Refs Rev Type Sw Trans Summ

211

Ball JD* Berry G* Clarke WG* Gilson JC* Thomas J*
A Controlled Trial of Anti-Tuberculosis Chemotherapy in the Early Complicated
Pneumoconiosis of Coalworkers
    Thorax 24 399-406, Jul 1969
    020 Refs Clin Type Eng

212

Sakamoto T* Lange G*
(Vestibular Hair Cell Changes in Guinea Pigs after Streptomycin-Ozothin)
    Arch Klin Exp Ohr Nas Kehlkopfheilk 195 (2) 169-178, 1969
    013 Refs Exp Histol Type Ger Trans Summ

213

Jawetz E*
Polymyxins, Colistin, Bacitracin, Ristocetin and Vancomycin
    Pediat Clin N Amer 15 85-94, Feb 1968
    027 Refs Art Type Eng

214

Riley HD,Jr*
Vancomycin and Novobiocin
    Med Clin N Amer 54 (5) 1277-1289, Sep 1970
    025 Refs Art Type Eng

215

Martin WJ*
The Present Status of Streptomycin in Antimicrobial Therapy
    Med Clin N Amer 54 (5) 1161-1172, Sep 1970
    012 Refs Art Type Eng

216

Lange G*
(Quantitative Evaluation of Streptomycin Damage of the Vestibular Sensory
Cells with the Aid of Cytovestibulogram and Caloric Excitability Test)
    Arch Klin Exp Ohr Nas Kehlkopfheilk 192 (3) 249-257, 1968
    015 Refs Exp Type Ger Trans Summ

217

Kohonen A*
(Ototoxicity of Drugs)
    Sairaanhoitaja 3 124-125, 1970
    000 Refs Comment Type Fin Trans Summ

218

Witzel L*
(Reversible Exclusion of the Vestibular Apparatus after Gentamycin)
    Fortschr Med 88 (16) 705-706, 1970
    016 Refs Clin Type Ger

219

Sheffield PA* Turner JS,Jr*
Ototoxic Drugs -- A Review of Clinical Aspects, Histopathologic Changes and
Mechanisms of Action
    Southern Med J 64 (3) 359-363, Mar 1971
    031 Refs Rev Type Eng

220

Ehrensing RH* Stokes PE* Pick GR* Goldstone S* Lhamon WT*
Effect of Alcohol on Auditory and Visual Time Perception
    Quart J Stud Alcohol 31 (4A) 851-860, Dec 1970
    022 Refs Exp Type Eng

221

Colombi M* Capaccio A*
Accorgimenti nella Poliantibioticoterapia della Tubercolosi Urogenitale
(Polyantibiotic Treatment of Urogenital Tuberculosis)
    Urologia (Treviso) 35 (5) 689-692, 1968

026 Refs Clin Type It

222

Trendelenburg F*
Kontrollen der Nebenwirkungen Einer Chemotherapie der Tuberkulose (Control of
the Side Effects of a Form of Chemotherapy of Tuberculosis)
    Therapiewoche 19 (8) 379-381, 1969
    000 Refs Art Type Ger

223

Toyota B*
(Medical Suit)
    J Jap Med Ass 58 65-69, Jul 1 1967
    000 Refs Clin Type Jap Trans Summ

224

Garland H* Pearce J*
Neurological Complications of Carbon Monoxide Poisoning
    Quart J Med 36 (144) 445-455, Oct 1967
    021 Refs Clin Type Eng

225

Arcieri GM* Falco FG* Smith HM* Hobson LB*
Clinical Research Experience with Gentamicin. Incidence of Adverse Reactions
    Med J Aust 1 (24) Suppl 30-34, Jun 13 1970
    007 Refs Clin Type Eng

226

Duvall AJ,3* Quick CA*
Tracers and Endogenous Debris in Delineating Cochlear Barriers and Pathways.
An Experimental Study
    Ann Otol 78 1041-1057, Oct 1969
    028 Refs Exp Histol Type Eng

227

Ransome J* Ballantyne JC* Shaldon S* Bosher SK* Hallpike CS*
Perceptive Deafness in Subjects with Renal Failure Treated with Haemodialysis
and Polybrene. A Clinico-Pathological Study
    J Laryng 80 (7) 651-677, Jul 1966
    011 Refs Clin Histol Type Eng

228

Ilic C*
(Hearing Damage in Workers in Viscose Industry)
    Srpski Arh Celok Lek 96 151-155, Oct 1968
    000 Refs Clin Type Ser Trans Summ

229

Nora AH* Nora JJ*
The Use and Abuse of Antibiotics in Children
    Med Times 95 905-913, Sep 1967
    012 Refs Art Type Eng

230

Fokina KV*
(The Functional Status of the Olfactory and Vestibular Analyzers in Persons
Subjected to the Action of Chloride Derivatives of Methane)
    Gig Sanit 32 (2) 22-26, Feb 1967
    009 Refs Clin Type Rus Trans Summ

231

Metcalf RG* Poliner IJ*
Long-Term Neomycin Therapy
    J Maine Med Ass 59 133-139, Jul 1968
    036 Refs Clin Type Eng

232

Lindeman HH*

Regional Differences in Structure of the Vestibular Sensory Regions
    J Laryng 83 (1) 1-17, Jan 1969
    032 Refs Exp Histol Type Eng

                                                                        233
Mounier-Kuhn P* Roche L* Morgon A* Bernard PH*
(Vestibular Involvement Immediately Following Acute Carbon Monoxide Poi-
soning)
    J Franc Otorhinolaryng 17 (6) 512-515, Jun 1968
    000 Refs Clin Type Fr

                                                                        234
Wigand ME* Heidland A*
Akute, Reversible Horverluste durch Rasche, Hochdosierte Furosemidinfusionen
bei Terminaler Niereninsuffizienz (Acute, Reversible Hearing Loss due to
Rapid, High-Dosage Furosemide Infusions for Terminal Kidney Insufficiency)
    Arch Klin Exp Ohr Nas Kehlkopfheilk 196 (2) 314-319,   1970
    010 Refs Clin Type Ger

                                                                        235
Paintal AS*
Action of Drugs on Sensory Nerve Endings
    Ann Rev Pharmacol 11 231-240,   1971
    096 Refs Rev Type Eng

                                                                        236
Yow M,Mod*
Panel Discussion -- Kanamycin in Pediatric Practice with Special Reference to
Observations on Ototoxicity
    Ann NY Acad Sci 132 (2) 1037-1044,   1966
    006 Refs Clin Type Eng

                                                                        237
Eichenwald HF*
Some Observations on Dosage and Toxicity of Kanamycin in Premature and Full-
Term Infants
    Ann NY Acad Sci 132 (2) 984-991,   1966
    007 Refs Clin Type Eng

                                                                        238
Zelenka J* Tomes D* Jilkova B*
(Possibilities of Ototoxic Effects of Orally Administered Neomycin in Dyspep-
sia in Infants. Experimental and Audiometric Study)
    Pediatrie 21 (5) 573-583, Jul-Aug 1966
    034 Refs Clin Type Fr

                                                                        239
Kahrweg A* Schmidt J*
(Acute Quinine Poisoning with Transitory Blindness and Deafness (Attempted
Suicide))
    Nervenarzt 39 (10) 478-480, Oct 1968
    020 Refs Clin Type Ger

                                                                        240
Kupper K* Stupp H* Orsulakova A* Quante M*
Vergleichende Untersuchungen der Ototoxicitat Verschiedener Antibiotischer
Substanzen bei Lokaler Applikation am Innenohr des Meerschweinchens (Compara-
tive Study of the Ototoxicity of Various Antibiotic Substances by Local
Application to the Inner Ear of Guinea Pigs)
    Arch Klin Exp Ohr Nas Kehlkopfheilk 196 (2) 169-172,   1970
    005 Refs Exp Type Ger

                                                                        241
Simon HJ* Axline SG*
Clinical Pharmacology of Kanamycin in Premature Infants
    Ann NY Acad Sci 132 1020-1025,   1966
    001 Refs Art Clin Type Eng

242

Ouchi J* Ohtani I*
Studies on the Ototoxicity of Kanamycin. The Correlation between Electrophysiological Findings and Histopathological Changes
    Pract Otorhinolaryng (Basel) 31 218-233, 1969
    022 Refs Exp Histol Type Eng

243

Staudt N*
(On Vestibular Lesions Following Treatment with Preparations of the Streptomyces Antibiotic Group)
    HNO 15 139-141, May 1967
    028 Refs Rev Clin Type Ger

244

Lehnhardt E*
(Ototoxicity of Antibiotics)
    HNO 18 97-101, Apr 1970
    045 Refs Rev Type Ger

245

Darrouzet J*
(Ototoxicity of Dihydrostreptomycin and Kanamycin. Comparative Experimental
Study)
    Rev Laryng (Bordeaux) 88 133-134, Jan-Feb 1967
    000 Refs Exp Histol Type Fr

246

Wilson   KS* Juhn SK*
The Effect of Ethacrynic Acid on Perilymph Na and K. Preliminary Report
    Pract Otorhinolaryng (Basel) 32 (5) 279-287, 1970
    029 Refs Exp Type Eng

247

Manzo   E* Giugni M*
Ancora sull'Ototossicita da Amminosidina (More on the Ototoxicity of Aminosidine)
    Arch Ital Laring 76 (1) 17-23, Jan-Feb 1968
    009 Refs Exp Type It

248

Oosterveld WJ* Janeke JB* Jongkees LB*
On the Vestibular Threshold
    Advances Otorhinolaryng 17 180-190, 1970
    029 Refs Exp Type Eng

249

Jolicoeur G*
(Ototoxic Medications)
    Un Med Canada 95 (11) 1319-1321, Nov 1966
    008 Refs Art Type Fr

250

Okihiro MM*
Postoperative Neurological Complications of Antibiotic Therapy
    Surg Clin N Amer 50 (2) 485-491, Apr 1970
    033 Refs Art Clin Type Eng

251

Manzo E* Mea O*
Ototossicita da Amminosidina. Nota 2. Ricerche Istologiche in Cavia Cobaya
(Ototoxicity of Aminosidine. Note 2. Histological Study in the Guinea Pig)
    Arch Ital Laring 75 189-199, 1967
    018 Refs Exp Histol Type It

252

Manzo E* Giugni M*
Ricerche sull'Ototossicita dell'Amminosidina nell'Uomo (Study of the Ototoxi-

city of Aminosidine in Man)
   Arch Ital Laring 75 201-205, 1967
   006 Refs Clin Type It

253

Spoendlin H*
(On the Ototoxicity of Streptomycin)
   Pract Otorhinolaryng 28 (5) 305-322, 1966
   025 Refs Exp Histol Type Ger Trans Summ

254

Lindquist B* Meeuwisse G*
Should Gastroenteritis in Infancy Be Treated with Antibiotics?
   Acta Paediat Scand 60 (1) 110, Jan 1971
   000 Refs Comment Type Eng

255

Kozakow H* Potworowska M* Janowiec M* Klimkiewicz H* Niemirowski J*
Pszonicka A* Pecyna-Sielewicz J* Polaczek E* Rykowska Z* Frenkel A*
Results of Treatment with Ethambutol and Capreomycin in Chronic Pulmonary
Tuberculosis
   Pol Med J 9 (4) 876-885, 1970
   004 Refs Clin Type Eng

256

Anon*
Proceedings of the Royal Society of Medicine
   J Laryng 83 (1) 91-93, Jan 1969
   000 Refs Exp Type Eng

257

Kacker SK*
Neomycin-Induced Spiral Organ Degeneration in the Guinea Pig. A Study Using
the Surface Specimen Technique
   Laryngoscope 80 (3) 391-399, Mar 1970
   006 Refs Exp Histol Type Eng

258

Lawrence M*
Circulation in the Capillaries of the Basilar Membrane
   Laryngoscope 80 (9) 1364-1375, Sep 1970
   019 Refs Exp Type Eng

259

Beck C* Hoffman M* Holz E* Stange G*
Restriction of Ototoxic Effect of Streptomycin
   Eye Ear Nose Throat Monthly 49 (1) 13-15, Jan 1970
   008 Refs Exp Histol Type Eng

260

Brun JP* Stupp H* Lagler F* Sous H*
Antibioticaspiegel bei Lokaler Applikation Verschiedener Antibiotica am
Innenohr des Meerschweinchens (Antibiotic Level with Local Application of
Various Antibiotics to the Inner Ear of Guinea Pigs)
   Arch Klin Exp Ohr Nas Kehlkopfheilk 196 (2) 177-181, 1970
   000 Refs Exp Type Ger

261

Lindeman HH*
Regional Differences in Sensitivity of Vestibular Sensory Epithelia to Ototoxic Antibiotics
   Acta Otolaryng (Stockholm) 67 177-189, Feb-Mar 1969
   020 Refs Exp Histol Type Eng

262

Wolff D* Gross M*
Temporal Bone Findings in Alcoholics. Preliminary Report on Chronic Alcoholics

Arch Otolaryng (Chicago) 87 (4) 350-358, Apr 1968
005 Refs Exp Histol Type Eng

263

Collum LM* Bowen DI*
Ocular Side-Effects of Ibuprofen
   Brit J Ophthal 55 (7) 472-477, Jul 1971
   006 Refs Comment Type Eng

264

Kornblut AD* Shumrick DA*
Complications of Head and Neck Surgery
   Arch Otolaryng (Chicago) 94 (3) 246-254, Sep 1971
   055 Refs Clin Comment Type Eng

265

Brown AS*
Neuroleptanalgesia
   Int Anesth Clin 7 (1) 159-175, Spr 1969
   009 Refs Art Type Eng

266

Schatzle W* Von Westernhagen B*
(Influence of Local Pantocain Application on Enzymes of the Cochlea and
Peripheral Vestibular Apparatus)
   Arch Klin Exp Ohr Nas Kehlkopfheilk 194 (2) 583-588, 1969
   019 Refs Exp Type Ger

267

Kreis B*
Kanamycin Toxicity in Adults
   Ann NY Acad Sci 132 957-967, 1966
   032 Refs Art Exp Type Eng

268

Finegold SM,Mod*
Panel Discussion -- Toxicity of Kanamycin in Adults
   Ann NY Acad Sci 132 968-976, 1966
   000 Refs Art Type Eng

269

Ino H*
(Vertigo as a Result of Public Health Hazards)
   J Otolaryng Jap 72 657-658, Feb 20 1969
   000 Refs Art Type Jap Trans Summ

270

Kakizaki I*
(Experimental Studies on the Toxic Effects of Kanamycin on the Cochlea)
   J Otolaryng Jap 71 68-83, Jan 1968
   000 Refs Exp Type Jap Trans Summ

271

Yamamoto K* Nakamura K* Toyama T*
(Statistics on Acquired Perceptive Deafness Among Children)
   Otolaryngology (Tokyo) 40 607-612, Aug 1968
   000 Refs Art Type Jap Trans Summ

272

Kohonen A*
(Drugs and Hearing)
   Duodecim 85 80-87, 1969
   000 Refs Rev Type Fin Trans Summ

273

Khodanova RN* Oberyukhtina TN* Dmitriyeva KA*
(Deafness Following Local Application of Neomycin)
   Vestn Otorinolaring 33 (1) 109-110, 1971

000 Refs Clin Type Rus
Abstr. (dsh Abstr 11 277, 1971)

                                                                        274

Watanuki K* Rauch S*
Partial Recovery of the Organ of Corti after Kanamycin Ototoxicosis
    Pract Otorhinolaryng 31 (2) 84-91, 1969
    009 Refs Exp Histol Type Eng

                                                                        275

Watanuki K* Meyer zum Gottesberge A*
Toxic Effects of Streptomycin and Kanamycin upon the Sensory Epithelium of
the Crista Ampullaris
    Acta Otolaryng (Stockholm) 72 (1-2) 59-67, Jul-Aug 1971
    027 Refs Exp Histol Type Eng

                                                                        276

Shirabe S*
(Objective Registration of Rotatory and Optokinetic Nystagmus in Guinea Pigs
-- Effects of Streptomycin Sulfate and Dimorpholamin)
    Arch Klin Exp Ohr Nas Kehlkopfheilk 198 (2) 206-214, 1971
    012 Refs Exp Type Ger

                                                                        277

Federspil P*
Uber die Klinische Ototoxicitat des Gentamycins und ihre Reversibiltat
(Clinical Ototoxicity of the Gentamycins and its Reversibility)
    Arch Klin Exp Ohr Nas Kehlkopfheilk 196 (2) 237-243, 1970
    006 Refs Clin Type Ger

                                                                        278

Haubrich J* Schatzle W*
Zur Frage Histochemischer Veranderungen der Meerschweinchenschnecke unter dem
Einfluss von Diuretica (On the Problem of Histochemical Changes in the Guinea
Pig Cochlea under the Influence of Diuretica)
    Arch Klin Exp Ohr Nas Kehlkopfheilk 196 (2) 319-324, 1970
    014 Refs Exp Type Ger

                                                                        279

Harada Y* Musso E* Mira E*
(Inhibitory Action in Vitro of Antibiotics of the Streptomycin Group on
Ampullar Receptors in the Frog)
    Boll Soc Ital Biol Sper 43 345-348, Apr 15 1967
    010 Refs Exp Type It

                                                                        280

Mc Lean CE* Stoughton PV* Kagey KS*
Experiences with Beta-Adrenergic Blockade
    Vasc Surg 1 (2) 108-126, Jun 1967
    018 Refs Clin Type Eng

                                                                        281

Ricavi A* Drakulic K*
Toksicni Vestibularni Neuronitis (Toxic Vestibular Neuronitis)
    Vojnosanit Pregl 24 (4) 225-228, 1967
    000 Refs Clin Type Ser
    Abstr. (Excer Med Sect 11 20 676, 1967)

                                                                        282

Sasaki H*
(The Early, But Limited Effects of Kanamycin, Dihydrostreptomycin, or Chloramphenicol upon the Guinea Pig Cochlea)
    J Otolaryng Soc Jap 70 (10) 1716-1721, 1967
    000 Refs Exp Type Jap
    Abstr. (Excer Med Sect 11 21 362, 1968)

                                                                        283

Bergomi A* Bertazzoli C* Deffenu G*

(Further Research in the Field Ototoxicity of Antibiotics (Recording of
Cortical Action Potentials at the Level of the Primary Acoustic Area in Cats
Following Treatment with Streptomycin and Kanamycin))
    Rev Otoneurooftal 42 367-384, Sep-Oct 1967
    034 Refs Exp Type It

284

Mounier-Kuhn P* Morgon A* Haguenauer JP*
(When and How is It Ethical to Prescribe an Ototoxic Drug?)
    Rev Prat (Paris) 17 (21) 2971-2978, 1967
    000 Refs Art Type Fr
    Abstr. (Excer Med Sect 11 21 48, 1968)

285

Harada Y* Musso E* Mira E*
Action of Streptomycin, Dihydrostreptomycin, Neomycin, and Kanamycin on the
Ampullar Receptors of the Frog
    Acta Otolaryng (Stockholm) 64 (4) 327-337, 1967
    045 Refs Exp Type Eng

286

Tyberghein J*
(The Influence of Pantothenic Acid on the Ototoxicity of Kanamycin in the
Guinea Pig)
    Med Welt (Stuttgart) 3 (3) 2017-2020, 1967
    000 Refs Exp Type Ger
    Abstr. (Excer Med Sect 11 21 230, 1968)

287

Fujimori H*
(Safety Margin of Kanamycin in Newborn and Young Infants. Effect of Kanamycin
on Hearing)
    J Jap Med Ass 58 1448-1450, Dec 15 1967
    003 Refs Clin Type Jap Trans Summ

288

Sambe T*
(Application of Kanamycin in Otolaryngology and its Side Effects, Especially
in Hearing Disorders)
    J Jap Med Ass 58 1437-1440, Dec 15 1967
    005 Refs Clin Exp Type Jap Trans Summ

289

Ghitescu M*
Complicatiile Terapiei cu Cloramfenicol (Complications of Chloramphenicol
Therapy)
    Viata Med 16 (7) 481-484, 1969
    017 Refs Clin Type Rum

290

Horak J*
The Contribution of Cupulometry to the Prevention of Streptomycin Intoxication
    Acta Univ Caroli (Med) (Praha) 15 641-660, 1969
    043 Refs Clin Exp Type Eng

291

Hommer K*
(On Quinine Poisoning of the Retina. With a Remark on Experimental Chloroquine Poisoning)
    Klin Mbl Augenheilk 152 785-805, 1968
    072 Refs Clin Exp Type Ger Trans Summ

292

Ondrejicka M* Holly D* Duris I*
(Hoigne's Syndrome--Nonallergic Reaction to Depot Penicillin)
    Bratisl Lek Listy 52 703-708, 1969
    010 Refs Clin Type Sl Trans Summ

293

Radanov R* Dobrev P* Slavov G* Pasmakov IV* Savov N*
(Side Reactions in the Treatment of Pulmonary Tuberculosis with Various
Combinations of Tuberculostatic Drugs)
    Ftiziatria (Sofiya) 5 (4) 164-169, 1968
    033 Refs Clin Type Bul Trans Summ

294

Todorenko AD* Mel'Man NIA*
(Some Complications Following Antibacterial Therapy in Patients with Chronic
Renal Insufficiency)
    Vrach Delo 2 128-130, Feb 1968
    000 Refs Clin Type Rus Trans Summ

295

Anon*
(Ototoxicity of Ethacrynic Acid in Patients with Poor Renal Function)
    Arch Pharm Chem (Kbh) 77 (9) 385-386, 1970
    012 Refs Clin Type Dan

296

Georgieva K* Novkova A*
(Side Effects of Penicillin and Streptomycin)
    Stomatologiya (Sofiya) 52 (2) 158-161, 1970
    018 Refs Clin Type Bul Trans Summ

297

Anon*
New Drugs Against Tuberculosis
    Brit Med J 1 (5531) 37-38, Jan 7 1967
    001 Refs Comment Type Eng

298

Anon*
Gentamicin
    Brit Med J 1 (5533) 158-159, Jan 21 1967
    014 Refs Clin Comment Type Eng

299

Schirrmacher UOE*
Case of Cobalt Poisoning
    Brit Med J 1 (5539) 544-545, Mar 4 1967
    005 Refs Clin Type Eng

300

Anon*
Reports on Gentamicin
    Brit Med J 2 (5551) 522-523, May 27 1967
    004 Refs Comment Type Eng

301

Darrell JH* Waterworth PM*
Dosage of Gentamicin for Pseudomonas Infections
    Brit Med J 1 (5551) 535-537, May 27 1967
    007 Refs Clin Type Eng

302

Pines A* Raafat H* Plucinski K*
Gentamicin and Colistin in Chronic Purulent Bronchial Infections
    Brit Med J 1 (5551) 543-545, May 27 1967
    013 Refs Clin Type Eng

303

Morrison JC* Fort AT* Fish SA*
Diuretic Induced Ototoxicity in Preeclampsia
    J Tenn Med Ass 64 (1) 36-37, Jan 1971
    008 Refs Clin Type Eng

304

Stillman MT*
Ethacrynic Acid, a Potent Diuretic
    Minn Med 50 (4) 573-585, Apr 1967
    035 Refs Art Type Eng

305

Pinals RS* Frank S*
Relative Efficacy of Indomethacin and Acetylsalicylic Acid in Rheumatoid
Arthritis
    New Eng J Med 276 (9) 512-514, Mar 2 1967
    010 Refs Clin Type Eng

306

Jackson GG*
Gentamicin
    Practitioner 198 (1188) 855-866, Jun 1967
    020 Refs Clin Type Eng

307

Sanders DY* Eliot DS* Cramblett HG*
Retrospective Study for Possible Kanamycin Ototoxicity Among Neonatal Infants
    J Pediat 70 (6) 960-962, Jun 1967
    009 Refs Clin Exp Type Eng

308

Mitchell RS*
'Second-Line' Antituberculosis Drugs
    JAMA 201 (2) 147, Jul 10 1967
    000 Refs Comment Type Eng

309

Toma GA* Main BJ*
Investigation of Kanamycin Ototoxicity in Genito-Urinary Surgery
    Postgrad Med J Suppl 46-52, May 1967
    020 Refs Clin Type Eng

310

Christrup J* Holberg F*
(Depression of Vestibular Function with Dehydrobenzperidol and Fentanyl
Citrate)
    Nord Med 78 (32) 1019-1021, 1967
    009 Refs Clin Type Dan Trans Summ

311

Edens ET*
Gehoorstoornissen na het Gebruik van een Mengsel, Bestaande uit Gelijke Delen
Streptomycine en Dihydrostreptomycine
    Ned T Geneesk 111 (8) 388, Feb 25 1967
    000 Refs Comment Type Dut

312

Perlman LV*
Salicylate Intoxication from Skin Application
    New Eng J Med 274 (3) 164, Jan 20 1966
    002 Refs Letter Type Eng

313

Heidland A* Wigand ME*
Deafness from Furosemide
    Ann Intern Med 73 (5) 858, 1970
    003 Refs Letter Type Eng

314

Koide Y* Hando R*
Vulnerability of the Organ of Corti in Poisoning
    Int Audiol 5 (2) 166-168, 1966
    000 Refs Exp Type Eng

315

Sugiyama T* Kayaba M* Kono Y* Sugada M*
On Massive Treatment of Aspirin Aluminum for Rheumatic Diseases
    Asian Med J 10 (7) 483-490, Jul 1967
    007 Refs Clin Type Eng

316

Meuwissen HJ* Robinson GC*
The Ototoxic Antibiotics. A Survey of Current Knowledge
    Clin Pediat 6 (5) 262-269, May 1967
    051 Refs Rev Type Eng

317

Kuschinsky G*
(On the Indications for Use and So-Called Detoxication of Streptomycin (Dihydrostreptomycin))
    Deutsch Med Wschr 91 (25) 1150-1151, 1966
    007 Refs Art Type Ger

318

Naumann P*
(The Treatment of Bacterial Infections with Combinations of Streptomycin (or
Dihydrostreptomycin) and Penicillin)
    Deutsch Med Wschr 91 (25) 1152-1157, 1966
    038 Refs Rev Type Ger

319

Decher H*
(Comments on the Use of Penicillin-Streptomycin Combinations in the Treatment
of Diseases of the Ear, Nose, and Throat)
    Deutsch Med Wschr 91 (25) 1158-1159, 1966
    040 Refs Rev Type Ger

320

Schmidt P* Friedman IS*
Adverse Effects of Ethacrynic Acid
    NY J Med 67 1438-1442, Jun 1 1967
    023 Refs Clin Type Eng

321

Cutu G*
Electronistagmografia in Sindromul Vestibular Streptomicinic (Electronystagmography in the Streptomycin Vestibular Syndromes)
    Rev Med Chir Iasi 75 (1) 71-76, 1971
    004 Refs Clin Type Rum Trans Summ

322

Oury M* Tuchais E* Norval C* Carbonnelle B* Leroux MF* Corre C* Parvery
F*
Traitement de Tuberculoses Pulmonaires Inveterees. Place de la Capreomycine
dans les Regimes Therapeutiques avec Rifampicine et Ethambutol (Treatment of
Resistant Pulmonary Tuberculosis with Capreomycin, Rifomycin, and Ethambutol)
    Rev Tuberc (Paris) 34 (4) 519-530, Jun 1970
    000 Refs Clin Type Fr

323

Jelert H*
Severe Reduction of Hearing and Vestibular Involvement Caused by Vionactan
    J Laryng 81 (3) 317-323, Mar 1967
    015 Refs Clin Type Eng

324

Webster JC* Mc Gee TM* Carroll R* Benitez JT* Williams ML*
Ototoxicity of Gentamicin. Histopathologic and Functional Results in the Cat
    Trans Amer Acad Ophthal Otolaryng 74 (6) 1155-1165, Nov-Dec 1970
    009 Refs Exp Histol Type Eng

325

Lester   W* Fischer   DA* Dye   WE*
Evaluation of Capreomycin and Ethambutol in Retreatment of Pulmonary Tuberculosis
    Ann NY Acad Sci 135 (2) 890-900,   1966
    012 Refs Clin Type Eng

326

Justice   FK* Schwartz   WS*
Treatment of Original Cavitary Pulmonary Tuberculosis with Capreomycin (CM)
and Para-Aminosalicylic Acid (PAS)
    Ann NY Acad Sci 135 (2) 1007-1010,   1966
    000 Refs Clin Type Eng

327

Monroe   J* Pecora   DV* Yegian   D*
The Use of Capreomycin in Combined Antibacterial Therapy and Early Surgery in
So-Called Treatment Failures of Pulmonary Tuberculosis
    Ann NY Acad Sci 135 (2) 1074-1078,   1966
    000 Refs Clin Type Eng

328

Browning   RH* Donnerberg   RL*
Capreomycin-Experiences in Patient Acceptance and Toxicity
    Ann NY Acad Sci 135 (2) 1057-1064,   1966
    005 Refs Clin Type Eng

329

Schless   JM* Allison   RF* Inglis   RM* Topperman   S* Trapp   E*
Capreomycin-Ethionamide as a Retreatment Regimen for Pulmonary Tuberculosis
    Ann NY Acad Sci 135 (2) 1085-1097,   1966
    001 Refs Clin Type Eng

330

Welles   JS* Harris   PN* Small   RM* Worth   HM* Anderson   RC*
The Toxicity of Capreomycin in Laboratory Animals
    Ann NY Acad Sci 135 (2) 960-973,   1966
    006 Refs Exp Type Eng

331

Kass   I*
(Capreomycin and Ethambutol in Retreatment of Pulmonary Tuberculosis. Discussion)
    Ann NY Acad Sci 135 (2) 900-903,   1966
    002 Refs Clin Type Eng

332

Donomae   I*
Capreomycin in the Treatment of Pulmonary Tuberculosis
    Ann NY Acad Med 135 (2) 1011-1038,   1966
    025 Refs Clin Type Eng

333

Dunphy   EB*
Adverse Effects of Drugs on the Eye, Ear, Nose and Throat
    Trans Amer Acad Ophthal Otolaryng 70 (1) 9-16,   1966
    000 Refs Art Type Eng

334

Podvinec   S* Mihaljevic   B* Marcetic   A* Simonovic   M*
Schadigungen des Fotalen Cortischen Organs durch Streptomycin (Damage to
Fetal Organ of Corti by Streptomycin)
    Mschr Ohrenheilk 100 (6) 250,   1966
    000 Refs Exp Type Ger

335

Hutzler   RU*
Estreptomicina. Kanamicina. Neomicina. Gentamicina (Streptomycin. Kanamycin.
Neomycin. Gentamicin)

Rev Med (S Paulo) 54 (4) 78-86, Nov 1970
    024 Refs Art Type Sp

                                                                          336
Spoendlin H*
L'Ototoxicite de la Streptomycine (Ototoxicity of Streptomycin)
    Med Hyg (Geneve) 24 (752) 1059, Oct 26 1966
    008 Refs Art Type Fr

                                                                          337
Koide Y* Stern R* Roesler HK* Daly JF*
Studies on Susceptibility to Kanamycin. Histopathological and Electrophysio-
logical Observations
    Laryngoscope 76 (11) 1769-1785, Nov 1966
    016 Refs Exp Histol Type Eng

                                                                          338
Kohonen A* Tarkkanen JV*
Dihydrostreptomycin and Kanamycin Ototoxicity. An Experimental Study by
Surface Preparation Technique
    Laryngoscope 76 (10) 1671-1680, Oct 1966
    010 Refs Exp Histol Type Eng

                                                                          339
Cohn ES* Gordes EH* Brusilow SW*
Ethacrynic Acid Effect on the Composition of Cochlear Fluids
    Science 171 910-911, Mar 5 1971
    008 Refs Exp Type Eng

                                                                          340
Virsik K* Havelka C* Bajan A* Badalik L* Skutilova L* Taborska Z*
(Secondary Effects of Thiacetazone)
    Bratisl Lek Listy 55 (4) 470-475, 1971
    012 Refs Clin Type Sl Trans Summ

                                                                          341
Bochenek Z* Gromow L* Klott M*
(Electronystagmographic Investigations into the Effect of Streptomycin on the
Vestibular Organ)
    Gruzlica 39 (4) 289-295, 1971
    030 Refs Clin Type Pol Trans Summ

                                                                          342
Miller JD* Popplewell AG* Landwehr A* Greene ME*
Toxicology Studies in Patients on Prolonged Therapy with Capreomycin
    Ann NY Acad Sci 135 (2) 1047-1056, 1966
    011 Refs Clin Type Eng

                                                                          343
Garfield JW* Jones JM* Cohen NL* Daly JF* Mc Clement JH*
The Auditory, Vestibular, and Renal Effects of Capreomycin in Humans
    Ann NY Acad Sci 135 (2) 1039-1046, 1966
    000 Refs Clin Type Eng

                                                                          344
Sekitani T* Ryu JH* Mc Cabe BF*
Drug Effects on the Medial Vestibular Nucleus. Perrotatory Response
    Arch Otolaryng (Chicago) 94 (5) 401-405, Nov 1971
    017 Refs Exp Type Eng

                                                                          345
Lucente FE*
Aspirin and the Otolaryngologist
    Arch Otolaryng (Chicago) 94 (5) 443-446, Nov 1971
    015 Refs Art Type Eng

                                                                          346
Kluyskens P*

Specific Action of Some Drugs on Bechterew Nystagmus
    Acta Otorhinolaryng Belg 24 (5) 593-597, 1970
    006 Refs Art Exp Histol Type Eng

                                                                         347

Podvinec S* Stefanovic P*
Surdite par la Streptomycine et Predisposition Familiale (Deafness from
Streptomycin and Familial Predisposition)
    J Franc Otorhinolaryng 15 (1) 61-67, Jan-Feb 1966
    023 Refs Clin Type Fr

                                                                         348

Pannone T*
Sulla Terapia di Alcune Forme Flogistiche dell'Orecchio Mediante. Un'Associa-
zione di Fluocinolone Acetonide, Polimixina B e Neomicina (On Therapy of
Various Infections of the Middle Ear. A Combination of Fluocinolone Acetonide, Polymyxin B, and Neomycin)
    Boll Mal Orecch 88 65-77, 1970
    028 Refs Clin Type It

                                                                         349

Ouchi H* Ishida H* Otani I*
(Effects of Vitamin B1 Derivatives on the Hearing Disorders Caused by Kanamycin. 2)
    J Otolaryng Jap 73 Suppl 984-985, Jul 1970
    000 Refs Exp Type Jap Trans Summ

                                                                         350

Rempt E*
(Side Effects of Streptomycin and Kanamycin from the Otologic Standpoint)
    Z Erkrank Atm-Org 134 (2) 177-183, 1971
    036 Refs Clin Type Ger

                                                                         351

Ochs IL*
Topical Anesthesia for Myringotomy
    Trans Amer Acad Ophthal Otolaryng 71 918-922, Nov-Dec 1967
    000 Refs Clin Type Eng

                                                                         352

Marcus RE*
Reduced Incidence of Congenital and Prelingual Deafness
    Arch Otolaryng (Chicago) 92 343-347, Oct 1970
    029 Refs Art Type Eng

                                                                         353

Finch JS* De Kornfeld TJ*
Clonixin -- A Clinical Evaluation of a New Oral Analgesic
    J Clin Pharmacol and New Drugs 11 (5) 371-377, Sep-Oct 1971
    000 Refs Clin Type Eng

                                                                         354

Sutherland AM*
Genital Tuberculosis in Women
    Pak J Surg Gynaec Obstet 10 (10) 337-350, Oct 1968
    000 Refs Clin Type Eng

                                                                         355

Chalmers TM*
Clinical Experience with Ibuprofen in the Treatment of Rheumatoid Arthritis
    Ann Rheum Dis 28 (5) 513-517, Sep 1969
    004 Refs Clin Type Eng

                                                                         356

Tarasov DI* Kosacheva AP*
(Hearing Disorders in Early Childhood after the Employment of Some Antibiotics)
    Vestn Otorinolaring 33 (4) 10-13, Jul-Aug 1971

012 Refs Clin Type Rus Trans Summ

357

Gyulkhasyan AA*
(The State of the Auditory Function in Patients during Treatment with Some
Antibiotics)
    Vestn Otorinolaring 33 (4) 13-15, Jul-Aug 1971
    000 Refs Clin Type Rus Trans Summ

358

Petrova EI*
(The Function of the Vestibular Analyzer in Patients with Otosclerosis Occur-
ring after Treatment with Some Antibiotics)
    Vestn Otorinolaring 33 (4) 15-19, Jul-Aug 1971
    019 Refs Clin Type Rus Trans Summ

359

Dick-Smith JB*
Ibuprofen, Aspirin, and Placebo in the Treatment of Rheumatoid Arthritis--A
Double-Blind Clinical Trial
    Med J Aust 2 (17) 853-859, Oct 25 1969
    011 Refs Clin Type Eng

360

Boardman PL* Nuki G* Hart FD*
Ibuprofen in the Treatment of Rheumatoid Arthritis and Osteo-Arthritis
    Ann Rheum Dis 26 560-561, 1967
    005 Refs Clin Type Eng

361

Jasani MK* Downie WW* Samuels BM* Buchanan WW*
Ibuprofen in Rheumatoid Arthritis. Clinical Study of Analgesic and Anti-
Inflammatory Activity
    Ann Rheum Dis 27 457-462, 1968
    011 Refs Clin Type Eng

362

Shevtsov VM*
(The Prophylaxis and Treatment of Ototoxic Lesions Caused by Antibiotics)
    Vestn Otorinolaring 33 (4) 19-22, Jul-Aug 1971
    013 Refs Clin Type Rus Trans Summ

363

Senyukov MV*
(The Effectiveness of Treatment of Patients with a Disturbance of the Auditory Function Associated with Streptomycin Therapy)
    Vestn Otorinolaring 33 (4) 22-27, Jul-Aug 1971
    015 Refs Clin Type Rus Trans Summ

364

Ageeva AN* Evstratova LI* Lantsov AA* Osherovich AM* Rozenblyum AS*
Yushkova ZN*
(The Use of Unitiol in Toxic Lesions of the Auditory Analyzer)
    Vestn Otorinolaring 33 (4) 27-31, Jul-Aug 1971
    009 Refs Clin Exp Type Rus Trans Summ

365

Chum-Chantholl*
Interet de l'Association de l'Amino 4 Quinoleine et de la Sulfamethoxy-Pyri-
dazine dans le Traitement de la Maladie de Hansen, Forme Tuberculoide. Resultats Obtenus apres Cinq Ans d'Observation (Association of 4 Amino Quinolein
and Sulfamethoxy Pyridazin in the Treatment of Tuberculoid Lepra)
    Bull Soc Path Exot 61 (4) 504-510, 1968
    010 Refs Clin Type Fr

366

Exaire S* Cardenas M* Rotberg T*
Intoxicacion Quinidinica (Quinidine Intoxication)

Arch Inst Cardiol Mex 37 (3) 321-329, May-Jun 1967
011 Refs Clin Type Sp

367

Miller AB* Nunn AJ* Robinson DK* Ferguson GC* Fox W* Tall R*
A Second International Co-Operative Investigation into Thioacetazone Side-
Effects. 1. The Influence of a Vitamin and Antihistamine Supplement
   Bull World Health Org 43 (1) 107-125, 1970
   024 Refs Clin Type Eng

368

Bickel G*
Le Traitement Chimiotherapique de la Tuberculose (Chemotherapy of Tuberculosis)
   Med Hyg (Geneve) 27 (853) 22-26, Jan 8 1969
   000 Refs Art Type Fr

369

Bernabei L* Pierangeli CE* Di Brino M* Consalvo P*
(Experimental Labyrinth Damage by Gentamicin. 1. Functional Data)
   Atti Accad Fisiocr Siena (Medicofis) 16 445-467, 1967
   021 Refs Exp Type It

370

Bernabei L* Di Brino M* Consalvo P* Pierangeli CE*
(Experimental Labyrinth Damage Induced by Gentamicin. 2. Histo-Pathologic
Findings)
   Atti Accad Fisiocr Siena (Medicofis) 16 1221-1249, 1967
   000 Refs Exp Histol Type It

371

Brun JP* Stupp H*
(Quantitative Evaluation of Hair Cell Damage Following Treatment with Kanamycin Sulfate, Kanamycin Monopantothenate and Ozothin)
   Arch Klin Exp Ohr Nas Kehlkopfheilk 194 (2) 566-569, Dec 22 1969
   000 Refs Exp Histol Type Ger

372

Konishi T* Kelsey E*
Effect of Cyanide on Cochlear Potentials
   Acta Otolaryng (Stockholm) 65 (4) 381-390, Apr 1968
   025 Refs Exp Type Eng

373

Morrison AW* Booth JB*
Sudden Deafness -- An Otological Emergency
   Brit J Hosp Med 4 (3) 287-298, Sep 1970
   050 Refs Rev Clin Type Eng

374

Jung W* Machold W*
Zum Einfluss von Salidiuretica auf die Cochlea-Mikrophonpotentiale beim
Meerschweinchen (On the Effect of Salidiuretica on the Cochlear Microphonic
Potentials in Guinea Pigs)
   Arch Klin Exp Ohr Nas Kehlkopfheilk 196 (2) 307-314, 1970
   008 Refs Exp Type Ger

375

Baker SB* Davey DG*
The Predictive Value for Man of Toxicological Tests of Drugs in Laboratory
Animals
   Brit Med Bull 26 208-211, 1970
   011 Refs Rev Type Eng

376

Pluzhnikov MS* Teplitskaya TI*
(A Comparative Study of Neomycin Content in the Aural Lymph and Similar
Biological Fluids)

Vestn Otorinolaring 33 (1) 52-56,   1971
015 Refs Exp Type Rus Trans Summ

377

Obara K*
(A Case of Isolated Lesion of the Vestibular Apparatus in a Patient with
Pulmonary Tuberculosis Treated with Streptomycin)
    Otolaryng Pol 25 (1) 109-111,   1971
    011 Refs Clin Type Pol Trans Summ

378

Sellars SL*
Acute Deafness Associated with Depoprogesterone
    J Laryng 85 (3) 281-282, Mar 1971
    005 Refs Clin Type Eng

379

Gonzalez G* Istre C* Rubin W*
Labyrinthine Catastrophe -- Is It the Pill?
    J Louisiana Med Soc 120 (12) 487-494, Dec 1968
    015 Refs Clin Type Eng

380

Fairbanks DNF* Shimizu H* Warfield D*
Unilateral Vestibular Ablation with Streptomycin. A Study in Cats
    Arch Otolaryng (Chicago) 93 (6) 590-596, Jun 1971
    011 Refs Exp Type Eng

381

Schindel L*
(Clinically Observed Side Effects of More Recent Antibiotics. Amphotericin-B-
Bacitracin-Cycloserine-Neomycin-Novobiocin-Polymyxin)
    Ther Umsch 23 (7) 302-314, Jul 1966
    051 Refs Rev Type Ger

382

Von Ilberg C* Spoendlin H* Arnold W*
Autoradiographical Distribution of Locally Applied Dihydrostreptomycin in the
Inner Ear
    Acta Otolaryng (Stockholm) 71 (2-3) 159-165, Feb-Mar 1971
    015 Refs Exp Type Eng

383

Klaus W*
Risiken Moderner Arzneimitteltherapie (Kommentar Zueiner Unfrage an Padiatri-
schen Kliniken) (Risks in Modern Therapeutic Medicine (Comment on an Inquiry
in a Pediatric Clinic))
    Mschr Kinderheilk 119 (7) 392-401, Jul 1971
    060 Refs Rev Type Ger Trans Summ

384

Ballantyne J*
Iatrogenic Deafness
    J Laryng 84 (10) 967-1000, Oct 1970
    108 Refs Rev Clin Type Eng

385

Braun OH*
(Possible Adverse Effects of the Antibiotic Treatment of Infant Enteritis)
    Arch Kinderheilk 179 1-6, May 1969
    040 Refs Rev Type Ger

386

Breuninger H*
Nasentropfen, Ohrentropfen (Nosedrops and Eardrops)
    HNO 19 (3) 65-68, Mar 1971
    000 Refs Art Type Ger Trans Summ

387

Anon*
Neomycin -- A New Route for Therapy
    Med World News 12 (26) 52B, Jul 1 1971
    000 Refs Comment Type Eng

388

Mc Kinna   AJ*
Quinine Induced Hypoplasia of the Optic Nerve
    Canad J Ophthal 1 261-266,   1966
    014 Refs Clin Type Eng

389

Hoft   J*
Die Permeabilitat und die Beeinflussung der Permeabilitat der Membran des
Runden Fensters durch Pantocain (Tetracain) (The Permeability of the Round
Window Membrane and its Changes by Pantocain (Tetracain))
    Arch Klin Exp Ohr Nas Kehlkopfheilk 193 (2) 128-137,   1969
    010 Refs Exp Histol Type Ger Trans Summ

390

Gyulkhasyan   AA*
(Some Data on the Lesion of the Auditory Function in Patients with Tuberculosis of the Lungs Treated with Streptomycin)
    Zh Ushn Nos Gorl Bolez 2 13-16,   1969
    021 Refs Clin Type Rus
    Abstr. (dsh Abstr 10 37-38, 1970)

391

Fujimori   H*
The Effects of Kanamycin on the Acoustic Function
    Asian Med J 11 (5) 365-369, May 1968
    000 Refs Clin Exp Type Eng

392

Sambe   B*
Clinical Application of Kanamycin to the Otorhinolaryngological Field and its
Side-Effects, Especially Ototoxicity of Kanamycin
    Asian Med J 11 (5) 341-348, May 1968
    008 Refs Clin Exp Type Eng

393

Kato   T*
Kanamycin Excretion in Renal Failure
    Asian Med J 11 (5) 324-329, May 1968
    015 Refs Clin Type Eng

394

Teramatsu   T*
Pulmonary Tuberculosis Surgery and Kanamycin Introduction
    Asian Med J 11 (5) 390-398, May 1968
    000 Refs Clin Type Eng

395

Winther   FO*
Early Degenerative Changes in the Inner Ear Sensory Cells of the Guinea Pig
Following Local X-ray Irradiation. A Preliminary Report
    Acta Otolaryng (Stockholm) 67 (2-3) 262-268, Feb-Mar 1969
    009 Refs Exp Histol Type Eng

396

Laurini   F* Cosimo   W* Incutti   V* Galli   V*
Rilievi Audiovestibolari nel Corso della Somministrazione di 'Tofranil'
(Audiovestibular Findings Following Administration of 'Tofranil')
    Arch Ital Laring 74 325-345,   1966
    000 Refs Clin Type It
    Abstr. (dsh Abstr 8 9, 1968)

397

Nagoshi Y* Ohshita F* Hayakawa K* Nakayama T*
The Studies of Hearing Disorder on (sic) Diabetics
    Audiology (Japan) 12 (2) 155-159, 1969
    015 Refs Clin Type Eng
    Abstr. (dsh Abstr 10 150-151, 1970)

398

Torii H*
Experimental Study of Effect of Drugs on Acoustic Threshold and Cochlear
Blood Circulation in Dogs
    Otol Fukuoka 15 (1) 1-27, 1969
    091 Refs Exp Type Eng
    Abstr. (dsh Abstr 10 114, 1970)

399

Wirth K*
Zur Meningitis Behandlung beim Erwachsenen. 2 (Treatment of Meningitis in
Adults. 2)
    Fortschr Med 86 (21) 956-958, 1968
    025 Refs Art Type Ger

400

May P* Konig K*
(Experiences with the Newer Tuberculostatic Agents in the Treatment of Genitourinary Tuberculosis (Capreomycin, Ethambutol, Rifampicin))
    Z Urol Nephrol 62 (9) 657-662, 1969
    026 Refs Art Type Ger

401

Lawrence M* Gonzalez G* Hawkins JE,Jr*
Some Physiological Factors in Noise-Induced Hearing Loss
    Amer Industr Hyg Ass J 28 (5) 425-430, Sep-Oct 1967
    015 Refs Clin Exp Type Eng

402

Schiff M*
The 'Pill' in Otolaryngology
    Trans Amer Acad Ophthal Otolaryng 72 76-84, 1968
    018 Refs Art Type Eng

403

Howard PH*
Infection of the Central Nervous System. Advances in Treatment
    Mod Treatm 8 (2) 277-287, May 1971
    019 Refs Rev Type Eng

404

Morris AJ* Bilinsky RT*
Prevention of Staphylococcal Shunt Infections by Continuous Vancomycin Prophylaxis
    Amer J Med Sci 262 (2) 87-92, Aug 1971
    016 Refs Clin Type Eng

405

Chambers AH* Lucchina GG*
Effects of Dinitrophenol on Cochlear Potentials of the Cat. 1. Normal Ear
    J Aud Res 6 (1) 13-21, Jan 1966
    009 Refs Exp Type Eng

406

Lucchina GG* Chambers AH*
Effects of Dinitrophenol on Cochlear Potentials of the Cat. 2. Acoustically
Injured Ear
    J Aud Res 6 (1) 23-30, Jan 1966
    003 Refs Exp Type Eng

407
Anon*
Prevention des Surdites d'Origine Medicamenteuse (Prevention of Medicinal
Deafness)
    Rev Ouie Sourd Franc 43 132-133,   1967
    000 Refs Art Type Fr
    Abstr. (dsh Abstr 8 220, 1968)

408
Wagner P*
Conferences a La Chaux de Fonds (Suisse) en 1966 (Conference Held at La Chaux
de Fonds, Switzerland, in 1966)
    Rev Ouie Sourd Franc 43 101-114,   1967
    000 Refs Art Type Fr
    Abstr. (dsh Abstr 8 84, 1968)

409
Goldman JL*
What's New and Important in Otolaryngology?
    Med Trib 12 (39) 10, Oct 6 1971
    000 Refs Comment Type Eng

410
Mounier-Kuhn P* Morgon A* Charachon D*
Manifestations Otologiques des Embryopathies et des Foetopathies (Otological
Manifestations of Embryopathies and Fetopathies)
    J Franc Otorhinolaryng 15 759-763,   1966
    000 Refs Art Type Fr
    Abstr. (dsh Abstr 7 260, 1967)

411
Gignoux M* Martin H* Cajgfinger H*
(Cochleo-Vestibular Complaints after Attempted Suicide by Aspirin)
    J Franc Otorhinolaryng 15 (6) 631-635,   1966
    000 Refs Clin Type Fr
    Abstr. (dsh Abstr 7 256-257, 1967)

412
Khilov VS* Cherkasov VS*
(On So-Called Neuritis of the Auditory Nerve)
    Zh Ushn Nos Gorl Bolez 27 (2) 10-14,   1967
    014 Refs Exp Type Rus
    Abstr. (dsh Abstr 7 258, 1967)

413
Baru AV*
(Pecularities (sic) of the Detection of Acoustic Signals of Different Dura-
tion under the Action of Some Drugs)
    Zh Vyssh Nerv Deiat Pavlov 17 (1) 107-115,   1967
    034 Refs Exp Type Rus
    Abstr. (dsh Abstr 7 229-230, 1967)

414
Venkateswaran PS*
Transient Deafness from High Doses of Frusemide
    Brit Med J 4 (5779) 113-114, Oct 9 1971
    002 Refs Letter Clin Type Eng

415
Anderton JL* Kincaid-Smith P*
Diuretics. 2. Clinical Considerations
    Drugs 1 (2) 142-165,   1971
    113 Refs Rev Type Eng

416
Dale AJD* Love JG*
Thorium Dioxide Myclopathy
    JAMA 199 (9) 606-609, Feb 27 1967
    010 Refs Clin Type Eng

417

Wasson HW* Uncapher B*
Effects of Dextro-Amphetamine on Auditory Threshold in Man
    J Aud Res 6 (3) 351-355, Jul 1966
    012 Refs Exp Type Eng

418

Fruttero F* Sartoris A*
Recherches Experimentales sur l'Action Novocainique au Niveau de l'Appareil
Acoustique (Experimental Research on the Action of Novocaine at the Level of
the Acoustic Mechanism)
    J Franc Otorhinolaryng 15 805-808, 1966
    000 Refs Exp Type Fr
    Abstr. (dsh Abstr 7 224-225, 1967)

419

Rossberg G*
(Diseases Caused by Pharmacological Agents in the ENT Field)
    Arch Klin Exp Ohr Nas Kehlkopfheilk 188 201-210, 1967
    008 Refs Art Type Ger Trans Summ

420

Kupper K*
(Ototoxic Effect of Gentamicin in Humans)
    Arch Klin Exp Ohr Nas Kehlkopfheilk 194 569-573, Dec 22 1969
    006 Refs Clin Type Ger

421

Elin DM* Gruzdev AV*
(Toxic Effect of Preparations of the Streptomycin Series on Cochlear and
Vestibular Function)
    Voennomed Zh 4 82-83, Apr 1970
    000 Refs Clin Type Rus Trans Summ

422

Avksent'Eva TA*
(Complications in Obstetric-Gynecologic Practice from Antibiotic Therapy)
    Antibiotiki 13 1039, Nov 1968
    000 Refs Clin Type Rus Trans Summ

423

Martin H*
Les Facteurs Aggravants de la Senescence Auriculaire (Worsening Factors in
Aging Ear)
    J Franc Otorhinolaryng 17 (10) 803-805, Dec 1968
    000 Refs Art Type Fr

424

Vesely C* Faltynek L*
(The Function of Middle-Ear Muscles in Neomycin Intoxication of Guinea Pigs)
    Sborn Ved Prac Lek Fak Karlov Univ Suppl 12, 279-285, 1969
    000 Refs Exp Type Cz Trans Summ

425

Von Westernhagen B* Schatzle W*
(Enzyme Histochemical Studies on the Influence of Ozothin on the Ototoxic
Effect of Streptomycin in Guinea Pigs)
    Arch Klin Exp Ohr Nas Kehlkopfheilk 194 558-561, Dec 22 1969
    007 Refs Exp Type Ger

426

Evo NO*
Bacteriuria Again
    Brit Med J 2 (5756) 278, May 1 1971
    001 Refs Letter Type Eng

427

Gingell JC*

Bacteriuria Again
    Brit Med J 2 (5756) 278, May 1 1971
    002 Refs Letter Type Eng

                                                                    428
Leigh DA*
Bacteriuria Again
    Brit Med J 2 (5760) 527, May 29 1971
    012 Refs Letter Type Eng

                                                                    429
Pokotilenko AK* Gyulkhasyan AA*
(Ototoxic Effect of Colimycin)
    Tr Erevan Gos Inst Usoversh Vrachei 4 277-279, 1969
    000 Refs Exp Histol Type Rus Trans Summ

                                                                    430
Gyulkhasyan AA*
(Effect of Some Antibiotics on Auditory Function in Animals)
    Tr Erevan Gos Inst Usoversh Vrachei 4 281-282, 1969
    000 Refs Exp Type Rus Trans Summ

                                                                    431
Marks MI* Printice R* Swarson R* Cotton EK* Eickhoff TC*
Carbenicillin and Gentamicin -- Pharmacologic Studies in Patients with Cystic
Fibrosis and Pseudomonas Pulmonary Infections
    J Pediat 79 (5) 822-828, Nov 1971
    010 Refs Clin Type Eng

                                                                    432
Watanuki K* Meyer zum Gottesberge A*
Streptomycin and Kanamycin Effect upon the Vestibular Sensory Epithelia of
the Maculae Sacculi and Utriculi in the Guinea Pig
    Pract Otorhinolaryng 33 (3) 169-175, 1971
    009 Refs Exp Histol Type Eng

                                                                    433
Singapore Tuberculosis Services*
A Controlled Clinical Trial of the Role of Thiacetazone-Containing Regimens
in the Treatment of Pulmonary Tuberculosis in Singapore
    Tubercle 52 (2) 88-116, 1971
    028 Refs Clin Type Eng
    Abstr. (Biol Abstr 52 11731, 1971)

                                                                    434
Varpela E* Hietalahti J* Aro MJ*
Streptomycin and Dihydrostreptomycin Medication during Pregnancy and their
Effect on the Child's Inner Ear
    Scand J Resp Dis 50 101-109, 1969
    021 Refs Clin Type Eng

                                                                    435
Konishi T* Kelsey E* Singleton GT*
Negative Potential in Scala Media during Early Stage of Anoxia
    Acta Otolaryng (Stockholm) 64 (2) 107-118, Aug 1967
    021 Refs Exp Type Eng

                                                                    436
Kittel G* Theissing G*
(Histological Studies of the Cochlea on Cuticle Preparations and Scalariform
Sections Following Severe Protacted (sic) Hypoxia)
    Arch Klin Exp Ohr Nas Kehlkopfheilk 191 534-538, 1968
    010 Refs Exp Histol Type Ger Trans Summ

                                                                    437
Holz E* Hoffmann M* Beck C*
(Morphological and Bacteriological Findings on the Decrease of Ototoxicity of
Basic Streptomyces Antibiotics)

Arch Klin Exp Ohr Nas Kehlkopfheilk 188 236-242, 1967
015 Refs Exp Type Ger Trans Summ

438

Matsuura S* Ikeda K* Furukawa T*
Effects of Streptomycin, Kanamycin, Quinine, and Other Drugs on the Microphonic Potentials of Goldfish Sacculus
Jap J Physiol 21 (5) 579-590, Oct 1971
024 Refs Exp Type Eng

439

Aran JM*
(Electrophysiologic Control of the Function of the Organ of Corti Following
Exposure of Some Other Agents)
Acta Otolaryng (Stockholm) 63 Suppl 40-49, 1967
000 Refs Exp Type Fr Trans Summ

440

Andersen JB* Pederson CB*
A Method for the Determination of Transplacental Transmission of Drugs -- The
Distribution of Kanamycin in Pregnant Guinea-Pigs
Acta Pathol Microbiol Scand Sec B Microbiol Immunol 79 (2) 204-208, 1971
009 Refs Exp Type Eng
Abstr. (Biol Abstr 52 11200, 1971)

441

Kashkin PN* Bezborodov AM* Elinov NP* Tsyganov VA*
Antibiotiki (Antibiotics)
Leningrad, Meditsina 1970
718 Refs Monogr Type Rus
Abstr. (Biol Abstr 52 11175, 1971)

442

Lindsay JR*
Histopathologic Characteristics of Viral Labyrinthitis
Otologia Fukuoka (Tokyo) 13 77-78, 1967
000 Refs Art Type Eng
Abstr. (dsh Abstr 9 49, 1969)

443

Flach M* Knothe J* Seidel P*
Adaptationsverhalten des Cortischen Organs nach Einwirkung von Lokalanaesthe-
tica (Tetracain und Lidocain) (Adaptation in the Organ of Corti after Local
Anesthesia (Tetracain and Lidocain))
Arch Klin Exp Ohr Nas Kehlkopfheilk 192 (4) 325-332, 1968
012 Refs Exp Type Ger
Abstr. (dsh Abstr 9 210, 1969)

444

Buongiavanni S* De Michelis G* Fruttero F* Hahn R* Schindler O*
Modificazioni delle Funzioni Acustica e Vestibolare Indotte da Farmaci ad
Azione Neuropsicotropa (Modifications of the Acoustic and Vestibular Func-
tions Induced by Drugs with a Neuropsychotropic Action)
Boll Mal Orecch 85 (2) 1-109, 1967
284 Refs Rev Clin Exp Type It
Abstr. (dsh Abstr 9 154, 1969)

445

Swaiman KF* Flagler DG*
Mercury Poisoning with Central and Peripheral Nervous System Involvement
Treated with Penicillamine
Pediatrics 48 (4) 639-642, Oct 1971
011 Refs Clin Type Eng

446

East African-British Medical Research Council Retreatment Investigation
(1971)*
Streptomycin plus PAS plus Pyrazinamide in the Retreatment of Pulmonary

Tuberculosis in East Africa
    Tubercle 52 (3) 191-198, Sep 1971
    020 Refs Clin Type Eng

447
Pamra SP*
A Co-Operative Trial on the Toxicity and Efficacy of Thiacetazone
    Indian J Med Res 59 683-698, May 5 1971
    016 Refs Clin Type Eng

448
Krzanowski JJ,Jr* Matschinsky FM*
A Phosphocreatine Gradient Opposite to That of Glycogen in the Organ of Corti
and the Effect of Salicylate on Adenosine Triphosphate and P-creatine in
Cochlear Structures
    J Histochem Cytochem 19 (5) 321-323, May 1971
    012 Refs Exp Type Eng

449
Sekitani T*
(Jumping of Objects (Dandy's Symptom) and Vestibular Function Disorder due to
Streptomycin Intoxication)
    Otolaryngology (Tokyo) 42 93-100, Feb 1970
    000 Refs Clin Type Jap Trans Summ

450
Cocchi A* Invernizzi G*
(Electroencephalographic Research on Acute Quinine Poisoning)
    Riv Neurol 37 377-386, Jul-Aug 1967
    000 Refs Clin Type It

451
Stratford BC* Dixson S*
Results of Treatment of 104 Patients with Gentamicin
    Med J Aust 1 (21) 1107-1110, May 22 1971
    029 Refs Clin Type Eng

452
Telegdi I* Pinter G*
Streptomycinnel Kezelt Betegeink Hallasvizsgalata (Checkup of Hearing in
Patients Treated with Streptomycin)
    Orv Hetil 112 (28) 1638-1639, 1971
    006 Refs Clin Type Hun

453
Herpell R*
(Reinstatement of Labyrinthine Function after Damage Caused by Streptomycin)
    HNO 19 (9) 285, Sep 1971
    000 Refs Clin Type Ger

454
Lange G*
(Gentamicin Damage of the Vestibular Organs in Guinea Pigs (Cytovestibulo-
gram, Colorization) and after Therapeutic Use)
    Arch Klin Exp Ohr Nas Kehlkopfheilk 196 (2) 153-158, 1970
    000 Refs Clin Exp Type Ger

455
Watanuki K*
(Pathology of the Vestibular Sensory Epithelia in Streptomycin and Kanamycin
Ototoxicosis)
    J Otolaryng Jap 74 (6) 1028-1035, Jun 1971
    028 Refs Exp Histol Type Jap Trans Summ

456
Nagaba M*
Electron Microscopic Study of Semicircular Canal Organs and Otolith Organs of
Squirrel Monkeys after Administration of Streptomycin Sulfate

Acta Otolaryng (Stockholm) 66 541-552,   1968
028 Refs Exp Histol Type Eng

                                                               457

Nilges TC* Northern   JL*
Iatrogenic Ototoxic Hearing Loss
   Ann Surg 173 (2) 281-289, Feb 1971
   016 Refs Clin Type Eng

                                                               458

Ostyn F* Tyberghein J*
Influence of Some Streptomyces Antibiotics on the Inner Ear of the Guinea
Pig. Electrophysiological and Histological Study.   1. Introduction, Experi-
mental Techniques
   Acta Otolaryng (Stockholm) Suppl 234, 5-29, 1968
   074 Refs Exp Histol Type Eng

                                                               459

Ostyn F* Tyberghein J*
Influence of Some Streptomyces Antibiotics on the Inner Ear of the Guinea
Pig. Electrophysiological and Histological Study.   2. Kanamycin
   Acta Otolaryng (Stockholm) Suppl 234, 30-53, 1968
   074 Refs Exp Histol Type Eng

                                                               460

Ostyn F* Tyberghein J*
Influence of Some Streptomyces Antibiotics on the Inner Ear of the Guinea
Pig. Electrophysiological and Histological Study.   3. Streptomycin, Viomycin,
Capreomycin
   Acta Otolaryng (Stockholm) Suppl 234, 54-65, 1968
   074 Refs Exp Histol Type Eng

                                                               461

Ostyn F* Tyberghein J*
Influence of Some Streptomyces Antibiotics on the Inner Ear of the Guinea
Pig. Electrophysiological and Histological Study.   4. Neomycin
   Acta Otolaryng (Stockholm) Suppl 234, 66-73, 1968
   074 Refs Exp Histol Type Eng

                                                               462

Ostyn F* Tyberghein J*
Influence of Some Streptomyces Antibiotics on the Inner Ear of the Guinea
Pig. Electrophysiological and Histological Study.   5. General Discussion and
Conclusions, Summary
   Acta Otolaryng (Stockholm) Suppl 234, 74-91, 1968
   074 Refs Exp Histol Type Eng

                                                               463

Greiner GF* Collard   M* Conraux C* Haushalter G*
Les Modifications Electronystamographiques Provoquees par l'Alcool (Alcohol
Induced Electronystagmographic Modifications)
   Rev Otoneuroophtal 43 (4) 198-206, May-Jun 1971
   000 Refs Exp Type Fr

                                                               464

Madonia T* Conticello S*
(Protective Possibilities of a Citrobioflavonoid Complex on Experimental
Labyrinthine Damage Caused by Dihydrostreptomycin in Guinea Pigs)
   Clin Otorinolaring 20 416-434, Sep-Oct 1968
   000 Refs Exp Type It Trans Summ

                                                               465

Ino H*
(Vestibular and Hearing Disturbances in Organic Mercury Poisoning)
   Otolaryngology (Tokyo) 42 (3) 165-170, Mar 1970
   000 Refs Clin Type Jap Trans Summ

466

Darrouzet MJ*
(Attempt to Protect the Organ of Corti against the Ototoxicity of Antibiotics)
    Acta Otolaryng (Stockholm) 63 Suppl 49-64, 1967
    000 Refs Exp Type Fr

467

Von Westernhagen B*
(Chronic Lead Poisoning -- Enzyme Histochemical Studies of the Internal Ear
of the Guinea Pig)
    Arch Klin Exp Ohr Nas Kehlkopfheilk 188 231-236, 1967
    022 Refs Exp Type Ger

468

Daigneault EA* Pruett JR* Brown RD*
Influence of Ototoxic Drugs on Acetylcholine-Induced Depression of the Cochlear N1 Potential
    Toxic Appl Pharmacol 17 (1) 223-230, Jul 1970
    012 Refs Exp Type Eng

469

Supacek I*
(Toxic Deafness due to Neomycin)
    Voix Silence 10 (1-4) 111-114, 1966
    000 Refs Art Type Fr Trans Summ

470

Fabre J*
(Drugs and Kidney Function)
    Helv Med Acta 34 Suppl 24-41, 1967
    000 Refs Clin Type Fr

471

Bussien R*
(Precautions in the Use of Gentamycin)
    Munchen Med Wschr 112 2-3, Aug 14 1970
    000 Refs Clin Type Ger Trans Summ

472

Vol'Fovskaia RN* Makulova ID*
(On the Problem of the Course of Angiodystonic State with Arterial Hypertension of Toxic Etiology)
    Gig Tr Prof Zabol 12 12-15, Nov 1968
    000 Refs Clin Type Rus Trans Summ

473

Dyer JR* Carter JH,2* Van Wyk PJ*
Catalytic Hydrogenation of Viomycin and Capreomycin
    J Med Chem 14 (11) 1120-1121, 1971
    009 Refs Exp Type Eng

474

Gingell JC* Waterworth PM*
Dose of Gentamicin in Patients with Normal Renal Function and Renal Impairment
    Brit Med J 2 (5596) 19-22, Apr 6 1968
    014 Refs Clin Type Eng

475

Anon*
Bacteriuria Again
    Brit Med J 1 (5745) 361-362, Feb 13 1971
    019 Refs Comment Type Eng

476

Ukleja Z*
(Protective Importance of Vitamin A on Toxic Action of Streptomycin on the
Inner Ear)

Otolaryng Pol 21 (5) 715-719, 1967
000 Refs Exp Histol Type Pol
Abstr. (Excer Med Sect 11 21 293, 1968)

477

El-Mofty A* El-Serafy S*
The Effect of Ototoxic Antibiotics on the Oxygen Uptake of the Membranous
Cochlea
Ann Otol 75 (1) 216-224, 1966
011 Refs Exp Type Eng

478

Serles W*
(Subject -- Recent Developments in ENT. Streptomycin Damage in the Electrony-
stagmogram)
Mschr Ohrenheilk 100 (6) 251-255, 1966
006 Refs Clin Type Ger
Abstr. (Excer Med Sect 11 20 108, 1967)

479

Klotz PL*
(Dangerous Drugs for the Ears)
Infirmiere 45 34-35, Dec 1967
000 Refs Art Type Fr

480

Nakamura F*
(Electron Microscopic Studies of Acid Phosphatase Activity in the Vestibular
Apparatus (With Special Reference to the Damage Caused by Streptomycin Sul-
fate))
J Otolaryng Jap 71 294-299, Mar 1968
000 Refs Exp Type Jap Trans Summ

481

Citron KM* De Silva DJ*
The Results of Tuberculosis Chemotherapy in Chest Clinic Practice
Tubercle 52 31-36, Mar 1971
007 Refs Clin Type Eng

482

D'Avino A* De Maio M* Marmo E*
Ricerche Sperimentali sulla Ototossicita di Alcuni Farmaci (Experimental
Research on Ototoxicity of Some Pharmaceuticals)
Minerva Otorinolaring 21 (4) 156-161, Jul-Aug 1971
006 Refs Exp Type It

483

Philip JR*
Untoward Effects of Antimicrobial Drugs. Prevention and Control
Postgrad Med 50 (5) 193-200, Nov 1971
000 Refs Art Type Eng

484

Savini EC* Moulin MA* Herrou MFJ*
(Experimental Study of Effects of Quinine on Rat, Rabbit, and Dog Fetuses)
Therapie 26 (3) 563-574, May-Jun 1971
027 Refs Exp Type Fr

485

Stupp HF*
(Studies on the Concentration of Aminoglycoside Antibiotics in the Labyrin-
thine Fluids and their Significance for the Specific Ototoxicity of the
Aminoglycoside Antibiotics)
Acta Otolaryng (Stockholm) Suppl 262, 1970
203 Refs Monogr Exp Type Ger
Abstr. (Yearb Ear Nose Throat 50-52, 1971)

486

Iinuma T*
(The Possible Effects of Various Ototoxic Drugs upon the ATP-hydrolyzing
System in the Stria Vascularis and Spiral Ligament of Guinea Pigs)
    J Otorhinolaryng Soc Jap 69 (10) 1698-1703, 1966
    000 Refs Exp Type Jap
    Abstr. (Excer Med Sect 11 20 250, 1967)

487

Teubner E*
Zur Prophylaxe der Streptomycinschaden des Ohres. Praktische Erfahrungen mit
dem 3-Frequenzaudiometer, Typ MA 4 (Prophylaxis of Damage to the Ear by
Streptomycin. Practical Experience with the 3-Frequency Audiometer, Type MA
4)
    Z Tuberk 125 (1-2) 44-50, 1966
    078 Refs Clin Type Ger
    Abstr. (Excer Med Sect 11 20 300, 1967)

488

Bac E*
Ototoksicnost Streptomicina (Ototoxicity of Streptomycin)
    Med Arh 20 (3) 105-110, 1966
    007 Refs Clin Type Ser Trans Summ
    Abstr. (Excer Med Sect 11 20 249, 1967)

489

Lundquist P-G* Wersall J*
Kanamycin-Induced Changes in Cochlear Hair Cells of the Guinea Pig
    Z Zellforsch 72 (4) 543-561, 1966
    021 Refs Exp Histol Type Eng

490

Johnsonbaugh RE* Drexler HG* Sutherland JM* Light IJ*
Audiometric Study of Streptomycin-Treated Infants
    Amer J Dis Child 112 (1) 43-45, Jul 1966
    008 Refs Clin Type Eng

491

Pellant A*
Vliv Ototoxickych Antibiotik na Otocystu Slepicino Zarodku (Effect of Ototoxic Antibiotics on Otocyst of Chicken Embryo)
    Cesk Otolaryng 17 (2) 71-77, 1968
    016 Refs Exp Histol Type Cz
    Abstr. (Excer Med Sect 11 21 723, 1968)

492

Portmann M* Darrouzet J* Aran J*
Etude Experimentale sur la Cellule de l'Organe de Corti Conditions Normales
et Pathologiques (An Experimental Study of the Cell of the Organ of Corti
under Normal and Pathological Conditions)
    Int Audiol 6 (3) 380-385, 1967
    004 Refs Exp Histol Type Fr
    Abstr. (Excer Med Sect 11 21 417, 1968)

493

Shida S* Sugano T* Okamoto M*
Some Observations on the Ototoxic Effect of Kanamycin
    Int Aud 6 (3) 359-364, 1967
    000 Refs Exp Histol Type Eng

494

Hoshino T*
(Experimental Study on the Possible Pathways of Kanamycin into the Inner Ear)
    J Otorhinolaryng Soc Jap 70 (3) 641-648, 1967
    000 Refs Exp Type Jap
    Abstr. (Excer Med Sect 11 21 666, 1968)

495

Stange G* Soda T* Beck C*

Elektrophysiologische Ergebnisse bei Ototoxicitatsminderung Basischer Streptomyces Antibiotica (Electrophysiological Data in Connection with the Decrease in the Ototoxicity of Alkaline Streptomyces Antibiotics)
    Arch Klin Exp Ohr Nas Kehlkopfheilk 188 (2) 242-249, 1967
    010 Refs Exp Type Ger
    Abstr. (Excer Med Sect 11 21 416, 1968)

496

Stupp H* Rauch S* Sous H* Brun JP* Lagler F*
Kanamycin Dosage and Levels in Ear and Other Organs
    Arch Otolaryng (Chicago) 86 (5) 515-521, 1967
    012 Refs Exp Type Eng

497

Girardi G* Cis C* Piatti A*
La Sindrome Nucleo-Reticolare Cronica nelle Intossicazioni Professionali (The
Nucleo-Reticular Syndrome in Professional Intoxications)
    Arch Ital Otol 78 (6) 756-770, 1967
    038 Refs Clin Type It
    Abstr. (Excer Med Sect 11 21 610, 1968)

498

Ruben RJ* Daly JF*
Neomycin Ototoxicity and Nephrotoxicity. A Case Report Following Oral Administration
    Laryngoscope 78 (10) 1734-1737, Oct 1968
    016 Refs Clin Type Eng

499

Robin IG*
Clinical Management of Peripheral Sensori-Neural Deafness
    Sound 3 (1) 12-13, Feb 1969
    000 Refs Art Type Eng

500

Fraser GR*
The Spectrum of Causation of Profound Deafness in Childhood
    J Otolaryng Soc Aust 2 (3) 25-33, Mar 1968
    000 Refs Art Type Eng

501

Hellstrom PE* Repo UK* Mattson K*
New Drugs in Tuberculosis
    Drugs 1 (5) 349-353, 1971
    000 Refs Art Type Eng

502

Anon*
Rifampicin -- A Review
    Drugs 1 (5) 345-398, 1971
    113 Refs Rev Type Eng

503

Barjon P* Fourcade J* Mimran A*
Surdite Transitoire et Acide Ethacrynique, Role Eventuel des Modifications de
Composition des Liquides Cochleaires (Transient Hearing Loss and Ethacrynic
Acid, Possible Part of Modifications in the Composition of Cochlear Fluids)
    Presse Med 79 (40) 1757, Sep 25 1971
    002 Refs Letter Type Fr

504

Wojnarowska-Kulesza W*
Przpadek Calkowitego Wyleczenia Uszkodenia Ucha Wewnetrznego (A Case of
Complete Cure of Injury to Internal Ear)
    Otolaryng Pol 23 (2) 229-231, 1969
    000 Refs Clin Type Pol

505

Ruben   RJ*
Congenital Hearing Loss. Part 1
   Maico Audiol Lib Ser 7 (2)   1968
   000 Refs Art Type Eng

506

Wersall   J* Lundquist P-G*
Ototoxic Drugs
   In -- A Symposium on Drugs and Sensory Functions 142-151 London, J and A
   Churchill Ltd 1968
   022 Refs Clin Exp Type Eng
   Abstr. (Aerospace Med Biol NASA SP-7011 60 80, 1968)

507

Lloyd-Mostyn RH* Lord IJ*
Ototoxicity of Intravenous Frusemide
   Lancet 2 (7734) 1156-1157, Nov 20 1971
   006 Refs Letter Clin Type Eng

508

Schroeder   DJ*
Alcohol and Disorientation--Related Responses.   1. Nystagmus and 'Vertigo'
during Caloric and Optokinetic Stimulation
   Okla City, Civil Aeromedical Inst   Feb 1971
   000 Refs Exp Type Eng

509

Durska-Zakrzewska A* Zakrzewski A*
(Long Term Results of Investigations on Hearing of Patients Treated with High
Doses of Streptomycin)
   Otolaryng Pol Suppl 47-50, 1970
   000 Refs Clin Type Pol Trans Summ

510

Von Westernhagen B*
Histochemisch Nachweisbare Stoffwechselveranderungen am Innenohr des Meersch-
weinchens nach Chronischer Arsenvergiftung (Histochemical Demonstration of
Changes of Metabolism in the Inner Ear of Guinea-Pig after Chronic Arsenic
Poisoning)
   Arch Klin Exp Ohr Nas Kehlkopfheilk 197 (1) 7-13, 1970
   033 Refs Exp Type Ger

511

David   DS* Hitzig P*
Diuretics and Ototoxicity
   New Eng J Med 284 (23) 1328-1329, Jun 10 1971
   002 Refs Letter Type Eng

512

Homer   MJ*
Deafness after Ethacrynic Acid
   New Eng J Med 285 (20) 1152, Nov 11 1971
   000 Refs Letter Type Eng

513

Wigand ME* Heidland A*
Ototoxic Side-Effects of High Doses of Frusemide in Patients with Uraemia
   Postgrad Med J 47 Suppl 54-56, Apr 1971
   000 Refs Clin Type Eng

514

Cantarovich F* Locatelli A* Fernandez JC* Loredo JP* Cristhot J*
Frusemide in High Doses in the Treatment of Acute Renal Failure
   Postgrad Med J 47 Suppl 13-17, Apr 1971
   020 Refs Clin Type Eng

515

Muth   RG*

Frusemide in Severe Renal Insufficiency
    Postgrad Med J 47 Suppl 21-25, Apr 1971
    000 Refs Clin Type Eng

516

Sullivan JF* Kreisberger C* Mittal AK*
Use of Frusemide in the Oliguria of Acute and Chronic Renal Failure
    Postgrad Med J 47 Suppl 26-28, Apr 1971
    005 Refs Clin Type Eng

517

Morelli OH* Moledo LI* Alanis E* Gaston OL* Terzaghi O*
Acute Effects of High Doses of Frusemide in Patients with Chronic Renal
Failure
    Postgrad Med J 47 Suppl 29-35, Apr 1971
    019 Refs Clin Type Eng

518

Muraveiskaya VS*
(Histological Studies on Vascular Cavity and Epithelium of Outer Spiral
Fissure in Guinea Pigs with Impaired Hearing due to Neomycin Treatment)
    Antibiotiki 16 (10) 920-923, Oct 1971
    007 Refs Exp Histol Type Rus Trans Summ

519

Hellstrom P-E* Repo UK*
Capreomycin, Ethambutol and Rifampicin in Apparently Incurable Pulmonary
Tuberculosis
    Scand J Resp Dis Suppl 69, 69-74, 1969
    001 Refs Clin Type Eng

520

Precerutti G* Vidi I*
Rilievo delle Risposte Evocate (EEA) in Condizioni Basali e dopo Somministra-
zione di Antibiotici nella Cavia Albina (Evoked Audiometry Response in Albino
Guinea Pig after Antibiotic Administration)
    Boll Soc Ital Biol Sper 47 (8) 231-233, Apr 30 1971
    010 Refs Exp Type It

521

Velikorussova NV* Eidelstein SI*
(Antibiotics and Hearing)
    Antibiotiki 16 180-184, 1971
    013 Refs Clin Type Rus Trans Summ

522

Byalik IB*
(Kanamycin and Florimycin in Therapy of Lung Tuberculosis)
    Antibiotiki 16 184-188, 1971
    011 Refs Clin Type Rus Trans Summ

523

Anon*
(Ototoxic Antibiotics)
    T Nor Laegeforen 90 1894, Oct 15 1970
    000 Refs Comment Type Nor

524

Richet G* Lopez de Novales E* Verroust P*
Drug Intoxication and Neurological Episodes in Chronic Renal Failure
    Brit Med J 2 (5706) 394-395, May 16 1970
    019 Refs Clin Type Eng

525

Nakai Y* Nakai S*
Ototoxic Effect of Nitromin and Some Congenital Deaf Animal Cochlea. An
Electron Microscopical Study
    Arch Klin Exp Ohr Nas Kehlkopfheilk 198 325-338, 1971

023 Refs Exp Histol Type Eng

526

Pietruski J*
The Effect of Ethyl Alcohol on Permeation of NA-24 Sodium into the Perilymph
Acta Otolaryng (Stockholm) 71 494-499, 1971
013 Refs Exp Type Eng

527

Eidelberg E* Bond ML* Kelter A*
Effects of Alcohol on Cerebellar and Vestibular Neurones
Arch Int Pharmacodyn 192 213-219, 1971
018 Refs Exp Type Eng

528

Yuce K* Van Rooyen CE*
Carbenicillin and Gentamicin in the Treatment of Pseudomonas Aeruginosa
Infection
Canad Med Ass J 105 (9) 919-922, Nov 6 1971
025 Refs Clin Type Eng

529

Vernier VG* Alleva FR*
The Bioassay of Kanamycin Auditory Toxicity
Arch Int Pharmacodyn 176 (1) 59-73, Nov 1968
024 Refs Exp Type Eng

530

Haiat R*
(Clinical Experiences with Carbochromen in Almost 500 Patients)
Arzneimittelforschung 20 465-467, Mar 1970
000 Refs Clin Type Ger

531

Knotkova V* Vacek J* Beran M*
(Neurotoxic Effect of Lincomycin in a Patient after Bilateral Nephrectomy)
Bratisl Lek Listy 53 (4) 433-440, Apr 1970
003 Refs Clin Type Cz Trans Summ

532

Latkowski B* Radomska M* Szulc-Kuberska J*
(A Case of Acute Intoxication with 'Nitro' Solvent with Manifestations of
Damage to the Vestibular Organ)
Pol Tyg Lek 24 (7) 238-239, Feb 18 1969
005 Refs Clin Type Pol Trans Summ

533

Sliwowska W*
(Vestibulo-Cochlear Disturbances in the Course of Paroxysmal Atrial Fibrilla-
tion)
Pol Tyg Lek 25 (51) 1995-1996, Dec 21 1970
011 Refs Clin Type Pol Trans Summ

534

Line DH* Poole GW* Waterworth PM*
Serum Streptomycin Levels and Dizziness
Tubercle 51 (1) 76-81, Mar 1970
005 Refs Clin Type Eng

535

Stradling P* Poole GW*
Twice-Weekly Streptomycin plus Isoniazid for Tuberculosis
Tubercle 51 (1) 44-47, Mar 1970
005 Refs Clin Type Eng

536

Pande BR* Martischnig KM* Feinmann L*
A Two-Year Follow-Up of 181 Sputum-Positive Tuberculosis Patients Treated in

Gateshead between 1961 and 1966
   Tubercle 51 (1) 39-43, Mar 1970
   011 Refs Clin Type Eng

537

East African-British Medical Research Council Fifth Thiacetazone Investiga-
tion*
Isoniazid with Thiacetazone (Thioacetazone) in the Treatment of Pulmonary
Tuberculosis in East Africa--Fifth Investigation. A Co-Operative Study in
East African Hospitals, Clinics and Laboratories with the Collaboration of
the East African and British Medical Research Councils
   Tubercle 51 (2) 123-151, Jun 1970
   019 Refs Clin Type Eng

538

Newman R* Doster B* Murray FJ* Ferebee S*
Rifampin in Initial Treatment of Pulmonary Tuberculosis. A U.S. Public Health
Service Tuberculosis Therapy Trial
   Amer Rev Resp Dis 103 (4) 461-476, Apr 1971
   008 Refs Clin Type Eng

539

Federspil P*
Ubersicht uber die in Deutschland Beobachteten Falle von Gentamycin-Ototoxi-
citat (A Review of Gentamicin Ototoxicity Observed in Germany)
   HNO 19 (11) 328-331, Nov 1971
   000 Refs Rev Type Ger Trans Summ

540

Nakamura S* Murakami Y* Tsunoda Y* Katano A*
(Cytotoxic Effect of Nitrogen Mustard Compounds in the Cochlear Cells and the
Development of the Secondary Course)
   J Otolaryng Jap 72 370-371, Feb 20 1969
   000 Refs Exp Histol Type Jap Trans Summ

541

Gayford JJ* Redpath TH*
The Side-Effects of Carbamazepine
   Proc Roy Soc Med 62 615-616, Jun 1969
   016 Refs Art Type Eng

542

Khanna BK* Bhatia ML*
Congenital Deaf Mutism Following Streptomycin Therapy to Mother during Pregnancy. A Case of Streptomycin Ototoxicity in Utero
   Indian J Chest Dis 11 51-53, Jan 1969
   000 Refs Clin Type Eng

543

Bodi S* Palfalvi L*
(Temporary Hearing Disorders due to the Administration of Drugs)
   Mschr Ohrenheilk 103 (4) 156-161, 1969
   015 Refs Clin Type Ger Trans Summ

544

Delaude A* Albarede JL* Girard M* Dirat J* Puel J*
(Ethambutol in the Treatment of Pulmonary Tuberculosis (Experience of 70
Cases))
   Rev Tuberc (Paris) 31 (7) 1035-1053, Nov 1967
   081 Refs Rev Clin Type Fr

545

Cairella M* Marasa G*
Aggiornamenti in Tema di Terapia con Chemioantibiotici (Refresher Notes on
Antibiotic Therapy)
   Clin Ter 49 (2) 167-180, 1969
   000 Refs Rev Clin Type It Trans Summ

594   CITATION SECTION

546

Wersall J* Bjorkroth B* Flock A* Lundquist P-G*
Sensory Hair Fusion in Vestibular Sensory Cells after Gentamycin Exposure. A
Transmission and Scanning Electron Microscope Study
   Arch Klin Exp Ohr Nas Kehlkopfheilk 200 (1) 1-14, 1971
   011 Refs Exp Histol Type Eng

547

Matz GJ* Beal DD* Krames L*
Ototoxicity of Ethacrynic Acid. Demonstrated in a Human Temporal Bone
   Arch Otolaryng (Chicago) 90 152-155, Aug 1969
   003 Refs Clin Exp Histol Type Eng

548

Witzel L*
(Reversible Nonfunctioning of the Vestibular Apparatus Following Gentamicin)
   Munchen Med Wschr 112 Suppl 52, Dec 25 1970
   000 Refs Clin Type Ger Trans Summ

549

Vasiliev NA*
(Toxicity to the Cochleovestibular Apparatus during Antibiotic Therapy)
   Klin Med 47 (9) 61-65, 1969
   015 Refs Clin Type Rus Trans Summ

550

Mapelli A* Precerutti G*
(Studies on the Etiology of the Acoustic Damage after Anesthesia)
   Boll Mal Orecch Gola Naso 87 (5) 371-380, 1969
   015 Refs Exp Type It

551

Tsuiki T* Murai S*
Familial Incidence of Streptomycin Hearing Loss and Hereditary Weakness of
Cochlea
   Audiology 10 (5-6) 315-322, Sep-Dec 1971
   003 Refs Clin Type Eng

552

Mostyn RHL*
Tinnitus and Propranolol
   Brit Med J 2 (5659) 766, Jun 21 1969
   001 Refs Letter Clin Type Eng

553

Smith CA* Steinhaus JE* Haynes CD*
The Safety and Effectiveness of Intravenous Regional Anesthesia
   Southern Med J 61 1057-1060, Oct 1968
   015 Refs Exp Type Eng

554

Eggemann G* Roschig M* Matschiner H* Bruchmuller W*
(Inversvoltametric Lead Determination in the Inner Ear)
   Arch Klin Exp Ohr Nas Kehlkopfheilk 200 125-131, 1971
   023 Refs Exp Type Ger

555

Bloom C*
Capreomycin Laboratory Studies
   Antibiot Chemother 16 1-9, 1970
   005 Refs Exp Type Eng

556

Lucchesi M*
The Antimycobacterial Activity of Capreomycin
   Antibiot Chemother 16 27-31, 1970
   000 Refs Clin Exp Type Eng

557
Wilson TM*
Clinical Experience with Ethambutol
    Antibiot Chemother 16 222-229, 1970
    000 Refs Clin Type Eng

558
Krivinka R* Tousek J*
The First Clinical Experiences with Ethambutol in Chronic Pulmonary Tubercu-
losis and Basilar Meningitis
    Antibiot Chemother 16 215-221, 1970
    000 Refs Clin Type Eng

559
Pathy MS*
The Use, Action and Side Effects of Diuretics
    Geront Clin (Basel) 13 (5) 261-268, 1971
    020 Refs Rev Type Eng

560
Maekawa N*
(Side Effects of Antituberculosis Agents)
    Bull Chest Dis Res Inst Kyoto Univ 4 (2) 70-76, 51, Mar 1971
    020 Refs Clin Type Jap Trans Summ

561
Kanzaki J* Okada J* Saga J* Nameki H*
(A Longitudinal Study on Deafened Persons Treated in Tochigi Prefecture)
    Audiol Jap 13 (1) 25-36, 1970
    000 Refs Clin Type Jap
    Abstr. (Excer Med Sect 11 24 252, 1971)

562
Matsuura S* Furukawa T*
(The Effects of Metabolic Inhibitors and Some Other Drugs on the Microphonic
Potential of Goldfish Sacculus)
    J Physiol Soc Jap 32 (7) 414-415, 1970
    000 Refs Exp Type Jap
    Abstr. (Excer Med Sect 11 24 412, 1971)

563
Necker R*
(On the Origin of the Cochlear Potentials in Birds -- Effects of Oxygen
Deficiency, Cyanide Poisoning and Cooling as well as Observations on the
Spatial Distribution)
    Z Vergl Physiol 69 (4) 367-425, 1970
    074 Refs Exp Type Ger
    Abstr. (Excer Med Sect 11 24 351-352, 1971)

564
Goldman S* Brzakovic N* Muzikravic T*
Clinical and Bacteriological Results with Myambutol
    Antibiot Chemother 16 239-256, 1970
    019 Refs Clin Type Eng

565
Sato Y* Mizukoshi O* Daly JF*
Microrespirometry of the Membranous Cochlea and Ototoxicity in Vitro
    Ann Otol 78 (6) 1201-1209, Dec 1969
    020 Refs Exp Type Eng

566
Tanaka Y* Brown PG*
Action of Metabolic Inhibitors and Energy-Rich Phosphate Compounds on Coch-
lear Potentials
    Ann Otol 79 (2) 338-351, Apr 1970
    020 Refs Exp Type Eng

567

Van den Bercken J* Akkermans LMA*
Negative Temperature Coefficient of the Action of DDT in a Sense Organ
    Europ J Pharmacol 16 (2) 241-244, Oct 1971
    014 Refs Exp Type Eng

568

Kropp R* Jungbluth H* Radenbach KL*
Influence of Capreomycin on Renal Function. Preliminary Results
    Antibiot Chemother 16 59-68, 1970
    023 Refs Clin Type Eng

569

Schutz I* Radenbach KL* Bartmann K*
The Combination of Ethambutol, Capreomycin and a Third Drug in Chronic Pulmonary Tuberculosis with Bacterial Polyresistance
    Antibiot Chemother 16 43-58, 1970
    028 Refs Clin Type Eng

570

Anon*
Discussion on Capreomycin
    Antibiot Chemother 16 73-83, 1970
    000 Refs Clin Type Eng

571

Felgenhauer F* Lagler F*
Experimental Animal Investigations with Rifampicin on the Question of its
Influence on the Vestibular System and its Period of Retention in the Peri-
lymph of the Inner Ear
    Antibiot Chemother 16 361-368, 1970
    002 Refs Exp Type Eng

572

Collins WE* Schroeder DJ* Gilson RD* Guedry FE,Jr*
Effects of Alcohol Ingestion on Tracking Performance during Angular Acceleration
    J Applied Psychol 55 (6) 559-563, 1971
    010 Refs Exp Type Eng

573

Igarashi M* Lundquist P-G* Alford BR* Miyata H*
Experimental Ototoxicity of Gentamicin in Squirrel Monkeys
    J Infect Dis 124 Suppl 114-124, Dec 1971
    008 Refs Exp Histol Type Eng

574

Waitz JA* Moss EL,Jr* Weinstein MJ*
Aspects of the Chronic Toxicity of Gentamicin Sulfate in Cats
    J Infect Dis 124 Suppl 125-129, Dec 1971
    010 Refs Exp Type Eng

575

Jackson GG* Arcieri G*
Ototoxicity of Gentamicin in Man -- A Survey and Controlled Analysis of
Clinical Experience in the United States
    J Infect Dis 124 Suppl 130-137, Dec 1971
    018 Refs Clin Type Eng

576

Webster JC* Carroll R* Benitez JT* Mc Gee TM*
Ototoxicity of Topical Gentamicin in the Cat
    J Infect Dis 124 Suppl 138-144, Dec 1971
    004 Refs Exp Histol Type Eng

577

Cox CE* Harrison LH*
Comparison of Gentamicin and Polymyxin B-Kanamycin in Therapy of Bacteremia

due to Gram-Negative Bacilli
   J Infect Dis 124   Suppl 156-163, Dec 1971
   019 Refs Clin Type Eng

578

Mc Henry MC* Gavan TL* Van Ommen RA* Hawk WA*
Therapy with Gentamicin for Bacteremic Infections -- Results with 53 Patients
   J Infect Dis 124   Suppl 164-173, Dec 1971
   021 Refs Clin Type Eng

579

Haghbin M* Armstrong D* Murphy ML*
Intravenous Gentamicin for Infectious Complications in Children with Acute
Leukemia
   J Infect Dis 124   Suppl 192-197, Dec 1971
   016 Refs Clin Type Eng

580

Garfunkel JM*
Use of Gentamicin in Newborn Infants
   J Infect Dis 124   Suppl 247-248, Dec 1971
   002 Refs Clin Type Eng

581

Newman RL* Holt RJ*
Gentamicin in Pediatrics. 1. Report on Intrathecal Gentamicin
   J Infect Dis 124   Suppl 254-256, Dec 1971
   001 Refs Clin Type Eng

582

Holt RJ* Newman RL*
Gentamicin in Pediatrics. 2. Treatment of Severe Urinary-Tract Infections
Caused by Gram-Negative Bacilli and of Staphylococcal Infections
   J Infect Dis 124   Suppl 257-258, Dec 1971
   002 Refs Clin Type Eng

583

Howard JE* Donoso E* Mimica I* Zilleruelo G*
Gentamicin in Infections in Infants with Low Birthweights
   J Infect Dis 124   Suppl 232-233, Dec 1971
   001 Refs Clin Type Eng

584

Howard JE* Donoso E* Mimica I* Zilleruelo G*
Gentamicin for Urinary-Tract Infections in Infants
   J Infect Dis 124   Suppl 234-235, Dec 1971
   001 Refs Clin Type Eng

585

Riley HD,Jr* Rubio T* Hinz W* Nunnery AW* Englund J*
Clinical and Laboratory Evaluation of Gentamicin in Infants and Children
   J Infect Dis 124   Suppl 236-246, Dec 1971
   019 Refs Clin Type Eng

586

Abston S* Capen DA* Clement RL* Larson DL*
Gentamicin for Septicemia in Patients with Burns
   J Infect Dis 124   Suppl 275-277, Dec 1971
   000 Refs Clin Type Eng

587

Mac Millan BG*
Ecology of Bacteria Colonizing the Burned Patient Given Topical and Systemic
Gentamicin Therapy -- A Five-Year Study
   J Infect Dis 124   Suppl 278-286, Dec 1971
   007 Refs Clin Type Eng

588

Felarca AB* Laqui EM* Ibarra LM*
Gentamicin in Gonococcal Urethritis of Filipino Males -- Dosage and Response
    J Infect Dis 124 Suppl 287-292, Dec 1971
    007 Refs Clin Type Eng

589

Boxerbaum B* Pittman S* Doershuk CF* Stern RC* Matthews LW*
Use of Gentamicin in Children with Cystic Fibrosis
    J Infect Dis 124 Suppl 293-295, Dec 1971
    004 Refs Clin Type Eng

590

Rossi P* Matzeu M* Bracci C*
L'Attivita Antimicrobatterica in Vivo e in Vitro della Capreomicina (In Vivo
and in Vitro Antimycobacterial Activity of Capreomycin)
    Ann Ist Forlanini 28 (2) 116-125, 1968
    000 Refs Exp Type It

591

Wilson TM*
Capreomycin and Ethambutol
    Practitioner 199 (1194) 817-824, 1967
    000 Refs Clin Type Eng

592

Cada K*
(Side Effect of Some Drugs in Otolaryngology)
    Cesk Otolaryng 20 (1) 33-38, 1971
    000 Refs Art Type Cz Trans Summ

593

Boudin G* Pepin B* Decroix G* Vernant JC*
Intoxication par la Diphenylhydantoine Declenchee par un Traitement Antituberculeux (A Propos de Deux Observations) (Intoxication by Diphenylhydantoin
during Antituberculous Treatment (Concerning 2 Cases))
    Ann Med Interne 122 (8-9) 855-860, Aug-Sep 1971
    027 Refs Clin Type Fr

594

Katz N* Pellegrino J* Oliveira CA* Cunha AS*
Experimental Chemotherapy of Schistosomiasis. 2. Laboratory and Clinical
Trials with A-16612, a Piperazine Derivative
    J Parasit 53 (6) 1229-1232, Dec 1967
    006 Refs Clin Type Eng

595

Brun J* Perrin-Fayolle M* Sedallian A*
La Gentamycine en Pneumologie. Etude Clinique et Bacteriologique (Gentamicin
in Pneumology. A Clinical and Bacteriological Study)
    Lyon Med 218 (4) 1263-1270, 1967
    000 Refs Clin Type Fr

596

Done AK* Temple AR*
Treatment of Salicylate Poisoning
    Mod Treatm 8 (3) 528-551, Aug 1971
    017 Refs Art Type Eng

597

Arena JM*
General Principles of Treatment and Specific Antidotes
    Mod Treatm 8 (3) 461-502, Aug 1971
    016 Refs Art Type Eng

598

Lafaix C* Rey M* Diop Mar I* Nouhouayl A*
Essai de Traitement Curatif du Paludisme pour un Nouvel Antipaludique de
Synthese, le 16-126 RP (Test of Curative Treatment of Malaria with a New

Synthetic Antimalarial, 16-126 RP)
    Bull Soc Med Afr Noire Lang Franc 12 (3) 546-551, 1967
    000 Refs Clin Type Fr

599

Naumann P* Auwarter W*
(Pharmacologic and Therapeutic Properties of Gentamycin. Experimental Studies
on Drug Level, Excretion, Stability, and Therapeutic Indications)
    Arzneimittelforschung 18 (9) 1119-1123, 1968
    020 Refs Clin Exp Type Ger

600

Muller FE*
Chemotherapie der Pseudomonas-Infektion bei Schwerverbrannten
    Deutsch Med Wschr 93 (35) 1637-1641, 1968
    015 Refs Clin Type Ger

601

Ueda Y*
Indication for Kanamycin Therapy in Various Infections in Medicine
    Asian Med J 11 (5) 302-308, 1968
    000 Refs Clin Type Eng

602

Yad MI* Quraishi SM*
Streptomycin vs. Dihydrostreptomycin. A Comparative Study of Toxic Effects on
the Eighth Nerve
    Pak Med Rev 2 (9) 13-28, 1967
    000 Refs Clin Type Eng

603

Schroeder JM* Weeth JB*
Phase 2. Evaluation of Fluorometholone (NSC-33001)
    Cancer Chemother Rep 51 (7) 525-534, 1967
    019 Refs Clin Type Eng

604

Borg E* Moller AR*
Effect of Ethylalcohol and Pentobarbital Sodium on the Acoustic Middle Ear
Reflex in Man
    Acta Otolaryng (Stockholm) 64 (5-6) 415-426, 1967
    023 Refs Exp Type Eng

605

Wagman GH* Oden EM* Weinstein MJ* Irwin S*
Effect of Calcium on the Toxicity of Gentamicin
    Antimicrob Agents Chemother-1966 175-181, 1967
    011 Refs Exp Type Eng

606

Anon*
Discussion
    J Infect Dis 119 427-431, 1969
    000 Refs Clin Type Eng

607

Mc Kenzie IFC* Mathew TH* Bailie MJ*
Peritoneal Dialysis in the Treatment of Quinine Overdose
    Med J Aust 55 (2) 58-59, Jan 13 1968
    014 Refs Clin Type Eng

608

Lampe I* Szucs J*
(Some Problems of the Hearing Damaging Role of Ototoxic Antibiotics)
    Tuberk Tudobet (Budapest) 21 (6) 178-181, Jun 1968
    012 Refs Clin Type Hun Trans Summ

609

Naumann P* Hubmann R*
Zur Antibakteriellen Therapie Urologischer Infektionen (The Antibacterial
Therapy of Urinary Tract Infections)
    Urologie 7 (1) 16-23, Jan-Feb 1968
    047 Refs Rev Type Ger Trans Summ

610

Konig K* May P*
Die Behandlung der Urogenitaltuberkulose mit Neuren Medikamenten (The Treatment of Urogenital Tuberculosis with New Drugs)
    Urologie 7 (1) 23-29, Jan-Feb 1968
    047 Refs Art Type Ger Trans Summ

611

Draskovich E*
Adatok a Neomycin Ototoxicitasahoz (Data of (sic) the Ototoxicity of Neomycin)
    Orv Hetil 109 (18) 969-971,   1968
    017 Refs Clin Type Hun

612

Carrero N*
Las Sorderas Toxicas Estreptomicinicas (Continuacion) (Toxic Streptomycin
Deafness (Continuation))
    Galicia Clin 40 (4) 263-288, Apr 1968
    110 Refs Rev Type Sp

613

Knothe J* Flach M* Seidel P*
Die Wirkung von Kokain und Tetracain auf die Elektrische Aktivitat der Meers-
chweinchencochlea (MP.AP) (The Effect of Cocaine and Tetracaine on the Elec-
tric Activity of the Guinea Pig Cochlea (MP.AP))
    Z Laryng Rhinol Otol 47 (6) 434-441, Jun 1967
    013 Refs Exp Type Ger Trans Summ

614

Pines A* Raafat H* Plucinski K* Greenfield JSB* Solari M*
Antibiotic Regimens in Severe and Acute Purulent Exacerbations of Chronic
Bronchitis
    Brit Med J 2 (5607) 735-738, Jun 22 1968
    017 Refs Clin Type Eng

615

Miller AB*
Thiacetazone Toxicity -- A General Review
    Tubercle 49 Suppl 54-56, Mar 1968
    005 Refs Clin Type Eng

616

Wright IM*
An Experimental Study of Gentamicin Ototoxicity
    Int Aud 7 (4) 393-394,   1968
    000 Refs Exp Histol Type Eng

617

Fujii R*
The Present Appraisal of Kanamycin in Pediatrics
    Asian Med J 11 (3) 162-172,   1968
    006 Refs Clin Type Eng

618

Gomi J*
The Treatment of Pulmonary Tuberculosis with Kanamycin
    Asian Med J 11 (3) 173-180,   1968
    000 Refs Clin Type Eng

619

Cooperative Study Unit on Chemotherapy of Tuberculosis of the National Sana-

toria in Japan*
Comparison between High Daily Dosage of Isoniazid in Divided Doses and Low
Daily Dosage in a Single Dose in Triple-Drug Regimens
    Tubercle 49 (2) 170-179, 1968
    012 Refs Clin Type Eng

                                                                      620

Ukleja Z* Lipowska-Pawlak K*
(Toxic Effects of Streptomycin on the Nerve Cells of Vermis Cerebelli in
Pigeons)
    Otolaryng Pol 23 (5) 507-512, 1969
    028 Refs Exp Type Pol Trans Summ

                                                                      621

Suarez FJR* Calderon ED*
Evaluacion Critica de las Drogas Ototoxicas (Critical Evaluation of Ototoxic
Drugs)
    Rev Med Hosp Colonia 18 (100) 189-195, Nov-Dec 1969
    020 Refs Art Type Sp

                                                                      622

Anon*
Rifampin
    Med Lett Drugs Ther 12 (9) 37-38, May 1 1970
    008 Refs Art Type Eng

                                                                      623

Anon*
Nalidixic Acid
    Med Lett Drugs Ther 12 (11) 46-47, May 29 1970
    002 Refs Art Type Eng

                                                                      624

Anon*
Carbenicillin and Other Antibiotics for Therapy of Pseudomonas Infections
    Med Lett Drugs Ther 12 (25) 101-103, Dec 11 1970
    006 Refs Art Type Eng

                                                                      625

Muth RG*
Diuretic Response to Furosemide in the Presence of Renal Insufficiency
    JAMA 195 (12) 1066-1069, Mar 21 1966
    012 Refs Clin Type Eng

                                                                      626

Atlas E* Turck M*
Laboratory and Clinical Evaluation of Rifampicin
    Amer J Med Sci 256 247-254, Oct 1968
    011 Refs Clin Type Eng

                                                                      627

Hammond V*
Perceptive Deafness in Adults
    Brit Med J 2 (5708) 523-525, May 30 1970
    000 Refs Art Clin Exp Type Eng

                                                                      628

Bodey GP* Middleman E* Umsawasdi T* Rodriguez V*
Intravenous Gentamicin Therapy for Infections in Patients with Cancer
    J Infect Dis 124 Suppl 174-179, Dec 1971
    011 Refs Clin Type Eng

                                                                      629

Andrial M*
General Survey of Clinical Experience with Gentamicin. Study of 285 Patients
Treated in the USA
    Ther Umsch Suppl 1, 27-31, 1969
    004 Refs Art Type Eng

630

Okihiro MM*
Neurological Complications of Antibiotic Therapy
   Straub Clin Proc 34 (3) 72-77, 1968
   000 Refs Clin Type Eng

631

Aleksiev N* Cernev B* Geron E*
(Results and Side Reactions in the Treatment of Recent Cavernous Pulmonary
Tuberculosis with Bulgarian Streptomycin)
   Ftiziatria (Sofiya) 5 (4) 170-176, 1968
   000 Refs Clin Type Bul Trans Summ

632

Aufdermaur F* Tonz O* Mathis A* Graf K*
Wirkung und Nebenwirkungen von Gentamicin bei Schweren Erkrankungen des
Neugeborenen
   Helv Paediat Acta Suppl 21, 21, 1970
   000 Refs Clin Comment Type Ger

633

Hechtermans R*
Resultats de l'Utilisation de la Kanacillin dans le Traitement de Certains
Etats Infectieux en Gynecologie (Results of the Use of Kanamycin in the
Treatment of Certain Infectious Gynecologic Conditions)
   Bull Soc Roy Belg Gynec Obstet 39 (3) 181-202, 1969
   000 Refs Clin Type Fr

634

Grosset J* Benhassine M*
(Thiacetazone (Tb1) -- Recent Clinical and Experimental Data)
   Bibl Tuberc 26 107-153, 1970
   000 Refs Clin Exp Type Fr

635

Ohtani I* Ishida H* Ogawa Y* Ouchi J*
(The Experimental Study on the Effect of Thiamine Derivative on Kanamycin
Ototoxicity)
   Audiol Jap 13 (1) 49-53, 1970
   000 Refs Exp Type Jap Trans Summ

636

Harada Y*
The Influence of Quinine on the Ampullar Receptors of the Isolated Posterior
Semicircular Canal of the Frog
   Acta Otolaryng 69 (3) 200-205, Mar 1970
   012 Refs Exp Type Eng

637

Boehncke H* Wieczorek A*
Ertaubung nach Anwendung Eines Penizillin-Streptomyzin-Kombinationspraparates
   Chir Praxis 14 (3) 493-494, 1970
   009 Refs Art Clin Type Ger

638

Preobrazhensky BS* Tsukanova VN*
(General Therapeutic Use of Some Antibiotics as a Cause of Persistent Deafness and Impaired Hearing)
   Ter Arkh 42 (9) 48-52, 1970
   000 Refs Clin Type Rus Trans Summ

639

Delonca K*
Statistics on Injectable Gentamicin
   Paris, Unilaob 1967
   000 Refs Art Type Eng

Excer Med
  Excerpta Medica
Exp Neurol
  Experimental Neurology (New York)
Eye Ear Nose Throat Monthly
  Eye, Ear, Nose and Throat Monthly
  (Chicago)
Fed Proc
  Federation Proceedings (Bethesda)
Fortschr Med
  Fortschritte der Medizin
Ftiziatria (Sofiya)
  Ftiziatria (Sofiya)
Fysiat Reum Vestn
  Fysiatricky a Reumatologicky
  Vestnik (Praha)
Galicia Clin
  Galicia-Clinica
Geront Clin (Basel)
  Gerontologia Clinica (Basel)
Gig Sanit
  Gigiena i Sanitariia (Moskva)
Gig Tr Prof Zabol
  Gigiena Truda i Professional'nye
  Zabolevania (Moskva)
Gruzlica
  Gruzlica i Choroby Pluc (Warsza-
  wa)
Helv Med Acta
  Helvetica Medica Acta (Basel)
Helv Paediat Acta
  Helvetica Paediatrica Acta (Ba-
  sel)
Hiroshima J Med Sci
  Hiroshima Journal of Medical
  Sciences
HNO
  HNO -- Wegweiser fur die Fachaer-
  ztliche Praxis (Berlin)
Hospital (Rio)
  Hospital (Rio de Janeiro)
Indian J Chest Dis
  Indian Journal of Chest Diseases
  (Delhi)
Indian J Med Res
  Indian Journal of Medical Re-
  search (New Delhi)
Indian J Tuberc
  Indian Journal of Tuberculosis
Infirmiere
  Infirmiere
Int Anesth Clin
  International Anesthesiology
  Clinics (Boston)
Int Aud
  International Audiology (Leiden)
Int Audiol
  International Audiology (Leiden)
J Applied Psychol
  Journal of Applied Psychology
  (Washington)
J Aud Res
  Journal of Auditory Research
J Bone Joint Surg (Amer)
  Journal of Bone and Joint Sur-
  gery, American Volume (Boston)
J Clin Pharmacol and New Drugs
  Journal of Clinical Pharmacology

New Drugs (Stamford, Conn)
J Franc Otorhinolaryng
  Journal Francais d'Oto-Rhino-
  Laryngologie, Audio-Phonologie et
  Chirurgie Maxillo-Faciale (Lyon)
J Histochem Cytochem
  Journal of Histochemistry and
  Cytochemistry (Baltimore)
J Indian Med Ass
  Journal of the Indian Medical
  Association (Calcutta)
J Indiana Med Ass
  Journal of the Indiana Medical
  Association
J Infect Dis
  Journal of Infectious Diseases
  (Chicago)
J Jap Med Ass
  Journal of the Japanese Medical
  Association
J Laryng
  Journal of Laryngology and Otolo-
  gy (London)
J Louisiana Med Soc
  Journal of the Louisiana State
  Medical Society (New Orleans)
J Maine Med Ass
  Journal of the Maine Medical
  Association
J Med Bordeaux
  Journal de Medecine de Bordeaux
  et du Sud-Ouest
J Med Chem
  Journal of Medicinal Chemistry
  (Washington)
J Otolaryng Jap
  Journal of Otolaryngology of
  Japan (Tokyo)
J Otolaryng Jap Abstr
  Journal of Otolaryngology of
  Japan (Tokyo) Abstracts
J Otolaryng Soc Aust
  Journal of the Oto-Laryngological
  Society of Australia (Melbourne)
J Otorhinolaryng Soc Jap
  Journal of the Oto-Rhino-Laryngo-
  logical Society of Japan (Tokyo)
J Parasit
  Journal of Parasitology (Chicago)
J Path Bact
  Journal of Pathology and Bac-
  teriology (London)
J Pediat
  Journal of Pediatrics (St Louis)
J Physiol Soc Jap
  Journal of the Physiological
  Society of Japan (Tokyo)
J Speech Hear Dis
  Journal of Speech and Hearing
  Disorders (Danville, Ill)
J Tenn Med Ass
  Journal of the Tennessee Medical
  Association
JAMA
  Journal of the American Medical
  Association (Chicago)
Jap J Physiol
  Japanese Journal of Physiology

(Kyoto)
Klin Mbl Augenheilk
   Klinische Monatsblaetter fur
   Augenheilkunde (Stuttgart)
Klin Med
   Klinicheskaia Meditsina (Moskva)
Lakartidningen
   Lakartidningen (Stockholm)
Lancet
   Lancet (London)
Laryngoscope
   Laryngoscope (St. Louis)
Laval Med
   Laval Medical (Quebec)
Lyon Med
   Lyon Medical
Maico Audiol Lib Ser
   Maico Audiological Library Series
Maroc Med
   Maroc Medical (Casablanca)
Med Ann Dc
   Medical Annals of the District of
   Columbia
Med Arh
   Medicinski Arhiv (Sarajevo)
Med Clin N Amer
   Medical Clinics of North America
   (Philadelphia)
Med Hyg (Geneve)
   Medecine et Hygiene (Geneve)
Med J Aust
   Medical Journal of Australia
   (Sydney)
Med Lett Drugs Ther
   Medical Letter on Drugs and
   Therapeutics (New York)
Med Times
   Medical Times (Manhasset)
Med Trib
   Medical Tribune (New York)
Med Welt (Stuttgart)
   Medizinische Welt (Stuttgart)
Med World News
   Medical World News (New York)
Minerva Otolaring
   Minerva Otorinolaringologica
   (Torino)
Minerva Otorinolaring
   Minerva Otorinolaringologica
   (Torino)
Minn Med
   Minnesota Medicine (St Paul)
Mod Treatm
   Modern Treatment (New York)
Mschr Kinderheilk
   Monatsschrift fur Kinderheilkunde
   (Berlin)
Mschr Ohrenheilk
   Monatsschrift fur Ohrenheilkunde
   und Laryngo-Rhinologie (Wien)
Munchen Med Wschr
   Munchener Medizinische Wochensch-
   rift
Nature (London)
   Nature (London)
NEB St Med J
   Nebraska State Medical Journal
Ned T Geneesk

   Nederlands Tijdschrift voor
   Geneeskunde (Amsterdam)
Nervenarzt
   Der Nervenarzt (Berlin)
Neurol Neurochir Pol
   Neurologia i Neurochirurgia
   Polska (Warszawa)
New Eng J Med
   New England Journal of Medicine
   (Boston)
New Zeal Med J
   New Zealand Medical Journal
   (Wellington)
Nord Med
   Nordisk Medicin (Stockholm)
NY J Med
   New York State Journal of Medi-
   cine (New York)
Orv Hetil
   Orvosi Hetilap (Budapest)
Orvoskepzes
   Orvoskepzes
Otol Fukuoka
   Otologia Fukuoka (Tokyo)
Otolaryng Pol
   Otolaryngologia Polska (Warszawa)
Otolaryngology (Tokyo)
   Otolaryngology (Tokyo)
Otologia Fukuoka (Tokyo)
   Otologia Fukuoka (Japan)
Pak J Surg Gynaec Obstet
   The Pakistan Journal of Surgery.
   Gynaecology and Obstetrics
Pak Med Rev
   Pakistan Medical Review
Panminerva Med
   Panminerva Medica (Torino)
Pediat Clin N Amer
   Pediatric Clinics of North Ameri-
   ca (Philadelphia)
Pediatrics
   Pediatrics (Springfield, Ill)
Pediatrie
   Pediatrie (Lyon)
Pharmacologist
   The Pharmacologist
Pluc Bolest Tuberk
   Plucne Bolesti i Tuberkuloza
   (Beograd)
Pneumonologie
   Pneumonologie (Berlin)
Pol Med J
   Polish Medical Journal (Warszawa)
Pol Tyg Lek
   Polski Tygodnik Lekarski (Warsza-
   wa)
Postgrad Med
   Postgraduate Medicine (Minneapo-
   lis)
Postgrad Med J
   Postgraduate Medical Journal
   (London)
Pract Otorhinolaryng (Basel)
   Practica Oto-Rhino-Laryngologica
   (Basel)
Practitioner
   Practitioner (London)
Prax Pneumol

Praxis der Pneumologie vereinigt
mit der Tuberkulosearzt (Stutt-
gart)
Praxis
Praxis (Bern)
Presse Med
Nouvelle Presse Medicale (Paris)
Prezgl Lek
Przeglad Lekarski (Krakow)
Proc Roy Soc Med
Proceedings of the Royal Society
of Medicine (London)
Psychom Sci
Psychonomic Science
Public Health Rep
Public Health Reports (Washing-
ton)
Quart J Med
Quarterly Journal of Medicine
(Oxford)
Quart J Stud Alcohol
Quarterly Journal of Studies on
Alcohol (New Haven)
Rev Esp Otoneurooftal
Revista Espanola de Oto-Neuro-
Oftalmologia y Neurocirugia
(Valencia)
Rev Laryng (Bordeaux)
Revue de Laryngologie, Otologie-
Rhinologie (Bordeaux)
Rev Med (S Paulo)
Revista de Medicina (Sao Paulo)
Rev Med Chir Iasi
Revista Medico-Chirurgicala a
Societatii di Medici si Naturali-
sti din Iasi
Rev Med Hosp Colonia
Revista Medica del Hospital
Colonia
Rev Otoneurooftal
Revista Oto-Neuro-Oftalmologica
(Bologna)
Rev Otoneuroophtal
Revue d'Oto-Neuro-Ophtalmologie
(Paris)
Rev Ouie Sourd Franc
Revue de l' Ouie et le Sourd
Francais
Rev Prat (Paris)
La Revue du Praticieu (Paris)
Rev Tuberc (Paris)
Revue de Tuberculose et de Pneu-
mologie (Paris)
Riv Neurol
Rivista di Neurologia (Napoli)
S Afr Med J
South African Medical Journal
(Cape Town)
Sairaanhoitaja
Sairaanhoitaja
Saishin Igaku
Saishin Igaku (Osaka)
Sborn Ved Prac Lek Fak Karlov Univ
Sbornik Vedeckych Praci Lekarske
Fakulty Karlovy University (Hra-
dec Kralove)
Scand J Resp Dis
Scandinavian Journal of Respira-

tory Diseases (Kobenhavn)
Science
Science (Washington)
Sound
Sound, its Uses and Control
Southern Med J
Southern Medical Journal (Birmin-
gham)
Srpski Arh Celok Lek
Srpski Arhiv za Celokupno Lekars-
tvo (Beograd)
Stomatologiya (Sofiya)
Stomatologiya (Sofiya)
Straub Clin Proc
Straub Clinic Proceedings (Hono-
lulu)
Surg Clin N Amer
Surgical Clinics of North America
(Philadelphia)
T Nor Laegeforen
Tidsskrift for den Norske Laege-
forening (Oslo)
T Norsk Laegeforen
Tidsskrift for den Norske Laege-
forening (Oslo)
Ter Arkh
Terapevticheskii Arkhiv (Moskva)
Tex Med
Texas Medicine (Austin)
Ther Umsch
Therapeutische Umschau (Bern)
Therapeutique
Therapeutique (Paris)
Therapie
Therapie (Paris)
Therapiewoche
Therapie Woche
Thorax
Thorax (London)
Toxic Appl Pharmacol
Toxicology and Applied Pharmaco-
logy (New York)
Tr Erevan Gos Inst Usoversh Vrachei
Trudy Erevanskogo Gosuvarstvenno-
go Instituta Usovershenstvovaniya
Vrachei
Trans Amer Acad Ophthal Otolaryng
Transactions of the American
Academy of Ophthalmology and
Otolaryngology (Rochester, Minn)
Trans Amer Otol Soc
Transactions of the American
Otological Society, Inc
Tubercle
Tubercle (London)
Tuberk Tudobet (Budapest)
Tuberkulozis es Tudobetegsegek
Tuberkuloza
Tuberkuloza
Ugeskr Laeg
Ugeskrift for Laeger (Kobenhavn)
Un Med Canada
Union Medicale du Canada (Mon-
treal)
Urologia (Treviso)
Urologia (Treviso)
Urologie
Der Urologe

Vasc Surg
    Vascular Surgery (New York)
Vestn Otorinolaring
    Vestnik Oto-Rino-Laringologii
    (Moskva)
Viata Med
    Viata Medicala
Voennomed Zh
    Voenno-Meditsinskii Zhurnal
    (Moskva)
Voix Silence
    la Voix du Silence (Roma)
Vojnosanit Pregl
    Vojnosanitetski Pregled (Beograd)
Volta Rev
    Volta Review
Vrach Delo
    Vrachebnoe Delo (Kiev)
Yearb Ear Nose Throat
    Yearbook of Ear, Nose, and Throat
Z Erkrank Atm Org
    Zeitschrift fur Erkrankungen der
    Atmungsorgane mit Folia Broncho-
    logica (Leipzig)
Z Erkrank Atmung
    Zeitschrift fur Erkrankungen der
    Atmungsorgane mit Folia Broncho-
    logica (Leipzig)
Z Laryng Rhinol Otol
    Zeitschrift fur Laryngologie,
    Rhinologie, Otologie und ihre
    Grenzgebiete (Stuttgart)
Z Mikr Anat Forsch
    Zeitschrift fur Mikroskopisch-
    Anatomische Forschung (Leipzig)
Z Tuberk
    Zeitschrift fur Tuberkulo
Erkrankungen der Theraxorgane
Z Urol Nephrol
    Zeitschrift fur Urologia und
    Nephrologie (Leipzig)
Z Vergl Physiol
    Zeitschrift fur Vergleichende
    Physiologie
Z Zellforsch
    Zeitschrift fur Zellforschung und
    Mikroskopische Anatomie (Berlin)
Zdrav Vestn
    Zdravstveni Vestnik
Zh Ushn Nos Gorl Bolez
    Zhurnal Ushnykh, Nosovykh i
    Gorlovykh Boleznei (Kiev)
Zh Vyssh Nerv Deiat Pavlov
    Zhurnal Vysshei Nervnoi Deiatel-
    'Nosti Imeni I.P. Pavlova (Mosk-
    va)

Appendix II TRADE NAME INDEXES

GENERIC NAME TO TRADE NAME INDEX

Acetazolamide
  Diamox
Alcohol
  Ethanol
Ampicillin
  Polycillin (ampicillin trihy-
  drate)
Aspirin
  Hypyrin (aspirin aluminum)
Capreomycin
  Capastat
  Capastat Sulfate
  Ogostal
Carbamazepine
  Tegretol
Chloramphenicol
  Chloromycetin
Chlorophenothane
  DDT
Chloroquine
  Aralen Hydrochloride
  Aralen Phosphate
  Nivaquine (chloroquine sulfate)
Chromonar
  Intensain
Colistin
  Colimycin
  Coly-Mycin S (colistin sulfate)
Digitalis
  Cedilanid
Dimenhydrinate
  Dramamine
Diphenylhydantoin
  Dilantin
  Phenhydan
  Phenytoin (dephenylhydantoin
  sodium)
Ethacrynic acid
  Edecrin
  Hydromedin
  Lyovac (sodium ethacrynate)
  Mingit
Fentanyl and droperidol
  Innovar
Framycetin
  Sofradex
Furosemide
  Lasix
  Lasix-Furosemide
Gentamicin
  Cidomycin
  Garamicin (gentamicin sulfate)
  Garamycin (gentamicin sulfate)
  Garamycin Injectable
  Gentalline
  Genticin
  Refobacin

GENERIC NAME TO TRADE NAME INDEX

Hexadimethrine bromide
  Polybrene
Imipramine hydrochloride
  Tofranil
Indomethacin
  Indocin
Kanamycin
  Kanamytrex
  Kanendomycin
  Kantrex
  Kantrex Injection (kanamycin
  sulfate)
  Resistomycin
Lidocaine
  Xylocaine
Lincomycin
  Lincocin
Monophenylbutazone
  Mobutazone
Nalidixic acid
  NegGram
Neomycin
  Glaxo (neomycin sulfate)
  Mycifradin (neomycin sulfate)
  Mycifradin Sulfate
  Myciguent (neomycin sulfate)
  Neobiotic (neomycin sulfate)
  Quintess-N (neomycin sulfate)
  White's Otobiotic (neomycin
  sulfate)
Paromomycin
  Humatin (paromomycin sulfate)
Pentobarbital
  Nembutal (pentobarbital sodium)
Polymyxin B
  Polymyxin B Sulfate
Procaine
  Novocaine (procaine hydroch-
  loride)
Quinacrine
  Atabrine (quinacrine hydroch-
  loride)
Rifampicin
  Rifadin
  Rimactane
Ristocetin
  Spontin
Spectinomycin
  Trobicin
Streptomycin
  Streptothenat (streptomycin
  pantothenate)
Tetracaine
  Pantocaine (tetracaine hydroch-
  loride)
Thiabendazole
  Mintezol

620   TRADE NAME INDEXES

GENERIC NAME TO TRADE NAME INDEX

Thorium dioxide
   Thorotrast
Vancomycin
   Vancocin

GENERIC NAME TO TRADE NAME INDEX

Viomycin
   Vinactane
   Viocin
   Vionactan
   Viothenat

TRADE NAME TO GENERIC NAME INDEX

Aralen Hydrochloride
   Chloroquine (chloroquine hydroch-
   loride)
Aralen Phosphate
   Chloroquine (chloroquine phos-
   phate)
Atabrine
   Quinacrine (quinacrine hydroch-
   loride)
Capastat
   Capreomycin
Capastat Sulfate
   Capreomycin
Cedilanid
   Digitalis
Chloromycetin
   Chloramphenicol
Cidomycin
   Gentamicin
Colimycin
   Colistin
Coly-Mycin S
   Colistin (colistin sulfate)
Diamox
   Acetazolamide
Dilantin
   Diphenylhydantoin
Dramamine
   Dimenhydrinate
DDT
   Chlorophenothane
Edecrin
   Ethacrynic acid
Ethanol
   Alcohol
Garamicin
   Gentamicin (gentamicin sulfate)
Garamycin
   Gentamicin (gentamicin sulfate)
Garamycin Injectable
   Gentamicin
Gentalline
   Gentamicin
Genticin
   Gentamicin
Glaxo
   Neomycin (neomycin sulfate)
Humatin
   Paromomycin (paromomycin sulfate)
Hydromedin
   Ethacrynic acid
Hypyrin
   Aspirin (aspirin aluminum)

TRADE NAME TO GENERIC NAME INDEX

Indocin
   Indomethacin
Innovar
   Fentanyl and droperidol
Intensain
   Chromonar
Kanamytrex
   Kanamycin
Kanendomycin
   Kanamycin
Kantrex
   Kanamycin
Kantrex Injection
   Kanamycin (kanamycin sulfate)
Lasix
   Furosemide
Lasix-Furosemide
   Furosemide
Lincocin
   Lincomycin
Lyovac
   Ethacrynic acid (sodium etha-
   crynate)
Mingit
   Ethacrynic acid
Mintezol
   Thiabendazole
Mobutazone
   Monophenylbutazone
Mycifradin
   Neomycin (neomycin sulfate)
Mycifradin Sulfate
   Neomycin
Mycifradin Sulphate
   Neomycin
Myciguent
   Neomycin (neomycin sulfate)
NegGram
   Nalidixic acid
Nembutal
   Pentobarbital (pentobarbital
   sodium)
Neobiotic
   Neomycin (neomycin sulfate)
Nivaquine
   Chloroquine (chloroquine sulfate)
Novocaine
   Procaine (procaine hydrochloride)
Ogostal
   Capreomycin
Pantocaine
   Tetracaine (tetracaine hydroch-
   loride)

Appendix III   THE INDEX-HANDBOOK PROJECT

PURPOSE

The INDEX-HANDBOOK OF OTOTOXIC AGENTS is designed to provide comprehensive information succinctly and quickly to the research scientist, clinician, or student interested in the effects of ototoxic agents on the auditory system.

HISTORY

The project began in 1970 with the creation and development of new ways to analyze the published literature on ototoxic agents. Some of the procedures developed were derived from earlier experiments and studies in the field of information science. One of these was the Cardiovascular Literature Project, established in 1955, which resulted in four Index-Handbooks dealing with the effects of chemical agents upon the anatomy, physiology, and pathology of the cardiovascular system. This project demonstrated that detailed, lengthy, and informative index entries could effectively replace conventional abstracts.

The second information system, the TRACE METALS LITERATURE INDEX-HANDBOOK, carried the procedure two steps further by 1) development of brief, stylized index-abstracts in natural English, in which each word can be retrieved by computer and 2) use of a computer to prepare and store a file of such miniature or mini-abstracts. The file could then be searched according to specification and the results printed in the form of a handbook or in a customized printout for the individual who desired combinations of variables not available in the printed version. This information system showed that a carefully constructed sentence could contain both the index entries and the key facts and that such a sentence could be manipulated by computer to serve several purposes.

The preparation of the INDEX-HANDBOOK OF OTOTOXIC AGENTS involved the following steps:

1) Development of a detailed profile or list of items to follow in analyzing the body of literature collected for this project

2) Arrangement of the analyzed data in narrative form

3) Subsequent storage of such material in a form that can be used for computer search, retrieval, print, and display of data in tabular array.

The central purpose was to develop a systematic analysis procedure for a typical body of literature so that results of studies could be compared easily and that, once analyzed, such data would be available for other purposes. Such an analysis procedure may also provide a guide for the recording of data by clinicians and research scientists in a more uniform way.

SEARCH OF THE LITERATURE

To obtain a comprehensive list of published papers on ototoxic agents, a search of the literature was made covering the period 1966 through 1971. The following sources were used:

Adverse Reactions Titles	Vol. 1, 1966 - Vol. 6, 1971
Biological Abstracts	Vol. 47, 1966 - Vol. 52, 1971
dsh Abstracts	Vol. 6, 1966 - Vol. 11, 1971
Excerpta Medica, Section 11	Vol. 19, 1966 - Vol. 24, 1971
Index Medicus	Vol. 7, 1966 - Vol. 12, 1971

Toxicity Bibliography	Vol. 1, 1968 - Vol. 4, 1971
Yearbook of Drug Therapy	1966 - 1971
Yearbook of Ear, Nose, and Throat	1966 - 1971

In addition, the files of the following organizations were searched by computer:

Information Center for Hearing, Speech, and	
Disorders of Human Communication	1967 - Dec., 1971
National Library of Medicine (MEDLARS)	1968 - Dec., 1970
State University of New York (SUNY)	1966 - Oct., 1971

A weekly ASCA (Automated Subject Citation Alert) computer search was also conducted by the Institute for Scientific Information for the period April - December, 1971.

The search of the literature yielded 732 papers in 19 languages. The papers were read in their original languages whenever possible. The literature of many disciplines, including otolaryngology, audiology, pharmacology, neurology, surgery, and biochemistry, is represented.

PROFILE

A list was compiled containing all those features which one would expect to find in clinical studies or research findings reported in the literature. A sample of 25 papers was examined to see how well the data fit into this preliminary profile which was then revised on the basis of this pilot review. The final profile included these elements:

        Ototoxic agents
        Routes of administration of ototoxic agents
            Oral
            Parenteral
            Topical
        Dosage of ototoxic agents
            Daily dosage
            Total dosage
            Levels of ototoxic agents in blood and inner ear fluids
        Duration of administration of ototoxic agents
        Effects of ototoxic agents
            Physiological effects
            Cochlear function
            Vestibular function
            Cochleo-vestibular function
        Structural effects
            Cochlear findings
            Vestibular findings
            Cochleo-vestibular findings
        Species affected by ototoxic agents
            Humans
            Animals
        Controls
        Additional information

ANALYSIS PROCEDURE

Mini-Abstracts

The 732 papers were analyzed according to the profile, and mini-abstracts were written for each. A mini-abstract may be defined as a machine-searchable index-abstract consisting of key words which are part of a controlled vocabulary and which are arranged, with filler words such as AND OF FOR in a grammatical order that can be read as an English sentence.

Format of the Mini-Abstracts

The format devised for the order of the profile elements is as follows:

(EFFECTS) due to (ROUTES OF ADMINISTRATION) of (DOSAGE)

of (OTOTOXIC AGENT(S)) for (DURATION OF ADMINISTRATION)

in (SPECIES)

(CONTROLS)

(ADDITIONAL INFORMATION)

Such a format enables the abstractor to prepare a uniform input. It also reveals whether a paper contains all the information considered necessary for such a study. The reader can thus obtain some view of the design and content of the study.

As prepared for computer processing, the mini-abstract appears somewhat different from its printed form in the Index-Handbook. A mini-abstract written for computer input appears as follows:

/HEARING LOSS/DUE TO/PARENTERAL/,/INTRAMUSCULAR/,/ADMINISTRATION/

OF/4 MG PER KG EVERY 4 HOURS IN 4 DIVIDED DOSES/OF/ANTIBIOTIC/,/

GENTAMICIN/(GENTAMICIN SULFATE)/,/FOR/138 DAYS/,/IN/1/HUMAN/,/

ADULT/,/23 YEARS/AGE/,/FEMALE/,/WITH/INFECTION/SECONDARY/TO/BURN/S/

The key or substantive words, which are the searchable terms, as well as the filler words, are bounded by virgules (/). The key words were selected from a thesaurus of index terms developed for this project.

The same mini-abstract appears in the following form in the Index-Handbook. The virgules have been removed to make the text easier to read, the mini-abstracts have been printed in upper and lower case, and periods have been added at the end of each mini-abstract:

Hearing loss due to parenteral, intramuscular, administration of 4 mg per kg every 4 hours in 4 divided doses of antibiotic, gentamicin (gentamicin sulfate), for 138 days in 1 human, adult, 23 years age, female, with infection secondary to burns.

ORGANIZATION OF DATA IN THE INDEX-HANDBOOK

The mini-abstracts have been grouped under three headings: 1) ototoxic agents, 2) effects of ototoxic agents, and 3) species affected by ototoxic agents. Subject headings were selected that would be useful for clinicians and research scientists.

COMPUTER PROCESSING

The Information Package developed by the Computing Center of The Johns Hopkins University School of Medicine was used in the processing of the Index-Handbook. These programs were developed specifically for text handling, and provide for the establishment, editing, searching, and printing of a file. In addition, codes have been devised to obtain the search capacity and print format desired for this project. Additional computer programs were also developed for the manipulation of the data to produce from one file the various parts of the Index-Handbook in upper and lower case. The computer language used for these programs was Manipulator, designed at The Johns Hopkins University Computing Center for handling free text.

FUTURE PLANS

The computer-based data system devised may be easily updated. The Information Center plans to issue supplementary material or revisions as required.

REFERENCES

AMA Council on Drugs:
AMA Drug Evaluations, ed. 1,
     Chicago, American Medical Association, 1971.

American Pharmaceutical Association:
The National Formulary, ed. 13,
     Washington, D.C., American Pharmaceutical Association, 1970.

Goodman, L.S., and Gilman, A., ed.:
The Pharmacological Basis of Therapeutics,
     New York, The Macmillan Company, 1965.

Lunin, L.F.:
A Trace Metals, Radiobiology, and Cancer Information Retrieval System (TRA-CIRS),
     Methods of Information in Medicine 4: 120-125 (Sep) 1965.

Lunin, L.F.:
The Development of a Machine-Searchable Index-Abstract and Its Application to
Biomedical Literature,
     in Garner, R.; Lunin, L.; and Baker, L.:
     Three Drexel Information Science Studies,
     Philadelphia, Pa., Drexel Press, 1967.

Lunin, L.F.:
A New Indexing Method and a New Information Center,
     Drug Information Bulletin 1: 81-85 (Apr - Jun) 1967.

Lunin, L.F.; Worthington, E.L., and Catlin, F.I.:
System for Computer-Oriented Retrieval of Evaluated Data (SCORED) on Ototoxic
Drugs,
     Paper presented at the Drug Information Association Computer Workshop
     III: Information Processing System Support of Clinical Research,
     Chicago, Sep. 12-21, 1971.

Miller, A.B., publ.:
Physicians' Desk Reference to Pharmaceutical Specialties and Biologicals,
     Oradell, N.J., Medical Economics, Inc., 1970.

Modell, W.:
Drugs of Choice 1970-1971,
     St. Louis, The C. V. Mosby Company, 1970.

Pharmaceutical Society of Great Britain:
British Pharmaceutical Codex 1968,
     London, The Pharmaceutical Press, 1968.

Stecher, P.G.; Windholz, M.; Leahy, D.S.; Bolton, D.M., and Eaton, L.G.:
The Merck Index. An Encyclopedia of Chemicals and Drugs, ed. 8,
     Rahway, N. J., Merck and Company, Inc., 1968.

Welt, I.D., direc.:
Index-Handbook of Cardiovascular Agents,
     Washington, D.C., National Academy of Sciences National Research
     Council, 1960, Vol. I.

Wilson, C.O., and Jones, T.E.:
American Drug Index 1971,
     Philadelphia, J.B. Lippincott Company, 1971.

INDEX TO MINI-ABSTRACTS BY PAGE NUMBER

AUTHOR TO DOCUMENT NUMBER INDEX